International Agency for Research on Cancer

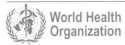
World Health
Organization

World Cancer Report 2014

Edited by BERNARD W. STEWART and CHRISTOPHER P. WILD

Lyon, 2014

Published by the International Agency for Research on Cancer,
150 cours Albert Thomas, 69372 Lyon Cedex 08, France

©International Agency for Research on Cancer, 2014

Distributed by
WHO Press, World Health Organization, 20 Avenue Appia, 1211 Geneva 27, Switzerland
(tel: +41 22 791 3264; fax: +41 22 791 4857; email: bookorders@who.int).

Cover images, from top to bottom: A woman in The Gambia prepares cereal, using scales to measure portions (Credit:
C.P. Wild/IARC). Next-generation gene sequencing equipment in use at the Joint Genome Institute in Walnut Creek,
California, USA (Credit: Joint Genome Institute, U.S. Department of Energy Genomic Science Program). Manhattan
plot of pooled genome-wide association study (GWAS) results (Credit: P. Brennan/IARC). A group of researchers
from the Epigenetics Group in the Section of Mechanisms of Carcinogenesis at IARC (Credit: R. Dray/IARC).
Representative example of high-grade serous carcinoma, one of the main types of ovarian carcinoma (Credit: J. Prat,
Autonomous University of Barcelona). Background image: The Blue Marble: Next Generation is a mosaic of satellite
data taken mostly from a NASA sensor called the Moderate Resolution Imaging Spectroradiometer (MODIS) that flies
aboard NASA's Terra and Aqua satellites (Credit: NASA/Goddard Space Flight Center/Reto Stöckli).

IARC Library Cataloguing in Publication Data

World cancer report / edited by Bernard W. Stewart and Christopher P. Wild

1. Neoplasms – etiology 2. Neoplasms – prevention and control 3. Neoplasms – genetics 4. Neoplasms by site
5. World Health
I. Stewart, B.W. II. Wild, C.P.

ISBN 978-92-832-0429-9   (NLM Classification: W1)

World Cancer Report 2014

Editors	Bernard W. Stewart
	Christopher P. Wild
Associate Editors	Freddie Bray
	David Forman
	Hiroko Ohgaki
	Kurt Straif
	Andreas Ullrich
Managing Editor	Nicolas Gaudin
English Editor	Karen Müller
Project Manager	Sylvia Lesage
Production Assistant	Solène Quennehen
Illustrations	Roland Dray
Layout	www.messaggio.eu.com
Printing	Naturaprint, France

IARC acknowledges generous assistance from the American Association for Cancer Research with the promotion of *World Cancer Report 2014*.

Contributors

Jean-Pierre Abastado (Singapore)

Cary Adams (Switzerland)

Isaac F. Adewole (Nigeria)

Hideyuki Akaza (Japan)

Naomi E. Allen (United Kingdom)

Marcella Alsan (USA)

Nada Al Alwan (Iraq)

Mahul B. Amin (USA)

Benjamin O. Anderson (USA)

Ahti Anttila (Finland)

Daniel A. Arber (USA)

Bruce K. Armstrong (Australia)

Héctor Arreola-Ornelas (Mexico)

Silvina Arrossi (Argentina)

Rifat Atun (United Kingdom and USA)

Robert A. Baan (France)

Yung-Jue Bang (Republic of Korea)

Emmanuel Barillot (France)

Jill Barnholtz-Sloan (USA)

Laura E. Beane Freeman (USA)

Rachid Bekkali (Morocco)

Agnès Binagwaho (Rwanda)

Elizabeth H. Blackburn (USA)

Evan Blecher (USA)

Ron Borland (Australia)

Fred T. Bosman (Switzerland)

Peter Bouwman (Netherlands)

Guledal Boztas (Turkey)

Elisabeth Brambilla (France)

Freddie Bray (France)

Paul Brennan (France)

Louise A. Brinton (USA)

Nathalie Broutet (Switzerland)

Michael P. Brown (Australia)

Heather Bryant (Canada)

Nikki Burdett (Australia)

Robert C. Burton (Australia)

Agnès Buzyn (France)

Kenneth P. Cantor (USA)

Federico Canzian (Germany)

Fátima Carneiro (Portugal)

Webster K. Cavenee (USA)

Eduardo L. Cazap (Argentina and Switzerland)

Frank J. Chaloupka (USA)

Stephen J. Chanock (USA)

Bob Chapman (USA)

Simon Chapman (Australia)

Chien-Jen Chen (Taiwan, China)

Il Ju Choi (Republic of Korea)

Rafael Moreira Claro (Brazil)

Hans Clevers (Netherlands)

Vincent Cogliano (USA)

Aaron J. Cohen (USA)

Carlo M. Croce (USA)

Min Dai (China)

Sarah C. Darby (United Kingdom)

Peter B. Dean (France)

Lynette Denny (South Africa)

Ethel-Michele de Villiers (Germany)

John E. Dick (Canada)

Joakim Dillner (Sweden)

Susan M. Domchek (USA)

Tandin Dorji (Bhutan)

Roland Dray (France)

Majid Ezzati (United Kingdom)

Lee Fairclough (Canada)

Jacques Ferlay (France)

David Forman (France)

Silvia Franceschi (France)

A. Lindsay Frazier (USA)

Christine M. Friedenreich (Canada)

Søren Friis (Denmark)

Tamara S. Galloway (United Kingdom)

Maurice Gatera (Rwanda)

Wentzel C.A. Gelderblom (South Africa)

Margaret A. Goodell (USA)

Sharon Lynn Grant (France)

Mel Greaves (United Kingdom)

Adèle C. Green (Australia and United Kingdom)

Murat Gultekin (Turkey)

Christine Guo Lian (USA)

Prakash C. Gupta (India)

Ezgi Hacikamiloglu (Turkey)

Andrew J. Hall (France)

Stanley R. Hamilton (USA)

Marianne Hammer (Norway)

Curtis C. Harris (USA)

Takanori Hattori (Japan)

Zdenko Herceg (France)

Hector Hernandez Vargas (France)

Rolando Herrero (France)

David Hill (Australia)

Martin Holcmann (Austria)

James F. Holland (USA)

Ralph H. Hruban (USA)

Thomas J. Hudson (Canada)

Peter A. Humphrey (USA)

Elaine S. Jaffe (USA)

Prabhat Jha (Canada)

Jos Jonkers (Netherlands)

Margaret R. Karagas (USA)

Michael Karin (USA)

Maria Sibilia (Austria)

Jack Siemiatycki (Canada)

Ronald Simon (Germany)

Pramil N. Singh (USA)

Rashmi Sinha (USA)

Nadia Slimani (France)

Avrum Spira (USA)

Gustavo Stefanoff (Brazil)

Eva Steliarova-Foucher (France)

Bernard W. Stewart (Australia)

Kurt Straif (France)

Simon B. Sutcliffe (Canada)

Rosemary Sutton (Australia)

Steven H. Swerdlow (USA)

Neil D. Theise (USA)

David B. Thomas (USA)

Lester D.R. Thompson (USA)

Michael J. Thun (USA)

Mark R. Thursz (United Kingdom)

Massimo Tommasino (France)

William D. Travis (USA)

Edward L. Trimble (USA)

Giorgio Trinchieri (USA)

Ugyen Tshomo (Bhutan)

Murat Tuncer (Turkey)

Andreas Ullrich (Switzerland)

Toshikazu Ushijima (Japan)

Carlos Vallejos (Peru)

Piet van den Brandt (Netherlands)

James W. Vardiman (USA)

Jim Vaught (USA)

Cesar G. Victora (Brazil)

Paolo Vineis (United Kingdom)

Lawrence von Karsa (France)

Melanie Wakefield (Australia)

Guiqi Wang (China)

Frank Weber (Germany)

Elisabete Weiderpass
(Norway and Sweden)

Zena Werb (USA)

Theresa L. Whiteside (USA)

Christopher P. Wild (France)

Walter C. Willett (USA)

Dillwyn Williams (United Kingdom)

Rena R. Wing (USA)

Deborah M. Winn (USA)

Martin Wiseman (United Kingdom)

Scott Wittet (USA)

Magdalena B. Wozniak (France)

Hai Yan (USA)

Teruhiko Yoshida (Japan)

Jiri Zavadil (France)

Harald zur Hausen (Germany)

For a complete list of contributors and their affiliations, see pages 596–605.

Contents

Foreword

The world has opened its eyes to the threat posed by cancer and other noncommunicable diseases (NCDs). Realization is growing, in global political circles and in civil society, that these diseases constitute a major obstacle to human development and well-being.

The United Nations General Assembly High-Level Meeting on the Prevention and Control of Noncommunicable Diseases, held in September 2011, marked a turning point in the awareness of political leaders and the international community of the need for urgent action to avert a worldwide crisis.

The new figures and projections of the global cancer burden presented in this edition of *World Cancer Report* starkly highlight the problem: the incidence of cancer has increased from 12.7 million in 2008 to 14.1 million in 2012, and this trend is projected to continue, with the number of new cases expected to rise a further 75%. This will bring the number of cancer cases close to 25 million over the next two decades. The greatest impact will unquestionably be in low- and middle-income countries, many of which are ill-equipped to cope with this escalation in the number of people with cancer.

Many developing countries find themselves in the grip of cancers from two vastly different worlds. Those associated with the world of poverty, including infection-related cancers, are still common, while those associated with the world of plenty are increasingly prevalent, owing to the adoption of industrialized lifestyles, with increasing use of tobacco, consumption of alcohol and highly processed foods, and lack of physical activity.

This rising burden of cancer and other NCDs places enormous strains on the health-care systems of developing countries. Coupled with ageing populations and the spiralling costs of cancer treatment, increasing demands are placed on the health-care budgets of even the wealthiest nations. As a result, prevention is central to reducing or reversing the rise in cancer burden. The central role of prevention was acknowledged in the Political Declaration adopted at the United Nations meeting, which described it as the cornerstone of the global response.

The United Nations Political Declaration gave WHO a clear mandate to coordinate the global response to this threat along with some important time-bound responsibilities captured within the Global Action Plan for the Prevention and Control of NCDs 2013–2020. IARC's contribution has been and will continue to be instrumental in this process. Independent, robust scientific evidence is the foundation of the formulation of sound public health policies. The high-quality research produced by IARC is essential for the development of evidence-based guidelines and policy by WHO, and for the adoption of regulatory decisions by national institutions to protect the health of their populations.

This new edition of *World Cancer Report* represents a timely update on the state of knowledge on cancer statistics, causes, and mechanisms, and on how this knowledge can be applied for the implementation of effective, resource-appropriate strategies for cancer prevention and early detection. I am confident that *World Cancer Report 2014*, like the previous editions, will constitute a key reference tool that will find extensive use among scientists, public health workers, and governments in supporting the implementation of national and regional plans for cancer prevention and control.

Dr Margaret Chan

Director-General
World Health Organization

Preface

Cancer is costly. First and foremost there is the human cost, comprising the uncertainty and suffering that a diagnosis of cancer brings in its wake. Behind each statistic of a new cancer case is an individual face, accompanied by the faces of family and friends drawn into this singular event. The harrowing experience of a cancer diagnosis is a truly universal one, played out in every community worldwide, every day.

In contrast, as a cancer patient moves beyond diagnosis, individual experiences diversify across the world. In fact, the future of a cancer patient depends in large part on where the person lives. In less economically developed countries, cancer is typically diagnosed at more advanced stages of disease, while access to effective treatment is limited or unavailable, as is palliative care. Even within more economically developed countries, there are disparities in access to care among different communities. The experiences of individual cancer patients all too frequently reflect the worst of global inequalities.

Cancer also has a societal cost; enormous human potential is lost, and treating and caring for an increasing number of cancer patients has an escalating economic impact. This too is a universal experience, but again the details differ greatly between countries. *World Cancer Report 2014* reveals a cancer burden that is projected to increase by about 70% worldwide in just two decades, but it is in the lowest-income countries with the least-developed cancer services that the impact will be greatest. Already, the early onset of some common cancers (e.g. cervix, liver) and generally poorer survival in low- and middle-income countries mean that the burden of years of life lost to cancer in these countries is similar to that in higher-income countries. Given population growth, ageing, and the spread of risk factors, such as tobacco use, the situation will worsen in the next decades, posing a major challenge to health systems in low- and middle-income countries, so that this divide between the experiences of individual cancer patients will only broaden. Taken in isolation, this is a dark prediction.

It is time to take up the challenges posed by the markedly increasing number of cancer cases globally. The particularly heavy burden projected to fall on low- and middle-income countries makes it implausible to treat our way out of cancer; even the highest-income countries will struggle to cope with the spiralling costs of treatment and care. Therefore, elucidating the causes and devising effective prevention strategies are essential components of cancer control, as is the gathering of accurate data on cancer occurrence from population-based cancer registries. These approaches will complement the benefits in improved access to affordable and effective cancer treatment.

In parallel to work carried out on causes and prevention, remarkable progress has been made in understanding the molecular and cellular events that transform a normal functioning cell into part of a malignant growth that can kill its host. These exciting advances in basic science have ramifications that are evident throughout this edition of *World Cancer Report*, notably in classifying cancers, in providing new avenues for clues about their causes, in highlighting opportunities for early detection and prevention, and in laying a foundation for the development of new, targeted treatments in the clinic. As never before, there is an opportunity to bring together interdisciplinary cancer expertise so that the advances of basic science are translated into both improved treatment and more widespread prevention and early detection. This integrated and complementary approach reflects not only the duty of care to today's cancer patients but also the duty of care to the next generation, to free as many people as possible from the threat of this disease.

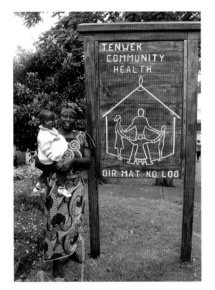

In the highlands of Kenya among the Kalenji people, who incidentally have provided some of the greatest middle- and long-distance runners in the world, there is a saying: "We should put out the fire while it is still small." It is this saying that greets patients arriving at the Tenwek Mission Hospital in the Western Highlands (see photo). We might adopt it as an idiom for cancer prevention. Since the middle of the last century, enormous progress has been made in identifying the causes of cancer, so that more than 50% of cases could be prevented based on current knowledge. These successes in identifying cancer causes must be complemented by an evaluation of the most effective interventions and an understanding of how best to support their implementation into specific health-care settings. Collectively, this knowledge provides huge potential for reducing the cancer burden; one can only imagine the interest that would follow an announcement of the availability of new cancer treatments able to cure 50% of all patients. Therefore, prevention must be writ large in cancer control plans if we are to defy the dark prediction of the statistics.

The International Agency for Research on Cancer (IARC) will play its part as it works for cancer prevention and control, with a particular commitment to low- and middle-income countries. IARC has a primary role in promoting international collaboration, and this role, acting as a catalyst for research, is increasingly proving to be vital because national questions can only be answered by international studies. Furthermore, the interdisciplinary approach taken by IARC is bearing fruit as knowledge about mechanisms of carcinogenesis casts new light on the causes and prevention of the disease.

The personal impact of cancer should never be far from the minds of all whose careers lead them to join in efforts to reduce the burden of suffering due to cancer. At the same time, cancer professionals from all disciplines need reliable knowledge on which to act, and the general public has the same need in order to make informed decisions. It is in this context that *World Cancer Report 2014* provides its up-to-date description of the occurrence, causes, underlying mechanisms, and prevention of cancer. My hope is that it will be a catalyst for collectively meeting the challenges of cancer in a way that benefits people in an inclusive way worldwide.

Dr Christopher P. Wild

Director
International Agency for Research on Cancer

Introduction

Research underpins the development and implementation of all measures calculated to reduce the cancer burden. In addressing cancer research developed over the five-year period since the previous edition of *World Cancer Report* was published, all the contributors to this volume faced the challenge of identifying the most pertinent developments. At the same time, an interval of five years represents a suitable time frame to reappraise the descriptive epidemiology of cancer occurrence worldwide – with this edition of *World Cancer Report* incorporating GLOBOCAN 2012 data as they became available in the weeks immediately before publication – and to assess cancer occurrence in relation to the broad and rapidly expanding knowledge available for cancer control.

Cancer etiology and biology

Specification of cancer incidence and mortality data with varying degrees of confidence for virtually all countries is fundamental to cancer control. These data – particularly as they relate to specific tumour types – not only establish the burden of disease as it may impinge upon public health and clinical services planning; they also indicate, in many instances, causative relationships, the impact of socioeconomic differences, and priorities that may be accorded to particular cancer control options.

In many cases, differences in cancer incidence between countries reflect the decades-old perception that cancer is a disease of affluence. But this perception is inadequate, having been displaced initially by the level of tobacco-induced lung cancer in China and some other Asian countries, and more recently as cancer rates are expected to grow due to the impact of rapid increases in the prevalence of obesity, which is not confined to high-income countries. Cancers associated with chronic infections remain a particularly important challenge in low- and middle-income countries. These differing and evolving profiles of risk factors are occurring against the background of marked demographic changes, characterized in many countries by an ageing and growing population, which will see the greatest proportional increases in cancer burden falling on some of the economically poorest regions of the world. *World Cancer Report* illustrates that cancer is truly a global problem.

The impacts of tobacco, obesity, and infections are just part of a broad spectrum of other agents and risk factors that contribute to cancer development and that, together, influence the striking geographical heterogeneity in incidence rates. Certain of these risk factors are non-modifiable, for example race, familial genetic background, and reproductive and hormonal history. Exposure to carcinogens may result from what are often characterized as lifestyle choices, which include alcohol consumption and behaviour in relation to avoidable sun exposure. Finally, people may be exposed to carcinogens in circumstances over which they have little or no control, which is the case in relation to occupational exposures, the effects of pollution (e.g. of ambient air or water), and exposures resulting from the use of particular foods, drugs, or consumer products. Priorities accorded to avoiding the impact of various causative agents may be influenced by attributable risk: the proportion of total cancers for which a particular agent or circumstance played a causal role in the development. Such quantitative determinations may vary markedly depending on which community or country is under consideration. The overarching principle, however, is that people should not be knowingly exposed to circumstances likely to increase their risk of developing cancer.

Analytical epidemiological studies, often incorporating molecular and biological measurements made possible through the availability of, for example, archived blood and/or tissue samples, increasingly identify key biological processes whose relevance is initially indicated through experimental studies. The past five years has witnessed the identity of many cancer pathways being derived from whole-genome sequencing for multiple cases of each major tumour type, and from analogous comprehensive data of the "–omics" sciences, which encompass genomics, transcriptomics, proteomics, metabolomics, and the like. These data have been generated through international collaboration. Genomic and similar data provide singular insight into the nature of cancer cell development within the context of normal tissue. These data offer, for example, the prospect of improved detection of early-stage disease, but also more refined molecular classification of malignancy with relevance to descriptive and etiological epidemiology. They also reveal perturbed signalling and other alterations in cancer cells, which, by definition, establish at least a basis for what is termed targeted therapy. Such opportunities are already being translated into clinical practice. The elucidation of biological changes that characterize cancer cells has been paralleled by observations at the cellular level to the effect that malignant tumours are inadequately understood as simply a mass of cancer cells: malignant tumours are also made up of fibrous, inflammatory, vascular, and immunological cell populations. Any one or more of these populations may be, at particular times, critical to tumour development and hence may offer an approach to prevention or therapy.

Reducing cancer incidence and mortality

Community awareness of the burden of cancer is inevitably focused on the development of improved therapies to the benefit of cancer patients, and media reports of "breakthroughs" are often the vehicle for reporting novel developments. The challenge posed by agent-specific resistance largely accounts for the reality of persistent disease despite incremental progress. This challenge highlights the certain benefits accruing from the adoption of measures to prevent cancer – benefits that accrue, however, in the longer term. For example, the impact of reduced cigarette consumption at the population level on lung cancer incidence came with a lag of some two to three decades. While smoking cessation is the most effective cancer preventive measure involving reduced exposure to proven carcinogens, cancer prevention involves a broad spectrum of initiatives, extending from vaccination – to ameliorate or prevent entirely the impact of relevant infections – through to screening tests aimed at detection, and consequently treatment, of early-stage disease.

National planning and international collaboration have emerged as critical to effective cancer control. Along with GLOBOCAN 2012 and the availability of genomic and related data, this edition of *World Cancer Report* highlights the WHO Framework Convention on Tobacco Control, the first international treaty negotiated under the auspices of WHO. As a response to the major recognized cause of cancer, tobacco control measures are almost universally applicable: what is effective in one country has been established as likely to be effective in most, if not all, countries. Although priorities must be accorded on a national basis, options for cancer control are increasingly available to countries and communities based on what has succeeded elsewhere. The inherent worth and benefit of collaboration across national boundaries is established for cancer control. Without doubt, national governments are seeking this internationally established evidence base, developed free from vested interests, for implementation at the local level.

The scope and design of *World Cancer Report*

Comprehensive texts on clinical oncology, often including sections on epidemiology, cancer biology, and public health matters, are published regularly and typically extend to thousands of pages. Likewise, annual reviews provide both researchers and clinicians with comprehensive coverage of recent publications in particular disciplines or concerning specified types of cancer or advances in therapies. *World Cancer Report* is readily distinguished from both these types of publication with reference to its scope and design. Concerning scope, emphasis on the global burden of cancer, and the environmental, lifestyle, and biological factors that might account for that burden, elevates the means of cancer prevention and their implementation to singular prominence. *World Cancer Report* does not address clinical care and the determination of optimal therapies, notwithstanding the exciting promise of these areas. Concerning design, *World Cancer Report* seeks to provide authoritative assessments through several different presentational approaches, while maintaining a publication of manageable length.

We, as editors, are grateful to the contributors to *World Cancer Report*, who, without exception, are aware of literally hundreds of publications that could be reasonably cited in the respective chapters were it not for length constraints that the present publication imposes. Because of these limitations, and the possibility that inevitable generalizations may preclude an appreciation of complexity, *World Cancer Report* features "boxes" in which a further group of investigators outline how certain precise issues are being elucidated with relevance to particular chapters.

The structure of *World Cancer Report 2014* is essentially in line with that adopted for earlier editions. However, *World Cancer Report 2014* is distinguished from its predecessors by the inclusion of a series of "Perspectives". Several prominent investigators have been invited to provide a personal viewpoint without the boundaries implicit in the headings of particular chapters. The perspectives offered are both distinctive and challenging, and serve to indicate the variety of issues immediately relevant to cancer control that either remain as challenges for further research or have yet to achieve their full potential by comprehensive implementation.

Cancer continues as a scourge of humankind. Increasingly, cancer is a particular burden on the populations of low- and middle-income countries. Cancer control may be achieved in large part through the insight gained from research, through detailed knowledge of how individuals and communities are affected, and through implementation of policies whose efficacy is often proven by the experience of other countries or groups of countries. The inclusion in this volume of several examples of national cancer control planning further demonstrates both the specific and general experiences from which lessons can be drawn in translating research-derived evidence into practice. *World Cancer Report 2014* therefore captures the dynamic state of both cancer research and cancer control worldwide with respect to what has been achieved, and what remains to be accomplished, to the benefit of the global community.

Bernard W. Stewart and Christopher P. Wild (Editors)
Lyon, December 2013

1

Cancer
worldwide

Cancer affects all of humankind, but there are marked differences across local, national, and regional boundaries, particularly when considering specific tumour types rather than cancer as a whole. Epidemiological data on incidence of cancer and deaths caused by cancer vary enormously in coverage and quality between countries and regions worldwide, ranging from complete coverage by national cancer registries to population-based registries covering a part of the country, hospital-based registries, or no available data at all on cancer occurrence. In the absence of data, inferences must be drawn from surrounding countries to provide the best estimate possible. This edition of *World Cancer Report* provides data

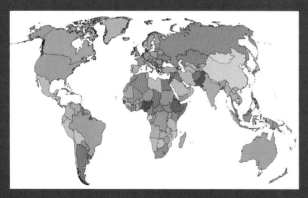

from GLOBOCAN 2012, the most current appraisal of the distribution of cancer worldwide. The findings show that high-resource countries have the highest incidence of cancer and also provide the best services for detection, diagnosis, and treatment, as may be inferred from mortality and survival data. The highest prevalence proportions of cancer also occur in these populations. The most common cancers include lung, breast, prostate, and colorectal cancers. In countries in epidemiological transition, these cancers are increasingly common but incidence of stomach, oesophageal, and liver cancers remains high. Data from low-resource countries show that cervical cancer is still often the most common cancer among women. In low- and middle-resource countries, incidence of particular tumours may be relatively low, but corresponding mortality data often reflect late-stage diagnosis as the norm and consequently poor clinical outcomes. Worldwide, differences in cancer incidence have been recognized for more than half a century as indicating different causes and, by inference, different opportunities for prevention. These lines of investigation have been greatly refined in recent years. Accordingly, cancer epidemiological data as now presented not only establish the burden of cancer but also underpin and very often confirm determinations of causation and opportunities for prevention, as elaborated in subsequent sections of this Report.

1.1 The global and regional burden of cancer

1 WORLDWIDE

David Forman
Jacques Ferlay

Bernard W. Stewart (reviewer)
Christopher P. Wild (reviewer)

Summary

- Cancer is a major cause of morbidity and mortality, with approximately 14 million new cases and 8 million cancer-related deaths in 2012, affecting populations in all countries and all regions. These estimates correspond to age-standardized incidence and mortality rates of 182 and 102 per 100 000, respectively.

- Among men, the five most common sites of cancer diagnosed in 2012 were the lung (16.7% of the total), prostate (15.0%), colorectum (10.0%), stomach (8.5%), and liver (7.5%). Among women, the five most common incident sites of cancer were the breast (25.2% of the total), colorectum (9.2%), lung (8.7%), cervix (7.9%), and stomach (4.8%).

- Among men, lung cancer had the highest incidence (34.2 per 100 000) and prostate cancer had the second highest incidence (31.1 per 100 000). Among women, breast cancer had a substantially higher incidence (43.3 per 100 000) than any other cancer; the next highest incidence was of colorectal cancer (14.3 per 100 000).

- Prevalence estimates for 2012 indicate that there were 8.7 million people (older than 15 years) alive who had had a cancer diagnosed in the previous year, 22.0 million with a diagnosis in the previous 3 years, and 32.6 million with a diagnosis in the previous 5 years.

- The worldwide estimate for the number of cancers diagnosed in childhood (ages 0–14 years) in 2012 is 165 000 (95 000 in boys and 70 000 in girls).

- For all cancers combined (excluding non-melanoma skin cancer) the highest incidence rates are associated with the high-income countries of North America and western Europe (together with Japan, the Republic of Korea, Australia, and New Zealand).

- More than 60% of the world's cancer cases occur in Africa, Asia, and Central and South America, and these regions account for about 70% of the cancer deaths.

- The distribution of cancer in world regions indicates marked, and sometimes extreme, differences with respect to particular tumour types. Such data are key to any understanding of causation, and hence the development of preventive measures.

Robust statistics on cancer occurrence and outcome are an essential prerequisite for national and regional programmes of cancer control and for informing the cancer research agenda. Since 1984, IARC has regularly published estimates of the global and regional burden of cancer in terms of both incidence and mortality [1]. Since 2001, such estimates have also been made available for all major countries of the world through the GLOBOCAN project [2,3]. These estimates are based on all sources of information available for any given country

Fig. 1.1.1. Fishermen in Bahia de Kino, Mexico. On a world scale, intermediate cancer incidence rates occur in Central and South America.

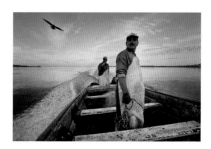

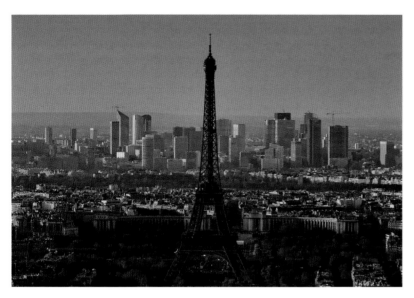

Fig. 1.1.2. A view of Paris. High-income countries, exemplified by countries in western Europe and North America, have the highest overall cancer rates in both sexes.

[4] and, where possible, make use of incidence data published in the IARC series *Cancer Incidence in Five Continents* [5–7] and mortality data made available by WHO [8]. For more details about the graphics presented in this chapter, see "A guide to the epidemiology data in *World Cancer Report*".

Global burden of cancer

Incidence and mortality

Results from GLOBOCAN [3] show that in 2012 there were an estimated 14.1 million new cases of cancer diagnosed worldwide (excluding non-melanoma skin cancer) and 8.2 million estimated deaths from cancer. These estimates correspond to age-standardized incidence and mortality rates of 182 and 102 per 100 000, respectively. There were slightly more incident cases (53% of the total) and deaths (57%) among men than among women. The estimated global annual numbers of new cases and cancer deaths for the most important types of cancer are shown in Figs 1.1.4 and 1.1.5, for both sexes combined and for men and women separately.

Among men, the five most common sites of cancer diagnosed in 2012 were the lung (16.7% of the total), prostate (15.0%), colorectum (10.0%), stomach (8.5%), and liver (7.5%). These sites also represented the most common causes of cancer death in men; the relative importance of lung cancer increased to 23.6% of the total, followed by liver cancer (11.2%) and stomach cancer (10.1%) as the second and third most common causes of cancer death.

Among women, the five most common incident sites of cancer were the breast (25.2% of the total), colorectum (9.2%), lung (8.7%), cervix (7.9%), and stomach (4.8%). These sites also represented the most common causes of cancer death in women; the relative importance of breast cancer decreased to 14.7% of the total, followed by lung cancer (13.8%) as the second most common cause of cancer death. In both sexes combined, the five most common incident sites of cancers were the lung (13.0% of the total), breast (11.9%), colorectum (9.7%), prostate (7.9%), and stomach (6.8%); together, cancers of these five sites constitute half of the overall global cancer burden.

Estimated age-standardized incidence and mortality rates for the 15 most common cancers worldwide for men and women in 2012 are shown in Fig. 1.1.6. Among men, lung cancer has the highest incidence and mortality rates (34.2 and 30.0 per 100 000, respectively). Prostate cancer has the second highest incidence rate (31.1 per 100 000), not far below that for lung cancer. However, the mortality rate for prostate cancer (7.8 per 100 000) is considerably lower than that for lung cancer. The differential between mortality and incidence for these two cancers reflects the much lower fatality rate (or improved survival) of prostate cancer compared with lung cancer. Stomach, liver, and oesophageal cancers are three of the other major cancers in men that, like lung cancer, have relatively poor survival and hence mortality rates that are close to the incidence rates (incidence and mortality of 17.4 and 12.7 per 100 000, respectively, for stomach cancer, 15.3 and 14.3 per 100 000 for liver cancer, and 9.0 and 7.7 per 100 000 for oesophageal cancer). The other major cancer in men is colorectal cancer, which has an incidence rate of 20.6 per 100 000 but a substantially lower mortality rate of 10.0 per 100 000.

Among women, breast cancer has a considerably higher incidence rate (43.3 per 100 000) than any other cancer. The next highest is cancer of the colorectum (14.3 per 100 000), and then cancers of the cervix (14.0), lung (13.6), corpus uteri (8.2), and stomach (7.5).

Fig. 1.1.3. Times Square, New York. The four major cancers that affect populations in North America are the same as those in Europe: cancers of the prostate, breast, lung, and colorectum.

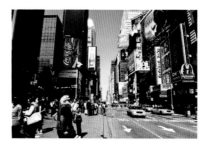

Fig. 1.1.4. Estimated world cancer incidence proportions by major sites, in both sexes combined, in men, and in women, 2012.

World

Both sexes
Estimated number of cancer cases, all ages (total:14 090 149)

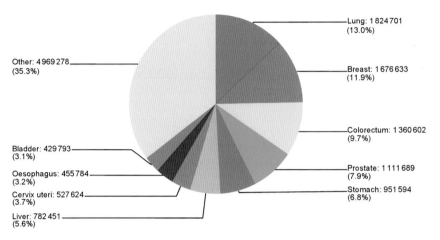

Men
Estimated number of cancer cases, all ages (total:7 427 148)

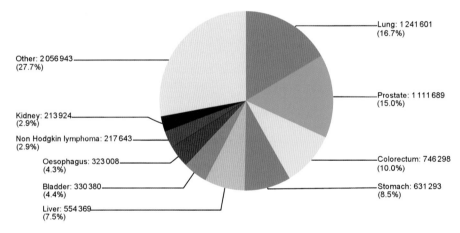

Women
Estimated number of cancer cases, all ages (total:6 663 001)

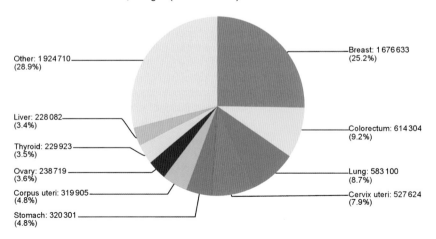

Fig. 1.1.5. Estimated world cancer mortality proportions by major sites, in both sexes combined, in men, and in women, 2012.

World

Both sexes
Estimated number of cancer deaths, all ages (total:8 201 030)

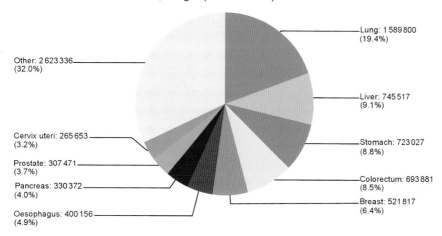

Other: 2 623 336 (32.0%)

Lung: 1 589 800 (19.4%)

Liver: 745 517 (9.1%)

Stomach: 723 027 (8.8%)

Colorectum: 693 881 (8.5%)

Breast: 521 817 (6.4%)

Oesophagus: 400 156 (4.9%)

Pancreas: 330 372 (4.0%)

Prostate: 307 471 (3.7%)

Cervix uteri: 265 653 (3.2%)

Men
Estimated number of cancer deaths, all ages (total:4 653 132)

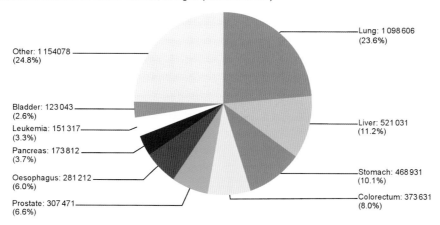

Other: 1 154 078 (24.8%)

Lung: 1 098 606 (23.6%)

Liver: 521 031 (11.2%)

Stomach: 468 931 (10.1%)

Colorectum: 373 631 (8.0%)

Prostate: 307 471 (6.6%)

Oesophagus: 281 212 (6.0%)

Pancreas: 173 812 (3.7%)

Leukemia: 151 317 (3.3%)

Bladder: 123 043 (2.6%)

Women
Estimated number of cancer deaths, all ages (total:3 547 898)

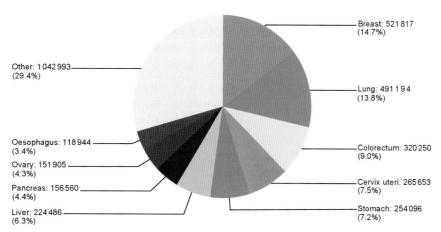

Other: 1 042 993 (29.4%)

Breast: 521 817 (14.7%)

Lung: 491 194 (13.8%)

Colorectum: 320 250 (9.0%)

Cervix uteri: 265 653 (7.5%)

Stomach: 254 096 (7.2%)

Liver: 224 486 (6.3%)

Pancreas: 156 560 (4.4%)

Ovary: 151 905 (4.3%)

Oesophagus: 118 944 (3.4%)

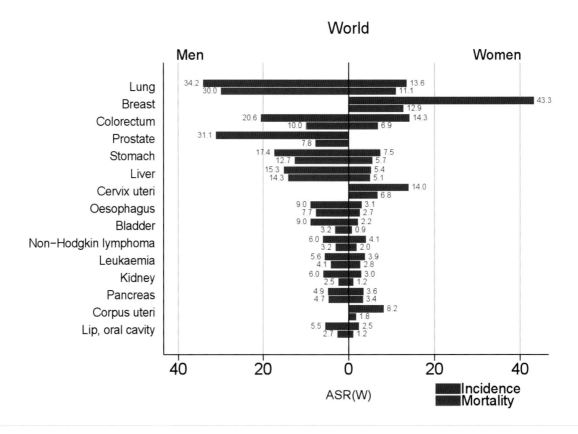

However, breast cancer has a relatively low fatality rate, and thus although it has the highest mortality rate of any cancer in women (12.9 per 100 000), this is less than one third of the incidence rate and not much higher than the lung cancer mortality rate (11.1 per 100 000), which is the next highest. As in men, the stomach cancer mortality rate (5.7 per 100 000) is not far below the incidence rate, but the mortality rates for the other major cancers in women – cancers of the colorectum (6.9 per 100 000), cervix (6.8) and, especially, corpus uteri (1.8) – are substantially lower than the corresponding incidence rates.

Prevalence

A further measure of cancer burden is prevalence: the number of people who have been diagnosed with cancer and are still alive at a specific time [9]. Prevalence estimates for 2012 show that there were 8.7 million people (older than 15 years) alive who had had a cancer diagnosed in the previous year, 22.0 million with a diagnosis in the previous 3 years, and 32.6 million with a diagnosis in the previous 5 years [3]. Estimates of 5-year prevalence for the nine most common cancer sites worldwide are shown in Fig. 1.1.7, for both sexes combined and for men and women separately. With 6.3 million survivors diagnosed within the previous 5 years, breast cancer is by far the most prevalent cancer, even when results for both sexes are combined. The second most prevalent is prostate cancer, with 3.9 million, and then colorectal cancer, with 3.5 million (1.9 million men and 1.6 million women), and lung cancer, with 1.9 million (1.3 million men and 0.6 million women). Prevalence reflects the integration of incidence and extent of survival, and for lung cancer, because of its very poor survival, the 5-year prevalence is very close to the annual mortality (1.6 million).

Incidence by age group

Cancer has a strong relationship with age, and Fig. 1.1.8 shows the GLOBOCAN estimated incidence rates for all cancers combined (excluding non-melanoma skin cancer) by age group for men and women. Rates in the youngest age group (0–14 years) are about 10 per 100 000, increasing to 150 per 100 000 by 40–44 years and to more than 500 per 100 000 by 60–64 years. Only in the youngest age group (0–14 years) are rates similar between the sexes. After childhood, rates are higher in women than in men until about the age of 50 years, when rates in men overtake those in women and then become substantially higher from the age of 60 years. The excess in women before the age of 50 years is due

Fig. 1.1.7. Estimated world cancer 5-year prevalence proportions by major sites, in both sexes combined, in men, and in women, 2012.

World

Both sexes
Estimated 5-year prevalent cancer cases, adult population (total: 32 544 633)

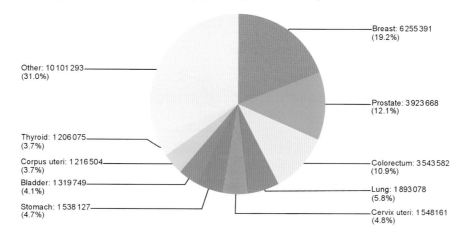

Other: 10 101 293 (31.0%)
Thyroid: 1 206 075 (3.7%)
Corpus uteri: 1 216 504 (3.7%)
Bladder: 1 319 749 (4.1%)
Stomach: 1 538 127 (4.7%)
Breast: 6 255 391 (19.2%)
Prostate: 3 923 668 (12.1%)
Colorectum: 3 543 582 (10.9%)
Lung: 1 893 078 (5.8%)
Cervix uteri: 1 548 161 (4.8%)

Men
Estimated 5-year prevalent cancer cases, adult population (total: 15 362 289)

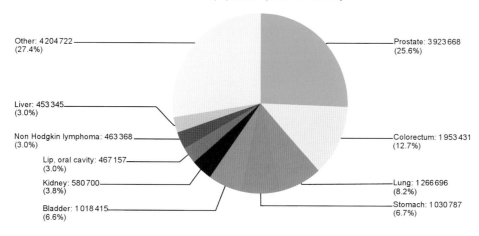

Other: 4 204 722 (27.4%)
Liver: 453 345 (3.0%)
Non Hodgkin lymphoma: 463 368 (3.0%)
Lip, oral cavity: 467 157 (3.0%)
Kidney: 580 700 (3.8%)
Bladder: 1 018 415 (6.6%)
Prostate: 3 923 668 (25.6%)
Colorectum: 1 953 431 (12.7%)
Lung: 1 266 696 (8.2%)
Stomach: 1 030 787 (6.7%)

Women
Estimated 5-year prevalent cancer cases, adult population (total: 17 182 344)

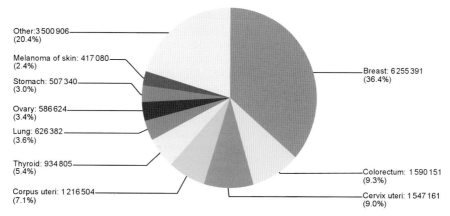

Other: 3 500 906 (20.4%)
Melanoma of skin: 417 080 (2.4%)
Stomach: 507 340 (3.0%)
Ovary: 586 624 (3.4%)
Lung: 626 382 (3.6%)
Thyroid: 934 805 (5.4%)
Corpus uteri: 1 216 504 (7.1%)
Breast: 6 255 391 (36.4%)
Colorectum: 1 590 151 (9.3%)
Cervix uteri: 1 547 161 (9.0%)

Fig. 1.1.8. Estimated world cancer incidence rates per 100 000 by 5-year age group, for all sites combined (excluding non-melanoma skin cancer), in men and women, 2012.

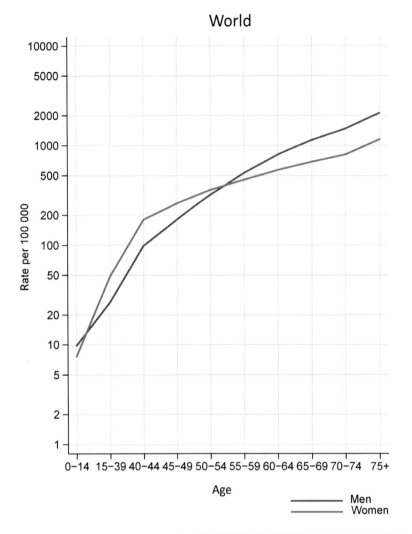

of the upper rate category is higher in men than in women. Intermediate rates are seen in Central and South America, eastern Europe, and much of South-East Asia (including China), and the lowest rates are seen in much of Africa and West and South Asia (including India). There are some interesting exceptions to this pattern. For example, Uruguay and Mongolia fall into the high-incidence category, Uruguay partly because of particularly high rates for lung cancer (and other smoking-related cancers), which are now being brought under control [10], and Mongolia because of the extraordinary high rate of liver cancer resulting from the particularly high prevalence of infection with hepatitis B and C viruses [11].

Mortality

Similar world maps are shown in Fig. 1.1.10 for age-standardized mortality rates. These also show extensive international variation, but the contrasts are less marked than those for incidence. For example, there is less variation between North and South America and between western and eastern Europe. In both cases, this is a result of the impact of clinical care and generally improved cancer survival in North America and western Europe, leading to lower mortality rates (relative to the incidence rates) than is observed in South America and eastern Europe [12]. In addition, and as described in the discussion of regional patterns of cancer below, cancers associated with a lifestyle typical of industrialized countries, including cancers of the breast, colorectum, and prostate, have a relatively good prognosis, whereas cancers of the liver, stomach, and oesophagus, which are more common in low-income countries, have a significantly poorer prognosis. In general, therefore, relatively more cancer deaths are seen for a given number of incident cases in the less economically developed countries, and cancer mortality rates are not very different from those in more developed countries.

to the relatively earlier age at onset of cervical cancer and, especially, breast cancer compared with other major cancers. Above the age of 60 years, prostate cancer and lung cancer in men become more common. The worldwide estimate for the number of cancers diagnosed in childhood (0–14 years) in 2012 is 165 000 (95 000 in boys and 70 000 in girls), and in teenagers and young adults (15–39 years), the estimate is just more than 1 million (380 000 in men and 670 000 in women). For more information on the descriptive epidemiology of cancer in these age groups, see Chapter 1.3.

Global distribution

Incidence

World maps of estimated age-standardized incidence rates for all cancers combined (excluding non-melanoma skin cancer) in 2012 are shown in Fig. 1.1.9 for men (Fig. 1.1.9A) and women (Fig. 1.1.9B). In general, and with some exceptions, the highest incidence rates are associated with the high-income countries of North America and western Europe (together with Japan, the Republic of Korea, Australia, and New Zealand). This is the case for both sexes, although the absolute level

Fig. 1.1.9. Global distribution of estimated age-standardized (World) cancer incidence rates (ASR) per 100 000, for all sites combined (excluding non-melanoma skin cancer), in (A) men and (B) women, 2012.

A

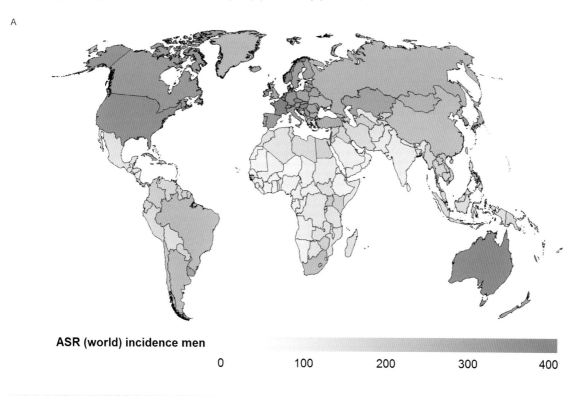

ASR (world) incidence men

0   100   200   300   400

B

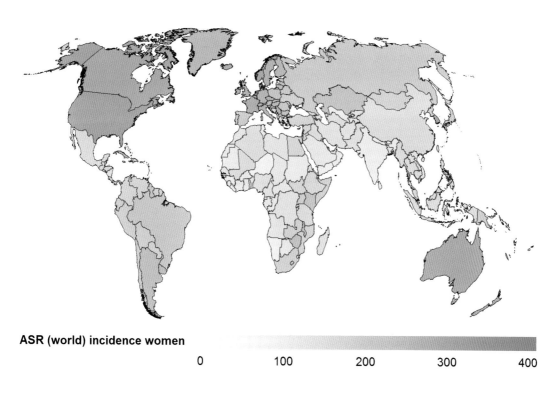

ASR (world) incidence women

0   100   200   300   400

Fig. 1.1.10. Global distribution of estimated age-standardized (World) cancer mortality rates (ASR) per 100 000, for all sites combined (excluding non-melanoma skin cancer), in (A) men and (B) women, 2012.

A

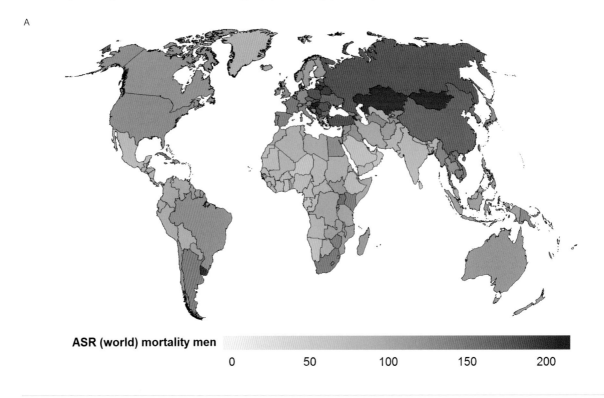

ASR (world) mortality men

0	50	100	150	200

B

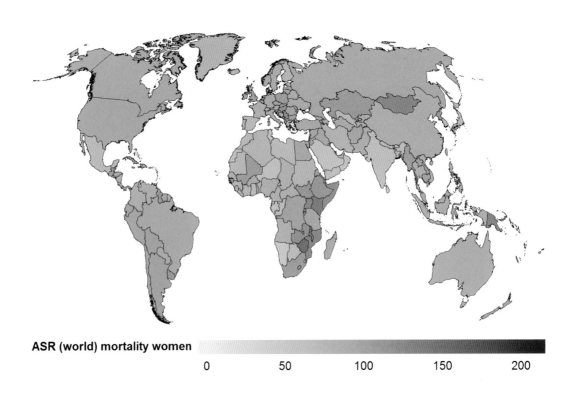

ASR (world) mortality women

0	50	100	150	200

Regional patterns of cancer

A regional breakdown of the global cancer incidence and mortality burden by continental region is provided in Fig. 1.1.11. About half of the incidence burden occurs in Asia, and almost a half of this, or 22% of the global total, arises in China, and 7% in India. A quarter of the incidence burden occurs in Europe, and the remainder is divided between the Americas and Africa (with 1% in Oceania). The mortality proportional distribution shows an increase in the proportion of cancer-related deaths occurring in Asia and Africa, together with a decrease in the proportions occurring in the economically more developed regions of Europe and North America.

Further analyses of the regional patterns are shown in Figs 1.1.12 to 1.1.39, in which, for each world region, a proportional breakdown is provided of the estimated 2012 numbers of cancer cases and deaths by sex, together with histograms showing the age-standardized incidence and mortality rates by cancer site and a chart showing the major 5-year prevalent cancers.

Europe

In Europe, the incidence pattern is dominated by prostate and breast cancers, which are the most common sites in men and women, respectively, together with lung and colorectal cancers (Fig. 1.1.12). In terms of mortality, lung cancer, because of its poor survival, is the most important cause of cancer death in men (Fig. 1.1.13). Bladder, stomach, and kidney cancers also contribute significantly to the burden in men, with incidence rates of more than 10 per 100 000, whereas in women, cancers of the corpus uteri and cervix also have incidence rates of more than 10 per 100 000 (Fig. 1.1.14). Breast, prostate, and colorectal cancers are the most prevalent; together, cancers of these three sites represent half of all the 5-year prevalent cases in Europe (Fig. 1.1.15).

North America

In North America, patterns of the four major cancers are very similar to those in Europe. Prostate and breast cancer are the most common

incident sites in men and women, respectively, and lung cancer is the most common cause of cancer death in both sexes (Figs 1.1.16, 1.1.17). However, unlike in Europe, lung cancer is also relatively more important than colorectal cancer in women in terms of incidence. Also, alongside bladder and kidney cancers, malignant melanoma, non-Hodgkin lymphoma, and leukaemia contribute significantly to the cancer burden in men, with incidence rates of more than 10 per 100 000 (Fig. 1.1.18). This is also evident for malignant melanoma, non-Hodgkin lymphoma, corpus uteri, and thyroid cancers in women. Compared with the European pattern, stomach cancer in men and cervical cancer in women are much less common, at least partially reflecting the greater heterogeneity in rates across Europe for these cancer sites. The prevalence pattern in North America is very similar to that in Europe, with prostate, breast, and colorectal cancers together accounting for half of all the 5-year prevalent cases (Fig. 1.1.19).

Fig. 1.1.11. Estimated world cancer incidence and mortality proportions by major world regions, in both sexes combined, 2012.

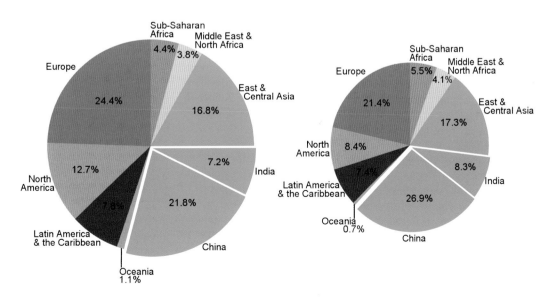

World

Incidence: 14.1 million estimated new cases   Mortality: 8.2 million estimated deaths

Oceania

In Oceania, one again sees the European and North American patterns in relation to prostate and breast cancers as the most common sites in men and women, respectively, and lung cancer as the most common cause of cancer death in men (Figs 1.1.20, 1.1.21). However, after colorectal cancer, malignant melanoma is the third most important incident cancer in both sexes, although it ranks relatively low in terms of mortality. Lung, kidney, and bladder cancers as well as non-Hodgkin lymphoma and leukaemia in men and cancers of the lung, corpus uteri, cervix, and thyroid in women are the other cancers with rates of more than 10 per 100 000 (Fig. 1.1.22). Malignant melanoma makes an important contribution to cancer prevalence in Oceania, as the third most prevalent type. Otherwise, the pattern of prevalence is similar to that in Europe and North America (Fig. 1.1.23).

Latin America and the Caribbean

For the region Latin America and the Caribbean, in common with Europe and North America, prostate and breast cancers are the most common incident sites in men and women, respectively (Fig. 1.1.24). Breast cancer is the most common cause of cancer death in women, whereas prostate and lung cancers make similar contributions to cancer mortality in men (Figs 1.1.25, 1.1.26). However, and unlike the situation in the more economically developed regions, cervical cancer makes a major contribution to the cancer burden in women, as the second most common incident cancer and cause of cancer death in women. The incidence rate for cervical cancer (21.2 per 100 000) is substantially larger than that estimated for Europe or North America (11.4 and 6.6 per 100 000, respectively) (Fig. 1.1.26). Stomach cancer is also important, especially in men, where it is the fourth most common incident cancer (with lung and colorectal cancers as second and third, respectively). Whereas the incidence rates for stomach cancer (12.8 and 7.1 per 100 000 in men and women, respectively) are of similar magnitude to those in Europe (13.2 and 6.4 per 100 000), these are much higher than those in North America (5.5 and 2.8 per 100 000). Cervical cancer also contributes to the pattern of cancer prevalence in the region, representing 8.6% of all 5-year prevalent cancers, third in importance after breast and prostate cancers (Fig. 1.1.27).

Middle East and North Africa

In the Middle East and North Africa region (Figs 1.1.28, 1.1.29), breast cancer again dominates the pattern of cancer in women, representing 30% of the cancer cases. Colorectal cancer is the next most common cancer in women, but breast cancer is the only type for which the incidence or mortality rates (43.0 and 16.2 per 100 000, respectively) exceed 10 per 100 000 (Fig. 1.1.30). Among men, lung cancer is the most important incident cancer and cause of cancer death, with incidence and mortality rates of 27.1 and 24.5 per 100 000, respectively (Fig. 1.1.30). Prostate, bladder, colorectal, and liver cancers are the next most common, all with incidence rates of more than 10 per 100 000. In this region, breast cancer represents a quarter of all 5-year prevalent cancers, and whereas prostate cancer is relatively less prevalent compared with other world regions, bladder and thyroid cancers make important contributions to the overall pattern (Fig. 1.1.31).

Sub-Saharan Africa

Sub-Saharan Africa provides several contrasts with other world regions. Among women, this is the only region where cervical cancer is equivalent to breast cancer in terms of incidence (each constitutes approximately a quarter of the total burden) and is the most common cause of cancer death in women (23.2% of the total) (Figs 1.1.32, 1.1.33). The incidence and mortality rates for cervical cancer are 34.8 and 22.5 per 100 000, respectively (Fig. 1.1.34), the highest of any world region. Among men, prostate and liver cancers are the most common forms of incident cancer and causes of cancer death. Although the leading role of prostate cancer in the cancer incidence pattern in men is shared with most other world regions, this region also has mortality rates comparable to incidence rates. The rates of 27.9 and 20.9 per 100 000 for prostate cancer incidence and mortality, respectively, stand in marked contrast to those in Europe (64.0 and 11.3 per 100 000, respectively) or North America (97.2 and 9.8 per 100 000, respectively), where incidence is much higher but mortality is much lower. The importance of liver cancer in this region should be emphasized; it is the second most common cancer in men and the third most common in women. Cervical and breast cancers in women and prostate and liver cancers in men are the only cancers with sex-specific incidence or mortality rates of more than 10 per 100 000, but the high rates of Kaposi sarcoma in sub-Saharan Africa, especially in men, should also be noted. Kaposi sarcoma is the third most common cancer in men and represents 9.2% of all cancer diagnoses, with an incidence rate of 7.2 per 100 000. This reflects the very high regional level of HIV infection and associated cancer sequelae before the advent of highly active antiretroviral therapy [13]. Cervical cancer and Kaposi sarcoma also make important contributions to the pattern of 5-year prevalence in the region (Fig. 1.1.35).

East and Central Asia

East and Central Asia is by far the most populous world region, containing 57% of the global population (19% in China and 18% in India). Among men, the most common cancers and causes of cancer death are cancers of the lung, stomach, liver, colorectum, and oesophagus (Figs 1.1.36, 1.1.37), sites with incidence rates of more than 10 per 100 000 (Fig. 1.1.38). Although relatively high, the incidence and mortality rates for lung cancer in men (35.1 and 31.5 per 100 000, respectively) are still substantively below those in Europe and North America. However, the corresponding rates for stomach cancer (23.3 and 16.9 per 100 000, respectively) and liver cancer (20.7 and 19.5 per 100 000, respectively) are the highest of any world region. Among women, breast cancer is the most common incident cancer, followed by cancers of the lung, cervix, colorectum, and stomach. Due to the varying fatality rates of these cancers, the mortality patterns are a little different in the region, and lung cancer is the leading cause of cancer death. As in other regions, breast cancer makes a substantial contribution to 5-year prevalence in East and Central Asia, but in contrast to elsewhere, cancers of the stomach and lung are also important contributors to the pattern of prevalence (Fig. 1.1.39).

Fig. 1.1.12. Europe. Estimated cancer incidence proportions by major sites, in both sexes combined, in men, and in women, 2012.

Europe

Both sexes
Estimated number of cancer cases, all ages (total:3 442 276)

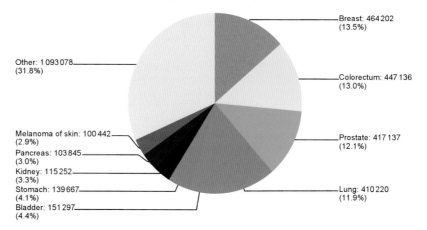

Breast: 464 202 (13.5%)
Colorectum: 447 136 (13.0%)
Prostate: 417 137 (12.1%)
Lung: 410 220 (11.9%)
Other: 1 093 078 (31.8%)
Melanoma of skin: 100 442 (2.9%)
Pancreas: 103 845 (3.0%)
Kidney: 115 252 (3.3%)
Stomach: 139 667 (4.1%)
Bladder: 151 297 (4.4%)

Men
Estimated number of cancer cases, all ages (total:1 830 541)

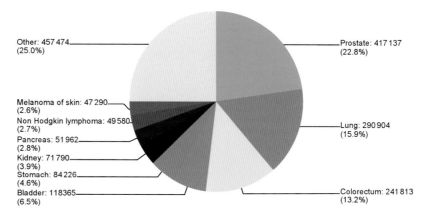

Prostate: 417 137 (22.8%)
Lung: 290 904 (15.9%)
Colorectum: 241 813 (13.2%)
Other: 457 474 (25.0%)
Melanoma of skin: 47 290 (2.6%)
Non Hodgkin lymphoma: 49 580 (2.7%)
Pancreas: 51 962 (2.8%)
Kidney: 71 790 (3.9%)
Stomach: 84 226 (4.6%)
Bladder: 118 365 (6.5%)

Women
Estimated number of cancer cases, all ages (total:1 611 735)

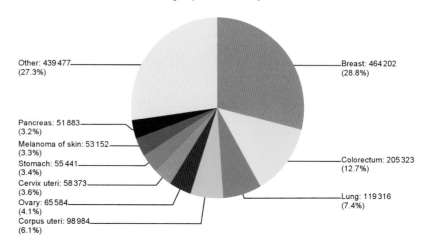

Breast: 464 202 (28.8%)
Colorectum: 205 323 (12.7%)
Lung: 119 316 (7.4%)
Other: 439 477 (27.3%)
Pancreas: 51 883 (3.2%)
Melanoma of skin: 53 152 (3.3%)
Stomach: 55 441 (3.4%)
Cervix uteri: 58 373 (3.6%)
Ovary: 65 584 (4.1%)
Corpus uteri: 98 984 (6.1%)

Fig. 1.1.13. Europe. Estimated cancer mortality proportions by major sites, in both sexes combined, in men, and in women, 2012.

Europe

Both sexes
Estimated number of cancer deaths, all ages (total:1 755 786)

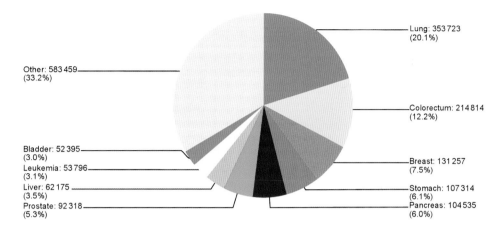

Other: 583 459 (33.2%)
Bladder: 52 395 (3.0%)
Leukemia: 53 796 (3.1%)
Liver: 62 175 (3.5%)
Prostate: 92 318 (5.3%)
Lung: 353 723 (20.1%)
Colorectum: 214 814 (12.2%)
Breast: 131 257 (7.5%)
Stomach: 107 314 (6.1%)
Pancreas: 104 535 (6.0%)

Men
Estimated number of cancer deaths, all ages (total:976 621)

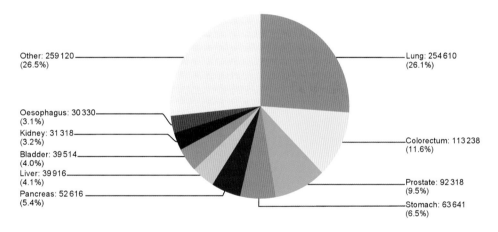

Other: 259 120 (26.5%)
Oesophagus: 30 330 (3.1%)
Kidney: 31 318 (3.2%)
Bladder: 39 514 (4.0%)
Liver: 39 916 (4.1%)
Pancreas: 52 616 (5.4%)
Lung: 254 610 (26.1%)
Colorectum: 113 238 (11.6%)
Prostate: 92 318 (9.5%)
Stomach: 63 641 (6.5%)

Women
Estimated number of cancer deaths, all ages (total:779 165)

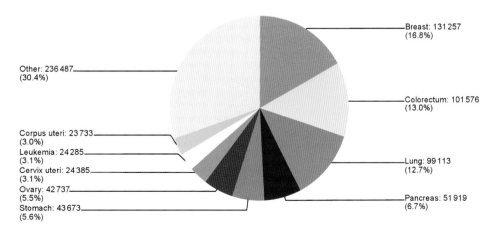

Other: 236 487 (30.4%)
Corpus uteri: 23 733 (3.0%)
Leukemia: 24 285 (3.1%)
Cervix uteri: 24 385 (3.1%)
Ovary: 42 737 (5.5%)
Stomach: 43 673 (5.6%)
Breast: 131 257 (16.8%)
Colorectum: 101 576 (13.0%)
Lung: 99 113 (12.7%)
Pancreas: 51 919 (6.7%)

Fig. 1.1.14. Europe. Estimated age-standardized (World) cancer incidence and mortality rates (ASR) per 100 000, by major sites, in men and women, 2012.

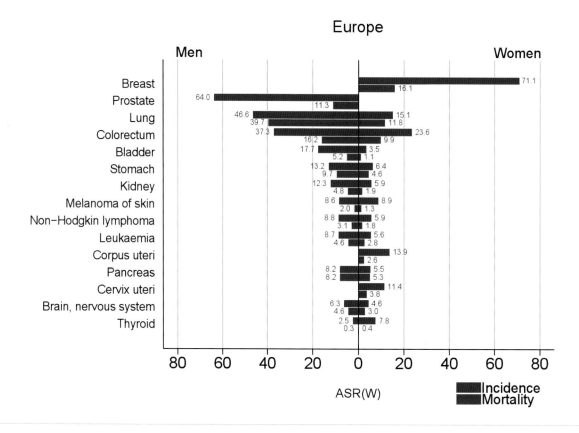

Fig. 1.1.15. Europe. Estimated cancer 5-year prevalence proportions by major sites, in both sexes combined, 2012.

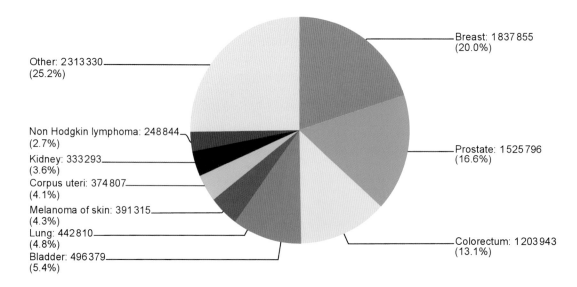

Fig. 1.1.16. North America. Estimated cancer incidence proportions by major sites, in both sexes combined, in men, and in women, 2012.

North America

Both sexes
Estimated number of cancer cases, all ages (total:1 786 369)

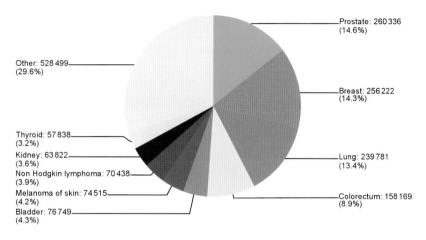

Men
Estimated number of cancer cases, all ages (total:920 629)

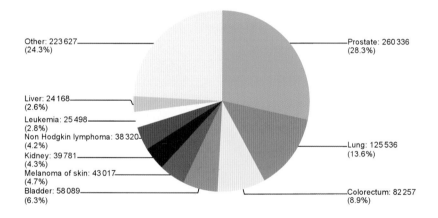

Women
Estimated number of cancer cases, all ages (total:865 740)

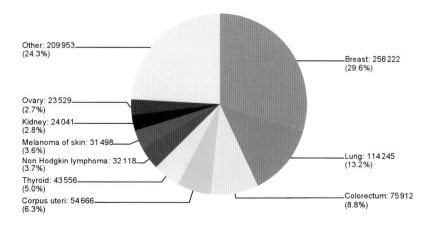

North America

Both sexes
Estimated number of cancer deaths, all ages (total:691 507)

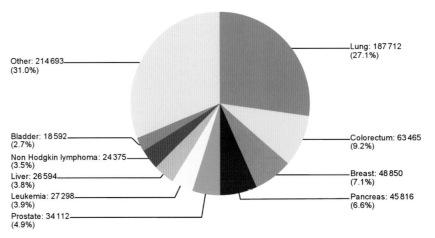

Other: 214 693 (31.0%)
Lung: 187 712 (27.1%)
Bladder: 18 592 (2.7%)
Non Hodgkin lymphoma: 24 375 (3.5%)
Liver: 26 594 (3.8%)
Leukemia: 27 298 (3.9%)
Prostate: 34 112 (4.9%)
Colorectum: 63 465 (9.2%)
Breast: 48 850 (7.1%)
Pancreas: 45 816 (6.6%)

Men
Estimated number of cancer deaths, all ages (total:362 823)

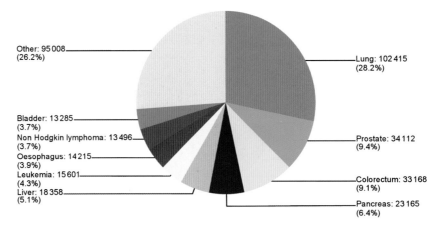

Other: 95 008 (26.2%)
Lung: 102 415 (28.2%)
Bladder: 13 285 (3.7%)
Non Hodgkin lymphoma: 13 496 (3.7%)
Oesophagus: 14 215 (3.9%)
Leukemia: 15 601 (4.3%)
Liver: 18 358 (5.1%)
Prostate: 34 112 (9.4%)
Colorectum: 33 168 (9.1%)
Pancreas: 23 165 (6.4%)

Women
Estimated number of cancer deaths, all ages (total:328 684)

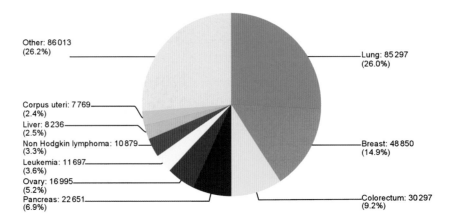

Other: 86 013 (26.2%)
Lung: 85 297 (26.0%)
Corpus uteri: 7 769 (2.4%)
Liver: 8 236 (2.5%)
Non Hodgkin lymphoma: 10 879 (3.3%)
Leukemia: 11 697 (3.6%)
Ovary: 16 995 (5.2%)
Pancreas: 22 651 (6.9%)
Breast: 48 850 (14.9%)
Colorectum: 30 297 (9.2%)

Fig. 1.1.18. North America. Estimated age-standardized (World) cancer incidence and mortality rates (ASR) per 100 000, by major sites, in men and women, 2012.

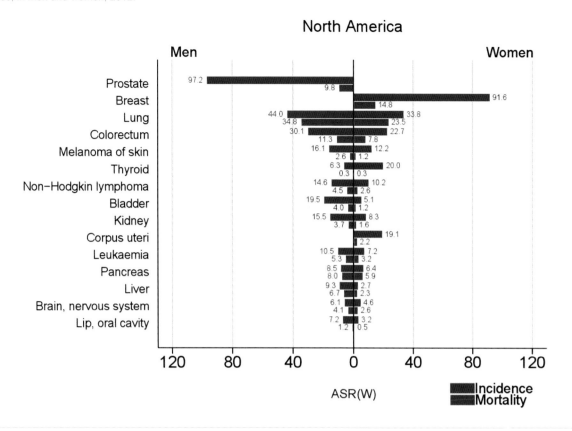

Fig. 1.1.19. North America. Estimated cancer 5-year prevalence proportions by major sites, in both sexes combined, 2012.

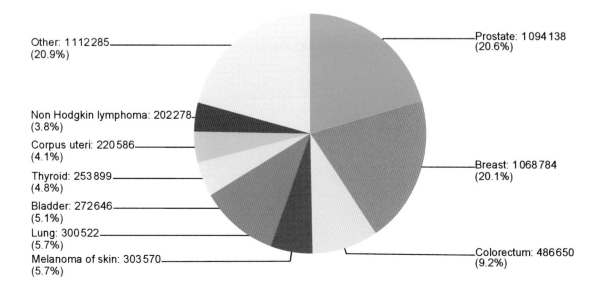

Fig. 1.1.20. Oceania. Estimated cancer incidence proportions by major sites, in both sexes combined, in men, and in women, 2012.

Oceania

Both sexes
Estimated number of cancer cases, all ages (total:155457)

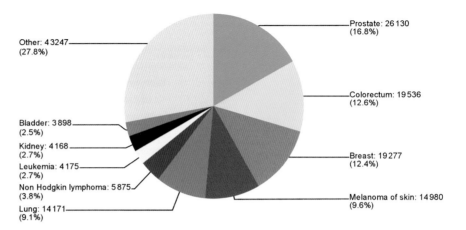

Other: 43247
(27.8%)

Bladder: 3898
(2.5%)

Kidney: 4168
(2.7%)

Leukemia: 4175
(2.7%)

Non Hodgkin lymphoma: 5875
(3.8%)

Lung: 14171
(9.1%)

Prostate: 26130
(16.8%)

Colorectum: 19536
(12.6%)

Breast: 19277
(12.4%)

Melanoma of skin: 14980
(9.6%)

Men
Estimated number of cancer cases, all ages (total:86035)

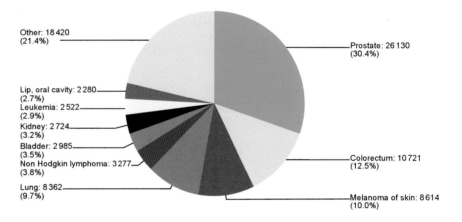

Other: 18420
(21.4%)

Lip, oral cavity: 2280
(2.7%)

Leukemia: 2522
(2.9%)

Kidney: 2724
(3.2%)

Bladder: 2985
(3.5%)

Non Hodgkin lymphoma: 3277
(3.8%)

Lung: 8362
(9.7%)

Prostate: 26130
(30.4%)

Colorectum: 10721
(12.5%)

Melanoma of skin: 8614
(10.0%)

Women
Estimated number of cancer cases, all ages (total:69422)

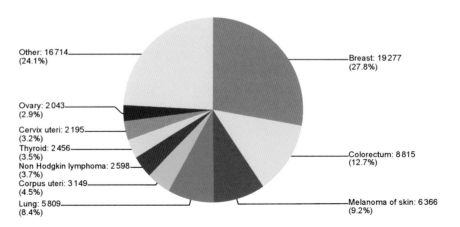

Other: 16714
(24.1%)

Ovary: 2043
(2.9%)

Cervix uteri: 2195
(3.2%)

Thyroid: 2456
(3.5%)

Non Hodgkin lymphoma: 2598
(3.7%)

Corpus uteri: 3149
(4.5%)

Lung: 5809
(8.4%)

Breast: 19277
(27.8%)

Colorectum: 8815
(12.7%)

Melanoma of skin: 6366
(9.2%)

Fig. 1.1.21. Oceania. Estimated cancer mortality proportions by major sites, in both sexes combined, in men, and in women, 2012.

Oceania

Both sexes
Estimated number of cancer deaths, all ages (total:59663)

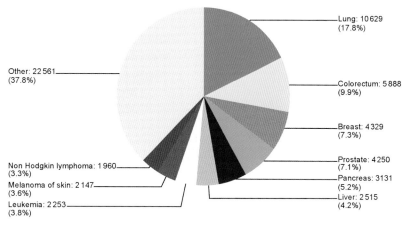

Other: 22561
(37.8%)

Lung: 10629
(17.8%)

Colorectum: 5888
(9.9%)

Breast: 4329
(7.3%)

Prostate: 4250
(7.1%)

Pancreas: 3131
(5.2%)

Liver: 2515
(4.2%)

Non Hodgkin lymphoma: 1960
(3.3%)

Melanoma of skin: 2147
(3.6%)

Leukemia: 2253
(3.8%)

Men
Estimated number of cancer deaths, all ages (total:32545)

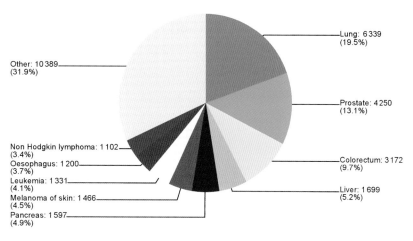

Other: 10389
(31.9%)

Lung: 6339
(19.5%)

Prostate: 4250
(13.1%)

Colorectum: 3172
(9.7%)

Liver: 1699
(5.2%)

Non Hodgkin lymphoma: 1102
(3.4%)

Oesophagus: 1200
(3.7%)

Leukemia: 1331
(4.1%)

Melanoma of skin: 1466
(4.5%)

Pancreas: 1597
(4.9%)

Women
Estimated number of cancer deaths, all ages (total:27118)

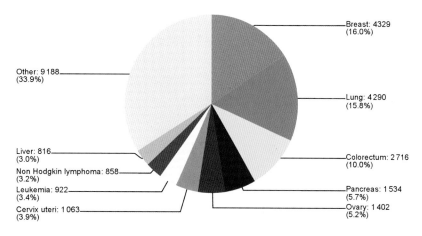

Other: 9188
(33.9%)

Breast: 4329
(16.0%)

Lung: 4290
(15.8%)

Colorectum: 2716
(10.0%)

Pancreas: 1534
(5.7%)

Ovary: 1402
(5.2%)

Liver: 816
(3.0%)

Non Hodgkin lymphoma: 858
(3.2%)

Leukemia: 922
(3.4%)

Cervix uteri: 1063
(3.9%)

Fig. 1.1.22. Oceania. Estimated age-standardized (World) cancer incidence and mortality rates (ASR) per 100 000, by major sites, in men and women, 2012.

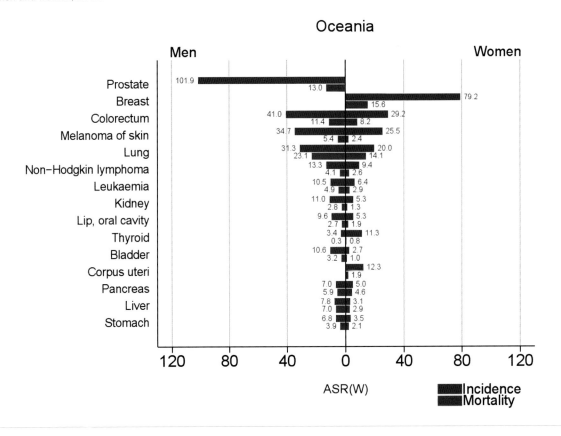

Fig. 1.1.23. Oceania. Estimated cancer 5-year prevalence proportions by major sites, in both sexes combined, 2012.

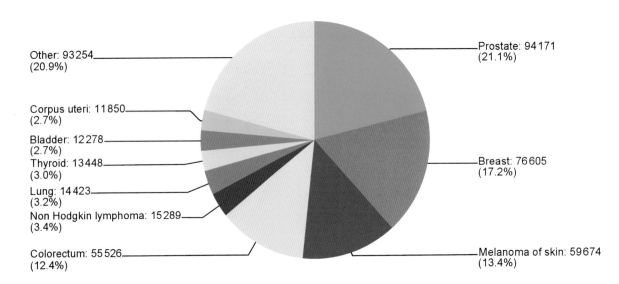

Fig. 1.1.24. Latin America and the Caribbean. Estimated cancer incidence proportions by major sites, in both sexes combined, in men, and in women, 2012.

Latin America & the Caribbean

Both sexes
Estimated number of cancer cases, all ages (total:1 096 056)

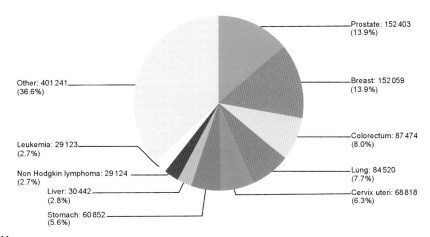

Men
Estimated number of cancer cases, all ages (total:533 049)

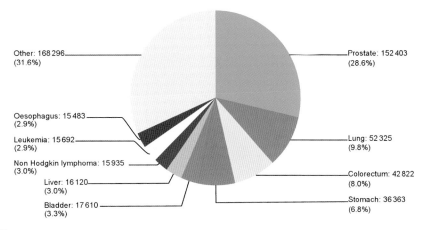

Women
Estimated number of cancer cases, all ages (total:563 007)

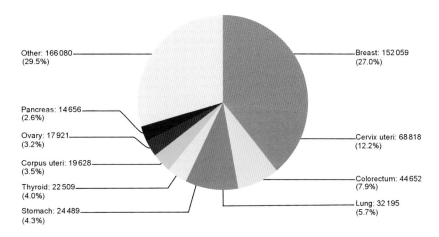

Fig. 1.1.25. Latin America and the Caribbean. Estimated cancer mortality proportions by major sites, in both sexes combined, in men, and in women, 2012.

Latin America & the Caribbean

Both sexes
Estimated number of cancer deaths, all ages (total:603 359)

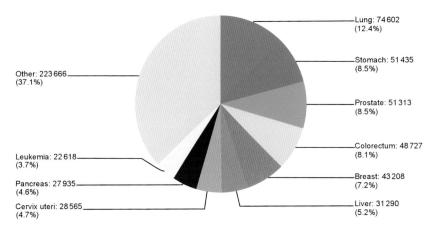

Other: 223 666 (37.1%)
Leukemia: 22 618 (3.7%)
Pancreas: 27 935 (4.6%)
Cervix uteri: 28 565 (4.7%)
Lung: 74 602 (12.4%)
Stomach: 51 435 (8.5%)
Prostate: 51 313 (8.5%)
Colorectum: 48 727 (8.1%)
Breast: 43 208 (7.2%)
Liver: 31 290 (5.2%)

Men
Estimated number of cancer deaths, all ages (total:313 822)

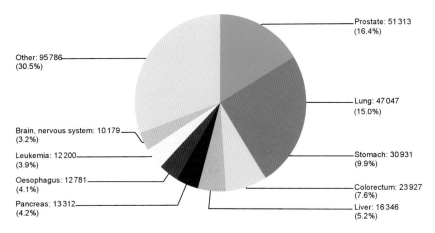

Other: 95 786 (30.5%)
Brain, nervous system: 10 179 (3.2%)
Leukemia: 12 200 (3.9%)
Oesophagus: 12 781 (4.1%)
Pancreas: 13 312 (4.2%)
Prostate: 51 313 (16.4%)
Lung: 47 047 (15.0%)
Stomach: 30 931 (9.9%)
Colorectum: 23 927 (7.6%)
Liver: 16 346 (5.2%)

Women
Estimated number of cancer deaths, all ages (total:289 537)

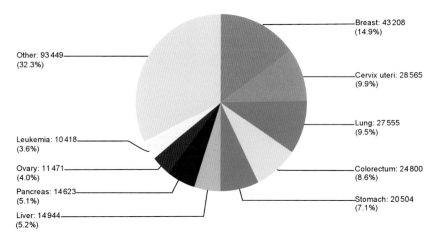

Other: 93 449 (32.3%)
Leukemia: 10 418 (3.6%)
Ovary: 11 471 (4.0%)
Pancreas: 14 623 (5.1%)
Liver: 14 944 (5.2%)
Breast: 43 208 (14.9%)
Cervix uteri: 28 565 (9.9%)
Lung: 27 555 (9.5%)
Colorectum: 24 800 (8.6%)
Stomach: 20 504 (7.1%)

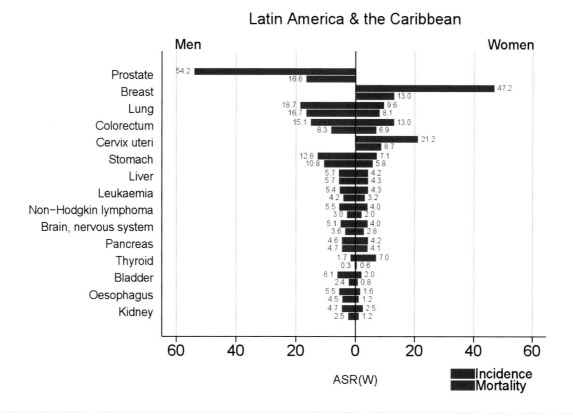

Fig. 1.1.26. Latin America and the Caribbean. Estimated age-standardized (World) cancer incidence and mortality rates (ASR) per 100 000, by major sites, in men and women, 2012.

Fig. 1.1.27. Latin America and the Caribbean. Estimated cancer 5-year prevalence proportions by major sites, in both sexes combined, 2012.

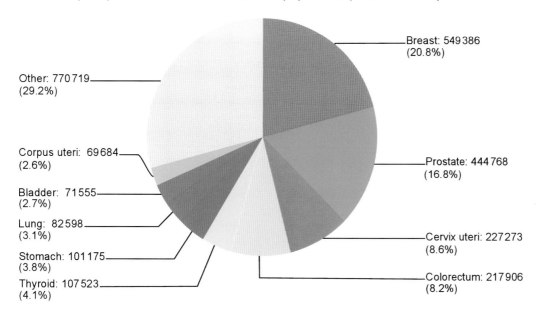

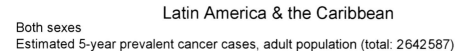

Fig. 1.1.28. Middle East and North Africa. Estimated cancer incidence proportions by major sites, in both sexes combined, in men, and in women, 2012.

Middle East & North Africa

Both sexes
Estimated number of cancer cases, all ages (total:538131)

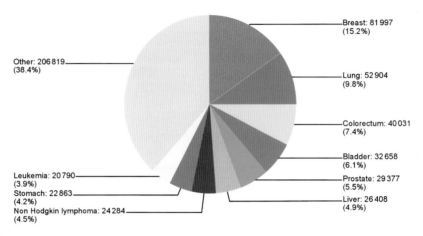

Other: 206819 (38.4%)
Breast: 81997 (15.2%)
Lung: 52904 (9.8%)
Colorectum: 40031 (7.4%)
Bladder: 32658 (6.1%)
Prostate: 29377 (5.5%)
Liver: 26408 (4.9%)
Leukemia: 20790 (3.9%)
Stomach: 22863 (4.2%)
Non Hodgkin lymphoma: 24284 (4.5%)

Men
Estimated number of cancer cases, all ages (total:274450)

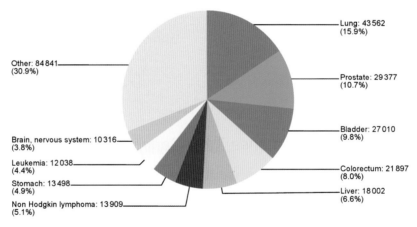

Other: 84841 (30.9%)
Lung: 43562 (15.9%)
Prostate: 29377 (10.7%)
Bladder: 27010 (9.8%)
Colorectum: 21897 (8.0%)
Liver: 18002 (6.6%)
Brain, nervous system: 10316 (3.8%)
Leukemia: 12038 (4.4%)
Stomach: 13498 (4.9%)
Non Hodgkin lymphoma: 13909 (5.1%)

Women
Estimated number of cancer cases, all ages (total:263681)

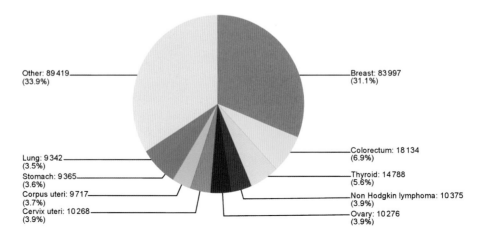

Other: 89419 (33.9%)
Breast: 83997 (31.1%)
Colorectum: 18134 (6.9%)
Thyroid: 14788 (5.6%)
Non Hodgkin lymphoma: 10375 (3.9%)
Ovary: 10276 (3.9%)
Lung: 9342 (3.5%)
Stomach: 9365 (3.6%)
Corpus uteri: 9717 (3.7%)
Cervix uteri: 10268 (3.9%)

Fig. 1.1.29. Middle East and North Africa. Estimated cancer mortality proportions by major sites, in both sexes combined, in men, and in women, 2012.

Middle East & North Africa

Both sexes
Estimated number of cancer deaths, all ages (total:332775)

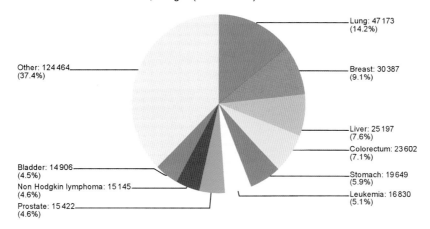

Other: 124464 (37.4%)

Bladder: 14906 (4.5%)
Non Hodgkin lymphoma: 15145 (4.6%)
Prostate: 15422 (4.6%)

Lung: 47173 (14.2%)
Breast: 30387 (9.1%)
Liver: 25197 (7.6%)
Colorectum: 23602 (7.1%)
Stomach: 19649 (5.9%)
Leukemia: 16830 (5.1%)

Men
Estimated number of cancer deaths, all ages (total:187090)

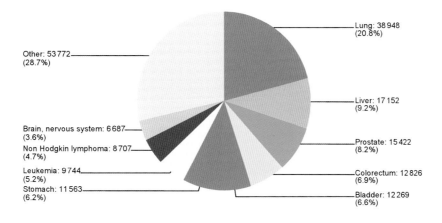

Other: 53772 (28.7%)

Brain, nervous system: 6687 (3.6%)
Non Hodgkin lymphoma: 8707 (4.7%)
Leukemia: 9744 (5.2%)
Stomach: 11563 (6.2%)

Lung: 38948 (20.8%)
Liver: 17152 (9.2%)
Prostate: 15422 (8.2%)
Colorectum: 12826 (6.9%)
Bladder: 12269 (6.6%)

Women
Estimated number of cancer deaths, all ages (total:145685)

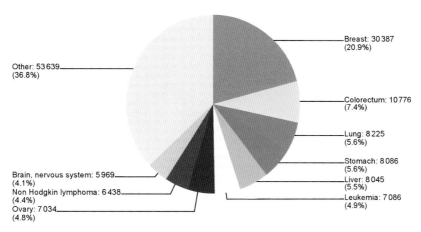

Other: 53639 (36.8%)

Brain, nervous system: 5969 (4.1%)
Non Hodgkin lymphoma: 6438 (4.4%)
Ovary: 7034 (4.8%)

Breast: 30387 (20.9%)
Colorectum: 10776 (7.4%)
Lung: 8225 (5.6%)
Stomach: 8086 (5.6%)
Liver: 8045 (5.5%)
Leukemia: 7086 (4.9%)

Fig. 1.1.30. Middle East and North Africa. Estimated age-standardized (World) cancer incidence and mortality rates (ASR) per 100 000, by major sites, in men and women, 2012.

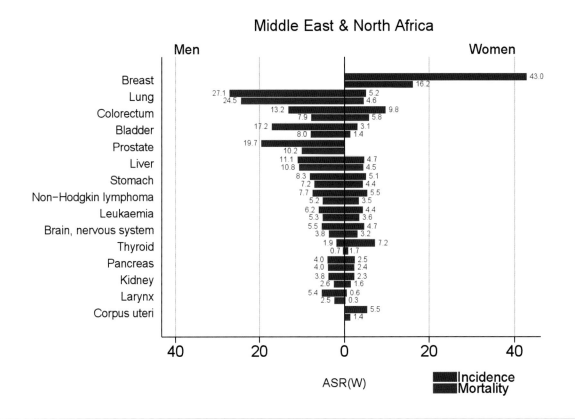

Fig. 1.1.31. Middle East and North Africa. Estimated cancer 5-year prevalence proportions by major sites, in both sexes combined, 2012.

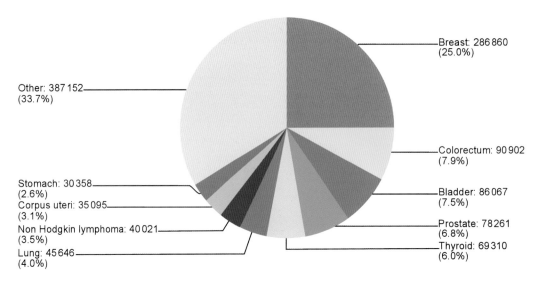

Fig. 1.1.32. Sub-Saharan Africa. Estimated cancer incidence proportions by major sites, in both sexes combined, in men, and in women, 2012.

Sub-Saharan Africa

Both sexes
Estimated number of cancer cases, all ages (total:626 399)

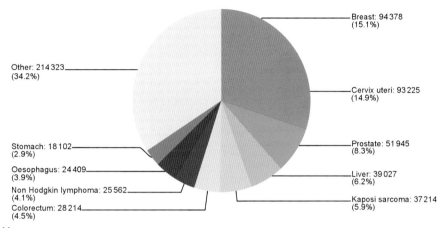

Breast: 94 378
(15.1%)

Cervix uteri: 93 225
(14.9%)

Prostate: 51 945
(8.3%)

Liver: 39 027
(6.2%)

Kaposi sarcoma: 37 214
(5.9%)

Other: 214 323
(34.2%)

Stomach: 18 102
(2.9%)

Oesophagus: 24 409
(3.9%)

Non Hodgkin lymphoma: 25 562
(4.1%)

Colorectum: 28 214
(4.5%)

Men
Estimated number of cancer cases, all ages (total:256 261)

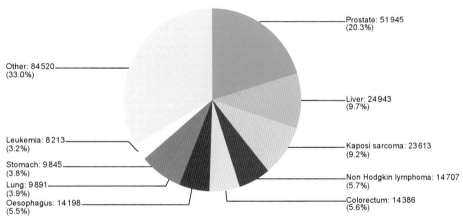

Prostate: 51 945
(20.3%)

Liver: 24 943
(9.7%)

Kaposi sarcoma: 23 613
(9.2%)

Non Hodgkin lymphoma: 14 707
(5.7%)

Colorectum: 14 386
(5.6%)

Other: 84 520
(33.0%)

Leukemia: 8 213
(3.2%)

Stomach: 9 845
(3.8%)

Lung: 9 891
(3.9%)

Oesophagus: 14 198
(5.5%)

Women
Estimated number of cancer cases, all ages (total:370 138)

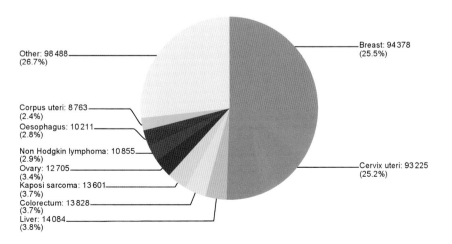

Breast: 94 378
(25.5%)

Cervix uteri: 93 225
(25.2%)

Other: 98 488
(26.7%)

Corpus uteri: 8 763
(2.4%)

Oesophagus: 10 211
(2.8%)

Non Hodgkin lymphoma: 10 855
(2.9%)

Ovary: 12 705
(3.4%)

Kaposi sarcoma: 13 601
(3.7%)

Colorectum: 13 828
(3.7%)

Liver: 14 084
(3.8%)

Fig. 1.1.33. Sub-Saharan Africa. Estimated cancer mortality proportions by major sites, in both sexes combined, in men, and in women, 2012.

Sub-Saharan Africa

Both sexes
Estimated number of cancer deaths, all ages (total:447 745)

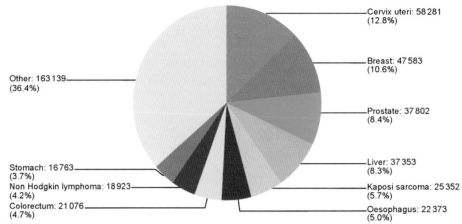

Cervix uteri: 58 281 (12.8%)
Breast: 47 583 (10.6%)
Prostate: 37 802 (8.4%)
Liver: 37 353 (8.3%)
Kaposi sarcoma: 25 352 (5.7%)
Oesophagus: 22 373 (5.0%)
Other: 163 139 (36.4%)
Stomach: 16 763 (3.7%)
Non Hodgkin lymphoma: 18 923 (4.2%)
Colorectum: 21 076 (4.7%)

Men
Estimated number of cancer deaths, all ages (total:200 881)

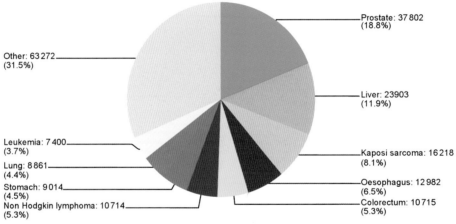

Prostate: 37 802 (18.8%)
Liver: 23 903 (11.9%)
Kaposi sarcoma: 16 218 (8.1%)
Oesophagus: 12 982 (6.5%)
Colorectum: 10 715 (5.3%)
Other: 63 272 (31.5%)
Leukemia: 7 400 (3.7%)
Lung: 8 861 (4.4%)
Stomach: 9 014 (4.5%)
Non Hodgkin lymphoma: 10 714 (5.3%)

Women
Estimated number of cancer deaths, all ages (total:246 864)

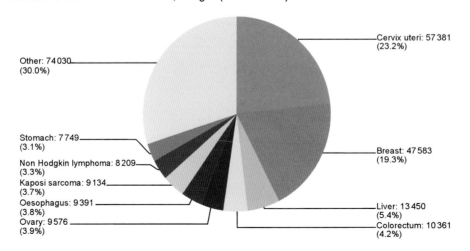

Cervix uteri: 57 381 (23.2%)
Breast: 47 583 (19.3%)
Liver: 13 450 (5.4%)
Colorectum: 10 361 (4.2%)
Other: 74 030 (30.0%)
Stomach: 7 749 (3.1%)
Non Hodgkin lymphoma: 8 209 (3.3%)
Kaposi sarcoma: 9 134 (3.7%)
Oesophagus: 9 391 (3.8%)
Ovary: 9 576 (3.9%)

Fig. 1.1.34. Sub-Saharan Africa. Estimated age-standardized (World) cancer incidence and mortality rates (ASR) per 100 000, by major sites, in men and women, 2012.

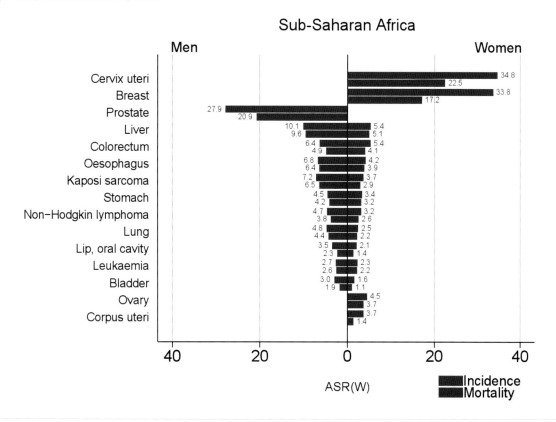

Fig. 1.1.35. Sub-Saharan Africa. Estimated cancer 5-year prevalence proportions by major sites, in both sexes combined, 2012.

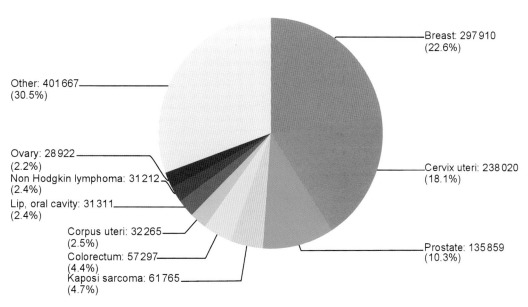

Fig. 1.1.36. East and Central Asia. Estimated cancer incidence proportions by major sites, in both sexes combined, in men, and in women, 2012.

East & Central Asia

Both sexes
Estimated number of cancer cases, all ages (total: 6 445 461)

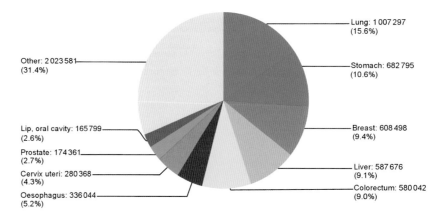

Other: 2 023 581 (31.4%)
Lip, oral cavity: 165 799 (2.6%)
Prostate: 174 361 (2.7%)
Cervix uteri: 280 368 (4.3%)
Oesophagus: 336 044 (5.2%)
Lung: 1 007 297 (15.6%)
Stomach: 682 795 (10.6%)
Breast: 608 498 (9.4%)
Liver: 587 676 (9.1%)
Colorectum: 580 042 (9.0%)

Men
Estimated number of cancer cases, all ages (total: 3 526 183)

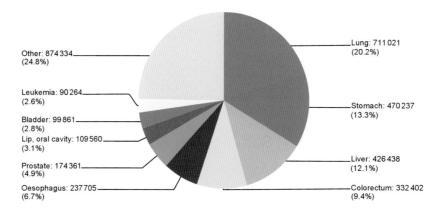

Other: 874 334 (24.8%)
Leukemia: 90 264 (2.6%)
Bladder: 99 861 (2.8%)
Lip, oral cavity: 109 560 (3.1%)
Prostate: 174 361 (4.9%)
Oesophagus: 237 705 (6.7%)
Lung: 711 021 (20.2%)
Stomach: 470 237 (13.3%)
Liver: 426 438 (12.1%)
Colorectum: 332 402 (9.4%)

Women
Estimated number of cancer cases, all ages (total: 2 919 278)

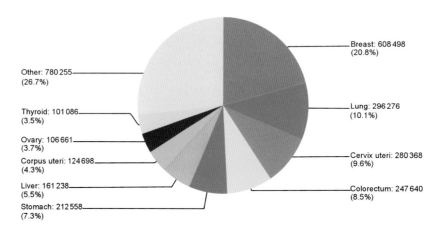

Other: 780 255 (26.7%)
Thyroid: 101 086 (3.5%)
Ovary: 106 661 (3.7%)
Corpus uteri: 124 698 (4.3%)
Liver: 161 238 (5.5%)
Stomach: 212 558 (7.3%)
Breast: 608 498 (20.8%)
Lung: 296 276 (10.1%)
Cervix uteri: 280 368 (9.6%)
Colorectum: 247 640 (8.5%)

Fig. 1.1.37. East and Central Asia. Estimated cancer mortality proportions by major sites, in both sexes combined, in men, and in women, 2012.

East & Central Asia

Both sexes
Estimated number of cancer deaths, all ages (total: 4 310 195)

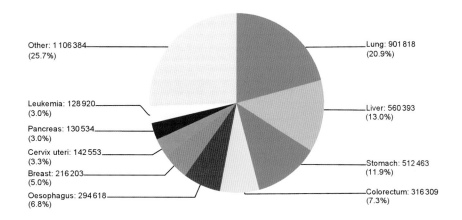

Other: 1 106 384
(25.7%)

Leukemia: 128 920
(3.0%)

Pancreas: 130 534
(3.0%)

Cervix uteri: 142 553
(3.3%)

Breast: 216 203
(5.0%)

Oesophagus: 294 618
(6.8%)

Lung: 901 818
(20.9%)

Liver: 560 393
(13.0%)

Stomach: 512 463
(11.9%)

Colorectum: 316 309
(7.3%)

Men
Estimated number of cancer deaths, all ages (total: 2 579 350)

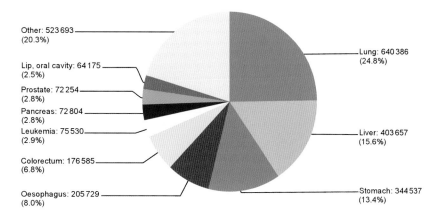

Other: 523 693
(20.3%)

Lip, oral cavity: 64 175
(2.5%)

Prostate: 72 254
(2.8%)

Pancreas: 72 804
(2.8%)

Leukemia: 75 530
(2.9%)

Colorectum: 176 585
(6.8%)

Oesophagus: 205 729
(8.0%)

Lung: 640 386
(24.8%)

Liver: 403 657
(15.6%)

Stomach: 344 537
(13.4%)

Women
Estimated number of cancer deaths, all ages (total: 1 730 845)

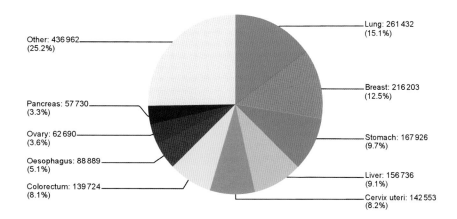

Other: 436 962
(25.2%)

Pancreas: 57 730
(3.3%)

Ovary: 62 690
(3.6%)

Oesophagus: 88 889
(5.1%)

Colorectum: 139 724
(8.1%)

Lung: 261 432
(15.1%)

Breast: 216 203
(12.5%)

Stomach: 167 926
(9.7%)

Liver: 156 736
(9.1%)

Cervix uteri: 142 553
(8.2%)

Fig. 1.1.38. East and Central Asia. Estimated age-standardized (World) cancer incidence and mortality rates (ASR) per 100 000, by major sites, in men and women, 2012.

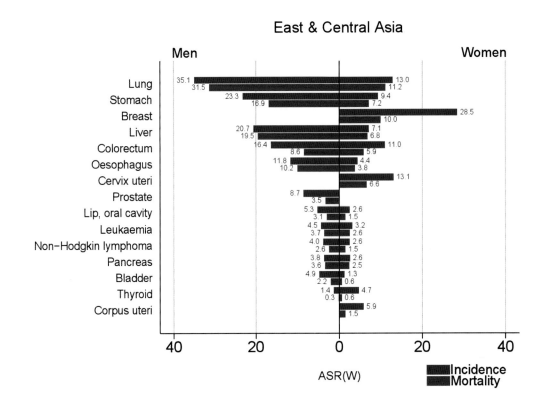

Fig. 1.1.39. East and Central Asia. Estimated cancer 5-year prevalence proportions by major sites, in both sexes combined, 2012.

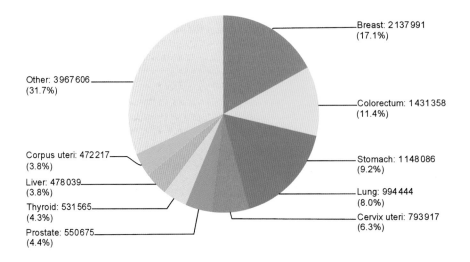

Fig. 1.1.40. Age-standardized (World) cancer incidence rates per 100 000 in selected cancer registry populations, for all cancers combined (excluding non-melanoma skin cancer) in men, 2003–2007.

Fig. 1.1.41. Age-standardized (World) cancer incidence rates per 100 000 in selected cancer registry populations, for all cancers combined (excluding non-melanoma skin cancer) in women, 2003–2007.

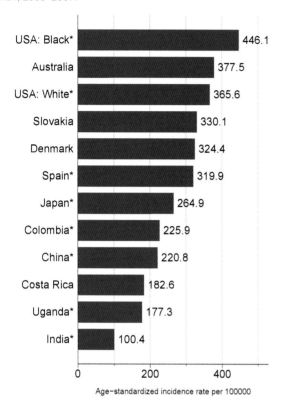

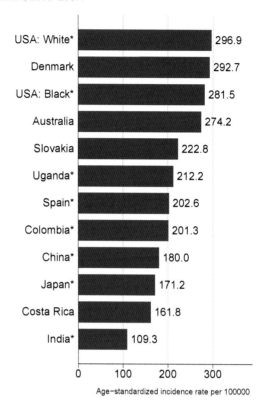

Country-specific patterns of cancer

The consideration of incidence and mortality rates in specific countries selected to be representative of the world regions provides a further degree of focus on the international variation in the cancer burden. Figs 1.1.40 and 1.1.41 show age-standardized incidence rates in men and women, respectively, in about 2005 for all cancers combined (excluding non-melanoma skin cancer) for a range of countries representative of different world regions and selected because of the high quality of their cancer incidence data. These data are derived from cancer registry data sets, and all of the registries have met the quality criteria for publication in *Cancer Incidence in Five Continents*, Volume X [7].

Comparable mortality data, where available from the WHO Mortality Database [8] or elsewhere [14], for

the same countries are shown in Figs 1.1.42 and 1.1.43. Cancer incidence and mortality information for the same set of countries is presented in the site-specific chapters later in this Report. It should be noted that cause-specific death certification is available for only a limited sample of the Chinese population and is not routinely undertaken in India and Uganda, and thus relevant mortality data are not available for India and Uganda.

Among men, incidence (Fig. 1.1.40) varies by approximately 4-fold, from 100 per 100 000 in Indian registries to more than 400 per 100 000 in the USA Surveillance, Epidemiology and End Results (SEER) Black population. Among women (Fig. 1.1.41), incidence varies by approximately 3-fold, from just more than 100 per 100 000 in Indian registries to about 300 per 100 000 in the USA SEER White population and in Denmark.

For both sexes there is, within this group of countries, a gradation in all-cancer incidence rates between the extremes and, especially in men, the higher rates are in economically more developed populations. Among women, while the association with economic development is also apparent, the rates in Japanese registries are at the lower end of the spectrum (170 per 100 000), whereas those in Uganda (212 per 100 000) are relatively high. As observed in the world maps, the between-country variation in mortality (Figs 1.1.42, 1.1.43) is less pronounced than that for incidence and, in both sexes, is less than 2-fold. Thus, in men (Fig. 1.1.42) the variation extends from 99 per 100 000 in Costa Rica to 203 per 100 000 in Slovakia, whereas in women (Fig. 1.1.43) it extends from 69 per 100 000 in Japan to 121 per 100 000 in Denmark.

Fig. 1.1.42. Age-standardized (World) cancer mortality rates per 100 000 by year in selected countries, for all cancers combined (excluding non-melanoma skin cancer) in men, 2003–2007.

Fig. 1.1.43. Age-standardized (World) cancer mortality rates per 100 000 by year in selected countries, for all cancers combined (excluding non-melanoma skin cancer) in women, 2003–2007.

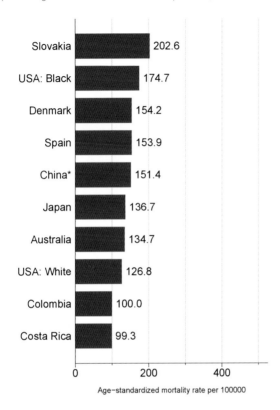

Age–standardized mortality rate per 100000

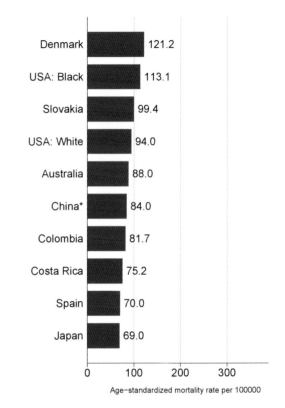

Age–standardized mortality rate per 100000

Data from the same populations and the same sources as used in Figs 1.1.40 to 1.1.43 are presented in terms of trends over time in Figs 1.1.44 and 1.1.45 (incidence) and Figs 1.1.46 and 1.1.47 (mortality) for all cancers combined (excluding non-melanoma skin cancer). It is difficult to discern any general consistent trends in incidence from country to country, although, with few exceptions (e.g. the decline in incidence among men in Chinese registries), rates have tended to increase from the 1980s to the present. In some cases, for example in Slovakia, Colombia, and Denmark, this has been a fairly constant increase over the entire time period, whereas elsewhere, for example in Japan and the USA, an initial period of increase has been followed by a drop in rates. Some of the observed effects can be readily explained. For example, the peak in the early 1990s among men in the USA

(Black and White) and Australia is explained by the rapid increase in the number of prostate cancer diagnoses after the introduction of testing for prostate-specific antigen [15]. Changes in the prevalence of smoking and hence, after a suitable lag period, in the incidence of lung cancer and other smoking-associated cancers, will also be important determinants of all-cancer incidence and mortality rates [16]. However, other trends require detailed consideration of country-specific patterns by type of cancer.

The mortality trends (Figs 1.1.46, 1.1.47) are more consistent in that, in both sexes, most populations have shown a substantive decline in age-standardized mortality, with the exception of China (although the Chinese data are for a much shorter time series). The mortality decline is evident in countries such as Denmark and Costa Rica, which have, respectively, relatively high

and low absolute levels of mortality. Such mortality decreases against a background of increase in incidence are indications of improved survival as a result of improved therapy and/ or earlier detection (including as a consequence of screening).

Nearly all cancer types show important variations between regions, subregions, and countries in terms of both contemporary incidence rates and their trends over time. The broad overview presented in this chapter inevitably masks some of these geographical associations. For example, the consideration given above, at the regional level, to East and Central Asia does not identify the extraordinarily high rates of thyroid cancer among women in the Republic of Korea, estimated as 89 per 100 000 – the most common cancer among women in the country, and the highest rate of any country in the world. It is currently unclear to what extent this

Fig. 1.1.44. Age-standardized (World) cancer incidence rates per 100 000 by year in selected populations, for all cancers combined (excluding non-melanoma skin cancer) in men, circa 1975–2012.

Fig. 1.1.45. Age-standardized (World) cancer incidence rates per 100 000 by year in selected populations, for all cancers combined (excluding non-melanoma skin cancer) in women, circa 1975–2012.

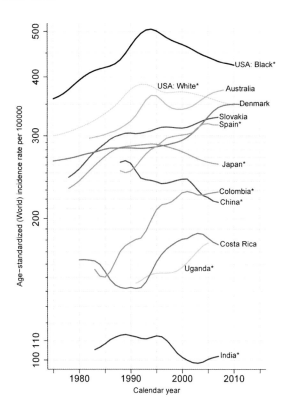

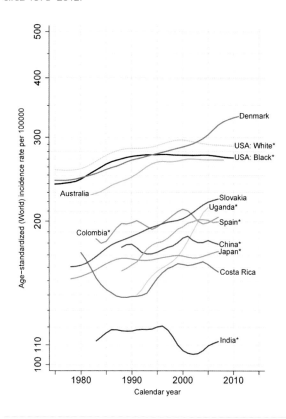

epidemic is driven by improved diagnostic technology [17]. Similarly, the estimated European incidence rate of cervical cancer (11.4 per 100 000) obscures the internal variation, ranging from 29 per 100 000 in Romania to 4 per 100 000 in Switzerland, due primarily to the impact of cytological screening programmes [18]. Likewise, in sub-Saharan Africa, the average incidence rate for oesophageal cancer in men is 6 per 100 000, ranging from 25 per 100 000 in Uganda and Malawi to less than 1 per 100 000 in Guinea and Nigeria. The reason for the variation in this case is little understood, which should act as a stimulus for research [19].

Conclusions

Monitoring geographical variation in disease prevalence and searching for an understanding of the underlying reasons is frequently an important starting point for cancer epidemiology [20]. The understanding of the causes of any specific cancer is not complete without an explanation of the geographical distribution, and cancer is especially complex, given the diversity in cancer types, with each type often having its own set of risk factors and giving rise to a unique geographical pattern. Such variations have significant implications for tailoring cancer control to region- or country-specific priorities [21]. This chapter has focused primarily on the current overall burden of cancer globally and in major world regions and serves as a backdrop to the consideration of specific types in later chapters of this Report. However, with approximately 14 million new cases and 8 million cancer-related deaths per year, cancer must be viewed as a major cause of morbidity and mortality that affects populations in all countries and all regions.

While there are some commonalities, such as breast cancer being the major type of cancer among women in all world regions, there are also important differences, and the variation in the relative importance of cervical cancer across different regions is one such example. Some of these differences relate to the level of economic development, for example the higher incidence of cancers associated with infections in less-developed economies [22], and the associations with development are considered in more detail in Chapter 1.2. The importance of genetic variation as a cause of between-population differences in risk, such as for prostate cancer, is also recognized.

At a more general level, understanding the pattern of cancer in a

Fig. 1.1.46. Age-standardized (World) cancer mortality rates per 100 000 by year in selected countries, for all cancers combined (excluding non-melanoma skin cancer) in men, circa 1975–2012.

Fig. 1.1.47. Age–standardized (World) cancer mortality rates per 100 000 by year in selected countries, for all cancers combined (excluding non-melanoma skin cancer) in women, circa 1975–2012.

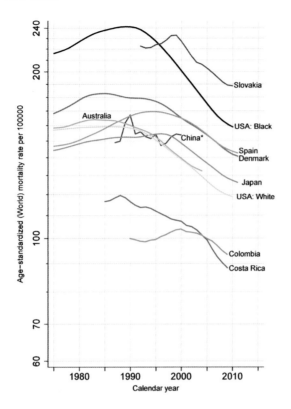

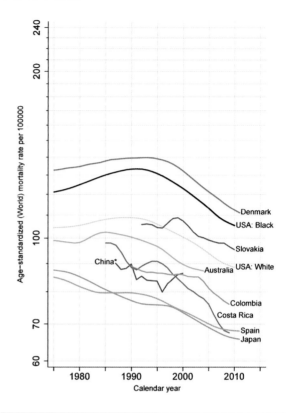

population is an essential prerequisite for planning any programme for cancer control. It is impossible to develop such plans without knowing which types of cancer are common and whether cancers are changing in incidence. Likewise, the impact of any control measures cannot be evaluated without monitoring the effect on cancer incidence or mortality in the years, or sometimes decades, after an intervention. To generate the relevant incidence data, as used extensively in this chapter, the work of cancer registries throughout the world is vital [23] and needs to be supported as part of any cancer control plans, especially in less-developed regions, where cancer registries are often absent or under-resourced [24].

The authors thank Joannie Lortet-Tieulent and Mathieu Laversanne for their assistance in producing the figures.

References

1. Parkin DM, Stjernswärd J, Muir CS (1984). Estimates of the worldwide frequency of twelve major cancers. *Bull World Health Organ*, 62:163–182. PMID:6610488

2. Ferlay J, Bray F, Pisani P, Parkin DM (2001). GLOBOCAN 2000: Cancer Incidence, Mortality and Prevalence Worldwide. IARC Cancer Base No. 5. Lyon: IARC.

3. Ferlay J, Soerjomataram I, Ervik M *et al.* (2013). GLOBOCAN 2012 v1.0, Cancer Incidence and Mortality Worldwide: IARC Cancer Base No. 11 [Internet]. Lyon: IARC. Available at http://globocan.iarc.fr.

4. Ferlay J, Shin HR, Bray F *et al.* (2010). Estimates of worldwide burden of cancer in 2008: GLOBOCAN 2008. *Int J Cancer*, 127:2893–2917. http://dx.doi.org/10.1002/ijc.25516 PMID:21351269

5. Parkin DM, Ferlay J, Curado MP *et al.* (2010). Fifty years of cancer incidence: CI5 I-IX. *Int J Cancer*, 127:2918–2927. http://dx.doi.org/10.1002/ijc.25517 PMID:21351270

6. Ferlay J, Parkin DM, Curado MP *et al.* (2010). *Cancer Incidence in Five Continents, Volumes I to IX: IARC Cancer Base No. 9* [Internet]. Lyon: IARC. Available at http://ci5.iarc.fr.

7. Forman D, Bray F, Brewster DH *et al.*, eds (2013). *Cancer Incidence in Five Continents*, Vol. X [electronic version]. Lyon: IARC. Available at http://ci5.iarc.fr.

8. WHO Mortality Database. Available at http://www.who.int/healthinfo/statistics/mortality_rawdata/en/index.html.

9. Bray F, Ren JS, Masuyer E, Ferlay J (2013). Global estimates of cancer prevalence for 27 sites in the adult population in 2008. *Int J Cancer*, 132:1133–1145. http://dx.doi.org/10.1002/ijc.27711 PMID:22752881

10. Abascal W, Esteves E, Goja B *et al.* (2012). Tobacco control campaign in Uruguay: a population-based trend analysis. *Lancet*, 380:1575–1582. http://dx.doi.org/10.1016/S0140-6736(12)60826-5 PMID:22981904

11. Dondog B, Lise M, Dondov O *et al.* (2011). Hepatitis B and C virus infections in hepatocellular carcinoma and cirrhosis in Mongolia. *Eur J Cancer Prev*, 20:33–39. http://dx.doi.org/10.1097/CEJ.0b013e32833f0c8e PMID:21166097

12. Edwards BK, Brown ML, Wingo PA *et al.* (2005). Annual report to the nation on the status of cancer, 1975–2002, featuring population-based trends in cancer treatment. *J Natl Cancer Inst*, 97:1407–1427. PMID:16204691

13. Geng EH, Hunt PW, Diero LO *et al.* (2011). Trends in the clinical characteristics of HIV-infected patients initiating antiretroviral therapy in Kenya, Uganda and Tanzania between 2002 and 2009. *J Int AIDS Soc*, 14:46. http://dx.doi.org/10.1186/1758-2652-14-46 PMID:21955541

14. National Center for Health Statistics, Centers for Disease Control and Prevention. Available at http://www.cdc.gov/nchs/.

15. Center MM, Jemal A, Lortet-Tieulent J *et al.* (2012). International variation in prostate cancer incidence and mortality rates. *Eur Urol*, 61:1079–1092. http://dx.doi.org/10.1016/j.eururo.2012.02.054 PMID:22424666

16. Jha P, Ramasundarahettige C, Landsman V *et al.* (2013). 21st-century hazards of smoking and benefits of cessation in the United States. *N Engl J Med*, 368:341–350. http://dx.doi.org/10.1056/NEJMsa1211128 PMID:23343063

17. Pellegriti G, Frasca F, Regalbuto C *et al.* (2013). Worldwide increasing incidence of thyroid cancer: update on epidemiology and risk factors. *J Cancer Epidemiol*, 2013:965212. http://dx.doi.org/10.1155/2013/965212 PMID:23737785

18. Anttila A, Ronco G; Working Group on the Registration and Monitoring of Cervical Cancer Screening Programmes in the European Union; within the European Network for Information on Cancer (EUNICE) (2009). Description of the national situation of cervical cancer screening in the member states of the European Union. *Eur J Cancer*, 45:2685–2708. http://dx.doi.org/10.1016/j.ejca.2009.07.017 PMID:19744852

19. Hendricks D, Parker MI (2002). Oesophageal cancer in Africa. *IUBMB Life*, 53:263–268. http://dx.doi.org/10.1080/15216540212643 PMID:12121007

20. Doll R (1967). *Prevention of Cancer: Pointers from Epidemiology*. London: Nuffield Provincial Hospitals Trust.

21. Wild CP (2012). The role of cancer research in noncommunicable disease control. *J Natl Cancer Inst*, 104:1051–1058. http://dx.doi.org/10.1093/jnci/djs262 PMID:22781435

22. de Martel C, Ferlay J, Franceschi S *et al.* (2012). Global burden of cancers attributable to infections in 2008: a review and synthetic analysis. *Lancet Oncol*, 13:607–615. http://dx.doi.org/10.1016/S1470-2045(12)70137-7 PMID:22575588

23. Brewster DH, Coebergh JW, Storm HH (2005). Population-based cancer registries: the invisible key to cancer control. *Lancet Oncol*, 6:193–195. http://dx.doi.org/10.1016/S1470-2045(05)70071-1 PMID:15811615

24. Global Initiative for Cancer Registry Development in Low- and Middle-Income Countries. Available at http://gicr.iarc.fr/

1.2

Transitions in human development and the global cancer burden

Freddie Bray

Bernard W. Stewart (reviewer)
Christopher P. Wild (reviewer)

Summary

- From a global perspective, the cancer burden for each country, and the most common tumour types, are associated with the value of the Human Development Index (HDI) for that country. Transitions towards higher levels of human development have the effect of increasing the burden of cancer overall, and of specific types.

- Cancers of the lung, breast, prostate, and colorectum are the major incident cancers in countries with high or very high HDI. In countries with low or medium HDI, cancers of the colorectum, breast, and lung have become rather more frequent, although there remains an excess of poverty- and infection-related cancers, notably cancers of the stomach, liver, cervix, and oesophagus.

- In countries in transition, declines in the incidence of cervical cancer tend to be offset by concomitant increases in the incidence of female breast cancer. In countries with low or medium HDI, incidence rates of colorectal cancer increase markedly as HDI rises in a given country.

- The predicted global cancer burden is expected to exceed 20 million new cancer cases annually by 2025, compared with the estimated 14.1 million new cases worldwide in 2012.

This chapter reviews the evolution of the cancer burden worldwide in relation to transitions in human development. Societal, economic, and lifestyle changes in a rapidly globalizing world continue to have profound effects on the scale and profile of the cancer burden and the need for tailored and effective strategies for cancer control and prevention. The increasing magnitude of the cancer problem is partly the consequence of population growth and ageing. Such demographic transitions mean that by 2030, well over 20 million new cancer cases will be diagnosed every year. The greatest impact will unquestionably be in countries presently in the midst of

Fig. 1.2.1. In India, an information technology business park stands where agricultural fields previously existed, indicative of the transition towards a higher Human Development Index rating.

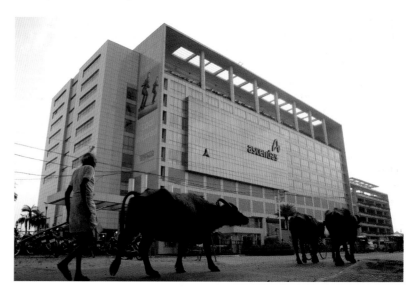

this developmental transition, many of which are ill-equipped to deal with the escalating numbers of cancer patients expected over the next decades.

As countries transition to higher levels of human development, the underlying populations tend to increasingly adopt behavioural and lifestyle habits that have become conventional in prosperous and industrialized countries. A changing prevalence and distribution of several reproductive, dietary, and hormonal risk factors has the effect of increasing the risk at the population level of certain cancers associated with affluence; these include female breast cancer, prostate cancer, and colorectal cancer in both sexes. The net effect of this shift to lifestyles typical of industrialized countries – occurring largely in countries traditionally classified as "developing" – is a steady increase in the overall incidence rates of cancer, as well as a change in the spectrum of the most common cancers towards those observed in most of the highly developed industrialized countries.

This chapter explores the link between developmental trends and these dual aspects of *cancer transition* using the Human Development Index, an indicator introduced through the United Nations Development Programme [1]. The geographical and temporal patterns of cancer-specific incidence, mortality, and prevalence are examined at the national, regional, and global level. The combined demographic and epidemiological impact of a rising and transforming cancer burden in the many countries undergoing transition has, of course, major implications for public health and clinical services planning. Some of the main characteristics of this global phenomenon emphasize the need for an increasing focus on the cancers associated with affluence, which invariably rank within the "top five" most frequent cancers presently observed in high-income countries.

Fig. 1.2.2. The 10 leading causes of death worldwide in 2011. COPD, chronic obstructive pulmonary disease.

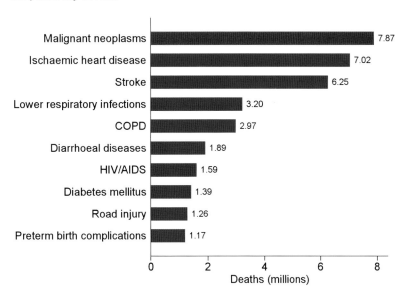

Epidemiological transitions, noncommunicable diseases, and cancer

Omran's theory of epidemiological transition focused on how changing health and disease patterns interact with complex demographic, social, and economic determinants [2]. Omran described how, in the third stage of transition, "pandemics of infection" are superseded by "degenerative and man-made diseases" as the major causes of morbidity and mortality. Thus, there is some analogy with the rather recent documentation of the increasing burden of noncommunicable diseases, which are displacing infection-related diseases as major causes of morbidity and mortality in many parts of the world. Noncommunicable diseases are the foremost cause of total mortality in the world today, responsible for two thirds of the estimated 57 million deaths worldwide in 2008 [3]. This shift in disease burden has been gaining political momentum and, subsequent to the United Nations Resolution on noncommunicable diseases in 2011, governments have approved a global monitoring framework and an updated Global Action Plan 2013–2020 for the prevention and control of

noncommunicable diseases, aimed at tackling the four major diseases – cardiovascular disease, diabetes, chronic respiratory disease, and cancer – at the national, regional, and global level.

That cancer has emerged as such an important cause of death in human populations is, and remains, striking [4]. Yet in compilations of global mortality by cause, the common practice of distinguishing between neoplasms according to the major anatomical sites has tended to obscure cancer's importance as a leading cause of death, in some instances almost to the point of its exclusion. As an example, WHO statistics for 2011 place ischaemic heart disease, stroke, lower respiratory infections, chronic obstructive pulmonary disease, diarrhoea, and HIV/AIDS above lung cancer as leading causes of death worldwide [5]. However, when presented as a single entity, the 7.9 million deaths due to cancer outrank deaths from every other major cause of death, as estimated, in that year (Fig. 1.2.2).

Countries in rapid societal, economic, and lifestyle transition are journeying towards an ever-greater impact of cancer. A global view of cancer patterns and trends in relation to national level of development becomes a vital consideration as a matter subject to understanding, prediction, and planning in relation to anticipated changes in the cancer burden and the spectrum of major cancer causes.

The Human Development Index: a marker of growth and development

Before studying cancer patterns and trends against socioeconomic markers, it is important to consider what constitutes human development, how it may be measured, and how it is changing with time. There is no automatic link between economic growth and human progress; thus, policy issues concern the exact process through which growth translates, or fails to translate, into human development under different developmental conditions. The Human Development Index (HDI) is a summary measure developed by the United Nations Development Programme and first published in 1990 [1]. For the 2012 estimates, the HDI is a composite index of three basic dimensions of human development – a long and healthy life, education, and a decent standard of living – combined into a unit-free index with a value between 0 and 1. The first dimension is measured by life expectancy at birth. This component is calculated using a minimum value of 20 years and a maximum value of 83.57 years; these are the observed extremes of this determination for countries over the period 1980–2012. Access to knowledge, the educational component, is indicated by the average duration of schooling that has been provided to adults aged 25 years and the expected years of schooling for children of school-entry age. The third component, a decent standard of living, is measured by gross national income per capita (in purchasing power parity in United States dollars).

Using country-specific HDI values, one can go beyond the historical construct of characterizing the

Fig. 1.2.3. Global map of development level of individual countries. (A) Historical approach: developing and developed countries. (B) Two levels of Human Development Index (HDI): countries with high or very high HDI versus those with low or medium HDI, 2012. (C) Four levels of HDI: countries with low, medium, high, and very high HDI, 2012.

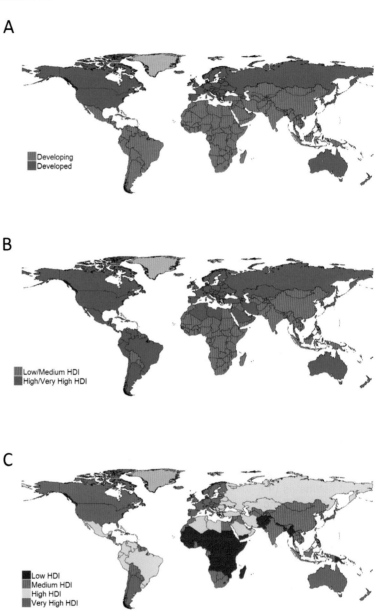

dichotomy between a "developed" and a "developing" country or area (Fig. 1.2.3A). A two-level construct based on HDI estimates for 2012 is shown in Fig. 1.2.3B. This still represents a rather crude dichotomy; therefore, to provide greater discrimination, four levels of HDI are used. The 2012 HDI is divided into quartiles, indicating "very high", "high", "medium", and "low" levels of human development. The global breakdown of countries according to the HDI quartiles is shown in Fig. 1.2.3C. The low HDI category is concentrated within sub-Saharan Africa, although several African countries have transitioned to the medium HDI category, as have many Asian countries, including the very densely populated countries of India and China. Many countries in Latin America and Central Asia now lie within the high HDI band.

Without exception, all countries worldwide have a higher HDI in 2012 than they had in 2000 (Fig. 1.2.4). Most countries experienced steady rises in the HDI determination over time. Highlighted are temporal patterns in eight countries that represent a broad spectrum of HDI values. The rates of change are such that a HDI of 0.4 was reached in Uganda 24 years after China, a value of 0.7 was attained in China 22 years after Argentina, and a value of 0.8 was reached in Argentina 30 years after Norway. In these examples, two to three decades were required to transition from one HDI category to the next.

Global cancer statistics by human development level in 2012

To examine cancer patterns in 2012 by levels of socioeconomic development, the country-specific GLOBOCAN estimates from IARC [6] were linked to the corresponding HDI, as estimated for 2012 by the United Nations Development Programme [7]. Methodological details of the data sources and methods of estimation used to compile global estimates of incidence, mortality, and prevalence are well documented, alongside more detailed presentation of these results [6,8–10]; the methods are largely dependent on the availability and the accuracy of the data sources locally. Generally, there is a paucity of high-quality cancer incidence and mortality data in areas with low and medium HDI. For example, there are national or regional population-based cancer registries in slightly more than one third of the 184 countries examined here; less than 20 of these systems are in countries with low or medium HDI, whereas there are no vital statistics available in more than 80 countries, predominantly those with low or medium HDI.

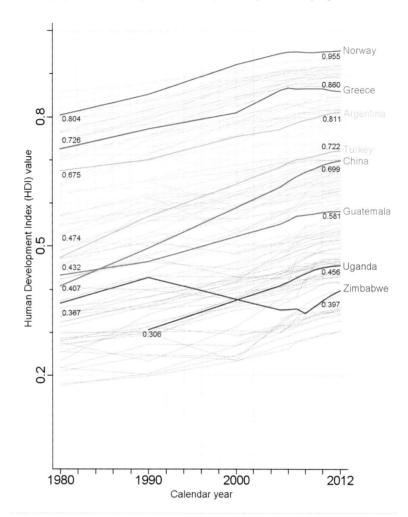

Fig. 1.2.4. Trends in Human Development Index (HDI) in 1980–2012, colour-coded by HDI category: red, low; orange, medium; turquoise, high; blue, very high.

Cancer burden by two-level Human Development Index

The most common cancers in terms of new cases and deaths according to two levels of HDI – high and very high HDI versus low and medium HDI – are shown in Fig. 1.2.5 for 2012. After lung cancer, breast, prostate, and colorectal cancers are the most frequent cancers in countries with high or very high HDI. Whereas colorectal, breast, and lung cancers have also become rather more frequent in countries with low or medium HDI, there remains a large excess of poverty- and infection-related cancers in these countries, notably cancers of the stomach, liver, cervix, and oesophagus.

Lung cancer is the major cause of cancer death in both HDI areas, and colorectal cancer ranks a clear second in countries with high or very high HDI. Liver and stomach cancers remain as major causes of cancer death in areas with low or medium HDI, a result of a high incidence of these cancers in these areas as well as an extremely poor prognosis for patients after diagnosis.

The extent to which cancers more strongly associated with lifestyles typical of industrialized countries (colorectal, breast, and prostate cancers combined) dominate the distribution of tumour types compared with those cancers wholly or partly related to infectious causes (cervical, liver, and stomach cancers

Fig. 1.2.5. Total burden of the 27 most common cancers in 2012: (A) incidence and (B) mortality according to two-level Human Development Index (HDI).

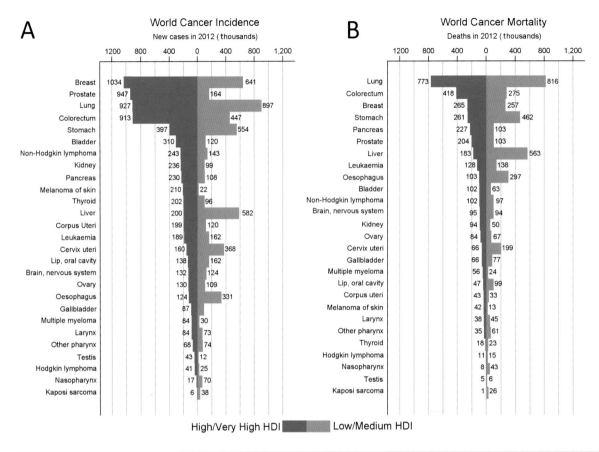

and Kaposi sarcoma combined) is captured in Fig. 1.2.6. Colorectal, breast, and prostate cancers constitute more than one third of the 7.9 million new cancers annually in countries with high or very high HDI, whereas cervical, liver, and stomach cancers and Kaposi sarcoma in combination constitute less than 10% of the total cancer burden in these areas. Conversely, in countries with low or medium HDI, infection-related cancers form a greater proportion of the 6.2 million estimated new cases annually, with one quarter due to infection – a higher relative proportion than the one fifth due to cancers of the colorectum, breast, and prostate.

Cancer burden by four-level Human Development Index

A closer examination of the five most common cancers contributing to incidence, mortality, and 5-year prevalence by sex and by four levels of HDI is depicted in Fig. 1.2.7. Overall, in countries with high or very high HDI, the same five neoplasms rank as the five most frequently diagnosed cancers: lung and stomach cancers and the so-called cancers of affluence, breast, prostate, and colorectal cancers. Lung cancer occupies a high rank in terms of incidence and is the most frequent cause of cancer death in all HDI categories except low HDI. The disease has a lesser rank in terms of prevalence, however, because of poor survival after diagnosis.

Incidence rates of breast, prostate, and colorectal cancers in 2012 are a function of level of development, and risk of developing these cancers increases as countries transition to higher HDI levels, while risk of mortality varies considerably less, because of proportionately higher case fatality in countries with lower HDI (Fig. 1.2.8). For female breast cancer, there is a gradient in the magnitude of the cumulative incidence with HDI level (Fig. 1.2.8A), with cumulative risks of 2.7%, 4.9%, and 8.4% estimated in 2012 in countries with medium, high, and very high HDI, respectively; cumulative risk is also relatively high in areas with low HDI (3.4%). However, this gradient is much less consistent for corresponding mortality; the estimates of 1.6% and 1.5% in areas with high and very high HDI, respectively, are elevated compared with those for countries with medium HDI. Risk of breast cancer death is highest in countries with low HDI (1.8%), due to incidence combined with a predominantly poorer survival prospect

Fig. 1.2.6. Percentage of cancers related to industrialized lifestyles (colorectal cancer, female breast cancer, and prostate cancer), infection-related cancers (cervical, liver, and stomach cancers and Kaposi sarcoma), and all other cancers (A) in countries with high or very high Human Development Index (HDI) and (B) in countries with low or medium HDI, 2012.

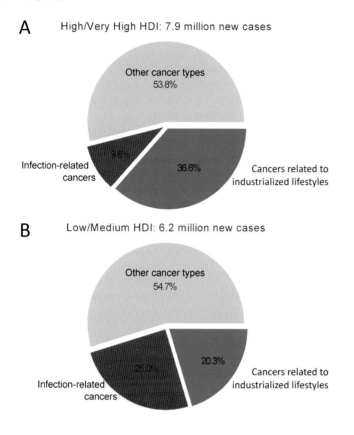

A   High/Very High HDI: 7.9 million new cases

Other cancer types
53.8%

9.6%

Infection-related cancers

36.6%   Cancers related to industrialized lifestyles

B   Low/Medium HDI: 6.2 million new cases

Other cancer types
54.7%

25.0%

20.3%

Infection-related cancers

Cancers related to industrialized lifestyles

after diagnosis in these areas. Despite affecting women almost exclusively, breast cancer (close to 1.7 million new cases worldwide in 2012) is among the five most common incident and prevalent cancers in each of the four HDI categories, and it is also the leading cause of cancer death in women in countries with low HDI (Fig. 1.2.7).

Similarly, prostate cancer also shows rapidly diverging incidence rates at medium to very high HDI, with lifetime risk of diagnosis ranging from 0.7% to 9.3% in countries with medium to very high HDI (Fig. 1.2.8B). As with breast cancer, the cumulative incidence of prostate cancer is higher in countries with low HDI than in those with medium HDI, while the corresponding risk of death in areas with low HDI (1.1%) is comparable to the risk estimated

in countries with high HDI (1.3%), which is elevated relative to countries with medium or very high HDI.

Perhaps the clearest gradient of increasing risk of cancer with human development is for colorectal cancer, with almost a 2-fold increment in cumulative incidence in both sexes combined: from 0.6% in countries with low HDI to 1.3%, 2.1%, and 3.6% in countries with medium, high, and very high HDI, respectively. A similar gradient emerges for mortality, although the estimated risk of death from colorectal cancer is close to equal in countries with high and very high HDI. Colorectal cancer now ranks within the five most frequent cancers in countries with medium, high, or very high HDI, is the second most common cause of cancer death in countries with high and

very high HDI, and ranks among the top five prevalent cancers in all four HDI areas (Fig. 1.2.7).

Stomach cancer appears within the top five cancers in term of both incidence and mortality in all four HDI categories (Fig. 1.2.7). Whereas stomach cancer is the fifth most frequent cancer in countries with high or very high HDI, it is the third most common cancer in countries with medium HDI. Liver cancer ranks above stomach cancer in countries with medium HDI, surpassed only by lung cancer, with the impact of cancers common in China influencing the cancer profile in this HDI category. Cervical cancer is the second most common cause of cancer incidence and mortality burden in countries with low HDI, where it is the cause of almost one in five of the cancer deaths estimated among women.

Evidence of cancer transitions: some temporal examples

Colorectal cancer as a marker of development

Fig. 1.2.9 shows trends in colorectal cancer incidence rates plotted concomitantly with HDI levels for men in selected countries with high-quality population-based cancer registries. Across most countries, increasing incidence rates have paralleled increases in HDI. However, the magnitude of the rates does not necessarily correspond with HDI levels attained by a given year: for example, rates are much lower in Colombia than in China in recent years, when their respective HDI levels were broadly similar. HDI has also increased in some countries where increases in colorectal cancer incidence are not evident, as is the case in Uganda. Finally, it is notable that rates tend to eventually stabilize and decline in countries that have attained very high HDI, as can be observed in the USA from 1985, Japan from the early 1990s, and Australia from 1995.

Fig. 1.2.7. The five most frequent cancers in terms of incident cases, cancer deaths, and 5-year cancer prevalence in 2012 (ages 15 years and older), according to four-level Human Development Index (HDI).

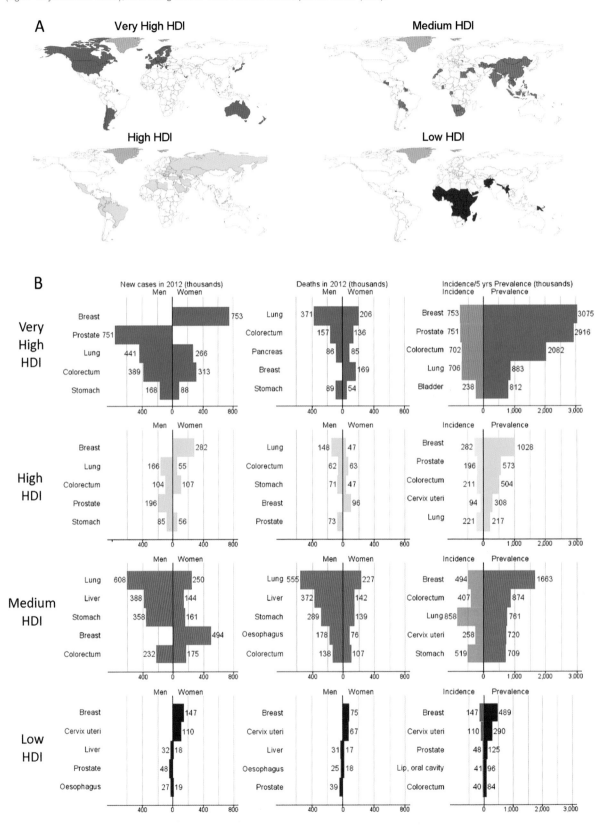

Fig. 1.2.8. Cumulative risk of (A) female breast cancer, (B) prostate cancer, and (C) colorectal cancer incidence and mortality (ages 0–74 years) in 2012, according to four-level Human Development Index (HDI).

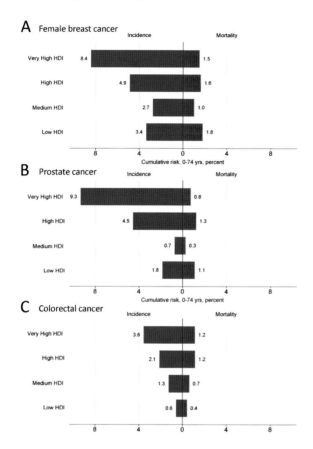

Mozambique to about 0.7 in Botswana and Gabon, with the highest values in the North African countries of Algeria, the Libyan Arab Jamahiriya, and Tunisia. Rates of cervical cancer tend to be very high in countries with the lowest HDI (< 0.4), including Mali, Malawi, Mozambique, and Zimbabwe, yet rates are low in Niger, the country with the lowest HDI ranking worldwide in 2012, as well as among the highest HDI ranked countries on the continent, in North Africa.

For breast cancer, the situation tends to be reversed, with the highest rates observed where HDI is high and cervical cancer rates are low, as in Algeria and Egypt, or intermediate, as in Ethiopia and Nigeria. Yet breast cancer incidence rates are relatively low in countries with elevated cervical cancer rates, such as Malawi and Mozambique, whereas in Botswana breast cancer rates are low and cervical cancer rates intermediate, contrasting with the country's relatively high HDI. Of course, this observation may partly relate to heterogeneity in the prevalence and distribution of risk factors for breast cancer within these countries, as well as the considerable lag between average changes in human development in the national population and anticipated increases in breast cancer incidence, linked to the etiological factors and the natural history of the disease.

For prostate cancer, rates tend to be less driven by HDI levels, with rates elevated in countries with low to intermediate HDI, such as the United Republic of Tanzania, Uganda, Zimbabwe, Guinea, and the Republic of the Congo, but also in countries with higher HDI, such as South Africa; rates are consistently low in North Africa.

In Latin America, the HDI does not vary as much as on the African continent, from about 0.6, as in Guatemala and Nicaragua, to just over 0.8, as in Chile and Argentina. However, some of the disparities in burden are in line with cancer transitions, with relatively low rates of cervical cancer, and relatively high

The rise of cancer in women: breast cancer compared with cervical cancer

The evolution of cancers in women shows a consistent and very striking pattern during the epidemiological transition, with rapid declines in the incidence of cervical cancer offset by concomitant increases in the incidence of breast cancer (Fig. 1.2.10). The year in which the two cancers are equally common, with one trending up and the other down, is a marker of the extent of transition in a given country; this time is in the distant past for Australia, Spain, and the USA and is much more recent for Colombia, Costa Rica, and India. However, the picture in Uganda is markedly different, with rates of both cancers still rising, and cervical cancer incidence rates twice those of breast cancer. This is in major

contrast to the 10–20-fold variations in breast and cervical cancer incidence rates in countries with very high HDI across Europe, Oceania, and North America.

Regional cancer profiles and human development

Chapter 1.1 includes a regional and inter-regional analysis of the geographical variations in the cancer burden according to continent. To link such variations to level of human development, the ecological comparisons of the levels of HDI in the countries of Africa and Latin America and the corresponding age-standardized rates of cervical, breast, and prostate cancer are presented in Fig. 1.2.11.

In Africa, the HDI varies from about 0.3 in the Democratic Republic of the Congo, Niger, and

Fig. 1.2.9. Trends in age-standardized (World) incidence rates (ASR) for colon cancer in men in 1978–2010 in 12 countries versus concomitant trends in Human Development Index (HDI) in 1980–2012. Incidence is smoothed using Loess regression.

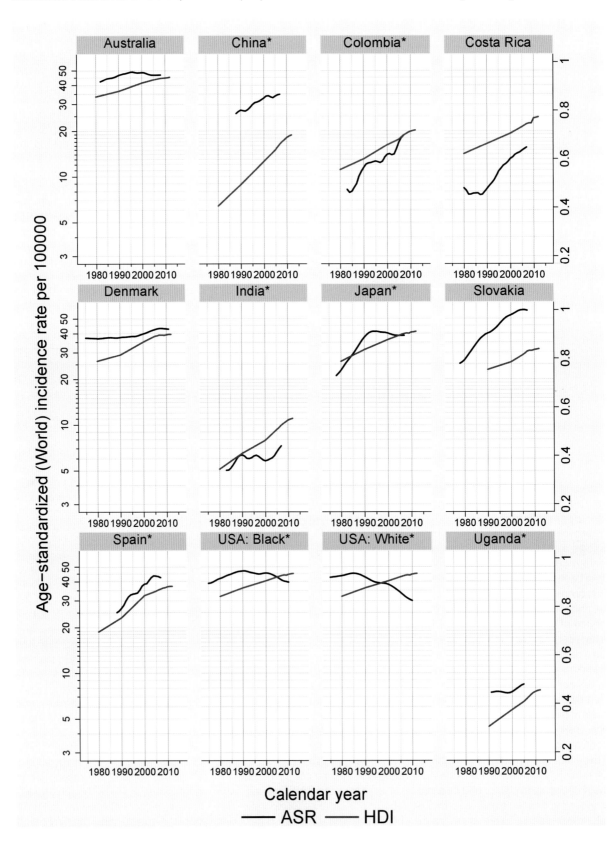

Fig. 1.2.10. Trends in age-standardized (World) incidence rates (ASR) for breast cancer versus cervical cancer in 1978–2010 in 12 countries. Incidence is smoothed using Loess regression.

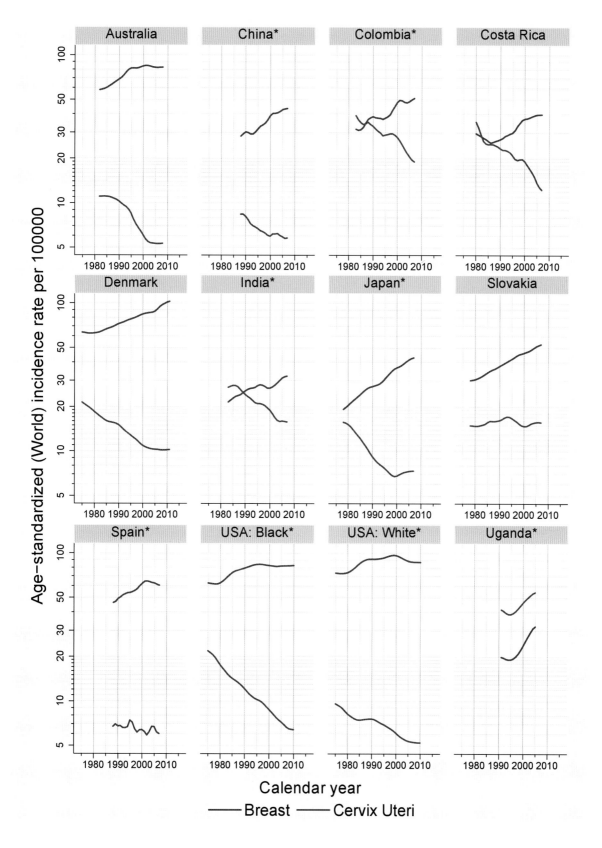

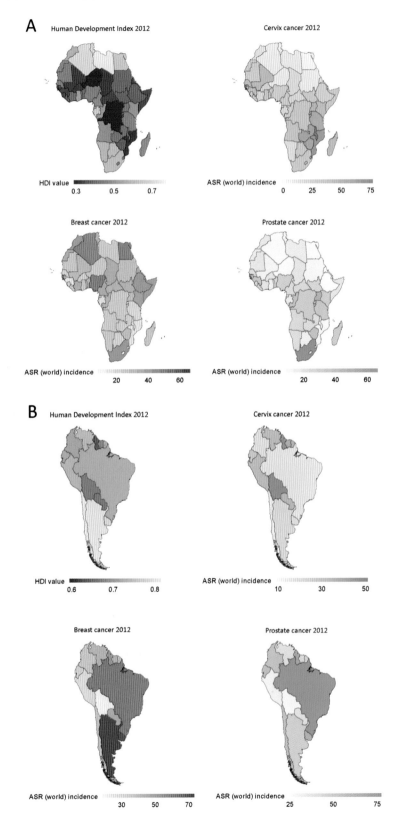

rates of breast cancer, in countries with high HDI, such as Argentina, Uruguay, and Brazil, and the opposite situation in countries with lower HDI, such as Nicaragua and Bolivia. Yet for other Latin American countries such simple relations appear not to hold: the rates of both cancers are relatively low in Chile, while for cervical cancer, rates in Peru are twice those of neighbouring Brazil, despite approximately similar HDI levels in 2012. Prostate cancer incidence is high in countries with higher HDI such as Brazil and Costa Rica, but in countries with analogous development levels such as Argentina and Peru, rates are intermediate to low in relative terms, respectively.

This description of the cancer burden for the three cancers by region and level of human development provides some evidence of cancer transition at the continental level but reveals the complexity limiting a broad interpretation, given the counter-intuitive examples provided above, and indeed the possible lag between HDI transitions and cancer risk. Certainly, the extent and modalities of early detection and screening vary from country to country and between and within the two regions examined. Increasing levels of screening at the population level are linked to human development, and where precursor lesions are not the target of the intervention, such interventions have the potential to artificially increase the incidence burden of female breast cancer due to mammographic screening programmes and, particularly, prostate cancer due to prostate-specific antigen testing of asymptomatic individuals.

The extent to which cytological screening of the cervix has been introduced is partly linked to development levels and national cancer control policies and will have had an impact on the rates of cervical cancer in some countries, while other factors may explain some of the variation, including rates of high-risk human papillomavirus infection at the population level, as influenced by religious and cultural practices in given countries.

Fig. 1.2.12. A woman in China tends a farm with her child at her side. Generally, there is a relative paucity of cancer incidence and mortality data in areas with low and medium Human Development Index.

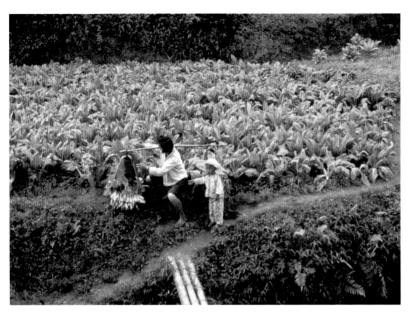

increasing life expectancy are having a major impact on population growth and ageing in countries in developmental transition, with the greatest increases in cancer burden in the very same countries where trends in overall cancer rates are also rising. Updating an exercise based on the observed time trends in cancer-specific incidence by HDI level [9], with annual increases in rates of colorectal cancer, female breast cancer, and prostate cancer worldwide – and, in areas with high to very high HDI, for lung cancer in women – alongside annual decreases in rates of stomach cancer and cervical cancer worldwide – and, in areas with high to very high HDI, for lung cancer in men – a predicted global burden of more than 20 million new cancer cases can be anticipated by 2025. Countries with medium HDI and, particularly, those with low HDI will experience the greatest proportional population growth during this time, and thus the greatest increases in the future cancer burden (Fig. 1.2.14). Notably, this scenario predicts an excess of almost 2 million cancers in men over cancers in women.

There are regional determinants for prostate cancer. Incidence rates are influenced by the diagnosis of latent cancers mainly in countries with higher HDI, while the distribution of mortality rates is less affected by the effects of early diagnosis. Evidently the elevated mortality rates in several sub-Saharan countries, such as Uganda and Zimbabwe, suggest that prostate cancers commonly diagnosed in these populations are developed as a result of largely unknown inherited or environmental factors linked to the underlying risk of invasive disease, rather than being determined by interventions aimed at revealing evidence of asymptomatic cancers.

As with breast cancer, differences within countries in the unknown determinants and the extensive delay between developmental changes and an increasing risk of prostate cancer may help to illuminate the apparent paradoxes. The inherent lack of high-quality registry data underpinning national incidence estimation, most notably in Africa, is likely to have hampered the inference attempted here.

Cancer incidence by 2025: demographic and trend-based predictions

The global population, 7 billion in 2012, will reach 8.3 billion by 2025 [11]. Slow changes in fertility and

Fig. 1.2.13. Children look out at Kampala's skyline during a celebration of Uganda's 50th anniversary of independence. Currently, all countries worldwide have a higher Human Development Index (HDI) than they had in 2000, but countries differ in the rate of transition to a higher HDI level.

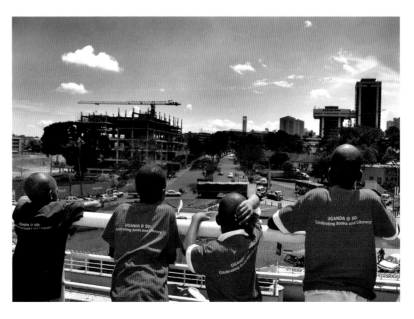

Overview

The predicted global burden is expected to surpass 20 million new cancer cases by 2025, compared with an estimated 14.1 million new cases in 2012. Demographic changes are the key drivers of the unprecedented growth in the cancer burden, but the profiles of cancer are changing as populations increasingly adopt behavioural and lifestyle habits that are common in affluent, industrialized countries. Elevated rates of female breast cancer, prostate cancer, and colorectal cancer incidence are linked to an attainment of higher levels of human development, with colorectal cancer the most markedly associated with HDI. A close to 2-fold increase in cumulative incidence of colorectal cancer is estimated as countries transition from low to higher categories of HDI. This, coupled with the increases in incidence rates of colorectal cancer in countries where HDI is rapidly rising, may be related to the increasing prevalence of unhealthy dietary habits and decreased levels of physical activity in populations undergoing developmental transition.

Lung cancer is the leading cause of cancer death in countries with medium, high, and very high HDI and is determined very largely by tobacco smoking, with risk being influenced by the number of cigarettes smoked, the duration of the habit, and the composition of the tobacco used. Given the limited nature of long-term data accumulation on tobacco-related cancer incidence and mortality in countries with low and medium HDI, alongside the relatively recent smoking histories in these populations, current lung cancer rates are often low and not indicative of impending epidemics in either sex. The extent of the projected increases in lung cancer and other tobacco-related diseases is, however, inextricably linked to the global tactics of tobacco companies aiming to expand their sales [12]. A smoking epidemic is unfolding in many countries with lower HDI that are in transition,

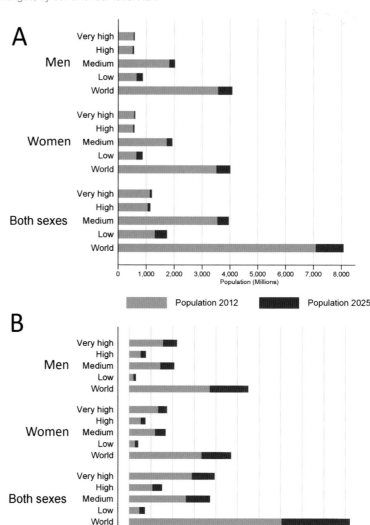

Fig. 1.2.14. Population estimates for 2012 and predictions for 2025: (A) changes in total population size by four-level Human Development Index (HDI); (B) incident cancer burden based on demographic changes and demographic + incidence rate changes, by sex and four-level HDI.

potentially impeding human development by consuming scarce resources, increasing pressures on already weak health-care systems, and inhibiting national productivity. Discernible increases in smoking-attributable risks have recently been reported in Bangladesh [13], China [14], India [15], and South Africa [16]. In many countries, in keeping with the tobacco epidemic model, the habit has been acquired relatively recently in women; in some countries, in a departure from this model, women have not acquired the habit at all. Perhaps there is more encouraging evidence of the latter scenario, at least in China where a recent epidemiological study of asbestos workers reported

Fig. 1.2.15. Ranking of premature mortality from cancer compared with cardiovascular disease and diabetes (combined) and chronic obstructive pulmonary disease (ages 30–69 years, both sexes), estimated for 2011.

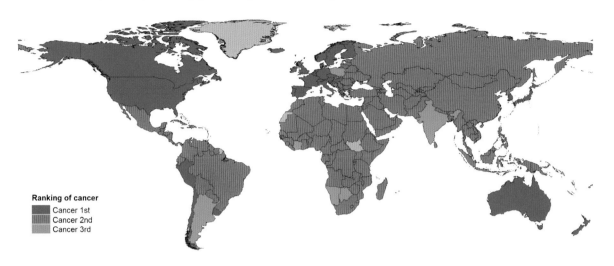

Ranking of cancer
- Cancer 1st
- Cancer 2nd
- Cancer 3rd

that of the relevant workforce, 79% of men smoked compared with less than 1% of women [17].

Cancer is becoming the major cause of premature deaths among noncommunicable diseases. A rapid assessment of the ranking of premature mortality (ages 30–69) from major noncommunicable diseases (Fig. 1.2.15) reveals how cancer has surpassed cardiovascular disease (here combined with diabetes) and chronic obstructive pulmonary disease in countries with very high HDI. It can therefore be expected that cancer will become a leading cause of premature death not only compared with other noncommunicable diseases but across the spectrum of causes, as countries head towards the higher human development threshold. In turn, therefore, noncommunicable diseases are recognized as a barrier to human development and as such should be a central part of the post-2015 agenda, after the target date for the Millennium Development Goals.

The author thanks Mathieu Laversanne for statistical analysis and generation of the graphics.

References

1. United Nations Development Programme (1990). *Human Development Report 1990. Concept and Measurement of Human Development.* New York: UNDP. Available at http://hdr.undp.org/en/reports/global/hdr 1990/.

2. Omran AR (1971). The epidemiologic transition. A theory of the epidemiology of population change. *Milbank Mem Fund Q*, 49:509–538. http://dx.doi.org/10.2307/3349375 PMID:5155251

3. WHO (2011). *Global Status Report on Non-Communicable Diseases 2010.* Geneva: WHO. Available at http://www.who.int/nmh/publications/ncd_report2010/en/.

4. Gersten O, Wilmoth JR (2002). The cancer transition in Japan since 1951. *Demogr Res*, 7:271–306. http://dx.doi.org/10.4054/DemRes.2002.7.5

5. WHO (2013). The top 10 causes of death. Available at http://www.who.int/mediacentre/factsheets/fs310/en/.

6. Ferlay J, Soerjomataram I, Ervik M *et al.* (2013). GLOBOCAN 2012 v1.0, Cancer Incidence and Mortality Worldwide: IARC Cancer Base No. 11 [Internet]. Lyon: IARC. Available at http://globocan.iarc.fr.

7. United Nations Development Programme (2013). *Human Development Report 2012. The Rise of the South: Human Progress in a Diverse World.* New York: UNDP. Available at http://www.undp.org/content/undp/en/home/librarypage/hdr/human-development-report-2013/.

8. Bray F, Ren JS, Masuyer E, Ferlay J (2013). Global estimates of cancer prevalence for 27 sites in the adult population in 2008. *Int J Cancer*, 132:1133–1145. http://dx.doi.org/10.1002/ijc.27711 PMID:22752881

9. Bray F, Jemal A, Grey N *et al.* (2012). Global cancer transitions according to the Human Development Index (2008–2030): a population-based study. *Lancet Oncol*, 13:790–801. http://dx.doi.org/10.1016/S1470-2045(12)70211-5 PMID:22658655

10. Ferlay J, Shin HR, Bray F *et al.* (2010). Estimates of worldwide burden of cancer in 2008: GLOBOCAN 2008. *Int J Cancer*, 127:2893–2917. http://dx.doi.org/10.1002/ijc.25516 PMID:21351269

11. United Nations Population Division (2007). *World Population Prospects: The 2008 Revision.* New York: United Nations. Available at http://www.un.org/en/development/desa/population/publications/trends/population-prospects.shtml.

12. O'Connor RJ, Wilkins KJ, Caruso RV *et al.* (2010). Cigarette characteristic and emission variations across high-, middle- and low-income countries. *Public Health*, 124:667–674. http://dx.doi.org/10.1016/j.puhe.2010.08.018 PMID:21030055

13. Alam DS, Jha P, Ramasundarahettige C *et al.* (2013). Smoking-attributable mortality in Bangladesh: proportional mortality study. *Bull World Health Organ*, 91:757–764. http://dx.doi.org/10.2471/BLT.13.120196 PMID:24115799

14. Gu D, Kelly TN, Wu X *et al.* (2009). Mortality attributable to smoking in China. *N Engl J Med*, 360:150–159. http://dx.doi.org/10.1056/NEJMsa0802902 PMID:19129528

15. Jha P, Jacob B, Gajalakshmi V *et al.*; RGI-CGHR Investigators (2008). A nationally representative case-control study of smoking and death in India. *N Engl J Med*, 358:1137–1147. http://dx.doi.org/10.1056/NEJMsa0707719 PMID:18272886

16. Sitas F, Egger S, Bradshaw D *et al.* (2013). Differences among the coloured, white, black, and other South African populations in smoking-attributed mortality at ages 35–74 years: a case-control study of 481,640 deaths. *Lancet*, 382:685–693. http://dx.doi.org/10.1016/S0140-6736(13)61610-4 PMID:23972813

17. Wang X, Lin S, Yu I *et al.* (2013). Cause-specific mortality in a Chinese chrysotile textile worker cohort. *Cancer Sci*, 104:245–249. http://dx.doi.org/10.1111/cas.12060 PMID:23121131

1.3 Childhood cancer

1 WORLDWIDE

Eva Steliarova-Foucher
A. Lindsay Frazier

Bernard W. Stewart (reviewer)
Christopher P. Wild (reviewer)

Summary

- Childhood cancers are distinct entities from cancers occurring in adults. Overall annual incidence rates vary between 50 and 200 per million in children and between 90 and 300 per million in adolescents. Reliable data on cancer in children and adolescents are available for only a small fraction of the world's population.

- Over the past 50 years, 5-year survival has improved in high-income countries from less than 30% to more than 80%, although this trend may have plateaued recently. Treatment and follow-up must be adapted to the age of the patient and must embrace the patient's family and its circumstances.

- The growing population of survivors requires specialized follow-up and care. Innovation in clinical research is required to ensure continued improvement of prognosis and reduced occurrence and severity of the late effects of treatment.

- The mortality-to-incidence ratio remains high in countries with low human development index, although some diagnoses are highly curable at low cost. National investment and international collaboration are required to improve outcomes.

Incidence rates

The term "childhood cancer" is most commonly used to designate cancers that arise before the age of 15 years. Cancer in childhood represents between 0.5% and 4.6% of the total number of cancer cases in a population (Fig. 1.3.1) [1]. The proportion of cancers that occur in children is higher in countries with low Human Development Index (HDI) than in countries with high HDI. This is

Fig. 1.3.1. Cancer cases and deaths in children (aged < 15 years) as a proportion of the total numbers in the population, in 2012. HDI, Human Development Index.

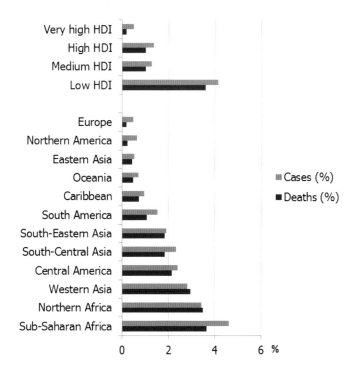

because children make up a larger percentage of the overall population (up to 50%) and concomitantly the elderly population, which exhibits the highest risk of cancer, is quite small in countries with low HDI.

Population-based cancer registries around the world report overall incidence rates that vary between 50 and 200 per million children per year. The spectrum of tumour types differs across populations (Fig. 1.3.2) [2–12]. Acute lymphoblastic leukaemia is the most common diagnosis, except in sub-Saharan Africa, where children are more prone to develop non-Hodgkin lymphomas (most commonly Burkitt lymphoma) and Kaposi sarcoma, due to the specific infectious exposures in that region (notably *Plasmodium*, Epstein–Barr virus, and HIV) [11]. Brain tumours are the second most common malignancy in regions that can afford to implement non-invasive diagnostic technologies [13]. Improved diagnostics may also influence the incidence of neuroblastoma; incidental findings of indolent tumours discovered in the countries with highly developed medical surveillance may account for observed increases in incidence.

All childhood cancers are individually rare, with incidence rates varying from 1 per million for a very rare cancer such as hepatoblastoma to 50 per million for the most common subgroup, lymphoid leukaemia. Haematological malignancies represent 40–60% of tumours in the first 15 years of life. Embryonal tumours (e.g. retinoblastoma, neuroblastoma, nephroblastoma) constitute about 20% of childhood malignancies and virtually never occur except in children. Carcinomas represent less than 5% of childhood tumours, while these are the most frequent histologies in adults. The characteristic morphological appearances imply a distinct developmental origin and etiology for tumours in childhood. Because of the age-specific histology, the International Classification of Childhood Cancer [14] is used to describe the occurrence and outcomes of cancer in childhood.

Increasingly, adolescents (aged 15–19 years) and young adults (aged 20–24 years) with cancer are being considered as a group requiring special consideration, similar to childhood cancer, due to the unique composition of cancer types (Fig. 1.3.3) [15] and their health-care requirements. Although embryonal neoplasms in adolescents are rare, haematological neoplasms continue to be common, and most are lymphomas. Central nervous system tumours still represent a large proportion of cancers, and bone tumours peak in the adolescent age group in many populations. Malignant melanoma is more common than in children, particularly in female adolescents. The leading cancer site in male adolescents is the testis, with age-specific rates rising until ages in the early forties. The prominent types in female adolescents are thyroid cancer, ovarian germ cell tumours, and cervical cancer. The worldwide incidence rates vary approximately 3-fold in male (9–30 per 100 000) and in female (9–27 per 100 000) adolescents [16].

Fig. 1.3.2. Incidence rates of cancer in children (aged 0–14 years) in the 1990s and 2000s. CNS, central nervous system; PNET, primitive neuroectodermal tumours; SEER, Surveillance, Epidemiology and End Results national statistics; SNS, sympathetic nervous system.

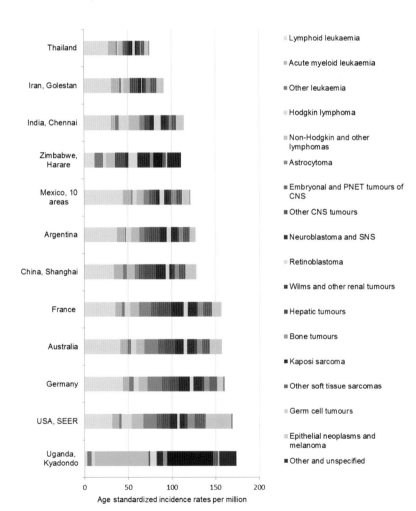

Fig. 1.3.3. Cancer incidence rates in (A) male and (B) female adolescents (aged 15–19 years) and young adults (aged 20–24 years) in Europe, in 2003–2007. Data from 84 cancer registries contributing data for the selected calendar years were retrieved from the European Cancer Observatory on 18 November 2013. CNS, central nervous system.

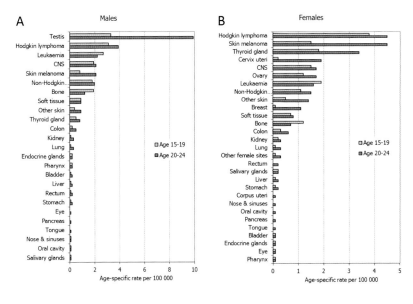

However, from the international data it appears that the rate of childhood leukaemia, the most common cancer in many childhood populations, is positively correlated with socio-economic status [23], and several hypotheses suggest that the risk factors associated with a high level of development, such as delayed exposure to common infections, population mixing, and changes in reproductive behaviour, influence the incidence of acute lymphoblastic leukaemia. In sub-Saharan African countries, where childhood leukaemia is reported relatively rarely, significant increases in rates of childhood leukaemia may be expected in the near future, both due to improving diagnostic facilities and due to adoption of industrialized lifestyles.

Outcomes

Over the past 40 years, outcomes of cancer in children have improved dramatically. In the United Kingdom, the 5-year survival rate increased from less than 30% to almost 80% on average, thus reducing the risk of death by 68% overall (Fig. 1.3.5) [24], and similar changes were observed in other high-income countries. These spectacular

The overall incidence of childhood cancer increased by about 1% per year over the last three decades of the 20th century in Europe, North America, Australia, and elsewhere, although the rate of increase seems to have levelled off over the most recent decade [10,17–19]. Among adolescents, incidence has also increased (Fig. 1.3.4), at a similar rate [17,20]. The observed temporal trends might partly reflect improved diagnosis and reporting of cancers [13], but the impact of changes in exposures and lifestyles over the same period may have also contributed to the changes in incidence. For example, the recent study that showed a reduction of incidence rates of Wilms tumour and some other rare childhood tumours in the USA after supplementation of the food supply with folic acid [21] provides hope that the predisposing environmental factors will be identified and childhood cancers prevented.

It is estimated that by 2035 the annual number of new cancers across all ages will grow by 70% compared with 2012 estimates [1] (see also Chapter 1.2). In comparison, the annual numbers of cancer cases and deaths among children are expected to increase by only 7%, based on the assumption of a medium fertility variant of the population growth [22] and stable incidence and mortality rates.

Fig. 1.3.4. Cancer trends in adolescents and young adults (aged 15–24 years) in Europe. Pooled data from the European Cancer Observatory from all cancer registries with data covering the period shown: Finland, Germany (Saarland), Iceland, Italy (Varese), Norway, Slovakia, Sweden, Switzerland (Geneva, St Gallen-Appenzell) and the United Kingdom (Scotland).

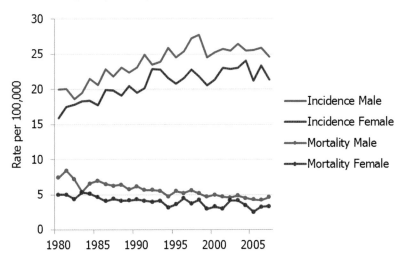

Fig. 1.3.5. Five-year survival rates of children diagnosed before the age of 15 years in Britain during the indicated periods.

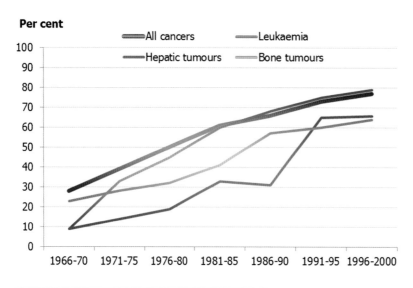

Per cent

The spectacular improvement in outcomes is, however, limited to high-income countries. The results from rare reports of childhood cancer survival in middle-income countries are compared with data from Australia in Table 1.3.1 [7,9,18,27]. Despite the different reporting periods, it is evident that the proportion of 5-year survivors in India is much lower than that seen in high-income countries. The low survival figures may be explained by late presentation at diagnosis, treatment abandonment, and the absence of sophisticated multidisciplinary care and adequate resources.

In the absence of globally comparable data on cancer patient survival, estimates are used to describe the ultimate cancer burden in terms of mortality. Compared with the estimated 163 000 new cancers in children worldwide in 2012, the 80 000 deaths represented about a half of the new cases. In 2012, 82% of the new cases and 93% of the deaths occurred in the less developed countries [1]. In Africa, the mortality represents 60% of the incidence, while in North America this ratio is less than 15% (Fig. 1.3.6) [1,16]. National investment and international collaborations are required to improve this situation.

improvements are the results of therapeutic advances, fostered through worldwide collaboration of childhood cancer study groups and the International Society of Paediatric Oncology (www.siop-online.org).

Because of the age proximity, the overlapping spectrum of tumours, and the need for a very sensitive approach, adolescent patients with selected malignancies are managed within a paediatric oncology practice. Indeed, adolescents may benefit from inclusion in paediatric therapeutic protocols compared with those developed for adults, at least for "paediatric-like" cancers such as acute lymphoblastic leukaemia [25]. The overall 5-year survival of adolescents is similar to that of children, reaching 84% [4,26].

Table 1.3.1. Five-year survival rates (%) in children (aged 0–14 years) with cancer diagnosed during the indicated periods

Cancer type	Location (period) [source of data]			
	Australia (1997–2006) [18]	Shanghai, China (2002–2005) [27]	Chennai, India (1990–2001) [9]	Thailand (2003–2004) [7]
All cancers	79.6	55.7	40.0	54.9
Leukaemias	80.6	52.2	36.3	57.4
Lymphomas	89.9	58.8	55.3	59.5
Central nervous system tumours	71.0	41.2	26.8	41.7
Neuroblastoma	67.8	—	36.9	33.6
Retinoblastoma	98.4	75.0	48.1	73.1
Renal cancers	88.6	86.7	58.0	70.4
Liver cancers	76.0	33.3	10.5	44.5
Malignant bone tumours	68.9	52.6	30.6	33.7
Soft tissue sarcomas	72.1	54.1	36.3	50.1
Germ cell tumours	89.4	78.4	38.0	70.6
Carcinomas and melanoma	93.3	88.9	35.1	—
Other	72.2	—	—	—

Fig. 1.3.6. Estimated mortality-to-incidence ratio for cancer in children (aged 0–14 years) in 2012, and percentage of population coverage by cancer registration (all ages).

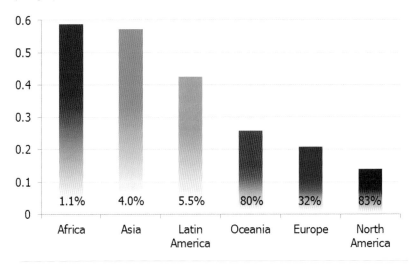

Whereas low- and middle-income countries need to build capacity to reach the 80% 5-year survival currently achievable in the countries with the most resources, the reduction in mortality observed in Europe and the USA has plateaued over the most recent period (Fig. 1.3.7) [28,29]. There remains, therefore, an urgent need for new major breakthroughs in therapies to re-accelerate the current rate of improvement in survival [30].

The greatly improved survival in high-income countries has given rise to a growing population of survivors of cancer in childhood or adolescence, a large proportion of whom face significant late effects of their primary disease and cancer treatment. Survivors experience an excess risk of death and second primary cancer long past their diagnosis. In a Nordic study of 21 984 5-year survivors of childhood cancer,

the overall standardized mortality ratio was 8.3 and the absolute excess risk was 6.2 per 1000 person-years. The causes of death included primary cancer (60%), subsequent malignant neoplasms (12%), and non-cancer causes (27%) [31]. Other sequelae of cancer treatment include neurocognitive impairment, cardiovascular disease, and other organ dysfunction, but also the psychosocial impact of the disease and its treatment on patients, their family members, and their future lives. It is clear that the usual 5-year survival statistics reflect a short-term, rather than a long-term, prognosis for children with cancer. Lifelong follow-up is important and has to take into account the inevitable transition into the non-specialized, and often unaware, primary health-care system.

Data sources

Worldwide, there are approximately 50 countries with established *national* population-based cancer registries, which provide their data for comparative international studies. Most of these registries collect data on cancers occurring in individuals of all ages (a general cancer registry), but some countries are also covered by a separate, national paediatric cancer registry. Paediatric cancer registries often collect more details on the patient, diagnosis, treatment, and outcome. *Regional* population-based cancer registries operate in other countries and provide valuable information on cancer burden, including that in children. Comparative incidence data on childhood cancer were reported in the two volumes of the IARC Scientific Publications series *International Incidence of Childhood Cancer*; a third volume of the series, describing incidence in children and adolescents over the past two decades, is in preparation (http://iicc.iarc.fr/).

Childhood cancer is a rare disease, requiring that large populations are covered to collect sufficient numbers of cases for meaningful analyses. National cancer registration is the ideal option for rare cancers such

Fig. 1.3.7. Cancer mortality in children (aged 0–14 years) in three European countries (Ireland, the Netherlands, and the United Kingdom combined) for 1950–2009 and in the USA for 1950–2007.

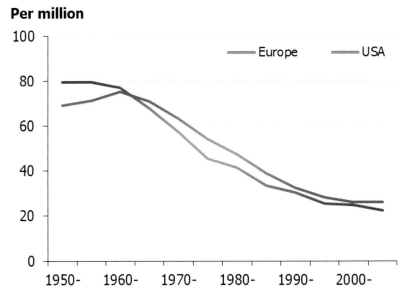

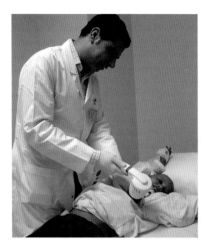

Fig. 1.3.8. A young patient is treated at the 57357 Children's Cancer Hospital in Cairo, Egypt.

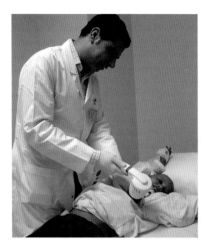

as those occurring in childhood and possibly also in adolescence, and is a workable model, as shown by the examples of Argentina, South Africa, and the Islamic Republic of Iran. In low-income settings, however, a more appropriate strategy would be to start a regional population-based cancer registry. In this respect, existing hospital-based cancer registries may aim to become population-based if they succeed in determining the relevant geographically defined population at risk. It is no coincidence that population coverage by cancer registration is correlated with high incidence rates and low mortality rates (Fig. 1.3.6). Although founding a cancer registry will not automatically reduce the mortality rates in a population, cancer registration is an essential element of a cancer control plan, and is bound to serve as the evidence base that will inform other services to cancer patients and eventually lead to improvements in survival.

The value of the statistics produced by cancer registries depends on the quality, accuracy, and completeness of the data generated in clinical practice. The better the cooperation between the partners, the more useful the produced output will be. For optimal functioning of cancer registries, it is essential to

ensure access to the relevant data. Regulations imposing requirements of informed consent, trusted third parties, or various encryption techniques would make it virtually impossible to use data from a cancer registry and thus hinder the achievement of better outcomes for current survivors and future patients.

Several initiatives have been undertaken in Europe recently to enlarge the information base available within population-based cancer registries and allow a more specific interpretation of the outcome in addition to a description of the geographical and temporal patterns. This work is funded by the European Union within the Seventh Framework Programme of the European Commission. The European Network for Cancer Research in Children and Adolescents is a Network of Excellence with the overall aims to improve survival and quality of life for children and adolescents with cancer, to facilitate access to the best therapies, to develop biology-guided therapies, and to efficiently structure and enhance collaboration within the field of paediatric oncology in Europe (http://www.encca.eu/). PanCare Childhood and Adolescent Cancer Survivor Care and Follow-up is a research project of the PanCare Network with a

mission to provide every childhood and adolescent cancer survivor with better access to care and better long-term health (http://www.pancaresurfup.eu/). The member registries of the European Network of Cancer Registries (http://www.encr.com.fr/) are involved in the European Network for Cancer Research in Children and Adolescents and in PanCare Childhood and Adolescent Cancer Survivor Care and Follow-up to investigate the feasibility of collecting additional clinically relevant information on children and adolescents with cancer to facilitate routine short-term clinical follow-up and long-term follow-up for selected late effects. The additional variables of interest may include pre-existing patient conditions (e.g. genetic syndrome), diagnostic data (e.g. biological markers or stage), information on treatment received (e.g. inclusion in clinical trials), referral and follow-up (e.g. date of relapse), and possible late effects in long-term survivors (e.g. cause of death, cardiac condition). Sharing expertise between clinical and population-based research will simultaneously enhance the potential of data collected in both types of resources and provide a cost-effective solution to advance research in paediatric oncology.

Fig. 1.3.9. A child receiving chemotherapy at the Uganda Cancer Institute (Lymphoma Treatment Centre). Burkitt lymphoma is common in Uganda.

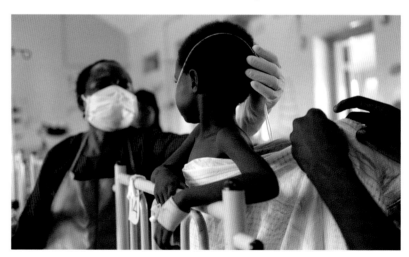

References

1. Ferlay J, Soerjomataram I, Ervik M et al. (2013). GLOBOCAN 2012 v1.0, Cancer Incidence and Mortality Worldwide: IARC CancerBase No. 11 [Internet]. Lyon: IARC. Available at http://globocan.iarc.fr.

2. Moreno F, Loria D, Abriata G, Terracini B; ROHA network (2013). Childhood cancer: incidence and early deaths in Argentina, 2000–2008. Eur J Cancer, 49:465–473. http://dx.doi.org/10.1016/j.ejca.2012.08.001 PMID:22980725

3. Moradi A, Semnani S, Roshandel G et al. (2010). Incidence of childhood cancers in Golestan province of Iran. Iran J Pediatr, 20:335–342. PMID:23056726

4. Howlader N, Noone AM, Krapcho M et al., eds (2013). SEER Cancer Statistics Review, 1975–2010. Bethesda, MD: National Cancer Institute. Available at http://www.seer.cancer.gov/csr/1975_2010/browse_csr.php?section=29&page=sect_29_table.02.html.

5. Lacour B, Guyot-Goubin A, Guissou S et al. (2010). Incidence of childhood cancer in France: National Children Cancer Registries, 2000–2004. Eur J Cancer Prev, 19:173–181. http://dx.doi.org/10.1097/CEJ.0b013e32833876c0 PMID:20361423

6. Kaatsch P, Spix C (2012). German Childhood Cancer Registry Annual Report 2011 (1980–2010). Mainz: Institute of Medical Biostatistics, Epidemiology and Informatics at the University Medical Center of the Johannes Gutenberg University. Available at http://www.kinderkrebsregister.de/extern/veroeffentlichungen/jahresberichte/aktueller-jahresbericht/index.html?L=1.

7. Wiangnon S, Veerakul G, Nuchprayoon I et al. (2011). Childhood cancer incidence and survival 2003–2005, Thailand: study from the Thai Pediatric Oncology Group. Asian Pac J Cancer Prev, 12:2215–2220. PMID:22296359

8. Fajardo-Gutiérrez A, Juárez-Ocaña S, González-Miranda G et al. (2007). Incidence of cancer in children residing in ten jurisdictions of the Mexican Republic: importance of the Cancer registry (a population-based study). BMC Cancer, 7:68. PMID:17445267

9. Swaminathan R, Rama R, Shanta V (2008). Childhood cancers in Chennai, India, 1990–2001: incidence and survival. Int J Cancer, 122:2607–2611. http://dx.doi.org/10.1002/ijc.23428 PMID:18324630

10. Baade PD, Youlden DR, Valery PC et al. (2010). Trends in incidence of childhood cancer in Australia, 1983–2006. Br J Cancer, 102:620–626. http://dx.doi.org/10.1038/sj.bjc.6605503 PMID:20051948

11. Parkin DM, Ferlay J, Hamdi-Chérif M et al. (2003). Cancer in Africa: Epidemiology and Prevention. Chapter 5: Childhood cancer. Lyon: IARC (IARC Scientific Publications Series, No. 153), pp. 381–396.

12. Bao PP, Zheng Y, Wang CF et al. (2009). Time trends and characteristics of childhood cancer among children age 0–14 in Shanghai. Pediatr Blood Cancer, 53:13–16. http://dx.doi.org/10.1002/pbc.21939 PMID:19260104

13. Kroll ME, Carpenter LM, Murphy MF, Stiller CA (2012). Effects of changes in diagnosis and registration on time trends in recorded childhood cancer incidence in Great Britain. Br J Cancer, 107:1159–1162. http://dx.doi.org/10.1038/bjc.2012.296 PMID:22898786

14. Steliarova-Foucher E, Stiller CA, Lacour B, Kaatsch P (2005). International Classification of Childhood Cancer, third edition. Cancer, 103:1457–1467. http://dx.doi.org/10.1002/cncr.20910 PMID:15712273

15. Steliarova-Foucher E, O'Callaghan M, Ferlay J et al. (2012). European Cancer Observatory: Cancer Incidence, Mortality, Prevalence and Survival in Europe, version 1.0. European Network of Cancer Registries, IARC. Available at http://eco.iarc.fr.

16. Curado MP, Edwards B, Shin HR et al. (2007). Cancer Incidence in Five Continents, Vol. IX. Lyon: IARC (IARC Scientific Publications Series, No. 160).

17. Kohler BA, Ward E, McCarthy BJ et al. (2011). Annual report to the nation on the status of cancer, 1975–2007, featuring tumors of the brain and other nervous system. J Natl Cancer Inst, 103:714–736. http://dx.doi.org/10.1093/jnci/djr077 PMID:21454908

18. Baade PD, Youlden DR, Valery PC et al. (2010). Population-based survival estimates for childhood cancer in Australia during the period 1997–2006. Br J Cancer, 103:1663–1670. http://dx.doi.org/10.1038/sj.bjc.6605985 PMID:21063404

19. Baba S, Ioka A, Tsukuma H et al. (2010). Incidence and survival trends for childhood cancer in Osaka, Japan, 1973–2001. Cancer Sci, 101:787–792. http://dx.doi.org/10.1111/j.1349-7006.2009.01443.x PMID:20132215

20. Stiller CA, Desandes E, Danon SE et al. (2006). Cancer incidence and survival in European adolescents (1978–1997). Report from the Automated Childhood Cancer Information System project. Eur J Cancer, 42:2006–2018. http://dx.doi.org/10.1016/j.ejca.2006.06.002 PMID:16919767

21. Linabery AM, Johnson KJ, Ross JA (2012). Childhood cancer incidence trends in association with US folic acid fortification (1986–2008). Pediatrics, 129:1125–1133. http://dx.doi.org/10.1542/peds.2011-3418 PMID:22614769

22. UN World Population Prospects, 2010 revision. Available at http://www.un.org/esa/population/unpop.htm.

23. Kroll ME, Stiller CA, Richards S et al. (2012). Evidence for under-diagnosis of childhood acute lymphoblastic leukaemia in poorer communities within Great Britain. Br J Cancer, 106:1556–1559. http://dx.doi.org/10.1038/bjc.2012.102 PMID:22472883

24. Stiller CA, Kroll ME, Eatock EM (2007). Survival from childhood cancer. In: Stiller CA, ed. Childhood Cancer in Britain: Incidence, Survival, Mortality. Oxford: Oxford University Press, pp. 131–204.

25. Ram R, Wolach O, Vidal L et al. (2012). Adolescents and young adults with acute lymphoblastic leukemia have a better outcome when treated with pediatric-inspired regimens: systematic review and meta-analysis. Am J Hematol, 87:472–478. http://dx.doi.org/10.1002/ajh.23149 PMID:22388572

26. Gatta G, Zigon G, Capocaccia R et al.; EUROCARE Working Group (2009). Survival of European children and young adults with cancer diagnosed 1995–2002. Eur J Cancer, 45:992–1005. http://dx.doi.org/10.1016/j.ejca.2008.11.042 PMID:19231160

27. Bao PP, Zheng Y, Wu CX et al. (2012). Population-based survival for childhood cancer patients diagnosed during 2002–2005 in Shanghai, China. Pediatr Blood Cancer, 59:657–661. http://dx.doi.org/10.1002/pbc.24043 PMID:22302759

28. WHO Mortality Database. Available at http://www.who.int/healthinfo/mortality_data/en/ and http://www-dep.iarc.fr.

29. Pritchard-Jones K, Pieters R, Reaman GH et al. (2013). Sustaining innovation and improvement in the treatment of childhood cancer: lessons from high-income countries. Lancet Oncol,14:e95–e103. http://dx.doi.org/10.1016/S1470-2045(13)70010-X PMID:23434338

30. Sullivan R, Kowalczyk JR, Agarwal B et al. (2013). New policies to address the global burden of childhood cancers. Lancet Oncol, 14:e125–e135. http://dx.doi.org/10.1016/S1470-2045(13)70007-X PMID:23434339

31. Garwicz S, Anderson H, Olsen JH *et al.*; Association of the Nordic Cancer Registries; Nordic Society for Pediatric Hematology Oncology (2012). Late and very late mortality in 5-year survivors of childhood cancer: changing pattern over four decades–experience from the Nordic countries. *Int J Cancer*, 131:1659–1666. http://dx.doi.org/10.1002/ijc.27393 PMID:22170520

Websites

CANCER*Mondial*: http://www-dep.iarc.fr

European Cancer Observatory: http://eco.iarc.fr

European Network for Cancer Research in Children and Adolescents: http://www.encca.eu/

European Network of Cancer Registries: http://www.encr.com.fr/

German Childhood Cancer Registry Annual Report 2011 (1980–2010): http://www.kinderkrebsregister.de/extern/veroeffentlichungen/jahresberichte/aktueller-jahresbericht/index.html?L=1

GLOBOCAN: http://globocan.iarc.fr

International Incidence of Childhood Cancer: http://iicc.iarc.fr/

International Society of Paediatric Oncology: www.siop.nl

PanCare Childhood and Adolescent Cancer Survivor Care and Follow-up: http://www.pancaresurfup.eu/

Surveillance, Epidemiology and End Results Program: http://seer.cancer.gov/

UN Department of Economic and Social Affairs, Population Division: http://www.un.org/esa/population/unpop.htm

WHO Mortality Data and Statistics: http://www.who.int/healthinfo/statistics/mortality/en/index.html

Elizabeth H. Blackburn

Reconciling stress and cancer: insights from telomeres

*Elizabeth H. Blackburn,
a professor at the University of
California San Francisco, was
awarded the Nobel Prize in Physiology
or Medicine 2009 for her discovery
of how chromosomes are protected
by telomeres and the enzyme
telomerase. The pioneering work
of Dr Blackburn and her colleagues
has far-reaching implications and
has advanced the knowledge of the
impact of telomeres and telomerase in
human health and disease, particularly
in cancer, inherited diseases,
and ageing. Born in Australia,
Dr Blackburn earned B.Sc. and M.Sc.
degrees in biochemistry from the
University of Melbourne, received
her Ph.D. in molecular biology from
the University of Cambridge, and
completed postdoctoral work in
molecular and cell biology at Yale
University. Beyond the laboratory,
Dr Blackburn's contemplation of the
implications of scientific research for
society underpins her recognized
contributions to bioethics and
public policy discourse.*

Summary

Various conditions throughout geographically and societally diverse parts of the world share in common the potential to inflict severe, often prolonged, psychological stresses on human populations. Telomere maintenance, which is emerging as a central biological process that plays roles in both prevention and progression of human cancers and other ageing-related diseases, is adversely affected by psychological stress. Telomeres are the dynamic structures that cap and protect chromosome ends. Telomeric DNA attrition commonly occurs in human cells during ageing or because of inherited "telomere syndromes". If unchecked, such attrition can eventually lead to cellular malfunctioning. This in turn contributes to multiple, often co-morbid, diseases of ageing, including a spectrum of cancers. Clear links already are known to exist between stress, telomere attrition, and several other common diseases of ageing besides cancers. Therefore, the lessons already learned from such studies should inform strategies and policies in efforts to intercept human cancers and reduce their worldwide burden.

Telomeres, the protective terminal regions of our chromosomes, are dynamic structures that play multiple roles to ensure correct cellular functions and prevent genomic instability. Both biologically internal and external factors that influence human conditions can compromise telomere maintenance, and as I discuss in this Perspective, this knowledge has implications for reducing cancer risks.

First, a short background on telomeres and telomerase. Telomeres, found at every end of every stable eukaryotic chromosome, form "caps" made up of elaborately controlled DNA–protein complexes. The telomere structure consists of a scaffold of a thousands-of-base-pairs-long stretch of a simple repeated DNA sequence at the extreme end of the chromosome that directly binds a suite of telomeric, DNA sequence-specific, protective proteins. These proteins in turn interact with several other proteins that, through multiple mechanisms (collectively called capping), aid in protecting the telomeres (reviewed in [1]).

Crucially, a minimum length of telomeric DNA is required to sustain chromosome stability and cellular functions. However, net telomere erosion commonly occurs in humans over the lifespan [2]. Action of the cellular enzyme telomerase (a specialized ribonucleoprotein reverse transcriptase) can elongate telomeric DNA and thus counteract telomere erosion, replenishing telomere length and functional integrity. The telomeric complex is a dynamic entity, with the capacity to be constantly shortened, built, shortened, and rebuilt. Yet the general rule in humans as they age appears to be that telomerase action overall in somatic cells is insufficient to guarantee continued telomere maintenance in the face of attrition throughout the human lifetime.

If the telomeric repeat DNA tract becomes too short, the chromosome end behaves as though it is a broken DNA end and becomes subject to inappropriate responses in the cell. These responses include premature cessation of cell division as well as reprogramming of transcriptional and other pathways to produce pro-inflammatory and tumour-promoting factors (reviewed in [3]). Furthermore, deleterious attempts by the cell to repair the telomere lead to genomic instabilities of various kinds that can promote cancers [4]. In humans the net result is to cause or spur various disease processes, including cancer progression [3,5].

Telomere maintenance and telomerase

Clinical, genetic, cellular, and molecular research of the past several years has recently converged to show that either too much or too little telomerase, even over quite a narrow range, can greatly increase lifetime risks of a range of different cancers, including many common cancers. Such findings indicate that humans appear to live on a knife-edge with respect to the telomere maintenance machinery and cancer risks. Therefore, external factors that influence telomere maintenance and telomerase constitute potentially significant contributors to cancer risks. Importantly, these factors include psychosocial inputs that bear on chronic psychological

stress. In this Perspective, I briefly discuss current understanding of these issues, and their implications.

Can telomere shortening contribute to diseases of ageing, including cancers? The answer is yes. Inherited disorders that compromise telomere maintenance establish a causal relationship between functional compromise of telomeres (usually caused by their over-shortening to below-functional lengths) and a wide range of diseases, collectively dubbed "telomere syndromes" [3]. These inherited syndromes include pulmonary fibrosis, diabetes, compromised cardiovascular function, and immune system disorders such as aplastic anaemia. They also include high risks for various haematological malignancies and gastrointestinal tract and squamous cell cancers, which can account for about 10% of the overall mortality in individuals with such syndromes. Such telomere maintenance mutations have cropped up sporadically in individual families from different parts of the world and are often well studied, as are mouse genetic models of telomere deficiency. Therefore, the causal link between this large inherited risk of cancers and very short, and hence non-functional, telomeres (caused by inadequate telomerase action) is compelling.

Can there be too much telomerase? Again the answer is yes, in abnormal situations. In addition to the cancer-causing mutations that diminish telomerase and cause overly short telomeres, even small changes in telomerase activity in the upward as well as the downward direction can greatly augment risks for some cancers and appear to act early in cancer progression. Point mutations (somatic or inherited) that increase expression of a telomerase component by only about 2-fold were recently shown to be associated with dramatically increased risks of melanoma in humans and are highly recurrent in sporadic melanomas [6,7]. Similar mutations were found also in liver and bladder cancers. It has been

known for many years that highly upregulated telomerase is a hallmark of many advanced (especially highly malignant) human cancers. This upregulation can be rationalized primarily as the need for cancer cells to maintain their telomeres to sustain their continued proliferation, a central property of cancer cells. However, interestingly, the melanoma-causing mutations described above bear the hallmarks of sunlight-induced mutations. This suggests that small but abnormal increases in telomerase may drive melanoma at even early stages [6,7].

Risks of age-related diseases

In human populations as well as patients with inherited telomere maintenance diseases, telomere shortness is linked to risks of some cancers. Indeed, in multiple population and cohort studies, the degree of telomere shortness is quantitatively linked to future risks of acquiring many age-related diseases, including some (but not all) cancers [8]. Impaired telomere maintenance leading to eventual over-shortening of telomeres has defined cellular and pathogenic consequences, as shown by laboratory research and the inherited telomere syndromes described above. Strikingly, these early-onset telomere syndrome diseases echo the diseases that become common with ageing in general human populations. After correcting for age and many other factors, links repeatedly have been found between shortness of telomeres in normal cells and the most common diseases of ageing – poor immune function, various forms of cardiovascular disease, diabetes, pulmonary disease, certain cancers, dementia, depression, and some other mental disorders. Such conditions are often co-morbid. Thus, it is plausible and indeed likely that in general populations, telomere shortening can contribute a causal role (but obviously not the sole role) in the development and pathogenesis of these diseases. Being systemic, and hence common across all organs and tissues, telomere shortening (with eventual loss of telomere function) begins to provide a compelling explanation for the co-morbidity of many age-related diseases and conditions.

Since most cancers in general populations are not obviously inherited, and since compromised telomere maintenance can increase cancer risks, factors that can affect telomere maintenance are of great interest. Although telomeres generally shorten with age in humans, chronological age can account for only 10% or less of the total variance in telomere length in the general population [9]. While telomere length shows some degree of heritability, common genetic variations in populations (as opposed to rare mutations) account for only a very limited portion of variability in telomere length. Furthermore, the heritability of telomere length diminishes with age. In a telling example, an interaction between smoking history and a common single-nucleotide polymorphism associated with telomere length has been reported for risk of bladder cancer (reviewed in [10]). Hence, it is important to understand other influences on telomere maintenance, and eventually to understand how genetic and non-genetic influences interact to affect cancer risks.

Effects of psychological stress

One important factor is severe psychological stress. This can have many inputs, including societal conditions of poverty, war, and social strife, and childhood abuse, trauma, and neglect [11]. Psychological stress has long been established as an important risk factor for some common diseases of ageing – prominently including cardiovascular disease, diabetes, and depression – but its relationship to cancers is

less well understood. Chronic psychological stress is also associated with telomere shortness. A growing body of studies links various types of chronic psychological stress, distress, and poor lifestyle (e.g. smoking and lack of exercise) to shorter telomeres [12,13]. In addition, social factors that cause chronic psychological stress are also established as risk factors for at least some chronic diseases of ageing and are also linked to telomere shortness in both adults and children. Some of these studies indicate that the psychological stress causes the telomere shortening, but this does not exclude two-way effects. Hence, stress, telomere shortness, and disease risks are quantifiably related through three pairwise links: stress with telomere shortness, stress with disease risks, and telomere shortness with risks of these same diseases (reviewed in [14]). The fact that telomere compromise is linked to (and in some situations is known to cause) diseases similar to those linked to (and in some cases caused by) stress leads directly to the hypothesis that telomere shortness at least partly explains how stress causes many common, often comorbid, diseases of ageing.

Effects of severe stress on telomere shortness can begin even early in life, as shown in direct studies of children exposed to adverse socioeconomic situations and violence. Significantly, the effects can be lasting: past histories of childhood adversity, and even exposure of developing fetuses to maternal stress, have been quantitatively related to telomere shortness in human adults (reviewed in [14]). It is also well established that adverse events that occurred in childhood predict early onset of chronic diseases, including mental disorders, in adults. Thus, it will be important to understand how much telomere compromise underlies or contributes

to the effects of childhood stressors on risks of diseases that continue to reverberate throughout life. An important unanswered question is whether such diseases include cancers. While compromised telomere maintenance has been linked to cancer risks, less is known about the impact of chronic psychological stress on cancer. Nonetheless, because both telomere shortness and chronic stress have independently been linked to several other chronic diseases of ageing, it will be important to extend the lessons learned from these other chronic diseases into a fuller understanding of cancer risks and cancer progression. Going forward, policies aimed at lessening the burden of cancer and other diseases throughout the world [15] cannot afford to ignore these connections.

Conclusions

A tsunami of overwhelming health and social issues is looming for the world's ageing population, cancers being prominent among them. We need to know how stress affects cancers. Basic biomedical research has identified telomeres, and correctly controlled telomere maintenance mechanisms, as crucial for replenishment of cells and tissues and prevention of cancers. Compromised telomere maintenance is emerging as a potential root factor underlying and interacting with mechanisms and etiologies of multiple co-morbid diseases of ageing. Psychological stress, including that related to societal and life factors, has independently been linked to these same chronic diseases and to telomere compromise. What we have learned about this underlying disease process should be applied to strategies to mitigate cancer risks, intercept cancer progression, and improve cancer survival.

References

1. Sfeir A, de Lange T (2012). Removal of shelterin reveals the telomere end-protection problem. *Science*, 336:593–597. http://dx.doi.org/10.1126/science.1218498 PMID:22556254

2. Aubert G, Lansdorp PM (2008). Telomeres and aging. *Physiol Rev*, 88:557–579. http://dx.doi.org/:10.1152/physrev.00026.2007 PMID:18391173

3. Armanios M, Blackburn EH (2012). The telomere syndromes. *Nat Rev Genet*, 13:693–704. http://dx.doi.org/10.1038/nrg3246 PMID:22965356

4. Chin L, Artandi SE, Shen Q et al. (1999). p53 deficiency rescues the adverse effects of telomere loss and cooperates with telomere dysfunction to accelerate carcinogenesis. *Cell*, 97:527–538. http://dx.doi.org/10.1016/S0092-8674(00)80762-X PMID:10338216

5. Hills M, Lansdorp PM (2009). Short telomeres resulting from heritable mutations in the telomerase reverse transcriptase gene predispose for a variety of malignancies. *Ann N Y Acad Sci*, 1176:178–190. http://dx.doi.org/10.1111/j.1749-6632.2009.04565.x PMID:19796246

6. Huang FW, Hodis E, Xu MJ et al. (2013). Highly recurrent TERT promoter mutations in human melanoma. *Science*, 339:957–959. http://dx.doi.org/10.1126/science.1229259 PMID:23348506

7. Horn S, Figl A, Rachakonda PS et al. (2013). TERT promoter mutations in familial and sporadic melanoma. *Science*, 339:959–961. http://dx.doi.org/10.1126/science.1230062 PMID:23348503

8. Willeit P, Willeit J, Kloss-Brandstätter A et al. (2011). Fifteen-year follow-up of association between telomere length and incident cancer and cancer mortality. *JAMA*, 306:42–44. http://dx.doi.org/10.1001/jama.2011.901 PMID:21730239

9. Lin J, Epel ES, Blackburn EH (2009). Telomeres, telomerase, stress, and aging. In: Berntson GG, Cacioppo JT, eds. *Handbook of Neuroscience for the Behavioral Sciences*. Hoboken, NJ: Wiley, pp. 1280–1295.

10. Blackburn EH (2011). Walking the walk from genes through telomere maintenance to cancer risk. *Cancer Prev Res (Phila)*, 4:473–475. http://dx.doi.org/10.1158/1940-6207.CAPR-11-0066 PMID:21460394

11. Adler N, Pantell MS, O'Donovan A et al. (2013). Educational attainment and late life telomere length in the Health, Aging and Body Composition Study. *Brain Behav Immun*, 27:15–21. http://dx.doi.org/10.1016/j.bbi.2012.08.014 PMID:22981835

12. Surtees PG, Wainwright NW, Pooley KA et al. (2011). Life stress, emotional health, and mean telomere length in the European Prospective Investigation into Cancer (EPIC)-Norfolk population study. *J Gerontol A Biol Sci Med Sci*, 66:1152–1162. http://dx.doi.org/10.1093/gerona/glr112 PMID:21788649

13. Lin J, Epel E, Blackburn E (2012). Telomeres and lifestyle factors: roles in cellular aging. *Mutat Res*, 730:85–89. http://dx.doi.org/10.1016/j.mrfmmm.2011.08.003 PMID:21878343

14. Blackburn EH, Epel ES (2012). Telomeres and adversity: too toxic to ignore. *Nature*, 490:169–171. http://dx.doi.org/10.1038/490169a PMID:23060172

15. Marmot M, Friel S, Bell R et al.; Commission on Social Determinants of Health (2008). Closing the gap in a generation: health equity through action on the social determinants of health. *Lancet*, 372:1661–1669. http://dx.doi.org/10.1016/S0140-6736(08)61690-6 PMID:18994664

2

Cancer
etiology

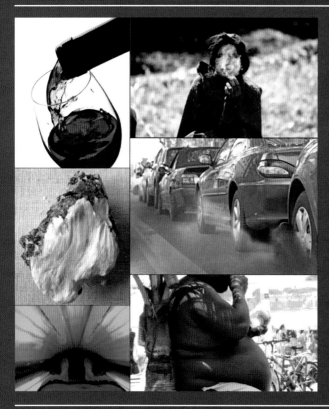

Most cancers are associated with risks from environmental, lifestyle, or behavioural exposures. Comparing the highest with the lowest incidence recorded for different communities or examining changes over time provides clues as to which factors determine the distribution of cancer globally and how they differ in their impact. For the most important factor – tobacco smoking – differences worldwide reflect timing. The epidemic of lung cancer has peaked in high-income countries, whereas in China, for example, the epidemic is starting. Chronic infections continue to play a major role in common cancers in parts of Africa and Asia but are far less common in Europe and North America. Diet exerts an influence on cancer development; in parts of Africa and Asia, this is sometimes related to the impact of potent carcinogens such as aflatoxins, but in high-income countries this is primarily because of energy-rich food intake and associated overweight or obesity, linked in part to low levels of physical activity. Personal choices about alcohol intake and deliberate sun exposure are reflected in the incidence of particular cancer types. Worldwide, exposure to hazardous workplaces and environmental pollution causes cancer in low- and middle-income countries despite experience that may have been gained from other communities.

2.1

The global tobacco epidemic

Michael J. Thun
Jane R. Nilson
Alex C. Liber
Evan Blecher

Prabhat Jha (reviewer)
Pramil N. Singh (reviewer)

Summary

- Worldwide, tobacco use kills approximately 6 million people annually, from cancer and other diseases.

- Consumption of manufactured cigarettes has peaked and is declining in most high-income countries but is increasing or persisting at high levels in many low- and middle-income countries.

- The historical progression of the cigarette epidemic that unfolded first in high-income countries is now occurring worldwide, especially in men.

- The application of effective tobacco control measures such as large periodic increases in excise taxes and the elimination of advertising can provide unparalleled opportunities for the prevention of cancer and other diseases worldwide.

At least 1.3 billion people worldwide use some form of tobacco [1]. In 2000, 4.83 million (uncertainty range, 3.94–5.93 million) premature deaths globally were attributable to smoking, 2.41 million (1.80–3.15 million) in low- and middle-income countries and 2.43 million (2.13–2.78 million) in high-income countries. Of these deaths, 3.84 million were in men. The leading causes of death from smoking were cardiovascular diseases (1.69 million deaths), chronic obstructive pulmonary disease (0.97 million deaths), and lung cancer (0.85 million deaths) [2]. By 2013, the total number of deaths worldwide attributable to tobacco use was approximately 6 million [3].

Manufactured cigarettes are the predominant tobacco product used globally; nearly 20% of the world's adult population (about 800 million men and 200 million women) smoke cigarettes [4]. Other smoked products (cigars, pipes, bidis, kreteks, and water pipes) and smokeless forms of tobacco (snuff, chewing tobacco, betel quid, and paan) are also commonly used regionally [5]. Reliable nationally representative data on smoking prevalence have been available for certain high-income countries since the mid-20th century, but coverage of low- and middle-income countries has expanded only during the past decade. The Global Adult Tobacco

Fig. 2.1.1. In Togo, a group of schoolboys huddle together on a street to smoke cigarettes.

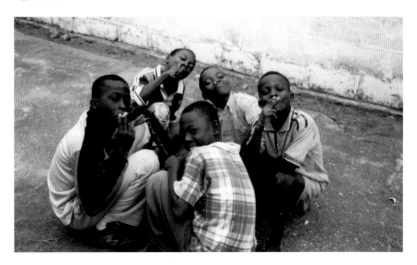

Fig. 2.1.2. Stages of the tobacco epidemic in (A) men and (B) women. For details, see text.

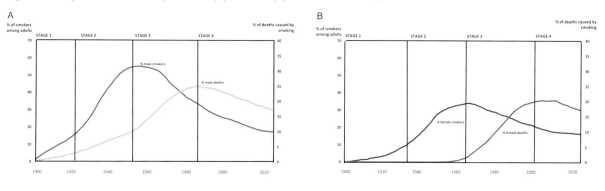

Survey has now surveyed 19 countries that include half of the world's adult population [6]; the Global Youth Tobacco Survey has studied students aged 13–15 years in more than 160 countries [7]. Whereas in most high-income countries cigarette smoking has now peaked and is declining, in many low- and middle-income countries it has become entrenched, especially in men. More than 80% of all smokers reside in low- and middle-income countries; more than 60% live in just 10 countries (in decreasing order): China, India, Indonesia, the Russian Federation, the USA, Japan, Brazil, Bangladesh, Germany, and Turkey [8].

Historical progression

The large geographical and temporal variations in tobacco use observed currently are best understood in terms of the historical progression that unfolded first in high-income countries such as the United Kingdom and the USA [9,10] and that is now occurring worldwide, especially in men. Manufactured cigarettes were introduced early in the 20th century in the USA and the United Kingdom. They rapidly displaced traditional tobacco products such as cigars, pipes, hand-rolled cigarettes, and snuff and by 1920 were the product of choice among new users. The distribution of free cigarettes to soldiers in the First and Second World Wars, combined with mass advertising, greatly increased cigarette sales. Women did not begin smoking regularly until the Second World War, when advertising targeted to women and the entry of women into the workforce overcame social and cultural norms against female smoking.

Successive birth cohorts of men, and later women, smoked more cigarettes per day and initiated smoking at progressively earlier ages. Cigarette sales continued to increase sharply in the United Kingdom until the 1950s and in the USA until the early 1960s, when studies of smoking and mortality and authoritative government reports increased concern about the health hazards of smoking, causing a decline in consumption and smoking prevalence [10,11]. Continuing publicity about the harmful effects of smoking and the introduction of effective tobacco control policies such as smoke-free laws and increased taxes on cigarettes further discouraged smoking. However, the number of deaths caused by smoking continued to increase for several decades after the decline in cigarette sales, due to the ageing of continuing smokers with the greatest lifetime exposure to actively inhaled tobacco smoke.

Stages of the epidemic

The progression of the cigarette epidemic, first observed in developed countries, has been conceptualized as a sequence of four stages that apply more broadly worldwide. These stages (Fig. 2.1.2) are conventionally defined by increasing or decreasing trends in smoking prevalence, and then in smoking-attributable deaths, in a given country. However, most low- and middle-income countries have only cross-sectional data on smoking prevalence and no formal estimates of smoking-attributable deaths. In these countries, the stages can be approximated using cross-sectional measures of adult prevalence in relation to longitudinal trends in per capita cigarette sales. The staging of countries discussed below refers only to cigarettes or cigarette-like

Fig. 2.1.3. Smoking home-grown tobacco wrapped in green leaves or stuffed in a pipe is a tribal tradition in Phak Nam in north-eastern Cambodia, among members of the Kreung ethnic minority.

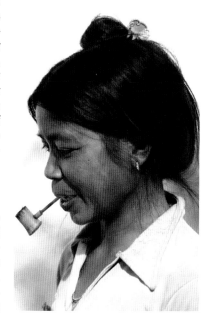

Fig. 2.1.4. Tobacco advertising has always been common in Formula One racing. However, as tobacco advertising bans take effect, teams have started using an alternative livery that alludes to the tobacco sponsor or eliminates its name entirely.

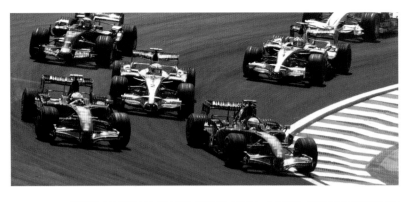

products such as bidis, although other tobacco products are also discussed. The stages typically differ for men and women in their severity and timing.

Stage 1 represents the beginning of the epidemic. At this stage, the prevalence of cigarette smoking in adult men or women is low (< 20%), and as yet few deaths can be attributed to smoking. Per capita consumption is flat or only beginning to increase, and there is no history of greater smoking in the past. In stage 2, the prevalence of cigarette smoking in adults rises above 20% and may increase to a peak of between 40% and 80%. Per capita cigarette consumption also rises. In countries where estimates of tobacco-attributable deaths are available, this percentage begins to rise as a fraction of all deaths. Stage 3 is characterized by a flattening or downturn in smoking prevalence (and usually in per capita consumption), coinciding with a continuing steep increase in smoking-attributable deaths. Stage 4 is characterized by a decline in both smoking prevalence and smoking-attributable deaths [11].

Several factors influence the stage of the epidemic within a given country or region. These include the affordability and availability of cigarettes and the intensity of tobacco industry marketing efforts. The uptake of smoking among women may be deterred, possibly indefinitely, by religious and social norms that discourage female smoking, hence limiting the applicability of the stages of the epidemic model to countries that observe a significant increase in female smoking prevalence. Public education about the harmful effects of smoking and second-hand smoke and implementation of effective tobacco control policies also curtail tobacco use. Even within a given region there may be considerable variation in tobacco use because of these factors.

Geographical variations

Most of the stages of the cigarette epidemic can be observed in Africa. Women in all countries are in stage 1, as are men in many countries in sub-Saharan Africa [12]. Men in several sub-Saharan African countries, such as Namibia, Botswana, and Sierra Leone, are in stage 2 (adult prevalence > 20%), as are men in all countries in North Africa [4]. The prevalence of cigarette smoking among adult men in North Africa ranges from 28% in Morocco to 53% in Tunisia (stage 2 or 3), not counting the use of water pipes (shisha and hookah) [4]. In Egypt, 38% of adult men smoke cigarettes, and per capita consumption has nearly doubled over the past 20 years [13,14]. Most sub-Saharan African countries, with the exception of South Africa, are positioned on the upslope rather than the downslope of the epidemic curve and remain especially vulnerable to industry marketing [12,15].

In Central and South America, the prevalence of cigarette smoking in men generally increases from north to south, ranging from 3% in Suriname and Belize to 30% in Chile [4]. The smoking prevalence in individual countries does

Fig. 2.1.5. Preparation of paan in Varanasi, India. Paan is a stimulating, psychoactive preparation of betel leaf combined with areca nut and/or cured tobacco. It is chewed and then spat out or swallowed.

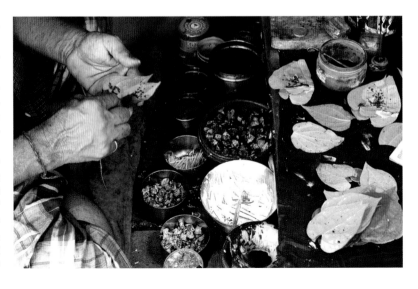

not necessarily follow this general pattern. Male smoking prevalence exceeds 40% in Cuba, Peru, and Bolivia and exceeds 30% in Venezuela, Uruguay, and Argentina [4]. Brazil is the only country in South America that may be in stage 4 for men, with decreases in per capita consumption and smoking prevalence in men (22%) and women (13%) due to rigorous tobacco control efforts [13,16]. Cuba has the highest female smoking prevalence in the Caribbean (29%) [4] and also has higher lung cancer death rates in women than those in most of Europe [17].

In North America, northern Europe, Australia, and New Zealand, men are in stage 4 of the epidemic, whereas women are generally transitioning from stage 3 to stage 4. In all of these countries, male cigarette smoking prevalence exceeded 50% in past decades [16]. Currently, Sweden has the lowest smoking prevalence in men (13%) and is the only country in Europe where prevalence is higher

in women (16%) than in men [4]. The use of smokeless tobacco (snus) is most common in Sweden but is also seen in other Scandinavian countries [4]. Greece has the highest smoking prevalence in men (63%), and Austria has the highest prevalence in women (45%) [4].

Countries in the former Soviet Union have some of the highest male cigarette smoking prevalence rates in the world, whereas smoking prevalence in men has decreased substantially in some countries in eastern Europe. Male smoking prevalence exceeds 50% in the Russian Federation (59%) and Georgia (57%) and remains at 50% in Latvia [4]. Smoking prevalence among men has decreased in Poland and Ukraine [13]. Although female prevalence does not generally exceed 25% in these countries, it is increasing rapidly in the Russian Federation and to a lesser extent in Ukraine [4]. Per capita consumption in the Russian Federation has almost doubled in the past 20 years [14].

Tobacco smoking is uncommon among women in the Middle East, except in Lebanon [4]. Men are in stage 1 in Qatar, Oman, Saudi Arabia, and the United Arab Emirates and in stage 3 or late stage 2 in Turkey (48%) [14], Jordan (42%) [4], and the Syrian Arab Republic (36%) [4]. Use of water pipes (shisha, hookah, and narghile) is common throughout the region.

Smoking is uncommon (< 10%) among women in nearly all countries in East and South-East Asia [4]. Among men the highest smoking prevalence estimates are in Indonesia (57%) [4] and China (53%) [13]. Per capita cigarette consumption is still increasing in many countries (China, Bangladesh, Nepal, Viet Nam, Indonesia, and the Philippines) where men account for most of the smoking [14]. Smoking prevalence is decreasing among older women in China. A concern, based on limited anecdotal information, is that smoking prevalence may be beginning to increase

Fig. 2.1.6. Cigarette consumption and prices in (A) France (1980–2011), (B) Thailand (1990–2011), and (C) South Africa (1961–2009). THB, Thai baht; ZAR, South African rand.

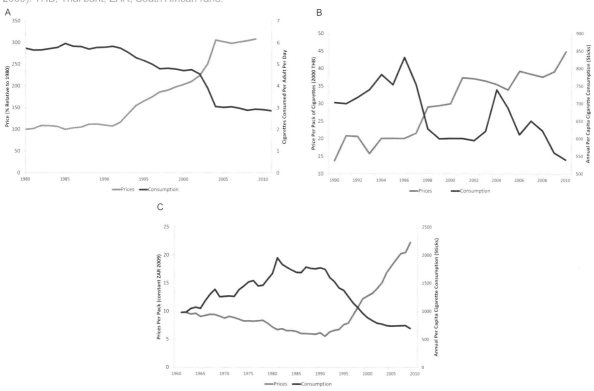

among young urban Chinese women [18]. Smoking typically begins at young ages, and Chinese women represent a vast untapped market for the tobacco companies.

Tobacco smoking is rare among women in India, Pakistan, and Bangladesh, but the use of smokeless tobacco by women in these countries is the highest in the world [4]. Nearly half of adult men in Bangladesh (45%) smoke either cigarettes or bidis [13]. The prevalence of male tobacco smoking is lower in India (24%) and Pakistan (28%) [4], but the use of smokeless products (paan, gutkha, and betel quid) exceeds 30% [13]. Per capita consumption of manufactured cigarettes is low in all three countries [14].

Strategies to curtail the epidemic

Education about the harms of tobacco use and policy interventions advocated by the WHO Framework Convention on Tobacco Control have reduced tobacco use in many countries. For example, increases in excise taxes on cigarettes consistently decrease cigarette sales [19,20]. This is exemplified by the decrease in per capita cigarette consumption in Thailand, South Africa, and France, which coincided with large increases in the real price of cigarettes (Fig. 2.1.6) [14,21–26]. Other important strategies that promote cessation and decrease initiation include smoke-free laws, public service counter-advertising, and restrictions on or banning of tobacco industry advertising [27]. Many countries have implemented graphic health warnings on cigarette packs. Australia is leading the way on plain packaging (removal of all graphic branding from cigarette packs). The widespread application of a few powerful tobacco control interventions could prevent a large proportion of the anticipated 450 million deaths from tobacco over the next few decades by enabling those who are current smokers to quit and by persuading youth to never start smoking in the first place [28].

In conclusion, tobacco use remains an enormous health problem worldwide. Use is currently decreasing in most high-income countries but increasing or persisting at high levels in many low- and middle-income countries. Effective tobacco control strategies such as large periodic increases in excise taxes and the elimination of advertising provide unparalleled opportunities for cancer prevention worldwide.

References

1. Glynn T, Seffrin JR, Brawley OW et al. (2010). The globalization of tobacco use: 21 challenges for the 21st century. *CA Cancer J Clin*, 60:50–61. http://dx.doi.org/10.3322/caac.20052 PMID:20097837

2. Ezzati M, Lopez AD (2003). Estimates of global mortality attributable to smoking in 2000. *Lancet*, 362:847–852. http://dx.doi.org/10.1016/S0140-6736(03)14338-3 PMID:13678970

3. WHO (2013). *WHO Report on the Global Tobacco Epidemic, 2013: Enforcing Bans on Tobacco Advertising, Promotion and Sponsorship.* Geneva: WHO. Available at http://apps.who.int/iris/bitstream/10665/85380/1/9789241505871_eng.pdf.

4. Eriksen M, Mackay J, Ross H (2012). *The Tobacco Atlas*, 4th ed. Atlanta, GA: American Cancer Society, World Lung Foundation. Available at http://www.tobaccoatlas.org/.

5. IARC (2012). Personal habits and indoor combustions. *IARC Monogr Eval Carcinog Risks Hum*, 100E:1–575. PMID:23193840

6. WHO (2012). Global Adult Tobacco Survey. Available at http://www.who.int/tobacco/surveillance/survey/gats/en/index.html.

7. WHO (2012). Global Youth Tobacco Survey. Available at http://www.who.int/tobacco/surveillance/gyts/en/index.html.

8. WHO (2008). *MPOWER: A Policy Package to Reverse the Tobacco Epidemic.* Geneva: WHO. Available at http://www.who.int/tobacco/mpower/mpower_english.pdf.

9. Pirie K, Peto R, Reeves GK et al.; Million Women Study Collaborators (2013). The 21st century hazards of smoking and benefits of stopping: a prospective study of one million women in the UK. *Lancet*, 381:133–141. http://dx.doi.org/10.1016/S0140-6736(12)61720-6 PMID:23107252

10. U.S. Public Health Service (1964). *Smoking and Health: Report of the Advisory Committee to the Surgeon General of the Public Health Service.* Washington, DC: U.S. Department of Health, Education, and Welfare, Public Health Service (Public Health Service Publication No. 1103).

11. Thun M, Peto R, Boreham J, Lopez AD (2012). Stages of the cigarette epidemic on entering its second century. *Tob Control*, 21:96–101. http://dx.doi.org/10.1136/tobaccocontrol-2011-050294 PMID:22345230

12. Pampel F (2008). Tobacco use in sub-Sahara Africa: estimates from the demographic health surveys. *Soc Sci Med*, 66:1772–1783. http://dx.doi.org/10.1016/j.socscimed.2007.12.003 PMID:18249479

13. Giovino GA, Mirza SA, Samet JM et al.; GATS Collaborative Group (2012). Tobacco use in 3 billion individuals from 16 countries: an analysis of nationally representative cross-sectional household surveys. *Lancet*, 380:668–679. http://dx.doi.org/10.1016/S0140-6736(12)61085-X PMID:22901888

14. ERC (2010). *World Cigarette Reports 2010.* Suffolk, UK: ERC Group.

15. Blecher E (2010). Targeting the affordability of cigarettes: a new benchmark for taxation policy in low-income and middle-income countries. *Tob Control*, 19:325–330. http://dx.doi.org/10.1136/tc.2009.030155 PMID:20530141

16. OECD (2012). Non-medical determinants of health. OECD Health Statistics database. Paris: Organisation for Economic Co-operation and Development. http://dx.doi.org/10.1787/20758480

17. WHO (2012). Cancer Mortality Database. Available at http://www-dep.iarc.fr/WHOdb/WHOdb.htm.

18. Ho MG, Ma S, Chai W et al. (2010). Smoking among rural and urban young women in China. *Tob Control*, 19:13–18. http://dx.doi.org/10.1136/tc.2009.030981 PMID:19822528

19. WHO (2003). *WHO Framework Convention on Tobacco Control.* Available at http://www.who.int/fctc/en/.

20. IARC (2011). IARC Handbooks of Cancer Prevention, Vol. 14: *Tobacco Control: Effectiveness of Tax and Price Policies for Tobacco Control.* Lyon: IARC.

21. Economist Intelligence Unit (2011). Worldwide Cost of Living Survey. London: The Economist Group.

22. Economist Intelligence Unit (2011). Marlboro cigarette and local cigarette prices, Worldwide Cost of Living Survey. London: The Economist Group.

23. International Monetary Fund (2011). World Economic Outlook Database, April 2011 edition. Available at http://www.imf.org/external/pubs/ft/weo/2011/01/weodata/index.aspx.

24. Levy DT, Benjakul S, Ross H, Ritthiphakdee B (2008). The role of tobacco control policies in reducing smoking and deaths in a middle income nation: results from the Thailand SimSmoke simulation model. *Tob Control*, 17:53–59. http://dx.doi.org/10.1136/tc.2007.022319 PMID:18218810

25. Blecher EH (2011). *The Economics of Tobacco Control in Low- and Middle-Income Countries* [thesis]. Cape Town, South Africa: School of Economics, University of Cape Town.

26. Guérin S, Hill C (2010). Cancer epidemiology in France in 2010: comparison with the USA [in French]. *Bull Cancer*, 97:47–54. http://dx.doi.org/10.1684/bdc.2010.1013 PMID:19995688

27. Blecher E (2008). The impact of tobacco advertising bans on consumption in developing countries. *J Health Econ*, 27:930–942. http://dx.doi.org/10.1016/j.jhealeco.2008.02.010 PMID:18440661

28. Jha P (2009). Avoidable global cancer deaths and total deaths from smoking. *Nat Rev Cancer*, 9:655–664. http://dx.doi.org/10.1038/nrc2703 PMID:19693096

2.2 Tobacco smoking and smokeless tobacco use

Jonathan M. Samet
Prakash C. Gupta
Cecily S. Ray

Catherine Sauvaget (reviewer)
Deborah M. Winn (reviewer)

Summary

• Tobacco smoke contains more than 7000 chemical compounds, of which many are known carcinogens. Components of tobacco smoke contribute to carcinogenesis through multiple pathways, including DNA binding and mutations, inflammation, oxidative stress, and epigenetic changes.

• Smokeless tobacco products contain more than 3000 chemicals and numerous carcinogens. DNA binding and mutations are among the mechanisms clearly implicated in carcinogenesis due to smokeless tobacco use.

• Epidemiological studies have shown causal associations between tobacco smoking and at least 14 different types of cancer to date. Accumulated evidence from epidemiological studies so far has been sufficient to show that smokeless tobacco causes cancers of the oral cavity and pancreas.

• Comprehensive tobacco control strategies are in place at the global level through provisions in the WHO Framework Convention for Tobacco Control to combat the epidemic of tobacco use.

Worldwide, tobacco is used in diverse smoked or smokeless products, all delivering nicotine to their users. The worldwide epidemic of tobacco-caused diseases comes largely from widespread smoking of manufactured cigarettes, now mostly manufactured and distributed by a small number of multinational corporations and, in the case of China, the China National Tobacco Corporation. In some countries, particularly India and Bangladesh, smokeless tobacco use is prominent, especially among women, even though smoking is rare among them. The potency of tobacco products, particularly cigarettes, as a cause of cancer and their role in causing cardiovascular and lung diseases make tobacco use the leading cause of avoidable premature mortality worldwide, causing an estimated 6 million deaths annually [1].

Tobacco smoking

Manufactured cigarettes are highly engineered for the purpose of delivering nicotine-containing smoke to their users. They burn at high temperature, generating thousands of chemicals, and consequently smokers inhale a highly toxic mixture containing many known carcinogens and toxins, such as benzo[a]pyrene and other polycyclic aromatic hydrocarbons, tobacco-specific nitrosamines (N-nitroso derivatives of nicotine and its metabolites), benzene (a cause of leukaemia), formaldehyde (an irritant and carcinogen), carbon monoxide and cyanide (asphyxiants), acrolein (an irritant), and polonium (a radioactive carcinogen) [2]. The smoke inhaled by the smoker is referred to as mainstream smoke, and that emitted from the smouldering cigarette is called sidestream smoke. In the presence of smoking, nonsmokers inhale second-hand smoke, made up largely of sidestream smoke and also some exhaled mainstream smoke. Pipes, cigars, and water pipes deliver smoke with mixtures of components comparable to those from cigarettes, although there are differences in smoke characteristics across products.

Smokeless tobacco

Smokeless tobacco is consumed in ways apart from the tobacco being burnt; relevant products are most commonly used orally and sometimes nasally. Oral smokeless tobacco use delivers nicotine more slowly than cigarette smoking does – the peak increase in plasma levels of nicotine in smokeless tobacco users is 30 minutes after intake – but the level remains higher longer because it declines slowly while the product is held in the mouth. Over the course of a day, a smokeless tobacco user may ingest twice as much nicotine as a smoker. Smokeless tobacco comes in many forms, with names specific to the countries of origin, but the products may be generally classified as loose leaf for chewing or twist (sweetened, flavoured strands), flakes, shredded or fine-cut tobacco for chewing or holding in the mouth, solid compressed tobacco products in the form of chunks or sticks, viscous pastes, dry or moist ground tobacco (snuff) for oral or nasal use, liquid snuff (an extract) for nasal use in Eastern Africa, and tobacco-smoke water for gargling in South Asia. Newer products include fine-cut or powdered tobacco (i.e. snuff) in teabag-like pouches, dissolvable tobacco lozenges, and tobacco toothpicks.

Some smokeless tobacco products are plain tobacco leaf. Most products are flavoured: sweetened with sugar, molasses, or artificial sweeteners, salted, and/or aromatized with substances like essences, spices, and perfumes. Menthol is often used to prevent irritation. Smokeless tobacco is used along with areca nut by many people of South-East Asia, both in their countries of origin and wherever they have migrated. The user may mix tobacco with areca nut or may purchase a pre-mixed product. Areca nut contributes its own set of carcinogens, mainly through areca nut-specific nitrosamines [3].

Tobacco-specific nitrosamines are relevant to both smoking and smokeless tobacco use but are of particular prominence in the use of smokeless tobacco because polycyclic aromatic hydrocarbons are generated by combustion and are therefore not implicated in smokeless tobacco carcinogenesis. These compounds are formed by the nitrosation of nicotine and its metabolites. The nature and amount of these compounds depends on the tobacco species, the growing conditions, the amount of fermentation and ageing, and how finely the tobacco is cut or powdered. Smokeless tobacco

products, as with many cigarette brands, usually have an ingredient that increases the pH, to promote the availability of nicotine for absorption. Such agents include ammonia, ammonium carbonate, calcium hydroxide, potassium hydroxide, potassium carbonate, and sodium carbonate. Nicotine availability also increases with finer powdering of the tobacco [3]. Products with different levels of free nicotine are marketed to different types of users; novices usually start with low-nicotine products and may graduate to brands with higher levels [4].

Patterns of use

Cigarettes

The Global Adult Tobacco Survey and the Global Youth Tobacco Survey, both implemented by WHO and the United States Centers for Disease Control and Prevention in collaboration with participating countries, track the use of tobacco worldwide. The first global report based on the Global Adult Tobacco Survey was published in 2012, drawing on findings from 14 low- and middle-income countries and from the USA and the United Kingdom [5]. The findings showed a wide range

of smoking prevalence among the 19 countries and far higher rates of smoking among men than women, although in several countries the prevalence of smoking among women approached that among men (Fig. 2.2.1). In some countries, exemplified by China and India, only a small percentage of ever-smokers had stopped smoking. This survey, which covered most of the high-burden countries, documented tobacco use by about 850 million people. Among those aged 24–35 years who were interviewed for this survey, the mean age of smoking initiation was 17.7 years in men and 18.0 years in women [5]. For those aged 35 years or older, the average age of initiation was generally older in women than men.

The Global Youth Tobacco Survey data collected from adolescents aged 13–15 years in schools in most countries show that youth continue to smoke worldwide [6]. In some countries more than 30% of boys and girls in this age range have smoked in the past month and the prevalence of smoking among girls is approaching that among boys. Countries with the highest rate of smoking among boys include Papua New Guinea (50.6% prevalence), Timor-Leste

Fig. 2.2.1. Prevalence of current tobacco smoking among male and female adults aged ≥ 15 years in 14 Global Adult Tobacco Survey countries, the United Kingdom, and the USA.

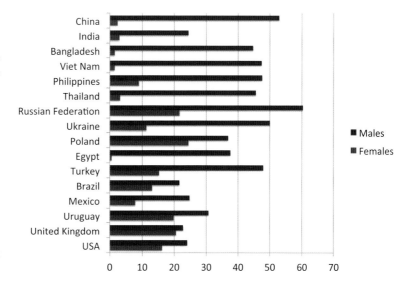

(50.6%), and Tonga (37.5%), whereas the highest rates of smoking among girls were reported in Chile (39.9%), Papua New Guinea (35.8%), and the Czech Republic (32.7%) [6].

Smokeless tobacco

Smokeless tobacco is used orally in all regions of the world, but its use is most prevalent in the Pacific Islands, South and South-East Asia, Africa, and Europe [6]. Countries with the highest known prevalence of smokeless tobacco use include Marshall Islands, Myanmar, Bangladesh, India, and Madagascar (prevalence 20% and above). These are followed by Bhutan, Nepal, Sweden, Sri Lanka, Sudan, Turkmenistan, Federated States of Micronesia, Uzbekistan, Yemen, and Norway (prevalence 10–19%). Fig. 2.2.2 shows the relative position of countries according to national prevalence of adult smokeless tobacco use. Such data are not yet available for many countries, especially in Africa. Products are exported from the USA, Sweden, and India to many destinations around the world. Several of the largest cigarette manufacturers are now marketing smokeless tobacco products to smokers as extensions of their cigarette brands, pitching them as products to be used in smoke-free environments [6]. Prevalence figures for youth who use smokeless tobacco are not available from most countries at present. However, the Global Youth Tobacco Survey shows a high proportion of non-cigarette tobacco use among youth in many countries, and a large part of this use is believed to be smokeless tobacco [7]. In Congo in 2006, 18.0% of youth aged 13–15 years had used smokeless tobacco in the previous 30 days [8]. In India in 2006, the corresponding prevalence was 8.1% [9].

Tobacco as a cause of cancer

Mechanisms of cancer causation

Tobacco smoking

Tobacco smoke is a mixture of gases and particles sufficiently small to reach and deposit in the bronchioles and alveoli. Tobacco smoke components, including nicotine, move from the lungs into the circulation and reach throughout the body, resulting in various tissues being exposed to differing levels of carcinogens, not simply in organs where primary absorption occurs but throughout most of the body.

Tobacco smoke contains more than 7000 chemical compounds, including numerous known carcinogens, as evaluated for carcinogenicity by IARC [10]. Broad classes of carcinogens in tobacco smoke include polycyclic aromatic hydrocarbons, N-nitrosamines, and aromatic amines, together with a range of tobacco-specific toxins, including volatile aldehydes and phenolic amines.

Fig. 2.2.3 provides a general schema for the causation of cancer by the carcinogens in tobacco smoke. There are both specific and nonspecific pathways by which smoking causes cancer, and there is very extensive experimental evidence documenting these pathways [2,10]. The figure begins with initiation of cigarette smoking and addiction; it is the maintained contact with tobacco smoke carcinogens resulting from addiction that leads to the very high risk of cancer in those who smoke daily throughout their lives, the general pattern of the addicted smoker. It is not necessary to smoke across the full lifetime to have excess risk of cancer from smoking. Even a decade or two of smoking increases risk, and cancer risk for former smokers, although reduced, does not drop to that of never-smokers. The figure highlights the multiple processes that lead to uncontrolled cell growth and malignancy and the multiple points in these processes at which tobacco smoke components contribute to carcinogenesis. The major pathway to cancer is considered to be DNA binding and consequent mutations (central pathway), but tobacco smoke also contributes to increased cancer risk through inflammation (top pathway) and epigenetic mechanisms (bottom pathway) [10].

Smokeless tobacco

Smokeless tobacco contains more than 3000 chemicals and at least 28 carcinogens, many the same as those contained in cigarette smoke, and the general scheme of Fig. 2.2.3 is applicable. Smokeless tobacco use results in exposure to tobacco-specific nitrosamines, volatile N-nitrosamines, N-nitrosamino acids, and volatile aldehydes such as formaldehyde and acetaldehyde, as well as metals including cadmium, lead, arsenic, nickel, and chromium, and radioactive elements. Certain tobacco-related nitrosamines (e.g. nicotine-derived nitrosamine ketone and N'-nitrosonornicotine), their metabolites, and benzo[a]pyrene are

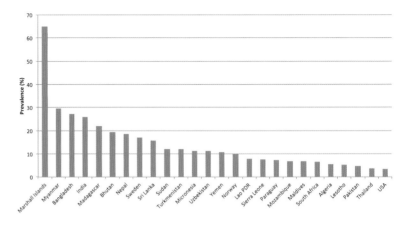

Genetic susceptibility to tobacco-related cancers

James D. McKay

The first-degree relatives of patients with tobacco-related cancers have an excess risk of developing the same type of cancer. While a shared environmental exposure such as tobacco could influence such observations, this finding also suggests a role for genetic susceptibility [1]. Susceptibility genes have indeed been identified and encompass both rare and common genetic variants.

Several rare cancer syndromes, such as Li–Fraumeni syndrome (OMIM 151623) and dyskeratosis congenita (OMIM 127550), linked with mutations in the *TP53* and *TERT* genes, respectively, include tobacco-related cancers in their disease spectrum, which implicates such genes in genetic susceptibility. Similarly, a rare familial form of lung adenocarcinoma appears to be linked with germline mutations in *EGFR* [2].

Genome-wide association study (GWAS) approaches have identified several other intriguing loci with much more common population frequencies (Fig. B2.2.1). At chromosome 15q25, a locus that contains several nicotinic acetylcholine receptors, the same variants linked with lung cancer are also linked with propensity to smoke, leading to the debated suggestion that this association could be mediated by behavioural changes [3,4]. Two independent common variants at 5p15.33, a region containing the *TERT* gene, have been linked with

lung cancer [5]. These variants, although in close proximity, appear to differ in their effects in terms of histology, with one being more relevant to adenocarcinoma [6]. This same locus has been subsequently linked with genetic susceptibility to many other cancer types [7].

GWAS and other approaches have identified genetic variants at several other lung cancer susceptibility loci; the chromosome 6 major histocompatibility complex (MHC) region [3], which is critical to immune response; and several genes involved in DNA repair and cell-cycle regulation, notably *CHEK2* [8], *RAD52* [9], and *CDNK2A* [9], all of which appear particularly relevant to lung squamous cell carcinoma (Fig. B2.2.1). Several additional lung cancer susceptibility loci have been identified in Asian populations [10], although their involvement in lung cancer in other populations remains unclear. Within cancers of the head and neck, the genes involved in alcohol metabolism (*ADH* and *ALDH2*) appear particularly relevant [11].

It is also notable that the genetic studies carried out so far have identified fewer susceptibility loci in tobacco-related cancers compared with other common cancers, despite the comparably sized genetic studies and similar estimations of hereditary components. The reason for this remains unclear, but some of the unexplained risk may be explained by components of genetic

variation not tested extensively to date, such as rare population frequencies and copy number repeats, with the latter potentially important particularly for metabolism genes. Further studies are also required on gene–environment interactions.

References

1. Brennan P et al. (2011). Lancet Oncol, 12:399–408. http://dx.doi.org/10.1016/S1470-2045(10)70126-1 PMID:20951091

2. Ohtsuka K et al. (2011). J Clin Oncol, 29:e191–e192. http://dx.doi.org/10.1200/JCO.2010.31.4492 PMID:21172876

3. Hung RJ et al. (2008). Nature, 452:633–637. http://dx.doi.org/10.1038/nature06885 PMID:18385738

4. Chen D et al. (2011). Cancer Epidemiol Biomarkers Prev, 20:658–664. http://dx.doi.org/10.1158/1055-9965.EPI-10-1008 PMID:21335511

5. McKay JD et al. (2008). Nat Genet, 40:1404–1406. http://dx.doi.org/10.1038/ng.254 PMID:18978790

6. Truong T et al. (2010). J Natl Cancer Inst, 102:959–971. http://dx.doi.org/10.1093/jnci/djq178 PMID:20548021

7. Zou P et al. (2012). BMC Cancer, 12:7. http://dx.doi.org/10.1186/1471-2407-12-7 PMID:22221621

8. Brennan P et al. (2007). Hum Mol Genet, 16:1794–1801. http://dx.doi.org/10.1093/hmg/ddm127 PMID:17517688

9. Timofeeva MN et al. (2012). Hum Mol Genet, 21:4980–4995. http://dx.doi.org/10.1093/hmg/dds334 PMID:22899653

10. Dong J et al. (2013). PLoS Genet, 9:e1003190. http://dx.doi.org/10.1371/journal.pgen.1003190 PMID:23341777

11. McKay JD et al. (2011). PLoS Genet, 7:e1001333. http://dx.doi.org/10.1371/journal.pgen.1001333 PMID:21437268

Fig. B2.2.1. Manhattan plot of lung cancer genome-wide association study results, overall (A) and restricted to adenocarcinoma (B) and squamous cell carcinoma (C).

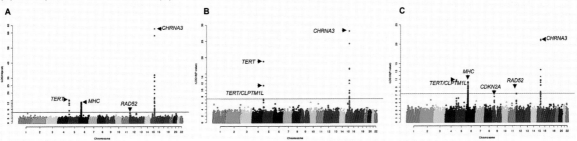

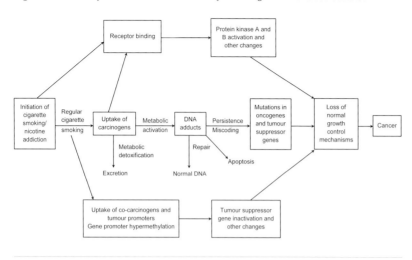

known to attach to cellular DNA, leading to certain mutations in oncogenes and tumour suppressor genes, which are found in oral premalignant lesions associated with smokeless tobacco use. Smokeless tobacco also generates reactive oxygen species, oxidative stress, and associated DNA fragmentation in laboratory experiments. Inflammation of the oral mucosa at the site of tobacco quid placement may begin as early as 2–7 days after the initial application by regular users on a new site. A precise role for inflammation caused by smokeless tobacco use is not clear at present.

Epidemiological evidence

Tobacco smoking

The epidemiological evidence on smoking and cancer comes from numerous case–control and cohort studies carried out since the mid-20th century. The epidemiological evidence on smoking and cancer is consistent in identifying cigarette smoking as a cause of many types of cancer [11,12]. Fig 2.2.4 identifies the cancer sites and types for which IARC [12] and/or the United States Surgeon General [11] have concluded that the relationship is causal. The affected sites include those where smoke is directly deposited (e.g. the oropharynx and lung) and distal sites that are reached by circulating tobacco smoke components (e.g. the pancreas and

urinary bladder). Overall, risks of cancers caused by smoking increase with duration of smoking and with number of cigarettes smoked daily; cancer risk falls after successful cessation of smoking, but for longer-term smokers, the risks do not completely drop to those of never-smokers [11]. Associations between active smoking and breast cancer continue to be investigated [13].

Fig. 2.2.4. Cancer sites and types for which IARC [12] and/or the United States Surgeon General [11] have concluded that the relationship with tobacco smoking is causal. Note: For cancers of the liver, colon, rectum, ovary (mucinous), and paranasal sinuses, causal conclusions reached by IARC only.

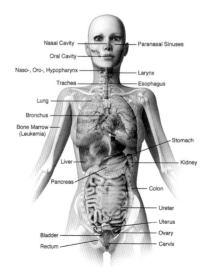

Table 2.2.1 provides estimates of relative risks of death from smoking-related cancers for major sites in two cohort studies carried out in the USA by the American Cancer Society: Cancer Prevention Study I (CPS-I) (enrolment in 1959, follow-up through 1965) and CPS-II (enrolment in 1982, follow-up through 1988) [14]. Questionnaires administered at enrolment provided the data on participants' smoking status. Several general findings are notable: (i) the relative risks for current and former smokers compared with never-smokers are remarkably high for some sites (e.g. lung and laryngeal cancer), (ii) former smokers uniformly have decreased relative risks compared with current smokers, (iii) relative risks have tended to be lower in women than in men, and (iv) relative risks tended to increase for women over the two decades between the two studies [14]. Findings of more recent studies suggest that relative risks have continued to rise as more recent cohorts of women have started to smoke at a similarly young age as men and have smoked at comparable rates for similar periods [15]. The relative risks in Table 2.2.1 reflect those in high-income countries. In low- and middle-income countries, the relative risks tend to be lower because heavy smoking beginning at a young age – the pattern in high-income countries – has not been typical of smokers to date.

Epidemiological evidence also shows that involuntary smoking, the inhalation of second-hand smoke by nonsmokers, causes cancer. The first epidemiological studies on involuntary smoking and lung cancer risk in nonsmokers were published in 1981; by 1986, there was sufficient evidence, particularly in the context of the already extensive literature on active smoking, to conclude that involuntary smoking causes lung cancer in nonsmokers [16,17]. Exposure to involuntary smoking increases lung cancer risk by about 25%, a finding replicated worldwide [10].

Smokeless tobacco

Numerous epidemiological studies, including cohort and case–control

Table 2.2.1. Age-adjusted relative risks of death from smoking-related cancers from the Cancer Prevention Study I (CPS-I) and CPS-II, adults aged ≥ 35 years

Disease category (ICD-9 code)	CPS-I (1959–1965)				CPS-II (1982–1988)			
	Men		Women		Men		Women	
	CS	FS	CS	FS	CS	FS	CS	FS
Lip, oral cavity, pharynx (140–149)	6.3	2.7	2.0	1.9	10.9	3.4	5.1	2.3
Oesophagus (150)	3.6	1.3	1.9	2.2	6.8	4.5	7.8	2.8
Stomach (151)	1.8	1.7	1.0	1.0	2.0	1.5	1.4	1.3
Pancreas (157)	2.3	1.3	1.4	1.4	2.3	1.2	2.3	1.6
Larynx (161)	10.0	8.6	3.8	3.1	14.6	6.3	13.0	5.2
Trachea, bronchus, lung (162)	11.4	5.0	2.7	2.6	23.3	8.7	12.7	4.5
Cervix uteri (180)	NA	NA	1.1	1.3	NA	NA	1.6	1.1
Urinary bladder (188)	2.9	1.8	2.9	2.3	3.3	2.1	2.2	1.9
Kidney, other urinary (189)	1.8	1.8	1.4	1.5	2.7	1.7	1.3	1.1
Acute myeloid leukaemia (204–208)	1.6	1.6	1.0	1.0	1.9	1.3	1.1	1.4

CS, current smokers; FS, former smokers; ICD-9, *International Classification of Diseases, 9th Revision*; NA, not applicable.

studies adjusted or stratified for smoking and alcohol intake, have also shown a causal relationship of smokeless tobacco use with cancer [3]. At this time, the evidence is strongest for cancers of the oral cavity and pancreas. Traditional products from the USA, South Asia, and Sudan have been found to contain very high amounts of tobacco-specific nitrosamines, and users have high risk of oral cancer, as shown in several studies. The level of risk experienced by users depends largely on the type of product they are using. Risk estimates for cancer associated with smokeless tobacco use in case–control studies increase with frequency of use per day and with duration of use in years, and women smokeless tobacco users tend to have higher risks, compared with non-users, than men. Smokeless tobacco users often have pre-cancerous oral mucosal lesions, such as leukoplakia. These white lesions tend to disappear within 1–2 months after discontinuation of tobacco use. These lesions are more common in smokers who also use smokeless tobacco, and such individuals also have a higher risk of cancer.

Prevention

Tobacco smoking

Tobacco control has had a lengthy evolution that has been closely linked to the increasing evidence on the health effects of active and involuntary smoking and on which tobacco control modalities are efficacious [4,18]. Historically, the initial findings on lung cancer and smoking were followed by efforts to educate the public about the risks of smoking, with the expectation that they would stop. Since then, we have learned that tobacco control requires far more complex approaches that acknowledge the hierarchy of factors that determine the use of tobacco and the interplay of these factors across the life-course, as health is damaged by smoking from conception onward. At each age, the emphasis of tobacco control shifts, moving from preventing initiation to promoting successful cessation. Particular issues include avoiding exposure to second-hand smoke and discouraging pregnant women from smoking. In addition, tobacco control efforts need to be dynamic in time, changing as the tobacco industry attempts to counter control measures.

Many nations have now implemented tobacco control programmes.

Most importantly, there is now the WHO Framework Convention on Tobacco Control (FCTC), the first treaty negotiated under the auspices of WHO, which brings a global approach to the global epidemic of tobacco use. The WHO FCTC has been in force since 2005, and most nations of the world have become Parties. Key elements of most national tobacco control policies coincide with core WHO FCTC provisions, including a comprehensive ban on tobacco advertising, promotion, and sponsorship; a ban on misleading descriptors such as "light"; and a mandate to place rotating warnings that cover at least 30% of tobacco packaging and encouragement for even larger, graphic

Fig. 2.2.5. Chewing tobacco has been proven to cause oesophageal, oral, bladder, and pancreatic cancers.

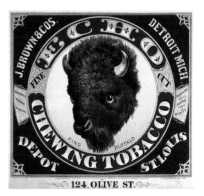

warnings. The WHO FCTC also has provisions requiring Parties to implement smoke-free workplace laws, address tobacco smuggling, and increase tobacco taxes.

In 2008, WHO identified six evidence-based tobacco control measures that are the most effective in reducing tobacco use [19]. Known as "MPOWER", these measures correspond to one or more of the demand reduction provisions included in the WHO FCTC: Monitor tobacco use and prevention policies, Protect people from tobacco smoke, Offer help to quit tobacco use, Warn people about the dangers of tobacco, Enforce bans on tobacco advertising, promotion, and sponsorship, and Raise taxes on tobacco. WHO is tracking in-country implementation of MPOWER and coverage of the world's population by its provisions. To date, its reach is still limited, although increasing coverage of the world's population by its elements can be anticipated [1]. Global tobacco control has been supported by governments as well as from nongovernment sources, including funding from the Bloomberg Family Foundation and the Bill & Melinda Gates Foundation, first made available in 2007 and now slated to continue through 2016.

Information about the impact of initiatives designed to encourage individuals to cease smoking is presented in Chapter 4.1.

Smokeless tobacco

Tobacco control needs to include smokeless tobacco in its purview. Each aspect of tobacco control has to take into consideration both smoking and smokeless tobacco use. Hence, taxation needs to cover both forms equally so that people do not simply switch over to cheaper smokeless forms after an increase in cigarette taxation, as has happened in some countries. Information campaigns need to explicitly address the dangers of both types of tobacco, so that smokeless tobacco is not seen as risk-free. The risk of oral cancer is very high for smokeless tobacco users, especially if use is initiated at an early age or if the same individuals are also smokers. The impact of unbranded products has been recognized in several countries and warrants action. Prohibition of spitting in public places, prohibition of smokeless tobacco use at the workplace, and bans on the sale of all tobacco products in and around educational institutions are options to control smokeless tobacco use. The same stringent requirements on health warnings and prohibition of advertisements, including use of tobacco-related imagery and extending the tobacco brand to other products (i.e. brand stretching), are appropriate for smokeless tobacco as for smoked products. Health-care providers may be informed on how to encourage and support smokeless tobacco users to quit. Bans on import of smokeless tobacco and control of smuggling are also appropriate and required to control smokeless tobacco use.

In areas where smokeless tobacco is widely used, such as South-East Asia, the acceptance of tobacco use as "normal" needs to be addressed along with raising public awareness of the health hazards and offering help for quitting [20]. For example, successful interventions with student youth in India have been formulated based on a study of the characteristics and needs of target groups. These targeted interventions have been able to engage the students' interest. The interventions have involved the students in interactive classroom and home-based activities (with parents) as well as in activism for tobacco control. Significantly reduced indicators of tobacco use compared with non-intervention schools have been achieved [21,22]. Researchers have been sharing their systematically tested and well-documented concepts and materials with the government for application across the country in government schools [21]. In community interventions, use of multiple types of media with pretested messages to diffuse information at mass level and in small groups as well as by one-to-one interaction with

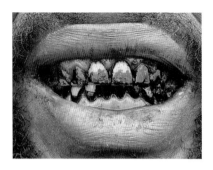

Fig. 2.2.6. Areca nut chewing is popular in Papua New Guinea. When the nut's fibrous inner core is chewed, a red colour is produced that stains the teeth.

health educators has been found to be reinforcing and effective [23,24]. Inclusion of oral examination in community and worksite interventions has also been found to be effective for promoting cessation and reduction of tobacco use among adults, as well as for implementing interventions that lead to regression of leukoplakia in tobacco users [25,26].

Conclusion

Tobacco use in both smoked and smokeless forms remains the world's leading cause of cancer morbidity and mortality. Numerous mechanistic pathways have been implicated in tobacco-induced carcinogenesis. For multiple sites, including lung cancer in smokers and oral cancer in smokeless tobacco users, risks are remarkably high compared with other circumstances involving cancer development, and causality is proven. Thus, tobacco control provides a tremendous opportunity for cancer prevention. A global public health treaty, the WHO FCTC, calls for the ratifying nations to implement a set of effective tobacco control policies. In force since 2005 and ratified by 176 nations to date, the FCTC has created a global tobacco control movement that continues to work towards preventing initiation and promoting successful cessation of tobacco use.

References

1. WHO (2011). *WHO Report on the Global Tobacco Epidemic, 2011: Warning about the Dangers of Tobacco.* Geneva: WHO.

2. U.S. Department of Health and Human Services (2010). *How Tobacco Smoke Causes Disease: The Biology and Behavioral Basis for Smoking-Attributable Disease: A Report of the Surgeon General.* Atlanta, GA: U.S. Department of Health and Human Services, Centers for Disease Control and Prevention, National Center for Chronic Disease Prevention and Health Promotion, Office on Smoking and Health.

3. IARC (2007). Smokeless tobacco and some tobacco-specific N-nitrosamines. *IARC Monogr Eval Carcinog Risks Hum*, 89:1–592. PMID:18335640

4. U.S. Department of Health and Human Services (2000). *Reducing Tobacco Use: A Report of the Surgeon General.* Atlanta, GA: U.S. Department of Health and Human Services, Centers for Disease Control and Prevention, National Center for Chronic Disease Prevention and Health Promotion, Office on Smoking and Health.

5. Giovino GA, Mirza SA, Samet JM *et al.*; GATS Collaborative Group (2012). Tobacco use in 3 billion individuals from 16 countries: an analysis of nationally representative cross-sectional household survey. *Lancet*, 380:668–679. http://dx.doi.org/10.1016/S0140-6736(12)61085-X PMID:22901888

6. Eriksen M, Mackay J, Ross H (2012). *The Tobacco Atlas*, 4th ed. Atlanta, GA: American Cancer Society, World Lung Foundation.

7. Sinha DN, Palipudi KM, Rolle I *et al.* (2011). Tobacco use among youth and adults in member countries of South-East Asia region: review of findings from surveys under the Global Tobacco Surveillance System. *Indian J Public Health*, 55:169–176. http://dx.doi.org/10.4103/0019-557X.89946 PMID:22089684

8. Rudatsikira E, Muula AS, Siziya S (2010). Current use of smokeless tobacco among adolescents in the Republic of Congo. *BMC Public Health*, 10:16. http://dx.doi.org/10.1186/1471-2458-10-16 PMID:20074362

9. Sinha DN, Gupta PC, Gangadharan P (2007). Tobacco use among students and school personnel in India. *Asian Pac J Cancer Prev*, 8:417–421. PMID:18159980

10. IARC (2004). Tobacco smoke and involuntary smoking. *IARC Monogr Eval Carcinog Risks Hum*, 83:1–1438. PMID:15285078

11. U.S. Department of Health and Human Services (2004). *The Health Consequences of Smoking: A Report of the Surgeon General.* Atlanta, GA: U.S. Department of Health and Human Services, Centers for Disease Control and Prevention, National Center for Chronic Disease Prevention and Health Promotion, Office on Smoking and Health.

12. IARC (2012). Personal habits and indoor combustions. *IARC Monogr Eval Carcinog Risks Hum*, 100E:1–575. PMID:23193840

13. Gaudet MM, Gapstur SM, Sun J *et al.* (2013). Active smoking and breast cancer risk: original cohort data and meta-analysis. *J Natl Cancer Inst*, 105:515–525. http://dx.doi.org/10.1093/jnci/djt023 PMID:23449445

14. National Cancer Institute (1997). *Changes in Cigarette-Related Disease Risks and Their Implications for Prevention and Control.* Smoking and Tobacco Control Monograph No. 8. Bethesda, MD: U.S. Department of Health and Human Services, National Institutes of Health, National Cancer Institute (NIH Publication No. 97-4213).

15. Thun MJ, Carter BD, Feskanich D *et al.* (2013). 50-year trends in smoking-related mortality in the United States. *N Engl J Med*, 368:351–364. http://dx.doi.org/10.1056/NEJMsa1211127 PMID:23343064

16. IARC (1986). Tobacco smoking. *IARC Monogr Eval Carcinog Risk Chem Hum*, 38:1–421. PMID:3460963

17. U.S. Department of Health and Human Services (1986). *The Health Consequences of Involuntary Smoking: A Report of the Surgeon General.* Washington, DC: U.S. Department of Health and Human Services, Public Health Service, Office on Smoking and Health.

18. Wipfli H, Samet JM (2009). Global economic and health benefits of tobacco control: part 1. *Clin Pharmacol Ther*, 86:263–271. http://dx.doi.org/10.1038/clpt.2009.93 PMID:19536067

19. WHO (2008). *WHO Report on the Global Tobacco Epidemic, 2008: The MPOWER Package.* Geneva: WHO.

20. Kakde S, Bhopal RS, Jones CM (2012). A systematic review on the social context of smokeless tobacco use in the South Asian population: implications for public health. *Public Health*, 126:635–645. http://dx.doi.org/10.1016/j.puhe.2012.05.002 PMID:22809493

21. Arora M, Stigler MH, Reddy K (2011). Effectiveness of health promotion in preventing tobacco use among adolescents in India: research evidence informs the National Tobacco Control Programme in India. *Glob Health Promot*, 18:9–12. http://dx.doi.org/10.1177/1757975910393163 PMID:21721292

22. Sorensen G, Gupta PC, Nagler E, Viswanath K (2012). Promoting life skills and preventing tobacco use among low-income Mumbai youth: effects of Salaam Bombay Foundation intervention. *PLoS One*, 7:e34982. http://dx.doi.org/10.1371/journal.pone.0034982 PMID:22523567

23. Aghi MB, Gupta PC, Bhonsle RB, Murti PR (1992). Communication strategies for intervening in the tobacco habits of rural populations in India. In: Gupta PC, Hamner JE III, Murti PR, eds. *Control of Tobacco-Related Cancers and Other Diseases.* Proceedings of an International Symposium, TIFR, Bombay, January 15–19, 1990. Bombay: Oxford University Press, pp. 303–306.

24. Anantha N, Nandakumar A, Vishwanath N *et al.* (1995). Efficacy of an anti-tobacco community education program in India. *Cancer Causes Control*, 6:119–129. http://dx.doi.org/10.1007/BF00052772 PMID:7749051

25. Gupta PC, Mehta FS, Pindborg JJ *et al.* (1986). Intervention study for primary prevention of oral cancer among 36 000 Indian tobacco users. *Lancet*, 1:1235–1239. http://dx.doi.org/10.1016/S0140-6736(86)91386-3 PMID:2872391

26. Mishra GA, Shastri SS, Uplap PA *et al.* (2009). Establishing a model workplace tobacco cessation program in India. *Indian J Occup Environ Med*, 13:97–103. http://dx.doi.org/10.4103/0019-5278.55129 PMID:20386628

Websites

American Cancer Society. Tobacco and Cancer: http://www.cancer.org/cancer/cancercauses/tobaccocancer/index

Framework Convention Alliance: http://www.fctc.org/

The Tobacco Atlas: http://www.tobaccoatlas.org/

U.S. Centers for Disease Control and Prevention. Smoking & Tobacco Use: http://www.cdc.gov/tobacco/index.htm

WHO. MPOWER measures: http://www.who.int/tobacco/mpower/en/

WHO. Tobacco Free Initiative (TFI): http://www.who.int/tobacco/en/

2.3 Alcohol consumption

Jürgen Rehm
Kevin Shield

Naomi E. Allen (reviewer)
Min Dai (reviewer)
Elisabete Weiderpass (reviewer)

Summary

- The relationship between alcohol consumption and cancer risk has been known since the beginning of the 20th century. Epidemiological and biological research on the association has established that alcohol consumption causes cancers of the mouth, pharynx, larynx, oesophagus, liver, colorectum, and female breast.

- Typically, for cancer types caused by alcohol consumption, a dose–response association has been established.

- For 2010, alcohol-attributable cancers were estimated to be responsible for 337 400 deaths worldwide, predominantly among men, with liver cancer accounting for the largest proportion of deaths among the different tumour types.

- Alcoholic beverages are complex mixtures, but ethanol, mediating a genotoxic effect upon metabolism to acetaldehyde, is recognized as the agent predominantly accounting for carcinogenesis.

- The burden of alcohol-attributable cancer can be reduced through alcohol policy measures such as reduction of availability, increases in price, and marketing bans.

The association between alcohol consumption and risk of cancer was known as early as the beginning of the 20th century, when Lamy observed that approximately 8 out of 10 patients with either cancer of the oesophagus or cancer of the cardiac region of the stomach were alcohol misusers [1]. This observation was followed by an ecological study indicating that people who were more likely to consume alcohol (such as people involved in the production and distribution of alcoholic beverages) had a higher risk of head and neck cancers compared with people who abstained from drinking for religious reasons, and that such abstainers had a markedly lower risk of these forms of cancers compared with the population as a whole [2]. After these early observations, several thousand more analytical studies followed to explore the biology and epidemiology of the relationship between alcohol consumption and risk of cancer. As a result, alcoholic beverages were declared "carcinogenic to humans" (Group 1) by the IARC Monographs Programme, first in 1988 [2] and then again in 2007 and in 2010

[3–5]. Tumour types caused by drinking alcoholic beverages include cancers of the oral cavity, pharynx, larynx, oesophagus, liver, colorectum, and female breast. For renal cell carcinoma and non-Hodgkin lymphoma, there is "evidence suggesting lack of carcinogenicity" for alcohol consumption [4,5].

Most cultures throughout the world have traditionally consumed some form of alcoholic beverages, and local specialty alcoholic beverages still account for the majority. Only a small number have evolved into commodities that are produced commercially on a large scale, such as beer from barley, wine from grapes, and certain distilled beverages. Further known beverages are other fruit wines, cider, and a broad range of very diverse spirits, including shochu, sake, lotus- or agave-based spirits, and various types of country-made liquor in India. In many developing countries, various types of home-made or locally produced alcoholic beverages, such as sorghum beer, palm wine, or sugar-cane spirits, continue to be the main available beverage types. Alcopops – flavoured, often sweet, alcoholic beverages – have received special attention mainly in a European context.

A large variety of substances that are not intended for human

Table 2.3.1. Cancers where alcohol consumption may be a component cause

Disease	ICD-10 code	Effect[a]	Epidemiological evidence[a]
Malignant neoplasms			
Cancers of the upper aerodigestive tract			
Cancer of the oral cavity and pharynx	C00–C13	Detrimental	Causally related
Cancer of the larynx	C32	Detrimental	Causally related
Cancer of the oesophagus	C15	Detrimental	Causally related
Cancer of the colorectum	C18–C21	Detrimental	Causally related
Cancer of the liver and hepatobiliary tract	C22	Detrimental	Causally related
Cancer of the stomach	C16	Detrimental	Insufficient causal evidence
Cancer of the pancreas	C25	Detrimental	Causality may need to be re-evaluated
Cancer of the lung	C33–C34	Detrimental	Insufficient causal evidence
Cancer of the female breast	C50	Detrimental	Causally related
Cancer of the prostate	C61	Detrimental	Insufficient causal evidence
Cancer of the kidney and cancer of the urinary bladder	C64–C66, C68 (except C68.9)	Beneficial[b]/no association[a] (renal cell carcinoma only)	Insufficient causal evidence
Cancers of the lymphatic and haematopoietic system			
Hodgkin lymphoma	C81	Beneficial[c]/no association[a]	Insufficient causal evidence
Non-Hodgkin lymphoma	C82–C85, C96	Beneficial[d]/no association[a]	Insufficient causal evidence

ICD-10, *International Classification of Diseases, 10th Revision.*
[a] For more information, see [4].
[b] For more information, see [4,9–11].
[c] For more information, see [4,6].
[d] For more information, see [4,7,8].

consumption are nevertheless being consumed as alcohol (surrogate alcohol such as hairspray, aftershaves, lighter fluid, medicines, or alcohol-containing mouthwash). They often contain very high concentrations of ethanol and may also contain higher alcohols and toxic concentrations of methanol and other chemicals [5].

Epidemiological evidence

Since the association between alcohol and various forms of cancer is relatively modest at lower levels of consumption, there have been multiple individual observational studies, where the majority of participants consume low to moderate amounts of alcohol, that have found a significant positive association, an absence of a significant association, or a significant negative association between alcohol consumption and the risk of mortality and morbidity from certain cancers. To determine whether an association exists between alcohol

consumption and various forms of cancer, the results of numerous case–control and cohort studies have been combined using meta-analytical techniques. These meta-analyses establish that a significant positive dose–response association exists between alcohol consumption and cancers of the mouth, pharynx, oesophagus, colorectum, liver, larynx, pancreas, female breast, and prostate, while a significant negative association or no association have been observed for each of Hodgkin lymphoma [4,6], non-Hodgkin lymphoma [4,7,8], and renal cell carcinoma [4,9–11]. When epidemiological criteria were examined for causality [12], the association between alcohol consumption and cancers of the mouth, pharynx, oesophagus, colorectum, liver, larynx, and female breast was found to be causal [4,5,13]. Table 2.3.1 provides a list of cancers that have been found to be associated with alcohol consumption through at least one meta-analysis

and shows the level of evidence supporting these associations.

The relationship between average daily alcohol consumption and the risk of mortality from cancers of the upper digestive tract (except cancers of the mouth and oral cavity) and from cancer of the female breast is exponential. The relationship between alcohol consumption and the risk of mortality from cancers of the lower digestive tract and from cancers of the mouth and oral cavity is linear. For cancers of the upper digestive tract, lower digestive tract, mouth, oral cavity, and female breast, former drinkers (people who have not consumed alcohol within the past year but who have consumed it before in their lifetime) were found to have a higher risk of cancer compared with lifetime abstainers. It should be noted that there is evidence that the risk of head and neck cancers decreases with time since cessation of drinking [14]; however, more data are needed to explore the effect of drinking

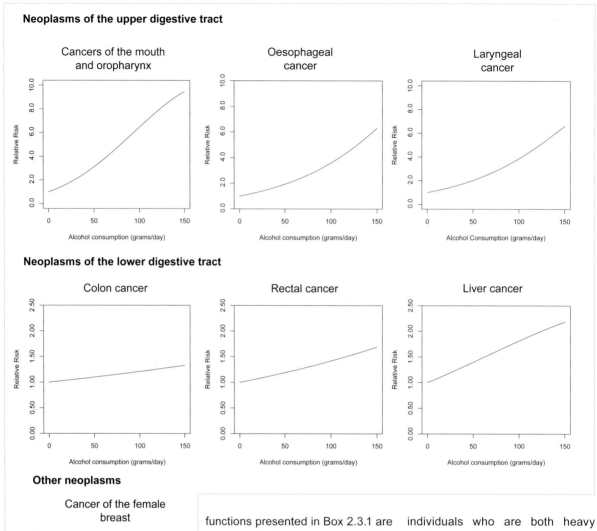

Neoplasms of the upper digestive tract

Neoplasms of the lower digestive tract

Other neoplasms

cessation on risk over time for other alcohol-related cancer sites. Box 2.3.1 provides plots of the relative risk functions for all cancers that are currently determined to be causally associated with alcohol consumption [13]. The relative risk functions presented in Box 2.3.1 are not separated by cancer mortality and incidence. However, the relative risk functions for alcohol-related cancers may be different for mortality and incidence (as a difference between relative risks of mortality and incidence has been observed for other alcohol-related diseases, such as liver cirrhosis [15]). Thus, more research is needed to systematically determine whether there is a difference between the relative risks of incidence and mortality for alcohol-related cancers.

Evidence suggests a synergistic effect of tobacco smoking and consumption of alcoholic beverages on the risk of cancer of the oral cavity, pharynx, larynx, and oesophagus, with very high risks observed in individuals who are both heavy drinkers and heavy smokers [4].

Observational research has suggested that there is a significant positive dose–response association between alcohol consumption and risk of prostate cancer, with multiple meta-analyses confirming this relationship. Biological pathways indicating how alcohol consumption may increase the risk of prostate cancer are currently unknown (see below), and thus additional research is needed to clarify a possible causal association.

Conflicting epidemiological evidence exists for the association between alcohol consumption and cancers of the bladder, lung, and stomach. A nonsignificant positive association has been observed between alcohol consumption and cancers of the endometrium and ovary [13].

One pooled analysis and one meta-analysis found that in cohort and case–control studies, heavy alcohol consumption – drinking more than 30 g of pure alcohol per day – has been consistently related to an increase in the risk of pancreatic cancer (cited in [4]); however, as mentioned in [4], confounding of smoking could not be excluded as a possible explanation of these results.

Meta-analyses have found no association or a significant negative association between alcohol consumption and the risk of renal cell carcinoma, Hodgkin lymphoma, and non-Hodgkin lymphoma [5,6]. These apparently protective observed effects should be interpreted with caution since the biological mechanisms are not understood and confounding and/or misclassification of abstainers may be responsible for the observations that have been made.

Associations have been reported between alcohol consumption and

cancer of the cervix, endometrium, ovary, vulva and vagina, testis, brain, thyroid, and skin (malignant melanoma, basal cell carcinoma, and squamous cell carcinoma) as well as leukaemia and multiple myeloma [5]; however, few studies have examined these associations. Epidemiological research is required to support previous study results, and biological studies are needed to determine the mechanisms by which alcohol intake affects the risk of developing these cancers.

Global rates of alcohol-attributable cancers

The number of deaths and number of disability-adjusted life years (DALYs) lost (a measure that combines years of life lost due to premature mortality and years of healthy life lost due to disability) from cancers that are currently determined to be causally associated with alcohol consumption and from other disease conditions and injuries, in each case

for 2010, can be calculated using mortality and morbidity data (see the WHO Global Information System on Alcohol and Health for global alcohol exposure estimates since 1960), with reference to the alcohol-attributable fraction methodology of the 2010 Global Burden of Disease study (see [16]).

In 2010, 337 400 deaths (91 500 of women and 245 900 of men) and 8 670 000 DALYs lost (2 252 000 for women and 6 418 000 for men) were caused by malignant neoplasms attributable to alcohol consumption. This burden represents 0.6% of all deaths (0.4% of all deaths of women and 0.8% of all deaths of men) and 0.3% of all DALYs lost (0.2% of all DALYs lost for women and 0.5% of all DALYs lost for men) in 2010. It should be noted that alcohol-attributable cancer data for 2010 reflect the level of drinking in the early 1990s, due to the long time it takes for cancer to develop [17].

The rates of alcohol-attributable cancer deaths and of alcohol-

Fig. 2.3.1. Percentage of deaths from various forms of cancer attributable to alcohol consumption, in 2010.

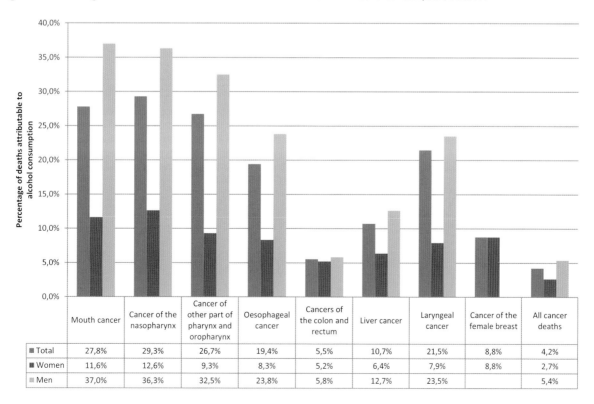

	Mouth cancer	Cancer of the nasopharynx	Cancer of other part of pharynx and oropharynx	Oesophageal cancer	Cancers of the colon and rectum	Liver cancer	Laryngeal cancer	Cancer of the female breast	All cancer deaths
■ Total	27,8%	29,3%	26,7%	19,4%	5,5%	10,7%	21,5%	8,8%	4,2%
■ Women	11,6%	12,6%	9,3%	8,3%	5,2%	6,4%	7,9%	8,8%	2,7%
■ Men	37,0%	36,3%	32,5%	23,8%	5,8%	12,7%	23,5%		5,4%

Fig. 2.3.2. Percentage of disability-adjusted life years (DALYs) lost from various forms of cancer attributable to alcohol consumption, in 2010.

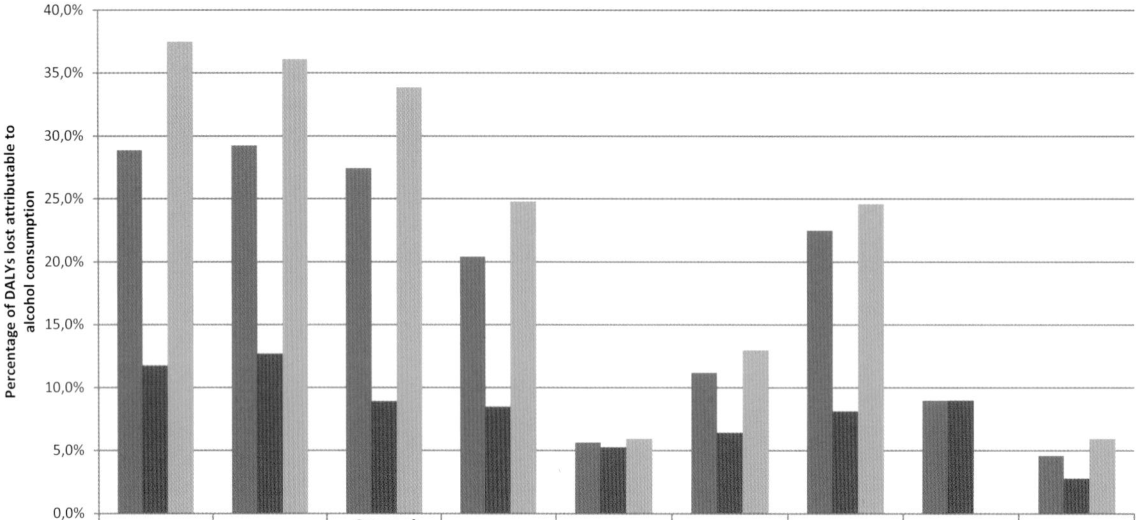

	Mouth cancer	Cancer of the nasopharynx	Cancer of other part of pharynx and oropharynx	Oesophageal cancer	Cancers of the colon and rectum	Liver cancer	Laryngeal cancer	Cancer of the female breast	All cancer DALYs lost
■ Total	28,9%	29,3%	27,4%	20,4%	5,6%	11,2%	22,5%	9,0%	4,6%
■ Women	11,8%	12,7%	8,9%	8,5%	5,3%	6,4%	8,2%	9,0%	2,8%
▪ Men	37,5%	36,1%	33,9%	24,8%	6,0%	13,0%	24,6%		6,0%

attributable DALYs lost varied globally with reference to regions defined by WHO as Global Burden of Disease regions (see [23]). The number of deaths and the number of DALYs lost per 100 000 people are shown in Tables 2.3.2 and 2.3.3, respectively, by Global Burden of Disease region for 2010. The Eastern Europe region experienced the highest alcohol-attributable cancer burden, with 8.7 cancer deaths per 100 000 people (5.7 per 100 000 women and 12.9 per 100 000 men) and 242.5 DALYs lost per 100 000 people (153.9 per 100 000 women and 357.4 per 100 000 men), while the North Africa/Middle East region experienced the lowest alcohol-attributable cancer burden, with 0.6 cancer deaths per 100 000 people (0.5 per 100 000 women and 0.8 per 100 000 men) and 18.5 DALYs lost per 100 000 people (14.8 per 100 000 women and 22.0 per 100 000 men).

In 2010, the largest contributors to the burden of alcohol-attributable cancer deaths were: overall, liver cancer (responsible for 23.9% of all such deaths); for women, breast cancer (responsible for 42.0% of these deaths); and for men, oesophageal cancer (responsible for 27.4% of these deaths). In 2010, the largest contributors to DALYs lost caused by alcohol-attributable cancer were: overall, liver cancer (responsible for 24.7% of all such DALYs lost); for women, breast cancer (responsible for 48.1% of these DALYs lost); and for men, liver cancer (responsible for 28.2% of these DALYs lost).

The percentage of cancer deaths and the percentage of cancer DALYs lost attributable to alcohol consumption are shown in Figs 2.3.1 and 2.3.2, respectively, by cause. In 2010, 4.2% of all deaths caused by cancer were attributable to alcohol consumption (2.7% for women and 5.4% for men) and 4.6% of all DALYs lost caused by cancer were attributable to alcohol consumption (2.8% for women and 6.0% for men). In 2010, alcohol consumption was responsible for the largest percentage of the total deaths and DALYs lost

from nasopharyngeal cancer compared with other cancer types; was responsible for 29.3% of all deaths from cancers of the mouth and oropharynx (12.6% for women and 36.3% for men); and was responsible for 29.3% of all DALYs lost from cancers of the mouth and oropharynx (12.7% for women and 36.1% for men).

Contribution of cancer to the total alcohol-attributable burden of disease

Alcohol consumption is related to more than 200 three-digit ICD-10 (*International Classification of Diseases, 10th Revision*) code diseases, conditions, and injuries, such as infectious diseases, malignant neoplasms, diabetes, neuropsychiatric conditions, cardiovascular disease, digestive diseases, conditions arising during the prenatal period, and injuries (for an overview of the conditions related to alcohol consumption, see [16]). In 2010, alcohol consumption was responsible for 2 734 200 deaths (910 800 of

Table 2.3.2. Cancer deaths attributable to alcohol consumption, by sex and by Global Burden of Disease region, for 2010[a]

Global Burden of Disease region[b]	Female		Male		Total	
	Deaths	Deaths per 100 000 people	Deaths	Deaths per 100 000 people	Deaths	Deaths per 100 000 people
Asia Pacific, high-income	4 000	2.4	13 400	8.1	17 400	5.2
Asia, Central	1 200	3.3	2 000	6.2	3 300	4.6
Asia, East	20 300	2.7	99 800	11.8	120 100	7.5
Asia, South	6 300	1.1	27 200	4.2	33 400	2.7
Asia, South-East	4 700	1.9	12 200	4.7	16 900	3.3
Australasia	800	4.1	1 200	5.6	2 000	4.9
Caribbean	400	2.0	1 000	4.4	1 400	3.2
Europe, Central	3 600	3.7	9 900	11.2	13 500	7.2
Europe, Eastern	10 400	5.7	17 300	12.9	27 700	8.7
Europe, Western	18 300	4.8	29 700	8.2	48 000	6.5
Latin America, Andean	400	2.0	300	1.4	700	1.7
Latin America, Central	1 800	1.8	2 800	3.0	4 600	2.4
Latin America, Southern	1 700	4.4	2 200	6.3	3 900	5.3
Latin America, Tropical	2 800	2.8	5 900	6.2	8 600	4.4
North Africa/Middle East	800	0.5	1 300	0.8	2 100	0.6
North America, high-income	8 500	3.4	11 300	4.4	19 800	3.9
Oceania	100	4.6	200	5.6	300	5.1
Sub-Saharan Africa, Central	400	1.8	700	2.9	1 100	2.3
Sub-Saharan Africa, Eastern	2 500	2.8	3 300	3.7	5 900	3.3
Sub-Saharan Africa, Southern	600	2.1	1 600	6.8	2 200	4.3
Sub-Saharan Africa, Western	1 700	2.0	2 700	2.9	4 400	2.4
World	91 500	2.7	245 900	7.1	337 400	4.9

[a] Numbers have been rounded.
[b] For definitions of regions, see [23].

women and 1 823 400 of men) and 97 118 000 DALYs lost (22 523 000 for women and 74 595 000 for men). Of the total deaths and DALYs lost attributable to alcohol consumption in 2010, alcohol-attributable cancers were responsible for 12.3% of all alcohol-attributable deaths (10.0% for women and 13.5% for men) and 8.9% of all alcohol-attributable DALYs lost (10.0% for women and 8.6% for men).

Possible biological mechanisms

As indicated above, alcohol consumption is carcinogenic and causes a variety of human cancers, and there may be different biological pathways depending on the anatomical site. Alcoholic beverages are multicomponent mixtures containing several carcinogenic compounds, such as ethanol, acetaldehyde, aflatoxins, and ethyl carbamate (see [18]), and all of these compounds may contribute to increase the risk of cancer due to alcohol consumption reported in observational studies. A recent chemical risk analysis concluded that ethanol is the most important carcinogen in alcoholic beverages, with all other carcinogenic compounds contained in alcoholic beverages increasing the risk of cancer below the threshold normally acceptable for food contaminants [18].

The biological mechanisms by which alcohol intake increases the risk of cancer are not fully understood, but the main mechanisms are likely to include a genotoxic effect of acetaldehyde, the induction of cytochrome P450 2E1 and associated oxidative stress, increased estrogen concentration, a role as a solvent for tobacco carcinogens, changes in folate metabolism, and changes in DNA repair [4,5].

For cancers of the digestive tract, especially those of the upper digestive tract, acetaldehyde from alcohol metabolism in the body and from

Table 2.3.3. Cancer disability-adjusted life years (DALYs) lost attributable to alcohol consumption, by sex and by Global Burden of Disease region, for 2010[a]

Global Burden of Disease region[b]	Sex					
	Female		Male		Total	
	DALYs lost	DALYs lost per 100 000 people	DALYs lost	DALYs lost per 100 000 people	DALYs lost	DALYs lost per 100 000 people
Asia Pacific, high-income	81 000	60.8	284 000	196.5	365 000	128.5
Asia, Central	38 000	98.5	58 000	170.9	95 000	132.1
Asia, East	530 000	69.3	2 690 000	318.9	3 221 000	200.0
Asia, South	182 000	28.8	782 000	115.3	964 000	73.9
Asia, South-East	113 000	41.8	342 000	124.7	455 000	82.7
Australasia	17 000	101.3	24 000	129.6	42 000	115.9
Caribbean	12 000	53.6	25 000	113.2	36 000	83.5
Europe, Central	90 000	103.8	253 000	302.9	342 000	199.6
Europe, Eastern	250 000	153.9	461 000	357.4	711 000	242.5
Europe, Western	374 000	121.5	649 000	206.5	1 023 000	163.9
Latin America, Andean	11 000	48.9	9 000	38.0	20 000	43.4
Latin America, Central	47 000	45.9	66 000	67.1	112 000	56.6
Latin America, Southern	38 000	106.8	49 000	144.4	86 000	124.4
Latin America, Tropical	76 000	75.4	167 000	172.7	243 000	122.7
North Africa/Middle East	28 000	14.8	42 000	22.0	70 000	18.5
North America, high-income	205 000	90.0	263 000	112.0	468 000	100.8
Oceania	4 000	124.0	5 000	153.4	9 000	138.7
Sub-Saharan Africa, Central	13 000	47.6	21 000	81.9	34 000	64.4
Sub-Saharan Africa, Eastern	72 000	71.3	98 000	97.9	170 000	84.3
Sub-Saharan Africa, Southern	17 000	56.6	47 000	182.8	63 000	114.9
Sub-Saharan Africa, Western	54 000	53.0	85 000	80.7	139 000	66.9
World	2 252 000	66.0	6 418 000	184.8	8 670 000	125.9

[a] Numbers have been rounded.
[b] For definitions of regions, see [23].

ingestion as a component of alcoholic beverages [19] has been highlighted as a likely and important causal pathway [4,5]. For colorectal cancer, in addition to the genotoxic effect of acetaldehyde, there may be the involvement of folate: alcohol may act through folate metabolism or synergistically with low folate intake (see [5]). The biological mechanisms accounting for how alcohol intake may cause pancreatic cancer are currently unclear; however, potential mechanisms include pancreatitis and the accumulation of fatty acid esters in the pancreas, which may induce inflammatory responses and fibrosis [4].

The biological effects of alcohol intake on the risk of digestive tract cancers are also dependent on the genotype of the consumer; individuals with the *ALDH2* Lys487 allele (and therefore a deficiency of ALDH2) experience a higher risk of oesophageal cancer for the same amount of alcohol consumed. The *ALDH2* Lys487 allele is thought to modify the risk of all cancers that are caused by the metabolites of alcohol [4,5].

In relation to breast cancer, alcohol intake has been shown to increase levels of estrogen and plasma insulin-like growth factor produced by the liver, to enhance mammary gland susceptibility to carcinogenesis (by altering mammary gland structural development and by stimulating cell proliferation), to increase mammary DNA damage, and to facilitate the ability of breast cancer cells to migrate [20].

Implications for prevention

The relationship between alcohol consumption and cancer has been observed as monotonic and without threshold (see above and

[3,4]). Thus, as the amount of alcohol consumed increases, the risk of developing cancer increases. This means that any reduction in alcohol consumption will be beneficial for health through the reduction of cancer risk. There are cost-effective ways to reduce alcohol consumption: most notably, restrictions in availability; increases in price for alcoholic beverages, which could be achieved by increasing taxation or increasing minimum prices; and marketing bans [21]. In addition, the risk of cancer for high-risk heavy alcohol consumers can be reduced by providing more opportunities for brief interventions and treatment for alcohol use disorders [22].

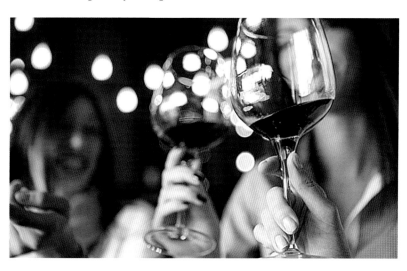

Fig. 2.3.3. Female drinking has risen steadily for the past 20 years, with more women than men drinking heavily on single occasions.

References

1. Lamy L (1910). Clinical and statistical study of 134 cases of cancer of the oesophagus and of the cardia [in French]. *Arch Mal Appar Dig Mal Nutr*, 4:451–475.

2. IARC (1988). Alcohol drinking. *IARC Monogr Eval Carcinog Risks Hum*, 44:1–378. PMID:3236394

3. Baan R, Straif K, Grosse Y et al.; WHO IARC Monograph Working Group (2007). Carcinogenicity of alcoholic beverages. *Lancet Oncol*, 8:292–293. http://dx.doi.org/10.1016/S1470-2045(07)70099-2 PMID:17431955

4. IARC (2012). Personal habits and indoor combustions. *IARC Monogr Eval Carcinog Risks Hum*, 100E:1–575. PMID:23193840

5. IARC (2010). Alcohol consumption and ethyl carbamate. *IARC Monogr Eval Carcinog Risks Hum*, 96:1–1428. PMID:21735939

6. Tramacere I, Pelucchi C, Bonifazi M et al. (2012). A meta-analysis on alcohol drinking and the risk of Hodgkin lymphoma. *Eur J Cancer Prev*, 21:268–273. http://dx.doi.org/10.1097/CEJ.0b013e328350b11b PMID:22465910

7. Tramacere I, Pelucchi C, Bonifazi M et al. (2012). Alcohol drinking and non-Hodgkin lymphoma risk: a systematic review and a meta-analysis. *Ann Oncol*, 23:2791–2798. PMID:22357444

8. Morton LM, Zheng T, Holford TR et al.; InterLymph Consortium (2005). Alcohol consumption and risk of non-Hodgkin lymphoma: a pooled analysis. *Lancet Oncol*, 6:469–476. http://dx.doi.org/10.1016/S1470-2045(05)70214-X PMID:15992695

9. Bellocco R, Pasquali E, Rota M et al. (2012). Alcohol drinking and risk of renal cell carcinoma: results of a meta-analysis. *Ann Oncol*, 23:2235–2244. http://dx.doi.org/10.1093/annonc/mds022 PMID:22398178

10. Song DY, Song S, Song Y, Lee JE (2012). Alcohol intake and renal cell cancer risk: a meta-analysis. *Br J Cancer*, 106:1881–1890. http://dx.doi.org/10.1038/bjc.2012.136 PMID:22516951

11. Cheng G, Xie L (2011). Alcohol intake and risk of renal cell carcinoma: a meta-analysis of published case-control studies. *Arch Med Sci*, 7:648–657. http://dx.doi.org/10.5114/aoms.2011.24135 PMID:22291801

12. Rothman KJ, Greenland S, Lash TL, eds (2008). *Modern Epidemiology*, 3rd ed. Philadelphia, PA: Lippincott Williams & Wilkins.

13. Shield KD, Parry C, Rehm J (2013). Chronic diseases and conditions related to alcohol use. *Alcohol Res*, (in press).

14. Lubin JH, Purdue M, Kelsey K et al. (2009). Total exposure and exposure rate effects for alcohol and smoking and risk of head and neck cancer: a pooled analysis of case-control studies. *Am J Epidemiol*, 170:937–947. http://dx.doi.org/10.1093/aje/kwp222 PMID:19745021

15. Rehm J, Taylor B, Mohapatra S et al. (2010). Alcohol as a risk factor for liver cirrhosis: a systematic review and meta-analysis. *Drug Alcohol Rev*, 29:437–445. http://dx.doi.org/10.1111/j.1465-3362.2009.00153.x PMID:20636661

16. Rehm J, Baliunas D, Borges GLG et al. (2010). The relation between different dimensions of alcohol consumption and burden of disease: an overview. *Addiction*, 105:817–843. http://dx.doi.org/10.1111/j.1360-0443.2010.02899.x PMID:20331573

17. Holmes J, Meier PS, Booth A et al. (2012). The temporal relationship between per capita alcohol consumption and harm: a systematic review of time lag specifications in aggregate time series analyses. *Drug Alcohol Depend*, 123:7–14. http://dx.doi.org/10.1016/j.drugalcdep.2011.12.005 PMID:22197480

18. Lachenmeier DW, Przybylski MC, Rehm J (2012). Comparative risk assessment of carcinogens in alcoholic beverages using the margin of exposure approach. *Int J Cancer*, 131:E995–E1003. http://dx.doi.org/10.1002/ijc.27553 PMID:22447328

19. Lachenmeier DW, Kanteres F, Rehm J (2009). Carcinogenicity of acetaldehyde in alcoholic beverages: risk assessment outside ethanol metabolism. *Addiction*, 104:533–550. http://dx.doi.org/10.1111/j.1360-0443.2009.02516.x PMID:19335652

20. Singletary KW, Gapstur SM (2001). Alcohol and breast cancer: review of epidemiologic and experimental evidence and potential mechanisms. *JAMA*, 286:2143–2151. http://dx.doi.org/10.1001/jama.286.17.2143 PMID:11694156

21. Babor T, Caetano R, Casswell S et al. (2010). *Alcohol: No Ordinary Commodity: Research and Public Policy*, 2nd ed. Oxford: Oxford University Press. http:dx.doi.org/10.1093/acprof:oso/9780199551149.001.0001

22. Rehm J, Shield KD, Gmel G et al. (2013). Modeling the impact of alcohol dependence on mortality burden and the effect of available treatment interventions in the European Union. *Eur Neuropsychopharmacol*, 23:89–97. http://dx.doi.org/10.1016/j.euroneuro.2012.08.001 PMID:22920734

23. Murray CJL, Ezzati M, Flaxman AD et al. (2012). GBD 2010: design, definitions, and metrics. *Lancet*, 380: 2063–2066. http://dx.doi.org/10.1016/S0140-6736(12)61899-6 PMID:23245602

Website

WHO Global Information System on Alcohol and Health: http://apps.who.int/ghodata/?theme=GISAH

2.4 Infections

2 ETIOLOGY

Silvia Franceschi
Rolando Herrero

Andrew J. Hall (reviewer)
Robert Newton (reviewer)
You-Lin Qiao (reviewer)

Summary

- Infections with viruses, bacteria, and macroparasites have been identified as strong risk factors for specific cancers.

- Overall, about 2 million (16%) of the total of 12.7 million new cancer cases in 2008 are attributable to infections. This fraction varies 10-fold by region; it is lowest in North America, Australia, and New Zealand (≤ 4%) and highest in sub-Saharan Africa (33%).

- *Helicobacter pylori*, hepatitis B and C viruses, and human papillomaviruses are responsible for 1.9 million cancer cases globally, including mainly gastric, liver, and cervical cancer, respectively.

- Infection with HIV substantially increases the risk of virus-associated cancers, through immunosuppression.

- Application of existing methods for infection prevention, such as vaccination, safe injection practices, and safe sexual behaviour, or antimicrobial and antiparasite treatments could have a major impact on the future burden of cancer worldwide.

Few aspects of cancer etiology have undergone as much progress in the past three decades as the relationship between a selected number of chronic infections and the risk of cancer. When Doll and Peto [1] estimated in 1981 the proportion of cancer cases attributable to different causes, only the relationships of hepatitis B virus (HBV) with liver cancer and of Epstein–Barr virus (EBV) with Burkitt lymphoma were relatively well understood, and the attribution to infections was very uncertain (> 1%, but the upper confidence interval limit was not reported). About 30 years later, the IARC Monographs Volume 100B Working Group [2] declared 11 infectious agents as well-established human carcinogenic agents (Table 2.4.1). In addition, de Martel *et al.* [3] considered infectious agents classified by IARC as carcinogenic to humans and calculated corresponding population attributable fractions (PAFs) worldwide and in eight geographical regions, using statistics on estimated cancer incidence from 2008 [4] (Fig. 2.4.1). In this chapter, we use the term "developed regions" to include Japan, North America, Europe, Australia, and New Zealand, i.e. high-income countries, and the term "developing regions" to include all other countries, i.e. low- and middle-income countries. In this context, the PAF is an estimate of the proportion of cases of a cancer that could theoretically be avoided if exposure to a specific infection were avoided or if the infection were detected early and treated before the development of cancer.

The associations of infections with cancer are nearly always very strong (relative risk > 10), and therefore calculations can often be based on the prevalence of infection in cancer cases (e.g. DNA of human papillomavirus [HPV] or EBV in cancer tissue biopsies) rather than on the less-often-available prevalence in the general population [3]. Estimates of prevalence of infection and relative risks are extracted from published data, and a short description of the rationale for each cancer site is presented here for each infectious agent in relation to its associated cancer. HIV infection greatly increases the risk of some infection-associated cancer types, especially Kaposi sarcoma and lymphomas, through immunosuppression [2]. To avoid double attribution, the fraction of cancer due to HIV will not be reported separately, but HIV will be mentioned when the infection is strongly implicated in the increase of certain cancer types.

Helicobacter pylori

Non-cardia gastric adenocarcinoma

A causal association between chronic gastric infection with *Helicobacter*

Table 2.4.1. Major cancer sites related to infectious agents classified as carcinogenic to humans

Cancer site	Well-established human carcinogenic agents
Stomach	*Helicobacter pylori*
Liver	Hepatitis B virus Hepatitis C virus *Opisthorchis viverrini* *Clonorchis sinensis*
Cervix	Human papillomavirus, with or without HIV
Anogenital (penis, vulva, vagina, anus)	Human papillomavirus, with or without HIV
Nasopharynx	Epstein–Barr virus
Oropharynx	Human papillomavirus, with or without tobacco use/alcohol consumption
Non-Hodgkin lymphoma	*Helicobacter pylori* Epstein–Barr virus, with or without HIV Hepatitis C virus Human T-cell lymphotropic virus type 1
Kaposi sarcoma	Kaposi sarcoma herpesvirus, with or without HIV
Hodgkin lymphoma	Epstein–Barr virus, with or without HIV
Bladder	*Schistosoma haematobium*

pylori and development of gastric adenocarcinoma is well established [2]. The risk is restricted to the non-cardia part (i.e. body) of the stomach; adenocarcinoma of the gastric cardia shares risk factors with oesophageal cancer and is not associated with *H. pylori* [2,5]. Although environmental factors such as the dietary habits of the host or the genetic make-up of both the host and the bacterium can modulate the strength of the causal relation between the bacterium and the cancer, no risk factors for non-cardia gastric adenocarcinoma as strong as *H. pylori* have been recognized.

A well-known difficulty in estimating the prevalence of *H. pylori* infection is the gradual decline in bacterial load with increasing gastric atrophy – a precursor lesion of gastric adenocarcinoma – and the consequent lack of sensitivity of serological markers at the time of cancer diagnosis. Studies in which *H. pylori* antibodies were measured well before the onset of cancer are considered the most reliable for calculating the true prevalence in cases and controls and therefore for estimating the relative risk. A review of such studies in 2001 reported that the average prevalence of *H. pylori* infection in cases is 90%, a figure that was quite homogeneous across studies in various continents despite a highly variable background rate in population-based controls [5]. A pooled analysis of 11 of these studies yielded a common relative risk of 5.9 (95% confidence interval [CI], 3.4–10.3) for patients who developed cancer more than 10 years after blood draw [5]. This yields a PAF of 75% for *H. pylori* in non-cardia gastric adenocarcinoma [3] (Table 2.4.2).

Fig. 2.4.1. Number of new cancer cases in 2008 attributable to infection, by infectious agent and development status.

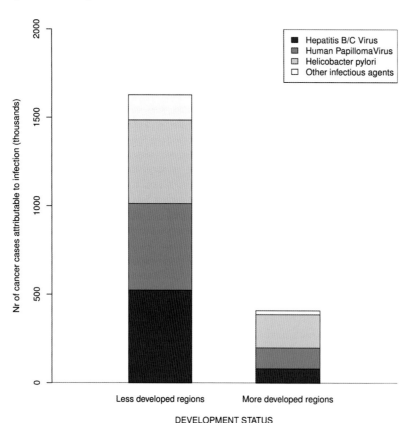

Inflammation and cancer

Curtis C. Harris

Inflammation has long been associated with cancer, and it is one of the hallmarks of cancer [1]. Whereas acute inflammation protects against infectious pathogens, chronic inflammation is associated with DNA and tissue damage, including genetic and epigenetic changes leading to cancer [2]. This association can be both inherited and acquired (Table B2.4.1). Both single-gene inheritance (e.g. haemochromatosis) and complex multiple-gene inheritance (e.g. inflammatory bowel disease) have been defined by genetic analysis. Infections by viruses, bacteria, and parasites are well-known examples of acquired etiology. Tobacco smoke contains more than 60 chemical carcinogens and also induces an inflammatory response that may facilitate lung carcinogenesis [3]. The inflammatory response to gastric acid reflux in Barrett disease may be responsible for the increased incidence of oesophageal cancer. Obesity has been recognized as a chronic inflammatory condition predisposing to cardiovascular disease and cancer [4]. The cellular and molecular basis of this predisposition involves the accumulation of macrophages in the adipose tissue, with the establishment of pro-inflammatory feedback loops among macrophages, pre-adipocytes, and adipocytes to generate inflammatory cytokines and free radicals [5]. The prevention of colon polyps and cancer by aspirin and other anti-inflammatory agents strengthens the

Table B2.4.1. Chronic inflammation or infection increases cancer risk

Disease	Type of cancer
Auto-inflammatory/non-infectious	
Crohn disease	Colon cancer
Ulcerative colitis	Colon cancer
Chronic pancreatitis	Pancreatic cancer
Endometriosis	Endometrial cancer
Haemochromatosis	Liver cancer
Thyroiditis	Thyroid cancer
α-1-Anti-trypsin deficiency	Liver cancer
Acquired	
Viral	
Hepatitis B virus	Liver cancer
Hepatitis C virus	Liver cancer
Epstein–Barr virus	Hodgkin lymphoma and Burkitt lymphoma
Bacterial	
Helicobacter pylori	Gastric cancer
Pelvic inflammatory disease	Ovarian cancer
Chronic prostatitis	Prostate cancer
Parasitic	
Schistosoma haematobium	Bladder cancer
Schistosoma japonicum	Colon cancer
Liver fluke	Cholangiocarcinoma and liver cancer
Chemical/physical/metabolic	
Alcohol	Multiple cancers (including cancers of the liver, pancreas, and head and neck)
Asbestos	Mesothelioma
Obesity	Multiple cancers
Tobacco smoke and inhalation of other noxious chemicals	Lung cancer (and multiple other cancers)
Gastric reflux, Barrett oesophagus	Oesophageal cancer

causal link between inflammation and cancer in humans [6].

The Human Microbiome Project is defining the microbes on the external and internal epithelial surfaces of the host in health and disease [7]. The gut microbiota is clearly implicated in intestinal inflammation and possibly human colon cancer [8]. Loss of the epithelial barrier integrity, due to mutations or other factors, allows translocation of the microbiota into the mucosa to elicit a cellular inflammatory response and release of cytokines. For example, microbes can elicit a TH17 response promoting IL-17 expression [9] and increase STAT3, which transcribes both coding and non-coding genes to signal proliferation of epithelial cells and their acquisition of epigenetic and genetic changes [10]. Current research focuses on the mechanistic connections among obesity, the microbiome, chronic inflammation, and cancer risk.

The molecular mechanisms of chronic inflammation driving cancer are being discovered [11]. The tumour microenvironment, including macrophages and senescent stromal cells, can facilitate tumour progression and metastasis [12]. Significant advances include identifying pro- and anti-inflammatory cytokines and their cellular signal transduction pathways, such as the NF-κB pathway [11]. Discoveries in the chemistry of free radicals generated by inflammation provide insight into their contribution to carcinogenesis. Mutations to DNA by both direct and indirect damage lead to activation of oncogenes and inactivation of tumour suppressor genes [13,14]. Animal models are helping to identify the oncogenic function of specific cytokines and free radicals [11,12]. Future research on inflammation will continue to improve prevention and treatment of cancer.

References

1. Hanahan D, Weinberg RA (2011). *Cell*, 144:646–674. http://dx.doi.org/10.1016/j.cell.2011.02.013 PMID:21376230

2. Rook GA, Dalgleish A (2011). *Immunol Rev*, 240:141–159. http://dx.doi.org/10.1111/j.1600-065X.2010.00987.x PMID:21349092

3. Hecht SS (2012). *Int J Cancer*, 131:2724–2732. http://dx.doi.org/10.1002/ijc.27816 PMID:22945513

4. Chaturvedi AK *et al.* (2013). *Am J Epidemiol*, 177:14–19. http://dx.doi.org/10.1093/aje/kws357 PMID:23171878

5. Weisberg SP *et al.* (2003). *J Clin Invest*, 112:1796–1808. http://dx.doi.org/10.1172/JCI19246 PMID:14679176

6. Thun MJ *et al.* (2012). *Nat Rev Clin Oncol*, 9:259–267. http://dx.doi.org/10.1038/nrclinonc.2011.199 PMID:22473097

7. Hooper LV *et al.* (2012). *Science*, 336:1268–1273. http://dx.doi.org/10.1126/science.1223490 PMID:22674334

8. Gallimore AM, Godkin A (2013). *N Engl J Med*, 368:282–284. http://dx.doi.org/10.1056/NEJMcibr1212341 PMID:23323906

9. Honda K, Littman DR (2012). *Annu Rev Immunol*, 30:759–795. http://dx.doi.org/10.1146/annurev-immunol-020711-074937 PMID:22224764

10. Tosolini M *et al.* (2011). *Cancer Res*, 71:1263–1271. http://dx.doi.org/10.1158/0008-5472.CAN-10-2907 PMID:21303976

11. Ben-Neriah Y, Karin M (2011). *Nat Immunol*, 12:715–723. http://dx.doi.org/10.1038/ni.2060 PMID:21772280

12. Qian BZ *et al.* (2011). *Nature*, 475:222–225. http://dx.doi.org/10.1038/nature10138 PMID:21654748

13. Lonkar P, Dedon PC (2011). *Int J Cancer*, 128:1999–2009. http://dx.doi.org/10.1002/ijc.25815 PMID:21387284

14. Hussain SP *et al.* (2003). *Nat Rev Cancer*, 3:276–285. http://dx.doi.org/10.1038/nrc1046 PMID:12671666

Gastric lymphoma

Non-Hodgkin lymphoma (NHL) in the stomach represents approximately 5% of all NHL and less than 2% of all gastric cancers. Nearly all

Fig. 2.4.2. *Helicobacter pylori* bacterium. *H. pylori* infection plays a key role in the genesis of gastric cancer.

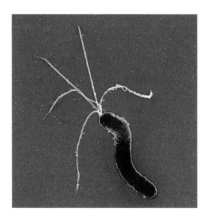

mucosa-associated lymphoid tissues and an unknown proportion of diffuse large B-cell lymphomas in the stomach are related to *H. pylori* infection [6]. Based on these limited data, the pooled prevalence of *H. pylori* in gastric lymphoma is 86% and the pooled relative risk estimate is 7.2, giving a PAF of 74% [3] (Table 2.4.2).

Hepatitis B and C viruses

Hepatocellular carcinoma

Chronic infection with HBV and/or HCV is the most common risk factor for hepatocellular carcinoma worldwide. Some non-viral exposures are also important risk factors for hepatocellular carcinoma, including heavy alcohol consumption and dietary aflatoxin contamination. The contribution of viral and non-viral risk factors, alone or in association, varies greatly in different geographical regions. For hepatitis viruses, HBV infection is found in the general population substantially more often than HCV in most Asian and African countries, while the opposite is true in Europe and the USA but also in Japan, Pakistan, and Mongolia [7]. In HBV-endemic areas, HBV is typically acquired in early life, and the prevalence of chronic HBV carriage tends to plateau after adolescence. In contrast, HCV infection can be acquired at any age through contaminated needles and blood, and HCV prevalence increases steadily with age due to the accumulating risk of exposure.

Estimates of HBV and HCV prevalence in hepatocellular carcinoma cases were derived from a 2007 review [7], which was updated using more recent papers [2]. However, there are few data on HBV and HCV

Table 2.4.2. Number of new cancer cases in 2008 attributable to infectious agents, by anatomical site

| Cancer site | Number of new cases in 2008[a] | PAF (%) | Number attributable to infection | | | |
| | | | By sex | | By development status[b] | |
			Male	Female	Developing regions	Developed regions
Carcinoma						
Non-cardia gastric	870 000	74.7	410 000	240 000	470 000	180 000
Liver[c]	750 000	76.9	400 000	170 000	510 000	69 000
Cervix	530 000	100.0	0	530 000	450 000	77 000
Vulva	27 000	43.0	0	12 000	4 100	7 500
Anus	27 000	88.0	11 000	13 000	12 000	12 000
Penis	22 000	50.0	11 000	0	7 600	3 200
Vagina	13 000	70.0	0	9 000	5 700	3 400
Oropharynx	85 000	25.6	17 000	4 400	6 400	15 000
Nasopharynx	84 000	85.5	49 000	23 000	66 000	5 900
Bladder	260 000	2.3	4 600	1 400	6 000	0
Lymphoma/leukaemia						
Hodgkin lymphoma	68 000	49.1	20 000	13 000	23 000	10 000
Non-Hodgkin gastric lymphoma	18 000	74.1	7 400	5 800	6 500	6 700
Burkitt lymphoma	11 000	62.5	4 000	2 800	6 300	530
HCV-associated non-Hodgkin lymphoma	360 000	8.2	17 000	13 000	18 000	11 000
Adult T-cell leukaemia/lymphoma	2 100	100.0	1 200	900	660	1 500
Sarcoma						
Kaposi sarcoma	43 000	100.0	29 000	14 000	39 000	4 100
Total from infections	3 200 000	64.4	990 000	1 100 000	1 600 000	410 000

HCV, hepatitis C virus; PAF, population attributable fraction.

[a] Numbers are rounded to two significant digits.

[b] Developed regions include Japan, North America, Europe, Australia, and New Zealand, i.e. high-income countries. Developing regions include all other countries, i.e. low- and middle-income countries.

[c] Including cholangiocarcinoma.

prevalence in large parts of eastern Europe and Central Asia. In HBV-endemic areas, almost all hepatocellular carcinomas in individuals younger than 50 years are due to HBV. The PAF for HCV is especially challenging as the infection does not show geographical clustering; high-prevalence countries may thus be geographically close to low-prevalence countries. For these reasons, regional prevalence estimates were derived by statistical modelling [3].

A meta-analysis of 32 case–control studies published in 1992–1997 yielded a summary relative risk of 22.5 (95% CI, 19.5–26.0) for HBV alone and of 17.3 (95% CI, 13.9–21.6) for HCV alone [8]. The dual impact of HBV and HCV infection on risk is not well quantified. Recent prospective and retrospective studies are consistent with previous studies in that they yield relative risks for hepatocellular carcinoma of a similar magnitude [2]. The estimated prevalence of either HBV or HCV in hepatocellular carcinoma cases varied from 42% in North America to 87% in Japan. Worldwide, the PAF for hepatocellular carcinoma is 77% (Table 2.4.2).

Non-Hodgkin lymphoma
HCV infection is a well-established cause of essential mixed cryoglobulinemia, a lymphoproliferative disease that can evolve into B-cell NHL. Several studies found a high prevalence of HCV seropositivity in patients with B-cell lymphoproliferative disorders, particularly B-cell NHL, including cases where essential mixed cryoglobulinemia was absent. A meta-analysis of studies of NHL and HCV seropositivity showed a pooled relative risk for NHL of 2.5 (95% CI, 2.1–3.1) based on 15 case–control studies and of 2.0 (95% CI, 1.8–2.2) in three cohort investigations [9]. The number of new cases of NHL attributable to HCV varies by country and therefore can be estimated very approximately. Based on a summary relative risk of 2.5 and the prevalence of HCV in cases from different regions [9], the HCV-associated PAF for NHL would be 8% (Table 2.4.2).

Fig. 2.4.3. Human papillomavirus (HPV)-mediated progression to cervical cancer. HPV is thought to access the basal cells through microabrasions in the cervical epithelium. After infection, the early HPV genes *E1*, *E2*, *E4*, *E5*, *E6*, and *E7* are expressed and the viral DNA replicates from episomal DNA. In the upper layers of epithelium (the midzone and superficial zone) the viral genome is replicated further, and the late genes *L1* and *L2*, and *E4* are expressed. L1 and L2 encapsidate the viral genomes to form progeny virions in the nucleus. LCR, long control region.

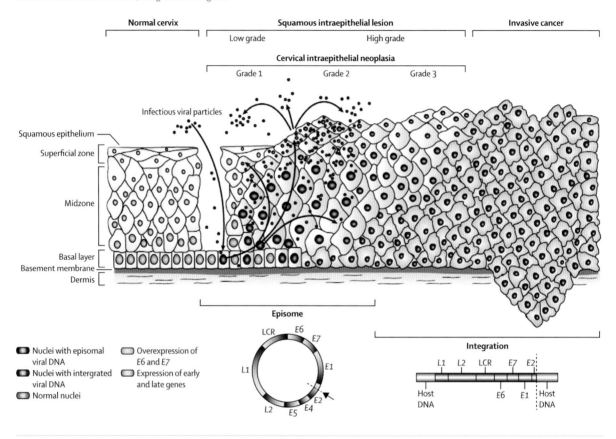

Human papillomaviruses

Cervical cancer and other anogenital cancers

HPV infection is a necessary cause of cervical cancer; its genome can be found in nearly all cervical cancers with the most sensitive detection methods [2]. Comprehensive mechanistic and epidemiological data have firmly established the chain of causality, with relative risks of more than 100 in many case–control studies [2]. It is generally acknowledged that 100% of cervical cancers are attributable to 13 high-risk HPV types classified as carcinogenic or probably carcinogenic (i.e. HPV16, 18, 31, 33, 35, 39, 45, 51, 52, 56, 58, 59, and 68) [2]. HPV16 and 18 are the most frequently involved types and together account for about 70% of cervical cancer in all world regions [10].

In contrast to the universal presence of HPV in cervical cancers, other anogenital cancer sites show a varying prevalence of HPV infection, depending on the cancer subtype, the age distribution, and the geographical region of the population studied [11]. High-risk HPVs were found in approximately 88% of anal cancers, 70% of vaginal cancers, 50% of penile cancers, and 43% of vulvar cancers [11]. Compared with cervical cancers, a stronger predominance of HPV16 is reported. PAFs for each anogenital site are reported in Table 2.4.2.

Head and neck cancers

Head and neck cancers represent a large and heterogeneous group of malignancies, for which tobacco use and alcohol consumption are considered the major causes. Over the past decade, HPV DNA has been reported to be present in a variable fraction of head and neck cancers (0–60%). Among HPV-positive cancers, HPV16 predominates (90% of HPV-positive carcinomas). HPV prevalence is notably high in oropharyngeal cancer [12], in which HPV16 is present at high copy number, localized to cell nuclei, frequently integrated into the cell genome, and actively transcribing viral oncoproteins E6 and E7 [13]. Survival differences by HPV DNA presence have also been consistently reported exclusively for oropharyngeal cancers. These features support, for the moment, a causal role of HPV infection in some oropharyngeal cancers, whose incidence is currently increasing in some developed

Do infections play a role in breast cancer?

James F. Holland

Human breast cancer has many phenotypes and, often modulated by estrogens, probably results from many different etiologies. Wide variation in the incidence of breast cancer globally is often ascribed to reproductive patterns, ethnicity, and diet. Breast cancer in feral and laboratory mice is caused by the mouse mammary tumour virus (MMTV), discovered in 1936. In the 1990s, molecular techniques not previously available were used to find a unique 660 bp sequence of MMTV that does not occur in the human genome or in any other organism. After this sequence was detected using polymerase chain reaction, the entire 9.9 kb viral structure of human mammary tumour virus (HMTV), which is 90–95% homologous to MMTV, was isolated [1].

The distribution of HMTV is similar to that of indigenous mouse species. *Mus domesticus*, the common house mouse, is dominant in countries in western Europe and in all of their former colonies, presumably distributed on sailing ships. *M.*

domesticus has abundant MMTV in its genome. In eastern Europe and Asia, different mouse species, with less MMTV in their genome, are indigenous. In six countries of western Europe and North and South America as well as in Australia, where breast cancer incidence is high, 30–40% of human breast cancer specimens contain HMTV sequences, but in four countries of Asia where breast cancer incidence is low, only 0–12% of specimens contain these sequences [2]. Normal tissues from the affected breast do not contain virus, thereby establishing that HMTV is acquired after conception and is not genetically inherited [3,4]. The possibility of MMTV contamination has been excluded in these analyses.

HMTV can be seen budding from breast cancer cells by electron microscopy, and can infect human mammary epithelial cells in vitro, causing changes in gene expression, morphology, and migration, suggesting malignant transformation. It also can infect B and T lymphocytes. In

mice, MMTV in breast milk infects lymphocytes, which transfer virus to the breast. HMTV has been detected in the breast milk of 8% of healthy American women; the virus has been passed from mother to daughter via breast milk perhaps for eons, extending the parallelism with mouse biology. These data raise the possibility that some breast cancers may have an infectious etiology, which would in turn open new perspectives on therapy and prophylaxis and raise questions about other "portable DNA" in the etiology of human cancer.

References

1. Liu B et al. (2001). *Cancer Res*, 61:1754–1759. PMID:11245493

2. Holland JF et al. (2004). *Clin Cancer Res*, 10:5647–5649. http://dx.doi.org/10.1158/1078-0432.CCR-04-1234 PMID:15355888

3. Pogo BG et al. (2010). *Cancer*, 116:2741–2744. http://dx.doi.org/10.1002/cncr.25179 PMID:20503403

4. Melana SM et al. (2010). *J Virol Methods*, 163:157–161. http://dx.doi.org/10.1016/j.jviromet.2009.09.015 PMID:19781575

countries [14]. The HPV-related PAF was, therefore, estimated only for cancers of the oropharynx including the tonsils and the base of the tongue (ICD-10 [*International Classification of*

Diseases, 10th Revision] codes C01 and C09–C10) [3].

High-risk HPVs were found in approximately half of oropharyngeal cancers in developed countries, but this weighted average prevalence varied in different areas; it was generally higher in North America and northern Europe than in southern Europe. In the few developing countries with available data, high-risk HPVs were found in 0–30% of oropharyngeal cancers [3]. The global PAF for oropharyngeal cancer is 26% (Table 2.4.2).

Epstein–Barr virus

Hodgkin lymphoma
EBV is more commonly associated with two Hodgkin lymphoma subtypes: nodular sclerosis and mixed cellular [2]. The EBV-related global PAF for Hodgkin lymphoma is 49% (Table 2.4.2); however, the PAF is

about 40% in adults in developed countries, whereas it is closer to 90% in children, and about 60% in adults in developing countries [3].

Burkitt lymphoma
In endemic areas of sub-Saharan Africa where malaria burden is very high, the EBV-related PAF for Burkitt lymphoma is more than 95% [2]. Outside endemic areas, EBV transcriptional gene products are detected much less frequently in Burkitt lymphoma. Sporadic forms of Burkitt lymphoma have been described elsewhere, but EBV was detected in only 20–30% of cases [3]. The EBV-related global PAF for Burkitt lymphoma is 63% (Table 2.4.2).

Nasopharyngeal carcinoma
Nasopharyngeal carcinoma is a rare cancer worldwide but has an exceptionally high incidence (10–30 per

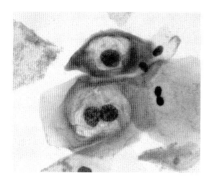

Fig. 2.4.4. Precancerous changes caused by human papillomavirus infection can be detected in cervical tissue. Micrograph (400×) of a Pap test showing a low-grade squamous intraepithelial lesion with effects of human papillomavirus.

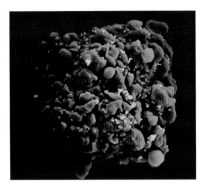

100 000 person-years in men) in southern China, Singapore, and Malaysia [2]. For the non-keratinizing subtype, EBV genome or gene products have been detected in virtually all cases, irrespective of geographical origin, and thus EBV appears to be a necessary step in the malignant process [2]. The EBV-associated PAF for nasopharyngeal carcinoma in areas of high or intermediate incidence is nearly 100%. This figure is probably less (possibly about 80%) in areas of low incidence [3], but the lack of published data does not allow a precise estimate (the global PAF is 86%) (Table 2.4.2).

Other non-Hodgkin lymphomas

Due to the heterogeneity of this group of tumours, even a crude estimation of the PAF is not possible from the published data, although most NHLs arising in HIV-positive individuals and organ transplant recipients are causally related to EBV [15].

Gastric carcinoma

Although EBV DNA has been found in 5–10% of gastric carcinomas, the IARC Monographs Volume 100B Working Group [2] concluded that there is insufficient epidemiological evidence for the involvement of the virus. Therefore, we have not calculated the PAF for EBV and gastric cancer.

Kaposi sarcoma herpesvirus

Kaposi sarcoma

Kaposi sarcoma herpesvirus is a causal factor for the development of Kaposi sarcoma and a few rare lymphoproliferative disorders, including primary effusion lymphoma and multicentric Castleman disease [2]. Although virtually all cases of Kaposi sarcoma are attributable to Kaposi sarcoma herpesvirus [3], various forms of the disease have been described and suggest that other factors, notably immunosuppression associated with HIV or organ transplantation, have an important contributory role in cancer development. In some regions of Europe and North America, after years of dramatically increasing Kaposi sarcoma incidence, a rapid decline of incidence has followed the introduction of highly active antiretroviral therapy in 1996 [16]. Conversely, with the large number of people with HIV/AIDS in sub-Saharan Africa and the still-limited access to treatment, the estimated incidence of Kaposi sarcoma is, for example, about 40 per 100 000 person-years in Zimbabwe, and it is the most common cancer in men in a few sub-Saharan African countries.

Human T-cell lymphotropic virus type 1

Adult T-cell leukaemia

A causal association between human T-cell lymphotropic virus type 1 (HTLV-1) and adult T-cell leukaemia, found nearly exclusively in Japan, has been firmly established. Thus, 100% of adult T-cell leukaemia cases in Japan are attributable to HTLV-1 [3] (Table 2.4.2), although the global PAF is unclear [3]. Restriction of the duration of breastfeeding has diminished the circulation of HTLV-1 and the corresponding cancer burden in Japan [2].

Macroparasite infections

Chronic infections with the liver flukes *Opisthorchis viverrini* and *Clonorchis sinensis* have long been associated with cholangiocarcinoma (cancer of the bile ducts). Human liver fluke infection is endemic in areas of China, the Republic of Korea, the Democratic People's Republic of Korea, Thailand, Lao People's Democratic Republic, Viet Nam, and Cambodia, where it is estimated that a total of 24.4 million people are infected [2]. Flukes are acquired from eating contaminated raw fish, either fresh or fermented. A total of

Fig. 2.4.6. Unsafe needle use during an immunization day in rural Sylhet, Bangladesh. Contaminated needles have been implicated in the spread of infections such as HIV/AIDS.

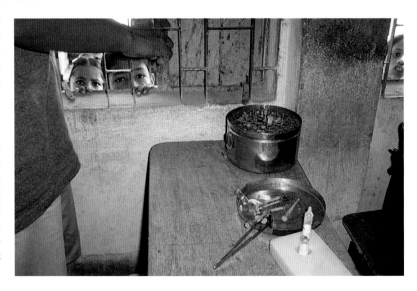

Table 2.4.3. Number of new cancer cases in 2008 attributable to infectious agents, by geographical region

Region	Number of new cases in 2008[a]	Number attributable to infection	PAF (%)
Africa			
Sub-Saharan Africa	550 000	180 000	32.7
North Africa and West Asia	390 000	49 000	12.7
Asia			
India	950 000	200 000	20.8
Other Central Asia	470 000	81 000	17.0
China	2 800 000	740 000	26.1
Japan	620 000	120 000	19.2
Other East Asia	1 000 000	230 000	22.5
Americas			
South America	910 000	150 000	17.0
North America	1 600 000	63 000	4.0
Europe			
Europe	3 200 000	220 000	7.0
Oceania			
Australia and New Zealand	130 000	4 200	3.3
Other Oceania	8 800	1 600	18.2
Developing regions[b]	7 100 000	1 600 000	22.9
Developed regions[b]	5 600 000	410 000	7.4
World	12 700 000	2 000 000	16.1

PAF, population attributable fraction.
[a] Numbers are rounded to two significant digits.
[b] Developed regions include Japan, North America, Europe, Australia, and New Zealand, i.e. high-income countries. Developing regions include all other countries, i.e. low- and middle-income countries.

2000 cases of cholangiocarcinoma were attributable to liver flukes [3] (included in liver cancer in Table 2.4.2).

The causal association between the macroparasite *Schistosoma haematobium* and bladder cancer is strong and consistent [2]. Endemic areas are found in sub-Saharan Africa, Sudan, Egypt, and Yemen, where the snail that transmits the macroparasite is present. The number of people infected with *S. haematobium* in sub-Saharan Africa is estimated to be 112 million, and the number of bladder cancers per year attributable to *S. haematobium* was estimated to be about 6000 [3]. The global PAF for bladder cancer is 2% (Table 2.4.2).

HIV

HIV-positive individuals have an increased cancer risk. Advanced HIV infection is characterized by immunosuppression, which is a risk factor for many malignancies [16]. There are three AIDS-defining cancers: Kaposi sarcoma, NHL, and cervical cancer. In contrast to the general population, almost all NHLs in HIV-infected people are caused by EBV. HIV-infected people also have elevated risks of other virus-related cancers, notably anal cancer, hepatocellular carcinoma, and Hodgkin lymphoma. As HIV typically coexists with oncogenic viruses, the inclusion of HIV-associated malignancies in the computation of global PAF would mean that some infection-associated cancers would be counted twice. However, HIV-infected people also have a higher prevalence of lifestyle-associated risk factors, including smoking and alcohol consumption, leading to increased risks of cancers of the head and neck and lung.

Overall, in HIV-infected people the risk of non-AIDS-defining cancers is double that in the general population [16]. The advent of antiretroviral therapy led to a striking increase in the life expectancy of HIV-infected people. The cancer burden is set to increase as they age, and cancer prevention strategies need to be put in place in parallel with efforts to detect and treat HIV infection early enough to prevent immunosuppression.

Conclusions

Conservative estimates indicate that about 2 million of the new cancer cases per year (16% of the global cancer burden) are attributable to a few chronic infections [3]. This fraction is substantially larger in developing countries (26%) than in developed countries (8%) (Fig. 2.4.1). Large variations are also seen by continent and country (Table 2.4.3). The fraction of cancer attributable to infections is largest in sub-Saharan Africa (33%) and smallest in Australia, New Zealand, and North America (≤ 4%). A better understanding of the association between NHL and infectious agents would lead to a substantial increase in the infection-associated PAF, especially in developed countries.

Prevention or eradication of these infections is a key tool to overcome inequalities in cancer incidence between populations in high-income countries and those in low- and middle-income countries. Of note, substantial reductions in the occurrence of many cancer-associated infections are now achievable and, in many instances, affordable. Control measures include avoidance of contaminated blood and needles (HBV, HCV, HIV), safe sex practices (HBV and HIV), and early detection and treatment of the infection (e.g. detection and treatment of HPV-related precancerous cervical lesions in screening programmes, antibiotic treatment of *H. pylori*, and praziquantel against liver flukes). Very efficacious vaccines against HBV and HPV are currently available (see Chapter 4.6). Historically, only clean water has performed better than vaccination to reduce disease burden. If high coverage can be achieved, vaccines can reduce inequalities in health more than other medical interventions can. Clinicians and public health professionals should better appreciate the importance of infections that cause cancer and support the implementation of currently available prevention strategies, especially in developing countries.

References

1. Doll R, Peto R (1981). The causes of cancer: quantitative estimates of avoidable risks of cancer in the United States today. *J Natl Cancer Inst*, 66:1191–1308. PMID:7017215

2. IARC (2012). Biological agents. *IARC Monogr Eval Carcinog Risks Hum*, 100B: 1–441. PMID:23189750

3. de Martel C, Ferlay J, Franceschi S *et al.* (2012). Global burden of cancers attributable to infections in 2008: a review and synthetic analysis. *Lancet Oncol*, 13:607–615. http://dx.doi.org/10.1016/S1470-2045(12)70137-7 PMID:22575588

4. Ferlay J, Shin HR, Bray F *et al.* (2010). Estimates of worldwide burden of cancer in 2008: GLOBOCAN 2008. *Int J Cancer*, 127:2893–2917. http://dx.doi.org/10.1002/ijc.25516 PMID:21351269

5. *Helicobacter* and Cancer Collaborative Group (2001). Gastric cancer and *Helicobacter pylori*: a combined analysis of 12 case control studies nested within prospective cohorts. *Gut*, 49:347–353. http://dx.doi.org/10.1136/gut.49.3.347 PMID:11511555

6. Parsonnet J, Hansen S, Rodriguez L *et al.* (1994). *Helicobacter pylori* infection and gastric lymphoma. *N Engl J Med*, 330:1267–1271. http://dx.doi.org/10.1056/NEJM199405053301803 PMID:8145781

7. Raza SA, Clifford GM, Franceschi S (2007). Worldwide variation in the relative importance of hepatitis B and hepatitis C viruses in hepatocellular carcinoma: a systematic review. *Br J Cancer*, 96:1127–1134. http://dx.doi.org/10.1038/sj.bjc.6603649 PMID:17406349

8. Donato F, Boffetta P, Puoti M (1998). A meta-analysis of epidemiological studies on the combined effect of hepatitis B and C virus infections in causing hepatocellular carcinoma. *Int J Cancer*, 75:347–354. http://dx.doi.org/10.1002/(SICI)1097-0215(19980130)75:3<347::AID-IJC4>3.0.CO;2-2 PMID:9455792

9. Dal Maso L, Franceschi S (2006). Hepatitis C virus and risk of lymphoma and other lymphoid neoplasms: a meta-analysis of epidemiologic studies. *Cancer Epidemiol Biomarkers Prev*, 15:2078–2085. http://dx.doi.org/10.1158/1055-9965.EPI-06-0308 PMID:17119031

10. Li N, Franceschi S, Howell-Jones R *et al.* (2011). Human papillomavirus type distribution in 30,848 invasive cervical cancers worldwide: variation by geographical region, histological type and year of publication. *Int J Cancer*, 128:927–935. http://dx.doi.org/10.1002/ijc.25396 PMID:20473886

11. De Vuyst H, Clifford GM, Nascimento MC *et al.* (2009). Prevalence and type distribution of human papillomavirus in carcinoma and intraepithelial neoplasia of the vulva, vagina and anus: a meta-analysis. *Int J Cancer*, 124:1626–1636. http://dx.doi.org/10.1002/ijc.24116 PMID:19115209

12. Herrero R, Castellsagué X, Pawlita M *et al.*; IARC Multicenter Oral Cancer Study Group (2003). Human papillomavirus and oral cancer: the International Agency for Research on Cancer multicenter study. *J Natl Cancer Inst*, 95:1772–1783. http://dx.doi.org/10.1093/jnci/djg107 PMID:14652239

13. Begum S, Cao D, Gillison M *et al.* (2005). Tissue distribution of human papillomavirus 16 DNA integration in patients with tonsillar carcinoma. *Clin Cancer Res*, 11:5694–5699. http://dx.doi.org/10.1158/1078-0432.CCR-05-0587 PMID:16115905

14. Chaturvedi AK, Engels EA, Pfeiffer RM *et al.* (2011). Human papillomavirus and rising oropharyngeal cancer incidence in the United States. *J Clin Oncol*, 29:4294–4301. http://dx.doi.org/10.1200/JCO.2011.36.4596 PMID:21969503

15. Hjalgrim H, Engels EA (2008). Infectious aetiology of Hodgkin and non-Hodgkin lymphomas: a review of the epidemiological evidence. *J Intern Med*, 264:537–548. http://dx.doi.org/10.1111/j.1365-2796.2008.02031.x PMID:19017178

16. Franceschi S, Lise M, Clifford GM *et al.*; Swiss HIV Cohort Study (2010). Changing patterns of cancer incidence in the early- and late-HAART periods: the Swiss HIV Cohort Study. *Br J Cancer*, 103:416–422. http://dx.doi.org/10.1038/sj.bjc.6605756 PMID:20588274

2.5 Reproductive and hormonal factors

2 ETIOLOGY

Louise A. Brinton

Silvia Franceschi (reviewer)
David B. Thomas (reviewer)

Summary

- Reproductive and menstrual factors are relevant to the etiology of breast, endometrial, and ovarian cancers.

- Obesity is a risk factor for these cancers in women as well as for some cancers in men; its influence is most likely mediated through hormonal mechanisms, as further supported by the influence of obesity on the effects of exogenous and endogenous hormones.

- Use of oral contraceptives substantially reduces the risk of endometrial and ovarian cancers but appears to increase the risk of breast and of cervical cancers, consistent with growing evidence for a possible role of hormonal factors in cervical carcinogenesis.

- Reproductive and hormonal factors appear to have particular associations for different subtypes of cancers in women, including those defined by either histology or hormone receptor status.

- The role of hormonal factors in the etiology of some cancers in men is being revealed, although

risk relationships remain to be clarified.

Reproductive and hormonal factors are well recognized to play a major role in the etiology of many cancers in women. This is particularly true for breast, endometrial, and ovarian cancers, where such factors likely explain large proportions of disease occurrence. A few cancers in men may also be influenced by hormonal factors, although the relationships are less well defined.

Female breast cancer

The role of reproductive factors in the etiology of breast cancer has been recognized for more than 100 years, beginning with the observation by Ramazzini of a high incidence of the disease in nuns. It is now well established that nulliparous women have approximately twice the risk of parous women, and that multiparity may be associated with further decreases in risk. Women with early age at first childbirth are at lowest risk, and risk rises steadily with later ages at first birth [1]. Interestingly, women with a first birth at age 30 or later are generally at higher risk than nulliparous women, presumably because of promotional effects of pregnancy on previously initiated

cells in older mothers. The effect of pregnancy on breast cancer risk is dependent on it being a full-term pregnancy; there is little evidence for relationships with short-term pregnancies, including miscarriages and abortions.

The reduced risk associated with parity may be further enhanced if a woman decides to breastfeed. However, protection is likely dependent on longer periods of breastfeeding; thus, in most developed countries, where numbers of births are limited and each child is breastfed for a relatively short period of time, there is little evidence of a relationship with breastfeeding. The most conclusive findings about the protective effects of breastfeeding derive from studies where women have given birth to multiple children who have been breastfed for long periods of time, leading to long durations of cumulative breastfeeding.

Menstrual factors are also predictive of risk; early age at menarche and later age at natural menopause are associated with the highest risks, presumably reflecting in part an influence of ovulatory activity (Fig. 2.5.1) [2]. Women who have an early surgical menopause involving removal of both ovaries are at low risk, and those who undergo this operation before the age of 40 have approximately half

Fig. 2.5.1. Relative risk of breast cancer by (A) age at menarche and (B) age at menopause, based on multiple studies. Calculated stratifying by study, age, year of birth, parity, age at first birth, smoking, alcohol consumption, height, and current body mass index. CI, confidence interval; g-s, group-specific; RR, relative risk.

A: Age at menarche

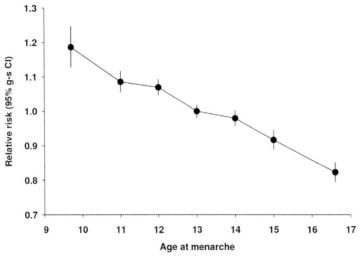

Age group (mean, years)	<11 (9.7)	11 (11.0)	12 (12.0)	13 (13.0)	14 (14.0)	15 (15.0)	16+ (16.6)
Cases/Controls	5511/11685	15855/37779	25806/61512	31759/83389	20599/53212	10576/31390	8858/27124
RR (95% g-s CI)	1.19 (1.13-1.25)	1.09 (1.06-1.12)	1.07 (1.05-1.09)	1.00 (0.98-1.02)	0.98 (0.96-1.00)	0.92 (0.89-0.95)	0.82 (0.79-0.85)

B: Age at menopause

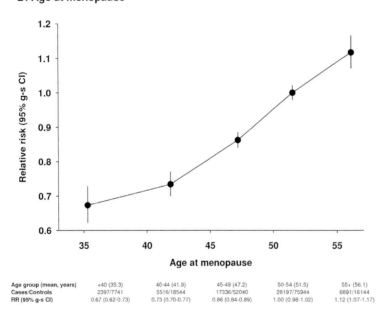

Age group (mean, years)	<40 (35.3)	40-44 (41.9)	45-49 (47.2)	50-54 (51.5)	55+ (56.1)
Cases/Controls	2397/7741	5516/18544	17336/52040	28197/75944	6891/16144
RR (95% g-s CI)	0.67 (0.62-0.73)	0.73 (0.70-0.77)	0.86 (0.84-0.89)	1.00 (0.98-1.02)	1.12 (1.07-1.17)

in endogenous hormonal profiles are involved, but additional research is needed to clarify effects. It is also unclear how hormonally induced changes in breast tissue are involved. Recent attention has focused on the effects of parity on involution of lobules, the structures from which the majority of breast cancers are thought to arise (Fig. 2.5.2) [3].

The relationship of obesity with breast cancer risk is complex; obesity is inversely related to risk of premenopausal-onset breast cancer and is directly associated with risk of postmenopausal breast cancer. Obesity-associated anovulation has been hypothesized as responsible for the decreased risk, while conversion of androgens to estrogens in adipose tissue appears to influence the increased risk. Menopausal hormone use has been associated with increased breast cancer risk among postmenopausal women, and the highest risks have been observed among thin women. The type of hormones used is also a major risk predictor, with higher risks observed for

Fig. 2.5.2. Terminal ductal lobular unit (TDLU) involution. (A) Minimal or no TDLU involution. (B) Marked involution demonstrating TDLUs containing few acini surrounded by dense collagen.

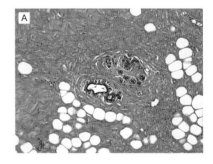

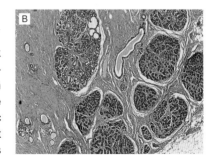

the risk of those who have a natural menopause after the age of 55.

Menstrual and reproductive factors are major risk factors and can be used to estimate individual risks via the Gail Model Breast Cancer Risk Assessment Tool (http://www. cancer.gov/bcrisktool/) and other risk prediction models. Despite the well-recognized role of these factors in breast cancer etiology, studies have been unable to relate them to specific underlying biological mechanisms. It is generally assumed that changes

Fig. 2.5.3. Sex steroid hormones and sex hormone-binding globulin (SHBG) levels in relation to estrogen receptor (ER) breast cancer subtypes, from the European Prospective Investigation into Cancer and Nutrition (EPIC) study. CI, confidence interval; OR, odds ratio. * Test for heterogeneity between ER-positive and ER-negative breast cancer was assessed using a log likelihood ratio test with and without an interaction term for breast cancer subtype outcome. ** Log2 continuous increase in circulating hormone level.

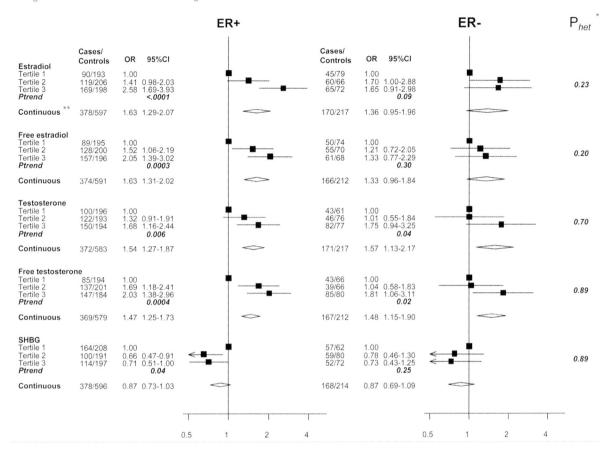

	ER+				ER-			P_{het}*
	Cases/ Controls	OR	95%CI		Cases/ Controls	OR	95%CI	
Estradiol								
Tertile 1	90/193	1.00			45/79	1.00		
Tertile 2	119/206	1.41	0.98-2.03		60/66	1.70	1.00-2.88	0.23
Tertile 3	169/198	2.58	1.69-3.93		65/72	1.65	0.91-2.98	
Ptrend			*<.0001*				*0.09*	
Continuous **	378/597	1.63	1.29-2.07		170/217	1.36	0.95-1.96	
Free estradiol								
Tertile 1	89/195	1.00			50/74	1.00		
Tertile 2	128/200	1.52	1.06-2.19		55/70	1.21	0.72-2.05	0.20
Tertile 3	157/196	2.05	1.39-3.02		61/68	1.33	0.77-2.29	
Ptrend			*0.0003*				*0.30*	
Continuous	374/591	1.63	1.31-2.02		166/212	1.33	0.96-1.84	
Testosterone								
Tertile 1	100/196	1.00			43/61	1.00		
Tertile 2	122/193	1.32	0.91-1.91		46/76	1.01	0.55-1.84	0.70
Tertile 3	150/194	1.68	1.16-2.44		82/77	1.75	0.94-3.25	
Ptrend			*0.006*				*0.04*	
Continuous	372/583	1.54	1.27-1.87		171/217	1.57	1.13-2.17	
Free testosterone								
Tertile 1	85/194	1.00			43/66	1.00		
Tertile 2	137/201	1.69	1.18-2.41		39/66	1.04	0.58-1.83	0.89
Tertile 3	147/184	2.03	1.38-2.96		85/80	1.81	1.06-3.11	
Ptrend			*0.0004*				*0.02*	
Continuous	369/579	1.47	1.25-1.73		167/212	1.48	1.15-1.90	
SHBG								
Tertile 1	164/208	1.00			57/62	1.00		
Tertile 2	100/191	0.66	0.47-0.91		59/80	0.78	0.46-1.30	0.89
Tertile 3	114/197	0.71	0.51-1.00		52/72	0.73	0.43-1.25	
Ptrend			*0.04*				*0.25*	
Continuous	378/596	0.87	0.73-1.03		168/214	0.87	0.69-1.09	

use of estrogen plus estrogen than for unopposed estrogen therapy. This has been hypothesized as being due to mitotic influences of progestins on breast tissues.

Combined estrogen–progestogen oral contraceptives are associated with an increased risk of breast cancer, notably among young women (see Chapter 2.10). Endogenous hormones clearly are important predictors of breast cancer risk, although it has been difficult for studies to fully define relationships with either breast cancer risk or patterns of risk factors. This most likely reflects difficulties in measuring hormones or the complexity of patterns of many interrelated markers, including not only estrogens but also androgens, progesterone, prolactin, and insulin-like growth factors. In addition, the importance of large inter-individual differences in metabolism, which may have etiological implications, is being increasingly recognized. Recent pooling efforts have provided evidence that estrogens and androgens are directly related to both hormone-receptor-positive and -negative breast cancers (Fig. 2.5.3) [4], but

Fig. 2.5.4. Endogenous estrogen metabolism in women.

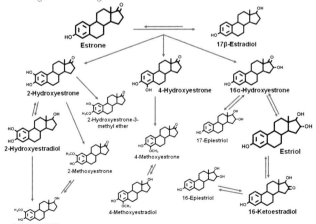

Fig. 2.5.5. Age-standardized incidence of endometrial cancer by menopausal hormone therapy use and body mass index, from the United States National Institutes of Health-American Association of Retired Persons (NIH-AARP) Diet and Health Study. EPT, estrogen plus progestin therapy; ET, unopposed estrogen therapy; MHT, menopausal hormone therapy.

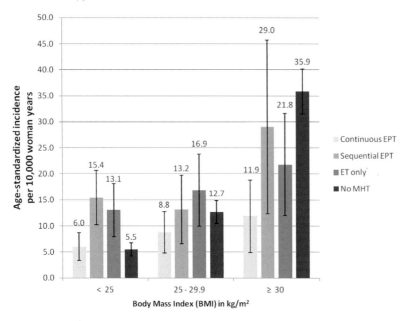

cancer is believed to arise as a result of estrogen stimulation that is unopposed by progestins. Both obesity and menopausal hormone therapy are strong risk predictors. Particularly high risks have been noted for unopposed estrogen use, which has been associated with 2–10-fold increases in risk, depending on the duration of use and the woman's body size (with higher relative risks observed among thin women).

Much lower risks have been noted for estrogen plus progestin hormone use; in fact, some studies suggest that relative risks may actually be lower among users than among non-users. These risks also appear to be modified by body mass, although in contrast to unopposed estrogens the greatest reductions in relative risks are seen among heavier women. Because of these complexities, more meaningful insights can be derived by a focus on absolute risks. The lowest risks are seen among thin women (either non-hormone users or users of continuous estrogen plus progestin therapy; these two groups are at similar risk), while the highest risks are observed among obese non-hormone users (who are at higher risk than obese users of continuous estrogen plus progestin therapy) (Fig. 2.5.5) [7]. Combination therapy may also be influenced by how it is prescribed (estrogens given sequentially vs

further clarity about relationships may derive from additional analyses that use more precise hormone measurement techniques. Recently developed liquid chromatography-mass spectrometry assays are now allowing measurements of 15 individual estrogen metabolites (Fig. 2.5.4) [5], which are showing different effects on breast cancer risk. A recent analysis within the Prostate, Lung, Colorectal, and Ovarian Cancer Screening Trial indicated that although total estrogens were predictive of risk, further risk discrimination was dependent on hydroxylation pathways [6].

Endometrial cancer
Endometrial tissue is extremely hormonally responsive, and endometrial

Table 2.5.1. Associations between history of endometriosis and the histological subtypes of ovarian cancer

Histological subtype	Stratified and adjusted OR[a] (95% CI)	P value
Invasive	1.46 (1.31–1.63)	< 0.0001
Clear cell	3.05 (2.43–3.84)	< 0.0001
Endometrioid	2.04 (1.67–2.48)	< 0.0001
Mucinous	1.02 (0.69–1.50)	0.93
High-grade serous	1.13 (0.97–1.32)	0.13
Low-grade serous	2.11 (1.39–3.20)	< 0.0001
Borderline	1.12 (0.93–1.35)	0.24
Mucinous	1.12 (0.84–1.48)	0.45
Serous	1.20 (0.95–1.52)	0.12

CI, confidence interval; OR, odds ratio.
[a] Stratified by age (5-year categories) and ethnic origin (non-Hispanic White, Hispanic White, Black, Asian, other) and adjusted for duration of oral contraceptive use (never, < 2 years, 2–4.99 years, 5–9.99 years, ≥ 10 years) and parity (0, 1, 2, 3, ≥ 4). Pooled analysis of 13 ovarian cancer case–control studies: 1 in Australia, 3 in Europe, and 9 in the USA.

Table 2.5.2. Associations between menopausal hormone therapy and ovarian cancer risk in the United States National Institutes of Health-American Association of Retired Persons (NIH-AARP) Diet and Health Study cohort, 1995–2006

	Number of cancers	Person-years	RR[a] (95% CI)
Use of ET only, among 23 584 women with a hysterectomy at baseline			
No MHT use	23	55 868	1.00 (reference)
ET only	76	116 139	1.69 (1.05–2.71)
Duration of use of ET only (years)			
< 10	27	58 393	1.25 (0.71–2.20)
≥ 10	49	55 878	2.15 (1.30–3.57)
Use of EPT only, among 68 596 women with an intact uterus at baseline			
No MHT use	150	316 239	1.00 (reference)
ET only	98	170 556	1.43 (1.09–1.86)
Duration of use of EPT only (years)			
< 10	67	126 465	1.33 (0.98–1.79)
≥ 10	31	43 752	1.68 (1.13–2.49)

CI, confidence interval; EPT, estrogen plus progestin therapy; ET, unopposed estrogen therapy; MHT, menopausal hormone therapy; RR, hazard rate ratio.
[a] RR adjusted for continuous age (years), race (White, other/unknown), parity (nulliparous, 1, 2, ≥ 3, unknown), duration of oral contraceptive use (none, < 10 years, ≥ 10 years, unknown), and body mass index (< 25 kg/m^2, 25–29 kg/m^2, ≥ 30 kg/m^2, unknown); models included terms for use of other MHT formulations.

continuously), although studies are only beginning to pursue this issue.

Whereas nulliparous women have high risks and multiparous women the lowest risks of developing endometrial cancer, no effect on risk has been demonstrated according to age at first birth. Instead, age at or interval since last birth may be an important contributor to risk, although studies are still attempting to understand these relationships. Early age at menarche and late age at menopause are even stronger risk factors for endometrial cancer than for breast cancer, presumably because these parameters indicate an enhanced opportunity for circulating estrogens to influence risk. Despite these patterns of risk, current understanding of the effects of endogenous hormones on endometrial cancer is still imprecise. Studies are needed to assess the independence of endogenous hormones from the strong effects on risk of obesity and of exogenous hormone use. Further study of estrogen metabolism patterns may also provide some clarity.

Whereas use of sequential oral contraceptives (estrogen-only pills followed by a limited number of days of progestin pills) has been related to elevated risks of endometrial cancer in premenopausal women, for the more commonly used oral contraceptives, a combination of estrogen and progestin, use has been related to substantial risk reductions. Long-term users have the lowest risk, and reduced risk persists for some time after discontinuation of use. Although the progesterone content of the pills used might affect risk, studies have not been able to definitely confirm this hypothesis.

Despite the recognition of a strong role for hormonal factors in the etiology of endometrial cancers, relatively few studies have undertaken the assessment of the role of endogenous hormones. There is suggestive evidence that both estrogens and androgens deserve specific further attention. In such studies, it will be important to distinguish patterns of risk according to specific tumour subtypes (e.g. type 1 vs type 2 endometrial cancers), which have been shown to be etiologically heterogeneous.

Ovarian cancer

Nulliparity is a well-recognized risk factor for ovarian cancers, as is infertility. Although there has been extensive controversy about potential effects of fertility drugs, the latest studies show that the indications for use are more important than the drugs themselves. Endometriosis is a well-established predictor of certain types of ovarian cancers, including clear cell and endometrioid cancers (Table 2.5.1) [8].

Some studies suggest elevated risks with early age at menarche and late age at menopause, but the results are not entirely consistent. Substantially reduced risks have been observed among women who have had a simple hysterectomy or tubal ligation. Although this finding might reflect detection of abnormalities and removal of ovaries during either of these procedures, more recent attention has focused on the effects of partial devascularization or partial removal of tubes, given increasing evidence of the tubal origin of many serous cancers.

Use of oral contraceptives is related to substantial reductions in the risk of ovarian cancer, particularly when long-term use is involved. However, use of menopausal hormones has been linked with increases in risk. This has been most clearly demonstrated for unopposed

Fig. 2.5.6. Estrogen signalling pathways (A) and process of cervical carcinogenesis (B). (A) Estrogen-bound receptors dimerize and translocate to the nucleus, where they activate or repress target genes by binding to estrogen response elements (ERE) or to AP1 or Sp1 transcription factors. Estrogen also binds to the membrane receptor GPR30 and transduces various signalling pathways, including phosphatidylinositol 3-kinase (PI3K), mitogen-activated protein kinase (MAPK), and Ca^{2+} signalling. (B) High-risk human papillomaviruses (HR-HPVs), such as HPV16, infect and persist in multipotent reserve cells, resulting in atypical squamous metaplasia (ASM), which gives rise to cervical intraepithelial neoplasia (CIN) grades 1–3 and eventually cervical cancer. This progressive neoplastic disease process usually takes more than a decade after initial HPV infection.

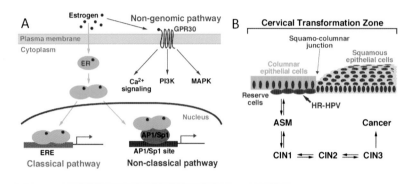

estrogen therapy, but there is growing evidence that combination estrogen plus progestin therapy may also be linked with elevated risk (Table 2.5.2) [9].

Although many of the identified risk factors for ovarian cancer are consistent with a protective effect of reduced ovulation, this does not appear to entirely explain all of the identified risk factors. Recent attention has focused on the possible role of hormonal and immunological factors [10]. Conflicting results have emerged about the respective role of estrogens, androgens, follicle-stimulating hormone, sex hormone-binding globulin, and insulin-like growth factor. Further investigation appears warranted, especially with respect to specific ovarian cancer subtypes, for which there is growing evidence of etiological heterogeneity.

Cervical cancer

Although infection with the human papillomaviruses is recognized as a necessary cause of cervical cancer, other co-factors are clearly important. Epidemiological studies have for some time implicated a variety of factors that could increase risk through hormonal mechanisms,

such as oral contraceptive use and multiparity, but the role of hormonal factors in the etiology of cervical cancer is not well understood. Transgenic mice models have recently provided evidence that estrogen and its nuclear receptor promote cervical cancer in combination with human papillomavirus oncogenes (Fig. 2.5.6) [11]. If future studies can

demonstrate that human cervical cancers are dependent on estrogens, it may be possible to develop hormonal agents to prevent or treat cervical cancers.

Testicular cancer

Hormonal factors clearly play a role in the etiology of testicular cancer, as evidenced by the rise in incidence starting at adolescence and a variety of risk factors including height, subfertility, and possibly exposure to endocrine disrupters. Several risk factors also support an influence of exposures received in utero, including cryptorchidism, hypospadias, inguinal hernia, low birth weight, short gestational age, and being a twin, some of which may reflect the influence of endogenous hormones [12]. Recent studies have attempted to assess the role of endogenous hormones in the etiology of testicular cancer, but further studies are needed to fully understand relationships.

Male breast cancer

The incidence of breast cancers in men is only about 1% of the rate in women, complicating the evaluation of etiological factors. The few available studies, however, appear

Fig. 2.5.7. Risk factors for male breast cancer, from the United States National Institutes of Health-American Association of Retired Persons (NIH-AARP) Diet and Health Study. RR, relative risk.

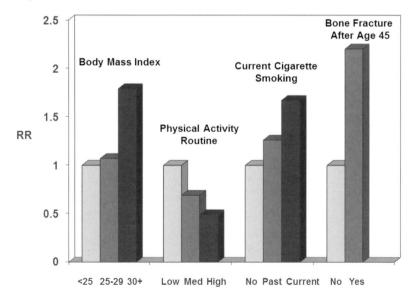

Fig. 2.5.8. Association between risk of prostate cancer and increasing fifths of hormone concentrations. The position of each square indicates the magnitude of the relative risk (RR), and the area of the square is proportional to the amount of statistical information available. The length of the horizontal line through the square indicates the 95% confidence interval (CI). The chi-square 1 degree of freedom statistic for linear trend is calculated by replacing the categorical variables with a continuous variable scored as 0, 0.25, 0.5, 0.75, and 1. The P value was two-sided for statistical significance of the chi-square linear trend statistic. DHEA-S, dehydroepiandrosterone sulfate; DHT, dihydrotestosterone; SHBG, sex hormone-binding globulin.

Hormone	Fifth	Cases/Controls	RR (95% CI)	RR & 95% CI	χ_1^2 for trend
Testosterone	1	784/1302	1.00		
	2	761/1309	0.97 (0.85-1.11)		0.17
	3	837/1287	1.08 (0.95-1.23)		P = 0.68
	4	792/1281	1.03 (0.90-1.17)		
	5	712/1259	0.94 (0.82-1.07)		
Free testosterone	1	691/1181	1.00		
	2	684/1165	1.01 (0.88-1.16)		2.89
	3	750/1155	1.13 (0.98-1.29)		P = 0.09
	4	707/1162	1.09 (0.95-1.25)		
	5	718/1152	1.11 (0.96-1.27)		
DHT	1	240/298	1.00		
	2	192/284	0.83 (0.65-1.07)		1.19
	3	188/282	0.82 (0.63-1.06)		P = 0.28
	4	194/295	0.83 (0.64-1.08)		
	5	196/286	0.86 (0.66-1.11)		
Androstanediol glucuronide	1	484/626	1.00		
	2	474/605	1.01 (0.85-1.21)		2.31
	3	497/600	1.07 (0.90-1.28)		P = 0.13
	4	465/601	1.03 (0.87-1.22)		
	5	533/603	1.15 (0.97-1.37)		
DHEA-S	1	255/393	1.00		
	2	212/374	0.92 (0.73-1.17)		3.24
	3	223/372	1.04 (0.81-1.32)		P = 0.07
	4	244/380	1.12 (0.89-1.42)		
	5	220/351	1.17 (0.92-1.50)		
Androstenedione	1	388/496	1.00		
	2	341/484	0.89 (0.73-1.09)		0.04
	3	341/484	0.91 (0.75-1.11)		P = 0.84
	4	353/485	0.95 (0.78-1.16)		
	5	358/481	1.00 (0.82-1.22)		
Estradiol	1	469/648	1.00		
	2	459/610	1.02 (0.86-1.21)		0.91
	3	431/606	0.96 (0.80-1.15)		P = 0.34
	4	425/580	0.97 (0.81-1.17)		
	5	402/595	0.93 (0.77-1.11)		
Free estradiol	1	438/563	1.00		
	2	384/550	0.90 (0.75-1.08)		0.09
	3	435/549	1.02 (0.85-1.22)		P = 0.77
	4	395/536	0.93 (0.77-1.12)		
	5	391/537	0.95 (0.79-1.15)		
SHBG	1	772/1211	1.00		
	2	773/1212	0.99 (0.87-1.13)		6.09
	3	756/1197	0.96 (0.84-1.10)		P = 0.01
	4	728/1195	0.92 (0.80-1.05)		
	5	675/1183	0.86 (0.75-0.98)		

0.5 0.75 1.0 1.5 2.0

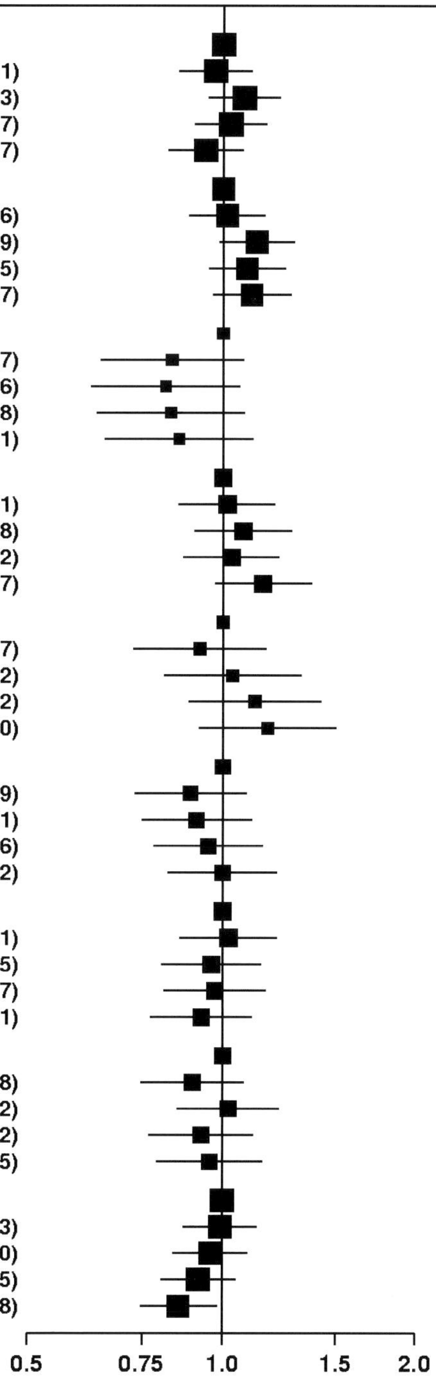

Fig. 2.5.9. One mother helps another to breastfeed her baby in Kolkata, India. Generally, reduced risk of breast cancer is associated with prolonged rather than short-term breastfeeding.

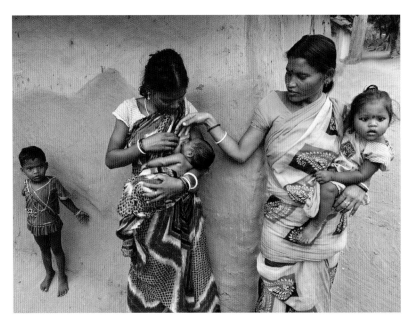

to implicate several hormonally related risk factors, with suggestions of increased risks related to gynaecomastia and Klinefelter syndrome and, in the most recent prospective study [13], to obesity, lack of physical activity, prior bone fractures, and current cigarette smoking (Fig. 2.5.7). Studies have not been undertaken to assess relationships with endogenous hormones.

Prostate cancer

Prostate cancers respond well to anti-androgen therapies, and both surgical and medical castration results in substantial reductions in risk of metastatic disease. Although it has also been assumed that androgens would play a role in the etiology of the disease, studies to date have not provided evidence of a role for any hormones as risk predictors. This includes an absence of association in a large pooling project (Fig. 2.5.8) [14] of testosterone, calculated free testosterone, and conversion products; the major conversion product is dihydrotestosterone, to which testosterone is converted within the prostate by 5α-reductase. The only evidence of association observed was an inverse relationship with sex hormone-binding globulin.

Finasteride use reduces prostate cancer risk by blocking the conversion of testosterone to dihydrotestosterone; use has also been associated with increases in estradiol levels. The Prostate Cancer Prevention Trial has shown substantial reductions in prostate cancer incidence associated with exposure to finasteride (http://www.cancer.gov/clinicaltrials/noteworthy-trials/pcpt/Page1). This has raised concern as to whether estrogen levels might play a role in prostate cancer etiology. As with androgens, however, no relationships of prostate cancer risk with estrogen levels have been observed. Data from the trial, however, have shown that participants who developed prostate cancer while taking finasteride experienced higher-grade tumours. Thus, it may be worthwhile for future studies to consider effects of estrogens and androgens on subgroups of prostate cancers as well as to consider effects on risk of combined measures or estrogens and androgens as well as hormone metabolites.

Other cancers

Although colorectal cancer is not classically considered as a hormonally related cancer, there is evidence supporting the possibility of inverse associations of colorectal cancer risk with use of both oral contraceptives and menopausal hormones. Oral contraceptives have also been noted to be a risk factor for liver cancer in the absence of infection with hepatitis B virus, an important cause of this disease.

References

1. Bernstein L (2002). Epidemiology of endocrine-related risk factors for breast cancer. *J Mammary Gland Biol Neoplasia*, 7:3–15. http://dx.doi.org/10.1023/A:1015714305420 PMID:12160084

2. Collaborative Group on Hormonal Factors in Breast Cancer (2012). Menarche, menopause, and breast cancer risk: individual participant meta-analysis, including 118 964 women with breast cancer from 117 epidemiological studies. *Lancet Oncol*, 13:1141–1151. http://dx.doi.org/10.1016/S1470-2045(12)70425-4 PMID:23084519

3. Yang XR, Figueroa JD, Falk RT *et al.* (2012). Analysis of terminal duct lobular unit involution in luminal A and basal breast cancers. *Breast Cancer Res*, 14:R64. http://dx.doi.org/10.1186/bcr3170 PMID:22513288

4. James RE, Lukanova A, Dossus L *et al.* (2011). Postmenopausal serum sex steroids and risk of hormone receptor-positive and -negative breast cancer: a nested case-control study. *Cancer Prev Res (Phila)*, 4:1626–1635. http://dx.doi.org/10.1158/1940-6207.CAPR-11-0090 PMID:21813404

5. Ziegler RG, Rossi SC, Fears TR *et al.* (1997). Quantifying estrogen metabolism: an evaluation of the reproducibility and validity of enzyme immunoassays for 2-hydroxyestrone and 16alpha-hydroxyestrone in urine. *Environ Health Perspect*, 105 Suppl 3:607–614. PMID:9168003

6. Fuhrman BJ, Schairer C, Gail MH *et al.* (2012). Estrogen metabolism and risk of breast cancer in postmenopausal women. *J Natl Cancer Inst*, 104:326–339. http://dx.doi.org/10.1093/jnci/djr531 PMID:22232133

7. Trabert B, Wentzensen N, Yang HP *et al.* (2013). Is estrogen plus progestin menopausal hormone therapy safe with respect to endometrial cancer risk? *Int J Cancer*, 132:417–426. http://dx.doi.org/10.1002/ijc.27623 PMID:22553145

8. Pearce CL, Templeman C, Rossing MA *et al.*; Ovarian Cancer Association Consortium (2012). Association between endometriosis and risk of histological subtypes of ovarian cancer: a pooled analysis of case-control studies. *Lancet Oncol*, 13:385–394. http://dx.doi.org/10.1016/S1470-2045(11)70404-1 PMID:22361336

9. Trabert B, Wentzensen N, Yang HP *et al.* (2012). Ovarian cancer and menopausal hormone therapy in the NIH-AARP Diet and Health Study. *Br J Cancer*, 107:1181–1187. http://dx.doi.org/10.1038/bjc.2012.397 PMID:22929888

10. Ness RB, Cottreau C (1999). Possible role of ovarian epithelial inflammation in ovarian cancer. *J Natl Cancer Inst*, 91:1459–1467. http://dx.doi.org/10.1093/jnci/91.17.1459 PMID:10469746

11. Chung SH, Franceschi S, Lambert PF (2010). Estrogen and ERalpha: culprits in cervical cancer? *Trends Endocrinol Metab*, 21:504–511. http://dx.doi.org/10.1016/j.tem.2010.03.005 PMID:20456973

12. McGlynn KA, Trabert B (2012). Adolescent and adult risk factors for testicular cancer. *Nat Rev Urol*, 9:339–349. http://dx.doi.org/10.1038/nrurol.2012.61 PMID:22508459

13. Brinton LA, Richesson DA, Gierach GL *et al.* (2008). Prospective evaluation of risk factors for male breast cancer. *J Natl Cancer Inst*, 100:1477–1481. http://dx.doi.org/10.1093/jnci/djn329 PMID:18840816

14. Roddam AW, Allen NE, Appleby P, Key TJ; Endogenous Hormones and Prostate Cancer Collaborative Group (2008). Endogenous sex hormones and prostate cancer: a collaborative analysis of 18 prospective studies. *J Natl Cancer Inst*, 100:170–183. http://dx.doi.org/10.1093/jnci/djm323 PMID:18230794

2.6 Diet, obesity, and physical activity

2 ETIOLOGY

Walter C. Willett
Tim Key
Isabelle Romieu

Martin Wiseman (reviewer)

Summary

- Excess body fat increases risk of cancers of the oesophagus, colon, pancreas, endometrium, and kidney, as well as postmenopausal breast cancer.

- Regular physical activity reduces risks of multiple cancers by contributing to weight control, and risks of colorectal and breast cancer by additional mechanisms.

- Among dietary factors related to excess body weight, reduction of consumption of sugar-sweetened beverages should be a high priority.

- High consumption of red meat, especially processed meat, is associated with risk of colorectal cancer.

- A diet high in fruits and vegetables and whole grains does not appear to be as strongly protective against cancer as initially believed. However, this dietary pattern is still advisable because of the benefits for diabetes and cardiovascular diseases, and some possible reductions in cancer incidence.

- Additional research is needed on many aspects of diet and physical activity in relation to cancer, including the effects of these behaviours during childhood and in early adult life.

Interest in diet as contributing to the cause and prevention of cancer emerged from observations that cancer rates vary greatly between countries and are correlated with dietary factors, and that nutrition can modify cancer incidence in animals. To provide more specific information for human cancer, many retrospective case–control studies, some prospective cohort studies, and a few randomized trials have been conducted. These studies have limitations: measurement of diet and physical activity is always imperfect, the diagnosis of cancer can distort the recall of diet in the retrospective studies, and adherence to the assigned diet is often poor in randomized trials (see "Challenges of measuring diet in cancer epidemiological studies and new perspectives"). In addition, initial nutritional status may affect response to changes in dietary intake. Despite the many methodological challenges, much has been learned during the past 30 years about the relation of diet, obesity, and physical activity to cancer; major findings are briefly described here. Because prospective cohort studies are least susceptible to biases, findings from these studies are emphasized, together with the findings from the small number of randomized trials.

Diet

Fat

Among dietary factors, fat has received the greatest attention due to strong international correlations with rates of several cancers common in developed countries. However, prospective studies have consistently shown little relationship of fat intake with breast cancer risk [1], even with up to 20 years of follow-up. In two large randomized trials of low-fat

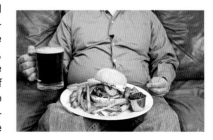

Fig. 2.6.1. A man eats a hamburger and fried potato chips and drinks a pint of beer. Drinking alcohol, consumption of red and processed meats, and a high caloric dietary intake are variously associated with increased risk of cancer at several anatomical sites.

Challenges of measuring diet in cancer epidemiological studies and new perspectives

Nadia Slimani

Among the different environmental and lifestyle risk factors, diet is one of the most complex exposures to investigate in relation to diseases, particularly cancer. Indeed, diet is a universal exposure, and foods are consumed in combinations and with preparation methods that vary greatly between individuals and over the whole lifespan. In addition, the several thousand chemicals (including contaminants) present in foods may have complex synergistic or antagonistic bioactive effects, making it difficult to disentangle individual chemical effects and remove confounding completely when investigating diet–disease relationships and underlying biological mechanisms [1]. Finally, diet has strong social, religious, and psychological aspects that affect study designs and the dietary outcomes of individuals [2].

In addition, the nutrition transition, a phenomenon occurring with an accelerated pace worldwide [3,4], is another under-evaluated challenge to measuring diet–cancer associations. The nutrition transition is the shift in dietary patterns from traditional diets (high in cereal and fibre) to diets more typical of developed countries and characterized by an increased contribution of (highly) industrially processed foods (high in sugars, fats, and animal sources) [4].

Cancer is a multiphase and multifactorial disease that essentially occurs late in life but that might be affected by different (early) exposure windows, which are difficult to evaluate. Most cancer epidemiological studies involve middle-aged populations and use single or limited repeated dietary measurements, which are not able to approximate lifelong dietary exposure [5]. Furthermore, the food frequency questionnaire (FFQ) assessment method predominantly used in epidemiology has been challenged with respect to its validity and reliability [6,7]. The FFQ is a retrospective method that asks respondents to report their usual frequency of consumption of each food from a list of foods for a specific period (several months or a year). In contrast, repeated 24-hour dietary recalls

Fig. B2.6.1. Integrative approaches for measuring diet in large-scale epidemiological studies. 24-HDRs, 24-hour dietary recalls; DQ, dietary questionnaire; FFQ, food frequency questionnaire; FPQ, food propensity questionnaire (non-quantitative FFQ).

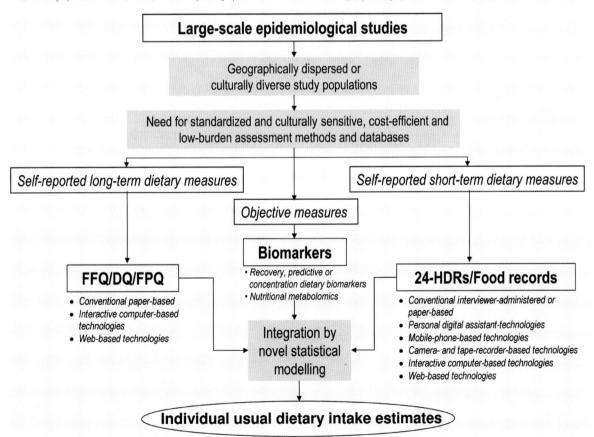

(24-HDRs) or food records (FRs), considered to be more precise and reliable than FFQs, are increasingly used or recommended in nutritional cancer research [8]. The 24-HDR is a retrospective assessment method in which an interviewer prompts a respondent to recall and describe all foods and beverages consumed during the preceding 24 hours or the preceding day. The FR is used to record food intake at the time of consumption, over a number of days that are not necessarily sequential.

Based on decades of methodological research [9], front-line nutritional research increasingly favours approaches that integrate traditional and more innovative measurements of dietary exposure: (i) repeated 24-HDRs or FRs benefiting from cost-effective new innovative (web) technologies [10,11]; (ii) the FFQ or food propensity questionnaire (FPQ) approach, designed to rank individuals and/or identify foods infrequently consumed, to complement 24-HDRs and other open-ended methods; and (iii) the use of recovery and/or concentration nutritional biomarkers

as independent observations or as substitute estimates of dietary exposure [12,13] (Fig. B2.6.1). In addition, the rapid development of metabolomic research opens a promising perspective for a more holistic approach to measure dietary exposure through individual and population-specific metabolomic profiles (or phenotypes) [14]. These approaches will be maximized when applied in large studies with wide variations in dietary exposures and disease outcomes.

References

1. Penn L et al. (2010). Genes Nutr, 5:205–213. http://dx.doi.org/10.1007/s12263-010-0175-9 PMID:21052527

2. Gibney MJ et al., eds (2004). Public Health Nutrition. Oxford: Blackwell Science.

3. Popkin BM et al. (2002). Public Health Nutr, 5:947–953. http://dx.doi.org/10.1079/PHN2002370 PMID:12633520

4. Popkin BM (2006). Am J Clin Nutr, 84:289–298. PMID:16895874

5. Kristal AR, Lampe JW (2011). Cancer Epidemiol Biomarkers Prev, 20:725–726. http://dx.doi.org/10.1158/1055-9965.EPI-10-1349 PMID:21546363

6. Kristal AR, Potter JD (2006). Cancer Epidemiol Biomarkers Prev, 15:1759–1760. http://dx.doi.org/10.1158/1055-9965.EPI-06-0727 PMID:17021349

7. Willett WC, Hu FB (2006). Cancer Epidemiol Biomarkers Prev, 15:1757–1758. http://dx.doi.org/10.1158/1055-9965.EPI-06-0388 PMID:17021351

8. Schatzkin A et al. (2009). Cancer Epidemiol Biomarkers Prev, 18:1026–1032. http://dx.doi.org/10.1158/1055-9965.EPI-08-1129 PMID:19336550

9. Thompson FE, Subar AM (2008). Dietary assessment methodology. In: Coulston AM, Boushey CJ, eds. Nutrition in the Prevention and Treatment of Disease, 2nd ed. San Diego: Elsevier, pp. 3–39.

10. Subar AF et al. (2012). J Acad Nutr Diet, 112:1134–1137. http://dx.doi.org/10.1016/j.jand.2012.04.016 PMID:22704899

11. Touvier M et al. (2011). Br J Nutr, 105:1055–1064. http://dx.doi.org/10.1017/S0007114510004617 PMID:21080983

12. Freedman LS et al. (2011). Am J Epidemiol, 174:1238–1245. http://dx.doi.org/10.1093/aje/kwr248 PMID:22047826

13. Illner AK et al. (2012). Int J Epidemiol, 41:1187–1203. http://dx.doi.org/10.1093/ije/dys105 PMID:22933652

14. Kaput J, Rodriguez RL (2004). Physiol Genomics, 16:166–177. PMID:14726599

diets, there was no significant effect on risk of breast cancer. Prospective studies of colorectal cancer have also not supported the positive relationship with fat intake suggested by international comparisons of cancer rates [1,2]. Prospective studies of dietary fat and prostate cancer are fewer but do not generally support a relation with total or specific types of dietary fat [1,3].

For patients with cancer, the effect of diet after diagnosis on survival is of great interest. Two randomized trials of low-fat diets have been conducted among women with breast cancer. In one study, a marginally significantly lower risk of breast cancer was seen, but this might have been explained by a greater weight loss compared with the control group. In the other trial, no effect of the dietary intervention was observed [4].

Meat and dairy products

Higher intake of red meat, especially processed meat, has been associated with greater risk of colorectal cancer in many prospective studies and in a meta-analysis of these studies [1] (see "Single-nucleotide polymorphisms relevant to meat consumption and cancer risk"). Although consumption of meat during midlife or later has generally not been associated with risk of breast cancer, a positive relation has been seen with intake in adolescence and early adult life [5]. Studies of red meat and risk of prostate cancer have been limited and results inconsistent [1].

Higher consumption of milk or dairy products has been associated with lower risk of colorectal cancer [1]. In contrast, higher consumption of dairy products has been associated with increased risks

of total or fatal prostate cancer in many studies [1]; the fat component of milk does not appear to account for these associations.

Fruits, vegetables, and phytochemicals

Higher intakes of essential nutrients and other biologically active constituents of plants have reduced cancer incidence in laboratory animals and appear to have benefits in isolated cells. Although higher intakes of fruits and vegetables were associated with lower risks of many cancers in retrospective studies, these findings have generally not been strongly supported by prospective studies [1].

A large protective role for total intake of fruits and vegetables against overall cancer risk now appears unlikely, but specific phytochemical or botanical subgroups may reduce risks of some cancers. Promising leads include carotenoid-containing vegetables and estrogen-receptor-negative breast cancer, cruciferous vegetables and several cancer sites including prostate, bladder, and lung; allium vegetables and stomach cancer; and folate-rich fruits and vegetables and colon cancer. High consumption of soy products, rich in anti-estrogenic compounds, during adolescence, but not during midlife or later, has been associated with lower risk of breast cancer [6]. More research is needed on these associations, and currently none of them is firmly established.

Dietary fibre

Fibre has long been hypothesized to reduce risk of colorectal cancer by providing bulk to dilute potential carcinogens and speed their transit through the colon, by binding and thus inactivating carcinogens, or by altering the flora and biochemical environment of the colon (see "Diet and the gut microbiome"). Several large prospective cohort studies of dietary fibre and colon cancer risk have not supported an association [7], although an inverse relation was seen in the large European Prospective Investigation into Cancer and Nutrition (EPIC)

study and a recent meta-analysis [8]. The variation in findings from prospective studies needs to be better understood; dietary fibre is complex and heterogeneous, and the relation with colorectal cancer could differ by dietary source [9].

Higher intake of fibre has also been hypothesized to reduce risk of breast cancer by interrupting the enterohepatic circulation of estrogens. Although no relation with breast cancer has been seen in most prospective studies, a weak inverse relation was seen in a recent meta-analysis [10] and a new analysis from the large EPIC study [11].

Vitamins and minerals

Calcium

In a pooled analysis of large cohort studies, persons with the highest calcium intake had a 22% lower risk of colorectal cancer [12]; most of the benefit was achieved with about 800 mg/day. This benefit is supported by reductions in recurrence of colorectal adenomas with calcium supplementation in some randomized trials [1], but not all [13]. However, higher calcium intake has also been associated with a greater risk of total or advanced prostate cancer in several studies [1]. The

possibility of competing risks and benefits associated with higher intake of dairy products and calcium has made recommendations about consumption difficult in relation to cancer, but adequate intakes of calcium are essential for bone growth and other aspects of health.

Vitamin D

Higher blood levels of vitamin D, which reflect both intakes and sunlight exposure, have been consistently associated with lower risk of colorectal cancer [14], and recently with survival [15], but more research is needed to determine whether this reflects a true protective effect. Inconsistent associations have been seen with other specific cancers.

Folate

Folate is important for DNA methylation, repair, and synthesis, and in some prospective studies, higher intakes have been associated with lower risk of colorectal and several other cancers [16]. In a recent analysis, a lag of at least 12–14 years was seen between low folate intake and increased risk of colorectal cancer [4]. A role of folate in colorectal carcinogenesis is supported by the confirmed association between a genetic polymorphism in MTHFR, an enzyme involved in folate metabolism, and risk of colorectal cancer [17].

In randomized trials among patients with a history of colorectal adenomas, supplements of folic acid have not reduced recurrent adenomas, and in one trial an increased risk of recurrent advanced adenoma or multiple adenomas was seen [18]. These studies suggest that supplemental folic acid is unlikely to be beneficial for those with existing colonic neoplasia and adequate folate intake, and might even be harmful. This concern was heightened by a report suggesting a small and transient increase in incidence of colorectal cancer in the USA almost immediately after the initiation of folic acid fortification of grain products, but this transient increase was likely to have been an artefact

Fig. 2.6.2. In a remote semi-arid region of Laikipia North in Kenya, Masai warriors have exchanged their spears for cricket bats. Physical activity is associated with reduced risk of colorectal and other cancers.

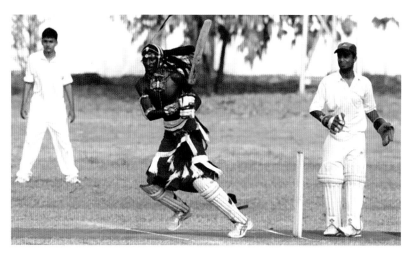

Single-nucleotide polymorphisms relevant to meat consumption and cancer risk

Rashmi Sinha

Meat is a source of a variety of carcinogens, including heterocyclic amines (HCAs) and polycyclic aromatic hydrocarbons (PAHs), which are formed in meats cooked at high temperatures, and N-nitroso compounds (NOCs), which are found in processed meats as a result of nitrate or nitrite added during processing, and are formed endogenously from haem iron. HCAs, PAHs, and NOCs undergo extensive metabolism by phase I (cytochrome P450s) and phase II (sulfotransferases, glucuronosyltransferases, N-acetyltransferases) xenobiotic metabolizing enzymes (XMEs). Single-nucleotide polymorphisms (SNPs) in the genes encoding these XMEs can modify the ability of these enzymes to activate or detoxify these meat carcinogens (Fig. B2.6.2).

While many studies have observed modifying effects of SNPs in XME genes on the association between meat carcinogen intake and colorectal cancer, the evidence for primary associations and interactions between XME polymorphisms, meat consumption, and the risk of colorectal adenomas or carcinomas has been mixed. One of the largest analyses to investigate these associations conducted to date, a study of 1205 advanced colorectal adenoma cases and 1387 controls, revealed only one statistically significant interaction. The study reported an interaction between intake of the HCA 2-amino-3,8-dimethylimidazo[4,5-f]quinoxaline (MeIQx) and the NAT1 polymorphism rs6586714 ($P_{interaction}$ = 0.001); among individuals carrying a GG genotype, high MeIQx intake was positively associated with colorectal adenoma (odds ratio [OR], 1.43; 95% confidence interval [CI], 1.11–1.85; P_{trend} = 0.07), whereas those with the A variant had a decreased risk (OR, 0.50; 95% CI, 0.30–0.84; P_{trend} = 0.01) [1]. The study also investigated substrate-oriented pathway-based approaches, incorporating a range of XME genes involved in both the activation and detoxification of xenobiotics, but there was no strong evidence for associations.

Two SNPs related to the xenobiotic MDRI, thought to restrict intestinal absorption of HCAs and PAHs, were associated with colorectal cancer in one study [2]. In contrast, 8 genes involved in uptake, absorption, and metabolism of dietary iron (TF, TFRC, HMOX1, SLC40A1, SLC11A2, HAMP, ACO1, HP01) were not associated with colorectal adenoma despite a statistically significant association between several SNPs and serum iron indices [3]. The PARP gene in the base excision repair pathway appeared to modify the association between intake of red meat cooked at high temperatures and risk of colorectal cancer as meat carcinogens may induce oxidative DNA damage [4].

Fig. B2.6.2. Simplified schematic of polymorphic genes coding for enzymes involved in metabolism of heterocyclic amines (HCAs), polycyclic aromatic hydrocarbons (PAHs), nitrate/nitrate, and iron. AHR, aryl hydrocarbon receptor.

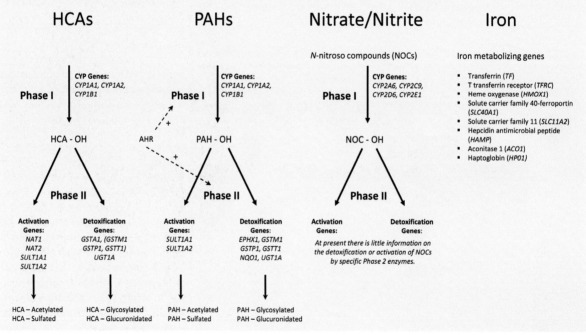

Overall, the inconsistent findings reflect several limitations of existing studies, including the inability to accurately estimate the intake of specific meat carcinogens, the limited number of well-characterized cases to ensure sufficient power by genotype, and our current limited understanding of the precise genetic variants that account for XME function.

Vitamin and mineral supplementation

The role of vitamin and mineral supplements in cancer prevention has been examined in both prospective cohort studies and randomized trials. Trials of β-carotene and other single supplements, including vitamin E and selenium, have not shown benefits [1]. In trials using combinations of multiple vitamins or minerals at lower doses than those in single supplements, reductions in cancer

Very large studies that include both comprehensive meat intake information and numerous markers across multiple XME genes are essential for studying this complex association.

References

1. Gilsing AM *et al.* (2012). *Carcinogenesis*, 33:1332–1339. http://dx.doi.org/10.1093/carcin/bgs158 PMID:22552404

rates have been seen in a Chinese population with multiple nutrient deficiencies [19,20], in French men but not women, and in physicians in the USA [21].The study of physicians in the USA was notable because this population was well nourished, and the modest benefit was detectable only after 10 years, which is a period longer than that used in virtually all other studies. Overall, supplements with multivitamins and minerals are likely to be beneficial in populations with multiple nutrient deficiencies, although improvements in general nutrition should be the long-term goal in such populations.

2. Andersen V *et al.* (2009). *BMC Cancer*, 9:407. http://dx.doi.org/10.1186/1471-2407-9-407 PMID:19930591

3. Cross AJ *et al.* (2011). *Cancer Prev Res (Phila)*, 4:1465–1475. http://dx.doi.org/10.1158/1940-6207.CAPR-11-0103 PMID:21685236

4. Brevik A *et al.* (2010). *Cancer Epidemiol Biomarkers Prev*, 19:3167–3173. http://dx.doi.org/10.1158/1055-9965.EPI-10-0606 PMID:21037106

Diet and excess adiposity

Because excess adiposity is associated with risk of many cancers [1], the relationship of diet to weight gain and obesity is important for cancer prevention. In trials with similar intensity of intervention and that have lasted at least 1 year, low-fat diets have not been effective in weight loss [22]. A diet low in rapidly absorbed carbohydrates (such as sugar, jam, and refined cereals) may facilitate weight loss [23]. A Mediterranean-style, restricted-calorie dietary pattern, which is high in cereals, fruits, and vegetables and low in animal products, has been effective in sustaining weight loss for as long as 6 years [24]. Reduced consumption of soda and other sugar-sweetened beverages has reduced weight among children and adults who were initially overweight [25].

In an analysis of long-term weight gain in three large cohort studies, foods associated with greater weight gain included potato chips, sugar-sweetened beverages, red meat, and processed meat, whereas fruits, vegetables, whole grains, nuts, and yogurt were associated with less weight gain [26]. Among beverages, sugar-sweetened beverages and fruit juices were associated with greater weight gain. Because they lack any nutritional value and are directly related to adiposity, diabetes, and cardiovascular disease, sugar-sweetened beverages are a high-priority focus area for weight control efforts in populations with substantial intakes.

Fig. 2.6.3. Relation of body mass index with risk of developing cancers of the oesophagus, colon, pancreas, breast, endometrium, and kidney.

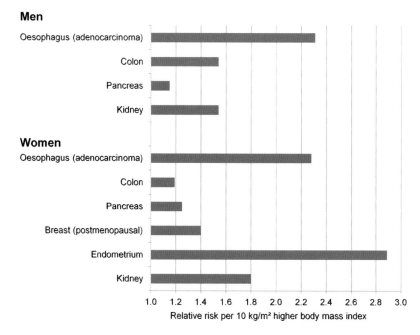

Fig. 2.6.4. Relation of body mass index with risk of death from cancer of any type in men and women who had never smoked.

Hazard ratio for death from cancer (95% CI)

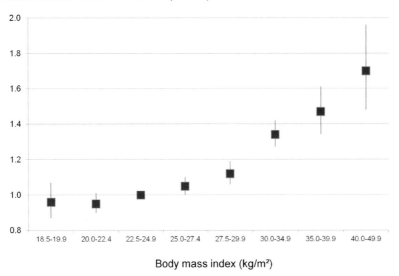

Body mass index (kg/m²)

Overweight and obesity

Overweight and obesity are important causes of several types of cancer. Body fatness is usually assessed using body mass index (BMI), which is calculated as the weight in kilograms divided by the square of the height in metres and thus provides a simple index of weight relative to height that can be measured easily in population studies. A BMI of 20–24.9 kg/m² is considered normal, whereas a BMI of 25–29.9 kg/m² is classed as overweight and a BMI of 30 kg/m² or more as obese. Waist circumference is another simple measure of adiposity, and shows associations with cancer risk similar to those for BMI.

Epidemiological studies have provided convincing evidence that obesity increases the risk of cancers of the oesophagus (adenocarcinoma), colon (in men), pancreas, breast (postmenopausal), endometrium, and kidney [27] (Fig. 2.6.3); these associations of BMI with cancer risk generally follow a dose–response relationship, so that as well as the increased risk with obesity, there is also a smaller increase in risk for people who are overweight but not obese.

The magnitude of the increase in risk varies between cancer sites. For an increase in BMI of 10 kg/m², relative risks are approximately 2.3 for adenocarcinoma of the oesophagus, 1.5 for colon cancer in men, 1.3 for pancreatic cancer in women, 1.4 for postmenopausal breast cancer, 2.9 for endometrial cancer, and more than 1.5 for kidney cancer.

There is also substantial evidence that obesity increases the risks of cancer of the gall bladder (in women), malignant melanoma, ovarian cancer, thyroid cancer, non-Hodgkin lymphoma, multiple myeloma, and leukaemia [1,28]. Cancer mortality (all sites combined) increases in a linear fashion with increasing BMI and is about 70% higher in people who are extremely obese than in people of normal weight (Fig. 2.6.4) [28].

Estimates of the percentage of cancers that can be attributed to excess body weight suggest that overweight and obesity are substantial causes of cancer in many developed countries [29], but the magnitude of attributable risk has varied depending on the prevalence of obesity and on other underlying assumptions. For example, estimates for the United Kingdom for 2007 suggested that 5% and 6% of all incident cancers in men and women, respectively, were attributable to overweight and obesity, with attributable risks of about 40% for cancers of the oesophagus (adenocarcinoma), gall bladder (in women), and endometrium [30], whereas estimates for the USA for 1999–2000 suggested that overweight and obesity were responsible for 4.2% and

Fig. 2.6.5. Children compete in a sack race in Banda Aceh, Indonesia. Such encouragement of physical activity may reduce the likelihood of overweight and obesity in childhood.

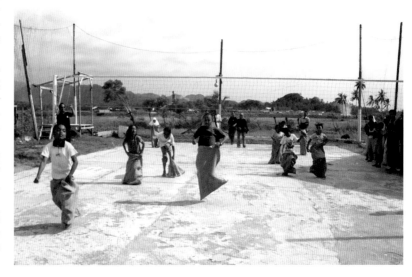

Diet and the gut microbiome

Johanna W. Lampe

The human gut is host to a large and diverse community of microbes that have physiological effects and carry out metabolic functions that can influence host health. Diet affects the amount and types of microbes present in the gut, and, in turn, actions of the gut microbiota on dietary constituents may shape cancer susceptibility. Bacteria metabolize xenobiotics, both potentially beneficial (e.g. phytochemicals) and detrimental (e.g. carcinogens), and harvest otherwise inaccessible nutrients and/or sources of energy from the diet.

Gut microbes carry out unique metabolic reactions that the host cannot. Metagenomic studies of the gut microbiome (i.e. the collective genomic content of a microbial community) have revealed the varied anaerobic reactions involved in fermentation and other processes. Enzymes specific to bacteria, and in some cases specific classes of bacteria, catalyse a range of metabolic reactions, such as hydrolysis of glycosides, amides, and esters, as well as reduction, ring cleavage, demethylation, and dehydroxylation. Plant polysaccharides (e.g. dietary fibre and resistant starch) are major dietary factors that mould the structure of the human gut microbial community [1]. Gut bacterial metabolism of non-digestible carbohydrates produces fermentation end-products, such as short-chain fatty acids, that act as signalling molecules, serve as fuel to gut epithelial cells (butyrate) and peripheral tissues (acetate and propionate), and modulate inflammation. Hydrolysis of plant glycosides typically results in metabolites that are more biologically active than the parent compounds. Further bacterial transformation of aglycones can produce lower-molecular-weight compounds that systemically may be more or less active. High inter-individual variation in circulating concentrations of phytochemicals and their metabolites is, in part, a reflection of variation in gut microbial activity [2]. Some microbial metabolites of dietary constituents are associated with increased risk of tumorigenesis. Ingested nitrate can be reduced to nitrite by bacterial nitrate reductase and produce N-nitroso compounds, which can form DNA adducts. Hydrogen sulfide, produced from sulfur-containing amino acids and inorganic sulfur sources by sulfate-reducing bacteria, has cytotoxic and genotoxic effects.

Gut microbes also promote the harvest of energy from the diet and contribute to fat deposition [3]. Thus, the gut microbiome may influence adiposity and adiposity-associated inflammation, and therefore, indirectly, cancers for which excess body fat is a risk factor. Studies in animal models suggest that gut microbes play an important role in energy regulation and adiposity. In humans, the gut microbial community is altered in obese individuals and can change with weight loss; however, whether the structure and function of the gut microbial community causes obesity in humans is unclear.

Understanding the complex and dynamic interaction between the gut microbiome and host diet may help elucidate mechanisms of carcinogenesis and guide future cancer prevention strategies.

References

1. Flint HJ (2012). *Nutr Rev*, 70 Suppl 1:S10–S13. http://dx.doi.org/10.1111/j.1753-4887.2012.00499.x PMID:22861801

2. Possemiers S *et al.* (2007). *FEMS Microbiol Ecol*, 61:372–383. http://dx.doi.org/10.1111/j.1574-6941.2007.00330.x PMID:17506823

3. Tremaroli V, Bäckhed F (2012). *Nature*, 489:242–249. http://dx.doi.org/10.1038/nature11552 PMID:22972297

14.3% of cancer mortality in men and women, respectively, rising to 14.2% and 19.8%, respectively, in men and women who had never smoked [31]. These proportions are predicted to grow in most countries due to the increasing prevalence of overweight and obesity.

Additional research is required on the possible associations of overweight and obesity with the risk of less common types of cancer. There is also a need to explore further the importance of obesity at different ages with lifetime risk of cancer, and to better understand whether the distribution of body fat is important.

Mechanisms

The mechanisms through which obesity increases cancer risk are only partially understood but appear to vary between different cancer sites. For adenocarcinoma of the oesophagus, the increase in cancer risk probably involves an increase in the prevalence of chronic acid reflux from the stomach into the oesophagus, which damages the oesophageal epithelium. For breast and endometrial cancers, the increased risk with obesity in postmenopausal women is probably caused by the increase in circulating estradiol, due to increased formation of estrogens from precursor hormones in the adipose tissue; obesity also increases the risk of endometrial cancer in premenopausal women, and this may be due to anovulation and therefore reduced production of progesterone in obese premenopausal women. For colon cancer in men, kidney cancer, and other cancers, the mechanisms by which obesity increases risk are less clear but may involve increases in insulin and other hormonal changes in obesity.

Reversing the effect of obesity on cancer risk

The clear evidence that overweight and obesity increase the risk of several types of cancer implies that weight loss should, to some extent, reverse this effect, and there is some direct evidence to support this understanding. Observational cohort studies and randomized controlled trials of both dietary interventions and bariatric surgery have shown reductions in cancer incidence occurring within a few years after intentional weight loss [32].

Obesity and cancer survival

Obesity may affect survival in cancer patients [33]. Several studies of breast cancer patients have shown that obesity is correlated with a poorer prognosis; this relationship is not well understood but may involve later diagnosis and also higher endogenous hormone levels in obese patients. Further research is needed on the effects of obesity on survival for breast cancer and for other types of cancer, including careful examination of relationships with stage at diagnosis and details of treatment.

Physical activity

Physical activity is difficult to measure in epidemiological studies, and understanding its relationship with cancer risk is complicated because it is generally inversely related to obesity and is also correlated with other factors that can affect cancer risk. Considering all the available evidence, it is likely that the most important impact of physical activity in relation to cancer prevention is through its contribution to protecting against weight gain and obesity. Thus, physical activity can contribute to reduction of risk of all types of cancer for which obesity increases risk. There is also evidence that physical activity reduces the risk of colon cancer and breast cancer and improves survival [34] independently of its effects on BMI, perhaps by acting through hormonal changes [1,27]. The type and amount of physical activity required to reduce cancer risk remains uncertain, but the general consensus among researchers is that activity should be of at least moderate intensity and should average at least 1 hour per day.

References

1. World Cancer Research Fund/American Institute for Cancer Research (2007). *Food, Nutrition, Physical Activity, and the Prevention of Cancer: A Global Perspective.* Washington, DC: American Institute for Cancer Research.

2. Liu L, Zhuang W, Wang RQ *et al.* (2011). Is dietary fat associated with the risk of colorectal cancer? A meta-analysis of 13 prospective cohort studies. *Eur J Nutr,* 50:173–184. http://dx.doi.org/10.1007/s00394-010-0128-5 PMID:20697723

3. Crowe FL, Allen NE, Appleby PN *et al.* (2008). Fatty acid composition of plasma phospholipids and risk of prostate cancer in a case-control analysis nested within the European Prospective Investigation into Cancer and Nutrition. *Am J Clin Nutr,* 88:1353–1363. PMID:18996872

4. Willett WC (2013). *Nutritional Epidemiology,* 3rd ed. New York: Oxford University Press.

5. Linos E, Willett WC, Cho E *et al.* (2008). Red meat consumption during adolescence among premenopausal women and risk of breast cancer. *Cancer Epidemiol Biomarkers Prev,* 17:2146–2151. http://dx.doi.org/10.1158/1055-9965.EPI-08-0037 PMID:18669582

6. Lee SA, Shu XO, Li H *et al.* (2009). Adolescent and adult soy food intake and breast cancer risk: results from the Shanghai Women's Health Study. *Am J Clin Nutr,* 89:1920–1926. http://dx.doi.org/10.3945/ajcn.2008.27361 PMID:19403632

7. Park Y, Hunter DJ, Spiegelman D *et al.* (2005). Dietary fiber intake and risk of colorectal cancer: a pooled analysis of prospective cohort studies. *JAMA,* 294:2849–2857. http://dx.doi.org/10.1001/jama.294.22.2849 PMID:16352792

8. Murphy N, Norat T, Ferrari P *et al.* (2012). Dietary fibre intake and risks of cancers of the colon and rectum in the European prospective investigation into cancer and nutrition (EPIC). *PLoS One,* 7:e39361. http://dx.doi.org/10.1371/journal.pone.0039361 PMID:22761771

9. Aune D, Chan DS, Lau R *et al.* (2011). Dietary fibre, whole grains, and risk of colorectal cancer: systematic review and dose-response meta-analysis of prospective studies. *BMJ,* 343:d6617. http://dx.doi.org/10.1136/bmj.d6617 PMID:22074852

10. Aune D, Chan DS, Greenwood DC *et al.* (2012). Dietary fiber and breast cancer risk: a systematic review and meta-analysis of prospective studies. *Ann Oncol,* 23:1394–1402. http://dx.doi.org/10.1093/annonc/mdr589 PMID:22234738

11. Ferrari P, Rinaldi S, Jenab M *et al.* (2013). Dietary fiber intake and risk of hormonal receptor-defined breast cancer in the European Prospective Investigation into Cancer and Nutrition study. *Am J Clin Nutr*, 97:344–353. http://dx.doi.org/10.3945/ajcn.112.034025 PMID:23269820

12. Cho E, Smith-Warner SA, Spiegelman D *et al.* (2004). Dairy foods, calcium, and colorectal cancer: a pooled analysis of 10 cohort studies. *J Natl Cancer Inst*, 96:1015–1022. http://dx.doi.org/10.1093/jnci/djh185 PMID:15240785

13. Neuhouser ML, Wassertheil-Smoller S, Thomson C *et al.* (2009). Multivitamin use and risk of cancer and cardiovascular disease in the Women's Health Initiative cohorts. *Arch Intern Med*, 169:294–304. http://dx.doi.org/10.1001/archinternmed.2008.540 PMID:19204221

14. Jenab M, Bueno-de-Mesquita HB, Ferrari P *et al.* (2010). Association between prediagnostic circulating vitamin D concentration and risk of colorectal cancer in European populations: a nested case-control study. *BMJ*, 340:b5500. http://dx.doi.org/10.1136/bmj.b5500 PMID:20093284

15. Fedirko V, Riboli E, Tjønneland A *et al.* (2012). Prediagnostic 25-hydroxyvitamin D, *VDR* and *CASR* polymorphisms, and survival in patients with colorectal cancer in western European populations. *Cancer Epidemiol Biomarkers Prev*, 21:582–593. http://dx.doi.org/10.1158/1055-9965.EPI-11-1065 PMID:22278364

16. Kim DH, Smith-Warner SA, Spiegelman D *et al.* (2010). Pooled analyses of 13 prospective cohort studies on folate intake and colon cancer. *Cancer Causes Control*, 21:1919–1930. http://dx.doi.org/10.1007/s10552-010-9620-8 PMID:20820900

17. Giovannucci E (2002). Modifiable risk factors for colon cancer. *Gastroenterol Clin North Am*, 31:925–943. http://dx.doi.org/10.1016/S0889-8553(02)00057-2 PMID:12489270

18. Cole BF, Baron JA, Sandler RS *et al.*; Polyp Prevention Study Group (2007). Folic acid for the prevention of colorectal adenomas: a randomized clinical trial. *JAMA*, 297:2351–2359. http://dx.doi.org/10.1001/jama.297.21.2351 PMID:17551129

19. Qiao YL, Dawsey SM, Kamangar F *et al.* (2009). Total and cancer mortality after supplementation with vitamins and minerals: follow-up of the Linxian General Population Nutrition Intervention Trial. *J Natl Cancer Inst*, 101:507–518. http://dx.doi.org/10.1093/jnci/djp037 PMID:19318634

20. Blot WJ, Li JY, Taylor PR *et al.* (1993). Nutrition intervention trials in Linxian, China: supplementation with specific vitamin/mineral combinations, cancer incidence, and disease-specific mortality in the general population. *J Natl Cancer Inst*, 85:1483–1492. http://dx.doi.org/10.1093/jnci/85.18.1483 PMID:8360931

21. Gaziano JM, Sesso HD, Christen WG *et al.* (2012). Multivitamins in the prevention of cancer in men: the Physicians' Health Study II randomized controlled trial. *JAMA*, 308:1871–1880. http://dx.doi.org/10.1001/jama.2012.14641 PMID:23162860

22. Sacks FM, Bray GA, Carey VJ *et al.* (2009). Comparison of weight-loss diets with different compositions of fat, protein, and carbohydrates. *N Engl J Med*, 360:859–873. http://dx.doi.org/10.1056/NEJMoa0804748 PMID:19246357

23. Larsen TM, Dalskov SM, van Baak M *et al.*; Diet, Obesity, and Genes (Diogenes) Project (2010). Diets with high or low protein content and glycemic index for weight-loss maintenance. *N Engl J Med*, 363:2102–2113. http://dx.doi.org/10.1056/NEJMoa1007137 PMID:21105792

24. Schwarzfuchs D, Golan R, Shai I (2012). Four-year follow-up after two-year dietary interventions. *N Engl J Med*, 367:1373–1374. http://dx.doi.org/10.1056/NEJMc1204792 PMID:23034044

25. Malik VS, Hu FB (2011). Sugar-sweetened beverages and health: where does the evidence stand? *Am J Clin Nutr*, 94:1161–1162. http://dx.doi.org/10.3945/ajcn.111.025676 PMID:21993436

26. Mozaffarian D, Hao T, Rimm EB *et al.* (2011). Changes in diet and lifestyle and long-term weight gain in women and men. *N Engl J Med*, 364:2392–2404. http://dx.doi.org/10.1056/NEJMoa1014296 PMID:21696306

27. IARC (2002). IARC Handbooks of Cancer Prevention, Vol. 6: *Weight Control and Physical Activity*. Lyon: IARC.

28. Renehan AG, Tyson M, Egger M *et al.* (2008). Body-mass index and incidence of cancer: a systematic review and meta-analysis of prospective observational studies. *Lancet*, 371:569–578. http://dx.doi.org/10.1016/S0140-6736(08)60269-X PMID:18280327

29. Berrington de Gonzalez A, Hartge P, Cerhan JR *et al.* (2010). Body-mass index and mortality among 1.46 million white adults. *N Engl J Med*, 363:2211–2219. http://dx.doi.org/10.1056/NEJMoa1000367 PMID:21121834

30. Key TJ, Spencer EA, Reeves GK (2010). Obesity and cancer risk. *Proc Nutr Soc*, 69:86–90. http://dx.doi.org/10.1017/S0029665109991698 PMID:19954565

31. Calle EE, Rodriguez C, Walker-Thurmond K, Thun MJ (2003). Overweight, obesity, and mortality from cancer in a prospectively studied cohort of U.S. adults. *N Engl J Med*, 348:1625–1638. http://dx.doi.org/10.1056/NEJMoa021423 PMID:12711737

32. Byers T, Sedjo RL (2011). Does intentional weight loss reduce cancer risk? *Diabetes Obes Metab*, 13:1063–1072. http://dx.doi.org/10.1111/j.1463-1326.2011.01464.x PMID:21733057

33. Parekh N, Chandran U, Bandera EV (2012). Obesity in cancer survival. *Annu Rev Nutr*, 32:311–342. http://dx.doi.org/10.1146/annurev-nutr-071811-150713 PMID:22540252

34. Ballard-Barbash R, Friedenreich CM, Courneya KS *et al.* (2012). Physical activity, biomarkers, and disease outcomes in cancer survivors: a systematic review. *J Natl Cancer Inst*, 104:815–840. http://dx.doi.org/10.1093/jnci/djs207 PMID:22570317

2.7 Occupation

2 ETIOLOGY

Jack Siemiatycki

Dana Loomis (reviewer)
Lesley Rushton (reviewer)

Summary

- To date, 32 occupational agents as well as 11 exposure circumstances are identified as carcinogenic to humans, and an additional 27 agents and 6 exposure circumstances primarily relevant to occupational exposure are probably carcinogenic to humans.

- Workplace exposure to several well-recognized carcinogens, such as asbestos, polycyclic aromatic hydrocarbons, heavy metals, diesel engine emissions, and silica, is still widespread.

- The burden of occupational cancer among exposed groups may be substantial.

- Prevention of occupational cancer is feasible and has taken place in industrialized countries during recent decades.

- Little information is available on occupational cancer risk in low-income countries, but it can be reasonably expected to become a large problem.

From the late 18th century until the early 20th century, remarkable numbers of cases of scrotal cancer were reported among chimney sweeps, coal tar and paraffin workers, shale oil workers, and mule spinners in the cotton textile industry. Remarkable numbers of lung cancer cases were reported among metal miners, and of bladder cancer cases among workers in a plant that produced dyestuffs from coal tar. During the first half of the 20th century, there were additional reports of cancer clusters among other identifiable occupational groups. Unexpectedly high numbers of occurrences of respiratory cancer were evident in such diverse occupational settings as nickel refineries, coal carbonization processes, chromate manufacture, manufacture of sheep dip containing inorganic arsenicals, and manufacture of asbestos products [1]. Each of these discoveries was typically based on astute observation of particular cases by a clinician, followed up with rather primitive retrospective cohort studies. In most of such instances of increased risk, the relevant information concerned a particular occupation or industry, with little or no information allowing risk to be attributed to particular chemicals. These high-risk occupations constituted virtually the only known causes of human cancer until the discovery in the 1950s of the cancer-causing effects of cigarette smoking.

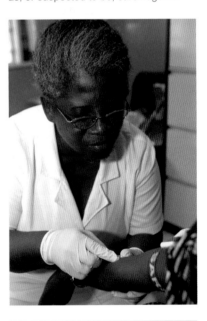

Fig. 2.7.1. A head nurse at a clinic outside Accra, Ghana, withdraws blood from a woman for an HIV test. In discharging their duties, nurses in a variety of clinical circumstances may be exposed to biological and chemical agents identified as, or suspected to be, carcinogenic.

After the discovery that cigarette smoking is a major cause of cancer, and the development of modern epidemiological and toxicological methods, much more systematic and widespread efforts were undertaken to determine the causes of cancer, and many more causes were identified, in both

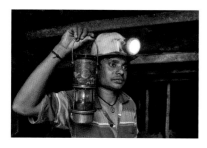

Fig. 2.7.2. A mine worker in Burdwan, India. Workers engaged in mining a range of products experience increased risk of lung cancer.

occupational and non-occupational settings. Even today, however, occupational carcinogens represent a large fraction of all known human carcinogens. Although the discovery of occupational carcinogens provides an immediate means for preventing occupational cancer, the potential benefit of such discoveries goes beyond the factory walls since most occupational carcinogens are also found in the general environment and in consumer products, sometimes at concentrations as high as those encountered in the workplace. Examples include polycyclic aromatic hydrocarbons in charcoal-broiled foods, 2-naphthylamine in tobacco smoke, asbestos fibres in poorly maintained buildings, and atmospheric pollution by diesel engine emissions, benzene, and polychlorinated biphenyls. Furthermore, research on occupational carcinogens can sometimes provide useful information for assessing risks incurred at levels found in the general environment.

Specifying occupational carcinogens

A large volume of epidemiological and experimental data concern cancer risks in different workplaces. This chapter includes a tabular summary of current knowledge on occupational carcinogens, the occupations and industries in which they are found, and their target organs [2].

Although seemingly simple, drawing up an unambiguous list of occupational carcinogens is difficult. The first source of ambiguity is the

definition of an "occupational carcinogen". Exposures to most occupational carcinogens also occur in the general environment and/or in the course of using consumer products, and reciprocally, most environmental exposures and those associated with using certain consumer products, including medications, foods, and others, also occur in some occupational context. The distinction between occupational and non-occupational exposures can be arbitrary. For instance, whereas exposures to tobacco smoke, sunlight, and immunosuppressive medications are generally not identified as occupational exposures, there are people whose occupation results in them being in contact with these agents to a degree that would not otherwise occur. Also, whereas asbestos, benzene, diesel engine emissions, and radon gas are considered to be occupational carcinogens, exposure to these agents is also experienced by the general population, and indeed many more people are probably exposed to these substances in the course of day-to-day life than are exposed at work. There is no simple criterion to distinguish "occupational" carcinogens from "non-occupational" carcinogens. Given this complexity, the following operational procedure is adopted: a carcinogen is considered to be "occupational" if the primary human exposure circumstance to the agent is in the workplace and/or if the main epidemiological studies that led to the identification of an elevated risk of cancer were undertaken among workers, and if notable numbers of workers are exposed to the agent. Even this operational definition is somewhat vague and requires judgement in its implementation.

Another source of ambiguity derives from the nature of the occupational circumstances that have been investigated. For instance, there is evidence that exposure to soot may cause skin tumours and that exposure to 2-naphthylamine may cause bladder tumours, and it is likely that the historical observations of excess risks of scrotal cancer in chimney sweeps and of bladder cancer in dye

factory workers were respectively related to these two carcinogens. If there is persuasive evidence that a given chemical or mixture is carcinogenic – soot and 2-naphthylamine, in the current example – then this may be considered a relatively established proposition, requiring consideration of the level of exposure but little else. However, the knowledge that an occupation or industry is associated with excess cancer risk is rooted in the specific time and place at which the research took place. In some instances, an occupationally characterized group may be shown to experience excess cancer risk but the causative agent is unknown, or at least unproven; examples are lung cancer among painters and bladder cancer among workers in the aluminium industry. An occupation does not in itself confer a carcinogenic risk; it is the exposures or conditions of work that may confer a risk. Thus, the statement that a given occupation involves a carcinogenic risk is potentially misleading and should be considered in light of the different exposure circumstances that may be associated with a given occupation in different times or places.

IARC Monographs

IARC Monographs provide authoritative information for compiling a list of occupational carcinogens [3]. The objective of the Monographs Programme, which has been operating

Fig. 2.7.3. A man in Uruguay wears a protective mask while spray-painting a car. Work as a painter is linked to increased risk of lung cancer and bladder cancer.

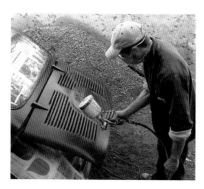

Evaluating carcinogens: dioxins and dioxin-like substances

Kurt Straif

Since 1997 [1], 2,3,7,8-tetrachlorodibenzo-*para*-dioxin (TCDD) has been classified by IARC as Group 1, carcinogenic to humans, based on limited evidence of carcinogenicity in humans, sufficient evidence in rodents, and strong evidence in humans and animals for a mechanism via initial binding to the aryl hydrocarbon receptor (AhR), which leads to changes in gene expression, cell replication, and apoptosis. Thus, TCDD was one of the first agents to be upgraded to Group 1 on the basis of mechanistic evidence (Table B2.7.1).

There is now sufficient evidence from epidemiological studies for all cancers combined, making TCDD the first agent to be classified as Group 1 initially based on strong mechanistic data and later confirmed by increased cancer risk in humans [2]. This highlights the ability of mechanistic information to provide robust evidence of carcinogenicity. Sufficient evidence for an increased risk for all cancers combined is mainly derived from heavily exposed occupational cohorts. In addition, there is limited evidence for an increased risk of lung cancer, soft-tissue sarcoma, and non-Hodgkin lymphoma.

Like TCDD, 2,3,4,7,8-pentachlorodibenzofuran and 3,3′,4,4′,5-pentachlorobiphenyl (PCB 126) are complete carcinogens in experimental animals, and there is strong evidence that they act through the same AhR-mediated mechanism. Therefore, in the context of the re-evaluation of TCDD, these two chemicals were classified as Group 1. Recognizing the complexity of the mechanistic evaluation, the IARC Monographs Volume 100F Working Group decided to make evaluations only for these two indicator chemicals, and suggested that future Monographs meetings be focused on other dioxin-like compounds.

PCB congeners can be categorized by their degree of chlorination, substitution pattern, and binding affinity to receptors. Twelve congeners with high affinity for AhR are referred to as dioxin-like PCBs. PCBs are readily absorbed and distributed in the body, and accumulate in adipose tissue. On the basis of sufficient evidence of carcinogenicity in experimental animals and humans (based on an increased risk of melanoma), PCBs were classified as Group 1 [3]. In addition, dioxin-like PCBs were also classified as Group 1 on the basis of extensive evidence of an AhR-mediated mechanism of carcinogenesis that is identical to that of TCDD, and sufficient evidence of carcinogenicity in experimental animals. It was noted that the carcinogenicity of PCBs cannot

Table B2.7.1. Evolution of evaluations of 2,3,7,8-tetrachlorodibenzo-*para*-dioxin (TCDD) and other dioxin-like compounds

IARC Monographs volume (V) or supplement (S) (year)	Agent	Degree of evidence of carcinogenicity		Overall evaluation of carcinogenicity to humans[a]
		In humans	In animals	
V7 (1974), V18 (1978), S1 (1979), S4 (1982)	Polychlorinated biphenyls	Inadequate	Sufficient	Group 2B
V15 (1977), S1 (1979)	TCDD	No overall evaluation		
V18 (1978)	Polybrominated biphenyls	No overall evaluation		
S4 (1982), S7 (1987)	TCDD	Inadequate	Sufficient	Group 2B
V41 (1986), S7 (1987)	Polybrominated biphenyls	Inadequate	Sufficient	Group 2B
S7 (1987)	Chlorinated dibenzodioxins (other than TCDD)	Inadequate	Inadequate	Group 3
S7 (1987)	Polychlorinated biphenyls	Limited	Sufficient	Group 2A
V69 (1997)	TCDD	Limited	Sufficient	Group 1[b]
V69 (1997)	Polychlorinated dibenzo-*para*-dioxins (other than TCDD)	No data	Inadequate or limited	Group 3
V69 (1997)	Polychlorinated dibenzofurans	Inadequate	Inadequate or limited	Group 3
V100F (2012)	TCDD	Sufficient	Sufficient	Group 1
V100F (2012)	3,3′,4,4′,5-Pentachlorobiphenyl (PCB 126)	Sufficient		Group 1[b]
V107 (2014)	Polychlorinated biphenyls	Sufficient	Sufficient	Group 1
V107 (2014)	Dioxin-like polychlorinated biphenyls[c]	Sufficient		Group 1[b]
V107 (2014)	Polybrominated biphenyls	Inadequate	Sufficient	Group 2A[b]

[a] Group 1, carcinogenic to humans; Group 2A, probably carcinogenic to humans; Group 2B, possibly carcinogenic to humans; Group 3, not classifiable as to its carcinogenicity to humans; Group 4, probably not carcinogenic to humans.
[b] Upgraded on the basis of mechanistic evidence.
[c] With a toxic equivalency factor (TEF) according to WHO (PCBs 77, 81, 105, 114, 118, 123, 126, 156, 157, 167, 169, 189).

be solely attributed to the carcinogenicity of the dioxin-like PCBs. Interestingly, particularly low-chlorinated PCBs also seem to act via a genotoxic mechanism. Polybrominated biphenyls (PBBs) were classified as Group 2A, probably carcinogenic to humans, taking into account

evidence of an AhR-mediated mechanism of carcinogenicity.

These evaluations refer to cancer hazard identification; the burden of cancer attributable to environmental exposures, for example via TCDD-contaminated food, is still controversial.

References

1. IARC (1997). IARC *Monogr Eval Carcinog Risks Hum*, 69:1–631. PMID:9379504

2. IARC (2012). IARC *Monogr Eval Carcinog Risks Hum*, 100F:1–599. PMID:23189753

3. Lauby-Secretan B *et al.* (2013). *Lancet Oncol*, 14:287–288. http://dx.doi.org/10.1016/S1470-2045(13)70104-9 PMID:23499544

since 1971, is to publish critical reviews of epidemiological and experimental data on carcinogenicity for chemicals, groups of chemicals, industrial processes, other complex mixtures, physical agents, and biological agents to which humans are known to be exposed, and to evaluate data indicative of carcinogenicity.

Agents are selected for evaluation on the basis of two criteria: humans are exposed to the agent, and there is reason to suspect that the agent may be carcinogenic. Direct evidence of carcinogenicity of an agent can be derived from epidemiological studies or from experimental studies of animals (usually rodents). Account may also be taken of chemical structure–activity relationships and data indicative of mechanism, including absorption and metabolism of the agent and physiological change induced, together with mutagenic, toxic, and other effects exhibited by the agent. Expert Working Groups are convened to evaluate all relevant data.

Over the past 40 years, more than 100 meetings have been convened by the IARC Monographs Programme and almost 1000 agents have been evaluated. Exposure to many such chemicals or mixtures occurs occupationally.

Occupational agents or exposure circumstances evaluated as carcinogenic or probably carcinogenic

Table 2.7.1 lists occupational agents, occupations, and industries that have been classified as Group 1, carcinogenic to humans. The table explicitly distinguishes 32 chemical or physical agents from 11 occupations and industries that involve an increased

risk of cancer but for which the responsible agent has not been specified. The overall burden of cancer caused by a given agent is a function of several factors, including the prevalence of the exposure, the type or types of cancer involved, and the relative risk of cancer induced as determined by each known exposure circumstance. Among the carcinogens listed in Table 2.7.1 that may induce the largest excess numbers of cases are asbestos, diesel engine emissions, silica, solar radiation, and second-hand tobacco smoke [4]. Some of the carcinogens listed occur naturally, such as wood dust or solar radiation, whereas some are man-made, such as 1,3-butadiene or vinyl chloride. Some are single chemical compounds, such as benzene or trichloroethylene; others are families of compounds that include some carcinogens, and still others are mixtures of varying chemical

composition, of which diesel engine emissions and mineral oils are examples. Most known human carcinogens have been established to induce only one or a few different types of cancer.

Among the occupations and industries shown in Table 2.7.1, most are industries in which the number of workers is relatively small, and so the population burden of any risk attributable to these industries would be limited, at least in developed countries. But one occupational group – painters – stands out as an occupation that is widespread on a population basis, and for which the agent or agents responsible for the excess risk of lung and bladder cancer have not been identified. Aromatic amines such as benzidine and 2-naphthylamine may be responsible for some of the excess bladder cancer risk, but the cause of excess lung cancer risk is not so readily suggested.

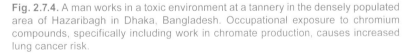

Fig. 2.7.4. A man works in a toxic environment at a tannery in the densely populated area of Hazaribagh in Dhaka, Bangladesh. Occupational exposure to chromium compounds, specifically including work in chromate production, causes increased lung cancer risk.

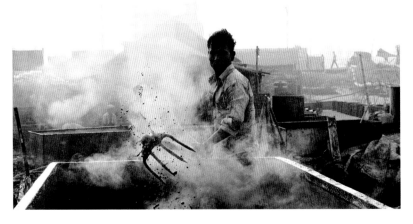

Table 2.7.1. Occupational exposures, occupations, industries, and occupational circumstances classified as definite carcinogenic exposures (Group 1) by the IARC Monographs, Volumes 1–106

Agent, occupation, or industry	Cancer site/Cancer	Main industry or use
Chemical or physical agent		
Acid mists, strong inorganic	Larynx	Chemical
4-Aminobiphenyl	Bladder	Rubber
Arsenic and inorganic arsenic compounds	Lung, skin, bladder	Glass, metals, pesticides
Asbestos (all forms)	Larynx, lung, mesothelioma, ovary	Insulation, construction, renovation
Benzene	Leukaemia	Starter and intermediate in chemical production, solvent
Benzidine	Bladder	Pigments
Benzo[a]pyrene	Lung, skin (suspected)	Coal liquefaction and gasification, coke production, coke ovens, coal-tar distillation, roofing, paving, aluminium production
Beryllium and beryllium compounds	Lung	Aerospace, metals
Bis(chloromethyl)ether; chloromethyl methyl ether	Lung	Chemical
1,3-Butadiene	Leukaemia and/or lymphoma	Plastics, rubber
Cadmium and cadmium compounds	Lung	Pigments, batteries
Chromium (VI) compounds	Lung	Metal plating, pigments
Coal-tar pitch	Lung, skin	Construction, electrodes
Diesel engine exhaust	Lung	Transportation, mining
Ethylene oxide	–	Chemical, sterilizing agent
Formaldehyde	Nasopharynx, leukaemia	Plastics, textiles
Ionizing radiation (including radon-222 progeny)	Thyroid, leukaemia, salivary gland, lung, bone, oesophagus, stomach, colon, rectum, skin, breast, kidney, bladder, brain	Radiology, nuclear industry, underground mining
Leather dust	Nasal cavity	Shoe manufacture and repair
4,4'-Methylenebis(2-chloroaniline) (MOCA)	–	Rubber
Mineral oils, untreated or mildly treated	Skin	Lubricant
2-Naphthylamine	Bladder	Pigments
Nickel compounds	Nasal cavity, lung	Metal alloy
Shale oils	Skin	Lubricant, fuel
Silica dust, crystalline, in the form of quartz or cristobalite	Lung	Construction, mining
Solar radiation	Skin	Outdoor work
Soot	Lung, skin	Chimney sweeps, masons, firefighters
2,3,7,8-Tetrachlorodibenzo-*para*-dioxin (TCDD)	–	Chemical
Tobacco smoke, second-hand	Lung	Bars, restaurants, offices
ortho-Toluidine	Bladder	Pigments
Trichloroethylene	Kidney	Solvent, dry cleaning
Vinyl chloride	Liver	Plastics
Wood dust	Nasal cavity	Wood
Occupation or industry, without specification of the responsible agent		
Aluminium production	Lung, bladder	–
Auramine production	Bladder	–
Coal gasification	Lung	–
Coal-tar distillation	Skin	–
Coke production	Lung	–
Haematite mining (underground)	Lung	–
Iron and steel founding	Lung	–
Isopropyl alcohol manufacture using strong acids	Nasal cavity	–
Magenta production	Bladder	–
Painter	Bladder, lung, mesothelioma	–
Rubber manufacture	Stomach, lung, bladder, leukaemia	–

Table 2.7.2 lists occupational agents, occupations, and industries that have been classified as Group 2A, probably carcinogenic to humans. The table explicitly distinguishes 27 chemical or physical agents from 5 occupations and industries that have been found to present a probable risk but for which a causative agent has not been identified, and the other singular occupational circumstance – shiftwork. Most agents in Table 2.7.2 are unequivocally carcinogenic in experimental animals, with little or no epidemiological evidence to confirm or contradict the evidence in animals. For a few of the agents, including lead compounds and creosotes, there is a reasonable body of epidemiological evidence. However, the evidence taken together provides *limited* evidence of carcinogenicity to humans by IARC Monographs criteria, i.e. because bias, confounding, or chance cannot be excluded as contributing to the association

Table 2.7.2. Occupational exposures, occupations, industries, and occupational circumstances classified as probable carcinogenic exposures (Group 2A) by the IARC Monographs, Volumes 1–106

Agent, occupation, or industry	Suspected target organ	Main industry or use
Chemical or physical agent		
Acrylamide	–	Plastics
Bitumens (combustion products during roofing)	Lung	Roofing
Captafol	–	Pesticide
α-Chlorinated toluenes (benzal chloride, benzotrichloride, benzyl chloride) and benzoyl chloride (combined exposures)	–	Pigments, chemicals
4-Chloro-*ortho*-toluidine	Bladder	Pigments, textiles
Cobalt metal with tungsten carbide	Lung	Hard-metal production
Creosotes	Skin	Wood
Diethyl sulfate	–	Chemical
Dimethylcarbamoyl chloride	–	Chemical
1,2-Dimethylhydrazine	–	Research
Dimethyl sulfate	–	Chemical
Epichlorohydrin	–	Plastics
Ethylene dibromide	–	Fumigant
Glycidol	–	Pharmaceutical industry
Indium phosphide	–	Semiconductors
Lead compounds, inorganic	Lung, stomach	Metals, pigments
Methyl methanesulfonate	–	Chemical
2-Nitrotoluene	–	Production of dyes
Non-arsenical insecticides	–	Agriculture
Polychlorinated biphenyls	–	Electrical components
Polycyclic aromatic hydrocarbons (several apart from benzo[a]pyrene)	Lung, skin	Coal liquefaction and gasification, coke production, coke ovens, coal-tar distillation, roofing, paving, aluminium production
Styrene-7,8-oxide	–	Plastics
Tetrachloroethylene (perchloroethylene)	–	Solvent
1,2,3-Trichloropropane	–	Solvent
Tris(2,3-dibromopropyl) phosphate	–	Plastics, textiles
Vinyl bromide	–	Plastics, textiles
Vinyl fluoride	–	Chemical
Occupation or industry, without specification of the responsible agent		
Art glass, glass containers, and pressed ware (manufacture of)	Lung, stomach	–
Carbon electrode manufacture	Lung	–
Food frying at high temperature	–	–
Hairdressers or barbers	Bladder, lung	–
Petroleum refining	–	–
Occupational circumstance, without specification of the responsible agent		
Shiftwork that involves circadian disruption	Breast	Nursing, several others

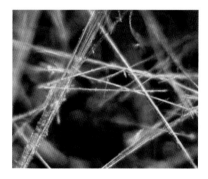

evident in epidemiological studies, or because different studies provide conflicting results.

Polycyclic aromatic hydrocarbons pose a particular challenge in the identification of occupational carcinogens. This class of chemicals includes several potent experimental carcinogens, such as benzo[a]pyrene, benz[a]anthracene, and dibenz[a,h]anthracene. However, humans are always exposed to *mixtures* of polycyclic aromatic hydrocarbons; several such mixtures are indicated in Tables 2.7.1 and 2.7.2, including coal tars, soots, and creosotes. Because of the difficulty of isolating the impact of specific polycyclic aromatic hydrocarbons in exposure assessment, it is difficult to evaluate human cancer risks associated with individual members of this class of chemicals. Only for benzo[a]pyrene has the evidence warranted a Group 1 evaluation, based on mechanistic data taken together with other available evidence, but there are probably many more individual polycyclic aromatic hydrocarbons that are carcinogenic to humans.

In the past, epidemiological research of occupational risk factors has largely focused on occupational exposures associated with "dirty" industrial environments. In recent decades, however, occupational hygiene in many industries has improved or different technology has been adopted such that the historical circumstances no longer apply, at least in developed countries. Increasing attention is now being paid to nonchemical agents in the work environment. Physical agents such as solar radiation and electromagnetic fields have been investigated, but behavioural and ergonomic characteristics of particular occupations, such as physical activity (or sedentary behaviour) are now also recognized as occupational cancer risk factors. Together with such factors may be included exposure to second-hand tobacco smoke at work. For almost all these risk factors, the distinction between occupational and non-occupational exposure is becoming more blurred. Although it is not of critical importance to maintain a clear distinction between occupational and non-occupational factors, it does facilitate communication and regulation to make this distinction, and the distinction may be critically relevant to controlling the exposure in question.

Industries and occupations are constantly evolving. Even if we knew all there was to know about the cancer risks in today's occupational environments – which we do not – continuing to monitor cancer risks in occupational settings would remain an important activity because occupational exposure circumstances change over time and novel exposures may be introduced; a recent example is exposure to nanoparticles.

Although the lists of occupational carcinogens and associated exposures shown in Tables 2.7.1 and 2.7.2 are long, they are not complete. There are likely many more occupational carcinogens that have not been discovered or properly documented. For many, if not most, occupational circumstances, there is no relevant epidemiological evidence about carcinogenic risk. One of the foremost problems in occupational epidemiology is to reveal as-yet-unrecognized carcinogens and carcinogenic risks.

Since the revolution in genetic research methods, there has been a shift in research resources on occupational cancer, from an attempt to assess the main effects of occupations and occupational exposures to an attempt to assess genetic risk factors or, at best, gene–environment interactions. This is an interesting and worthwhile pursuit, but it has not yet led to a proportionate increase in knowledge of new carcinogens. It remains the case that almost all the knowledge that has accrued about occupational risk factors has been gained without recourse to genetic data.

Estimates of the burden of occupational carcinogens

Over the years, there have been multiple attempts, sometimes accompanied by controversy, to estimate what proportion of cancer cases are attributable to occupation. Estimating attributable fractions is feasible when the exposure factor is well defined and there is a body of evidence to support estimates of the magnitude of risk associated with the risk factor and the prevalence of exposure to the risk factor in the population, such as is the case for cigarette smoking.

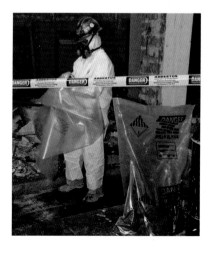

Preventing occupational cancer: successes and failures

Lesley Rushton

Approaches to preventing workplace exposures to occupational carcinogens and reduction of occupational cancer include eliminating the production or use of carcinogens and controlling exposure to below a minimal risk exposure level, for example an occupational exposure limit (OEL). Examples of potential control measures are given in Table B2.7.2. All routes of exposure need to be considered, and control measures should not themselves cause additional hazards.

Current occupational cancer is due to past exposures, sometimes over many years, and because of the long latency of many cancers, these (often high) exposures will contribute to substantial occupational cancers 20–30 years in the future [1]. Exposure to many established occupational carcinogens has gradually decreased over time in high-income countries due to an overall decline in heavy manufacturing industry and to regulatory activity and resulting risk reduction controls [2,3]. Some exposures will rapidly disappear in the future – for example, second-hand smoke, as the willingness of society to accept a ban on workplace smoking increases.

There has been mixed success in reducing other important exposures, such as asbestos, a major contributor to the total occupational cancer burden. Increasing calls for a total ban on asbestos production and use contrast with continuing mining and widespread use of products containing chrysotile asbestos (an IARC Group 1 carcinogen), particularly in developing countries.

In some circumstances, it can be demonstrated that certain risk reduction strategies, such as improvement of compliance with a current OEL (e.g. for silica exposure) and targeting small- and medium-sized industries, would be more effective than other measures, such as OEL reduction [1]. Similar strategies may be relevant in many rapidly industrializing countries.

Reduction of high levels of exposure to occupational carcinogens remains an urgent priority in low- and middle-income countries, where the newest technology may be unavailable, there is little or no regulation, and many may be employed in small workplaces, including children. Appropriate adaptation of effective regulation and control measures to different circumstances is required. However, the large numbers of workers who continue to be exposed to low levels of occupational carcinogens and who will contribute to the total occupational cancer burden must not be forgotten. Female workers are particularly affected; many are employed in service industries where low levels of many carcinogens, including asbestos, occur. Concurrent exposure to multiple carcinogens is of concern. Protection measures for one carcinogen may also simultaneously reduce others – for example, measures to reduce general dust; these will also potentially reduce non-malignant occupational disease, such as respiratory ill health. A concerted international effort is required to prioritize strategies to reduce occupational cancer in all workplaces where exposure to known carcinogens is still occurring.

References

1. Hutchings SJ et al. (2012). Cancer Prev Res (Phila), 5:1213–1222. http://dx.doi.org/10.1158/1940-6207.CAPR-12-0070 PMID:22961776

2. Cherrie JW (2009). Occup Med (Lond), 59:96–100. http://dx.doi.org/10.1093/occmed/kqn172 PMID:19233829

3. Symanski E et al. (1998). Occup Environ Med, 55:310–316. http://dx.doi.org/10.1136/oem.55.5.310 PMID:9764108

Table B2.7.2. Measures to control workplace exposures to occupational carcinogens

Reduction method	Examples of good practice
Worker education	Provide information and training on all workplace carcinogens and the use of appropriate control methods. Use information media (e.g. posters, leaflets, data sheets) imaginatively and strategically.
Safer occupational practices	Design and operate effective and reliable processes and activities to minimize exposure. Provide safe storage, handling, transportation, and disposal facilities. Use suitable personal protective equipment.
Surveillance	Design and use procedures for regular measuring and monitoring of carcinogens in the workplace, including accidental high exposures.

None of these conditions exist for the generic class of occupational exposures. Apart from the difficulty of establishing an unequivocal list of occupational carcinogens, there are many obstacles to deriving reliable estimates of attributable fractions for this class of carcinogens. These include the incompleteness of lists of occupational carcinogens, meagre information on quantitative relative risks associated with exposure to known carcinogens, and scant information on the prevalence of exposure, both historically and quantitatively, among workers. Furthermore, as with any estimates of attributable fractions, the results are rooted in the time and place at which estimates of exposure prevalence are estimated. Still, by way of illustration, recent estimates have been in the range of 4–8% of all cancers attributable to occupational cancer risk factors in developed countries [5,6,7], with higher fractions for lung cancer than for other cancers [6]. Estimates for other areas of the world are more speculative [8].

In developed countries, the heyday of dirty, smoky industrial workplaces was the first half of the 20th century. As a result of many social, economic, and technological forces in the past 50 years, in developed countries there have been declines both in the numbers of workers involved in "dirty" blue-collar work and in the concentration levels of pollutants in typical workplaces. In developing countries, however, the picture is reversed. There, industrial activities have undergone rapid growth, often in the absence of meaningful occupational hygiene control measures. Nor is there an infrastructure to conduct research into possible hazards in those environments. If the occupational environment in developing countries continues to be poorly regulated, a significant increase in occupational cancer

there may be expected in the coming decades.

Prevention

The designation of an agent as carcinogenic is an important public health statement, as well as a scientific one. Such a designation usually has implications for engineering and/or industrial hygiene measures to reduce or eliminate occupational exposure to the agent. There are many possible ways in which exposure to an agent may be prevented or at least reduced, depending on the agent and the nature of the industrial or occupational process in which the agent is used or produced (see "Preventing occupational cancer: successes and failures"). Sometimes one or another of the following classes of measures can be adopted: substitution of one type of raw material for another, modification or mechanization of an industrial process, and/or improved ventilation and/or the use of personal protective equipment. In addition to protecting workers, the designation of a carcinogen may trigger the need to exercise better control of emissions of that carcinogen into the atmo-

sphere, water, or soil, or changes to policies for marketing consumer and other products.

All of these policies and procedures would be facilitated through precise and reliable data on the magnitude of risks associated with different agents, and on the nature of dose–response relationships. Unfortunately, such information is not always available, or not in a form that facilitates intervention. Even the qualitative assessment of carcinogenicity is often rendered difficult by the fragility of data on exposure histories of workers. For quantitative risk estimation, the data sources are even more fragile, especially as the statistical modelling often requires an estimate of the exposure situation in the remote past. Thus, even if certain workers are known to have experienced an excess risk of cancer in the past, it is challenging to derive reliable estimates as to whether current workers, known to be exposed to different, often lower, levels of specified agents, would also be at risk. Equally challenging is the goal of determining a level of exposure such that carcinogenic risk is virtually eliminated.

References

1. Siemiatycki J, Richardson L, Boffetta P (2006). Occupation. In: Schottenfeld D, Fraumeni JF, Jr., eds. *Cancer Epidemiology and Prevention*, 3rd ed. New York: Oxford University Press, pp. 322–354.

2. Siemiatycki J, Richardson L, Straif K et al. (2004). Listing occupational carcinogens. *Environ Health Perspect*, 112:1447–1459. http://dx.doi.org/10.1289/ehp.7047 PMID:15531427

3. IARC Monographs on the Evaluation of Carcinogenic Risks to Humans. http://monographs.iarc.fr/

4. Rushton L, Bagga S, Bevan R et al. (2010). Occupation and cancer in Britain. *Br J Cancer*, 102:1428–1437. http://dx.doi.org/10.1038/sj.bjc.6605637 PMID:20424618

5. Nurminen M, Karjalainen A (2001). Epidemiologic estimate of the proportion of fatalities related to occupational factors in Finland. *Scand J Work Environ Health*, 27:161–213. http://dx.doi.org/10.5271/sjweh.605 PMID:11444413

6. Steenland K, Burnett C, Lalich N et al. (2003). Dying for work: the magnitude of US mortality from selected causes of death associated with occupation. *Am J Ind Med*, 43:461–482. http://dx.doi.org/10.1002/ajim.10216 PMID:12704620

7. Rushton L, Hutchings SJ, Fortunato L et al. (2012). Occupational cancer burden in Great Britain. *Br J Cancer*, 107 Suppl 1:S3–S7. http://dx.doi.org/10.1038/bjc.2012.112 PMID:22710676

8. Driscoll T, Nelson DI, Steenland K et al. (2005). The global burden of disease due to occupational carcinogens. *Am J Ind Med*, 48:419–431. http://dx.doi.org/10.1002/ajim.20209 PMID:16299703

2.8 Radiation: ionizing, ultraviolet, and electromagnetic

2 ETIOLOGY

Ausrele Kesminiene
Joachim Schüz

Bruce K. Armstrong (reviewer)
Sarah C. Darby (reviewer)

Summary

- Exposure to all types of ionizing radiation, from both natural and man-made sources, increases the risk of various types of malignancy; the risk is higher if the exposure occurs early in life.

- Cancer incidence rates among irradiated patients, workers in nuclear plants, and others underpin current consensus on the absence of a threshold for the induction of cancers by radiation and presumption of a linear dose–response relationship.

- Exposure to ultraviolet radiation – both from the sun and from tanning devices – is established to cause all types of skin cancers, including melanoma. Public health campaigns discourage deliberate sun exposure and specify options for sun protection.

- Associations between extremely low-frequency magnetic fields and cancer are restricted to increased risk of childhood leukaemia, where a causal relationship has not been recognized.

- Associations between heavy use of mobile phones and certain brain cancers have been observed, but causal interpretation is controversial; more data are needed, particularly on longer-term use of mobile phones.

Natural and man-made sources generate radiant energy in the form of electromagnetic waves. These are characterized by their wavelength, frequency, or photon energy. The electromagnetic spectrum extends from static (non-alternating) electric and magnetic fields to low-frequency electric and magnetic fields (low energy; long wavelength), intermediate and radiofrequency electromagnetic fields, microwaves, optical radiation

Fig. 2.8.1. The electromagnetic spectrum. The diagram shows several important divisions based on the properties and applications of the different frequencies: pale blue, extremely low-frequency; orange, radiofrequency; green, microwave; red, infrared; dark blue, ultraviolet; yellow, X-ray.

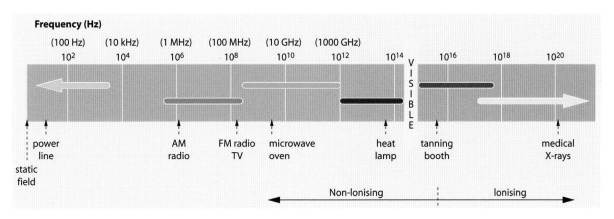

(infrared, visible light, ultraviolet radiation), and ionizing radiation (high energy; very short wavelength) (Fig. 2.8.1). The interaction of various types of radiation with biological systems is generally well understood on a cellular level and, when established, is determined by the intensity of the radiation, the related energy, and the energy absorbed by the exposed tissue. Ionizing radiation and ultraviolet radiation are known to cause cancer, but questions remain about dose-related effects, susceptibility, and mechanisms.

Ionizing radiation

By definition, ionizing radiation is sufficiently energetic to remove otherwise tightly bound electrons from atoms. Such radiation can be in the form of electromagnetic rays, such as X-rays or γ-rays, or in the form of subatomic or related particles, such as protons or neutrons, as well as α-particles and β-particles. Human exposure to environmental ionizing radiation is unavoidable [1].

Sources and exposures

Natural radiation

For the vast majority of people, exposure from natural sources accounts for most of the total annual dose of ionizing radiation (Fig. 2.8.2). The two major sources of natural radiation are cosmic rays and radionuclides originating from the Earth's crust, radiation from which is referred to as terrestrial radiation. Radionuclides are everywhere – in the ground, rocks, building materials, and drinking-water, as well as in the human body itself (sometimes designated as internal sources). Inhalation of radon gas, which arises from the decay of radium-226, is the leading source of natural ionizing radiation exposure in humans, and this source is responsible for nearly half of the average annual dose.

Man-made sources

The greatest contribution to ionizing radiation exposure from man-made sources is medical radiation. Other

Fig. 2.8.2. Annual per capita effective dose of ionizing radiation to the global population (1997–2007) due to all sources, in millisievert (mSv). Per caput, per unit of population.

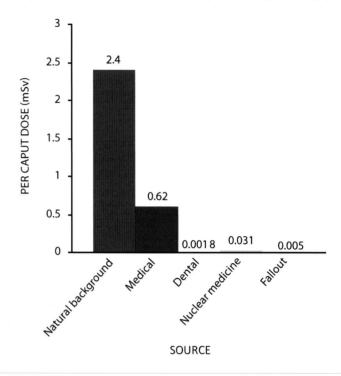

man-made sources of exposure include consumer products, fallout from weapons testing, nuclear accidents (as exemplified by the Chernobyl disaster), routine releases from nuclear installations, and occupational exposure. Exposures in the course of medical care arise from certain diagnostic procedures, such as radiography and computed tomography (CT), or as a consequence of treatment, most commonly during radiotherapy for cancer. In high-income countries, medical radiation exposure is increasing rapidly due to expansion in use of CT, angiography, and radiographically controlled interventional procedures. In some countries, average exposure from medical radiation now exceeds that from natural sources.

Cancer causation

Ionizing radiation is one of the most intensely studied carcinogens [1]. Evidence that ionizing radiation can cause human cancer has come from the follow-up of patients therapeutically irradiated for cancer

and for non-malignant conditions including ankylosing spondylitis and tinea capitis. This evidence is complemented by epidemiological studies involving people exposed to ionizing radiation as a result of nuclear accidents and atmospheric nuclear test sites and, most notably, thermonuclear warfare in the Japanese cities of Hiroshima and Nagasaki. Lately, evidence on the carcinogenic effects of ionizing radiation has emerged from studies on populations with protracted low-dose radiation exposures in occupational settings and also from patients who have undergone medical diagnostic procedures. These data are matched by tumorigenesis evident in animal bioassays.

A variety of mechanistic investigations have been made to evaluate the effects of different types of ionizing radiation, centred on the effects of variation in dose and exposure pattern, and with reference to cellular and molecular end-points. The energy-deposition characteristics of all sources of ionizing radiation cover a wide variety of molecular damage, specifically indicating DNA damage as the biological determinant of outcome from exposure [2,3]. However, only a small fraction of such changes result in malignant transformation. The processes through which cells harbouring DNA damage may give rise to neoplasia are not fully understood, although a basis for mutation is evident. However, demonstration of epigenetic effects and the role played by genomic instability and effects evident in surrounding cells not subject to radiation damage, so-called bystander effects, all attest to biological complexity. In addition, host factors such as age, sex, immune status, and genetic variations in specific genes may determine susceptibility.

X-radiation and γ-radiation
The study of the survivors of the thermonuclear bombings in Hiroshima and Nagasaki holds an important place in radiation epidemiology. The survivors were exposed primarily to γ-radiation, although there was also a neutron contribution. Leukaemia was the first cancer consequent upon the radiation exposure in this cohort [4] and exhibited the highest relative risk – more than 5-fold – of any cancer. Analyses of leukaemia mortality during 1950–2000 established that the excess risk was largest among those exposed at younger ages, but the risk decreased more rapidly than for those exposed later in life [5]. Approximately 11% of the solid cancer cases among survivors of detonations who were exposed to 0.005 Gy or more are thought to have been caused by the radiation. Significant radiation-associated increases in incidence occurred for multiple cancers, including those of the oral cavity, oesophagus, stomach, colon, lung, breast, bladder, nervous system, and thyroid, as well as non-melanoma skin cancer [6].

In a large IARC study of nuclear industry workers from 15 countries exposed to protracted low-dose radiation, a statistically significant positive dose–response association was evident for lung cancer mortality; no other specific cancer category demonstrated a statistically significant dose–response trend [7]. A study of the United Kingdom National Registry for Radiation Workers, which included many workers from the 15-country study but with a longer period of observation, found a positive association between radiation dose and mortality due to leukaemia excluding chronic lymphocytic leukaemia, and also between radiation dose and mortality due to all malignant neoplasms excluding leukaemia. Similar results were recorded in analyses of incidence of leukaemia and all malignant neoplasms [8].

Excesses of childhood leukaemia incidence in populations near nuclear installations in the United Kingdom, Germany, France, and other countries have been recorded [9], but in the absence of information on other major causes of childhood leukaemia, which might confound possible exposure to ionizing radiation in these environments, the correct interpretation of these findings is problematic [10].

Recent increases in the rates of CT use, which account for relatively high radiation doses in a broad cross-section of the community compared with doses attributable to conventional radiography, have raised health concerns despite the substantial immediate benefit of such scans to the individual patient when clinically indicated. In 2012, the first results were published from a historical cohort study of more than 175 000 patients without previous cancer diagnoses who were examined with CT scans in Great Britain [11]. The study reported a positive association between radiation dose from CT scans and leukaemia and brain tumours. Potential increases in future cancer risk, attributable to the rapid expansion in CT use, have encouraged the design of new CT scanners with dose-reduction options, as well as increased awareness among medical practitioners of the need to limit use of CT scans to situations involving a clear medical benefit and to optimize CT radiation doses, particularly for paediatric patients. Optimization involves keeping radiation exposure as low as reasonably achievable for every examination. Various modality- and procedure-specific techniques are available, although they are not always used.

Fig. 2.8.3. A technician at the University of Washington Medical Center, in Seattle, prepares a patient for a positron emission tomography-computed tomography (PET-CT) scan.

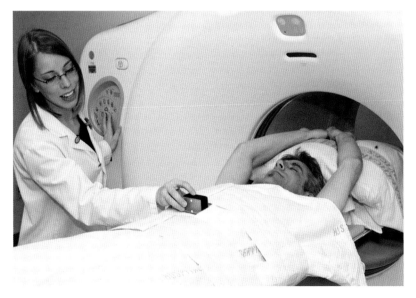

An IARC announcement that made waves

Robert A. Baan

In the early evening of Tuesday 31 May 2011, a Working Group of experts invited by the IARC Monographs Programme concluded what had become widely known as the "mobile phone radiation meeting". Although the Working Group decided on a broad evaluation of "radiofrequency electromagnetic fields" – placing this agent in Group 2B, possibly carcinogenic to humans – the post-meeting media attention was focused almost exclusively on two sets of epidemiological data that showed a slight increase in the risk for glioma – a malignant type of brain cancer – among heavy users of wireless and cordless telephones. With 6 billion such users across the globe, never in the history of the IARC Monographs had an evaluation touched so many.

Indeed, the highest human exposure to radiofrequency radiation comes from a functioning mobile phone held against the ear during a voice call. Holding a mobile phone against the head can result in relatively high exposures in the brain, depending on the position of the phone and its antenna, and the quality of the link with the base station: the better the connection, the lower the energy output from the phone. It is of interest to note that modern, third-generation (3G) phones emit, on average, about 1% of the energy emitted by the GSM (2G) phones that were in use when the above-mentioned epidemiological studies were conducted.

Also considered by the Working Group – but not mentioned in the media – were single-study findings of leukaemia or lymphoma among workers in plastic sealing and in radar maintenance, where exposures to radiofrequency fields are relatively high as well. In addition, studies in experimental animals showed effects with a variety of exposure scenarios and frequency ranges, which led the Working Group to decide not to limit the evaluation to the two narrow frequency bands used for wireless communication, but to define the agent as "radiofrequency electromagnetic fields". This being so, the hazard evaluation also encompasses exposures associated with, for example, base-station antennae, local area networks (Wi-Fi), radio or television broadcast antennae, and smart meters. Because exposures in these cases are 3–4 orders of magnitude lower than those from mobile phones, the ensuing risk from these sources is likely to be much less. Nonetheless, this latter point has remained a major issue in the continuing debate since the IARC evaluation was announced.

Prospective epidemiological studies – with accurate exposure assessment – still in progress now focus on possible effects of mobile phone use, also among youngsters. A large cancer bioassay in rodents is being conducted by the United States National Toxicology Program. Also, the search for a plausible mechanism continues, seeking complementary information to that from the epidemiological findings.

References

Baan R *et al.* (2011). *Lancet Oncol*, 12:624–626. http://dx.doi.org/10.1016/S1470-2045 (11)70147-4 PMID:21845765

IARC (2013). *IARC Monogr Eval Carcinog Risks Hum*, 102:1–460.

Internalized radionuclides
Internalized radionuclides that emit α-particles and β-particles are also carcinogenic to humans. For most people, exposure to ionizing radiation from inhaled and tissue-deposited radionuclides is mainly from naturally occurring radon-222. The epidemiological evidence that radon is a cause of lung cancer in humans is derived largely from cohort studies of underground miners who were exposed to high levels of radon in the past [12]. Evidence has subsequently emerged from case–control studies in North America, Europe [13], and China [14] that environmental radon exposure in buildings, and especially in homes, acts as a cause of lung cancer in the general population. Until recently, naturally occurring radiation was perceived as unalterable. However, it has now been shown that low radon concentrations can usually be achieved very cheaply if appropriate radon control measures are installed in new buildings. Several national programmes and international recommendations, including a WHO Handbook [15], were designed to provide recommendations on reducing cancer risk from radon, together with policy options.

Another source of exposure to internalized radionuclides for relevant workers and for the general community has been the occurrence of accidents and other releases from nuclear power plants. The largest nuclear accident in history occurred on 26 April 1986 at the Chernobyl nuclear plant in northern Ukraine. The Chernobyl accident resulted in a large release of radionuclides – of which the most important were iodine-131 and caesium-137 – that were deposited over a very wide area, particularly in Belarus, the western part of the Russian Federation, and Ukraine. In a large case–control study [16], exposure to iodine-131 in childhood was associated with an increased risk of thyroid cancer: for a dose of 1 Gy, the estimated odds ratio of thyroid cancer varied from 5.5 (95% confidence interval [CI], 3.1–9.5) to 8.4 (95% CI, 4.1–17.3), depending on the risk model.

Ultraviolet radiation

Sources and exposures
Solar radiation is the main source of human exposure to ultraviolet radiation. In addition to this natural source,

University of Chester Seaborne Library

Title: World cancer report 2014 / edited by
Bernard W. Stewart and Christopher P.
Wild
ID: 36200950
Due: 11 Jan 2016

Total items: 1
02/12/2015 16:1.

Renew online at
http://libcat.chester.ac.uk/patroninfo

Thank you for using Self Check

71

tanning lamps and beds are a common source of exposure. Ultraviolet radiation is conventionally classified into three types: UVA (wavelengths of 315–400 nm), UVB (280–315 nm), and UVC (100–280 nm). An intact ozone layer in the atmosphere absorbs almost all UVC, as well as approximately 90% of UVB. Because UVA radiation is less blocked by the ozone layer, the radiation reaching the Earth's surface is largely composed of UVA (95%), with just 5% UVB. The level of solar ultraviolet radiation exposure at the Earth's surface varies with latitude, altitude, time of day, time of year, cloud cover, other atmospheric factors (specifically including air pollution), and reflection from nearby surfaces (e.g. snow, water). Tanning lamps and beds emit mainly UVA, with less than 5% UVB. Powerful tanning equipment may be a source 10–15 times as intense as midday sunlight on the Mediterranean Sea [17].

The most common acute skin reaction induced by exposure to ultraviolet radiation is erythema (skin reddening), an inflammatory process in the skin, commonly called sunburn; tanning is another response. Tanning of the skin is predominantly triggered by DNA damage induced by ultraviolet radiation. UVB is far more efficient than UVA in inducing a deep, persistent tan and is 1000 times as potent as UVA in inducing sunburn. Individual reactions to ultraviolet radiation depend highly on skin type, as classified by individuals' susceptibility to sunburn and tanning. Generally, people with fair skin are more susceptible to sunburn and are less likely to develop a tan than people with olive or darker skin. A tan provides some protection against acute effects, and probably chronic effects, of sun exposure. Exposure to ultraviolet radiation also involves beneficial health effects. Photosynthesis mediated by sunlight is the most common source of vitamin D; however, it appears that rather modest amounts of sun exposure are needed to increase vitamin D levels sufficiently [18].

Cancer causation

Exposure to sunlight has been shown to be the main cause of skin cancer, including cutaneous malignant melanoma, basal cell carcinoma, and squamous cell carcinoma [19]. Epidemiological evidence has established that sunbed use also increases skin cancer risk [17]. In 2009, radiation from tanning devices was classified as carcinogenic to humans (Group 1) [1], the same as the earlier evaluation of solar radiation.

Although basal cell carcinoma and squamous cell carcinoma represent the most frequent types of skin cancer and contribute to the rising morbidity, cutaneous melanoma causes most skin cancer deaths because of its greater tendency to metastasize. Over the past 50 years, the incidence of all skin cancer types has steeply increased in Caucasian populations worldwide, with highest incidence rates where fair-skinned populations are exposed to intense ultraviolet radiation in countries such as Australia [20]. Individual risk varies widely, depending on environment, behaviour, and genetic constitution. In addition to ultraviolet radiation, a sun-sensitive phenotype and other genetically determined characteristics influence risk of skin cancer. Melanoma at younger ages occurs mainly at body sites with intermittent sun exposure, whereas in older people, who experience melanoma more frequently on the head and neck, risk is thought be more closely related to chronic exposure [21]. Findings from seminal migrant studies indicate that childhood is a susceptible period for ultraviolet carcinogenesis. Risk of squamous cell carcinoma occurrence is related to the total cumulative lifetime solar exposure, whereas that for basal cell carcinoma is more complicated and is suggested to be more strongly associated with intermittent exposure to ultraviolet radiation.

Prevention

The first sun protection activities were initiated in Australia in the 1960s. In the early 1980s, the primary prevention campaign "Slip! Slop!

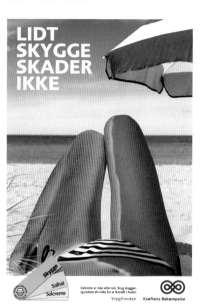

Fig. 2.8.4. Danish Cancer Society and TrygFonden campaign for the prevention of skin cancer (2013): "A little shade does not hurt. Reduce your sun between 12 and 3 pm. Sunscreen is not always enough. Use the shade and reduce your risk of skin cancer."

Slap!" was introduced, advising people to slip on a shirt, slop on the sunscreen, and slap on a hat. In 1988, the more comprehensive and broad-based skin cancer prevention programme SunSmart was implemented. Comparable activities, including education programmes and public awareness campaigns, were implemented starting in the mid-1980s in the USA and in several European countries (Fig. 2.8.4). Several organizations, including WHO, have developed recommendations about indoor tanning. Some jurisdictions have established laws banning provision of commercial sunbed services to those under 18 years old.

Electric, magnetic, and electromagnetic fields

Sources and exposures

Ubiquitous exposure occurs to extremely low-frequency electromagnetic fields due to power transmission and the use of electrical appliances, and to fields in the radiofrequency range due to communication

Fig. 2.8.5. Comparison of results from pooled analyses of epidemiological studies of residential exposure to extremely low-frequency magnetic fields and the risk of childhood cancer: (A) childhood leukaemia [23]; (B,C) childhood leukaemia [24], excluding (B) and including (C) a study from Brazil; and (D) childhood brain tumours [25]. Pooled odds ratios and their 95% confidence intervals (vertical axis) are shown by increasing levels of exposure to extremely low-frequency magnetic fields (reference category, < 0.1 µT).

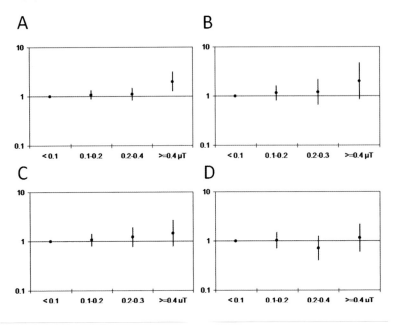

and broadcasting. Normal residential background exposure to extremely low-frequency magnetic fields is usually below 0.1 µT. A small fraction of households located very close to high-voltage power lines or other sources can have appreciably higher background exposures. Higher but short-term exposures occur when electrical devices are used and may also be experienced in particular categories of work, such as by electricians and electrical engineers. For most people, the highest exposure to radiofrequency electromagnetic fields occurs when using mobile (cell) phones because the source of emission is held close to the head. Much lower levels of exposure arise from transmitters, but field strength may exceed 1 V/m even at points several kilometres from high-output television or radio broadcast transmitters. The number of sources continues to increase with further use of the whole electromagnetic frequency spectrum.

Cancer risk

Studies have been conducted in residential settings by investigating cancer risk in relation to the nearest overhead high-voltage power lines and the resulting magnetic fields, as well as in occupational settings that involve electrical work. Epidemiological studies have consistently recorded a positive association of extremely low-frequency magnetic fields with childhood leukaemia, with an apparently 2-fold higher risk at average 24-hour exposure levels exceeding 0.3–0.4 µT (Fig. 2.8.5) [22–25]. However, a causal relationship has not been established due to the potential for bias and confounding in the observational studies and because supporting evidence from experimental studies and mechanistic data are lacking [26]. If a causal association did exist, it is estimated that < 1–4% of childhood leukaemia cases could be attributable to exposure to extremely low-frequency magnetic fields [27]. The 2001 IARC Monograph on extremely

low-frequency magnetic fields classified them as possibly carcinogenic to humans (Group 2B); the evidence for other types of malignancy was evaluated to be inadequate. Other reviews came to similar conclusions later [22,28]. Recent studies have not shown an effect of exposure to extremely low-frequency magnetic fields on survival after childhood leukaemia [29].

In the 2001 IARC Monograph evaluation, extremely low-frequency *electric* fields and static electric and magnetic fields were considered not classifiable as to their carcinogenicity to humans (Group 3). Since 2001, there have been few studies relevant to these evaluations and none suggest a basis for re-evaluation, as recently reflected by an expert panel of the European Commission [28].

Radiofrequency electromagnetic fields have been classified as possibly carcinogenic to humans (Group 2B) (see "An IARC announcement that made waves") (Fig. 2.8.6). Case–control studies on mobile phone use and cancer have reported increased risks of glioma and acoustic neuroma in heavy users of mobile phones [30]. A large Danish nationwide cohort study of mobile phone subscribers did not reveal any association with brain tumour risk. Such an increased risk was suggested from a series of interrelated case–control studies in 13 countries, Interphone, in which a 40% increased risk for glioma and also for acoustic neuroma was observed, restricted to the 10% of people who were the heaviest users of mobile phones. Several factors, including inaccuracy and evidence of bias in self-reported use, prevented causality being established by these studies [31]. Time trends in glioma incidence based on Nordic countries and the USA exclude any large increase in incidence attributable to mobile phone use, albeit with reference to a relatively short time from initiation of exposure. No association was observed between mobile phone use and other cancers. Several studies on occupational

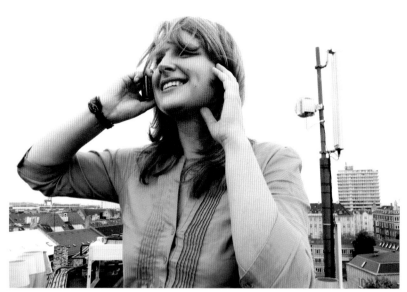

Fig. 2.8.6. Mobile phone use has become very popular over the past few decades. Studies have been done mainly in relation to mobile phone use causing radiofrequency electromagnetic field exposure to the head.

exposure to radiofrequency electromagnetic fields provide no consistent associations. With regard to environmental exposures from transmitters, including television, radio, and military transmissions as well as mobile phone networks, the evidence is inadequate due to lack of high-quality studies with accurate individual exposure assessment. Some large studies on childhood cancer and fields generated by high-output television and/or radio transmitters reported inconsistent or no associations [22]. Few data are available for electromagnetic fields in the intermediate frequency range [28].

References

1. IARC (2012). Radiation. IARC *Monogr Eval Carcinog Risks Hum*, 100D:1–437. PMID:23189752

2. UN Scientific Committee on the Effects of Atomic Radiation (UNSCEAR) (2000). *Sources and Effects of Ionizing Radiation, Vol. I: Sources*. New York: UN.

3. UN Scientific Committee on the Effects of Atomic Radiation (UNSCEAR) (2000). *Sources and Effects of Ionizing Radiation, Vol. II: Effects*. New York: UN.

4. Folley JH, Borges W, Yamawaki T (1952). Incidence of leukemia in survivors of the atomic bomb in Hiroshima and Nagasaki, Japan. *Am J Med*, 13:311–321. http://dx.doi.org/10.1016/0002-9343(52)90285-4 PMID:12985588

5. Preston DL, Pierce DA, Shimizu Y *et al.* (2004). Effect of recent changes in atomic bomb survivor dosimetry on cancer mortality risk estimates. *Radiat Res*, 162:377–389. http://dx.doi.org/10.1667/RR3232 PMID:15447045

6. Preston DL, Ron E, Tokuoka S *et al.* (2007). Solid cancer incidence in atomic bomb survivors: 1958–1998. *Radiat Res*, 168:1–64. http://dx.doi.org/10.1667/RR0763.1 PMID:17722996

7. Cardis E, Vrijheid M, Blettner M *et al.* (2007). The 15-country collaborative study of cancer risk among radiation workers in the nuclear industry: estimates of radiation-related cancer risks. *Radiat Res*, 167:396–416. http://dx.doi.org/10.1667/RR0553.1 PMID:17388693

8. Muirhead CR, O'Hagan JA, Haylock RG *et al.* (2009). Mortality and cancer incidence following occupational radiation exposure: third analysis of the National Registry for Radiation Workers. *Br J Cancer*, 100:206–212. http://dx.doi.org/10.1038/sj.bjc.6604825 PMID:19127272

9. Laurier D, Jacob S, Bernier MO *et al.* (2008). Epidemiological studies of leukaemia in children and young adults around nuclear facilities: a critical review. *Radiat Prot Dosimetry*, 132:182–190. http://dx.doi.org/10.1093/rpd/ncn262 PMID:18922823

10. Wakeford R (2013). The risk of childhood leukaemia following exposure to ionising radiation–a review. *J Radiol Prot*, 33:1–25. http://dx.doi.org/10.1088/0952-4746/33/1/1 PMID:23296257

11. Pearce MS, Salotti JA, Little MP *et al.* (2012). Radiation exposure from CT scans in childhood and subsequent risk of leukaemia and brain tumours: a retrospective cohort study. *Lancet*, 380:499–505. http://dx.doi.org/10.1016/S0140-6736(12)60815-0 PMID:22681860

12. BEIR VI (1999). *Health Effects of Exposure to Radon*. Washington, DC: National Academy Press.

13. Darby S, Hill D, Deo H *et al.* (2006). Residential radon and lung cancer – detailed results of a collaborative analysis of individual data on 7148 persons with lung cancer and 14,208 persons without lung cancer from 13 epidemiologic studies in Europe. *Scand J Work Environ Health*, 32 Suppl 1:1–83. PMID:16538937

14. Lubin JH, Wang ZY, Boice JD Jr *et al.* (2004). Risk of lung cancer and residential radon in China: pooled results of two studies. *Int J Cancer*, 109:132–137. http://dx.doi.org/10.1002/ijc.11683 PMID:14735479

15. WHO (2009). *WHO Handbook on Indoor Radon: A Public Health Perspective*. Geneva: WHO.

16. Cardis E, Kesminiene A, Ivanov V *et al.* (2005). Risk of thyroid cancer after exposure to ^{131}I in childhood. *J Natl Cancer Inst*, 97:724–732. http://dx.doi.org/10.1093/jnci/dji129 PMID:15900042

17. Boniol M, Autier P, Boyle P, Gandini S (2012). Cutaneous melanoma attributable to sunbed use: systematic review and meta-analysis. *BMJ*, 345:e4757. http://dx.doi.org/10.1136/bmj.e4757 PMID:22833605

18. Webb AR, Kift R, Durkin MT *et al.* (2010). The role of sunlight exposure in determining the vitamin D status of the U.K. white adult population. *Br J Dermatol*, 163:1050–1055. http://dx.doi.org/10.1111/j.1365-2133.2010.09975.x PMID:20716215

19. MacKie RM, Hauschild A, Eggermont AM (2009). Epidemiology of invasive cutaneous melanoma. *Ann Oncol*, 20 Suppl 6:vi1–vi7. http://dx.doi.org/10.1093/annonc/mdp252 PMID:19617292

20. Erdmann F, Lortet-Tieulent J, Schüz J *et al.* (2013). International trends in the incidence of malignant melanoma 1953–2008 – are recent generations at higher or lower risk? *Int J Cancer*, 132:385–400. http://dx.doi.org/10.1002/ijc.27616 PMID:22532371

21. Whiteman DC, Watt P, Purdie DM *et al.* (2003). Melanocytic nevi, solar keratoses, and divergent pathways to cutaneous melanoma. *J Natl Cancer Inst*, 95:806–812. http://dx.doi.org/10.1093/jnci/95.11.806 PMID:12783935

22. Schüz J, Ahlbom A (2008). Exposure to electromagnetic fields and the risk of childhood leukaemia: a review. *Radiat Prot Dosimetry*, 132:202–211. http://dx.doi.org/10.1093/rpd/ncn270 PMID:18927133

23. Ahlbom A, Day N, Feychting M *et al.* (2000). A pooled analysis of magnetic fields and childhood leukaemia. *Br J Cancer*, 83:692–698. http://dx.doi.org/10.1054/bjoc.2000.1376 PMID:10944614

24. Kheifets L, Ahlbom A, Crespi CM *et al.* (2010). Pooled analysis of recent studies on magnetic fields and childhood leukaemia. *Br J Cancer*, 103:1128–1135. http://dx.doi.org/10.1038/sj.bjc.6605838 PMID:20877339

25. Kheifets L, Ahlbom A, Crespi CM *et al.* (2010). A pooled analysis of extremely low-frequency magnetic fields and childhood brain tumors. *Am J Epidemiol*, 172:752–761. http://dx.doi.org/10.1093/aje/kwq181 PMID:20696650

26. IARC (2002). Non-ionizing radiation, part 1: static and extremely low-frequency (ELF) electric and magnetic fields. *IARC Monogr Eval Carcinog Risks Hum*, 80:1–395. PMID:12071196

27. WHO (2007). *Environmental Health Criteria 238: Extremely Low Frequency Fields*. Geneva: WHO.

28. European Commission Scientific Committee on Emerging and Newly Identified Health Risks (SCENIHR) (2009). *Health Effects of Exposure to EMF*. Brussels: European Commission – Directorate-General for Health and Consumers.

29. Schüz J, Grell K, Kinsey S *et al.* (2012). Extremely low-frequency magnetic fields and survival from childhood acute lymphoblastic leukemia: an international follow-up study. *Blood Cancer J*, 2:e98. http://dx.doi.org/10.1038/bcj.2012.43 PMID:23262804

30. IARC (2013). Non-ionizing radiation, part 2: radiofrequency electromagnetic fields. *IARC Monogr Eval Carcinog Risks Hum*, 102:1–460.

31. INTERPHONE Study Group (2010). Brain tumour risk in relation to mobile telephone use: results of the INTERPHONE international case-control study. *Int J Epidemiol*, 39:675–694. http://dx.doi.org/10.1093/ije/dyq079 PMID:20483835

2.9

Pollution of air, water, and soil

Aaron J. Cohen
Kenneth P. Cantor

Mark J. Nieuwenhuijsen (reviewer)
José Rogelio Pérez Padilla (reviewer)

Summary

- Many known, probable, and possible carcinogens can be found in the environment, and all people carry traces of these pollutants in their bodies.

- Air pollution from vehicle emissions, power generation, household combustion of solid fuels, and a range of industries includes known carcinogens such as diesel emissions, polycyclic aromatic hydrocarbons, benzene, and 1,3-butadiene, together with inorganic carcinogens such as asbestos, arsenic, and chromium compounds. Exposure to outdoor air pollution in general, and specifically to particulate matter, causes lung cancer. Household combustion of solid fuels causes lung cancer and is associated with other cancers in many low- and middle-income countries.

- In drinking-water, inorganic arsenic is a recognized carcinogen. Other contaminants, such as disinfection by-products, organic solvents, nitrates, nitrites, and some pesticides, may also contribute to an increased cancer burden.

- There are wide disparities in exposure, and pollution levels can be particularly high in newly and rapidly industrializing countries where environmental monitoring and regulation are less extensive and rigorous.

- Pollution of air, water, and soil contributes to the world's cancer burden to differing degrees depending on the geographical setting.

- Exposure to important sources of environmental pollution in water and air can be reduced by regulatory action and technological improvements, offering considerable promise for reduction of the burden of cancer and other adverse health outcomes.

The impact of pollution on cancer development is often described with reference to "environmental factors", which may lead to ambiguity. In a broad sense, environmental factors are implicated in the majority of human cancers. Environmental factors may be understood to encompass everything that is not specifically genetic in origin. The term therefore includes many significant causes of cancer – such as tobacco smoking, alcohol consumption, and diet – that are also considered lifestyle or behavioural factors. Evidence for the broad role of environmental factors comes from a variety of sources: from geographical variations in the distribution of the world cancer burden, from time trends showing increases or decreases in different forms of cancer, from studies of people migrating from one country to another, and from analytical studies within populations that have both high and low exposure to selected environmental factors.

However, the term "environment" may also identify a prominent subset of factors that are distinguished from lifestyle factors because the individual has little, if any, control over exposure to these factors. As affecting all in the community, exposure to pollution occurs because of the chemical contamination of the air breathed, the water and food consumed, and the soil, sediment, surface waters, and groundwater that surround living space. Some, such as polycyclic aromatic hydrocarbons generated by the combustion of fossil and biomass fuels, are the direct result of human activity, while others, such as aflatoxins that contaminate foods, are generated by natural processes involving little or no human activity (see Chapter 2.11). Regardless, many carcinogens occur in the environment, and all

Table 2.9.1. Environmental pollutants classified by IARC as Group 1, carcinogenic to humans

Agent	Cancer site/Cancer	Main context of pollution for general population
Arsenic and inorganic arsenic compounds	Lung, skin, bladder	Water
Asbestos (all forms)	Larynx, lung, mesothelioma, ovary	Atmosphere
Benzene	Acute non-lymphocytic leukaemia	Atmosphere (engine emissions)
1,3-Butadiene	Leukaemia, lymphoma	Atmosphere
Chromium (VI) compounds	Lung	Water, soil
Diesel engine exhaust	Lung	Atmosphere (engine emissions)
Erionite	Mesothelioma	Atmosphere (particular regions only)
Ethylene oxide[a]	Breast, lymphoid tumours	Atmosphere (indoor)
Formaldehyde	Nasopharynx, leukaemia	Atmosphere (indoor, outdoor)
Household coal combustion (indoor emissions)	Lung	Atmosphere (indoor)
Outdoor air pollution	Lung	Atmosphere
Particulate matter in outdoor air pollution	Lung	Atmosphere
Polychlorinated biphenyls	Skin	Food, atmosphere (indoor)
Radon and its decay products	Lung	Atmosphere (indoor)
Silica dust, crystalline	Lung	Atmosphere
2,3,7,8-Tetrachlorodibenzo-*para*-dioxin (TCDD)	All cancers combined	Food, soil
Tobacco smoke, second-hand	Lung	Atmosphere (indoor)
Trichloroethylene	Kidney	Water, food

[a] Upgraded to Group 1 based on mechanistic data; limited evidence of carcinogenicity in humans.

people carry traces of environmental pollutants in their bodies.

The cancer risks from environmental pollution are challenging to study. People are exposed to hundreds, if not thousands, of chemicals and other agents through their environment, and environmental exposure assessment, a necessary component of such studies, can be exceedingly complex. Some environmental pollutants are widely dispersed across the globe, while others are concentrated in small geographical areas near specific industrial sources. This results in wide disparities in the level of exposure to environmental pollutants. Some population groups may face high risks that do not have a noticeable impact on national cancer incidence statistics. IARC has identified environmental pollutants that are known to cause cancer in humans (Table 2.9.1) (http://monographs.iarc.fr/ENG/Classification/index.php).

Asbestos

Asbestos is one of the best characterized causes of human cancer in the workplace (see Chapter 2.7). The carcinogenic hazard associated with asbestos fibres has been recognized since the 1950s. Non-occupational exposure to asbestos may occur domestically and as a consequence of localized pollution. People who live with asbestos workers may be exposed to asbestos dust on clothes. The installation, degradation, removal, and repair of asbestos-containing products in the context of household maintenance represents another mode of residential exposure. Whole neighbourhoods may be exposed to asbestos as a result of local asbestos mining or manufacturing. Some parts of the world also experience asbestos exposure as a result of the erosion of asbestos or asbestiform rocks.

In common with occupational exposure, exposure to asbestos due to residential circumstances results in an increased risk of mesothelioma

[1]. Likewise, non-occupational exposure to asbestos may cause lung cancer, particularly among smokers [2]. A high incidence of mesothelioma as a consequence of neighbourhood exposure is evident among inhabitants of villages in Turkey where houses and natural surroundings contain the mineral erionite. All forms of asbestos are carcinogenic to humans [3], and stopping the use of all forms of asbestos is the most efficient way to eliminate asbestos-related diseases.

Outdoor air pollution

Emissions from multiple sources, including motor vehicles, industrial processes, power generation, and the combustion of household solid fuel, pollute the ambient and indoor air in all populated regions of the globe [4]. The precise chemical and physical features of air pollution, which comprises hundreds of individual chemical constituents, vary around the world, reflecting differences in the sources of pollution and

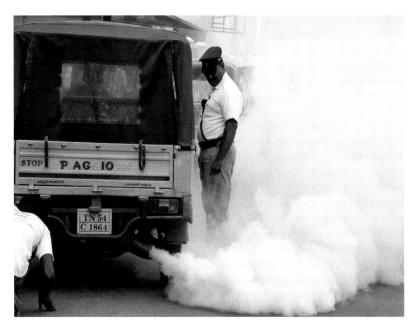

Fig. 2.9.1. A traffic police officer observes exhaust pouring from an automobile in Salem, Tamil Nadu, India. Motor vehicles are a recognized source of air pollution worldwide.

characterized by a relatively homogeneous concentration of the air pollution mixture or specific carcinogen. The actual dose of pollutants to the lung or other organs depends further on physiological characteristics such as pulmonary minute ventilation, metabolism, and rate of elimination. Typically, epidemiological studies rely solely on estimates of exposure to air pollution mixtures or specific carcinogens in single micro-environments, such as place of residence, to estimate the risk of cancer [5].

Ambient air contains a variety of known human carcinogens, including polycyclic aromatic hydrocarbons, 1,3-butadiene, benzene, inorganic compounds such as arsenic and chromium, and radionuclides. Some, such as polycyclic aromatic hydrocarbons, are present as part of complex mixtures such as diesel emissions, which are themselves carcinogenic [6]. Such mixtures often comprise carbon-based particles to which the organic compounds are adsorbed, sulfuric acid in particle form, and photochemical oxidants. Complex air pollution mixtures are characterized for purposes of both regulatory policy and scientific research in terms of indicators, for example, the mass

in meteorology, but these polluting mixtures contain specific chemicals or mixtures known to be carcinogenic to humans (Table 2.9.1) [5].

People are exposed to air pollution mixtures containing carcinogens that may cause lung cancer or cancers at other sites in a variety of settings, or micro-environments, both indoor and outdoor. A given individual's total personal exposure to such mixtures or to specific carcinogens is a function of the time spent in different micro-environments

Fig. 2.9.2. Estimated annual average atmospheric PM$_{2.5}$ (particulate matter < 2.5 μm in diameter) concentrations (μg/m³), for 2005. An estimated 89% of the world's population live in areas where the WHO air quality guideline (10 μg/m³ PM$_{2.5}$ annual average) is exceeded.

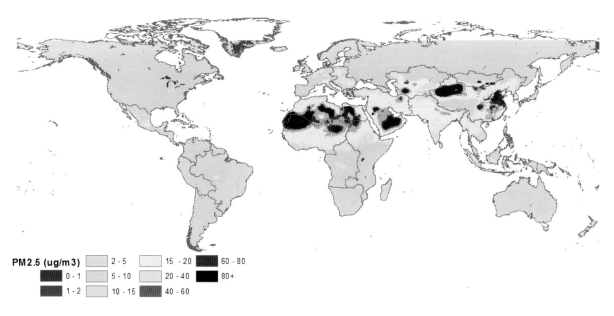

PM2.5 (ug/m3)
- 0 - 1
- 1 - 2
- 2 - 5
- 5 - 10
- 10 - 15
- 15 - 20
- 20 - 40
- 40 - 60
- 60 - 80
- 80+

Bisphenol A and cancer

David Melzer and Tamara S. Galloway

The rising incidence of certain reproductive cancers since the 1970s has been attributed to multiple possible factors, including exposure to endocrine disrupting agents in the environment. One widely studied compound is bisphenol A. This compound was first synthesized in the 1930s as an estrogen and is used as a loosely bound monomer in the production of polycarbonate plastic and in the epoxy resins lining food and beverage cans. More than 90% of people in the USA, Europe, and Asia are exposed to bisphenol A [1], probably through ingestion of bisphenol A-contaminated food and liquids. There is growing evidence from epidemiological and laboratory studies that exposure to this compound at levels found in the general population, about 0.2–20 ng/ml, may be associated with adverse human health effects. Exposure to bisphenol A in utero or during childhood has also been associated with reproductive and developmental abnormalities [2], whereas in adults there is prospective evidence of its association with cardiovascular disease [3].

Whether exposure to bisphenol A is linked to cancer incidence is far from clear. Work in the 1980s by the United States National Toxicology Program based on laboratory studies with rodents found that the compound was not a robust carcinogen in the context of adult exposure and supported a recommended maximum daily dose of 50 µg/kg/day as safe for humans (www.epa.gov/iris/subst/0356.htm). Since then, hundreds of studies have shown that bisphenol A disrupts the hormone system and causes changes that mirror properties of cancer cells at concentrations within current limits of exposure, although this evidence

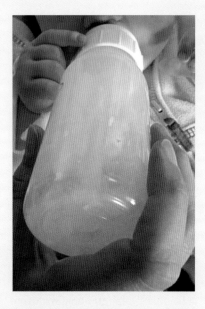

Fig. B2.9.1. Many food and liquid containers, including baby bottles, are made of polycarbonate or have a lining that contains bisphenol A. Studies have shown that bisphenol A may increase cancer risk.

is contested [4,5]. Potential modes of action proposed for a carcinogenic effect include estrogenic endocrine disruption, promotion of tumorigenic progression, genotoxicity, and developmental reprogramming that increases susceptibility to other carcinogenic events [6].

Bisphenol A binds to and activates both types of estrogen receptor (ERα and ERβ), albeit with weaker affinity than estradiol itself [7]. Additional cellular targets have emerged that may shed further light on the potential link between this pollutant and cancer induction. For example, binding of bisphenol A to G protein-coupled receptors has been implicated in the proliferation of breast cancer cells and

recruitment of cancer-associated fibroblasts [8]. Recent epidemiological studies have shown that exposure to bisphenol A is associated with enhanced expression of the orphan nuclear receptor estrogen-related receptor α (ERRα) in white blood cells in vivo [9]. ERRα is upregulated in advanced breast cancer cells and has been correlated with poor prognosis and the promotion of tumour growth [10].

References

1. Vandenberg LN *et al.* (2010). *Environ Health Perspect*, 118:1055–1070. http://dx.doi.org/10.1289/ehp.0901716 PMID:20338858

2. Diamanti-Kandarakis E *et al.* (2009). *Endocr Rev*, 30:293–342. http://dx.doi.org/10.1210/er.2009-0002 PMID:19502515

3. Melzer D *et al.* (2012). *Circulation*, 125:1482–1490. http://dx.doi.org/10.1161/CIRCULATIONAHA.111.069153 PMID:22354940

4. Vandenberg LN *et al.* (2009). *Endocr Rev*, 30:75–95. http://dx.doi.org/10.1210/er.2008-0021 PMID:19074586

5. Hengstler JG *et al.* (2011). *Crit Rev Toxicol*, 41:263–291. http://dx.doi.org/10.3109/10408444.2011.558487 PMID:21438738

6. Keri RA *et al.* (2007). *Reprod Toxicol*, 24:240–252. http://dx.doi.org/10.1016/j.reprotox.2007.06.008 PMID:17706921

7. Delfosse V *et al.* (2012). *Proc Natl Acad Sci U S A*, 109:14930–14935. http://dx.doi.org/10.1073/pnas.1203574109 PMID:22927406

8. Pupo M *et al.* (2012). *Environ Health Perspect*, 120:1177–1182. http://dx.doi.org/10.1289/ehp.1104526 PMID:22552965

9. Melzer D *et al.* (2011). *Environ Health Perspect*, 119:1788–1793. http://dx.doi.org/10.1289/ehp.1103809 PMID:21831745

10. Teng CT *et al.* (2011). In: Gunduz M *et al.*, eds. *Breast Cancer – Carcinogenesis, Cell Growth and Signalling Pathways*. InTech. pp. 313–330.

concentration of fine particles (particulate matter < 2.5 µm in diameter [$PM_{2.5}$]) and ozone. The combustion of fossil fuels and biomass for power generation, cooking, and transportation is the source of most of the

organic and inorganic compounds, acids, and oxidants, and contributes heavily to particulate air pollution in most populated areas [4,7].

Levels of ambient air pollutants, including $PM_{2.5}$, have been declining

steadily in high-income countries over the past 20 years, although air pollution levels remain elevated in many urban areas and current levels are associated with a range of adverse health outcomes [4,7].

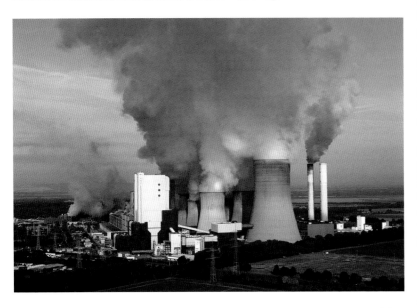

Fig. 2.9.3. The Niederaussem brown-coal power plant near Cologne, Germany. Coal-burning plants release carbon dioxide, fine particles, nitrogen oxide, and mercury, which can have a serious impact on public health. The coal ash produced by these plants contains contaminants such as arsenic, a known carcinogen.

weighted average annual levels of $PM_{2.5}$ in East Asia were 4 times those in high-income North America, and 89% of the world's population lived in areas where the WHO air quality guideline for exposure to $PM_{2.5}$ was exceeded (Fig. 2.9.2) [7]. In the USA, hazardous air pollutants, or air toxics, are reported to exceed applicable reference concentrations, and have been estimated to increase cancer risk [9].

Exposure to air pollution mixtures has effects at the genetic and cellular level that are considered likely to increase cancer risk. Urban air pollution mixtures are mutagenic in in vivo assays and carcinogenic in rodents, these effects being largely mediated by combustion products [10]. Studies in human populations have identified markers of genetic damage and cell mutation associated with exposure to combustion emissions [11].

Long-term exposure to ambient air pollution is associated with an increased risk of lung cancer. Populations in urban areas with elevated ambient levels of polycyclic aromatic hydrocarbons and other

Air quality has deteriorated, however, in some middle-income countries, including China and India, as a consequence of industrialization and an increased number of motor vehicles. The uncontrolled burning of low-quality biomass fuels and coal contributes to poor air quality in low- and middle-income countries [8]. In 2005, estimated population-

Fig. 2.9.4. Proportion of the national population (%) estimated by WHO to use solid fuels for cooking, for 2010. Common solid fuels include wood, charcoal, dung, and crop residues, which are not only environmentally unsustainable but also harmful to the local communities. In homes without proper ventilation, exposure to indoor smoke poses serious health threats.

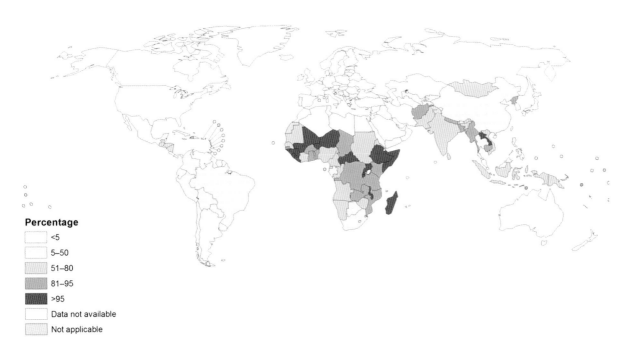

Percentage
- <5
- 5–50
- 51–80
- 81–95
- >95
- Data not available
- Not applicable

pollutants experience higher rates of lung cancer than rural populations, independent of tobacco smoking. Higher rates of lung cancer are also associated with long-term residence near stationary air pollution sources such as smelters, incinerators, and power plants, and with residential proximity to busy roads [5,12]. Increased risk has been reported in studies of populations both in Europe and the USA and in countries in Asia [5,8,13]. Large cohort studies of long-term exposure to $PM_{2.5}$ in the USA and Europe that controlled for tobacco smoking report 6–36% increases in lung cancer associated with each 10 µg/m³ increase in $PM_{2.5}$, an increment well within the range of exposure in North America and Europe, although the highest recorded levels occur in Saharan Africa, the Middle East, and Central Asia (Fig. 2.9.2). These studies also report an increased risk of lung cancer in never-smokers [14,15]. Biomarkers of air pollution exposure and genetic effects have been used in some epidemiological studies to link ambient exposure with lung cancer occurrence [16].

IARC recently reviewed the evidence summarized above and concluded that long-term exposure to outdoor air pollution, and specifically particulate matter in outdoor air, causes lung cancer. Exposure to outdoor air pollution is also associated with an increased risk of bladder cancer [17]. Exposure to ambient $PM_{2.5}$ has recently been estimated to have contributed to 3.2 million premature deaths worldwide in 2010, due largely to cardiovascular disease, and 223 000 deaths from lung cancer. More than half of the lung cancer deaths attributable to ambient $PM_{2.5}$ occurred in China and other countries in East Asia [18].

Comprehensive air quality management programmes, using regulatory approaches and adoption of cleaner technologies for transportation, power generation, industrial production, and waste management have led to improvements in population health [19,20].

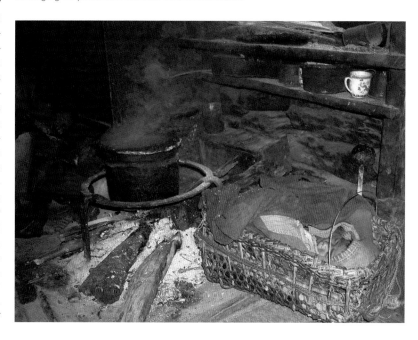

Fig. 2.9.5. On a cold day, a mother in Gatlang, a village in the Rasuwa district, Nepal, keeps her baby warm in front of a traditional wood stove. Indoor burning of solid fuels in unventilated homes results in exposures to levels of fine particles and other health-damaging air pollutants such as carbon monoxide.

Air pollution by chlorofluorocarbons is believed to be indirectly responsible for increases in skin cancer rates around the globe [21]. These chemicals, including carbon tetrachloride and methyl chloroform and other halons, are emitted from home air conditioners, foam cushions, and many other products. Chlorofluorocarbons are carried by winds into the stratosphere, where the action of strong solar radiation releases chlorine and bromine atoms that react with, and thereby eliminate, molecules of ozone. Depletion of the ozone layer is believed to be responsible for global increases in ultraviolet B (UVB) radiation (see Chapter 2.8).

Indoor air pollution

Household air pollution
Despite declines over the past 30 years in the percentage of the global population that burn solid fuels, either coal or biomass, for household cooking or heating, the number of people exposed has remained largely unchanged at 2.8 billion, due to population growth [22]. The proportion of the

population estimated by WHO to have been cooking with solid fuels in 2010 is highest in sub-Saharan Africa and South and East Asia (Fig. 2.9.4). Indoor burning of solid fuels in unventilated homes results in exposures to levels of fine particles ($PM_{2.5}$) and other health-damaging air pollutants, such as carbon monoxide, that are many times ambient levels, and the components of this indoor smoke include known human carcinogens such as polycyclic aromatic hydrocarbons, formaldehyde, and benzene. Household combustion of solid fuels also contributes to outdoor air pollution in settings where solid fuels are widely used [18].

Exposure to household air pollution from solid fuel use has recently been estimated to have contributed to 3.5 million premature deaths worldwide in 2010, due largely to cardiovascular disease and acute and chronic respiratory disease, and 126 000 deaths from lung cancer due to household coal burning [18]. Indoor burning of coal causes lung cancer in humans, and indoor burning of biomass may as well [23]. Exposure to emissions from indoor coal burning is

Pesticides and cancer

Laura E. Beane Freeman

Pesticides encompass a large and diverse number of chemicals designed to kill pests, including weeds, insects, rodents, algae, and moulds, for agricultural, residential, and public health purposes. These chemicals make important contributions to production and protection of agricultural commodities and control of insect disease vectors. They also present potential hazards to human health.

Unlike many other chemical agents, pesticides are designed for release into the environment, and exposure can occur occupationally, through environmental bystander exposure, and through ingestion of foods containing pesticides or pesticide residues. In 2007, the latest year for which estimates are available, 5.2 billion pounds (2.4 million tonnes) of pesticide active ingredient were applied in the world (http://www.epa.gov/opp00001/pestsales/07pestsales/usage2007.htm#3_1). Despite widespread potential exposure, cancer risks associated with long-term exposure to specific pesticides are generally not well characterized. Only one group of pesticides, inorganic arsenic compounds, and one pesticide contaminant, the dioxin TCDD, are classified by IARC as Group 1, carcinogenic to humans. The fungicide captafol and the fumigant ethylene dibromide are classified as Group 2A, probably carcinogenic to humans, as is occupational exposure in the application of non-arsenical insecticides. However, there are several pesticides that are listed as Group 3, not classifiable as

to their carcinogenicity to humans, largely due to inadequate evidence in humans, and many more that have been linked with cancer that require further investigation (http://monographs.iarc.fr/ENG/Classification/ClassificationsAlphaOrder.pdf).

A few areas where the evidence seems to be the strongest at this time are highlighted. Several organochlorine and organophosphate insecticides have been linked with an increased risk of prostate cancer. This is notable since farmers, an occupationally exposed group, have long been reported to have increased rates of prostate cancer [1]. Farmers also experience increased rates of lymphoma, and several reports have linked multiple pesticides to increased risk at this site, although confirmation is required [1]. Finally, a growing body of evidence suggests that parental exposure to pesticides, particularly of the mother during pregnancy, may increase the risk of leukaemia in children, although data on specific chemicals are largely lacking [2].

Developing accurate assessment of pesticide exposure is a major challenge in epidemiological studies but is essential for identifying hazards associated with these chemicals. Many studies of pesticides and cancer have focused on occupational exposures, where levels are likely to be highest, but it is also important for future research to assess effects of environmental exposures because of the widespread use of these chemicals. Future studies need to evaluate specific chemicals and to consider potential mechanisms of action to

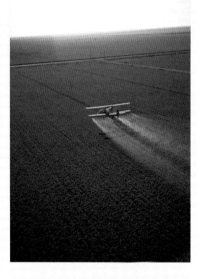

B2.9.2. A crop duster spraying pesticide in California.

support the biological plausibility of the epidemiological observations.

References

1. Blair A et al. (2009). J Agromedicine, 14:125–131. http://dx.doi.org/10.1080/10599240902779436 PMID:19437268

2. Van Maele-Fabry G et al. (2010). Cancer Causes Control, 21:787–809. http://dx.doi.org/10.1007/s10552-010-9516-7 PMID:20467891

Websites

Agents Classified by the IARC Monographs: http://monographs.iarc.fr/ENG/Classification/ClassificationsAlphaOrder.pdf

World and U.S. Pesticide Amount Used: http://www.epa.gov/opp00001/pestsales/07pestsales/usage2007.htm#3_1

associated with a 2-fold increase in lung cancer risk [24]. Women are the most heavily exposed, and nonsmoking women in some parts of China experience very high lung cancer rates due to indoor coal burning. Indoor exposure to cooking-oil emissions from high-temperature frying may cause lung cancer. Indoor burning of solid

fuels has also been associated with increased rates of cancer of the upper airways.

Improved ventilation of coal combustion emissions and the use of alternative types of stoves with lower emissions have been shown to reduce lung cancer rates in exposed women [24,25]. The use of cleaner

fuels, such as compressed natural gas, is associated with reduced rates of lung cancer and other adverse health outcomes relative to the use of coal and biomass.

Involuntary smoking
Tobacco smoke is an important source of indoor air pollution

worldwide, and involuntary smoking (exposure to second-hand or "environmental" tobacco smoke) is carcinogenic to humans (see Chapter 2.2).

Water pollution

Disinfection by-products

Access to clean water is one of the basic requirements of human health. Water quality is influenced by climate and weather, the geology of the soil, land use patterns, and discharges from agriculture and industry. The greatest and most immediate concern relates to infectious disease. Microbiological contamination of water is controlled by disinfection methods based on chlorine, chloramine, or ozone. As a result of the interaction of chlorine with organic chemicals already present, drinking-water typically contains chlorination by-products, some of which may present a carcinogenic risk. Chloroform and other trihalomethanes are among the by-products most commonly detected, but not necessarily the most threatening to health. Studies of bladder cancer and some other cancers have suggested increased risk associated with consumption of chlorinated drinking-water [26]. Given the large number of people exposed to chlorination by-products, however, even a small increase in risk would implicate a substantial number of cases. It is desirable to reduce such by-products without reducing the effectiveness of disinfection procedures.

Arsenic

Arsenic causes cancers of the skin, lung, bladder, and possibly other organs [27]. The main source of environmental exposure to arsenic for the general population is contaminated drinking-water. High exposure to arsenic from drinking-water is found around the world, including areas of Bangladesh, India, Mongolia, China, Argentina, Chile, Mexico, and the USA. In areas of high arsenic content, with concentrations typically above 100 µg/l, there is strong evidence of an increased risk of

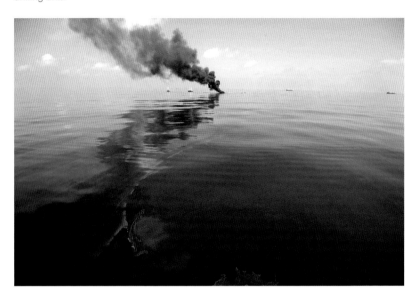

Fig. 2.9.6. Water pollution is usually identified with contaminants in water for domestic and agricultural use, but marine water may also be at risk. This oil spill occurred in the Gulf of Mexico in 2010 after an explosion on Deepwater Horizon, an offshore oil drilling unit.

cancers of the bladder, skin, and lung after consumption of water with high arsenic contamination [27]. The data for other cancers, such as those of the liver and kidney, are more limited but are consistent and suggestive of a systemic effect. Given the many difficulties of conducting studies in areas with arsenic concentrations below 100 µg/l, the risks at these markedly lower levels are not clear. However, given the demonstrated risk at higher levels, the possibility of increased risk of different types of cancer at low exposures is plausible.

Estimates of the cancer burden associated with arsenic in drinking-water have been made for some regions of the world. In northern Chile, where most of the population was exposed to very high levels of arsenic in drinking-water from 1955 to 1970, arsenic might still account for 7% of all deaths among those aged 30 years and older, given the long latency of the effect [27]. In Bangladesh, tens of millions of people have been exposed to elevated levels of arsenic in water, and an estimated 6% of all deaths, including cancer deaths, are due to these exposures [28]. West Bengal, India, which has a similar exposure

profile, may experience a similar burden of disease and death [29]. About 14 million people in Latin America are exposed to arsenic in drinking-water above the limit established by several national and international agencies [30].

Other drinking-water contaminants

Several other groups of pollutants of drinking-water have been investigated as possible sources of cancer risk in humans. These include organic compounds such as chlorinated solvents and pesticides from industrial, commercial, and agricultural activities, and chemicals leached from waste sites. Organic pollutants that persist in the environment and accumulate in fish, such as polychlorinated dibenzo-*para*-dioxin, polychlorinated biphenyls, and organochlorine pesticides, are of particular concern, as is contamination by nitrates and nitrites, radionuclides, hormonally active compounds, and asbestos. For most pollutants, the epidemiological studies are inconclusive; however, an increased risk of stomach cancer has been repeatedly reported in areas with high nitrate levels in drinking-water, and there is evidence of excess thyroid cancer [31].

Soil pollution

A variety of toxic agents, including heavy metals, solvents, and persistent organic pollutants such as dioxins, contaminate soil, sometimes at high concentrations [32]. In local regions, such pollution occurs by substances produced as waste or as other consequences of a particular mining or industrial process. The ranges of concentrations detected are specified for particular compounds in the corresponding IARC Monograph.

Soil contaminants present a carcinogenic risk as a result of being vaporized and consequently inhaled, or being leached from the soil to contaminate water supplies. Accordingly, risk of cancer has generally been studied in relation to consequential air or water pollution, rather than with primary reference to particular levels of contaminants in soil. However, accumulation of a variety of pollutants via the food-chain, and an estimate of any associated burden of disease, is being investigated through the WHO Foodborne Disease Burden Epidemiology Reference Group.

References

1. Boffetta P (2006). Human cancer from environmental pollutants: the epidemiological evidence. *Mutat Res*, 608:157–162. http://dx.doi.org/10.1016/j.mrgentox.2006.02.015 PMID:16843042

2. HEI Asbestos Literature Review Panel (1991). *Asbestos in Public and Commercial Buildings: A Literature Review and Synthesis of Current Knowledge*. Cambridge, MA: Health Effects Institute-Asbestos Research.

3. IARC (2012). Arsenic, metals, fibres, and dusts. *IARC Monogr Eval Carcinog Risks Hum*, 100C:1–499. PMID:23189751

4. WHO (2006). *Air Quality Guidelines. Global Update 2005*. Geneva: WHO. Available at http://www.euro.who.int/__data/assets/pdf_file/0005/78638/E90038.pdf.

5. Samet JM, Cohen AJ (2006). Air pollution. In: Schottenfeld D, Fraumeni JF, eds. *Cancer Epidemiology and Prevention*. New York: Oxford University Press, pp. 355–381.

6. IARC (2013). Diesel and gasoline engine exhausts and some nitroarenes. *IARC Monogr Eval Carcinog Risks Hum*, 105.

7. Brauer M, Amann M, Burnett RT *et al.* (2012). Exposure assessment for estimation of the global burden of disease attributable to outdoor air pollution. *Environ Sci Technol*, 46:652–660. http://dx.doi.org/10.1021/es2025752 PMID:22148428

8. HEI International Scientific Oversight Committee (2010). *Outdoor Air Pollution and Health in the Developing Countries of Asia: A Comprehensive Review*. HEI Special Report 18. Boston, MA: Health Effects Institute.

9. HEI Air Toxics Review Panel (2007). *Mobile-Source Air Toxics: A Critical Review of the Literature on Exposure and Health Effects*. HEI Special Report 16. Boston, MA: Health Effects Institute.

10. Claxton LD, Woodall GM Jr (2007). A review of the mutagenicity and rodent carcinogenicity of ambient air. *Mutat Res*, 636:36–94. http://dx.doi.org/10.1016/j.mrrev.2007.01.001 PMID:17451995

11. Lewtas J (2007). Air pollution combustion emissions: characterization of causative agents and mechanisms associated with cancer, reproductive, and cardiovascular effects. *Mutat Res*, 636:95–133. http://dx.doi.org/10.1016/j.mrrev.2007.08.003 PMID:17951105

12. HEI Panel on the Health Effects of Traffic-Related Air Pollution (2010). *Traffic-Related Air Pollution: A Critical Review of the Literature on Emissions, Exposure, and Health Effects*. HEI Special Report 17. Boston, MA: Health Effects Institute.

13. Cao J, Yang C, Li J *et al.* (2011). Association between long-term exposure to outdoor air pollution and mortality in China: a cohort study. *J Hazard Mater*, 186:1594–1600. http://dx.doi.org/10.1016/j.jhazmat.2010.12.036 PMID:21194838

14. Brunekreef B, Beelen R, Hoek G *et al.* (2009). *Effects of Long-Term Exposure to Traffic-Related Air Pollution on Respiratory and Cardiovascular Mortality in the Netherlands: The NLCS-AIR Study*. HEI Research Report 139. Boston, MA: Health Effects Institute.

15. Turner MC, Krewski D, Pope CA 3rd *et al.* (2011). Long-term ambient fine particulate matter air pollution and lung cancer in a large cohort of never-smokers. *Am J Respir Crit Care Med*, 184:1374–1381. http://dx.doi.org/10.1164/rccm.201106-1011OC PMID:21980033

16. Demetriou CA, Raaschou-Nielsen O, Loft S *et al.* (2012). Biomarkers of ambient air pollution and lung cancer: a systematic review. *Occup Environ Med*, 69:619–627. http://dx.doi.org/10.1136/oemed-2011-100566 PMID:22773658

17. Loomis D, Grosse Y, Lauby-Secretan B *et al.* (2013). The carcinogenicity of outdoor air pollution. *Lancet Oncol*, 14:1262–1263. http://dx.doi.org/10.1016/S1470-2045 (13)70487-X

18. Lim SS, Vos T, Flaxman AD *et al.* (2012). A comparative risk assessment of burden of disease and injury attributable to 67 risk factors and risk factor clusters in 21 regions, 1990–2010: a systematic analysis for the Global Burden of Disease Study 2010. *Lancet* 380:2224–2260. http://dx.doi.org/10.1016/S0140-6736(12)61766-8 PMID:23245609

19. Pope CA 3rd, Ezzati M, Dockery DW (2009). Fine-particulate air pollution and life expectancy in the United States. *N Engl J Med*, 360:376–386. http://dx.doi.org/10.1056/NEJMsa0805646 PMID:19164188

20. HEI Accountability Working Group (2003). *Assessing Health Impact of Air Quality Regulations: Concepts and Methods for Accountability Research*. HEI Communication 11. Boston, MA: Health Effects Institute. Available at http://pubs.healtheffects.org/view.php?id=153

21. IARC (2012). Radiation. *IARC Monogr Eval Carcinog Risks Hum*, 100D:1–437. PMID:23189752

22. Bonjour S, Adair-Rohani H, Wolf J *et al.* (2013). Solid fuel use for household cooking: country and regional estimates for 1980–2010. *Environ Health Perspect*, 121:784–790. http://dx.doi.org/10.1289/ehp.1205987 PMID:23674502

23. Hosgood HD 3rd, Boffetta P, Greenland S *et al.* (2010). In-home coal and wood use and lung cancer risk: a pooled analysis of the International Lung Cancer Consortium. *Environ Health Perspect*, 118:1743–1747. http://dx.doi.org/10.1289/ehp.1002217 PMID:20846923

24. Hosgood HD 3rd, Wei H, Sapkota A *et al.* (2011). Household coal use and lung cancer: systematic review and meta-analysis of case-control studies, with an emphasis on geographic variation. *Int J Epidemiol*, 40:719–728. http://dx.doi.org/10.1093/ije/dyq259 PMID:21278196

25. Lan Q, Chapman RS, Schreinemachers DM *et al.* (2002). Household stove improvement and risk of lung cancer in Xuanwei, China. *J Natl Cancer Inst*, 94:826–835. http://dx.doi.org/10.1093/jnci/94.11.826 PMID:12048270

26. Richardson SD, Plewa MJ, Wagner ED *et al.* (2007). Occurrence, genotoxicity, and carcinogenicity of regulated and emerging disinfection by-products in drinking water: a review and roadmap for research. *Mutat Res*, 636:178–242. http://dx.doi.org/10.1016/j.mrrev.2007.09.001 PMID:17980649

27. IARC (2004). Some drinking-water disinfectants and contaminants, including arsenic. *IARC Monogr Eval Carcinog Risks Hum*, 84:1–477. PMID:15645577

28. Flanagan SV, Johnston RB, Zheng Y (2012). Arsenic in tube well water in Bangladesh: health and economic impacts and implications for arsenic mitigation. *Bull World Health Organ*, 90:839–846. http://dx.doi.org/10.2471/BLT.11.101253 PMID:23226896

29. Chatterjee D, Halder D, Majumder S *et al.* (2010). Assessment of arsenic exposure from groundwater and rice in Bengal Delta Region, West Bengal, India. *Water Res*, 44:5803–5812. http://dx.doi.org/10.1016/j.watres.2010.04.007 PMID:20638702

30. Bundschuh J, Litter MI, Parvez F *et al.* (2012). One century of arsenic exposure in Latin America: a review of history and occurrence from 14 countries. *Sci Total Environ*, 429:2–35. http://dx.doi.org/10.1016/j.scitotenv.2011.06.024 PMID:21959248

31. Ritter L, Solomon K, Sibley P *et al.* (2002). Sources, pathways, and relative risks of contaminants in surface water and groundwater: a perspective prepared for the Walkerton inquiry. *J Toxicol Environ Health A*, 65:1–142. http://dx.doi.org/10.1080/152873902753338572 PMID:11809004

32. Porta D, Milani S, Lassarino A *et al.* (2009). Systematic review of epidemiological studies on health effects associated with management of solid waste. *Environ Health*, 8:60. http://dx.doi.org/10.1186/1476-069X-8-60 PMID:20030820

2.10 Pharmaceutical drugs

2 ETIOLOGY

Søren Friis
Jørgen H. Olsen

Margaret R. Karagas (reviewer)

Summary

- Pharmaceutical drugs may have the potential to induce or prevent cancer development.

- Antineoplastic agents used in cancer therapy can induce second cancers in patients who are apparently cured; this is most readily attributable to the genotoxicity of these agents.

- Apart from antineoplastic agents, drugs carcinogenic to humans include immunosuppressants, hormonal agents, and phenacetin.

- Some drugs are implicated, but not established, as carcinogenic to humans by limited epidemiological data or by data restricted to the results of bioassay in animals.

- Monitoring of possible carcinogenic risks associated with the use of pharmaceutical drugs is imperative.

- A few drugs have been approved for cancer preventive therapy, and several others are being evaluated as preventive agents, including aromatase inhibitors, aspirin, statins, and metformin.

Pharmaceutical drugs are chemicals that are developed and applied in medicine and dentistry for their ability to treat, prevent, or mitigate disease. Pharmaceutical drugs are invariably administered at levels that are biologically active, and thus may have side-effects in addition to their intended effects. A possible side-effect is modification of the likelihood of malignant transformation, which may involve either a risk-enhancing or a risk-reducing effect.

Hormonal agents are well established as drugs with carcinogenic potential. These agents include oral contraceptives, hormone replacement therapy, and anti-estrogens, such as tamoxifen. Other carcinogenic drugs include antineoplastic agents that – particularly among those that are genotoxic – cause second cancers. For many such agents the benefit–risk ratio, determined by reference to patients achieving increased survival or related outcome compared with those developing second cancers, is high and the continued use of these drugs is endorsed, although with intensive research to reduce dosage or develop safer and more effective replacement products. In contrast, a decision to prescribe and use drugs that are established, or considered likely, to be carcinogenic is more problematic in circumstances involving non-life-threatening conditions.

In the most recent review involving pharmaceuticals [1], the IARC Monographs Programme re-evaluated 23 agents or combination therapies categorized as carcinogenic to humans (Group 1). These predominantly include antineoplastic agents as well as a diverse range of drugs not used as cancer therapy.

Only a few drugs have been approved for cancer preventive therapy, including tamoxifen for women at risk of contralateral breast cancer.

Antineoplastic agents

Antineoplastic agents include multiple drugs that can induce second cancers in cancer patients who are apparently cured. Twelve such agents or combination therapies have been classified as carcinogenic to humans (Table 2.10.1) [1,2]. Of these, the majority, including busulfan, chlorambucil, cyclophosphamide, melphalan, semustine (methyl-CCNU), thiotepa, and treosulfan, are alkylating agents that exhibit genotoxic activity, commonly through alkylation of purine bases in DNA. Typically these agents cause acute myeloid leukaemia that often exhibits clonal loss of either chromosome 5 or 7, as distinct from acute myeloid leukaemia induced by topoisomerase II inhibitors, such as etoposide. Several such agents

Table 2.10.1. Antineoplastic drugs and other drugs evaluated by the IARC Monographs Programme

Group 1 agent	Cancer on which sufficient evidence in humans is based	Established mechanistic events
Antineoplastic agents		
Busulfan	Acute myeloid leukaemia	Genotoxicity (alkylating agent)
Chlorambucil	Acute myeloid leukaemia	Genotoxicity (alkylating agent)
Chlornaphazine	Bladder	Genotoxicity (alkylating agent, metabolism to 2-naphthylamine derivatives)
Cyclophosphamide	Acute myeloid leukaemia, bladder	Genotoxicity (metabolism to alkylating agents)
Etoposide (Group 2A in 2000)	–	Genotoxicity, translocations involving *MLL* gene
Etoposide in combination with cisplatin and bleomycin	Acute myeloid leukaemia	Genotoxicity, translocations involving *MLL* gene (etoposide)
Melphalan	Acute myeloid leukaemia	Genotoxicity (alkylating agent)
MOPP[a] combined chemotherapy	Acute myeloid leukaemia, lung	Genotoxicity
Semustine (methyl-CCNU)	Acute myeloid leukaemia	Genotoxicity (alkylating agent)
Thiotepa	Leukaemia	Genotoxicity (alkylating agent)
Treosulfan	Acute myeloid leukaemia	Genotoxicity (alkylating agent)
Immunosuppressive agents		
Azathioprine	Non-Hodgkin lymphoma, skin	Genotoxicity, immunosuppression
Ciclosporin	Non-Hodgkin lymphoma, skin, multiple other sites	Immunosuppression
Other carcinogenic agents		
Analgesic mixtures containing phenacetin	Renal pelvis, ureter	(See phenacetin)
Aristolochic acid (Group 2A in 2002)	–	Genotoxicity, DNA adducts in animals are the same as those found in humans exposed to plants, A:T → T:A transversions in *TP53*, *RAS* activation
Methoxsalen plus ultraviolet A radiation	Skin	Genotoxicity after photo-activation
Phenacetin (Group 2A in 1987)	Renal pelvis, ureter	Genotoxicity, cell proliferation
Plants containing aristolochic acid	Renal pelvis, ureter	Genotoxicity, DNA adducts in humans, A:T → T:A transversions in *TP53* in human tumours

[a] Chlormethine (mechlorethamine), vincristine (Oncovin), procarbazine, and prednisone.

have since been supplemented or superseded by newer drugs [3]. It is therefore imperative that these new drugs and combinations thereof are monitored for possible carcinogenic effects. Typically, the antineoplastic mechanisms of the replacement drugs are similar to those of the traditional drugs, and much insight can be gained from focusing on relevant mechanisms rather than the specific drugs. Since individual susceptibility is often a factor that emerges from relevant mechanistic analysis, this knowledge contributes to improved identification of patients who may be susceptible to drug-induced cancer [1].

Immunosuppressive agents

Immunosuppressive agents, such as azathioprine and ciclosporin (also known as cyclosporin, cyclosporine,

or cyclosporin A), are carcinogenic to humans because of immunosuppressive rather than genotoxic effects. Use of these agents may cause skin cancer and non-Hodgkin lymphoma; relevant evidence comes primarily from studies of patients who have undergone organ transplantation (Table 2.10.1) [1].

Hormone therapy

Female sex hormones, including estrogen-only and estrogen–progestogen agents, are used widely to achieve various outcomes, including contraception and the amelioration of menopausal symptoms, uterine bleeding, and endometriosis [1]. In addition, these agents have been used widely for prevention of osteoporosis and coronary heart disease among postmenopausal women, although the latter indication was

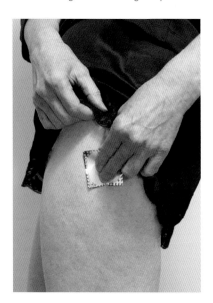

Fig. 2.10.1. A middle-aged woman sticks a hormone replacement therapy patch to her thigh. Hormonal agents are well established as drugs with carcinogenic potential.

Table 2.10.2. Hormonal agents assessed by the IARC Monographs Programme

Group 1 agent	Cancer on which sufficient evidence in humans is based	Sites where cancer risk is reduced	Established mechanistic events	Other likely mechanistic events
Combined estrogen–progestogen menopausal therapy	Endometrium (risk decreases with number of days per month of progestogen use), breast	–	Receptor-mediated events	Estrogen genotoxicity
Combined estrogen–progestogen oral contraceptives	Breast, cervix, liver	Endometrium, ovary	Receptor-mediated events	Estrogen genotoxicity, hormone-stimulated expression of human papillomavirus genes
Diethylstilbestrol	Breast (exposure during pregnancy), vagina and cervix (exposure in utero) Limited evidence: testis (exposure in utero), endometrium	–	Estrogen-receptor-mediated events (vagina, cervix), genotoxicity	Epigenetic programming
Estrogen-only menopausal therapy	Endometrium, ovary Limited evidence: breast	–	Estrogen-receptor-mediated events	Genotoxicity
Tamoxifen	Endometrium	Breast	Estrogen-receptor-mediated events, genotoxicity	–

abandoned in 2003 after publication of the Women's Health Initiative trial, which could not replicate the risk reduction for coronary heart disease reported in many observational studies [4]. There is consistent evidence that female sex hormones may influence the risk of cancers of the female reproductive organs and breast (Table 2.10.2) [1]. The mechanisms of carcinogenesis of female sex hormones include estrogen-receptor-mediated responses and potentially direct genotoxic effects of the estrogenic hormones or their associated by-products (Table 2.10.2) [1].

Estrogen-only menopausal therapy

Estrogen-only menopausal therapy refers to the use of estrogen without progestogen by perimenopausal and postmenopausal women, primarily for the treatment of menopausal symptoms [1]. After a substantial increase in the use of this regimen in the 1960s and early 1970s, the use declined after reports of a strong association between estrogen-only therapy and risk of endometrial cancer. Since then, estrogen-only menopausal agents have been prescribed predominantly to hysterectomized women. In the recent re-evaluation [1], IARC concluded that

estrogen-only menopausal therapy causes cancers of the endometrium and ovary (Table 2.10.2). Moreover, an increased risk of breast cancer was also noted.

Combined estrogen–progestogen menopausal therapy

Combined estrogen–progestogen menopausal therapy was initially developed to avoid the excess occurrence of endometrial cancer associated with estrogen-only therapy [1]. Estrogen–progestogen agents were used heavily in the 1990s and the beginning of the 2000s. However, in 2003 the Women's Health Initiative trial reported that use of combined estrogen–progestogen agents among women aged 50–79 years at baseline was associated with a hazard ratio for coronary heart disease of 1.24 (95% confidence interval, 1.00–1.54) after a mean follow-up of 5.2 years [4]. This study has affected the prescribing of combined estrogen–progestogen menopausal therapy substantially, resulting in rapidly declining use of these agents, restricted indications, and reduced duration of therapy. Based on a comprehensive amount of evidence, IARC has concluded that long-term combined estrogen–progestogen menopausal

therapy causes cancers of the breast and endometrium (Table 2.10.2) [1]. The increased risk of endometrial cancer decreases with the number of days per month that progestogens are added to the regimen. IARC has also noted an inverse association between the use of these agents and risk of colorectal cancer; however, this evidence is not conclusive. For several other sites, including cancers of the thyroid, lung, stomach, liver, urinary tract, pancreas, ovary, and cervix, as well as lymphoma, leukaemia, cutaneous melanoma, and central nervous system tumours, the current evidence does not point to an association with combined estrogen–progestogen menopausal therapy [1].

Fig. 2.10.2. Oral contraceptives are available in estrogen–progestogen combinations as well as in progestogen-only pills.

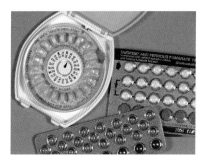

Breast implants and cancer

Eric Lavigne

The demand for breast implants among women has been rapidly increasing since the first mammary prosthesis was inserted into a woman's breast in the early 1960s [1]. Although breast implants are very popular for cosmetic purposes, considerable controversy remains about their long-term effects on cancer incidence. Concerns were initially raised about the possible carcinogenic effect of cosmetic breast implants, specifically for breast cancer [2]. However, the weight of epidemiological evidence based on large cohort studies with long follow-up periods showed no carcinogenic effect of breast augmentation on breast cancer [3–5].

Concerns about the carcinogenic effect of breast implants have also been characterized according to specific implant characteristics, such as the type of implant (saline-filled or silicone-gel-filled), implant placement (submuscular or subglandular), and implant envelope (with or without polyurethane coating). For the implant envelope, available laboratory studies show that 2,4-toluene-diamine, a biodegradation product of polyurethane, may promote the progression of already present mutated cells [6,7]. In addition, one epidemiological study showed an elevation in breast cancer incidence for women with polyurethane-coated subglandular implants compared with women with subglandular implants without polyurethane coating [3]. However, this finding is based on

only one study with a small number of cases, and further investigations are required before this interpretation can be used in clinical practice. No differences in breast cancer incidence have been reported between saline-filled and silicone-gel-filled implants [3,8]. In addition, one study found that women with subglandular implants had a reduced risk of breast cancer compared with women with submuscular implants [3].

Some studies have evaluated the relationship between breast implants and the incidence of cancers at sites other than the breast. No conclusive findings can be reported about risk of other types of cancers [3,5]. Although there is concern about a possible link between breast implants and anaplastic large T-cell lymphomas of the breast [9], no epidemiological cohort studies have reported any evidence for an association [3,5,10].

Another concern is that breast implants may obscure the visualization of breast tissue with mammography, which may impair the ability to identify breast cancer at an early stage, for which survival is generally more favourable. In fact, recent epidemiological evidence has suggested that breast cancers are diagnosed at more advanced stages among women with cosmetic breast implants and that breast cancer-specific survival is lower in these women [11]. However, further studies are warranted about breast cancer diagnosis and

prognosis among women with breast augmentation.

References

1. Love S, Lindsey K (2000). Variations in development. *Dr. Susan Love's Breast Book*, 3rd ed. Cambridge, MA: Perseus Publishing.

2. Deapen DM *et al.* (1986). *Plast Reconstr Surg*, 77:361–368. http://dx.doi.org/10.1097/00006534-198603000-00001 PMID:3952193

3. Pan SY *et al.* (2012). *Int J Cancer*, 131: E1148–E1157. http://dx.doi.org/10.1002/ijc.27603 PMID:22514048

4. Deapen DM, Brody GS (2012). *Plast Reconstr Surg*, 129:575e–576e. http://dx.doi.org/10.1097/PRS.0b013e31824199f1 PMID:22374025

5. Lipworth L *et al.* (2009). *Int J Cancer*, 124:490–493. http://dx.doi.org/10.1002/ijc.23932 PMID:19003966

6. Cunningham ML *et al.* (1991). *Toxicol Appl Pharmacol*, 107:562–567. http://dx.doi.org/10.1016/0041-008X(91)90319-A PMID:2000642

7. Shanmugam K *et al.* (2001). *Anal Sci*, 17:1369–1374. http://dx.doi.org/10.2116/analsci.17.1369 PMID:11783783

8. Friis S *et al.* (2006). *Int J Cancer*, 118:998–1003. http://dx.doi.org/10.1002/ijc.21433 PMID:16152592

9. Jewell M *et al.* (2011). *Plast Reconstr Surg*, 128:651–661. http://dx.doi.org/10.1097/PRS.0b013e318221db81 PMID:21865998

10. Lipworth L *et al.* (2009). *Plast Reconstr Surg*, 123:790–793. http://dx.doi.org/10.1097/PRS.0b013e318199edeb PMID:19319041

11. Lavigne E *et al.* (2012). *Cancer Epidemiol Biomarkers Prev*, 21:1868–1876. http://dx.doi.org/10.1158/1055-9965.EPI-12-0484 PMID:22850806

Combined estrogen–progestogen contraceptives

Numerous types of combined hormonal contraceptives have been marketed since these agents first became available in the late 1950s [1]. With reference to the IARC Monographs Programme evaluation, there is *sufficient* evidence that combined estrogen–progestogen oral contraceptives cause cancers of the breast (notably among young women),

cervix, and liver (Table 2.10.2) [1]. IARC has also concluded that these agents are protective against cancers of the endometrium and ovary (Table 2.10.2), and possibly also colorectal cancer, although the evidence is not conclusive for colorectal cancer [1]. For other sites, including cancers of the thyroid, lung, stomach, urinary tract, gall bladder, and pancreas, as well as lymphoma, cutaneous melanoma, and central nervous system

tumours, the available literature does not support an association with combined estrogen–progestogen contraceptives [1].

Diethylstilbestrol

This synthetic estrogen was first manufactured in 1938 [1]. Diethylstilbestrol was widely used, especially from the 1940s to the 1970s, to prevent potential miscarriages by stimulating the synthesis of estrogen and pro-gesterone in the placenta. In the USA alone, an estimated 5–10 million peo-ple received diethylstilbestrol during pregnancy or were exposed to the drug during fetal life. Subsequently, several adverse effects emerged (Table 2.10.2) [1]. First, slightly in-creased risks of breast cancer and possibly of endometrial cancer were observed among women exposed to diethylstilbestrol during pregnancy. Second, among female children of women who used diethylstilbestrol during pregnancy, a markedly in-creased risk of adenocarcinoma of the vagina or cervix was recorded, typically occurring during adoles-cence. Third, fetal exposure to di-ethylstilbestrol was associated with increased risks of squamous cell car-cinoma of the cervix among female offspring and testicular cancer among male offspring. Currently, evidence is accumulating of an increased risk of cancers of the female reproductive organs among third-generation off-spring of women who used diethyl-stilbestrol [1].

Tamoxifen

Tamoxifen is indicated as adjuvant therapy for treatment of postmen-opausal estrogen-receptor-positive or progesterone-receptor-positive breast cancer among both women and men, as well as ductal carci-noma in situ after breast surgery and radiotherapy among women [1]. Furthermore, tamoxifen has been approved as a breast cancer preventive agent among women at high risk of developing breast cancer (see below). Observational epide-miological studies and randomized trials have consistently shown that use of tamoxifen increases the risk of endometrial cancer whether given as adjuvant therapy among women with breast cancer or as preventive therapy among women at high risk of breast cancer (Table 2.10.2) [1]. There is also some indication that tamoxifen may be associated with an increased risk of some types of gas-trointestinal cancer; however, these results are not conclusive.

Phenacetin

The analgesic phenacetin and mix-tures containing phenacetin were until recently classified by IARC as probably carcinogenic to humans (Group 2A), since the available evidence had not been able to dis-criminate between potential carci-nogenic effects of phenacetin and those attributable to other analge-sics or components of analgesics used by the same patients. In the recent IARC re-evaluation [1], how-ever, phenacetin and phenacetin-containing mixtures were both clas-sified as carcinogenic to humans (Group 1), causing cancers of the renal pelvis and ureter (Table 2.10.1). Since phenacetin was withdrawn from the market in most countries in about 1980, the pool of patients with excess risk of cancers of the renal pelvis or ureter due to phenacetin therapy is probably limited now, although a long latency period for development of these cancer types cannot be excluded and relevant cancers may yet be diagnosed.

Miscellaneous agents

Use of *Aristolochia* plants contain-ing aristolochic acid has mainly

been limited to traditional Chinese drugs, weight-loss pills in Belgium, and cereals from Balkan fields [1]. Aristolochic acid induces DNA dam-age similar to that seen for antineo-plastic agents and is associated with nephropathy and an increased risk of cancers of the renal pelvis and ureter (Table 2.10.1). Genome-wide sequencing has established the mutational signature of aristolochic acid [5].

Methoxsalen, which is a pso-ralen produced naturally by vari-ous plants, is a photosensitizer: the agent increases skin reactivity to ul-traviolet radiation [1]. Methoxsalen is nowadays typically taken orally in conjunction with ultraviolet radiation as phototherapy for various condi-tions, notably psoriasis. The drug has been suspected to cause vari-ous types of skin cancer, but there is convincing evidence only for causa-tion of squamous cell carcinoma [1]. Some common vegetables naturally contain methoxsalen, and there have been reports of photosensitivity and skin lesions among grocery or farm workers.

Photosensitivity is also induced by frequently used drugs such as certain types of antihypertensives,

Fig. 2.10.3. A patient receives chemotherapy through a port located on his chest.

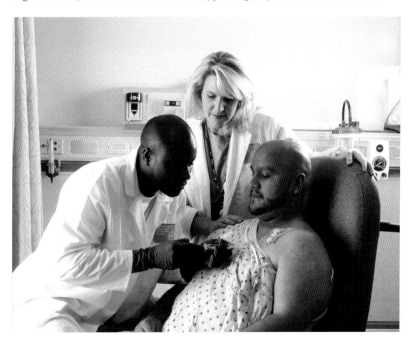

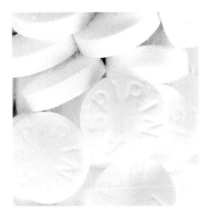

Fig. 2.10.4. Today, the evaluation of non-steroidal anti-inflammatory drugs as a potential cancer preventive measure is focused on aspirin.

for example hydrochlorothiazide and nifedipine. There is increasing evidence that these drugs increase the risk of lip and skin cancers [6].

Many of the drugs evaluated by IARC have been categorized as probably carcinogenic to humans (Group 2A) or possibly carcinogenic to humans (Group 2B) because the epidemiological evidence has not been definitive and is hence categorized as *limited* or because carcinogenicity has been demonstrated only in experimental animals. These agents include, for example, griseofulvin, metronidazole, phenytoin, chloramphenicol, iron-dextran complexes, phenoxybenzamine, phenobarbital, oxazepam, propylthiouracil, and anti-retroviral agents (e.g. zidovudine) [7].

Cancer preventive drugs

Hormone antagonists
Several drugs within the therapeutic groups of selective estrogen-receptor modulators and aromatase inhibitors have been approved for endocrine therapy among women with hormone-receptor-positive breast cancer. However, so far, only the two selective estrogen-receptor modulators tamoxifen and raloxifene have been approved for preventive therapy against breast cancer [8]. Tamoxifen reduces the risk of contralateral breast cancer and, when given as preventive therapy, reduces the risk of estrogen-receptor-positive breast cancers. Tamoxifen has greater efficacy than raloxifene and can be used in premenopausal women, but raloxifene has fewer side-effects and is not classified as carcinogenic to humans. Newer drugs within the class of selective estrogen-receptor modulators, for example lasofoxifene, also show efficacy, and possibly a better overall benefit–risk profile, but need further assessment. Aromatase inhibitors may be more efficacious, and drugs within this class, for example anastrozole and exemestane, are currently being evaluated as preventive agents among women with a history of carcinoma in situ of the breast or other women considered to be at high risk of developing breast cancer.

Aspirin and other non-steroidal anti-inflammatory drugs
Several observational epidemiological studies, randomized trials of colon adenoma recurrence, and randomized trials in patients with hereditary colorectal cancer syndromes have consistently shown that aspirin and other non-steroidal anti-inflammatory drugs (NSAIDs) reduce the risk of colorectal neoplasia and cancer [9,10]. A cancer preventive effect of aspirin or non-aspirin NSAIDs against other cancer types is less certain [9,10]. Despite the cancer preventive effect of non-aspirin NSAIDs, the use of these agents for prevention of colorectal cancer is hampered by their recently established association with cardiovascular events [10]. The evaluation of NSAIDs as a potential cancer preventive measure is thus focused on aspirin [10]. However, although the preventive effect of aspirin against colorectal neoplasia has been practically proven, aspirin cannot be recommended for cancer prevention in the general population of healthy individuals due to the risk of serious adverse events, notably upper gastrointestinal bleeding [10]. Moreover, uncertainty still remains as to the optimal dose and duration of aspirin therapy for cancer prevention [9]. The results of several current randomized trials will hopefully provide more confirmatory data on these issues.

Statins
HMG-CoA reductase inhibitors (statins) reduce serum levels of cholesterol and are widely used to manage and prevent cardiovascular and coronary heart disease. In addition, a growing body of experimental evidence has suggested that statins have cancer preventive properties [11]. To date, however, several randomized trials with cancer as secondary end-point have failed to demonstrate a reduced risk of cancer, overall or at specific sites, within statin treatment periods of 5–10 years. Likewise, observational epidemiological studies with longer follow-up have generally produced null results, with the exception of an inverse association between statin use and aggressive prostate cancer [12]. Statins have also been evaluated as adjuvant therapy to standard cancer therapy; however, to date this has yielded primarily null results [11]. Several current trials will hopefully clarify whether statins have a future role in cancer prevention or therapy.

Recent research issues
There is substantial evidence that female sex hormones are associated with a decreased risk of colorectal cancer and thus represent further hormonal agents associated with both carcinogenic and cancer preventive properties. Meta-analysis indicates significant duration-dependent reductions in ovarian cancer incidence associated with oral contraceptive use [13]. Observational epidemiological studies also indicate that metformin, a widely used oral antidiabetic drug, may reduce the risk of several cancer types; however, these associations require further assessment [14]. Several trials of metformin have recently been launched to assess whether this old drug may have a cancer preventive potential.

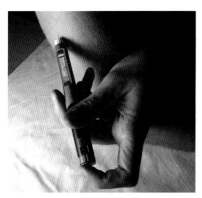

Some epidemiological studies indicate that insulin treatment is associated with increased risk of several cancer types; however, the results are equivocal [15]. Moreover, it has been suggested that insulin analogues are more prone to induce cancer, but this hypothesis also remains to be clarified. Several international research initiatives have recently been launched to clarify these issues. A recent single study indicated that long-term current use of calcium-channel blockers is associated with increased breast cancer risk among women aged 55–74 years [16].

Two large randomized trials have demonstrated that the two 5α-reductase inhibitors, finasteride and dutasteride, indicated for treatment of benign prostatic hyperplasia, reduce the risk of prostate cancer among men by 25%; however, both studies also revealed an increased risk of aggressive prostate cancer [17]. Whether the increased risk of aggressive prostate cancer is due to detection bias or a true biological association remains unclear [17]. Until this spurious phenomenon is resolved, these agents should not be recommended as cancer preventive agents.

Concerns have been raised about the new biological response modifiers for treatment of rheumatoid arthritis, which include tumour necrosis factor inhibitors. Tumour necrosis factor inhibitors have been suggested to increase the risk of certain cancers, including lymphoma in children and adolescents, and these agents currently carry a label warning against a possible risk of malignancy. A large meta-analysis of 61 randomized trials of tumour necrosis factor inhibitors, including a total of 29 423 patients, concluded that use of these drugs was not associated with an increased risk of cancer overall or at specific sites [18]. However, follow-up was short (24–156 weeks) in this analysis, and continued monitoring is warranted.

The carcinogenicity of some drugs was recently evaluated for Volume 108 of the IARC Monographs [19], and two drugs attracted particular attention. Pioglitazone, used for treatment of type 2 diabetes, was classified as probably carcinogenic to humans (Group 2A), with limited evidence that it causes bladder cancer in humans and evident carcinogenicity in experimental animals. Use of digoxin, which is widely prescribed for chronic heart failure and related conditions, is associated with an increased risk of breast cancer; causal interpretation of these data is precluded because of possible confounding, particularly in relation to obesity and alcohol consumption. In the absence of animal bioassay data, digoxin was categorized as possibly carcinogenic to humans (Group 2B).

References

1. IARC (2012). Pharmaceuticals. *IARC Monogr Eval Carcinog Risks Hum*, 100A: 1–437. PMID:23189749

2. Grosse Y, Baan R, Straif K *et al.*; WHO IARC Monograph Working Group (2009). A review of human carcinogens – Part A: pharmaceuticals. *Lancet Oncol*, 10:13–14. http://dx.doi.org/10.1016/S1470-2045(08)70286-9 PMID:19115512

3. WHO Collaborating Centre for Drug Statistics Methodology (2012). *Guidelines for ATC Classification and DDD Assignment.* Oslo: WHO. Available at http://www.whocc.no/atc_ddd_index/.

4. Manson JE, Hsia J, Johnson KC *et al.*; Women's Health Initiative Investigators (2003). Estrogen plus progestin and the risk of coronary heart disease. *N Engl J Med*, 349:523–534. http://dx.doi.org/10.1056/NEJMoa030808 PMID:12904517

5. Hoang ML, Chen C-H, Sidorenko VS *et al.* (2013). Mutational signature of aristolochic acid exposure as revealed by whole-exome sequencing. *Sci Transl Med*, 5:ra102. http://dx.doi.org/10.1126/scitranslmed.3006200 PMID:23926200

6. Friedman GD, Asgari MM, Warton EM *et al.* (2012). Antihypertensive drugs and lip cancer in non-Hispanic whites. *Arch Intern Med*, 172:1246–1251. http://dx.doi.org/10.1001/archinternmed.2012.2754 PMID:22869299

7. Friedman GD, Jiang SF, Udaltsova N *et al.* (2009). Epidemiologic evaluation of pharmaceuticals with limited evidence of carcinogenicity. *Int J Cancer*, 125:2173–2178. http://dx.doi.org/10.1002/ijc.24545 PMID:19585498

8. Cuzick J, DeCensi A, Arun B *et al.* (2011). Preventive therapy for breast cancer: a consensus statement. *Lancet Oncol*, 12:496–503. http://dx.doi.org/10.1016/S1470-2045(11)70030-4 PMID:21441069

9. Chan AT, Arber N, Burn J *et al.* (2012). Aspirin in the chemoprevention of colorectal neoplasia: an overview. *Cancer Prev Res (Phila)*, 5:164–178. http://dx.doi.org/10.1158/1940-6207.CAPR-11-0391 PMID:22084361

10. Umar A, Dunn BK, Greenwald P (2012). Future directions in cancer prevention. *Nat Rev Cancer*, 12:835–848. http://dx.doi.org/10.1038/nrc3397 PMID:23151603

11. Gazzerro P, Proto MC, Gangemi G *et al.* (2012). Pharmacological actions of statins: a critical appraisal in the management of cancer. *Pharmacol Rev*, 64:102–146. http://dx.doi.org/10.1124/pr.111.004994 PMID:22106090

12. Boudreau DM, Yu O, Johnson J (2010). Statin use and cancer risk: a comprehensive review. *Expert Opin Drug Saf*, 9:603–621. http://dx.doi.org/10.1517/14740331003662620 PMID:20377474

13. Havrilesky LJ, Moorman PG, Lowery WJ *et al.* (2013). Oral contraceptive pills as primary prevention for ovarian cancer: a systematic review and meta-analysis. *Obstet Gynecol*, 122:139–147. http://dx.doi.org/10.1097/AOG.0b013e318291c235 PMID:23743450

14. Kourelis TV, Siegel RD (2012). Metformin and cancer: new applications for an old drug. *Med Oncol*, 29:1314–1327. http://dx.doi.org/10.1007/s12032-011-9846-7 PMID:21301998

15. Onitilo AA, Engel JM, Glurich I *et al.* (2012). Diabetes and cancer II: role of diabetes medications and influence of shared risk factors. *Cancer Causes Control*, 23:991–1008. http://dx.doi.org/10.1007/s10552-012-9971-4 PMID:22527174

16. Li CI, Daling JR, Tang MT *et al.* (2013). Use of antihypertensive medications and breast cancer risk among women aged 55 to 74 years. *JAMA Intern Med*, http://dx.doi.org/10.1001/jamainternmed.2013.9071 PMID:23921840

17. Azzouni F, Mohler J (2012). Role of 5α-reductase inhibitors in prostate cancer prevention and treatment. *Urology*, 79:1197–1205. http://dx.doi.org/10.1016/j.urology.2012.01.024 PMID:22446342

18. Lopez-Olivo MA, Tayar JH, Martinez-Lopez JA *et al.* (2012). Risk of malignancies in patients with rheumatoid arthritis treated with biologic therapy: a meta-analysis. *JAMA*, 308:898–908. http://dx.doi.org/10.1001/2012.jama.10857 PMID:22948700

19. Grosse Y, Loomis D, Lauby-Secretan B *et al.* (2013). Carcinogenicity of some drugs and herbal products. *Lancet Oncol*, 14:807–808. http://dx.doi.org/10.1016/S1470-2045(13)70329-2

2.11 Naturally occurring chemical carcinogens

Ronald T. Riley

Wentzel C.A. Gelderblom (reviewer)
J. David Miller (reviewer)

Summary

- Natural products are chemicals from plants, fungi, lichens, and bacteria, some of which have unique pharmacological effects. Humans are primarily exposed to many of these bioactive naturally occurring chemicals through food and water; natural products are used as pharmaceuticals and herbal remedies.

- Natural products of bacteria that are possibly or probably carcinogenic to humans include antibiotics, chemotherapeutic agents, and the water contaminant microcystin-LR. Environmental exposure to cyanobacterial toxins is well documented.

- Mycotoxins are secondary metabolites of fungi that are known to cause sickness or death in humans or animals. Exposure to carcinogenic mycotoxins can be high in areas where a single commodity is consumed as a dietary staple.

- Several chemicals found in particular plants used as food, food additives, or herbal medicines have been classified as human or animal carcinogens. Some of these plants are weeds and are sometimes harvested with crop plants or are deliberately used as herbal medicines.

Information about possible, probable, and known carcinogens that are naturally occurring chemicals of microbial or plant origin is summarized in this chapter. Natural products are chemicals found in nature, which often have unique pharmacological effects. In the 2011 edition of the *Dictionary of Natural Products*, more than 230 000 natural products were described [1]. Cancer-causing chemicals produced by bacteria, fungi, and plants are discussed here. Compounds that are semisynthetic, such as etoposide and teniposide from podophyllotoxin, or are produced by a genetically modified organism, as illustrated by doxorubicin obtained from a genetically altered strain of *Streptomyces*, are not included. That said, these three agents do provide important insights into the potential of naturally occurring chemicals to be carcinogenic. "Natural products" from tobacco, betel quid, or areca nut (see Chapter 2.2), ethanol (see Chapter 2.3), or naturally occurring chemicals produced by anaerobic bacteria such as methylated arsenic species, which are environmental pollutants (see Chapter 2.9), are discussed elsewhere.

One of the striking attributes of nature is biodiversity. As might be expected, there are a large number of biologically active organic chemicals produced in nature by microbes and plants. Biologically produced naturally occurring organic compounds are structurally diverse. Not surprisingly, humans are exposed to many of these chemicals primarily through food and drinking-water. In addition, exposure to naturally occurring chemicals occurs because they are used as pharmaceuticals and herbal remedies useful in the treatment and/or prevention of diseases.

The discovery of naturally occurring chemicals with potentially useful or dangerous biological activity is still in progress and is often proprietary. The current edition of the *Dictionary of Natural Products* [1] is a comprehensive survey of the literature on natural product discovery. For example, from 1995 to 1997 more than 6000 new compounds were added to the dictionary. Making informed decisions about the carcinogenic risk to humans posed by exposure to each of these 230 000 (and growing) biologically active natural products is a daunting, if not impossible, task. However, considering bacteria, including actinomycetes, and fungi, there are only 45 000 compounds with known biological activity [2].

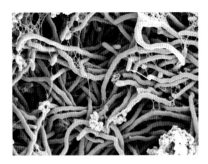

Fig. 2.11.1. *Streptomyces*, or soil bacteria, are commonly found in soil and water and are necessary for the decomposition of organic material.

The proportion of biologically active chemicals derived from plants that are used as therapeutic agents is quite low, despite some important examples [3].

Since 1971, the IARC Monographs Programme has evaluated more than 900 agents. More than 400 have been identified as carcinogenic, probably carcinogenic, or possibly carcinogenic to humans. The information gained from assessments of representative carcinogenic chemicals by IARC and the United States National Toxicology Program provides critical data for identifying which known or newly discovered chemicals may be carcinogenic hazards. For example, quantitative structure–activity relationships obtained from long-term feeding studies can be used to develop predictive models. These can be used for screening and prioritizing the carcinogenic hazards posed by naturally occurring chemicals when the data from animal studies are inadequate [4]. Accurate predictive modelling is dependent on the quality of the toxicology data rather than on the quantity of chemicals tested in long-term rodent carcinogenicity studies. Thus, it may be possible to predict which natural products are potential carcinogenic hazards without conducting long-term feeding studies on newly discovered natural products. This approach can be used effectively only if the toxicology database from long-term feeding studies represents all the relevant structures that have a high probability of contributing to cancer induction in humans. This task is also daunting, but not impossible, as would be testing every naturally occurring biologically active chemical.

Naturally occurring carcinogens produced by bacteria

Table 2.11.1 summarizes naturally occurring chemicals produced by bacteria evaluated by IARC as possibly or probably carcinogenic to humans. With the exception of microcystin-LR, human exposure to these agents occurs from treatment in a clinical setting. These six agents are produced by bacteria of the order *Actinomycetales*. The actinomycete genus *Streptomyces* produces a wide spectrum of natural products [5]. Actinomycetes are commonly found in soil and water and contribute to the decomposition of organic material [6]. The characteristic smell of wet soil is due in part to geosmin (meaning "earth smell"), a secondary metabolite produced by *Streptomyces*. *Streptomyces*-produced secondary metabolites

Table 2.11.1. Naturally occurring organic chemical carcinogens produced by bacteria

Agent (bacterial genera)[a]	Primary source of exposure[b]	Proposed mechanism of carcinogenicity[c]	Primary target or tumour sites[d]	IARC evaluation of carcinogenicity to humans[e]
Azacitidine (*Streptoverticillium*)	Chemotherapy	Cytidine analogue/DNA methylation inhibitor	Multiple sites	Group 2A
Chloramphenicol (*Streptomyces*)	Antibiotic	Inhibits mitochondrial protein synthesis → aplastic anaemia/bone-marrow depression	Blood	Group 2A
Azaserine (*Glycomyces*)	Antibiotic, chemotherapy	Glutamine/purine antagonist → inhibition of purine biosynthesis and glutamine-dependent enzymes	Pancreas, kidney	Group 2B
Daunomycin (*Streptomyces*)	Antibiotic, chemotherapy	DNA intercalation → inhibition of macromolecular biosynthesis → topoisomerase II inhibition	Mammary, kidney, local sarcomas	Group 2B
Microcystin-LR (*Microcystis*)	Water contaminant	Inhibition of protein phosphatases 1 and 2A → tumour promotion	Liver, colon	Group 2B
Mitomycin C (*Streptomyces*)	Antibiotic, chemotherapy	DNA/RNA alkylating agent → DNA/RNA damage Dithiol cross-linking agent → protein damage	Multiple sites	Group 2B
Streptozotocin (*Streptomyces*)	Antibiotic, chemotherapy	DNA alkylating agent → DNA damage Oxidative stress → diabetes	Liver, lung, kidney	Group 2B

[a] For all bacteria the most likely producing genera are given; the listing is not exhaustive.

[b] All of the agents listed can be produced by biosynthesis in situ, but for the antibiotics and chemotherapeutic agents exposure is in a controlled clinical setting.

[c] Where possible, the mechanism described is taken from the most recent IARC Monograph or IARC Scientific Publication.

[d] Includes reference to animal bioassay data. For some studies the route of exposure is oral, but in some studies exposure was intravenous, subcutaneous, or other.

[e] Group 1, carcinogenic to humans; Group 2A, probably carcinogenic to humans; Group 2B, possibly carcinogenic to humans; Group 3, not classifiable as to its carcinogenicity to humans; Group 4, probably not carcinogenic to humans. Only agents in Groups 1, 2A, and 2B are listed here. There are several naturally occurring agents classified by IARC as Group 3, but they are not included in this table.

may play important roles in bacterial–fungal, bacterial–plant, and bacterial–animal interactions in nature [6]. For example, *Streptomyces* are endosymbionts in wasps, and in the process of building cocoons the larvae incorporate nine different antibiotics on the surface of the cocoon for protection from microbial pathogens [7]. There are many other examples of actinomycetales secondary metabolites playing roles in symbiotic relationships with eukaryotic organisms [6]. Thus, environmental exposure to naturally produced antibiotics, including the six listed in Table 2.11.1, is possible, but the levels of human exposure would likely be quite low, given the nature of the environment where the producing organisms thrive (soil, compost, manure, fermenting hay).

In contrast, human environmental exposure to the cyanobacterial toxin microcystin-LR is well documented [8]. Exposure occurs most frequently through drinking-water or ingestion of water during recreational activities. Microcystin-LR contamination of dietary supplements produced using cyanobacteria has been demonstrated. In one documented case, exposure resulting from contamination of water used for renal dialysis has resulted in acute toxicity in humans [8]. Many countries have guidelines to minimize exposure from drinking-water and recreational exposure. In rodent studies, microcystin-LR was a promoter of preneoplastic lesions and persistent neoplastic nodules in the liver. Co-exposure to aflatoxin is a concern since in rats microcystin-LR promotes the formation of aflatoxin-induced glutathione *S*-transferase placental form-positive foci, which are considered preneoplastic lesions [8]. The inhibition of protein phosphatases 1 and 2A in vivo is consistent with microcystin promotion of liver tumours in animals. Inhibition of phosphatases causes hyperphosphorylation of intracellular proteins, disruption of intermediate filament assembly, altered expression of oncogenes and early response genes, and expression of tumour necrosis

factor α, leading to altered cell division, survival, and apoptosis [8].

Naturally occurring carcinogens produced by fungi

As with bacteria, the total number of naturally occurring fungal metabolites cannot be quantified; however, an estimate may be made. For example, all fungi produce secondary metabolites and there are approximately two unique secondary metabolites per fungal species [9]. Thus, the total number of unique fungal secondary metabolites can be estimated based on the estimated number of fungal species. In 2001, Hawksworth estimated that there were about 100 000 formally described fungal species, and that number was considered to represent 5% of the total worldwide [10]. However, this number is likely to be conservative since there are estimated to be 200 000 fungal species at the tip of Africa alone [11]. The recent completion of an online world catalogue of fungal names (http://www.indexfungorum.org/) has produced a more accurate figure of about 300 000 for the number of species names of fungi. Assuming two unique secondary metabolites per fungal species produces an estimate of about 600 000 secondary fungal metabolites. Some of these metabolites may be carcinogens. Currently, there are eight fungal compounds (excluding alcoholic beverages) that have been evaluated as having *sufficient* evidence of carcinogenicity in humans and/or animals (Table 2.11.2).

Human exposure to ciclosporin (also known as cyclosporin, cyclosporine, or cyclosporin A) and griseofulvin occurs exclusively in clinical settings. Nonetheless, environmental exposure is possible since the fungi that produce these agents are common in soil and other matrices [12]. The fungus most used for producing ciclosporin commercially, *Tolypocladium inflatum*, also produces fumonisins B_2 and B_4 [13]. Dietary exposure to griseofulvin is also possible since both *Penicillium*

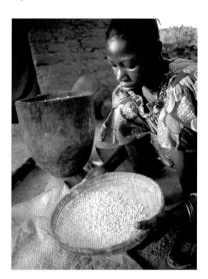

Fig. 2.11.2. A woman in sub-Saharan Mali sifts newly harvested grain. Cereal crops subject to storage under tropical conditions are susceptible to contamination by mycotoxins.

griseofulvum and griseofulvin have been isolated or detected in honey, service tree fruits, and cured meats. That said, it is unlikely that exposure outside clinical settings is of great significance.

Mycotoxins are secondary metabolites of microfungi that are known to cause sickness or death in humans or animals [14]. Of the toxins listed in Table 2.11.2, six are almost exclusively encountered as contaminants of food, although occupational exposure also occurs [14]. The foods most likely to be contaminated with high concentrations of mycotoxins are cereal grains and groundnuts, which are dietary staples in many developing countries [14]. The only fungal toxin for which there is *sufficient* evidence of carcinogenicity in humans is the group referred to as aflatoxins [14,15]. Aflatoxins include aflatoxins B_1, B_2, G_1, G_2, and M_1. In naturally contaminated food, aflatoxins B_1 and B_2 or aflatoxins G_1 and G_2 usually occur together; however, aflatoxins B_2 and G_2 are less biologically active and there is *limited* or *inadequate* evidence, respectively, of their carcinogenicity in experimental animals. Aflatoxin G_1 is less mutagenic than aflatoxin B_1, and forms fewer DNA adducts. Aflatoxin M_1

Table 2.11.2. Naturally occurring organic chemical carcinogens produced by fungi

Agent (fungal genera)[a]	Primary source of exposure[b]	Proposed mechanism of carcinogenicity[c]	Primary target or tumour sites[d]	IARC evaluation of carcinogenicity to humans (NTP class)[e]
Aflatoxins (*Aspergillus* sp.)	Food contaminant	Metabolism to DNA/protein-reactive epoxide → *TP53* mutations	Liver	Group 1 (K)
Ciclosporin (*Tolypocladium* and some *Fusarium* species)	Pharmaceutical	Binds cyclophilin, blocks calcineurin and inhibits its phosphatase activity → immune suppression	Skin, lymphoma, other sites	Group 1 (K)
Aflatoxin M_1 (*Aspergillus*)	Food contaminant	DNA-reactive epoxide → mutations	Liver	Group 2B
Fumonisin B_1 (*Fusarium* sp.)	Food contaminant	Inhibition of ceramide synthase → disruption of lipid metabolism and signalling pathways regulating cell growth/tumour promoter	Liver, kidney	Group 2B
Fusarium moniliforme toxins (*Fusarium* sp.)	Food contaminant	Inhibition of ceramide synthase → disruption of lipid metabolism and signalling pathways regulating cell growth/tumour promoter	Liver, kidney	Group 2B
Griseofulvin (*Penicillium* sp.)	Antifungal agent	Disruption of microtubule formation via tubulin binding/mitotic inhibitor	Liver, thyroid	Group 2B
Ochratoxin A (*Aspergillus* and *Penicillium* species)	Food contaminant	Phenylalanine analogue/disruption of signalling pathways regulating cell growth/DNA adducts?	Kidney, liver	Group 2B (R)
Sterigmatocystin (*Aspergillus* sp.)	Food contaminant	Metabolism to DNA-reactive epoxide → mutations	Liver, lung	Group 2B

[a] For all fungi the most likely producing genera are given; the listing is not exhaustive.

[b] All of the agents listed can be produced by biosynthesis in situ, but for ciclosporin and griseofulvin exposure is in a controlled clinical setting.

[c] Where possible, the mechanism described is taken from the most recent IARC Monograph or IARC Scientific Publication.

[d] For cancer studies, the route of exposure was usually oral.

[e] Group 1, carcinogenic to humans; Group 2A, probably carcinogenic to humans; Group 2B, possibly carcinogenic to humans; Group 3, not classifiable as to its carcinogenicity to humans; Group 4, probably not carcinogenic to humans. Only agents in Groups 1, 2A, and 2B are listed here. There are several naturally occurring agents classified by IARC as Group 3, but they are not included in this table. NTP, United States National Toxicology Program: K, known be a human carcinogen; R, reasonably anticipated to be a human carcinogen.

occurs almost exclusively in milk and milk products and is less carcinogenic than aflatoxin B_1. The mechanisms of action of aflatoxins B_1, G_1, and M_1 are similar in that they can be metabolized to *exo*-epoxides that can react with DNA, form chemical adducts, and modify genes. Less is known about the metabolism of sterigmatocystin to the *exo*-epoxide. For aflatoxins, one affected gene in humans is the tumour suppressor gene *TP53*, and there is a mechanistic link between levels of genetic biomarkers for aflatoxin exposure (codon 249-specific *TP53* mutations) and hepatocellular carcinoma.

Epidemiological studies of aflatoxin have provided strong evidence of a greater than multiplicative interaction between aflatoxin exposure and chronic infection with hepatitis B virus in relation to increased risk of hepatocellular carcinoma [14,15]. Other factors may potentiate the risk of aflatoxin-induced hepatocellular carcinoma. For example, many of the populations at high risk

for hepatocellular carcinoma are also consumers of large amounts of maize that is frequently co-contaminated with both aflatoxins and *Fusarium verticillioides* toxins, in particular fumonisin B_1 [14,16]. For example, fumonisin B_1 treatment was shown to synergistically increase the number of preneoplastic liver lesions in aflatoxin B_1-initiated rats and significantly increased liver tumours in a dose-dependent manner in aflatoxin B_1-initiated trout in a long-term fumonisin feeding study [14,16]. The mechanistic basis for fumonisin promotion of aflatoxin B_1 carcinogenicity in trout and preneoplastic lesions in rats is likely a result of inhibited biosynthesis of ceramide (a lipid mediator of cell death) and elevation in levels of the mitogenic sphingoid base metabolite sphinganine-1-phosphate, a ligand for the G protein-coupled extracellular receptors $S1P_1$–$S1P_5$ [16].

Ochratoxin A is a liver and kidney carcinogen in animals and is found in maize, many small grain cereals,

and other commodities such as grapes, coffee, and even some meat products [14]. The mechanistic basis for the carcinogenicity of ochratoxin A in animals is unclear. Ochratoxin A is a phenylalanine analogue that accumulates in the kidney via an organic anion transporter. Some of its biological effects are due to phenylalanine mimicry [14]. Like fumonisin, ochratoxin A causes changes in regulatory processes that affect cell survival and proliferation. There is also evidence for DNA adduct formation by ochratoxin A via both direct and indirect processes [14]. Ochratoxin A has, for many decades, been suspected as the cause of the high incidence of urinary tract tumours in the Balkans referred to as Balkan endemic nephropathy. However, epidemiological support for this is not clear. More recently, natural products and food contaminants derived from plants have also been implicated in the genesis of this disease [17].

Fig. 2.11.3. *Aspergillus flavus* (A) grown as colonies on Czapek yeast extract agar (left) and malt extract agar (right) at 25 °C for 7 days; (B,C) heads, bars = 20 µm; (D) conidia, bar = 5 µm. This organism produces aflatoxins.

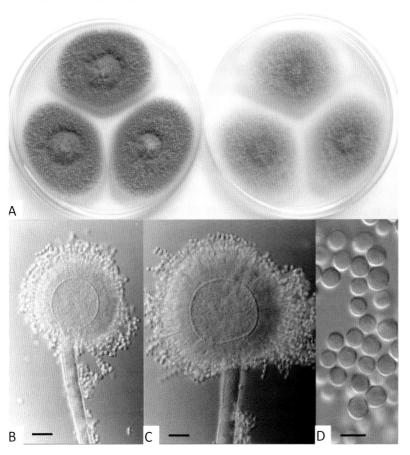

contributing to Balkan endemic nephropathy [19,20]. This suggestion is supported by mechanistic data involving aristolochic acid-derived DNA adducts detected in tumour tissue from people with Balkan endemic nephropathy. These same adducts are found in animals treated with aristolochic acid, and the same mutation in the *TP53* gene was seen in tumour tissues from patients with Balkan endemic nephropathy and in human *TP53* knock-in mouse fibroblasts treated with aristolochic acid [20]. More recently, whole-exome sequencing, based on urothelial carcinoma from 19 individuals with documented exposure to aristolochic acid, has established a mutational signature involving A:T → T:A transversions, indicating the power of this technique to reveal individual exposure to particular carcinogens [20].

Lasiocarpine, monocrotaline, and riddelliine (Table 2.11.3) are examples of pyrrolizidine alkaloids produced by plants growing in arid regions. For example, riddelliine-producing plants grow in desert areas of North America and are occasional contaminants of herbal products and food, but are most notable for poisoning of grazing

Naturally occurring carcinogens produced by plants

A large number of compounds produced by plants have been characterized as being dietary pesticides [18]. The number of so-called natural pesticides consumed (5000–10 000) and the amount (1.5 g/person/day) were also estimated, and it was speculated that many such biologically active compounds may exhibit carcinogenic activity in animal bioassays. Whether or not these estimates are correct, a large number of biologically active organic chemicals are biosynthesized by plants to deter a range of threats to their survival, and to promote successful competition with other plants and response to injury. Many may be carcinogenic

in rodent bioassays if administered at high levels.

Table 2.11.3 lists agents classified as human or animal carcinogens by IARC and produced by plants that have been used as food, food additives, or herbal medicines. A study conducted by the United States Centers for Disease Control and Prevention found that 10% of adults in the USA consumed herbal medicines in 1999 [19].

Herbal medicines containing extracts or preparations from plants producing aristolochic acid have been used since ancient times. Some herbal medicines and foods continue to be a source of intentional or inadvertent exposure to aristolochic acid. Contamination of wheat with seeds from *Aristolochia* species has been suggested as

Fig. 2.11.4. *Aristolochia manshuriensis*: (A) fruit twig, (B) flower, and (C) transverse section. *Aristolochia* species have been linked to endemic diseases of the kidney in the general population and in research.

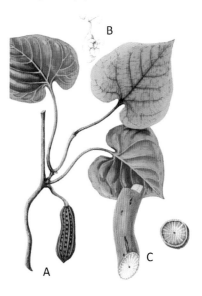

Table 2.11.3. Naturally occurring organic chemical carcinogens produced by plants that are used as herbal medicines, food, or food additives or contaminants

Agent/plants[a]	Primary source of exposure[b]	Proposed mechanism of carcinogenicity[c]	Primary target or tumour sites[d]	IARC evaluation of carcinogenicity to humans[e]
Aristolochic acid (*Aristolochia/Asarum* species)	Herbal medicine, food contaminant	Metabolism to DNA-reactive nitrenium ion → *TP53* mutations	Urothelium	Group 1
Plants containing aristolochic acid (Aristolochiaceae family)	Herbal medicine, food contaminant	Metabolism to DNA-reactive nitrenium ion → *TP53* mutations	Urothelium	Group 1
Bracken fern (*Pteridium* sp.)	Food, food contaminant	DNA alkylating activity (ptaquiloside?)	Bladder, gastrointestinal tract	Group 2B
Caffeic acid (Coffee, fruits, vegetables, grains, argan oil)	Herbal medicine, food component	Antioxidant/increased cell proliferation/ lipoxygenase inhibitor	Kidney, gastrointestinal tract	Group 2B
Carrageenan, degraded	Food additive	Oxidative stress/inflammation	Colorectum	Group 2B
Dihydrosafrole and safrole (*Sassafras*, essential oils, spices)	Food additive, food contaminant	Metabolism to DNA-reactive sulfo-oxy metabolites → mutations	Liver, lung, oesophagus	Group 2B
1-Hydroxyanthraquinone (*Tabebuia avellanedae*, *Morinda officinalis*, and many other plants)	Herbal medicine	Induces inflammation in the colon/oxidative stress/mutagen?	Large intestine	Group 2B
Lasiocarpine (Boraginaceae family)	Food contaminant	Metabolism to DNA-reactive dehydronecine → mutations	Liver, lymphoma, leukaemia	Group 2B
Methyleugenol (Essential oils, basil, tarragon, nutmeg, and others)	Food additive, food contaminant	Metabolism to DNA-reactive sulfo-oxy metabolites → mutations	Liver, stomach, kidney	Group 2B
Monocrotaline (Fabaceae family)	Food contaminant	Metabolism to DNA-reactive dehydronecine → mutations	Liver, multiple sites	Group 2B
Riddelliine (*Senecio* sp., Leguminosae family)	Herbal medicine	Metabolism to DNA-reactive dehydronecine → mutations	Liver, lung, leukaemia	Group 2B

[a] For all agents examples of natural sources of exposure are given; the listing is not exhaustive.

[b] All of the agents listed can be produced by biosynthesis in situ.

[c] Where possible, the mechanism described is taken from the most recent IARC Monograph or IARC Scientific Publication.

[d] For all cancer studies, including animal bioassays where relevant, the route of exposure was usually oral.

[e] Group 1, carcinogenic to humans; Group 2A, probably carcinogenic to humans; Group 2B, possibly carcinogenic to humans; Group 3, not classifiable as to its carcinogenicity to humans; Group 4, probably not carcinogenic to humans. Only agents in Groups 1, 2A, and 2B are listed here. There are several naturally occurring agents classified by IARC as Group 3, but they are not included in this table.

animals that consume the producing plants. Consumption of herbal teas prepared from plants that produce pyrrolizidine alkaloids has poisoned humans and caused death; however, there are no available human carcinogenicity data for riddelliine or any of the other pyrrolizidine alkaloids [21]. The mechanism of toxicity and carcinogenicity of pyrrolizidine alkaloids in animals involves their metabolism to DNA-reactive metabolites that bind DNA and cause mutations in specific genes, most notably *TP53* and the *K-ras* oncogene [21].

There are numerous other plant natural products classified by the IARC Monographs as being carcinogenic. However, exposure or production at levels sufficient to pose appreciable risk of biological effects is primarily through exposure in industrial/ occupational or clinical settings or by intake of the agent produced synthetically (Table 2.11.4). Examples are the pharmaceutical methoxsalen [17] and chemicals produced in an industrial setting that are also natural products of plant origin. Examples of agents that are natural products produced synthetically for industrial uses are listed in Table 2.11.4 [22].

Table 2.11.4. Naturally occurring organic chemical carcinogens derived from plants that are produced for industrial or medical uses but also can occur naturally in foods

Agent/plants[a]	Primary source of exposure[b]	Proposed mechanism of carcinogenicity[c]	Primary target or tumour sites[d]	IARC evaluation of carcinogenicity to humans[e]
Methoxsalen (plus ultraviolet A radiation) (Parsnip, parsley, other vegetables)	Pharmaceutical	Photo-activation, DNA reactivity → mutations	Skin	Group 1
5-Methoxypsoralen (Parsnip, parsley, other vegetables, bergamot and lime oils)	Pharmaceutical, cosmetic additive	Photo-activation, DNA reactivity → mutations	Skin	Group 2A
Acetaldehyde (Many fruits, vegetables, essential oils)	Industrial chemical	Irritant/DNA damage/protein binding	Upper respiratory tract	Group 2B[f]
Benzophenone (Grapes, black tea, papaya)	Industrial chemical	Endocrine disruption/oxidative stress	Liver, kidney, histiocytic sarcoma in multiple sites	Group 2B
Catechol (Fruits, vegetables, argan oil)	Industrial chemical	Metabolism to benzo-1,2-quinone, which binds to protein?	Stomach	Group 2B
Cumene (*Zingiber officinale*, fruits, vegetables, meat, many foods and beverages)	Industrial chemical	Metabolism to DNA-reactive α-methylstyrene oxide → mutations	Respiratory tract, spleen, liver, kidney	Group 2B
Dantron (danthron) (*Xyris semifuscata*, *Rheum palmatum*, some insects)	Industrial chemical	DNA damage? Tumour promoter	Liver, gastrointestinal tract	Group 2B
2,4-Hexadienal (Fruits, vegetables, meat, many foods and beverages)	Industrial chemical	Direct-acting DNA alkylating agent → mutations?	Forestomach, tongue, adrenal glands	Group 2B
Methyl isobutyl ketone (Fruits, vegetables, meat, beverages)	Industrial chemical	Cytotoxicity, regenerative cell proliferation	Liver, kidney (inhalation)	Group 2B

[a] For all agents examples of natural sources of exposure are given; the listing is not exhaustive.

[b] All of the agents listed can be produced by biosynthesis in situ.

[c] Where possible, the mechanism described is taken from the most recent IARC Monograph or IARC Scientific Publication.

[d] For cancer studies the route of exposure was most likely oral.

[e] Group 1, carcinogenic to humans; Group 2A, probably carcinogenic to humans; Group 2B, possibly carcinogenic to humans; Group 3, not classifiable as to its carcinogenicity to humans; Group 4, probably not carcinogenic to humans. Only agents in Groups 1, 2A, and 2B are listed here. There are several naturally occurring agents classified by IARC as Group 3, but they are not included in this table.

[f] Acetaldehyde associated with consumption of alcoholic beverages is classified as Group 1.

References

1. Buckingham J, ed. (2011). *Dictionary of Natural Products*. London: Chapman and Hall/CRC.

2. Kurtböke DI (2012). Biodiscovery from rare actinomycetes: an eco-taxonomical perspective. *Appl Microbiol Biotechnol*, 93:1843–1852. http://dx.doi.org/10.1007/s00253-012-3898-2 PMID:22297430

3. Newman DJ, Cragg GM (2012). Natural products as sources of new drugs over the 30 years from 1981 to 2010. *J Nat Prod*, 75:311–335. http://dx.doi.org/10.1021/np200906s PMID:22316239

4. Valerio LG Jr, Arvidson KB, Chanderbhan RF, Contrera JF (2007). Prediction of rodent carcinogenic potential of naturally occurring chemicals in the human diet using high-throughput QSAR predictive modeling. *Toxicol Appl Pharmacol*, 222:1–16. http://dx.doi.org/10.1016/j.taap.2007.03.012 PMID:17482223

5. Wink J. Compendium of Actinobacteria. Available at http://www.gbif-prokarya.de/microorganisms/wink.html

6. Seipke RF, Kaltenpoth M, Hutchings MI (2012). *Streptomyces* as symbionts: an emerging and widespread theme? *FEMS Microbiol Rev*, 36:862–876. http://dx.doi.org/10.1111/j.1574-6976.2011.00313.x PMID:22091965

7. Kroiss J, Kaltenpoth M, Schneider B *et al.* (2010). Symbiotic streptomycetes provide antibiotic combination prophylaxis for wasp offspring. *Nat Chem Biol*, 6:261–263. http://dx.doi.org/10.1038/nchembio.331 PMID:20190763

8. Paerl HW, Otten TG (2013). Harmful cyanobacterial blooms: causes, consequences, and controls. *Microb Ecol*, 65:995–1010. http://dx.doi.org/10.1007/s00248-012-0159-y PMID:23314096

9. Riley RT (1998). Mechanistic interaction of mycotoxins: theoretical considerations. In: Sinha KK, Bhatnagar D, eds. *Mycotoxins in Agriculture and Food Safety*. New York: Marcel Dekker, pp. 227–253.

10. Hawksworth DL (2001). The magnitude of fungal diversity: the 1.5 million species estimate revisited. *Mycol Res*, 105:1422–1432. http://dx.doi.org/10.1017/S0953756201004725

11. Crous PW, Rong IH, Wood A *et al.* (2006). How many species of fungi are there at the tip of Africa? *Stud Mycol*, 55:13–33. http://dx.doi.org/10.3114/sim.55.1.13 PMID:18490969

12. Rodríguez MA, Cabrera G, Godeas A (2006). Cyclosporine A from a nonpathogenic *Fusarium oxysporum* suppressing *Sclerotinia sclerotiorum*. *J Appl Microbiol*, 100:575–586. http://dx.doi.org/10.1111/j.1365-2672.2005.02824.x PMID:16478497

13. Mogensen JM, Møller KA, von Freiesleben P *et al.* (2011). Production of fumonisins B_2 and B_4 in *Tolypocladium* species. *J Ind Microbiol Biotechnol*, 38:1329–1335. http://dx.doi.org/10.1007/s10295-010-0916-1 PMID:21132348

14. Pitt J, Wild CP, Baan RA *et al.*, eds (2012). *Improving Public Health through Mycotoxin Control*. Lyon: IARC (IARC Scientific Publications Series, No. 158).

15. IARC (2012). Chemical agents and related occupations. *IARC Monogr Eval Carcinog Risks Hum*, 100F:1–599. PMID:23189753

16. Bulder AS, Arcella D, Bolger M *et al.* (2012). Fumonisins (addendum). In: *Safety Evaluation of Certain Food Additives and Contaminants: Prepared by the Seventy-fourth Meeting of the Joint FAO/WHO Expert Committee on Food Additives (JECFA)*. Geneva: WHO (WHO Food Additives Series, No. 65), pp. 325–794. Available at whqlibdoc.who.int/publications/2012/9789241660655_eng.pdf.

17. IARC (2012). Pharmaceuticals. *IARC Monogr Eval Carcinog Risks Hum*, 100A:1–437. PMID:23189749

18. Ames BN, Gold LS (2000). Paracelsus to parascience: the environmental cancer distraction. *Mutat Res*, 447:3–13. http://dx.doi.org/10.1016/S0027-5107(99)00194-3 PMID:10686303

19. Grollman AP (2013). Aristolochic acid nephropathy: harbinger of a global iatrogenic disease. *Environ Mol Mutagen*, 54:1–7. http://dx.doi.org/10.1002/em.21756 PMID:23238808

20. Hoang ML, Chen CH, Sidorenko VS *et al.* (2013). Mutational signature of aristolochic acid exposure as revealed by whole-exome sequencing. *Sci Transl Med*, 5:ra102. PMID:23926200

21. Chen T, Mei N, Fu PP (2010). Genotoxicity of pyrrolizidine alkaloids. *J Appl Toxicol*, 30:183–196. PMID:20112250

22. IARC (2012). Some chemicals present in industrial and consumer products, food and drinking-water. *IARC Monogr Eval Carcinog Risks Hum*, 101:1–610.

Cesar G. Victora

Early-life exposures, birth cohorts, and noncommunicable diseases (with special reference to cancer)

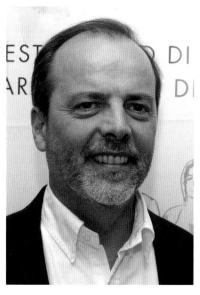

Cesar G. Victora is an emeritus professor of epidemiology at the Federal University of Pelotas in Brazil. He has conducted extensive research on maternal and child health and nutrition, on equity issues, and on the evaluation of health services.

Dr Victora obtained his medical degree from the Federal University of Rio Grande do Sul and a Ph.D. in health-care epidemiology from the London School of Hygiene and Tropical Medicine. His unit in Pelotas is a WHO Collaborating Centre in Maternal Health and Nutrition. He is a former international associate editor of the American Journal of Public Health *and was one of the coordinators of the 2008* Lancet *series on maternal and child undernutrition. Dr Victora was elected to the Brazilian Academy of Sciences in 2006. He is currently a visiting professor in the Department of International Health at the Johns Hopkins Bloomberg School of Public Health.*

Summary

There is strong evidence that several early-life factors influence the occurrence of different types of cancer as well as other noncommunicable diseases. Although stand-alone cohorts seldom have the statistical power to study cancer incidence directly, they can provide important information on how early-life exposures affect risk factors for common adult cancers, and thus contribute to their prevention. A potential solution is to pool several cohorts to increase sample size; such efforts have been limited by different definitions of exposures, outcomes, and confounders, as well as variable ages at ascertainment. Greater efforts should be made to coordinate data collection in cohorts that are still in early life so that, several decades from now, the problems that we are currently facing will have been overcome.

Why birth cohorts are important

The role of early influences in shaping adult life has long been recognized. Reviews of this topic often cite John Milton ("The childhood shows the man"; 1671) and William Wordsworth ("The Child is father of the Man"; 1802) as examples of the long-standing awareness of the importance of early factors.

In the 1960s the field was substantially advanced by René Dubos, who proposed the idea of "biological Freudianism" [1]. He built upon Sigmund Freud's work on the lasting effect of early behaviours, and expanded it to study the role of early stimuli in general, with special emphasis on nutritional and infectious exposures. Among many remarkable insights, Dubos highlighted the importance of the gut microbiota, a topic that is currently high on our research agenda. The work of Dubos, however, relied heavily on animal models instead of epidemiological studies.

Current interest in early exposures was boosted by the work of David Barker since the late 1970s. This evolved into the field of research that is currently known as developmental origins of health and disease [2,3], focusing on how several noncommunicable diseases (NCDs) – particularly cardiovascular disease (CVD) and metabolic diseases – may be programmed by early events. So far, research on developmental origins of health and disease has mainly addressed exposures related to nutrition and growth patterns, both in utero and during the first years of life, but the concept applies to many different types of risk factors.

Experimental studies on the long-term consequences of early-life exposures on NCDs are most often unethical, impracticable, or both. There are some remarkable exceptions, such as the nutrition supplementation trials carried out in Guatemala in the 1960s [4]. Other trials, such as the Belarus breast-feeding promotion trial [5] and the Hyderabad nutrition trial [6], are likely to eventually produce results, but their subjects are still too young.

As a result of the dearth of experimental studies, birth cohorts provide by far the largest amount of epidemiological evidence on early-life exposures. For most risk factors, prospective cohorts with primary data collection by trained and standardized field workers offer more reliable and complete information on exposures and confounders than do retrospective cohorts or case–control studies.

There are many more studies about early-life influences on CVD and related metabolic diseases than is the case for cancer. Two main reasons seem to explain this differential. First, incidence rates for CVD and metabolic conditions tend to be higher than those of most, if not all, cancers. Second, there are many well-established, easily measurable risk factors and biomarkers that may be used as surrogates for the risk of CVD and metabolic conditions, even among young adults. For example, studies of the associations between early growth patterns and adult body mass index, blood pressure, serum lipids, C-reactive protein, and so on are plentiful in the literature. The relatively high incidence of these diseases and the substantial prevalence of reliable risk markers mean that a relatively small sample size is adequate, and such associations may be investigated within cohorts with a few thousand participants, even if the subjects are still young adults.

The situation for cancer studies is more complex. Incidence rates are low compared with those for CVD or metabolic diseases, particularly among young adults. As a conse-

quence, large numbers of subjects must be followed up for several decades to study disease incidence. And while early determinants associated with common risk factors for cancer (e.g. smoking and high body mass index) may be studied in individual cohorts, there is a sharp contrast between the large number of easily measureable CVD biomarkers and the few that are currently available for cancer.

Research on the early determinants of cancer is therefore harder to carry out, as well as costlier, than similar studies for other NCDs, and will entail special requirements, which are addressed below.

Birth cohorts for studying NCDs: high-income countries

Existing prospective birth cohorts may be classified according to their sample size and duration of follow-up, as well as the level of economic development of the country where they take place.

A recent PubMed search for birth cohort studies produced about 6900 references. Of the 20 countries from which the largest number of articles originated, only Brazil (234 references) and India (47 references) do not fall into the high-income country category. (As far as I know, there is no comprehensive roster of birth cohorts, but there are ongoing attempts to register such studies on web sites – see http://www.birthco horts.net and http://www.chicospro ject.eu – as well as in the Cohort Profiles section in the *International Journal of Epidemiology*.)

Cohorts from high-income countries may be divided into two groups, according to duration of follow-up to the present time. The first group is made up of prospective cohorts with several decades of follow-up. The best-known examples include British and Scandinavian cohorts [7–12]. Typically, these studies have sample sizes of about 10 000 or fewer participants. While such numbers are sufficient for studying several CVDs, metabolic conditions, or mental illnesses, they are seldom large

enough for cancer outcomes. Few such analyses are therefore available in the literature – one example is a report on leukaemia [13] from the Jerusalem birth cohort, which started with more than 90 000 newborns recruited in the 1960s and 1970s [14].

A limitation of long-running cohorts is that – by definition – exposure information was collected many years ago. Few cohort studies collected biological samples, questionnaires were often very short and not standardized, and information on important exposures and confounders was not collected. An example is the Aberdeen Children of the 1950s Study, which failed to collect what is today regarded as essential information, such as parental smoking status [15]. This limitation restricts the ability of such studies to answer important questions on consequences of early risk factors.

The second group of cohorts from high-income settings includes young cohorts. Some of these cohorts have very large sample sizes, such as those launched in the past decade or two in Denmark, Norway, and the USA, among other countries [16]. Most include state-of-the-art exposure measurement tools, as well as collection and storage of biological samples. In terms of cancer epidemiology, early results from several of the new cohorts are already being pooled in the International Childhood Cancer Cohort Consortium [16], but unfortunately it will take many years before these can provide information on how early exposures affect risk factors for common adult cancers. A limitation of very large cohorts is that there is a trade-off between sample sizes and the frequency and intensity of measurements on individual participants. The most informative cohorts tend to be those with smaller sample sizes and more detailed measurements.

Birth cohorts for studying NCDs: low- and middle-income countries

As discussed above, most publications about birth cohort studies originate in high-income countries. Yet these countries account for only 11 million births a year, compared with 121 million births in low- and middle-income countries (LMICs) (http://www.unicef.org/sowc2012/statistics.php). Findings from high-income countries tend to influence global policies, and yet these may not be applicable to LMIC populations. As an example, concerns raised about the long-term consequences of higher birth weight or rapid weight gains in infancy, derived from cohorts where infant undernutrition is rare, do not apply to populations where poor nutrition and growth faltering are still highly prevalent [17]. In LMICs, rapid catch-up growth may be essential, not only for short-term survival but also for long-term health and human capital [18,19].

There are other reasons why more cohorts from LMICs are needed [20]. Risk factors may operate differently in each setting, as is the case for asthma [21]. The frequency of some exposures, including maternal and fetal undernutrition and infectious diseases, are markedly higher in LMICs. Even if exposures appear to have similar prevalence, their nature may vary; for example, in LMICs physical activity is mostly due to commuting and manual domestic labour, whereas in high-income countries leisure-time activities are the prevailing types of physical activity [22]. Last, confounders may operate in different directions in high-income countries and in LMICs, as was recently shown for the confounding effect of socioeconomic status on the association between breastfeeding duration and precursors for chronic diseases [23].

For these reasons there is a third relevant group of birth cohorts, comprising those from LMICs with long follow-up times [24]. The best-known of these studies are part of the Consortium of Health-Orientated Research in Transitioning Societies collaboration [25]. These five cohorts are providing important information on precursors for NCDs, particularly CVD and diabetes, sometimes

with conflicting results from those reported from high-income settings [26–30]. The Consortium of Health-Orientated Research in Transitioning Societies collaboration, however, is unlikely to provide direct evidence on cancer incidence. First, the total number of subjects under follow-up is close to 10 000, resulting in low statistical power for rare outcomes. Second, linkage studies are not possible because of inadequate sources of secondary data such as cancer registration and vital statistics. Another limitation is that none of these cohort studies collected biological samples in early life that could be analysed for biomarkers.

Other types of birth cohorts
The three categories of birth cohort studies discussed so far are not exhaustive. There are also several new, relatively small cohorts both in high-income countries and in LMICs. In LMICs, as far as I am aware, there is only one new cohort with more than a few thousand subjects: the China Children and Families Cohort Study, which started in 2006–2007 and plans to enrol 300 000 births [16].

There are also several retrospective cohorts, as well as cohorts that are fully based on record linkage, particularly in European countries. Most of these include subjects born in the 1970s or later, so that follow-up to the present time is about four decades. Also, because information on exposures is derived from routine records, available data are relatively restricted and their quality is variable. This is not to say that these cohorts cannot make important contributions to answering specific questions – for example, on the importance of birth weight – but their ability to address multiple risk factors and to control for confounding may be limited.

Famine studies, a special type of retrospective cohort, have led to important insights into the timing of nutritional insults and their effect on adult outcomes, including cancer [31–35]. However, these populations faced unusual hardship conditions

during relatively short time periods, and as such may not reflect the nature of exposures usually faced by populations, which tend to be less acute but have a longer duration.

Implications for future studies and collaborations
Birth cohorts have thus far provided invaluable amounts of evidence on the role of early-life exposures in adult diseases, but there is undoubtedly much more to be learned from existing and new cohorts.

A critical issue is that birth cohorts take a long time to produce results. Those launched several decades ago, whose members are now at the age of highest incidence for most NCDs, including cancers, tend to have limited information on most early-life exposures. Cohorts launched in the past two decades tend to have much better exposure data as well as larger sample sizes, but will take a long time to produce results. A second trade-off is that large cohorts have greater statistical power but tend to have less frequent and less detailed assessments of early-life exposures than do smaller cohorts.

An obvious solution, therefore, is to pool cohorts to increase sample size and enhance external validity. An excellent example is the Emerging Risk Factors Collaboration, with data from more than 100 prospective studies with more than 2 million participants (http://www.phpc.cam.ac.uk/ceu/research/erfc/). However, these cohorts recruited adults rather than pregnant women or newborns, and were assembled relatively recently, so that better and more standardized information on exposures is available, compared with what may be obtained from older birth cohorts. There are also several new initiatives for pooling birth cohorts to address specific health conditions, but these tend to be restricted to relatively young cohorts [16,36,37].

I am unaware of any successful initiatives in pooling several long-term birth cohorts from high-income countries, to study cancer outcomes or other NCDs. Even with large sample sizes, however, long-running cohorts are unlikely to have collected much information that is now considered as essential. For example, few if any cohorts have stored biological samples collected in childhood.

My own experience, and certainly that of others involved in such exercises, is that there are major gains from pooling cohorts, but there are also important difficulties. Pooling is easier said than done. We recently summarized the barriers we had to face in the Consortium of Health-Orientated Research in Transitioning Societies network [25]:

Some of the weaknesses include: (i) differences in variable definitions, or in measurement techniques across sites (this affects exposures, outcomes and confounding variables), which means that major effort has gone into producing a common data set; (ii) the different ages of individuals across the five cohorts and the different time periods they reflect; (iii) the different ages for which data are available throughout infancy and childhood; (iv) heterogeneity in the results for some of the analyses, for example, those on body composition. In order to overcome these limitations, we have restricted potential analyses to those including variables collected consistently across the cohorts; likewise, we have limited the analyses to ages with data available for all (or most) cohorts. In some analyses, different outcome variables have been used (e.g. pre-hypertension for adolescents and hypertension for adults) because of the different ages of the individuals across cohorts.

Similar difficulties have been reported by investigators involved in pooling younger birth cohorts from high-income countries [16].

Stand-alone, long-term birth cohorts also face important challenges. Attrition is possibly the most important issue. In the 1982 Pelotas (Brazil) birth cohort study, which I coordinate, we achieved relatively high follow-up rates (68% at the recently completed 30-year visit), but even so individuals who were lost to follow-up differ in many ways from those who came to the clinic. Ensuring consistency and standardization of exposure measures over time – when methods are constantly evolving – is another major challenge. Obtaining continued funding is also problematic, because donor fatigue affects even the most successful studies.

How can these challenges be overcome? Ideally, one would like to design an international birth cohort, involving multiple countries at different stages of development, with large sample sizes in each country. Measurements would take advantage of the variety of new tools that are now available, including genetic, epigenetic, microbiome, and exposome assessments [38], among others. This design would allow analyses not only at an individual level but also at an ecological level, because some exposures may affect most, if not all, subjects from a given site [39]. Information on exposures would be collected at similar ages at all sites, using similar methods, including questionnaires, biological samples, and environmental measurements. Obviously, this would be a massive undertaking with major practical difficulties, as has been shown by the long inception period that has been required for the United States National Children's Study (http://www.nationalchildrensstudy.gov/Pages/default.aspx). In addition to the major scientific challenges to be faced, finding sufficient financial resources for such a large cohort would require pooling funding agencies over an extended period of time – possibly an even harder task than pooling research teams.

A special plea must be made for multipurpose birth cohorts, addressing several different outcomes, related not only to health but also to human capital. This will allow us to investigate the full impact of early-life factors, because some exposures may positively affect some adult outcomes and have a detrimental effect on others. For example, adult height is largely determined by the linear growth velocity up to the age of 2 years [40]. Taller adults have greater incidence of several types of cancer [41] but also tend to be more intelligent, have higher schooling, and earn higher wages [19], as well as having lower all-cause mortality, largely due to protection against deaths due to CVD [42]. Only studies that capture multiple dimensions of human health and development can assess the overall effect of early-life exposures and growth patterns over the life-course.

In conclusion, there is strong evidence that several early-life factors influence the occurrence of different types of cancer as well as other NCDs. Whereas stand-alone cohorts seldom have the statistical power to study cancer incidence directly, they may provide important data on how early-life exposures affect the adult prevalence of risk factors for cancer, and thus contribute to their prevention. Pooling several cohorts to increase sample size is a potential solution, but so far such efforts have been limited by different definitions of exposures, outcomes, and confounders, as well as variable ages at ascertainment. Greater efforts should be made to coordinate data collection efforts in cohorts that are still in early life so that, several decades from now, the problems that we are currently facing will have been overcome.

I would like to thank Ezra Susser and Jørn Olsen for useful inputs to this Perspective.

References

1. Dubos R, Savage D, Schaedler R (2005). Biological Freudianism: lasting effects of early environmental influences. 1966. *Int J Epidemiol*, 34:5–12. http://dx.doi.org/10.1093/ije/dyh309 PMID:15649968

2. Barker DJ (1992). The fetal and infant origins of adult disease. *BMJ*, 301:1111. http://dx.doi.org/10.1136/bmj.301.6761.1111 PMID:2252919

3. Gluckman P, Hanson M, eds (2006). *Developmental Origins of Health and Disease*. Cambridge, UK: Cambridge University Press.

4. Stein AD, Melgar P, Hoddinott J, Martorell R (2008). Cohort Profile: the Institute of Nutrition of Central America and Panama (INCAP) Nutrition Trial Cohort Study. *Int J Epidemiol*, 37:716–720. PMID:18285366

5. Patel R, Oken E, Bogdanovich N et al. (2013). Cohort Profile: The Promotion of Breastfeeding Intervention Trial (PROBIT). *Int J Epidemiol*, 7:7. PMID:23471837

6. Kinra S, Rameshwar Sarma KV, Ghafoorunissa et al. (2008). Effect of integration of supplemental nutrition with public health programmes in pregnancy and early childhood on cardiovascular risk in rural Indian adolescents: long term follow-up of Hyderabad nutrition trial. *BMJ*, 337:a605. http://dx.doi.org/10.1136/bmj.a605 PMID:18658189

7. Kajantie E, Barker DJP, Osmond C et al. (2008). Growth before 2 years of age and serum lipids 60 years later: the Helsinki Birth Cohort study. *Int J Epidemiol*, 37:280–289. http://dx.doi.org/10.1093/ije/dyn012 PMID:18267964

8. Elliott J, Shepherd P (2006). Cohort Profile: 1970 British Birth Cohort (BCS70). *Int J Epidemiol*, 35:836–843. http://dx.doi.org/10.1093/ije/dyl174 PMID:16931528

9. Power C, Elliott J (2006). Cohort Profile: 1958 British Birth Cohort (National Child Development Study). *Int J Epidemiol*, 35:34–41. http://dx.doi.org/10.1093/ije/dyi183 PMID:16155052

10. Stenberg SA, Vågerö D (2006). Cohort Profile: the Stockholm Birth Cohort of 1953. *Int J Epidemiol*, 35:546–548. http://dx.doi.org/10.1093/ije/dyi310 PMID:16377656

11. Syddall HE, Aihie Sayer A, Dennison EM et al. (2005). Cohort Profile: the Hertfordshire Cohort Study. *Int J Epidemiol*, 34:1234–1242. http://dx.doi.org/10.1093/ije/dyi127 PMID:15964908

12. Rantakallio P (1988). The longitudinal study of the Northern Finland Birth Cohort of 1966. *Paediatr Perinat Epidemiol*, 2:59–88. http://dx.doi.org/10.1111/j.1365-3016.1988.tb00180.x PMID:2976931

13. Paltiel O, Harlap S, Deutsch L et al. (2004). Birth weight and other risk factors for acute leukemia in the Jerusalem Perinatal Study cohort. *Cancer Epidemiol Biomarkers Prev*, 13:1057–1064. PMID:15184264

14. Harlap S, Davies AM, Deutsch L et al. (2007). The Jerusalem Perinatal Study cohort, 1964–2005: methods and a review of the main results. *Paediatr Perinat Epidemiol*, 21:256–273. http://dx.doi.org/10.1111/j.1365-3016.2007.00799.x PMID:17439536

15. Leon DA, Lawlor DA, Clark H, Macintyre S (2006). Cohort Profile: the Aberdeen Children of the 1950s Study. *Int J Epidemiol*, 35:549–552. http://dx.doi.org/10.1093/ije/dyi319 PMID:16452107

16. Brown RC, Dwyer T, Kasten C et al.; International Childhood Cancer Cohort Consortium (I4C) (2007). Cohort Profile: the International Childhood Cancer Cohort Consortium (I4C). *Int J Epidemiol*, 36:724–730. http://dx.doi.org/10.1093/ije/dyl299 PMID:17255350

17. Black RE, Allen LH, Bhutta ZA et al.; Maternal and Child Undernutrition Study Group (2008). Maternal and child undernutrition: global and regional exposures and health consequences. *Lancet*, 371:243–260. http://dx.doi.org/10.1016/S0140-6736(07)61690-0 PMID:18207566

18. Victora CG, Barros FC (2001). Commentary: The catch-up dilemma – relevance of Leitch's 'low–high' pig to child growth in developing countries. *Int J Epidemiol*, 30:217–220. http://dx.doi.org/10.1093/ije/30.2.217 PMID:11369717

19. Victora CG, Adair L, Fall C et al.; Maternal and Child Undernutrition Study Group (2008). Maternal and child undernutrition: consequences for adult health and human capital. *Lancet*, 371:340–357. http://dx.doi.org/10.1016/S0140-6736(07)61692-4 PMID:18206223

20. Victora CG, Barros FC (2012). Cohorts in low- and middle-income countries: from still photographs to full-length movies. *J Adolesc Health*, 51 Suppl:S3–S4. http://dx.doi.org/10.1016/j.jadohealth.2012.09.003 PMID:23283157

21. Weinmayr G, Genuneit J, Nagel G et al.; ISAAC Phase Two Study Group (2010). International variations in associations of allergic markers and diseases in children: ISAAC Phase Two. *Allergy*, 65:766–775. http://dx.doi.org/10.1111/j.1398-9995.2009.02283.x PMID:20028376

22. Hallal PC, Andersen LB, Bull FC et al.; Lancet Physical Activity Series Working Group (2012). Global physical activity levels: surveillance progress, pitfalls, and prospects. *Lancet*, 380:247–257. http://dx.doi.org/10.1016/S0140-6736(12)60646-1 PMID:22818937

23. Brion MJ, Lawlor DA, Matijasevich A et al. (2011). What are the causal effects of breastfeeding on IQ, obesity and blood pressure? Evidence from comparing high-income with middle-income cohorts. *Int J Epidemiol*, 40:670–680. http://dx.doi.org/10.1093/ije/dyr020 PMID:21349903

24. Harpham T, Huttly S, Wilson I, De Wet T (2003). Linking public issues with private troubles: panel studies in developing countries. *J Int Dev*, 15:353–363. http://dx.doi.org/10.1002/jid.988

25. Richter LM, Victora CG, Hallal PC et al.; COHORTS Group (2012). Cohort Profile: the Consortium of Health-Orientated Research in Transitioning Societies. *Int J Epidemiol*, 41:621–626. http://dx.doi.org/10.1093/ije/dyq251 PMID:21224276

26. Adair LS, Fall CH, Osmond C et al.; COHORTS Group (2013). Associations of linear growth and relative weight gain during early life with adult health and human capital in countries of low and middle income: findings from five birth cohort studies. *Lancet*, 382:525–534. http://dx.doi.org/10.1016/S0140-6736(13)60103-8 PMID:23541370

27. Kuzawa CW, Hallal PC, Adair L et al.; COHORTS Group (2012). Birth weight, postnatal weight gain, and adult body composition in five low and middle income countries. *Am J Hum Biol*, 24:5–13. http://dx.doi.org/10.1002/ajhb.21227 PMID:22121058

28. Adair LS, Martorell R, Stein AD et al. (2009). Size at birth, weight gain in infancy and childhood, and adult blood pressure in 5 low- and middle-income-country cohorts: when does weight gain matter? *Am J Clin Nutr*, 89:1383–1392. http://dx.doi.org/10.3945/ajcn.2008.27139 PMID:19297457

29. Fall CH, Borja JB, Osmond C et al.; COHORTS Group (2011). Infant-feeding patterns and cardiovascular risk factors in young adulthood: data from five cohorts in low- and middle-income countries. *Int J Epidemiol*, 40:47–62. http://dx.doi.org/10.1093/ije/dyq155 PMID:20852257

30. Norris SA, Osmond C, Gigante D et al.; COHORTS Group (2012). Size at birth, weight gain in infancy and childhood, and adult diabetes risk in five low- or middle-income country birth cohorts. *Diabetes Care*, 35:72–79. http://dx.doi.org/10.2337/dc11-0456 PMID:22100968

31. Li QD, Li H, Li FJ et al. (2012). Nutrition deficiency increases the risk of stomach cancer mortality. *BMC Cancer*, 12:315. http://dx.doi.org/10.1186/1471-2407-12-315 PMID:22838407

32. Schouten LJ, van Dijk BAC, Lumey LH *et al.* (2011). Energy restriction during childhood and early adulthood and ovarian cancer risk. *PLoS One*, 6:e27960. http://dx.doi.org/10.1371/journal.pone.0027960 PMID:22132180

33. Hughes LA, van den Brandt PA, Goldbohm RA *et al.* (2010). Childhood and adolescent energy restriction and subsequent colorectal cancer risk: results from the Netherlands Cohort Study. *Int J Epidemiol*, 39:1333–1344. http://dx.doi.org/10.1093/ije/dyq062 PMID:20427463

34. Hughes LA, van den Brandt PA, de Bruïne AP *et al.* (2009). Early life exposure to famine and colorectal cancer risk: a role for epigenetic mechanisms. *PLoS One*, 4:e7951. http://dx.doi.org/10.1371/journal.pone.0007951 PMID:19956740

35. Elias SG, Peeters PH, Grobbee DE, van Noord PA (2005). The 1944–1945 Dutch famine and subsequent overall cancer incidence. *Cancer Epidemiol Biomarkers Prev*, 14:1981–1985. http://dx.doi.org/10.1158/1055-9965.EPI-04-0839 PMID:16103448

36. Gehring U, Casas M, Brunekreef B *et al.* (2013). Environmental exposure assessment in European birth cohorts: results from the ENRIECO project. *Environ Health*, 12:12–18. http://dx.doi.org/10.1186/1476-069X-12-8 PMID:23374669

37. Bousquet J, Anto J, Sunyer J *et al.* (2012). Pooling birth cohorts in allergy and asthma: European Union-funded initiatives - a MeDALL, CHICOS, ENRIECO, and GA²LEN Joint Paper. *Int Arch Allergy Immunol*, 161:1–10. http://dx.doi.org/10.1159/000343018 PMID:23258290

38. Wild CP (2005). Complementing the genome with an "exposome": the outstanding challenge of environmental exposure measurement in molecular epidemiology. *Cancer Epidemiol Biomarkers Prev*, 14:1847–1850. http://dx.doi.org/10.1158/1055-9965.EPI-05-0456 PMID:16103423

39. Rose G (1985). Sick individuals and sick populations. *Int J Epidemiol*, 14:32–38. http://dx.doi.org/10.1093/ije/14.1.32 PMID:3872850

40. Stein AD, Wang M, Martorell R *et al.*; COHORTS Group (2010). Growth patterns in early childhood and final attained stature: data from five birth cohorts from low- and middle-income countries. *Am J Hum Biol*, 22:353–359. http://dx.doi.org/10.1002/ajhb.20998 PMID:19856426

41. Green J, Cairns BJ, Casabonne D *et al.*; Million Women Study collaborators (2011). Height and cancer incidence in the Million Women Study: prospective cohort, and meta-analysis of prospective studies of height and total cancer risk. *Lancet Oncol*, 12:785–794. http://dx.doi.org/10.1016/S1470-2045(11)70154-1 PMID:21782509

42. Wormser D, Angelantonio ED, Kaptoge S *et al.*; Emerging Risk Factors Collaboration (2012). Adult height and the risk of cause-specific death and vascular morbidity in 1 million people: individual participant meta-analysis. *Int J Epidemiol*, 41:1419–1433. http://dx.doi.org/10.1093/ije/dys086 PMID:22825588

3

Cancer
biology

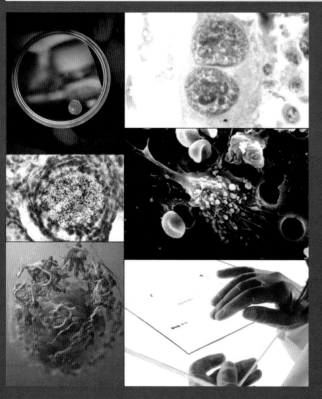

An understanding of cancer biology is critical to develop rationally designed therapy and offer preventive options. For decades, relevant knowledge has been sought by describing how cancer cells differ from normal cells – something being elucidated far more rapidly in the post-genomic era. Specification of the human genome has enabled the identification of how various types of tumour cells differ from normal cells in multiple parameters, including relevant somatic mutations and altered gene expression, which is often determined through epigenetic change such as alterations in DNA methylation patterns. Mutation or epigenetic change may mediate, amongst other effects, altered metabolism or modified intracellular signalling in response to growth-altering stimuli. In parallel, the roles of cancer stem cells and the tumour microenvironment have been recognized. Accordingly, description of how inflammation, growth of new blood vessels, and modification of the immune response mediate tumour growth now also enables options for cancer prevention and treatment to be identified.

3.1

Genomics

Thomas J. Hudson

James D. McKay (reviewer)
Teruhiko Yoshida (reviewer)

Summary

- All cancers harbour mutations in their genome, some of which have profound effects on the biology of the cancer cell by driving tumour growth that subsequently leads to cancer-related death.

- The types and subtypes of cancer, as well as the spectrum of cancer-causing mutations, differ considerably across world populations because of genetic diversity within communities and between individuals as well as diverse chemical exposures, infections, dietary components, and other factors that give rise to mutations.

- The International Cancer Genome Consortium was established to generate a catalogue of cancer mutations for more than 25 000 tumours representing 50 types of cancer that are variously of clinical and societal importance across the globe.

- The Consortium is making the data available to the research community as rapidly as possible to accelerate research into the etiology of cancer and development of tailored cancer treatment based on unique mutation profiles that are specific to individual tumours.

From the perspective of genome scientists, cancer is a disease of the genome. All cancers harbour mutations in their genome. Some of these mutations have profound effects on the biology of the cancer cell by driving tumour growth. Some mutations can inactivate genes that usually protect cells from abnormal proliferation; these are classically referred to as tumour suppressor genes. Other mutations can result in proteins with oncogenic functions that stimulate cell growth or provide other advantages to cancer cells, thus affecting biological pathways involved in the transformation of normal cells into cancer cells [1,2].

As the new millennium dawned, scientists working on the Human Genome Project revealed the first comprehensive view of the sequence of a "normal" human genome and its constituents: protein-coding genes, non-coding RNAs, and non-coding sequences conserved across species, providing clues to regulatory elements required for gene expression as well as catalogues of genetic variants (or polymorphisms) representing genomic diversity among individuals within and across populations [3]. When the first draft of the human genome sequence was released, it was estimated that more than 100 oncogenes and 30 tumour suppressor genes had been identified [4].

The types and subtypes of cancer, as well as the spectrum of cancer-causing mutations, vary considerably across world populations as a result of environmental differences, such as chemical exposures, infections, diet, and other factors, and population diversity in the genes encoding molecules that interact with the exogenous factors. In a new era of genome sciences and technologies [5,6], it became possible to conceive of systematic genome-wide searches of mutations in tumour genomes from a diversity of cancers originating in various organs of the body and affecting individuals in different parts of the world. This concept became a reality relatively quickly as it became clear that cancer-causing mutations could be used as biomarkers to inform clinical decisions. Thus, *KRAS* mutations may indicate non-responsiveness to drugs that inhibit a growth factor (EGFR) often found in colon cancer. Biomarkers may inform application of new targeted drugs such as trastuzumab, for breast cancers overexpressing the HER2 protein, and imatinib, a tyrosine kinase inhibitor effective in chronic myeloid leukaemia harbouring a specific mutation called the Philadelphia translocation

[7]. Understanding the mutational profiles of tumours in patients in different regions of the world is fundamental to translating genomic knowledge into diagnostic and treatment strategies, and for developing new targeted solutions for cancer control.

An international network was established to generate a catalogue of cancer mutations for more than 25 000 tumours representing 50 types of cancer [8]. This monumental effort came together in 2007 as the result of advances in genome sequencing technologies [6] and experience gained in pilot projects in the United Kingdom and the USA. International leaders in cancer and genome research convened in Toronto to establish a framework for an internationally coordinated effort that would generate comprehensive catalogues of cancer mutations [9]. With support from governmental and philanthropic granting agencies, teams of clinicians, scientists, ethicists, and computer scientists assumed responsibility for the comprehensive study of cancer genomes from one or more types of cancer under the auspices of the International Cancer Genome Consortium. This decade-long project will ultimately engage more than 1000 clinicians and scientists, who will be involved in generating data and analysing more than 25 000 cancer samples. Following the principles adopted by the Human Genome Project, the Consortium is making the data available to the research community as rapidly as possible, and with minimal restrictions, to accelerate research into the causes and control of cancer.

Between October 2008 and January 2013, there has been a steady increase in the number of tumour genome analyses undertaken by the International Cancer Genome Consortium, and the initial goal of 25 000 has now been surpassed (Fig. 3.1.1). As of January 2013, the halfway stage of the International Cancer Genome Consortium effort, 55 projects were under way in Asia, Australia, Europe, North America, and South America (Fig. 3.1.2). These projects will cover most of the common tumour types in participating countries (Fig. 3.1.3). At the halfway point in a decade-long initiative, the Consortium is providing cancer genome data sets from 7358 tumours (Fig. 3.1.4) to the international community via an Internet portal. To enable users to access the data and perform queries that will enable further cancer research, several data portals and search tools have been created by the Consortium and other organizations (Table 3.1.1). Despite this rapid growth of information, the task of completing the project and accelerating the translation of cancer genome information into clinically useful data will face several challenges, which are summarized below.

Biological challenges

Biological complexity results from many factors. One is that there are numerous types of cancer-causing mutations. The simplest mutations affect single DNA bases, such as the substitution of one nucleotide for another or the insertion or deletion of a nucleotide. Some mutations involve segments of a chromosome that are increased in number, typified by copy number gains and amplifications; others involve deletions of one or both copies of a gene, or sequences that are aligned in a direction opposite to their original orientations on normal chromosomes, referred to as inversions. Some mutations involve translocations between chromosomes. For example, the Philadelphia translocation mentioned previously results from the joining of chromosomes 9 and 22 and is observed in approximately 95% of patients with chronic myeloid leukaemia. In 2–3% of all cancers and more frequently in bone cancers and medulloblastomas, rearrangements are widespread and complex, a phenomenon called chromothripsis (or chromosome shattering) [10]. Cancer cells may also acquire DNA from viruses such as Epstein–Barr virus, hepatitis B virus, and human papillomavirus. In defining its guidelines, the International Cancer Genome Consortium established recommendations that will lead to all forms of mutations affecting DNA, RNA, and methylation being detected and catalogued. In practice, this usually requires the generation of different laboratory protocols for each mutation category, followed by parallel detection of normal and mutated constituents using high-throughput detection technologies [5–7].

A second reason for the biological complexity is the large number of mutations observed in every tumour. This is not unexpected given the frequent observations of chromosome anomalies revealed by cytogenetic

Fig. 3.1.1. Growth in the number of tumour genome analyses undertaken by International Cancer Genome Consortium members.

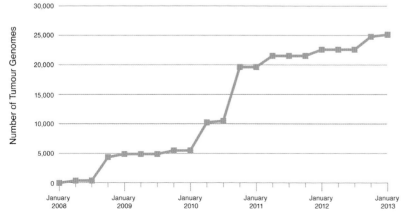

Fig. 3.1.2. National locations of International Cancer Genome Consortium projects as of January 2013.

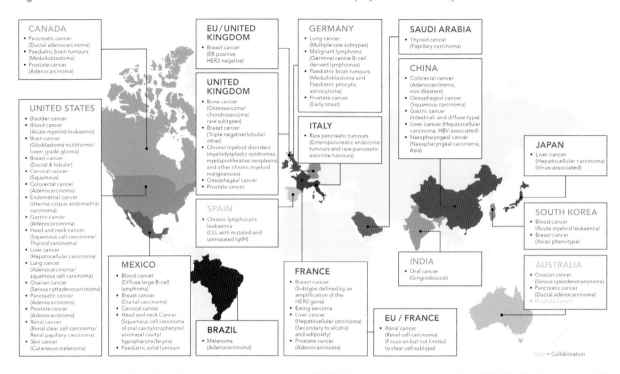

studies over many decades. The mutation spectra in cancer cells were further elucidated by whole cancer genome sequencing, which revealed an extensive number of putative somatic mutations in every cancer genome; for example, 33 345 somatic base substitutions were observed in the first melanoma genome and 22 910 in the first small cell lung cancer genome [11,12]. These large numbers of somatic mutations usually result from repeated exposure to carcinogens (e.g. tobacco smoke or ultraviolet radiation) and defective DNA repair pathways found in cancer cells [1], and thus occur randomly across the genome.

Some mutations occur in sequences that are functional and affect cellular mechanisms that provide growth advantages to cells, such as oncogenic mutations or inactivating mutations involving tumour suppressors. These are often referred to as driver mutations, while the remaining majority of somatic mutations with no biological consequence are called passenger mutations [5]. The large numbers of mutations also indicate the long

history between initiation of cancer and clinical manifestations for most cancers. There are exceptions to this, as some cancer types (usually paediatric) have low mutation rates. For example, rhabdoid tumours are highly aggressive cancers of

early childhood with extremely low numbers of mutations, including a characteristic driver mutation in the *SMARCB1* gene that is observed in all cases [13].

Heterogeneity of driver mutations among patients with similar forms

Fig. 3.1.3. Numbers of tumours, as indicated by numbers of donors, for each tumour type to undergo comprehensive genome analyses by International Cancer Genome Consortium members.

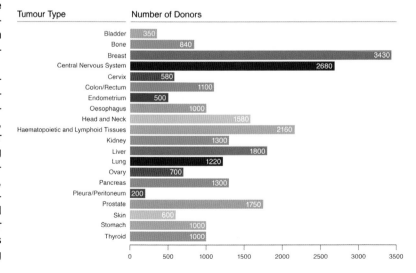

TP53 mutations and human cancer

Magali Olivier

The tumour suppressor gene *TP53* has been recognized as an important anticancer gene for more than 20 years because of its frequent alteration in most human cancers. *TP53* encodes a protein of 393 amino acids, p53, which plays an important role in the maintenance of cell integrity by responding to various forms of cellular stresses and acting as a multifunctional protein through the control of various cellular pathways. p53 has been shown to repress proliferative signalling, enhance the effects of growth suppressors, sensitize cells to apoptosis and autophagy, suppress replicative immortality through senescence, promote genetic and genomic stability, control inflammation, exert anti-angiogenic effects, and repress metastasis, thus counteracting a large panel of tumour-promoting cellular activities [1]. Because of this large spectrum of anti-tumour functions, inactivating p53 function is an essential step during cancer development, and this is most frequently achieved by mutating the *TP53* gene. *TP53* mutations are found in all cancer types with various frequencies, ranging from 5% to 90% (Fig. B3.1.1). Recent whole-genome and exome sequencing studies have confirmed that *TP53* is the most frequently mutated gene in most cancers.

IARC maintains a database that documents all *TP53* gene variations reported in the scientific literature (http://p53.iarc.fr). More than 30 000 somatic mutations are compiled, with annotations on tumour phenotype, patient characteristics, and structural and functional impacts of mutations [2]. Most *TP53* mutations are single-amino-acid substitutions that are located in the DNA-binding domain of p53 and disrupt the transcriptional activities of p53. Due to the three-dimensional structure of the p53 DNA-binding domain and its crucial function, most single-amino-acid substitutions would disrupt p53 function. As a result, mutations observed in cancers are very diverse and are scattered along the entire coding sequence, although some mutation hotspots are observed. Some hotspots, such as codons 175, 248, 273, 220, and 245, are found in all cancer types, while others are cancer-specific (such as codon 249 in liver cancer, or codons 280 and 285 in bladder cancer) (Fig. B3.1.1).

TP53 mutations may be used as diagnostic and prognostic markers in the clinic, and several drugs that target the p53 pathway are being developed [1]. *TP53* mutations are also informative markers for carcinogen exposure. Indeed, specific *TP53* mutation patterns have been described in relation with exposure to ultraviolet radiation in skin cancer, tobacco smoke in lung cancer, aflatoxins in liver cancer, or aristolochic acid in upper urinary tract cancers [3]. *TP53* mutations can thus be useful markers in molecular epidemiology studies to investigate tumour etiology.

References

1. Hainaut P *et al.* (2013). *TP53* somatic mutations: prognostic and predictive value in human cancers. *p53 in the Clinics*. New York: Springer.

2. Petitjean *A et al.* (2007). *Hum Mutat*, 28:622–629. http://dx.doi.org/10.1002/humu.20495 PMID:17311302

3. Olivier M *et al.* (2010). *Cold Spring Harb Perspect Biol*, 2:a001008. http://dx.doi.org/10.1101/cshperspect.a001008 PMID:20182602

Website

IARC TP53 Database: http://p53.iarc.fr

Fig. B3.1.1. Frequency of *TP53* mutations in various cancer types (histogram) and localization of mutation hotspots in the DNA-binding domain of the p53 protein (three-dimensional structure).

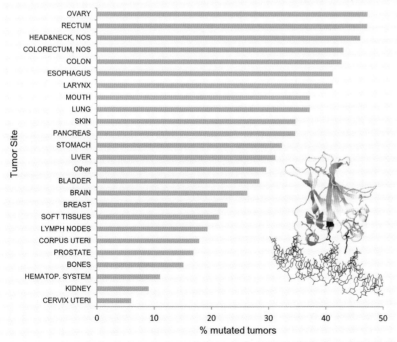

of cancer is an important source of complexity. In a survey of 100 breast tumours analysed for somatic mutations and copy number alterations, both gains and deletions, in approximately 21 500 protein-coding genes, also called an exome, 40 genes were implicated as driver mutations across the set, of which 7 were seen in more than 10% of cases and 33 were infrequent [14]. While some cells had more than one recognized driver mutation (the maximum seen in this study was six), 28 cases had only one. This study illustrates that most breast cancers differ from one another in the number of mutations and the set of driver mutations.

Another source of complexity is due to tumour masses usually being composed of different cancer cell subpopulations carrying related but distinct mutation profiles [15]. Over time and across metastatic lesions of a single patient, mutation spectra evolve. Although not surprising given the high mutation rates in patients, this evolution has many consequences, of which the most serious is the acquisition of drug resistance, either through new mutations in genes that alter critical drug receptors or pharmacogenomic pathways or through the ability of subclones that are insensitive to drugs to outcompete other clones that are not, after therapy. Thus, the dynamic evolution of cancer genomes is emerging as a critical factor in explaining disease relapse and, ultimately, cancer deaths.

Opportunities for research on etiology

The first melanoma and small cell lung cancer genomes [11,12] have revealed that genome-wide mutation patterns, or "mutation signatures", reflect exposure to environmental carcinogens (ultraviolet radiation, tobacco smoke). The mutation signatures found genome-wide in a single tumour were amazingly similar to those described in a single gene, *TP53* (see "*TP53* mutations and human cancer"). Similar striking mutation signatures have been reported

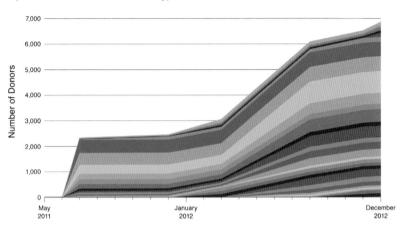

Fig. 3.1.4. Growth in the number of cancer genome data sets available via the International Cancer Genome Consortium Data Portal (http://dcc.icgc.org). Each colour represents a different tumour subtype.

in upper urinary tract cancers linked to exposure to aristolochic acid [16]. More systematic research on mutation signatures across cancer types has revealed recurrent mutation signatures in cancer genomes [17]. Through correlation of mutation signatures and exposures, the underlying mutagenic mechanisms causing some of these signatures could be deduced from previous knowledge (smoking, ultraviolet radiation, age, *BRCA1/2* germline mutations). However, many signatures remain unexplained and have led to new hypotheses about mutagenic mechanisms. For example, some signatures have been attributed to the APOBEC family of cytidine deaminases. As these enzymes are involved in the innate immune response to viruses and retrotransposons, the presence of these signatures might reflect an enhanced activity of APOBEC family members caused by a viral infection. These results may thus stimulate research on the potential role of viral infection in the development of new cancer types [18].

Research into associations between mutation signatures and exposures, through genomic epidemiology studies and model systems of induced mutagenesis, has great potential to uncover new causal links between the mutagenic processes and the influence of environmental

exposures. For these new research opportunities to have worldwide benefits, it is important for such genomic epidemiology studies to consider geographical heterogeneity in etiologies and to focus on exposures and cancer types relevant to low- and middle-income countries.

Technological challenges

Although genomic technologies are not discussed in detail in this Report, this topic is relevant to data generators, users of data available in International Cancer Genome Consortium and other databases, and future adoptees of genomic technologies for clinical applications. Given the recent development of most of these technologies, as well as the associated computational challenges, it is recognized that each data set contains false-positive results and is incomplete (i.e. contains false negatives). To facilitate the task of future users of Consortium data sets, various quality control metrics, including secondary validation of potentially deleterious mutations, are conducted and reported. It is thus essential for experts and non-experts to be aware that the technology has limitations and that potentially important mutations of clinical relevance require independent validation.

Table 3.1.1. Internet resources for cancer genomics data

Resource	Website	Description
International Cancer Genome Consortium (ICGC)	http://dcc.icgc.org/	The ICGC Data Portal provides access to cancer genome data and project data from ICGC members.
The Cancer Genome Atlas (TCGA)	https://tcga-data.nci.nih.gov/tcga/tcgaHome2.jsp	The TCGA Data Portal provides a platform for researchers to search, download, and analyse cancer genome data sets generated by institutions in the USA contributing to TCGA.
Catalogue of Somatic Mutations in Cancer (COSMIC)	http://www.sanger.ac.uk/genetics/CGP/cosmic	COSMIC stores and displays curated somatic mutation data and other information related to human cancers.
Broad Institute Integrative Genomics Viewer (IGV)	http://www.broadinstitute.org/igv/	IGV is a high-performance visualization tool for interactive exploration of large, integrated genomic data sets.
University of California Santa Cruz (USCS) Cancer Genomics Browser	https://genome-cancer.soe.ucsc.edu	The UCSC Cancer Genomics Browser is a suite of web-based tools to visualize, integrate, and analyse cancer genomics and its associated clinical data.
United States National Cancer Institute's Therapeutically Applicable Research to Generate Effective Treatments (TARGET)	http://target.nci.nih.gov/dataMatrix/TARGET_DataMatrix.html	TARGET data sets include genomic characterization, full clinical information, and sequencing files for five common types of childhood malignancies: acute lymphoblastic leukaemia, acute myeloid leukaemia, neuroblastoma, osteosarcoma, and Wilms tumour.

The rapid expansion of cancer genome data sets being generated is creating formidable challenges [19]. For each tumour, numerous types of primary data are collected, including clinical information, pathological data, DNA sequences (from normal and tumour tissues for the detection of several mutation categories, including simple base substitutions, copy number changes, and other structural alterations), methylation, and RNA expression. In addition, interpreted data such as functional consequences of mutations to protein structure and potential clinical correlates also need to be recorded in robust and user-friendly databases. As these individual-specific data sets become integrated at the project level and ultimately analysed across all tumour types, the computational challenges are daunting. Similarly, how this information is effectively disseminated to the wider scientific community (via descriptive databases or through transfer and analysis of the large amounts of

Fig. 3.1.5. Figurative depiction of somatic mutations present in a single cancer genome, part of a catalogue of somatic mutations in the small cell lung cancer cell line NCI-H2171. Individual chromosomes are depicted on the outer circle, followed by concentric tracks for point mutation, copy number, and rearrangement data relative to mapping position in the genome. Arrows indicate examples of the various types of somatic mutation present in this cancer genome.

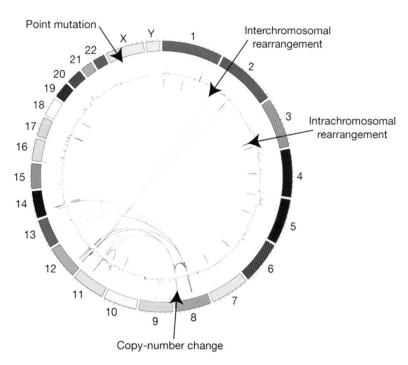

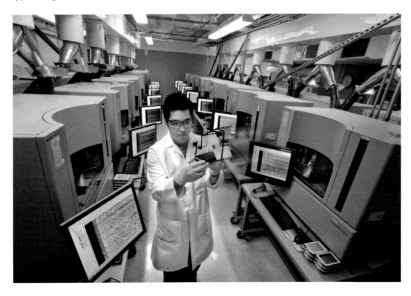

Fig. 3.1.6. Next-generation gene sequencing equipment in use at the Joint Genome Institute in Walnut Creek, California. Large-scale cancer genome studies are already applying next-generation sequencing technologies to tumours from 50 different cancer types to generate more than 25 000 cancer genomes.

raw data) also presents formidable challenges.

International issues
The most intense cancer genome research was initially concentrated in developed nations with a track record in large-scale genome research. When the International Cancer Genome Consortium was launched, a remarkable effort was made by funding agencies in many countries to participate, not only as a way of ensuring that cancers common in their respective populations were investigated but also to build capacity in next-generation sequencing technologies and allow their communities of scientists to be actively involved in cutting-edge research. For example, India established the National Institute of Biomedical Genomics in Kalyani, West Bengal, to conduct a Consortium project to study gingivo-buccal cancer. This form of oral cancer, which accounts for 30% of all cancers in India [20], is due to the habit of chewing tobacco with betel quid.

At the halfway mark in the Consortium's decade-long initiative, many types of cancer across the globe are being studied, but there are still obstacles (economic barriers, limited infrastructures for biobanking, paucity of skills, etc.) in analysing some forms of cancer that are common in some low- and middle-income countries (notably in Africa). Several approaches that may be considered to resolve this include collaborations between cancer care workers in these countries and international leaders in cancer research (including Consortium members), leveraging the expertise already established in these countries for conducting clinical trials for infectious diseases, and establishing a distributed model for tumour banking driven by standard operating procedures.

Legal and regulatory frameworks that differ among international jurisdictions have the potential to hinder the exchange of data among collaborating groups in different countries and also to limit the sharing of data via the Internet. Some valid reasons for placing restrictions on data include protection of privacy and the potential that misuse could harm individuals. For these reasons, the International Cancer Genome Consortium implemented robust governance procedures for handling data from human subjects, including the adoption of common bioethical elements and harmonized consent procedures [8]. Moreover, the Consortium structured its databases to classify data that cannot be used to identify individuals as "open", or unrestricted and publicly accessible. In parallel to this, the Consortium created mechanisms to classify more sensitive genetic and clinical information that could be misused by third parties to re-identify participants as "controlled", and available only to scientists and research institutions agreeing to conditions stipulated in an access agreement. Oversight of this process is conducted by an international committee [8,21].

Conclusions and next steps
Cancer genomics is a research field that is growing rapidly as a result of new genomic technologies. Given the fundamental role that mutations play in the development of cancer, cancer genomes will continue to be analysed and mined for additional clues that will increase our understanding of cancer cells, for biomarkers that will be used as indicators of prognosis and treatment response, and for targets that will be evaluated as substrates for new cancer drugs. The impact of this progress is apparent not only in the growing number of targeted agents being developed by biotechnology and pharmaceutical companies but also in the reduced time between identification of driver mutations and approval of a specific targeted therapy by regulatory agencies [7].

The diversity of mutational processes underlying development of cancer is evident from an analysis of 4 938 362 mutations from 7042 cancers. The prevalence of mutations varied over more than 5 orders of magnitude; childhood cancers carried the fewest, and cancers related to chronic mutagenic exposures, such as tobacco smoke or ultraviolet radiation, exhibited the most (> 400 per megabase of DNA). Mutations were categorized on the basis of 96 possible scenarios, and 21 distinct mutational signatures were defined in relation to 30 cancer classes [22].

It is expected that the growth in cancer genome information will continue exponentially, from thousands to millions of tumours in the next decade. Most of this growth is happening as a consequence of new sequencing technologies that are becoming easier to adapt to clinical laboratory environments. The feasibility of cancer clinical sequencing that is used in selecting therapies has been demonstrated in the clinical trials setting [23]. The challenges in converting cancer genome analyses into improved diagnosis, prognosis, and treatment are formidable, but the impact will be felt increasingly by health-care systems, clinicians, and patients [24].

Recently, the Cancer Genome Atlas Research Network documented point mutations and small insertions or deletions from 3281 tumours across 12 tumour types, including a clinical association analysis. Overall, mutations in several genes, including *BAP1*, *DNMT3A*, *KDM5C*, *FBXW7*, and *TP53*, correlated with poor prognosis, whereas mutations in two genes, *BRCA2* and *IDH1*, often correlated with improved prognosis [25].

References

1. Hanahan D, Weinberg RA (2000). The hallmarks of cancer. *Cell*, 100:57–70. http://dx.doi.org/10.1016/S0092-8674(00)81683-9 PMID:10647931

2. Hanahan D, Weinberg RA (2011). Hallmarks of cancer: the next generation. *Cell*, 144:646–674. http://dx.doi.org/10.1016/j.cell.2011.02.013 PMID:21376230

3. Lander ES, Linton LM, Birren B *et al.*; International Human Genome Sequencing Consortium (2001). Initial sequencing and analysis of the human genome. *Nature*, 409:860–921. http://dx.doi.org/10.1038/35057062 PMID:11237011

4. Futreal PA, Kasprzyk A, Birney E *et al.* (2001). Cancer and genomics. *Nature*, 409:850–852. http://dx.doi.org/10.1038/35057046 PMID:11237008

5. Stratton MR, Campbell PJ, Futreal PA (2009). The cancer genome. *Nature*, 458:719–724. http://dx.doi.org/10.1038/nature07943 PMID:19360079

6. Wong KM, Hudson TJ, McPherson JD (2011). Unraveling the genetics of cancer: genome sequencing and beyond. *Annu Rev Genomics Hum Genet*, 12:407–430. http://dx.doi.org/10.1146/annurev-genom-082509-141532 PMID:21639794

7. Chin L, Andersen JN, Futreal PA (2011). Cancer genomics: from discovery science to personalized medicine. *Nat Med*, 17:297–303. http://dx.doi.org/10.1038/nm.2323 PMID:21383744

8. Hudson TJ, Anderson W, Artez A *et al.*; International Cancer Genome Consortium (2010). International network of cancer genome projects. *Nature*, 464:993–998. http://dx.doi.org/10.1038/nature08987 PMID:20393554

9. Jennings J, Hudson TJ (2013). Reflections on the founding of the International Cancer Genome Consortium. *Clin Chem*, 59:18–21. http://dx.doi.org/10.1373/clinchem.2012.184713 PMID:23136248

10. Maher CA, Wilson RK (2012). Chromothripsis and human disease: piecing together the shattering process. *Cell*, 148:29–32. http://dx.doi.org/10.1016/j.cell.2012.01.006 PMID:22265399

11. Pleasance ED, Cheetham RK, Stephens PJ *et al.* (2010). A comprehensive catalogue of somatic mutations from a human cancer genome. *Nature*, 463:191–196. http://dx.doi.org/10.1038/nature08658 PMID:20016485

12. Pleasance ED, Stephens PJ, O'Meara S *et al.* (2010). A small-cell lung cancer genome with complex signatures of tobacco exposure. *Nature*, 463:184–190. http://dx.doi.org/10.1038/nature08629 PMID:20016488

13. Lee RS, Stewart C, Carter SL *et al.* (2012). A remarkably simple genome underlies highly malignant pediatric rhabdoid cancers. *J Clin Invest*, 122:2983–2988. http://dx.doi.org/10.1172/JCI64400 PMID:22797305

14. Stephens PJ, Tarpey PS, Davies H *et al.*; Oslo Breast Cancer Consortium (OSBREAC) (2012). The landscape of cancer genes and mutational processes in breast cancer. *Nature*, 486:400–404. http://dx.doi.org/10.1038/nature11017 PMID:22722201

15. Samuel N, Hudson TJ (2013). Translating genomics to the clinic: implications of cancer heterogeneity. *Clin Chem*, 59:127–137. http://dx.doi.org/10.1373/clinchem.2012.184580 PMID:23151419

16. Hoang ML, Chen CH, Sidorenko VS *et al.* (2013). Mutational signature of aristolochic acid exposure as revealed by whole-exome sequencing. *Sci Transl Med*, 5:197ra102. http://dx.doi.org/10.1126/scitranslmed.3006200 PMID:23926200

17. Alexandrov LB, Nik-Zainal S, Wedge DC *et al.* (2013). Signatures of mutational processes in human cancer. *Nature*, 500:415–421. http://dx.doi.org/10.1038/nature12477 PMID:23945592

18. Roberts SA, Lawrence MS, Klimczak LJ *et al.* (2013). An APOBEC cytidine deaminase mutagenesis pattern is widespread in human cancers. *Nat Genet*, 45:970–976. http://dx.doi.org/10.1038/ng.2702 PMID:23852170

19. Chin L, Hahn WC, Getz G, Meyerson M (2011). Making sense of cancer genomic data. *Genes Dev*, 25:534–555. http://dx.doi.org/10.1101/gad.2017311 PMID:21406553

20. Khan Z (2012). An overview of oral cancer in Indian subcontinent and recommendations to decrease its incidence. *Cancer*, 3:WMC003626.

21. Joly Y, Dove ES, Knoppers BM *et al.* (2012). Data sharing in the post-genomic world: the experience of the International Cancer Genome Consortium (ICGC) Data Access Compliance Office (DACO). *PLoS Comput Biol*, 8:e1002549. http://dx.doi.org/10.1371/journal.pcbi.1002549 PMID:22807659

22. Alexandrov LB, Nik-Zainal S, Wedge DC *et al.*; Australian Pancreatic Cancer Genome Initiative; ICGC Breast Cancer Consortium; ICGC MMML-Seq Consortium; ICGC PedBrain (2013). Signatures of mutational processes in human cancer. *Nature*, 500:415–412. http://dx.doi.org/10.1038/nature12477 PMID:23945592

23. Tran B, Brown AM, Bedard PL *et al.* (2013). Feasibility of real time next generation sequencing of cancer genes linked to drug response: results from a clinical trial. *Int J Cancer*, 132:1547–1555. http://dx.doi.org/10.1002/ijc.27817 PMID:22948899

24. Dancey JE, Bedard PL, Onetto N, Hudson TJ (2012). The genetic basis for cancer treatment decisions. *Cell*, 148:409–420. http://dx.doi.org/10.1016/j.cell.2012.01.014 PMID:22304912

25. Kandoth C, McLellan MD, Vandin F *et al.* (2013). Mutational landscape and significance across 12 major cancer types. *Nature*, 502:333–339. http://dx.doi.org/10.1038/nature12634

Website

International Cancer Genome Consortium: www.icgc.org

3.2 Genome-wide association studies

3 BIOLOGY

Stephen J. Chanock

Dongxin Lin (reviewer)
Paul Pharoah (reviewer)

Summary

- Cancer genome-wide association studies have successfully identified many new susceptibility alleles in the human genome, most of which are unique to each type of cancer.

- Cancer genome-wide association studies will continue to discover an increasing fraction of the common susceptibility alleles, and have uncovered distinct genetic architectures for specific cancer susceptibilities.

- Findings from cancer genome-wide association studies have provided new mechanistic insights into cancer etiology, including changes in the regulation of key genes and pathways. Investigations of the relationship between germline susceptibility alleles and somatic alterations should uncover new pathways and targets for therapeutic and preventive measures.

- Clinical cancer genetics will profit from the determination of a more comprehensive catalogue of susceptibility alleles, across a spectrum of frequencies and effect sizes, which could be implemented in precision medicine.

For nearly half a century, the heritable contribution to cancer has been investigated, beginning with studies of families in which multiple members developed the same type of cancer [1]. As the draft sequence of the human genome was completed [2,3], its annotation revealed a wide spectrum of genetic variation, from single base changes to large structural alterations and copy number variations [4]. Traditionally, investigators have focused on the single base substitution, known as the single-nucleotide polymorphism (SNP); the frequency of the alternative nucleotide is captured by the minor allele frequency (MAF). Differences in human populations are etched in the patterns of genetic variation; this includes both the correlation between nearby variants, known as linkage disequilibrium, and the actual frequencies of common variants, measured by the MAF. In turn, these differences have become attractive for investigating differences in incidence for distinct cancers, by either population or exposure.

Cancer susceptibility alleles can be discovered by different approaches, such as linkage and association analyses; the tools have improved substantively, shifting from genotyping of single tandem repeats and SNPs to whole-genome sequence analysis

using next-generation sequencing technologies. Not all alleles have comparable estimated effects (Fig. 3.2.1) [5]. Linkage analyses in family studies are used to discover highly penetrant mutations, as in BRCA1 or TP53, which are rare but have a strong predictive value. Due to the limitations in available tools, only a small fraction of pedigrees have been explained by mutations in "cancer susceptibility genes". These have provided a foundation for clinical cancer genetics.

Common susceptibility alleles are discovered by association studies, which compare allele frequencies between affected and unaffected individuals (Fig. 3.2.2). The estimated effect sizes are smaller for common variants and are neither necessary nor sufficient for cancer susceptibility (Fig. 3.2.1). Moreover, common variants contribute to a polygenic model for susceptibility, akin to complex diseases like diabetes and neurodegenerative disorders.

In 1996, Risch and Merikangas argued that linkage analysis for complex diseases would be less efficient than association analyses in populations for mapping common variants with smaller effect sizes [6]. The field turned towards association studies, initially using the candidate gene approach, in which investigators

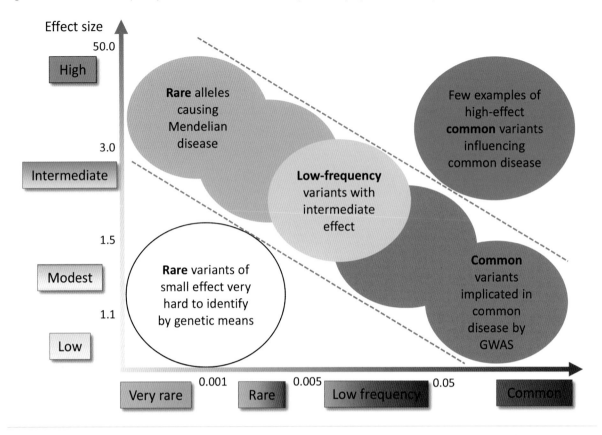

Fig. 3.2.1. Mapping genetic susceptibility. Distribution of susceptibility alleles by frequency and strength of genetic effect, illustrating the distribution of susceptibility alleles as well as the feasibility of identifying variants through GWAS and sequence analysis.

chose favourite genes or variants for testing, but with little success. Generally, reported findings failed to be replicated in subsequent studies, for a variety of reasons that included issues in study design, small sample sizes, and unrealistic expectations for effectively choosing functional variants. The candidate gene approach yielded less than a dozen conclusive variants that confer susceptibility to different cancers. Notable examples include the association of bladder cancer with *NAT2* variants or a common deletion of *GSTM1* [7] as well as of aerodigestive cancers with coding variants in alcohol dehydrogenase genes (*ADH1B* and *ADH7*) [8]. Still, what emerged was an appreciation of the value of robust replication together with the scaling of studies to a size that would provide adequate power to conclusively detect variants on statistical grounds.

Principles of cancer GWAS

The advent of genome-wide association studies (GWAS) has substantially accelerated discovery of common genetic susceptibility variants for a wide range of human diseases and traits. Advances in microarray technologies have enabled researchers to interrogate hundreds of thousands of SNPs in parallel using new analytical tools and standards. The underlying approach has been to conduct a statistical – or "agnostic" – analysis of commercial SNP microarrays designed to tag common variants across the entire genome. Consequently, GWAS find markers, or surrogates of susceptibility alleles, and rarely determine the "functional" variant, which can explain the association.

Many statistical tests are conducted, because the primary approach has been to identify common SNPs with a main effect using the trend test, thus raising the spectre of

false positives. The community has embraced a threshold of genome-wide significance for reporting GWAS results, defined as a trend association test with $P \leq 5 \times 10^{-8}$ after adjustment as per the GWAS study design. Because of the small effect sizes of most common SNPs conclusively associated with cancer risk, it is unlikely that the alleles incorporate a dominant effect. Follow-up studies or large meta-analyses are required to establish a conclusive finding [9]. Independent replication guards against the pursuit of false positives, which is important since the downstream cost of mapping and laboratory investigation is high with respect to time and resources [10]. The actual functional marker does not have to be tested; instead, a surrogate can be in linkage disequilibrium and thus replicated in follow-up [11]. Occasionally, a common genetic marker may point towards a less common variant with a

Fig. 3.2.2. Genetic analysis of GWAS. Multiple steps are conducted, including the choice of SNPs across the genome (usually included on a commercial SNP microarray) based on linkage disequilibrium in a region, enabling the selection of a surrogate to test for the region. Association analysis is conducted in a case–control setting, examining all SNPs in a Manhattan plot, followed by replication analyses that pinpoint markers on chromosomes, which are fine-mapped and investigated in the laboratory. MAF, minor allele frequency.

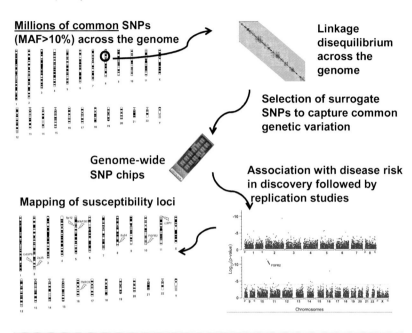

Millions of common SNPs (MAF>10%) across the genome

Genome-wide SNP chips

Mapping of susceptibility loci

Linkage disequilibrium across the genome

Selection of surrogate SNPs to capture common genetic variation

Association with disease risk in discovery followed by replication studies

stronger effect, known as a synthetic association. However, most GWAS signals map to common variants with direct functional effects on cancer susceptibility.

GWAS are scalable for discovery. For example, the Collaborative Oncological Gene-environment Study has pooled existing scans and conducted large-scale replication to discover new loci in three hormone-related cancers: breast, ovarian, and prostate cancers [12–14]. These studies have identified a larger fraction of the common variants that contribute to the comprehensive panel of independent loci. Since GWAS genotyping has been performed with different commercial and custom SNP microarrays, techniques for imputation of data have been developed to combine data sets. Several imputation programmes successfully infer untested and highly correlated SNPs based on reference data sets, such as the International HapMap Project, the 1000 Genome Project, or the Division of Cancer Epidemiology and Genetics (United States National Cancer Institute) imputation set [4,15,16].

Cancer GWAS discoveries

In the past 6 years, the pace of GWAS findings has accelerated (Box 3.2.1). Since the first cancer GWAS were published in 2007, nearly 400 distinct genetic loci have been conclusively identified for more than two dozen different cancers – including common cancers, such as breast, colon, and prostate cancers, as well as rarer paediatric cancers, like Ewing sarcoma and neuroblastoma [17–20]. Moreover, GWAS have identified susceptibility loci for specific subtypes of cancers, such as estrogen-negative breast cancer [21].

Reported cancer GWAS findings are associated with cancer susceptibility. With rare exceptions, the etiological markers are not associated with clinical outcomes, including metastatic disease or survival. Several neuroblastoma loci discriminate between aggressive and milder disease. Of the more than 75 independent loci identified for prostate cancer, not one accurately discriminates between aggressive and non-aggressive disease. Recently, variants in *SLC39A6* were conclusively associated with survival in individuals with oesophageal squamous cell carcinoma [22]. Still, the lack of correlation between etiological loci and clinical outcomes suggests that distinct regions of the genome may contribute to the development of cancer but not necessarily the progression of cancer.

Box 3.2.1. Current status of genome-wide association studies.

1. **Discovery of new regions in the genome associated with diseases/traits**
   - New candidate genes and regions

2. **Clues for mechanistic insights into the contribution of common genetic variation to cancer biology**
   - Etiology
   - Gene–environment/lifestyle interactions
   - Outcomes and pharmacogenomics

3. **Challenge of genetic markers for risk prediction for individual or public health decisions**
   - Common variants represent a fraction of the genetic contribution to risk
   - Polygenic risk models

Gene–environment interactions and breast cancer

Federico Canzian

GWAS have recently identified several genetic loci associated with risk of breast cancer. They are the latest addition to a list of established breast cancer risk factors, which are mainly environmental or lifestyle-related.

Exploring the possible interplay between genetic variants and established breast cancer risk factors can (i) provide hints on the function of the novel genetic loci, and in general on biological mechanisms of breast cancer etiology, and (ii) help in formulating better risk prediction models, with a potential impact on prevention.

Given the small risk modification conferred by each environmental and genetic risk factor, large-scale association studies, involving many thousands of cases and controls, are needed to explore gene–environment interactions. Several such studies have recently been published, on up to 26 000 breast cancer cases and 32 000 controls [e.g. 1–3]. They involved between 7 and 17 SNPs and established risk factors including age at menarche, parity, age at first live birth, breastfeeding, menopausal status, age at menopause, use of hormone replacement therapy, body mass index, height,

tobacco use, alcohol consumption, number of previous breast biopsies, and family history of breast cancer. Both prospective cohorts [1,2] and retrospective series of breast cancer cases and controls [3] were used. Most of the study subjects were Caucasians, with some studies done in Asian populations.

Results obtained so far [1–3] suggest that two-way interactions between known risk SNPs and established breast cancer risk factors are unlikely to be strong. None of the large-scale studies reported statistically significant gene–environment interactions, after correcting for multiple testing. These studies were well powered, having greater than 90% power to detect interaction odds ratios as low as 1.06. Higher-order interactions were not tested as they would require much larger sample sizes.

Previous reports suggested the existence of a few statistically significant gene–environment interactions, for example between SNPs in *FGFR2* and use of hormone replacement therapy, family history of breast cancer, age at menarche, and parity. None of these associations were observed in the larger

studies. Considering the relatively small sample size and the modest statistical significance of the interactions reported in the original studies, the most likely explanation is that these could be chance findings.

New GWAS on breast cancer risk, and meta-analyses of existing ones, are still being performed; therefore, more breast cancer susceptibility loci will be known in the near future. Consequently, new gene–environment interaction studies will be needed. Furthermore, all studies published so far assumed a multiplicative model of interaction. It remains to be seen whether significant gene–environment interactions can be detected by exploring different models, such as supra-additive interactions.

References

1. Travis RC et al. (2010). *Lancet*, 375:2143–2151. http://dx.doi.org/10.1016/S0140-6736(10)60636-8 PMID:20605201

2. Campa D et al. (2011). *J Natl Cancer Inst*, 103:1252–1263. http://dx.doi.org/10.1093/jnci/djr265 PMID:21791674

3. Milne RL et al. (2010). *Breast Cancer Res*, 12:R110. http://dx.doi.org/10.1186/bcr2797 PMID:21194473

Nearly all cancer GWAS markers have a MAF greater than 10%, with a handful in the 5–10% range [23]. This is a consequence of the design of the first-generation SNP microarray chips and the smaller sample sizes used. With larger meta-analyses and follow-up studies planned, further discovery in the MAF space between 2% and 10% will occur. An emerging concept is that there could be major differences in the underlying genetic architecture of different types of cancer [24]. For example, the range of effect sizes and allele frequencies varies between prostate cancer and breast cancer, which includes *BRCA1*, *BRCA2*, *TP53*, and a

set of moderately penetrant genetic mutations.

In the first wave of cancer GWAS, the per-allele estimated effect sizes were small, with odds ratios between 1.1 and 1.4. In paediatric cancer GWAS, estimates of 1.6–1.8 are not unusual, perhaps suggesting stronger drivers of cancer development. One notable exception for young adults is in testicular cancer GWAS, for which the per-allele effect estimate is greater than 2.5 for *KITLG* on chromosome 12 [25]. This is not surprising since testicular cancer has a high heritability in family studies. It is notable that as sample sizes increase, it is possible to find smaller estimated effect sizes.

The Collaborative Oncological Gene-environment Study consortium has discovered new breast and prostate cancer signals but with effect sizes of 1.05–1.15 (see "Gene–environment interactions and breast cancer").

Few of the cancer GWAS signals map to a coding change in a plausible candidate gene. Most signals map to non-coding regions. Approximately one quarter map to intergenic regions, in which there are no adjacent correlated markers that map to characterized genes. Together, these findings suggest that the majority of the common genetic variants contribute to cancer through perturbations of the regulation of known or novel pathways.

Most cancer GWAS signals are unique to a cancer type, but there are a few highly informative regions that harbour susceptibility alleles for multiple cancers, thus linking distinct cancers and suggesting shared pathways. A region flanking the *MYC* oncogene on 8q24 harbours at least five independent loci associated with prostate cancer as well as loci associated with four other cancers (breast, colon, and bladder cancers and chronic lymphocytic leukaemia) [23]. GWAS have detected strong signals for the human leukocyte antigen (HLA) regions for cancers of the immune system or those driven by viral infections (e.g. cervical, liver, and nasopharyngeal cancers) (see "DNA repair polymorphisms and human cancer").

A region on 5p15.33 containing the telomerase gene, *TERT*, harbours multiple susceptibility alleles for many cancers, including rare and common SNP alleles [26]. Rare mutations in *TERT* track with dyskeratosis congenita (an inherited bone-marrow failure syndrome) and idiopathic pulmonary fibrosis. Cancer GWAS have discovered susceptibility alleles for at least 10 different types over at least five independent signals. Moreover, a protective allele for one cancer can confer susceptibility to another cancer; notably, the same allele has inverse effects for two skin cancers, basal cell carcinoma and melanoma. The pleiotropy in this region hints at complex gene–gene or gene–environment interactions.

Whereas most of the initial GWAS were conducted in subjects of European ancestry, recently more have been conducted in subjects of Asian and African ancestry. Prostate cancer GWAS in men of African ancestry identified new independent loci on 8q24 as well as a new region on 17q21 [27]. Studies in Asia have concentrated on cancers notable for high incidence, such as gastric adenocarcinoma, oesophageal squamous cell carcinoma, and lung cancer in nonsmokers [28,29].

The underlying population genetic histories of distinct groups have important implications for the discovery of susceptibility alleles because the underlying linkage disequilibrium can vary greatly. In many regions of the genome, differences in MAFs between continental populations (e.g. European, Asian, and African descent) can account for variance in the detection of susceptibility alleles. For example, the MAF of a SNP is sufficiently high in men of African ancestry for the SNP to be detected in a GWAS of prostate cancer in African-American men, but because of its low MAF in Europeans, it is not easily detected in GWAS of European men [27].

Until recently, cancer GWAS lumped disparate study designs together and rarely addressed environmental exposures. Still, a handful of alleles have been shown to interact with specific exposures. In a study of oesophageal squamous cell carcinoma in China, a gene–environment interaction was observed between the variants in the *ADH*/*ALDH* genes and alcohol consumption [30]. In bladder cancer, a novel marker for *NAT2* interacts with smoking, correlating with low or intermediate acetylation status. In fact, common genetic variants have been shown to modify the effect of smoking on bladder cancer [31]. A GWAS of lung cancer in nonsmoking Asian women discovered regions not observed in lung cancer GWAS dominated by smokers [29]. Also, there was no signal in nonsmoking women across 15q24, a region strongly correlated with smoking behaviour and lung cancer in smokers, suggesting that the reported signals are primarily related to tobacco use.

Analysis of associated risk factors collected in cancer GWAS has been extremely informative for tobacco use, alcohol consumption, and anthropometric measures (e.g. height, weight, and waist size). Cross-disease consortia (e.g. diabetes and cardiovascular disease) have combined numbers to accelerate discovery of common risk factors. Already,

more than 200 independent loci have been identified for height [32].

Investigation of GWAS signals

Each region should be fine-mapped to determine optimal variants for functional analyses, mainly because of the large number of highly correlated variants. The pattern of linkage disequilibrium, often with apparent differences between ancestral populations, is examined to winnow down possible variants. Choosing the optimal ones also requires bioinformatics assessment using new public databases, such as the Encyclopedia of DNA Elements (ENCODE) project [33]. ENCODE has begun to systematically shed light on the biology of the regulation of the genome, specifically cataloguing signposts and markers of biological activity. This resource can be used for individual variants but also to look at patterns or pathways, as recently suggested for breast cancer susceptibility loci identified by GWAS [34]. A greater-than-expected fraction of cancer susceptibility alleles map to regulatory regions, suggesting that common variants confer susceptibility primarily through perturbations in regulatory events [23].

Laboratory investigation is required to explain the biological basis of the SNPs that directly associate with the cancer of interest. Each individual variant has to be studied separately, and a combination of different approaches and tools is required, which explains the markedly slower pace of characterization (Fig. 3.2.3). For example, investigation of a prostate cancer GWAS marker, which maps to the β-microseminoprotein gene (*MSMB*) on 10q11, revealed that the risk allele in the promoter region decreases transcriptional activity, lowering expression in prostate cancer tissue [35]. Expression decreases as prostate cancer progresses from early to late stages; loss of *MSMB* expression can be associated with disease recurrence after radical prostatectomy. Still, the finding may not be fully explained by

DNA repair polymorphisms and human cancer

Paolo Vineis

A wide range of DNA damage can be inflicted, both from extracellular agents – including environmental exposures – and via endogenous mechanisms. Genotoxic chemicals bind to DNA, forming adducts that in turn can be repaired by the DNA repair machinery (Fig. B3.2.1) or lead to permanent DNA damage. DNA damage can lead to cancer and other diseases. Therefore, it is plausible that inherited sequence variants in DNA repair genes are involved in cancer development.

Five main mechanisms are involved in DNA repair: base excision repair, which corrects non-bulky damage; nucleotide excision repair, which corrects lesions that disrupt the double helical structure of DNA; mismatch repair, which corrects replication errors; double-strand break repair, which corrects double-strand breaks through two different pathways, homologous and

non-homologous recombination; and direct repair, which corrects methylated or alkylated bases [1]. Rare, highly penetrant mutations of DNA repair genes (such as the XP family, involved in the heritable disease xeroderma pigmentosum) are associated with a high risk of cancer, whereas the evidence is weaker for common SNPs with low penetrance.

A systematic review and meta-analysis, based on systematic criteria, showed that out of 241 associations investigated, only three associations were graded as having strong epidemiological credibility of cumulative evidence [2]. These associations were between two SNPs – rs1799793 and rs13181 – in the *ERCC2* gene and lung cancer (recessive model), and between rs1805794 in the *NBN* gene and bladder cancer (dominant model). An update of this meta-analysis

has since been performed [3], and the authors found partially inconsistent results. In addition, none of the cancer GWAS published until 2011 showed highly statistically significant associations for any of the common DNA repair gene variants that would place DNA repair genes among the top 10–20 hits identified in GWAS. This suggests that it is unlikely that DNA repair gene polymorphisms per se play a major role. This is not surprising since in a multistep, multigenic process such as carcinogenesis, single polymorphisms in single genes are unlikely to alter the expression or function of specific proteins to the extent of producing a pathological phenotype. However, the combined effect of several SNPs in a gene or in multiple genes could have more impact.

Pathway approaches using novel genotyping technologies will enable more comprehensive studies of multiple SNPs in multiple genes, and it will be possible to investigate gene–environment interactions more rigorously than before, using novel statistical methodology. The combined effect of multiple SNPs in several genes in one or more relevant DNA repair pathways could have a greater impact on pathological phenotypes than SNPs in single genes, but this has been investigated only occasionally.

Fig. B3.2.1. DNA damage, repair mechanisms, and consequences. (A) Common DNA damaging agents (top), examples of DNA lesions induced (middle), and the most relevant DNA repair mechanisms responsible for the removal of those lesions (bottom). (B) Acute effects of DNA damage on cell-cycle progression, leading to transient arrest in the G1, S, G2, and M phases (top), and on DNA metabolism (middle). Long-term consequences of DNA injury (bottom) include point mutations or chromosome aberrations and their biological effects. *cis*-Pt, cisplatin; CPD, cyclobutane pyrimidine dimer; EJ, end joining; HR, homologous recombination; MMC, mitomycin C; (6-4)PP, 6-4 photoproduct; UV, ultraviolet.

References

1. Friedberg E *et al.* (2006). *DNA Repair and Mutagenesis*. Washington, DC: ASM Press.

2. Vineis P *et al.* (2009). *J Natl Cancer Inst*, 101:24–36. http://dx.doi.org/10.1093/jnci/djn437 PMID:19116388

3. Ricceri F *et al.* (2012). *Mutat Res*, 736:117–121. http://dx.doi.org/10.1016/j.mrfmmm.2011.07.013 PMID:21864546

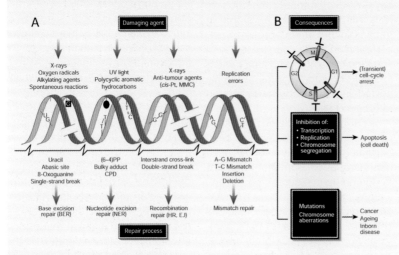

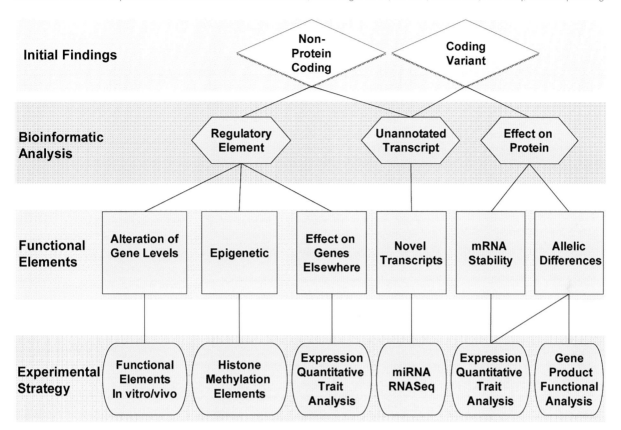

Fig. 3.2.3. Laboratory investigation of GWAS SNPs. Cartoon depiction of the steps after fine-mapping, beginning with the assessment of whether a marker resides in a coding region and continuing through the bioinformatics analysis and assessment of functional elements before the experimental studies are conducted. mRNA, messenger RNA; miRNA, microRNA, RNASeq, RNA sequencing.

MSMB alone. The gene on the other side of *MSMB*, *NCOA4*, is also upregulated by the GWAS promoter SNP, and *NCOA4* forms chimeric transcripts with *MSMB* [36,37]. Also promising is the relationship between the *MSMB* allele and urinary levels of β-microseminoprotein, which was validated as a serum biomarker of prostate cancer in previous investigations.

The value of fine-mapping is critical for exploring GWAS markers. Prokunina-Olsson *et al.* uncovered a novel gene, *IFNL4,* created by a complex dinucleotide variant (e.g. a single bp missense contiguous to a deletion) in strong linkage disequilibrium with the published marker on chromosome 19 associated with clearance of hepatitis C virus infection, a major risk factor for liver cancer [38]. Earlier investigators focused on variants upstream of the nearest gene, *IFNL3* (previously *IL28B*). The

deletion allele generates a frameshift, which leads to a novel protein that induces an interferon-type response, apparent on close inspection of RNA sequencing data in primary human hepatocytes. The complex *IFNL4* genetic variant has a strong effect on hepatitis C virus clearance, especially in individuals of African ancestry. The strength of the estimated effect on both spontaneous and treatment-induced clearance of hepatitis C virus is significantly larger than most cancer GWAS signals, prompting pursuit in clinical studies.

Understanding the biological basis of a GWAS signal can eventually lead to clinical translation. A bladder cancer GWAS locus maps to the prostate stem cell antigen gene (*PSCA*) [39]. Based on RNA sequencing followed by functional analysis, a promoter SNP, characterized in fine-mapping, influences messenger RNA (mRNA) PSCA

expression [40]. The creation of an alternative translation start site leads to increased expression of *PSCA* on the cell surface [41]. The actual genotype could predict PSCA protein expression and identify bladder cancer patients harbouring the PSCA variant, who may benefit from immunotherapy with anti-PSCA humanized antibody, an emerging therapy for different cancers.

SNP markers have yet to be incorporated into clinical practice, despite the opinions of some commercial groups. Adequate testing and validation have not been conducted in the clinical setting. Once a catalogue approaching a comprehensive set of common susceptibility alleles has been defined for a given cancer, it will be possible to explore applications in large validation studies. Already, it is possible to begin to develop the models to design and conduct the validation studies [42].

In a recent analysis of ovarian cancer, it appears that women harbouring germline mutations in *BRCA1* or *BRCA2* may actually have improved survival, partly due to increased sensitivity to standard chemotherapeutic agents [43]. So far, analyses of small numbers of cancer susceptibility SNPs have failed to confirm their utility using receiver operator curves [44]. Continued discovery is required to generate the comprehensive set of common and uncommon variants per disease, which could be used to reclassify risk status for either prevention or early intervention.

Future directions

Cancer GWAS will continue to discover susceptibility alleles but are now poised to investigate pharmacogenomics and outcome analyses, particularly with large studies on the horizon that are well phenotyped. The major discoveries of cancer GWAS represent an important transition in the development of integrative scientific collaborations because they have relied on a network of epidemiologists, geneticists, and analysts, who have uncovered genetic markers for risk. The next frontier lies in the investigation of the underlying biology that can explain the contribution of susceptibility alleles to disease pathogenesis or progression, which in turn could lead to more effective strategies for prevention or treatment.

The development of next-generation sequence analysis tools represents a major opportunity to map common and uncommon susceptibility alleles as well as highly penetrant mutations in families. There are daunting challenges in quality control of genome sequence data, including a substantively larger number of variants for testing, which compounds the challenge of distinguishing true signal from background noise [45]. To define the comprehensive set of uncommon variants (with a MAF between 0.5% and 5%), hybrid approaches will be required. Recently, two groups converged on susceptibility mutations in *MITF* for melanoma based on not only family- and population-based association studies but also laboratory insights into the underlying biology of disruption of sumoylation of MITF protein [46,47].

The next generation of studies will focus on two major extensions of the GWAS approach: (i) investigation of the interrelationship between germline susceptibility alleles and somatic alterations [43]; and (ii) testing the clinical and public health applicability of the full spectrum of cancer susceptibility alleles identified through GWAS, which includes rare, highly penetrant mutations, less common alleles with moderate penetrance, and the common alleles with small effect sizes. The susceptibility alleles discovered by cancer GWAS are not yet ready for clinical implementation. To develop accurate and useful recommendations for genetic counselling in the new age of complex disease, more discovery is needed that extends into the fraction of the uncommon variants and rare mutations. New paradigms for implementing susceptibility alleles in precision medicine represent long-term goals and are expected to be applied to classification of risk groups that could be offered early detection or intervention.

References

1. Knudson AG (2000). Chasing the cancer demon. *Annu Rev Genet*, 34:1–19. http://dx.doi.org/10.1146/annurev.genet.34.1.1 PMID:11092820

2. Lander ES, Linton LM, Birren B *et al.*; International Human Genome Sequencing Consortium (2001). Initial sequencing and analysis of the human genome. *Nature*, 409:860–921. http://dx.doi.org/10.1038/35057062 PMID:11237011

3. Venter JC, Adams MD, Myers EW *et al.* (2001). The sequence of the human genome. *Science*, 291:1304–1351. http://dx.doi.org/10.1126/science.1058040 PMID:11181995

4. Frazer KA, Ballinger DG, Cox DR *et al.*; International HapMap Consortium (2007). A second generation human haplotype map of over 3.1 million SNPs. *Nature*, 449:851–861. http://dx.doi.org/10.1038/nature06258 PMID:17943122

5. Manolio TA, Collins FS, Cox NJ *et al.* (2009). Finding the missing heritability of complex diseases. *Nature*, 461:747–753. http://dx.doi.org/10.1038/nature08494 PMID:19812666

6. Risch N, Merikangas K (1996). The future of genetic studies of complex human diseases. *Science*, 273:1516–1517. http://dx.doi.org/10.1126/science.273.5281.1516 PMID:8801636

7. Moore LE, Baris DR, Figueroa JD *et al.* (2011). *GSTM1* null and *NAT2* slow acetylation genotypes, smoking intensity and bladder cancer risk: results from the New England bladder cancer study and *NAT2* meta-analysis. *Carcinogenesis*, 32:182–189. http://dx.doi.org/10.1093/carcin/bgq223 PMID:21037224

8. Hashibe M, McKay JD, Curado MP *et al.* (2008). Multiple *ADH* genes are associated with upper aerodigestive cancers. *Nat Genet*, 40:707–709. http://dx.doi.org/10.1038/ng.151 PMID:18500343

9. Chanock SJ, Manolio T, Boehnke M *et al.*; NCI-NHGRI Working Group on Replication in Association Studies (2007). Replicating genotype-phenotype associations. *Nature*, 447:655–660. http://dx.doi.org/10.1038/447655a PMID:17554299

10. Burton PR, Clayton DG, Cardon LR *et al.*; Wellcome Trust Case Control Consortium (2007). Genome-wide association study of 14,000 cases of seven common diseases and 3,000 shared controls. *Nature*, 447:661–678. http://dx.doi.org/10.1038/nature05911 PMID:17554300

11. Orr N, Chanock S (2008). Common genetic variation and human disease. *Adv Genet*, 62:1–32. http://dx.doi.org/10.1016/S0065-2660(08)00601-9 PMID:19010252

12. Eeles RA, Olama AA, Benlloch S *et al.*; COGS–Cancer Research UK GWAS– ELLIPSE (part of GAME-ON) Initiative; Australian Prostate Cancer Bioresource; UK Genetic Prostate Cancer Study Collaborators/British Association of Urological Surgeons' Section of Oncology; UK ProtecT (Prostate testing for cancer and Treatment) Study Collaborators; PRACTICAL (Prostate Cancer Association Group to Investigate Cancer-Associated Alterations in the Genome) Consortium (2013). Identification of 23 new prostate cancer susceptibility loci using the iCOGS custom genotyping array. *Nat Genet*, 45:385–391, e1–e2. http://dx.doi.org/10.1038/ng.2560 PMID:23535732

13. Michailidou K, Hall P, Gonzalez-Neira A *et al.*; Breast and Ovarian Cancer Susceptibility Collaboration; Hereditary Breast and Ovarian Cancer Research Group Netherlands (HEBON); kConFab Investigators; Australian Ovarian Cancer Study Group; GENICA (Gene Environment Interaction and Breast Cancer in Germany) Network (2013). Large-scale genotyping identifies 41 new loci associated with breast cancer risk. *Nat Genet*, 45:353–361, e1–e2. http://dx.doi.org/10.1038/ng.2563 PMID:23535729

14. Pharoah PD, Tsai YY, Ramus SJ *et al.*; Australian Cancer Study; Australian Ovarian Cancer Study Group (2013). GWAS meta-analysis and replication identifies three new susceptibility loci for ovarian cancer. *Nat Genet*, 45:362–370, e1–e2. http://dx.doi.org/10.1038/ng.2564 PMID:23535730

15. Abecasis GR, Altshuler D, Auton A *et al.*; 1000 Genomes Project Consortium (2010). A map of human genome variation from population-scale sequencing. *Nature*, 467:1061–1073. http://dx.doi.org/10.1038/nature09534 PMID:20981092

16. Wang Z, Jacobs KB, Yeager M *et al.* (2012). Improved imputation of common and uncommon SNPs with a new reference set. *Nat Genet*, 44:6–7. http://dx.doi.org/10.1038/ng.1044 PMID:22200770

17. Chung CC, Magalhaes WC, Gonzalez-Bosquet J, Chanock SJ (2010). Genome-wide association studies in cancer – current and future directions. *Carcinogenesis*, 31:111–120. http://dx.doi.org/10.1093/carcin/bgp273 PMID:19906782

18. Hindorff LA, Gillanders EM, Manolio TA (2011). Genetic architecture of cancer and other complex diseases: lessons learned and future directions. *Carcinogenesis*, 32:945–954. http://dx.doi.org/10.1093/carcin/bgr056 PMID:21459759

19. Maris JM, Mosse YP, Bradfield JP *et al.* (2008). Chromosome 6p22 locus associated with clinically aggressive neuroblastoma. *N Engl J Med*, 358:2585–2593. http://dx.doi.org/10.1056/NEJMoa0708698 PMID:18463370

20. Postel-Vinay S, Véron AS, Tirode F *et al.* (2012). Common variants near *TARDBP* and *EGR2* are associated with susceptibility to Ewing sarcoma. *Nat Genet*, 44:323–327. http://dx.doi.org/10.1038/ng.1085 PMID:22327514

21. Garcia-Closas M, Couch FJ, Lindstrom S *et al.*; Gene ENvironmental Interaction and breast CAncer (GENICA) Network; kConFab Investigators; Familial Breast Cancer Study (FBCS); Australian Breast Cancer Tissue Bank (ABCTB) Investigators (2013). Genome-wide association studies identify four ER negative-specific breast cancer risk loci. *Nat Genet*, 45:392–398, e1–e2. http://dx.doi.org/10.1038/ng.2561 PMID:23535733

22. Wu C, Li D, Jia W *et al.* (2013). Genome-wide association study identifies common variants in *SLC39A6* associated with length of survival in esophageal squamous-cell carcinoma. *Nat Genet*, 45:632–638. http://dx.doi.org/10.1038/ng.2638 PMID:23644492

23. Chung CC, Chanock SJ (2011). Current status of genome-wide association studies in cancer. *Hum Genet*, 130:59–78. http://dx.doi.org/10.1007/s00439-011-1030-9 PMID:21678065

24. Park JH, Gail MH, Weinberg CR *et al.* (2011). Distribution of allele frequencies and effect sizes and their interrelationships for common genetic susceptibility variants. *Proc Natl Acad Sci U S A*, 108:18026–18031. http://dx.doi.org/10.1073/pnas.1114759108 PMID:22003128

25. Kanetsky PA, Mitra N, Vardhanabhuti S *et al.* (2009). Common variation in *KITLG* and at 5q31.3 predisposes to testicular germ cell cancer. *Nat Genet*, 41:811–815. http://dx.doi.org/10.1038/ng.393 PMID:19483682

26. Rafnar T, Sulem P, Stacey SN *et al.* (2009). Sequence variants at the *TERT-CLPTM1L* locus associate with many cancer types. *Nat Genet*, 41:221–227. http://dx.doi.org/10.1038/ng.296 PMID:19151717

27. Haiman CA, Chen GK, Blot WJ *et al.* (2011). Genome-wide association study of prostate cancer in men of African ancestry identifies a susceptibility locus at 17q21. *Nat Genet*, 43:570–573. http://dx.doi.org/10.1038/ng.839 PMID:21602798

28. Abnet CC, Freedman ND, Hu N *et al.* (2010). A shared susceptibility locus in *PLCE1* at 10q23 for gastric adenocarcinoma and esophageal squamous cell carcinoma. *Nat Genet*, 42:764–767. http://dx.doi.org/10.1038/ng.649 PMID:20729852

29. Lan Q, Hsiung CA, Matsuo K *et al.* (2012). Genome-wide association analysis identifies new lung cancer susceptibility loci in never-smoking women in Asia. *Nat Genet*, 44:1330–1335. http://dx.doi.org/10.1038/ng.2456 PMID:23143601

30. Wu C, Kraft P, Zhai K *et al.* (2012). Genome-wide association analyses of esophageal squamous cell carcinoma in Chinese identify multiple susceptibility loci and gene-environment interactions. *Nat Genet*, 44:1090–1097. http://dx.doi.org/10.1038/ng.2411 PMID:22960999

31. Garcia-Closas M, Rothman N, Figueroa JD *et al.* (2013). Common genetic polymorphisms modify the effect of smoking on absolute risk of bladder cancer. *Cancer Res*, 73:2211–2220. http://dx.doi.org/10.1158/0008-5472.CAN-12-2388 PMID:23536561

32. Lango Allen H, Estrada K, Lettre G *et al.* (2010). Hundreds of variants clustered in genomic loci and biological pathways affect human height. *Nature*, 467:832–838. http://dx.doi.org/10.1038/nature09410 PMID:20881960

33. Bernstein BE, Birney E, Dunham I *et al.*; ENCODE Project Consortium (2012). An integrated encyclopedia of DNA elements in the human genome. *Nature*, 489:57–74. http://dx.doi.org/10.1038/nature11247 PMID:22955616

34. Li Q, Seo JH, Stranger B *et al.* (2013). Integrative eQTL-based analyses reveal the biology of breast cancer risk loci. *Cell*, 152:633–641. http://dx.doi.org/10.1016/j.cell.2012.12.034 PMID:23374354

35. Lou H, Yeager M, Li H *et al.* (2009). Fine mapping and functional analysis of a common variant in *MSMB* on chromosome 10q11.2 associated with prostate cancer susceptibility. *Proc Natl Acad Sci U S A*, 106:7933–7938. http://dx.doi.org/10.1073/pnas.0902104106 PMID:19383797

36. Lou H, Li H, Yeager M *et al.* (2012). Promoter variants in the *MSMB* gene associated with prostate cancer regulate *MSMB/NCOA4* fusion transcripts. *Hum Genet*, 131:1453–1466. http://dx.doi.org/10.1007/s00439-012-1182-2 PMID:22661295

37. Pomerantz MM, Shrestha Y, Flavin RJ *et al.* (2010). Analysis of the 10q11 cancer risk locus implicates *MSMB* and *NCOA4* in human prostate tumorigenesis. *PLoS Genet*, 6:e1001204. http://dx.doi.org/10.1371/journal.pgen.1001204 PMID:21085629

38. Prokunina-Olsson L, Muchmore B, Tang W *et al.* (2013). A variant upstream of *IFNL3* (*IL28B*) creating a new interferon gene *IFNL4* is associated with impaired clearance of hepatitis C virus. *Nat Genet*, 45:164–171. http://dx.doi.org/10.1038/ng.2521 PMID:23291588

39. Wu X, Ye Y, Kiemeney LA *et al.* (2009). Genetic variation in the prostate stem cell antigen gene *PSCA* confers susceptibility to urinary bladder cancer. *Nat Genet*, 41:991–995. http://dx.doi.org/10.1038/ng.421 PMID:19648920

40. Fu YP, Kohaar I, Rothman N *et al.* (2012). Common genetic variants in the *PSCA* gene influence gene expression and bladder cancer risk. *Proc Natl Acad Sci U S A*, 109:4974–4979. http://dx.doi.org/10.1073/pnas.1202189109 PMID:22416122

41. Kohaar I, Porter-Gill P, Lenz P *et al.* (2013). Genetic variant as a selection marker for anti-prostate stem cell antigen immunotherapy of bladder cancer. *J Natl Cancer Inst*, 105:69–73. http://dx.doi.org/10.1093/jnci/djs458 PMID:23266392

42. Burton H, Chowdhury S, Dent T *et al.* (2013). Public health implications from COGS and potential for risk stratification and screening. *Nat Genet*, 45:349–351. http://dx.doi.org/10.1038/ng.2582 PMID:23535723

43. Bolton KL, Chenevix-Trench G, Goh C *et al.*; EMBRACE; kConFab Investigators; Cancer Genome Atlas Research Network (2012). Association between *BRCA1* and *BRCA2* mutations and survival in women with invasive epithelial ovarian cancer. *JAMA*, 307:382–390. http://dx.doi.org/10.1001/jama.2012.20 PMID:22274685

44. Wacholder S, Hartge P, Prentice R *et al.* (2010). Performance of common genetic variants in breast-cancer risk models. *N Engl J Med*, 362:986–993. http://dx.doi.org/10.1056/NEJMoa0907727 PMID:20237344

45. Mardis ER (2011). A decade's perspective on DNA sequencing technology. *Nature*, 470:198–203. http://dx.doi.org/10.1038/nature09796 PMID:21307932

46. Bertolotto C, Lesueur F, Giuliano S *et al.*; French Familial Melanoma Study Group (2011). A SUMOylation-defective *MITF* germline mutation predisposes to melanoma and renal carcinoma. *Nature*, 480:94–98. http://dx.doi.org/10.1038/nature10539 PMID:22012259

47. Yokoyama S, Woods SL, Boyle GM *et al.* (2011). A novel recurrent mutation in *MITF* predisposes to familial and sporadic melanoma. *Nature*, 480:99–103. http://dx.doi.org/10.1038/nature10630 PMID:22080950

Website

A Catalog of Published Genome-Wide Association Studies:
http://www.genome.gov/gwastudies

3.3

Gene expression

3 BIOLOGY

Magdalena B. Wozniak
Paul Brennan

Emmanuel Barillot (reviewer)
Dongxin Lin (reviewer)

Summary

- Expression of coded genetic information contained in DNA determines an organism's phenotype through synthesis of functional gene products; the synthesis of such proteins and RNA is regulated at the transcriptional and translational levels.

- In cancer, malignant transformation of normal cells results from structural changes in DNA and is mediated by aberrant expression of multiple genes.

- By reference to gene expression profiles, tumours have been subclassified into categories with distinct biological and clinical properties; this process sometimes identifies genetic changes and gives rise to therapeutic targets.

- The human genome is estimated to encode for more than 1000 microRNAs that regulate the translation of more than 60% of genes and hence determine gene expression.

- Currently, large-scale international collaborative cancer studies, based on next-generation sequencing technology, are generating a comprehensive catalogue of oncogenic alterations evident in particular tumour types.

Gene expression is the process of translating the information specified through the sequence of bases in DNA into functional products, including proteins and non-coding RNA, such as ribosomal RNA, transfer RNA, microRNA (miRNA), and small nuclear RNA, among others (Fig. 3.3.1). In eukaryotes, transcription is performed by three types of RNA polymerases, each of which requires a promoter DNA sequence and a set of DNA-binding transcription factors to initiate the process. The promoter sequence is almost always located just upstream of the transcription start site, which corresponds to the 5′ end. Binding of regulatory proteins to an enhancer sequence results in a shift in chromatin structure, which either promotes or inhibits RNA polymerase and transcription factor binding. Euchromatin, which has a more open structure, is associated with transcription, whereas heterochromatin is associated with transcriptional inactivity (Fig. 3.3.2A).

Only a fraction of the genes in a particular cell are expressed at a given time. The variety of gene expression profiles is determined by distinct sets of transcription regulators. Transcription creates precursor messenger RNA (pre-mRNA), which further undergoes a series of modifications, leading to mature mRNA. These modifications include the enzymatic reactions of 5′ capping and 3′ cleavage and polyadenylation. Protein-coding sequences in DNA account for only 1–2% of the human genome [1]. The increased diversity at the level of primary mRNA and proteins can be accounted for by alternative RNA splicing, which creates a series of different transcripts originating from a single gene by removing or retaining some introns or exons in particular mature mRNAs. The resulting transcripts can potentially be translated into different proteins. Each mRNA is composed of three parts: a 5′ untranslated region, an open reading frame, and a 3′ untranslated region.

Regulation of gene expression

Regulation of gene expression can occur at any step of expression and includes various systems that control and determine which genes are switched on or off and to what extent the genes are expressed. Transcriptional regulation of gene expression levels occurs in three main ways: genetic (involving direct interaction with DNA), modulation

Fig. 3.3.1. Schematic overview of the protein-coding gene expression pathway in eukaryotic organisms. E, enhancer sequence; T, terminator (transcription termination site); m⁷G, 7-methylguanylate cap.

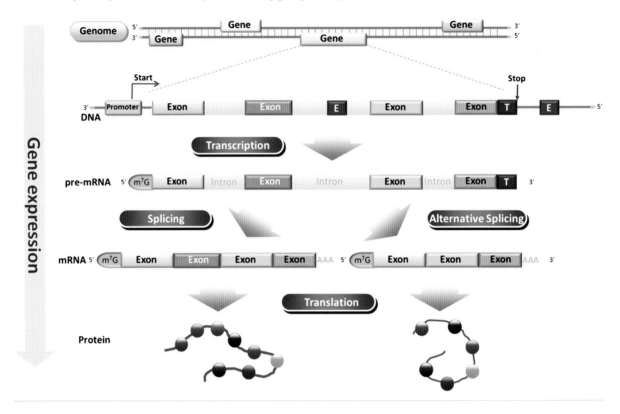

(involving interaction with transcription machinery), and epigenetic (involving non-sequence changes in DNA). Genes contain in their sequence several protein-binding sites around the coding regions, such as enhancers, insulators, and silencers. These sites facilitate binding of transcription factors, resulting in blocking or activation of transcription. Furthermore, the activity of transcription factors can also be modulated by post-translational protein modifications such as acetylation, phosphorylation, or glycosylation (Fig. 3.3.2B).

Epigenetic changes, and specifically DNA methylation, modulate transcription by altering the accessibility of DNA to proteins. Particularly important for regulation of gene expression levels are post-transcriptional modifications, including 5′ capping and 3′ polyadenylation, which protect mRNA from degradation during nuclear export. Once generated, mature RNA isoforms are subject to many levels of regulation, including the regulation of translation by

miRNAs and regulatory factors, the use of alternative translation start sites, RNA localization, and mRNA stability and turnover. Direct inhibition of protein translation by toxins and antibiotics is less frequent. In addition, a substantial number of isoforms can be an effect of single-nucleotide polymorphisms (SNPs), small genetic differences between alleles of the same gene. Finally, protein expression can also be reduced by degradation, in which unneeded, damaged, and improperly folded proteins are labelled for degradation by ubiquitination.

Dysregulation of gene expression in cancer

Malignant transformation is accompanied and characterized by disruption of genetic information and aberrant expression of multiple genes. These changes enhance the survival of tumour cells and alter their proliferative capacity, leading to tumour formation. The fact that the majority

of cells within a tumour mass share a common gene expression profile has encouraged systematic analyses of differential gene expression in human tumour samples to provide an estimate of the degree of genetic and epigenetic dysregulation.

Measurement of gene expression

To monitor gene expression, ideally the amount of each final gene product, which is in most cases a protein, should be measured. However, due to the limitations of protein-based assays, pre-mRNA expression is frequently studied. Several methods have been developed for quantification of mRNA levels. These include northern blotting, quantitative reverse transcription polymerase chain reaction (qRT-PCR), RNase protection assays, microarrays, serial analysis of gene expression (SAGE), and next-generation RNA sequencing (RNA-seq). While northern blotting and qRT-PCR are often used to

Therapeutic implications of dysregulated DNA damage signalling

Peter Bouwman and Jos Jonkers

The intimate link between cancer and DNA damage signalling is clear from the fact that many tumour suppressor genes are involved in DNA repair [1,2]. Well-known examples are *BRCA1* and *BRCA2*, which are important for DNA repair by homologous recombination. In addition, many known carcinogens such as tobacco smoke, alcohol, ultraviolet radiation, and ionizing radiation are known to cause DNA damage.

Paradoxically, tumours can also be treated by DNA-damaging irradiation or chemical compounds. Although DNA damage also affects normal cells, tumour cells are often more vulnerable because of defects in DNA repair pathways or critical cell-cycle checkpoints. Especially defects in homology-directed repair (HDR) of DNA double-strand breaks can be exploited therapeutically. It has recently become clear that this is possible not only by directly damaging the DNA but also via inhibition of PARP enzymes. Inhibition of PARP1 and PARP2 can block alternative repair pathways and result in trapping of PARP to DNA, which is detrimental for HDR-deficient cells [3].

Fig. B3.3.1. DNA damage response (DDR)-related mechanisms of therapy resistance. Loss of function of DNA repair genes can cripple the affected pathway to the extent that tumour cells become highly sensitive to certain types of DNA damage. In addition, the remaining repair pathways may become essential for survival. Resistance to chemotherapy can be a result of partial activity of mutated alleles. Such hypomorphic mutations can be sufficiently affected to lead to tumour formation, yet too active to result in hypersensitivity to targeted therapy. In case mutations lead to a completely inactivated (null) allele, chemotherapy may select for mutations that revert the original defect or select for mutations in other DDR genes that result in pathway rewiring. Crosses symbolize inactivation. Tumour cells with wild-type levels of DDR activity are indicated in green, cells with a partially active DDR pathway are shown in beige, and cells with impaired DDR are shown in purple.

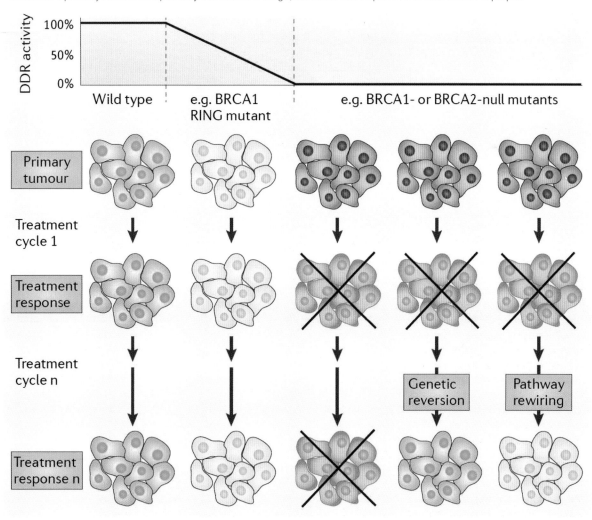

Despite their exquisite sensitivity to DNA damage, tumours with HDR defects can eventually become resistant to therapy. Apart from mechanisms that result in decreased intracellular drug concentrations, resistance may also be caused by altered DNA damage signalling [1,2]. Of note, tumours with mutations in a specific DNA repair gene do not always show the same response to therapy; missense mutations in a specialized region will have different effects compared with mutations that completely abolish expression. Furthermore, tumours often consist of heterogeneous populations of cells that may share a common ancestor but have acquired different additional mutations or epigenetic alterations. Data from preclinical models suggest that this may result in increased capacity to repair DNA damage, and hence resistance to therapy. It has also been shown that therapy-resistant BRCA1- and BRCA2-associated tumours may restore their HDR defect by genetic reversion. Secondary mutations may overcome the original defect, resulting in the expression of (partially) functional BRCA1 or BRCA2 protein. Alternatively, DNA repair pathways may be perturbed to withstand DNA-damaging therapy. Recent data suggest that this is possible in respect of the two major pathways for repair of DNA double-strand breaks, error-free homologous recombination and intrinsically error-prone non-homologous end joining (NHEJ). The HDR defect of BRCA1-deficient cells can, for instance, be suppressed by loss of the NHEJ protein 53BP1. Stratification of patients with specific DNA repair defects and combinations of targeted therapeutics will be required to maximize the likelihood of successful treatment. To avoid resistance, the development of biomarkers for the activity of factors involved in DNA damage response will be of critical importance.

References

1. Bouwman P, Jonkers J (2012). *Nat Rev Cancer*, 12:587–598. http://dx.doi.org/10.1038/nrc3342 PMID:22918414

2. Lord CJ, Ashworth A (2012). *Nature*, 481:287–294. http://dx.doi.org/10.1038/nature10760 PMID:22258607

3. Helleday T (2011). *Mol Oncol*, 5:387–393. http://dx.doi.org/10.1016/j.molonc.2011.07.001 PMID:21821475

verify the results for particular genes or for some low-expression genes, microarrays, SAGE, and RNA-seq are used to obtain broad coverage of the genome. Now that identification of genome-wide sets of protein-coding genes is feasible, combined with the discovery of miRNAs, many researchers have taken advantage of array-based approaches to search for gene expression patterns within most cancer types.

In the context of cancer, gene expression profiling with DNA microarrays has been used to identify individual transcripts and regulatory gene networks mediating disease pathogenesis, to discover molecular targets for drug development, to more accurately classify tumours, and to identify molecular markers useful for disease diagnosis and prognosis or as predictors of clinical outcomes. In addition to detecting changes in transcriptional levels, the recently developed RNA-seq technique can detect other abnormalities in the cancer transcriptome, such as SNPs, alternative splice variants, novel coding and non-coding transcripts, and gene fusions. Due to decreasing costs, RNA-seq is becoming more common as a method for cancer gene expression profiling. RNA-seq is also superior to microarray techniques, given its unbiased approach in probe selection. However, the requirement for increased amounts of sample RNA and the challenging bioinformatics analyses of generated data remain limitations of this technique.

Fig. 3.3.2. (A) Representation of "closed" and "open" chromatin structures. (B) Overview of major post-translational modifications that may play essential roles in the regulation of gene expression and be altered in the course of disease processes. Modifications are specified in relation to part of the N-terminal tail of a histone protein; the single letters indicate specific amino acid residues that may be subject to particular modifications.

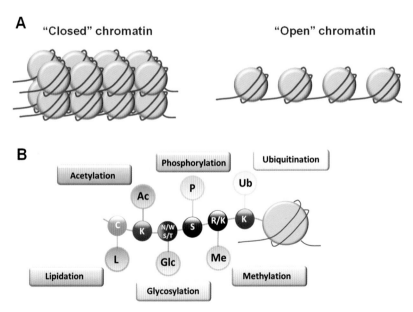

Gene expression microarray studies in cancer

Microarray profiling technology, which has been most widely used to study gene expression in cancer, represents an important development in genomic marker research and has been evaluated as a tool for decision-making in clinical practice. Microarray studies aim to identify genes that are differentially expressed between known groups of samples (class comparison), to discover unknown patterns of gene expression (class discovery), and to develop classifiers associated with disease or treatment outcome (class prediction). For that purpose, both supervised and unsupervised methods of analysis have been used to search for molecular signatures associated with known classes and to discover new classes of a disease. Even though diagnosis and tumour subclassification are still dominated by histological analysis for most cancers, these methods have proven to be insufficient to distinguish between subclasses in several types of cancer.

Specifically, consistent definition of diffuse large B-cell lymphoma has proven difficult due to discrepancies between inter- and intra-observer reproducibility [2]. Gene expression profiling has enabled the subclassification of diffuse large B-cell lymphoma tumours into categories with distinct biological properties and prognoses. This has led to the identification of two subtypes: germinal centre B-like and activated B-like diffuse large B-cell lymphoma [3]. For patients with germinal centre B-like disease, the 10-year survival rate was about 80%, whereas for those with activated B-like disease, the 8-year survival rate was about 40%.

In some tumour types, such as breast cancer [4] and leukaemia [5], molecular markers have been adjuncts to histological classification for decades. Perhaps the best known example is the contribution of expression profiling to the classification of breast tumours, which has resulted in the development of the PAM50 Breast Cancer Intrinsic Classifier, which sorts breast cancer into the major molecular subtypes of basal-like, human epidermal growth factor receptor 2 (HER2)-positive, luminal A, and luminal B (Fig. 3.3.3A). Gene expression signature studies performed in melanoma have also led to the development of a protein-based test measuring expression of five genes that can distinguish malignant melanoma from benign tissue [6].

The use of gene expression signatures has also enabled the identification of prognostic subclasses. The more successful examples of gene expression profiles as prognostic indicators have been their use to define the risk of relapse in patients with early-stage breast cancer. Three profiles have proven prognostic ability: the MammaPrint 70-gene profile, the Oncotype DX 21-gene recurrence score, and the Rotterdam 76-gene prognostic signature [7–9]. These profiles were obtained using tumour-derived mRNA either applied on DNA microarrays or by RT-PCR assay. All three tests are used in clinical practice to predict prognosis and assist therapeutic intervention. Using a similar approach, a 12-gene expression signature has been developed for colon cancer as an independent predictor of recurrence in patients with stage II disease, which aids the more accurate identification of patients who will not benefit from chemotherapy [10]. In addition, other studies have identified a 133-gene prognostic signature in adult acute myeloid leukaemia with normal karyotype as well as new prognostic subtypes in diffuse large B-cell lymphoma [11,12]. Gene expression signatures to assess the risk of recurrence in patients with non-small cell lung cancer [13] and in several other cancer types have also been proposed.

Involvement of non-coding RNAs in cancer

Recently, the functional relevance of the non-protein-coding portion of the genome became evident in the context of both normal development and disease pathogenesis. Currently, a total of 9173 small RNAs are annotated by the GENCODE project (version 16) [14], the majority of which correspond to four major classes: small nuclear RNAs, small nucleolar RNAs, miRNAs, and transfer RNAs. Other classes of short and midsize non-coding RNAs include PIWI-interacting RNAs (piRNAs), transcription initiation RNAs, promoter-associated small RNAs, transcription start site-associated RNAs, and promoter upstream transcripts. GENCODE also contains 13 220 long non-coding RNA genes, a heterogeneous group of non-coding transcripts longer than 200 nucleotides encompassing mainly large intergenic non-coding RNAs and transcribed ultraconserved regions (T-UCRs).

The most widely studied class of non-coding RNAs with functional importance are miRNAs. miRNAs are small RNA polymers, of approximately 21 nucleotides, that mediate post-transcriptional gene silencing through translational repression [15]. The human genome is estimated to encode for more than 1000 miRNAs that regulate the translation of more than 60% of protein-coding genes. The biogenesis of miRNAs involves a multistep process (Fig. 3.3.4). miRNAs are implicated in essentially all biological processes, given that a single miRNA can target hundreds of mRNAs. Aberrant miRNA expression has been observed in many diseases, including cancer, where miRNAs can operate as either oncogenes or tumour suppressor genes. In addition to single miRNAs, such as *miR-21* and *miR-10b*, clusters of miRNAs, such as the *miR-17-92* cluster, have been reported as oncogenes that are upregulated in cancers and that regulate tumour cell proliferation and metastasis. In contrast, members of the *let-7* and *miR-34* families are tumour suppressors, which are downregulated in many cancers. Under normal circumstances, these miRNAs inhibit cancer growth by targeting various oncogene-encoding mRNAs for degradation. Notably, some miRNAs can

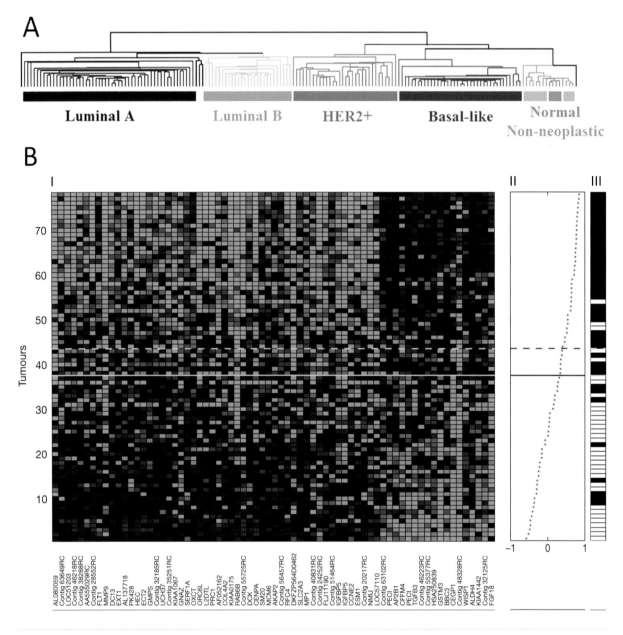

Fig. 3.3.3. Successful gene expression profiling applications in breast cancer. (A) Hierarchical clustering for the PAM50 classifier genes normalized to the 5 control genes using 171 formalin-fixed, paraffin-embedded procured breast samples. The cluster dendrogram shows the five significant groups previously identified and designated as luminal A, luminal B, HER2-positive, basal-like, and normal. (B) Expression data matrix of 70 prognostic marker genes from sporadic breast tumours from 78 patients diagnosed at age less than 55 years with tumour size less than 5 cm and no lymph node involvement (I). Each row represents a tumour and each column a gene. Genes are ordered according to their correlation coefficient with the two prognostic groups. Tumours are ordered by the correlation to the average profile of the good prognosis group (II). Solid line, prognostic classifier with optimal accuracy; dashed line, with optimized sensitivity. Above the dashed line, patients have a good prognosis signature; below the dashed line, the prognosis signature is poor. The metastasis status for each patient is also shown (III): white indicates patients who developed distant metastases within 5 years after the primary diagnosis; black indicates patients who continued to be disease-free for at least 5 years.

function as both an oncogene and a tumour suppressor, depending on the cell and cancer type; hence, miRNA expression profiles should be identified in each cancer type.

Genome-wide miRNA expression profiling microarray studies have shown that effectively all cancers present an altered miRNA profile. In one of the first studies, two

miRNAs were identified as tumour suppressors controlling the pathogenesis of B-cell chronic lymphocytic leukaemia. Both *miR-15a* and *miR-16-1* were found in a region of chromosome 13 (13q14) that is frequently deleted in chronic lymphocytic leukaemia cells [16]. In solid tumours, specific miRNA expression profiles were also investigated, including colon adenocarcinoma, breast carcinoma, glioblastoma, hepatocellular carcinoma, thyroid carcinoma, and lung cancer. A large miRNA profiling analysis of 540 samples covering 6 solid tumours (breast, lung, stomach, prostate, colon, and pancreas) identified 43 dysregulated miRNAs compared with normal tissues [17]. Attempts have been made to assess the correlation of outcome and relapse with miRNA expression levels in lung [18], colon [19], and liver [20] cancers. These findings, together with the high stability of miRNAs in serum samples, make miRNAs attractive candidates as both diagnostic and prognostic indicators in the clinical setting.

Several studies have demonstrated an association of circulating miRNAs with overall survival and early detection. A group of four miRNAs – *miR-486*, *miR-30d*, *miR-1*, and *miR-499* – are related to decreased overall survival of patients with non-small cell lung cancer [21]. In a study of ovarian cancer, *miR-21*,

Fig. 3.3.4. Model for the biogenesis and post-transcriptional suppression of microRNAs (miRNAs). The nascent primary miRNA (pri-miRNA) transcripts are first processed into precursor miRNAs (pre-miRNAs) of approximately 70 nucleotides by the RNase III enzyme Drosha inside the nucleus. Pre-miRNAs are transported to the cytoplasm by exportin 5 and are processed into miRNA:miRNA* duplexes by another RNase III enzyme, Dicer. Only one strand of the miRNA:miRNA* duplex is preferentially assembled into the RNA-induced silencing complex (RISC), which subsequently acts on its target by translational repression or messenger RNA (mRNA) cleavage, depending, at least in part, on the level of complementarity between the small RNA and its target. ORF, open reading frame; UTR, untranslated region.

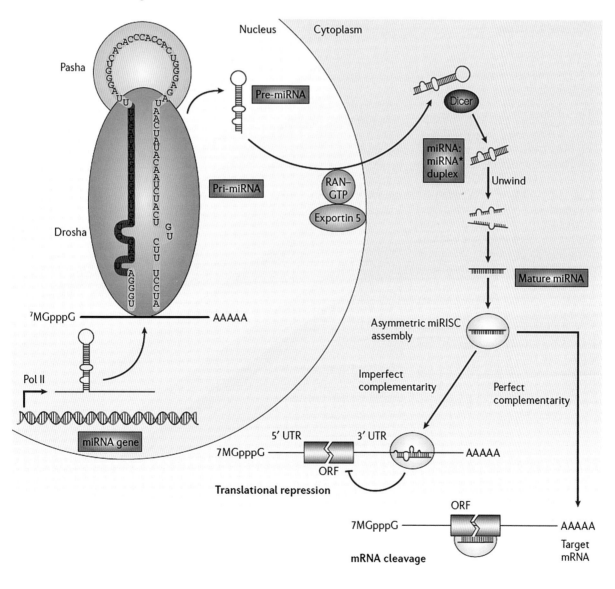

Fig. 3.3.5. Schematic overview of the process of formation and structure of fusion genes. The two vertical red lines at the top of the panel indicate break points on each of two chromosomes, to generate, as one product, a fused chromosome giving rise to a messenger RNA encoding the corresponding fusion protein.

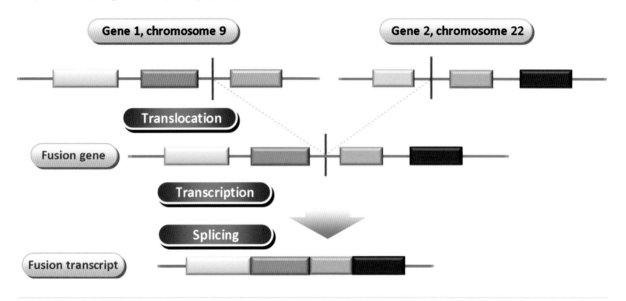

miR-92, miR-93, miR-126, and *miR-29a* were found to be overexpressed in cancer patients before therapy compared with healthy controls. The same study suggested *miR-21, miR-92,* and *miR-93* as potential early-detection biomarkers for ovarian cancer [22]. Other classes of non-coding RNAs, such as small nucleolar RNAs, piRNAs, and piRNA-like transcripts, have been found to be implicated in malignant processes in a range of tumour types, although the mechanisms underlying the oncogenic effects of these non-coding RNAs are largely unknown. The differential expression of small nucleolar RNAs has recently been demonstrated in non-small cell lung cancer [23]. T-UCRs and large intergenic non-coding RNAs have also been shown to be relevant in tumorigenesis. Many large intergenic non-coding RNAs are differentially expressed in cancers with different clinical outcomes. Aberrant expression signatures of T-UCRs have been described for chronic lymphocytic leukaemia, colorectal cancer, and hepatocellular carcinoma [24]. In addition, many T-UCRs show important complementarity to specific miRNAs, suggesting that T-UCRs could act as miRNA targets [25].

One of the best understood examples of the involvement of large intergenic non-coding RNAs in cancer is the overexpression of homeobox transcript antisense RNA (*HOTAIR*) in human neoplasia. This large intergenic non-coding RNA may have an active role in modulating the cancer epigenome and in mediating cell transformation [25,26].

Gene fusions

Fusion genes are hybrid genes formed through translocations, interstitial deletions, or chromosomal inversions of two previously separate genes (Fig. 3.3.5). Gene fusions are a known mechanism for oncogene activation in several malignancies, such as haematological cancers (e.g. leukaemia and lymphoma), sarcoma, and prostate cancer [27]. Oncogenic gene fusions may lead to a gene product with a different function from those of the two fusion partners. Examples of note include the oncogenic gene fusions *BCR-ABL* in chronic myeloid leukaemia [28], *TEL-AML1* in acute lymphoblastic leukaemia [29], recurrent translocations involving ETS family members such as *TMPRSS2-ERG* in prostate cancer [30], *EWS-FLI1* in

Ewing sarcoma [31], and *EML4-ALK* in lung cancer [32]. Even though gene fusions have been widely described in rare haematological malignancies and sarcomas [27], the discovery of recurrent gene fusions in prostate [30], lung [32], and breast cancer [33] suggests a putative role in other solid tumours.

Clinical relevance

Despite great advances in molecular profiling of cancers, only a few findings have been successfully translated into clinical applications. Many studies have shown the ability of gene expression profiling to identify diagnostic, prognostic, and predictive molecular markers or signatures. However, a substantial proportion of these biomarkers, identified in retrospective studies, have failed in subsequent validation studies. Also, many of the signatures were developed without a clear focus on the intended clinical use, and proper independent validation studies establishing their medical utility have rarely been performed. Indeed, the contribution that expression signatures may make to clinical practice has been questioned [34].

Of all the gene expression signatures identified for cancer, only a few have become commercially available. These include the MammaPrint 70-gene signature for breast cancer prognosis (Fig. 3.3.3B) [35], which is the only assay for breast cancer management that has been cleared by the United States Food and Drug Administration (FDA), in February 2007, and the Oncotype DX 21-gene signature for breast cancer [36].

Since then, some academic institutions in the Netherlands and the USA have initiated translation of these gene expression profiles into clinical practice. There is still concern about incorporation of gene expression signatures into routine clinical practice before confirmation of their efficacy from suitably powered randomized controlled trials. This has resulted in the initiation of large prospective clinical trials called MINDACT and TAILORx, to test the efficacy of MammaPrint and Oncotype DX, respectively, in predicting the benefit of adjuvant chemotherapy in breast cancer patients. Interestingly, a recent multicentre study showed that the medical oncologist's treatment recommendation was changed for almost one third of patients on the basis of the Oncotype DX 21-gene assay [37].

Development of targeted therapy

Gene expression profiling can contribute to more effective therapy through its diagnostic, prognostic, and predictive value as well as through target discovery. Accurate diagnosis will minimize the side-effects from non-beneficial treatments. Perhaps most revealing is the fact that 70–80% of breast cancer patients who receive chemotherapy based on traditional predictors would have survived without it. Since the early 1990s, targeted therapies have been developed, such as inhibitors targeted to proteins encoded by mutated or overexpressed cancer genes. One of the most remarkable examples is imatinib, a potent inhibitor of ABL kinase in chronic

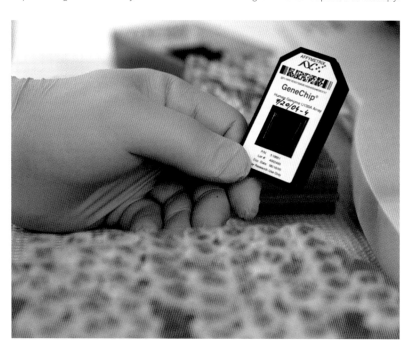

Fig. 3.3.6. A GeneChip loaded with RNA from a single tumour, to identify mutations in expressed genes that may account for the tumour's growth and response to therapy.

myeloid leukaemia, which was approved as the first-line treatment for this disease by the FDA in 2001 [38]. Imatinib was discovered in 1992 and is regarded as the first generation of targeted drugs. Furthermore, trastuzumab, a monoclonal antibody that targets HER2, was a groundbreaking drug in the treatment of HER2-positive breast cancer.

Recently, non-coding RNAs and the proteins involved in their biogenesis and activity have become targets of new therapeutic approaches. Therapies inhibiting miRNA function based on base-pair complementarity have been developed and include three main classes: locked nucleic acids, anti-miRNA oligonucleotides, and antagomirs. Several strategies, called miRNA replacement therapy, have also been proposed to restore the function of downregulated tumour suppressor miRNAs. However, these therapies are currently in the early stages of development and have been studied mostly in mouse models and non-human primates. Finally, an approach aimed at restoring the "global miRNAome" entails the use of histone deacetylase inhibitors and

DNA demethylating agents. These agents, even without target specificity, have been shown to release the epigenetic silencing of tumour suppressor non-coding RNAs, such as miRNAs and T-UCRs [25,39].

Large-scale cancer genome studies, such as the International Cancer Genome Consortium and the Cancer Genome Atlas, are already applying next-generation sequencing technologies to tumours from 50 different cancer types to generate more than 25 000 cancer genomes at the genomic, epigenomic, and transcriptomic levels and should generate a complete catalogue of oncogenic alterations. In addition, initiatives such as the Encyclopedia of DNA Elements integrate multiple technologies to encode all known functional elements of the genome, including the study of novel RNA transcripts, protein-coding regions, transcription factor binding sites, and chromatin structure such as DNA methylation patterns. These will provide a comprehensive catalogue of oncogenic alterations, some of which may prove to be new therapeutic targets.

Strengths and limitations

The advent of high-throughput gene expression technologies such as microarrays and RNA-seq has made it possible to assess the expression of tens of thousands of genes in a single experiment. Initial microarray studies raised concerns about reproducibility. To prevent common procedural failures and to establish high-quality tools for the microarray community, the FDA initiated the MicroArray Quality Control project in 2005 [40]. In addition, to standardize all microarray (and now RNA-seq) data, every new publication in the field is required to follow MIAME (Minimum Information About a Microarray Experiment) guidelines and to deposit expression profile data in an open database. The largest publicly accessible repositories of microarray and other high-throughput functional genomics data are the Gene Expression Omnibus at the United States National Center for Biotechnology Information [41] and ArrayExpress [42].

Microarray technology allows the identification of both single genes and multigene alterations at the level of molecular pathways and networks, providing a broader view of a disease. However, gene expression profiling studies, both microarray and RNA-seq, often generate immense amounts of data that are challenging to interpret and need to be subjected to more advanced bioinformatics data analysis. Furthermore, even though changes at the transcriptional level are important, it is essential to keep in mind that they are just a part of the bigger picture. The majority of cellular functions are carried out by proteins, and biological changes can be modulated not only through alterations at the protein level but also by post-translational modifications such as glycosylation, methylation, acetylation, and phosphorylation. These modifications could change protein conformation and lead to changes in activity. Several consortia are systematically studying the genome, the transcriptome, the epigenome, and the proteome. The key to making the best use of this information lies in the integration of these data. These technological advances coupled with systems biology promise exciting prospects of understanding the basis of cancer and developing improved diagnostic tools and therapies.

References

1. Claverie JM (2005). Fewer genes, more noncoding RNA. *Science*, 309:1529–1530. http://dx.doi.org/10.1126/science.1116800 PMID:16141064

2. The Non-Hodgkin's Lymphoma Classification Project (1997). A clinical evaluation of the International Lymphoma Study Group classification of non-Hodgkin's lymphoma. *Blood*, 89:3909–3918. PMID:9166827

3. Alizadeh AA, Eisen MB, Davis RE *et al.* (2000). Distinct types of diffuse large B-cell lymphoma identified by gene expression profiling. *Nature*, 403:503–511. http://dx.doi.org/10.1038/35000501 PMID:10676951

4. Sørlie T, Perou CM, Tibshirani R *et al.* (2001). Gene expression patterns of breast carcinomas distinguish tumor subclasses with clinical implications. *Proc Natl Acad Sci U S A*, 98:10869–10874. http://dx.doi.org/10.1073/pnas.191367098 PMID:11553815

5. Haferlach T, Kohlmann A, Wieczorek L *et al.* (2010). Clinical utility of microarray-based gene expression profiling in the diagnosis and subclassification of leukemia: report from the International Microarray Innovations in Leukemia Study Group. *J Clin Oncol*, 28:2529–2537. http://dx.doi.org/10.1200/JCO.2009.23.4732 PMID:20406941

6. Kashani-Sabet M, Rangel J, Torabian S *et al.* (2009). A multi-marker assay to distinguish malignant melanomas from benign nevi. *Proc Natl Acad Sci U S A*, 106:6268–6272. http://dx.doi.org/10.1073/pnas.0901185106 PMID:19332774

7. Paik S, Shak S, Tang G *et al.* (2004). A multigene assay to predict recurrence of tamoxifen-treated, node-negative breast cancer. *N Engl J Med*, 351:2817–2826. http://dx.doi.org/10.1056/NEJMoa041588 PMID:15591335

8. van 't Veer LJ, Dai H, van de Vijver MJ *et al.* (2002). Gene expression profiling predicts clinical outcome of breast cancer. *Nature*, 415:530–536. http://dx.doi.org/10.1038/415530a PMID:11823860

9. Wang Y, Klijn JG, Zhang Y *et al.* (2005). Gene-expression profiles to predict distant metastasis of lymph-node-negative primary breast cancer. *Lancet*, 365:671–679. PMID:15721472

10. Gray RG, Quirke P, Handley K *et al.* (2011). Validation study of a quantitative multigene reverse transcriptase-polymerase chain reaction assay for assessment of recurrence risk in patients with stage II colon cancer. *J Clin Oncol*, 29:4611–4619. http://dx.doi.org/10.1200/JCO.2010.32.8732 PMID:22067390

11. Dave SS, Fu K, Wright GW *et al.*; Lymphoma/Leukemia Molecular Profiling Project (2006). Molecular diagnosis of Burkitt's lymphoma. *N Engl J Med*, 354:2431–2442. http://dx.doi.org/10.1056/NEJMoa055759 PMID:16760443

12. Rosenwald A, Wright G, Chan WC *et al.*; Lymphoma/Leukemia Molecular Profiling Project (2002). The use of molecular profiling to predict survival after chemotherapy for diffuse large-B-cell lymphoma. *N Engl J Med*, 346:1937–1947. http://dx.doi.org/10.1056/NEJMoa012914 PMID:12075054

13. Potti A, Mukherjee S, Petersen R *et al.* (2006). A genomic strategy to refine prognosis in early-stage non-small-cell lung cancer. *N Engl J Med*, 355:570–580. http://dx.doi.org/10.1056/NEJMoa060467 PMID:16899777

14. Djebali S, Davis CA, Merkel A *et al.* (2012). Landscape of transcription in human cells. *Nature*, 489:101–108. http://dx.doi.org/10.1038/nature11233 PMID:22955620

15. He L, Hannon GJ (2004). MicroRNAs: small RNAs with a big role in gene regulation. *Nat Rev Genet*, 5:522–531. http://dx.doi.org/10.1038/nrg1379 PMID:15211354

16. Croce CM (2009). Causes and consequences of microRNA dysregulation in cancer. *Nat Rev Genet*, 10:704–714. http://dx.doi.org/10.1038/nrg2634 PMID:19763153

17. Volinia S, Calin GA, Liu CG et al. (2006). A microRNA expression signature of human solid tumors defines cancer gene targets. *Proc Natl Acad Sci U S A*, 103:2257–2261. http://dx.doi.org/10.1073/pnas.0510565103 PMID:16461460

18. Yu SL, Chen HY, Chang GC et al. (2008). MicroRNA signature predicts survival and relapse in lung cancer. *Cancer Cell*, 13:48–57. http://dx.doi.org/10.1016/j.ccr.2007.12.008 PMID:18167339

19. Schetter AJ, Leung SY, Sohn JJ et al. (2008). MicroRNA expression profiles associated with prognosis and therapeutic outcome in colon adenocarcinoma. *JAMA*, 299:425–436. http://dx.doi.org/10.1001/jama.299.4.425 PMID:18230780

20. Chung GE, Yoon JH, Myung SJ et al. (2010). High expression of microRNA-15b predicts a low risk of tumor recurrence following curative resection of hepatocellular carcinoma. *Oncol Rep*, 23:113–119. PMID:19956871

21. Cortez MA, Bueso-Ramos C, Ferdin J et al. (2011). MicroRNAs in body fluids – the mix of hormones and biomarkers. *Nat Rev Clin Oncol*, 8:467–477. http://dx.doi.org/10.1038/nrclinonc.2011.76 PMID:21647195

22. Resnick KE, Alder H, Hagan JP et al. (2009). The detection of differentially expressed microRNAs from the serum of ovarian cancer patients using a novel real-time PCR platform. *Gynecol Oncol*, 112:55–59. http://dx.doi.org/10.1016/j.ygyno.2008.08.036 PMID:18954897

23. Liao J, Yu L, Mei Y et al. (2010). Small nucleolar RNA signatures as biomarkers for non-small-cell lung cancer. *Mol Cancer*, 9:198. http://dx.doi.org/10.1186/1476-4598-9-198 PMID:20663213

24. Calin GA, Liu CG, Ferracin M et al. (2007). Ultraconserved regions encoding ncRNAs are altered in human leukemias and carcinomas. *Cancer Cell*, 12:215–229. http://dx.doi.org/10.1016/j.ccr.2007.07.027 PMID:17785203

25. Esteller M (2011). Non-coding RNAs in human disease. *Nat Rev Genet*, 12:861–874. http://dx.doi.org/10.1038/nrg3074 PMID:22094949

26. Gupta RA, Shah N, Wang KC et al. (2010). Long non-coding RNA HOTAIR reprograms chromatin state to promote cancer metastasis. *Nature*, 464:1071–1076. http://dx.doi.org/10.1038/nature08975 PMID:20393566

27. Mitelman F, Johansson B, Mertens F (2007). The impact of translocations and gene fusions on cancer causation. *Nat Rev Cancer*, 7:233–245. http://dx.doi.org/10.1038/nrc2091 PMID:17361217

28. de Klein A, van Kessel AG, Grosveld G et al. (1982). A cellular oncogene is translocated to the Philadelphia chromosome in chronic myelocytic leukaemia. *Nature*, 300:765–767. http://dx.doi.org/10.1038/300765a0 PMID:6960256

29. Golub TR, Barker GF, Bohlander SK et al. (1995). Fusion of the *TEL* gene on 12p13 to the *AML1* gene on 21q22 in acute lymphoblastic leukemia. *Proc Natl Acad Sci U S A*, 92:4917–4921. http://dx.doi.org/10.1073/pnas.92.11.4917 PMID:7761424

30. Tomlins SA, Rhodes DR, Perner S et al. (2005). Recurrent fusion of *TMPRSS2* and ETS transcription factor genes in prostate cancer. *Science*, 310:644–648. http://dx.doi.org/10.1126/science.1117679 PMID:16254181

31. Delattre O, Zucman J, Plougastel B et al. (1992). Gene fusion with an *ETS* DNA-binding domain caused by chromosome translocation in human tumours. *Nature*, 359:162–165. http://dx.doi.org/10.1038/359162a0 PMID:1522903

32. Choi YL, Takeuchi K, Soda M et al. (2008). Identification of novel isoforms of the *EML4-ALK* transforming gene in non-small cell lung cancer. *Cancer Res*, 68:4971–4976. http://dx.doi.org/10.1158/0008-5472.CAN-07-6158 PMID:18593892

33. Edgren H, Murumagi A, Kangaspeska S et al. (2011). Identification of fusion genes in breast cancer by paired-end RNA-sequencing. *Genome Biol*, 12:R6. http://dx.doi.org/10.1186/gb-2011-12-1-r6 PMID:21247443

34. Chibon F (2013). Cancer gene expression signatures – the rise and fall? *Eur J Cancer*, 49:2000–2009. http://dx.doi.org/10.1016/j.ejca.2013.02.021 PMID:23498875

35. van de Vijver MJ, He YD, van 't Veer LJ et al. (2002). A gene-expression signature as a predictor of survival in breast cancer. *N Engl J Med*, 347:1999–2009. http://dx.doi.org/10.1056/NEJMoa021967 PMID:12490681

36. Perou CM, Sørlie T, Eisen MB et al. (2000). Molecular portraits of human breast tumours. *Nature*, 406:747–752. http://dx.doi.org/10.1038/35021093 PMID:10963602

37. Lo SS, Mumby PB, Norton J et al. (2010). Prospective multicenter study of the impact of the 21-gene recurrence score assay on medical oncologist and patient adjuvant breast cancer treatment selection. *J Clin Oncol*, 28:1671–1676. http://dx.doi.org/10.1200/JCO.2008.20.2119 PMID:20065191

38. O'Brien SG, Guilhot F, Larson RA et al.; IRIS Investigators (2003). Imatinib compared with interferon and low-dose cytarabine for newly diagnosed chronic-phase chronic myeloid leukemia. *N Engl J Med*, 348:994–1004. http://dx.doi.org/10.1056/NEJMoa022457 PMID:12637609

39. Lujambio A, Portela A, Liz J et al. (2010). CpG island hypermethylation-associated silencing of non-coding RNAs transcribed from ultraconserved regions in human cancer. *Oncogene*, 29:6390–6401. http://dx.doi.org/10.1038/onc.2010.361 PMID:20802525

40. Shi L, Reid LH, Jones WD et al.; MAQC Consortium (2006). The MicroArray Quality Control (MAQC) project shows inter- and intraplatform reproducibility of gene expression measurements. *Nat Biotechnol*, 24:1151–1161. http://dx.doi.org/10.1038/nbt1239 PMID:16964229

41. Barrett T, Troup DB, Wilhite SE et al. (2009). NCBI GEO: archive for high-throughput functional genomic data. *Nucleic Acids Res*, 37:D885–D890. http://dx.doi.org/10.1093/nar/gkn764 PMID:18940857

42. Parkinson H, Kapushesky M, Shojatalab M et al. (2007). ArrayExpress – a public database of microarray experiments and gene expression profiles. *Nucleic Acids Res*, 35:D747–D750. http://dx.doi.org/10.1093/nar/gkl995 PMID:17132828

Websites

ArrayExpress:
http://www.ebi.ac.uk/arrayexpress/

Gene Expression Omnibus:
http://www.ncbi.nlm.nih.gov/geo/

International Cancer Genome Consortium:
www.icgc.org/

The Cancer Genome Atlas:
http://cancergenome.nih.gov/

The Encyclopedia of DNA Elements:
http://encodeproject.org/ENCODE/

3.4

Epigenetics

3 BIOLOGY

Toshikazu Ushijima
Zdenko Herceg

Saverio Minucci (reviewer)

Summary

- Epigenetics refers to all heritable changes in gene expression and associated phenotypic traits that are not coded in the DNA sequence itself, and these changes are mediated by DNA methylation, histone modifications, and non-coding RNAs.

- Epidemiological and laboratory-based studies either confirm or implicate that epigenetic changes are induced by environmental and lifestyle factors and that they are involved in a variety of human cancers, and possibly in other chronic disorders.

- Epigenetic changes in cancer provide unique biomarkers, and those in non-cancer tissues can reflect past exposure to carcinogenic factors.

- The suppression of epigenetic changes can, in principle, be used for cancer prevention, and reversibility of these changes is now exploited in cancer treatment.

Recent advances in the field of epigenetics have had a tremendous impact on our understanding of biological processes and complex human diseases. As a result, academic, medical, and public attention has turned to the potential application of these new advances in medicine and various fields of biomedical research. In addition to conceptual advances, the emergence of powerful technologies that enable the detection of epigenetic changes in high-throughput and genome-wide settings has dramatically accelerated cancer research and opened up new perspectives, resulting in a broader appreciation of the importance of epigenetics in the etiology of human cancer.

In the past, the term "epigenetics" was used to describe all biological phenomena that do not follow normal genetic principles; nowadays, the term refers to the study of all changes in gene expression transmitted across cell generations that do not involve changes in DNA sequence, i.e. mutations. One of the most remarkable recent discoveries is that different epigenetic phenomena share common underlying molecular mechanisms. There are three main epigenetic mechanisms: DNA methylation, histone modifications, and non-coding RNAs (Fig. 3.4.1), all of which are known to be critical for high-fidelity propagation of gene activity states in a cell type-specific manner.

Consistent with the importance of epigenetic mechanisms in critical cellular processes, dysregulation of epigenetic mechanisms has been linked to disease, most notably cancer. Virtually all critical processes found in cancer cells, such as silencing of tumour suppressor genes, activation of oncogenes, aberrant cell-cycle regulation, and defects in DNA repair, can be caused not only by genetic changes, including mutation, but also by epigenetic alterations. Accordingly, exploiting epigenetics may have potential in the prevention and treatment of cancer.

Epigenetic mechanisms

The three main epigenetic mechanisms (DNA methylation, histone modifications, and RNA-mediated gene silencing) have been studied primarily in the context of gene expression. However, they are increasingly recognized as important for other chromatin-based processes, such as DNA repair and replication, as well as in the integration of environmental signals [1]. The patterns of DNA methylation and histone modifications are cell type-specific and are propagated autonomously and with high fidelity over many cell generations.

The best-studied epigenetic mechanism is DNA methylation. The methylation of DNA refers to the

Fig. 3.4.1. Different types of epigenetic information. DNA methylation, histone modifications, and RNA-mediated gene silencing constitute three distinct mechanisms of epigenetic regulation. DNA methylation (Me) is a covalent modification of the cytosine (C) that is located 5′ to a guanosine (G) in a CpG dinucleotide. Histone (chromatin) modifications refer to covalent post-translational modifications of N-terminal tails of four core histones (H3, H4, H2A, and H2B). The most recently discovered mechanism of epigenetic inheritance involves RNAs, which in the form of microRNA (miRNA) acting with messenger RNA (mRNA) can alter gene expression states in a heritable manner.

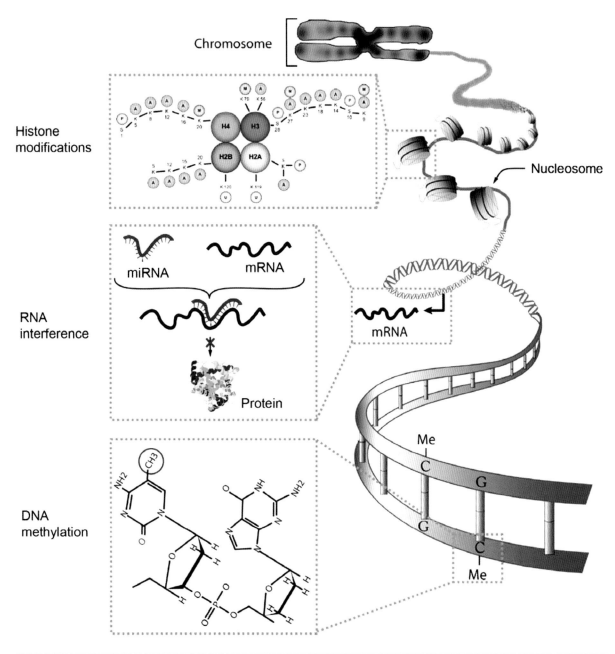

covalent addition of a methyl group to the 5-carbon position of cytosine in a CpG dinucleotide. DNA methylation has long been considered a highly stable epigenetic modification; however, it is now accepted that DNA methylation marks may be more dynamic than previously thought. Indeed, recent studies showed that the Tet family of proteins may be involved in active DNA demethylation. The capacity of Tet proteins to hydrolyse methyl cytosines (producing 5-hydroxymethylcytosine) and to act on fully methylated or hemi-methylated DNA has been reported [2].

The second epigenetic mechanism encompasses various histone modifications. These are post-translational alterations of histone proteins that interact with DNA to

The non-coding RNA revolution in medical research

Pier Paolo Pandolfi

The existence of a previously unrecognized RNA language by which all RNA transcripts communicate in extensive interconnected networks has been proposed. The lone code currently available to decipher gene function, the triplet amino acid code described almost 50 years ago, can be applied to only 2% of the human genome. Recent work by several groups of investigators has challenged the traditional view of RNAs as solely templates for protein synthesis, and suggested instead a model in which these complex molecules have important protein-independent functions, including a crucial role in post-transcriptional gene regulation. It may now be possible to systematically functionalize the entire transcriptome, which encompasses both protein-coding and non-coding transcripts. Notably, the transcriptome represents the majority of the human genome and is heavily dysregulated in cancer.

A proposed RNA language is based on the hypothesis that transcripts regulate and communicate with each other by competing for common microRNAs. Transcripts acting in this fashion are termed competing endogenous RNAs (ceRNAs). CeRNA-mediated regulation may involve cross-talk between multiple unrelated RNA molecules in complex networks. This ceRNA language imparts a novel transregulatory function to transcripts independent of their protein-coding function, and may shed light on regulatory networks that have been overlooked by conventional protein-coding studies.

This hypothesis was ultimately confirmed by studying the interaction between the messenger RNA (mRNA) encoding for the *PTEN* tumour suppressor gene and its closely related pseudogene, *PTENP1*, which acts as a tumour suppressor through this new mechanism.

Extending the analysis to mRNAs has identified several new regulators of *PTEN*, such *ZEB2* and *VAPA*, which are novel tumour suppressor molecules whose function was not previously associated with the proto-oncogenic PI3K/AKT pathway. More recently, work has focused on the *BRAF* pseudogene *BRAFps* and its role in promoting *MAPK* activation through regulation of its parental gene, *BRAF*. *BRAFps* is overexpressed in human cancers and is oncogenic in mice engineered to express high levels of it. This transformative new dimension of gene regulation has significant implications for the systematic functionalization of the entire transcriptome, and represents a paradigm shift for biomedical research at large.

Reference

Karreth FA *et al.* (2011). *Cell*, 147:382–395. http://dx.doi.org/10.1016/j.cell.2011.09.032 PMID:22000016

form a complex known as chromatin. Histone modifications include acetylation, methylation, phosphorylation, and ubiquitination of specific residues in the N-terminal tails of histones. Histone modifications regulate several cellular processes, including gene transcription, DNA repair, and DNA replication [3]. There is growing evidence that aberrant histone modifications and the dysregulation of gene products involved in these modifications are implicated in human neoplasms, and thus the importance of histone modifications in cancer and other diseases is becoming increasingly recognized [4].

The third class of epigenetic mechanisms is mediated by non-coding RNAs, in the form of either long non-coding RNAs or small RNAs (microRNAs), which also participate in the stable maintenance of gene activity states over cell divisions [5] (see "The non-coding RNA revolution in medical research"). Experimental evidence suggests that there is intimate and mutually reinforcing cross-talk between the three epigenetic mechanisms in setting up and maintaining the genome-wide expression programme in a tissue-specific and lineage-specific manner.

Epigenome changes in cancer

Consistent with the critical role of epigenetic mechanisms in the control of cellular processes, a plethora of studies have revealed that the epigenome is markedly dysregulated in virtually all malignancies [6]. Two forms of aberrant DNA methylation are found in human cancer: the overall loss of 5-methylcytosine (global hypomethylation) and gene promoter-associated (CpG island-specific) hypermethylation [7]. While the precise consequences of genome-wide

hypomethylation, including activation of cellular proto-oncogenes and induction of chromosome instability, are still debated, hypermethylation of gene promoters is associated with gene inactivation. When hypermethylated, gene promoters become unable to bind the factors that are responsible for gene expression [8], and therefore the gene is not transcribed. A large number of studies have indicated that the silencing of tumour suppressor genes and other cancer-related genes may occur through hypermethylation of their promoters.

Histone modifications are also dysregulated in cancers. The identification and functional characterization of chromatin modifying and remodelling complexes have revealed an important role for histone modifications in normal cellular processes and cancer development. Histone modification patterns have been found to modulate accessibility

Fig. 3.4.2. Epigenetics as an interface between the genetic code and the environment. Epigenetic mechanisms regulate many cellular processes directly or indirectly and play critical roles in cellular responses to environmental and endogenous stimuli. There is intimate and self-reinforcing cross-talk between different types of epigenetic information. This is proposed to constitute the "epigenetic code" that modulates the genetic code in response to endogenous and environmental cues. The epigenetic code is important to maintain gene expression profiles and chromatin structure in a heritable manner over many cell generations and may dictate cellular outcomes by regulating cellular processes such as gene transcription, proliferation, and DNA repair. Dysregulation of epigenetic mechanisms may promote the development of abnormal phenotypes and diseases, including cancer.

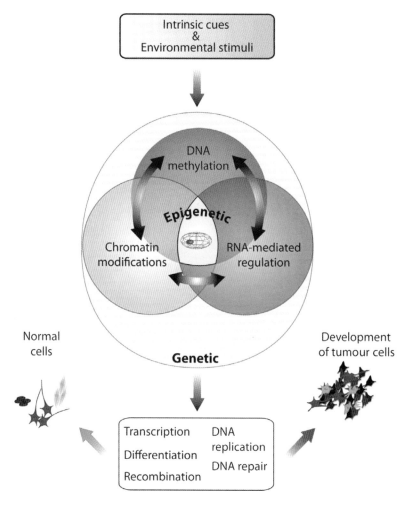

epigenetic changes, which may be referred to as "drivers" in the same way this term is used for mutations, and hence differentiated from "passenger" events, which are evident but not functionally important. Current epigenetic studies, including major international sequencing projects, are expected to generate information establishing the comprehensive epigenomic profiles of human cancers. These findings seem likely to facilitate mechanistic studies, leading to the development of epigenetic therapies and new biomarkers.

Environmental factors

Unlike the genome, which is replicated identically in every single cell of an organism, the epigenome shows wide-ranging variability across different cell types, and may also vary within populations of the same cell type under the influence of environmental stressors. Epigenetic mechanisms have been suggested to play critical roles in physiological responses to environmental exposures (Fig. 3.4.2). Different changes in the epigenome are involved in mediating gene expression programmes required for an organism's adaptation to environmental exposures. Studies in different model systems have provided important information on the role of epigenetic mechanisms in response to environmental stresses [1,9–12].

Many physical and chemical carcinogens and relevant infectious agents, to which individuals are environmentally exposed, are considered to promote cancer development through disruption of epigenetically maintained gene expression programmes. In addition, studies on monozygotic twins have highlighted epigenomic changes in response to environmental factors and associated disease susceptibility. While the importance of environment in the development of a wide variety of cancers is well supported by both epidemiological and laboratory-based studies, the mechanisms by which environmental exposures dysregulate

to DNA during gene transcription and DNA repair. Dysregulation of histone modifications may promote induction of mutations and genomic instability in cancer. Interestingly, a recent study revealed that chromatin organization has a major impact on regional mutation rates in human cancer. Furthermore, recent sequencing efforts have revealed that many genes involved in histone modifications and chromatin

remodelling are recurrently mutated in a wide range of human cancers. Many recent studies have also provided evidence that the dysregulation of non-coding RNAs is involved in the development of human neoplasia [6].

Although epigenetic changes have been implicated in different stages of tumour development and progression, the challenge is to identify functionally important the epigenome remain poorly characterized [1,9–13].

An interesting connection between the epigenome and metabolism in cancer has recently emerged. For example, cells with mutations in the isocitrate dehydrogenase genes *IDH1* and *IDH2* (events that frequently occur in human gliomas) exhibit accumulation of the oncometabolite D-2-hydroxyglutarate, resulting in inhibition of α-ketoglutarate dependent dioxygenases involved in DNA and histone demethylation [14]. Therefore, dysregulation of IDH1/ IDH2 represents a novel oncogenetic mechanism linking cellular metabolism and epigenome dysregulation in cancer.

The development of powerful epigenomic technologies and the availability of large population-based cohorts offer excellent opportunities to test the role of repeated and chronic exposure to environmental epimutagens and aberrant changes in the epigenome in the etiology of specific cancers. Prospects for epigenetic testing in the context of carcinogen identification and evaluation may be discerned [15].

Epigenetic changes as novel biomarkers

Epigenetic changes, especially DNA methylation, are expected to be useful as novel biomarkers. Before a tumour develops, DNA methylation changes can accumulate at high levels in normal-appearing tissues, unlike mutations [16], and methylation patterns often reflect past exposure to carcinogenic stimuli [17]. Also, the accumulation level of aberrant DNA methylation can be correlated with risk of cancer development [18]. Such a correlation has been well documented for gastric cancers, and has been implicated for many other cancers, including liver, colorectal, oesophageal, breast, and renal cancers. Therefore, DNA methylation profiles and patterns of methylation in non-cancer tissues can be used as a unique biomarker for past exposure to carcinogens and the risk of future cancers (Fig. 3.4.3).

Sites of DNA methylation in particular cancers can be used as a biomarker to detect cancer cells or cancer cell-derived DNA and also to elucidate the pathophysiology of tumours. DNA methylation can be sensitively detected by technologies based on polymerase chain reaction; DNA itself is more stable than RNA or proteins. In addition, most cancer cells have an ample number of aberrantly methylated genes [16]. Therefore, DNA methylation has multiple advantages as a biomarker to detect cancer cells or cancer cell-derived DNA. Once specificity of DNA methylation of a given gene in a population of cancer cells is established, such aberrant DNA methylation can be detected sensitively and stably. Such cancer detection systems are already commercially available, and multiple targets are under development [19,20].

The pathophysiology of tumours, as determining or relevant to patient prognosis, responsiveness to therapy, and the presence of lymph node

Fig. 3.4.3. DNA methylation as a biomarker for past exposure and future risk of cancers. Exposure to specific carcinogens, such as *Helicobacter pylori* infection and tobacco smoke, is known to induce aberrant DNA methylation of specific genes in normal-appearing tissue, which can be used as biomarkers for past exposure. The degree of epigenome damage, measured as the level of aberrant DNA methylation (the fraction of cells with methylation), correlates with risk of cancer development for some types of cancers, and can be used as a cancer risk marker.

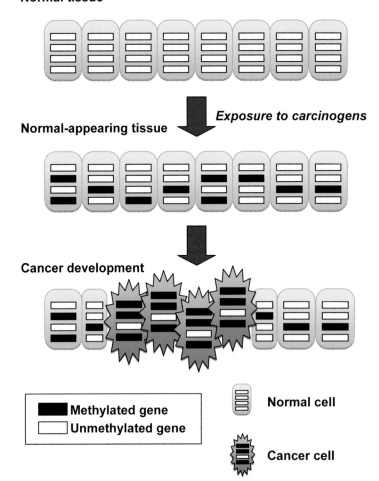

Normal tissue

Exposure to carcinogens

Normal-appearing tissue

Cancer development

■ **Methylated gene**
□ **Unmethylated gene**

Normal cell

Cancer cell

Fig. 3.4.4. Detection of inability to be expressed. The statuses of being unable to be expressed and of not being expressed are different. For example, expression of the DNA repair protein O^6-methylguanine methyltransferase can be repressed by DNA methylation or by the lack of its transcriptional activation. If O^6-methylguanine methyltransferase expression was repressed by DNA methylation at the time of biopsy, it cannot be induced even by implementation of chemotherapy with an alkylating agent. In contrast, if expression of the gene was repressed by lack of transcriptional activation, it can be induced by chemotherapy. Since O^6-methylguanine methyltransferase repairs DNA damage introduced by the alkylating agent, the effect of chemotherapy is diminished by its induction. DNA methylation can predict whether such induction of gene expression will happen. Pol II, RNA polymerase II.

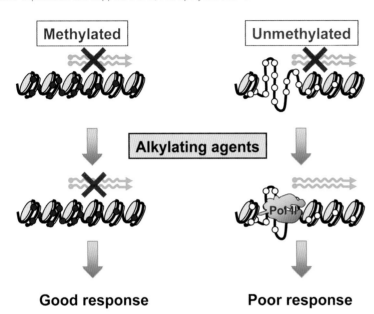

metastasis, can also be characterized using DNA methylation. In sharp distinction from patterns of gene expression, DNA methylation may indicate that a particular gene cannot be expressed even if its expression is induced in the future (Fig. 3.4.4). For example, if the promoter region of O^6-methylguanine methyltransferase is determined to be methylated at biopsy of a brain tumour, this gene will never be expressed even after future chemotherapy involving an alkylating agent, and in the absence of such repair, such chemotherapy will be effective. In contrast, if the same gene is not expressed simply because of the lack of its induction at biopsy, its expression can be induced upon chemotherapy, and the chemotherapy may be ineffective [21].

DNA methylation of multiple genes (the CpG island methylator phenotype) is associated with patient prognosis in several types of cancers, including colorectal and gastric malignancies, as well as neuroblastomas. Specifically, the CpG island methylator phenotype in neuroblastoma provides prognostic information that is more precise than amplification of the *MYCN* oncogene, one of the clearest prognostic indicators in clinical oncology [22].

Epigenetic therapy and prevention

One of the most important aspects of epigenetic change, which distinguishes such change from mutation, is reversibility induced by drugs [23,24]. DNA methylation can be reversed by the action of DNA demethylating agents, and two such drugs have been approved by the United States Food and Drug Administration and are used for treatment of haemato-

logical disorders [25]. Notably, using these two drugs, clinical responses were achieved in patients with myelodysplastic syndrome, for whom blood transfusions used to be the sole effective treatment. Histone deacetylation can be reversed by histone deacetylase inhibitors, and in this context two drugs have been approved for treatment of cutaneous lymphoma [26]. The mode of action of epigenetic drugs is different from that of cytotoxic drugs, and low-dose and long-term administration is seen to be important, especially for DNA demethylating agents [23]. Recent cancer genome studies have revealed previously unknown mutations of epigenetic regulators, and these mutated regulators are expected to provide novel therapeutic targets in the future [24]. Other potential targets for therapy may be microRNAs (see "Causes and consequences of microRNA dysregulation in cancer").

The reversibility of epigenetic changes is also useful for cancer prevention. As a proof of concept, in experimental animals tumours such as those of the colon and prostate have been suppressed by DNA demethylating agents [27,28]. However, it must be recognized that DNA methylation is physiologically essential to repress some genes, and nonspecific demethylation is expected to lead to long-term adverse effects [29]. Therefore, to render epigenetic cancer prevention practicable for the human population, the specificity of preventive agents for genes with aberrant epigenetic modifications must be improved. Also, it is now possible to identify individuals at extremely high risk of some cancers by assessing accumulation levels of aberrant DNA methylation. These individuals represent a population likely to benefit from effective chemoprevention. Since epigenetic cancer prevention has great potential, multiple relevant studies are required in a timely manner.

Causes and consequences of microRNA dysregulation in cancer

Carlo M. Croce

Since the discovery of *miR-15a* and *miR-16-1* deletions in chronic lymphocytic leukaemia, many laboratories around the world have shown microRNA (miRNA) dysregulation in all tumours studied, including the most common, such as lung, breast, prostate, and gastrointestinal cancers. Such dysregulation, like the dysregulation of oncogenes and tumour suppressor genes, can be caused by multiple mechanisms, such as deletion, amplification, mutation, transcriptional dysregulation, and epigenetic changes.

Since miRNAs have multiple targets, their function in tumorigenesis could be due to their regulation of a few specific targets – possibly of even one – or of many. A future challenge will be identifying all of the targets of the miRNAs involved in cancer and establishing their contributions to malignant transformation. An additional challenge will be identifying all of the miRNAs that are dysregulated by pathways that are consistently dysregulated in various types of human cancers. This point is of particular importance because instead of focusing on specific alterations in protein-coding oncogenes or tumour suppressor genes – which may be difficult to treat – the focus may be on their downstream miRNA targets. If these miRNA targets are crucial for the expression of the malignant phenotype and the cancer cells depend on their dysregulation for proliferation and survival, the use of miRNAs or anti-miRNAs may be expected to result in tumour regression.

Genomic analyses for alterations in miRNA genes or for copy number alterations in various human tumours by deep sequencing are in progress but have not been completed. These studies could provide additional information about the involvement of miRNAs in cancer and in many other diseases. Over the past few years, a shift from conventional chemotherapy to targeted therapies has occurred, and miRNAs and anti-miRNAs will contribute extensively to targeted therapies.

Reference

Iorio MV *et al.* (2012). *Cancer J*, 18:215–222. http://dx.doi.org/10.1097/PPO.0b013e318250c001 PMID:22647357

References

1. Feil R, Fraga MF (2011). Epigenetics and the environment: emerging patterns and implications. *Nat Rev Genet*, 13:97–109. http://dx.doi.org/10.1038/nrg3142 PMID:22215131

2. Tahiliani M, Koh KP, Shen Y et al. (2009). Conversion of 5-methylcytosine to 5-hydroxymethylcytosine in mammalian DNA by MLL partner TET1. *Science*, 324:930–935. http://dx.doi.org/10.1126/science.1170116 PMID:19372391

3. Bannister AJ, Kouzarides T (2011). Regulation of chromatin by histone modifications. *Cell Res*, 21:381–395. http://dx.doi.org/10.1038/cr.2011.22 PMID:21321607

4. Sawan C, Herceg Z (2010). Histone modifications and cancer. *Adv Genet*, 70:57–85. http://dx.doi.org/10.1016/B978-0-12-380866-0.60003-4 PMID:20920745

5. Pauli A, Rinn JL, Schier AF (2011). Non-coding RNAs as regulators of embryogenesis. *Nat Rev Genet*, 12:136–149. http://dx.doi.org/10.1038/nrg2904 PMID:21245830

6. Rodríguez-Paredes M, Esteller M (2011). Cancer epigenetics reaches mainstream oncology. *Nat Med*, 17:330–339. http://dx.doi.org/10.1038/nm.2305 PMID:21386836

7. Sinčić N, Herceg Z (2011). DNA methylation and cancer: ghosts and angels above the genes. *Curr Opin Oncol*, 23:69–76. http://dx.doi.org/10.1097/CCO.0b013e3283412eb4 PMID:21119515

8. Vaissière T, Sawan C, Herceg Z (2008). Epigenetic interplay between histone modifications and DNA methylation in gene silencing. *Mutat Res*, 659:40–48. http://dx.doi.org/10.1016/j.mrrev.2008.02.004 PMID:18407786

9. Herceg Z (2007). Epigenetics and cancer: towards an evaluation of the impact of environmental and dietary factors. *Mutagenesis*, 22:91–103. http://dx.doi.org/10.1093/mutage/gel068 PMID:17284773

10. Herceg Z, Vaissière T (2011). Epigenetic mechanisms and cancer: an interface between the environment and the genome. *Epigenetics*, 6:804–819. http://dx.doi.org/10.4161/epi.6.7.16262 PMID:21758002

11. Herceg Z, Paliwal A (2011). Epigenetic mechanisms in hepatocellular carcinoma: how environmental factors influence the epigenome. *Mutat Res*, 727:55–61. http://dx.doi.org/10.1016/j.mrrev.2011.04.001 PMID:21514401

12. Hou L, Zhang X, Wang D, Baccarelli A (2012). Environmental chemical exposures and human epigenetics. *Int J Epidemiol*, 41:79–105. http://dx.doi.org/10.1093/ije/dyr154 PMID:22253299

13. Ushijima T, Hattori N (2012). Molecular pathways: involvement of *Helicobacter pylori*-triggered inflammation in the formation of an epigenetic field defect, and its usefulness as cancer risk and exposure markers. *Clin Cancer Res*, 18:923–929. http://dx.doi.org/10.1158/1078-0432.CCR-11-2011 PMID:22205689

14. Xu W, Yang H, Liu Y et al. (2011). Oncometabolite 2-hydroxyglutarate is a competitive inhibitor of α-ketoglutarate-dependent dioxygenases. *Cancer Cell*, 19:17–30. http://dx.doi.org/10.1016/j.ccr.2010.12.014 PMID:21251613

15. Herceg Z, Lambert MP, van Veldhoven K et al. (2013). Towards incorporating epigenetic mechanisms into carcinogen identification and evaluation. *Carcinogenesis*, 34:1955–1967. http://dx.doi.org/10.1093/carcin/bgt212 PMID:23749751

16. Ushijima T, Asada K (2010). Aberrant DNA methylation in contrast with mutations. *Cancer Sci*, 101:300–305. http://dx.doi.org/10.1111/j.1349-7006.2009.01434.x PMID:19958364

17. Takeshima H, Ushijima T (2010). Methylation destiny: Moira takes account of histones and RNA polymerase II. *Epigenetics*, 5:89–95. http://dx.doi.org/10.4161/epi.5.2.10774 PMID:20160507

18. Ushijima T (2007). Epigenetic field for cancerization. *J Biochem Mol Biol*, 40:142–150. http://dx.doi.org/10.5483/BMB Rep.2007.40.2.142 PMID:17394762

19. Liloglou T, Bediaga NG, Brown BR et al. (2012). Epigenetic biomarkers in lung cancer. *Cancer Lett*, http://dx.doi.org/10.1016/j.canlet.2012.04.018 PMID:22546286

20. Nogueira da Costa A, Herceg Z (2012). Detection of cancer-specific epigenomic changes in biofluids: powerful tools in biomarker discovery and application. *Mol Oncol*, 6:704–715. http://dx.doi.org/10.1016/j.molonc.2012.07.005 PMID:22925902

21. Jacinto FV, Esteller M (2007). Mutator pathways unleashed by epigenetic silencing in human cancer. *Mutagenesis*, 22:247–253. http://dx.doi.org/10.1093/mutage/gem009 PMID:17412712

22. Abe M, Ohira M, Kaneda A et al. (2005). CpG island methylator phenotype is a strong determinant of poor prognosis in neuroblastomas. *Cancer Res*, 65:828–834. PMID:15705880

23. Boumber Y, Issa JP (2011). Epigenetics in cancer: what's the future? *Oncology (Williston Park)*, 25:220–226, 228. PMID:21548464

24. Dawson MA, Kouzarides T (2012). Cancer epigenetics: from mechanism to therapy. *Cell*, 150:12–27. http://dx.doi.org/10.1016/j.cell.2012.06.013 PMID:22770212

25. Fahy J, Jeltsch A, Arimondo PB (2012). DNA methyltransferase inhibitors in cancer: a chemical and therapeutic patent overview and selected clinical studies. *Expert Opin Ther Pat*, 22:1427–1442. http://dx.doi.org/10.1517/13543776.2012.729579 PMID:23033952

26. Batty N, Malouf GG, Issa JP (2009). Histone deacetylase inhibitors as anti-neoplastic agents. *Cancer Lett*, 280:192–200. http://dx.doi.org/10.1016/j.canlet.2009.03.013 PMID:19345475

27. McCabe MT, Low JA, Daignault S et al. (2006). Inhibition of DNA methyltransferase activity prevents tumorigenesis in a mouse model of prostate cancer. *Cancer Res*, 66:385–392. http://dx.doi.org/10.1158/0008-5472.CAN-05-2020 PMID:16397253

28. Yoo CB, Chuang JC, Byun HM et al. (2008). Long-term epigenetic therapy with oral zebularine has minimal side effects and prevents intestinal tumors in mice. *Cancer Prev Res (Phila)*, 1:233–240. http://dx.doi.org/10.1158/1940-6207.CAPR-07-0008 PMID:19138966

29. Bojang P Jr, Ramos KS (2013). The promise and failures of epigenetic therapies for cancer treatment. *Cancer Treat Rev*, http://dx.doi.org/10.1016/j.ctrv.2013.05.009 PMID:23831234

3.5

Metabolic change and metabolomics

3 BIOLOGY

Augustin Scalbert
Isabelle Romieu

James R. Krycer (reviewer)

Summary

- Cancers are increasingly seen as metabolic diseases, as exemplified by several oncogenes coding for metabolic enzymes and the impact of metabolic imbalance associated with obesity and other lifestyle factors known to increase cancer risk.

- The metabolome is the sum of low-molecular-weight metabolites in a particular sample and at a given time. Metabolomics is the systematic study of variations in the metabolome in particular situations, consequent upon various environmental or health conditions.

- Metabolomics provides a global view of metabolism and facilitates discovery of the role of metabolic pathways essential for cancer cell proliferation and the identification of new biomarkers for cancer diagnosis, prognosis, and recurrence.

- Metabolomics applied to cohorts in the context of metabolome-wide association studies should contribute to the identification of novel risk factors for cancer.

Genetic alterations have been considered as critical to the development of cancers. However, close connections also exist between metabolic change and cancer development. From one perspective, the metabolism of tumour cells differs from that of normal cells, and several oncogenes code for metabolic enzymes or alter the expression of these enzymes. From another perspective, associations between lifestyle, metabolism, and cancer risk are increasingly being reported. Obesity, which results in major metabolic imbalance, increases the risk of several malignancies, including colon, postmenopausal breast, endometrial, kidney, liver, pancreatic, thyroid, and oesophageal cancers. Cancers are thus increasingly seen as metabolic diseases. However, the contribution of metabolic dysfunction to the onset or development of cancer remains poorly understood.

The development of metabolomics and major progress in related analytical techniques have contributed to an improved understanding of the links between metabolism and cancer. Hundreds or thousands of metabolites can now be measured simultaneously in biospecimens to give a highly detailed picture of metabolic profiles in tumour tissues or biofluids. Metabolomics combines these highly sensitive analytical techniques with powerful methods for data analysis to characterize subtle metabolic changes associated with cancer. This approach has already led to the discovery of new biomarkers for cancer and to a better understanding of the mechanisms underlying the etiology of cancers.

Metabolism and cancer

Salient features of cancer cells compared with normal cells are their high rates of glycolysis and glutamine metabolism, which allow malignant cells to meet their high energy and anabolic requirements. Production of lactic acid from glucose, even under non-hypoxic conditions, as commonly exhibited by tumour tissue is a feature that has been recognized for more than 70 years and is known as the Warburg effect. Such metabolism offers several advantages to cancer cells, including a high rate of adenosine triphosphate (ATP) production and the production of intermediate metabolites like citrate in a truncated tricarboxylic acid cycle to feed biosynthetic pathways and support the production of macromolecules for cell proliferation, often resulting in a fine-tuning of these metabolic pathways. Otto Warburg sought to explain this effect as the result of damage to respiratory processes. However, it is now known

Fig. 3.5.1. Campaign poster from the Collectif National des Associations d'Obèses (France): "Obesity kills. Do you still think it's funny? Obesity is a serious condition that kills 55 000 people per year in France. It is neither a fault nor an inevitability, still less a joke." Obesity has been shown to increase susceptibility to diabetes and cancer.

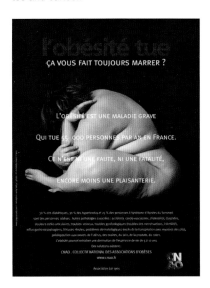

that dysregulation of glycolysis is a better explanation [1].

Connections between some major oncogenes or tumour suppressor genes and metabolism have been identified, and this finding has focused attention on metabolic dysregulation as a possible key mechanism leading to cancer. Mutations in the tumour suppressor gene *TP53* enhance glucose transport and metabolism, whereas mutations in the oncogenic transcription factor MYC enhance the expression of most glycolytic enzymes, lactase dehydrogenase A, and enzymes required for nucleotide biosynthesis and one-carbon metabolism [2].

Oncogenes also play a key role in enabling cancer cells to adapt to environmental changes and adjust their metabolism accordingly. At an early stage of tumorigenesis, the oncogene *ERBB2* was demonstrated to commit the metabolism of cancer cells detached from their normal matrix towards proliferation rather than apoptosis [3]. Detached cells usually undergo apoptosis and autophagy,

but overexpression of this oncogene rescues the cancer cells, restores glucose transport and the pentose phosphate pathway, and improves the redox status of the cells.

Metabolic genes associated with aggressive cancer and stem cell character were systematically investigated within a list of about 2700 genes encoding all known human metabolic enzymes and transporters [4]. Some of these genes had previously been shown to be highly expressed in tumours compared with normal tissues and also highly expressed in stem cells as assessed in a human breast cancer xenograft model. Sixteen of these genes were demonstrated to be required for tumorigenesis, including genes encoding transporters for mitochondrial ATP and for lactate as well as enzymes contributing to the glycolysis, pentose phosphate, and nucleotide biosynthesis pathways. This study also established the key role played by phosphoglycerate dehydrogenase, the first enzyme in the serine biosynthetic pathway, which drives the conversion of glutamine to tricarboxylic acid cycle intermediates for anabolic processes.

The role of metabolic alterations and adaptations in tumorigenicity is thus increasingly recognized. These metabolic alterations are now considered a new hallmark of cancer [5]. This has led to the development of new therapeutic approaches targeted at the modulation of corresponding signalling pathways or at the direct inhibition of some of the enzymes in the metabolic pathways involved in tumorigenicity. These approaches include inhibition of glycolysis, amino acid biosynthesis, and the mTOR and phosphatidylinositol 3-kinase (PI3K) signalling pathways [6].

Understanding the interactions between altered metabolism and cancer biology is important not only for therapeutic intervention for cancer but also for prevention of malignant development. Obesity and certain metabolic characteristics (the metabolic syndrome) are well-established risk factors for several

cancers, and various mechanisms have been proposed to explain such interactions [7]. These include the direct effects of adiposity on the secretion of pro-inflammatory cytokines and adipokines, and indirect effects such as insulin resistance and high insulinaemia commonly associated with obesity or an increase in the levels of steroid hormones. Alterations of metabolic profiles associated with obesity (e.g. excess circulating free fatty acids), other lifestyle factors, or some genetic factors may also increase cancer risk.

Metabolomics, through an in-depth characterization of metabolic profiles in cells, tissues, and human biofluids, may help elucidate both mechanisms of carcinogenesis and those underlying associations between lifestyle and cancer risk. Metabolomics can also be used to identify novel early biomarkers for cancer and to characterize new risk factors for cancer.

Metabolomics to better understand mechanisms of carcinogenesis

The metabolome – the sum of low-molecular-weight metabolites at a given time – is the most fundamental biochemical indicator of biological systems and is an indicator of both genetic and environmental conditions (Fig. 3.5.2). Metabolomics has been defined as the systematic study of variations of the metabolome under particular conditions [7] and involves assessing the metabolome in blood, urine, or tissues using modern and powerful analytical techniques based on mass spectrometry or nuclear magnetic resonance (NMR) spectroscopy. The sensitivity of these analytical techniques and the large number of metabolites detected allow the characterization of biological phenotypes with unprecedented precision, the identification of novel biomarkers for diseases and exposure to disease risk factors, and a better understanding of the etiology of diseases (Fig. 3.5.3).

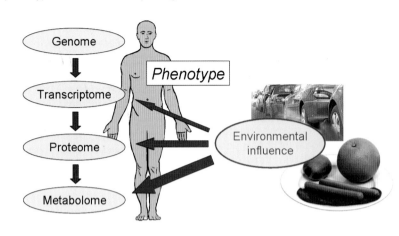

Fig. 3.5.2. The metabolome is the most downstream biochemical expression of the phenotype and is influenced by both genetic and environmental factors.

Two different metabolomic approaches can be distinguished. In the targeted approach, sets of tens or hundreds of metabolites identified a priori are quantified simultaneously in a single analytical operation, most often by mass spectrometry. In the untargeted approach, hundreds (with NMR spectroscopy) or thousands (with mass spectrometry) of metabolites are detected in individual profiles from large sets of samples (Fig. 3.5.4). Metabolites overexpressed or underexpressed in different groups of samples (e.g. plasma samples from case and control subjects) are identified using multivariate statistics and their structures established a posteriori by comparing their spectra to those stored in large metabolite databases.

When applied to tumour cells or animal models of cancers, metabolomics, through the wealth of data generated in a typical experiment, allows the formulation of novel hypotheses, which can then be tested in hypothesis-driven targeted experiments. Two recent publications show how metabolomics contributed to establishing the oncogenicity of glycine and glycine decarboxylase. In a metabolic survey of 60 primary human cancer cell lines from 9 common tumour types, 111 metabolites were measured in the cell culture medium [8]. About two thirds of the metabolites were found to be secreted and one third consumed during cell growth. Hierarchical clustering analysis of the metabolites permitted the recognition of several clusters related to different metabolic pathways (glycolysis, tricarboxylic acid cycle, nucleotide and polyamine metabolism) with no major distinction according to tissue of origin. Glycine consumption was found to be highly correlated to proliferation of transformed cells. This unique observation led to the recognition of the key role played by the mitochondrial glycine synthesis pathway in cancer cell proliferation.

Further confirmation of the role of glycine in cell proliferation was derived from another study, on stem cells from human lung tumours [9]. In this investigation, metabolomics was applied to characterize the role of a specific enzyme, glycine decarboxylase, in overall metabolism. Glycine decarboxylase was demonstrated to be one of the most upregulated genes in stem cells compared with other lung tumour cells. This enzyme catalyses the breakdown of glycine to the methyl donor 5,10-methylenetetrahydrofolate, which is required for the synthesis of nucleotides. Comparison of metabolic profiles of several cell lines overexpressing glycine decarboxylase or with this enzyme knocked down revealed alterations in the glycine pathway, glycolysis, and pyrimidine synthesis. The oncogenic character of glycine decarboxylase was further confirmed by higher mortality among non-small cell lung cancer patients exhibiting high expression of this enzyme in their tumours.

Metabolomics to identify novel biomarkers for cancer

Metabolomics has been used in various case–control studies to identify novel biomarkers for cancer

Fig. 3.5.3. The human metabolomes and the applications of metabolomics to cancer research.

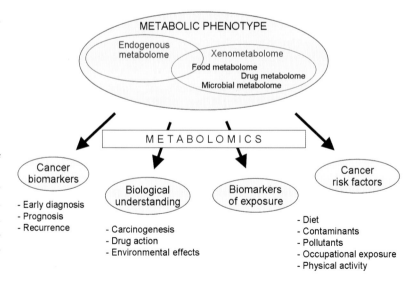

diagnosis, prognosis, or recurrence. New biomarkers were discovered by comparing metabolic profiles in tumours and benign adjacent tissues or blood or urine samples from patients and matched controls. Good examples of these novel biomarkers include hydroxylated ultra long-chain fatty acids for colorectal cancer [10] and 27-nor-5β-cholestane-3,7,12,24,25 pentol glucuronide for ovarian cancer [11]. In these two particular studies, serum samples were analysed by high-resolution mass spectrometry to detect features in metabolic profiles that provided for clearest discrimination between cases and controls. Relevant chemical structures were established by mass spectrometry and NMR spectroscopy.

The potential presented by metabolomics may be evident with reference to particular tumours. Because of its asymptomatic nature, hepatocellular carcinoma is usually diagnosed at late and advanced stages. For this tumour type, emerging high-throughput metabolomics technologies have been applied to the discovery of candidate biomarkers for cancer staging, prediction of recurrence and prognosis, and treatment selection [12].

Certain novel biomarkers are relatively rare metabolites. More common metabolites, when assembled in marking sets (metabolic signatures), may also constitute powerful biomarkers for cancer. Such marking sets characteristic of particular cancers have also been identified using metabolomics. Amino acid profiles in plasma were shown to permit the discrimination of patients with five different cancers from matched controls regardless of disease stage [13]. These characteristic profiles were also evident at an early stage, showing the value of these amino acids as biomarkers for detection of disease. Some of these amino acids were systematically increased or decreased independent of the cancer site, suggesting the existence of a generic metabolic signature for cancer. Other metabolomic studies also showed consistent alteration in the level of other metabolites.

A systematic analysis of metabolic signatures from 117 preclinical and clinical metabolomic studies revealed that, besides alterations in amino acids, metabolism of glutathione, bile acids, galactose, triglycerides, phospholipids, and nucleotides as well as ammonia recycling and the glycolytic and gluconeogenic pathways were consistently affected in cancers [14].

In all such metabolomic studies, a key step is biomarker validation. The large number of metabolic variables and the low number of subjects (commonly 50–200, depending on the study) increase the risk of false discovery. It is therefore essential to validate the new biomarkers in an independent population. Unfortunately, validation has been largely overlooked in most metabolomic studies published thus far. The identification of sarcosine as a biomarker for prostate cancer [15] raised expectations of a possible way to improve diagnosis, but this result could not be validated in a later study [16]. Examples of good

study design for biomarker validation can be recognized in a few metabolomic studies [10,11]. To limit the risk of false discovery and better appraise the value of biomarkers, it will be important to gain further insight into the potential confounding effects of factors such as body mass, age, gender, postmenopausal status, microbiome, drug treatment, or smoking – all known to affect the metabolome – and then conduct studies taking into account the influence of these factors.

Metabolomics to identify risk factors for cancer in cohort studies

Metabolomics is a powerful means to compare individual phenotypes in populations. A good illustration of the power of the approach is given by its application to the identification of the invariant part of the metabolome in a given individual. The analyses of the metabolome by NMR spectroscopy in a small set of urine samples from 22 subjects allowed the recognition, with 100% confidence, of

Fig. 3.5.4. Metabolomic workflow. MS, mass spectrometry; NMR, nuclear magnetic resonance spectroscopy.

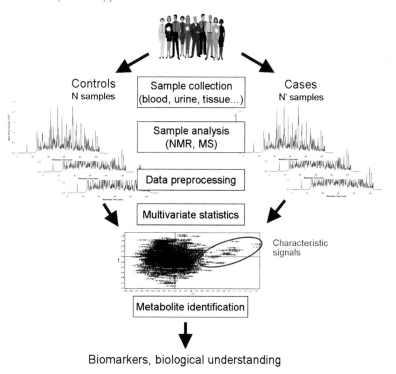

the donor of the samples [17]. The rapid development of more sensitive mass spectrometry techniques now permits the generation of metabolite profiles with much greater detail and the comparison of individual phenotypes in large groups of subjects, as is done in most epidemiological studies.

Several thousands of different metabolites constituting the human metabolome have been described in diverse biospecimens. So far, this considerable amount of metabolic information has been exploited to a very limited extent. The human metabolome includes both a stable and an unstable fraction. These were characterized by NMR spectroscopy in repeated plasma and urine samples collected 4 months apart, and the stable fraction was found to account for 60% and 47% of the plasma and urine metabolomes, respectively [18]. The unstable fraction reflects exposures to environmental and lifestyle factors, which occur only episodically. This fraction is not easily exploited in epidemiological studies unless repeated samples are available.

In contrast, the stable fraction captures both genetic and environmental variations of individual phenotypes, and its evolution over a lifetime can be described. Its measurement opens up wide perspectives to study the prevalence and risk of diseases in cohort studies. The

first metabolome-wide association studies (MWAS) (to be compared to the well-established genome-wide association studies) have recently been published. These studies are aimed at identifying the metabolites and metabolic pathways most strongly associated with a disease or with intermediate end-points. In a case–control study nested in the Framingham Offspring cohort, 61 metabolites were measured in plasma samples collected at baseline (average follow-up, 12 years; 189 cases and 189 controls), and 5 amino acids were identified that were strongly associated with the risk of type 2 diabetes [19]. These amino acids include three branched-chain amino acids previously known for their ability to promote insulin resistance. No such MWAS studies have yet been published on cancer.

The fraction of the human metabolome that varies with environmental exposure rather than genetic factors has been called the exposome [20]. The exposome notably reflects dietary exposure. Characteristic metabolic features could be identified in vegetarians and in low and high meat consumers, or in subjects consuming specific foods [21]. Variations in the urinary metabolome across countries as measured in the International Population Study on Macro/Micronutrients and Blood Pressure (INTERMAP) cohort were found to be partly explained

by metabolites directly derived from foods consumed in various amounts in these countries [22,23]. Measurement of the exposome in exposome-wide association studies (EWAS) should enable the identification of the environmental factors most strongly associated with cancer risk [21].

The few examples given here show the great potential of metabolomics for cancer research. Such studies have already contributed to elucidating the role of unexpected metabolic pathways of major importance in carcinogenesis. Investigation of metabolic processes has enabled the identification of novel biomarkers for cancer diagnosis. The application of metabolomics to molecular epidemiology also shows great potential to identify novel risk factors for cancer.

Metabolomics, among all "omics" technologies, is the one most recently introduced into biological and medical research. Techniques for metabolomics, although not yet fully mature, have considerably improved over the past few years, and there is now little doubt that metabolomics will emerge as an essential tool, complementary to the well-established genomics, transcriptomics, and proteomics approaches, to identify novel biomarkers for cancer and to better understand the etiology of the disease.

References

1. Koppenol WH, Bounds PL, Dang CV (2011). Otto Warburg's contributions to current concepts of cancer metabolism. *Nat Rev Cancer*, 11:325–337. http://dx.doi.org/10.1038/nrc3038 PMID:21508971

2. DeBerardinis RJ (2008). Is cancer a disease of abnormal cellular metabolism? New angles on an old idea. *Genet Med*, 10:767–777. http://dx.doi.org/10.1097/GIM.0b013e31818b0d9b PMID:18941420

3. Schafer ZT, Grassian AR, Song L *et al.* (2009). Antioxidant and oncogene rescue of metabolic defects caused by loss of matrix attachment. *Nature*, 461:109–113. http://dx.doi.org/10.1038/nature08268 PMID:19693011

4. Possemato R, Marks KM, Shaul YD *et al.* (2011). Functional genomics reveal that the serine synthesis pathway is essential in breast cancer. *Nature*, 476:346–350. http://dx.doi.org/10.1038/nature10350 PMID:21760589

5. Hanahan D, Weinberg RA (2011). Hallmarks of cancer: the next generation. *Cell*, 144:646–674. http://dx.doi.org/10.1016/j.cell.2011.02.013 PMID:21376230

6. Dang NH, Singla AK, Mackay EM *et al.* (2013). Targeted cancer therapeutics: biosynthetic and energetic pathways characterized by metabolomics and the interplay with key cancer regulatory factors. *Curr Pharm Des*, [epub ahead of print]. PMID:23859615

7. Khandekar MJ, Cohen P, Spiegelman BM (2011). Molecular mechanisms of cancer development in obesity. *Nat Rev Cancer*, 11:886–895. http://dx.doi.org/10.1038/nrc3174 PMID:22113164

8. Jain M, Nilsson R, Sharma S *et al.* (2012). Metabolite profiling identifies a key role for glycine in rapid cancer cell proliferation. *Science*, 336:1040–1044. http://dx.doi.org/10.1126/science.1218595 PMID:22628656

9. Zhang WC, Shyh-Chang N, Yang H *et al.* (2012). Glycine decarboxylase activity drives non-small cell lung cancer tumor-initiating cells and tumorigenesis. *Cell*, 148:259–272. http://dx.doi.org/10.1016/j.cell.2011.11.050 PMID:22225612

10. Ritchie SA, Ahiahonu PWK, Jayasinghe D *et al.* (2010). Reduced levels of hydroxylated, polyunsaturated ultra long-chain fatty acids in the serum of colorectal cancer patients: implications for early screening and detection. *BMC Med*, 8:13. http://dx.doi.org/10.1186/1741-7015-8-13 PMID:20156336

11. Chen J, Zhang X, Cao R *et al.* (2011). Serum 27-nor-5β-cholestane-3,7,12,24,25 pentol glucuronide discovered by metabolomics as potential diagnostic biomarker for epithelium ovarian cancer. *J Proteome Res*, 10:2625–2632. http://dx.doi.org/10.1021/pr200173q PMID:21456628

12. Wang X, Zhang A, Sun H (2013). Power of metabolomics in diagnosis and biomarker discovery of hepatocellular carcinoma. *Hepatology*, 57:2072–2077. http://dx.doi.org/10.1002/hep.26130 PMID:23150189

13. Miyagi Y, Higashiyama M, Gochi A *et al.* (2011). Plasma free amino acid profiling of five types of cancer patients and its application for early detection. *PLoS One*, 6:e24143. http://dx.doi.org/10.1371/journal.pone.0024143 PMID:21915291

14. Ng DJY, Pasikanti KK, Chan ECY (2011). Trend analysis of metabonomics and systematic review of metabonomics-derived cancer marker metabolites. *Metabolomics*, 7:155–178. http://dx.doi.org/10.1007/s11306-010-0250-7

15. Sreekumar A, Poisson LM, Rajendiran TM *et al.* (2009). Metabolomic profiles delineate potential role for sarcosine in prostate cancer progression. *Nature*, 457:910–914. http://dx.doi.org/10.1038/nature07762 PMID:19212411

16. Jentzmik F, Stephan C, Miller K *et al.* (2010). Sarcosine in urine after digital rectal examination fails as a marker in prostate cancer detection and identification of aggressive tumours. *Eur Urol*, 58:12–18, discussion 20–21. http://dx.doi.org/10.1016/j.eururo.2010.01.035 PMID:20117878

17. Assfalg M, Bertini I, Colangiuli D *et al.* (2008). Evidence of different metabolic phenotypes in humans. *Proc Natl Acad Sci U S A*, 105:1420–1424. http://dx.doi.org/10.1073/pnas.0705685105 PMID:18230739

18. Nicholson G, Rantalainen M, Maher AD *et al.*; The MolPAGE Consortium (2011). Human metabolic profiles are stably controlled by genetic and environmental variation. *Mol Syst Biol*, 7:525. http://dx.doi.org/10.1038/msb.2011.57 PMID:21878913

19. Wang TJ, Larson MG, Vasan RS *et al.* (2011). Metabolite profiles and the risk of developing diabetes. *Nat Med*, 17:448–453. http://dx.doi.org/10.1038/nm.2307 PMID:21423183

20. Wild CP (2005). Complementing the genome with an "exposome": the outstanding challenge of environmental exposure measurement in molecular epidemiology. *Cancer Epidemiol Biomarkers Prev*, 14:1847–1850. http://dx.doi.org/10.1158/1055-9965.EPI-05-0456 PMID:16103423

21. Stella C, Beckwith-Hall B, Cloarec O *et al.* (2006). Susceptibility of human metabolic phenotypes to dietary modulation. *J Proteome Res*, 5:2780–2788. http://dx.doi.org/10.1021/pr060265y PMID:17022649

22. Holmes E, Loo RL, Stamler J *et al.* (2008). Human metabolic phenotype diversity and its association with diet and blood pressure. *Nature*, 453:396–400. http://dx.doi.org/10.1038/nature06882 PMID:18425110

23. Lloyd AJ, Favé G, Beckmann M *et al.* (2011). Use of mass spectrometry fingerprinting to identify urinary metabolites after consumption of specific foods. *Am J Clin Nutr*, 94:981–991. http://dx.doi.org/10.3945/ajcn.111.017921 PMID:21865330

3.6

Stem cells and cancer stem cells

3 BIOLOGY

Zdenko Herceg
Hector Hernandez Vargas

Gianpaolo Papaccio (reviewer)

Summary

- Stem cells are defined by their capacity to self-renew, which is essential for the maintenance of a stem cell pool, and to differentiate according to different lineages, as required for the integrity and functioning of particular tissues.

- Because of their long half-life, stem or progenitor cells may be particularly affected by genetic and epigenetic changes, and may thereby contribute to cancer development.

- "Cancer stem cell" is an operational term used to define a distinct subpopulation of tumour cells functionally, with reference to aberrant renewal potential and the capacity to confer tumour heterogeneity.

- Although the origin of cancer stem cells has not been established, cancer stem cells as currently identified share many key properties with embryonic stem cells, including unlimited proliferative potential and the capacity to migrate.

- Research on stem cells and cancer stem cells may indicate novel approaches to cancer therapy.

The pace of discovery in the field of stem cells has drawn academic, political, and public attention to stem cells as tools for innovation in medicine and biomedical research. Stem cells are found in all multicellular organisms and are likely to be present as a discrete population in most tissues. Stem cells can be grown in culture and differentiated into specialized cells that exhibit properties specific to various tissues. The landmark discovery by Takahashi and Yamanaka that induced pluripotent stem cells, which have properties in common with embryonic stem cells, could be derived from differentiated cells – notably, skin fibroblasts [1] – led to the award of the Nobel Prize in Physiology or Medicine 2012 and has been reproduced using a variety of human cell types [2]. Furthermore, several studies have described the generation of induced pluripotent stem cell lines from individuals harbouring both simple and complex genetic diseases [3]. Therefore, stem cells have been seen as an essential resource in cloning and regenerative medicine.

Stem cells share important characteristics with malignant cells. A better understanding of the behaviour and properties of stem cells could be exploited to devise a range of novel agents for and/or approaches to cancer therapy. Although technical advances that enable the isolation and manipulation of embryonic stem cells, and hence the possibility of human cloning, have provoked intense ethical debate, these concerns should not detract from a recognition of the tremendous potential of stem cells for the treatment of various human diseases, such as neurodegenerative disorders and cancer [4,5].

Embryonic and tissue-specific stem cells

All cells in the body are descended from a single cell: the fertilized egg or zygote. From the moment of fertilization of an egg until death, an organism passes through several developmental stages (Fig. 3.6.1). Multiplication of cells from the fertilized egg gives rise to different cell types, as evident in complex organisms. This process involves populations of stem cells that can be propagated indefinitely in culture under adequate conditions. These cells are designated embryonic stem cells and can give rise to any cell type and reconstitute the entire embryo. In addition, many adult tissues contain a discrete population of undifferentiated cells with properties of stem cells. These cells are described as tissue-specific stem cells, also called somatic stem cells or adult stem cells. Haematopoietic stem cells are the best-characterized

Fig. 3.6.1. Embryonic stem cells, derived from the inner cell mass of the blastocyst, are pluripotent and can give rise to all cell types of the body. Somatic stem cells, sometimes termed adult stem cells, are also capable of self-renewal and, with appropriate signals, differentiate into various cell types of the organ from which they are derived. The extent to which somatic stem cells are capable of differentiating into cell types from alternative lineages is controversial.

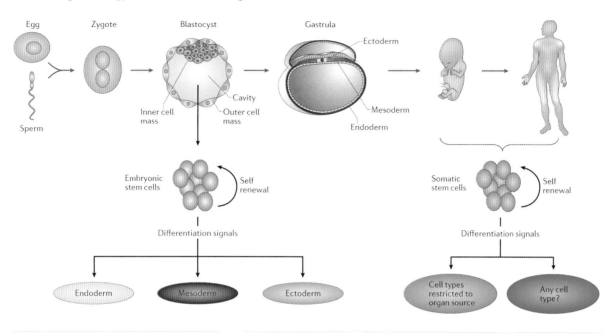

tissue-specific stem cells and can generate all blood lineages and mature blood elements. Adult stem cells have been identified in many other tissues, such as the brain, skin, and liver. Although only a few types of tissue-specific stem cells have undergone rigorous identification and characterization, stem cells are likely present in any tissue that is able to undergo renewal.

Tissue-specific stem cells also have the capacity to perpetuate themselves through self-renewal and to produce the various mature cells of a particular tissue through differentiation [6]. Tissue-specific stem cells constitute a very minor cell population in adult tissues, but this population is essential for the maintenance of tissue homeostasis. Dysregulation of tissue-specific stem cells may initiate diseases, most notably cancer.

The two characteristics of stem cells that distinguish them from all other cells are self-renewal and multipotency. Self-renewal is the capacity of a cell to divide and produce identical daughter cells over a long time period. This crucial property allows stem cells to persist for the lifetime of an organism. Multipotency is the capacity of stem cells to differentiate into many highly specialized cells, such as neurons, muscle fibres, and blood elements. Multipotency is necessary for the maintenance of integrity and functionality of many

Fig. 3.6.2. Embryonic skin-derived progenitor cells. Cancer stem cells share many properties with embryonic stem cells.

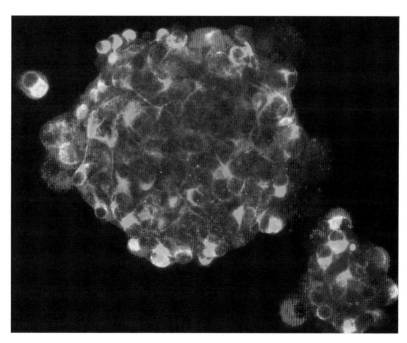

Stem cells in cancer: determinants of clinical outcome?

John E. Dick

The cellular and molecular basis for intratumour heterogeneity is poorly understood. Tumour cells can be genetically diverse due to mutations and clonal evolution, resulting in intratumour functional heterogeneity. Cancer stem cell models postulate that tumours are cellular hierarchies sustained by cancer stem cell heterogeneity due to epigenetic differences; that is, all cells present after long-term tumour growth are derived from cancer stem cells. There is strong evidence for the cancer stem cell model in acute myeloid leukaemia (AML). Examination of the gene signatures specific to either AML stem cells or normal haematopoietic stem cells indicates that they share a set of genes that define a common stemness programme. Only these stem cell-related gene signatures were significant independent predictors of patient survival in large clinical databases. Thus, determinants of stemness influence clinical outcome of AML, establishing that leukaemia stem cells are clinically relevant and not artefacts of xenotransplantation.

In an effort to determine whether the clonal evolution and stem cell models of cancer can be unified, two different studies were performed examining cancer stem cells at both the functional and the genetic level.

In Philadelphia chromosome-positive B-cell acute lymphoblastic leukaemia (B-ALL), diagnostic patient samples had extensive subclonal genetic diversity, and through the use of xenotransplant assays, this diversity was established to have originated from within the leukaemia-initiating cells. Reconstruction of their genetic ancestry showed that multiple leukaemia-initiating cell subclones were related through a complex branching evolutionary process, indicating that genetic and functional heterogeneity are closely connected. This research highlights the need to develop effective therapies to eradicate all genetic subclones to prevent further evolution and recurrence.

In a related functional and genetic study, a highly reliable xenograft assay was used for primary colorectal cancer. With a combination of DNA copy number alteration profiling, targeted and exome sequencing, and lentiviral lineage tracing, the repopulation dynamics of many single lentivirus-marked lineages from colorectal cancers were followed through serial xenograft passages. The xenografts were genetically stable on serial transplantation. Despite this genetic stability, the proliferation, persistence, and chemotherapy tolerance of lentivirus-marked lineages were variable within each clone. Thus, apart from genetic diversity, tumour cells display inherent functional variability in tumour propagation potential, a mechanism that maximizes tumour fitness, contributing to both tumour survival and therapy tolerance.

References

Notta F et al. (2011). Nature, 469:362–367.
http://dx.doi.org/10.1038/nature09733
PMID:21248843

Kreso A et al. (2013). Science, 339:543–548.
http://dx.doi.org/10.1126/science.1227670
PMID:23239622

tissues. Stem cells are essential for the development of each organism and thus can be considered to be a critical resource from the beginning of embryonic life until death. Given the potential of stem cells, their function and proliferation are subject to a range of control processes. Dysregulation of the surveillance mechanisms for proliferation and differentiation of stem cells may initiate a shift in the balance between self-renewal and differentiation, leading to either stem cell loss, which is associated with degenerative disorders, or abnormal proliferation of stem cells, which may be a source of malignant cells.

Cancer stem cells

Stem cells were discovered more than 30 years ago and have been exploited extensively for the generation of genetically modified animal models, such as knockout mice, which are essential in cancer research. However, the first identification of human stem cells and, in particular, so-called cancer stem cells resulted in the cancer research community giving almost unprecedented attention to these entities. Tumours have long been considered to be derived

Fig. 3.6.3. Genetic and epigenetic changes in susceptible cells may be an early event in the development of cancer and give rise to cancer stem cells and contribute to tumour heterogeneity. The origin of cancer stem cells may be early stem or progenitor cells, or differentiated cells distinguished by abnormal expression and function of a set of genes that may contribute to reprogramming into a pluripotent state.

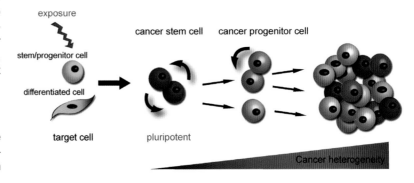

Table 3.6.1. Surface marker phenotypes commonly used to identify cancer stem cells

Tumour type [source of data]	Cancer stem cell marker
Acute myeloid leukaemia [12]	CD34+/CD38−
Breast cancer [13,14]	CD44+/CD24lo, CD133+
Gall bladder cancer [15]	CD44+/CD133+
Gastric cancer [16]	CD44+
Glioblastoma [17,18]	CD133+
Head and neck cancer [19]	CD44+
Hepatocellular carcinoma [20–23]	CD133+, CD13+, CD90+, EpCAM+
Lung cancer [24]	CD133+
Melanoma [25]	CD20+
Oesophageal cancer [26,27]	CD90+, CD44+
Ovarian cancer [28]	CD133+
Pancreatic cancer [29]	CD133+
Prostate cancer [30]	CD133+/CD44+/$\alpha_2\beta_1$hi

from a single cell that has been subject to transformation into a cancer-initiating cell through a series of genetic and epigenetic lesions. These initial events allow for the expansion of transformed cells and the formation of a population of altered cells, or a clone, with the capacity to grow and divide in defiance of normal cellular control. Continuing selection of "fitter" and more aggressive cells results in a generation of cancer clones capable of invading and destroying neighbouring tissues and migrating to distant organs to form metastatic tumours. The identity of that original "target cell" is not known (Fig. 3.6.3). However, recent studies indicate that many genetic and epigenetic changes underlying the aggressive and destructive behaviour of cancer are orchestrated by a discrete population of cancer cells with stem cell properties. These cells are known as cancer stem cells.

The cancer stem cell hypothesis states that cancer clones are maintained exclusively by a fraction of rare cells with stem cell properties [7]. A hierarchical organization has been established for several human cancers. In those cases, tumours are organized into undifferentiated cells that can drive disease progression

and differentiated cells with less capacity to drive disease progression, consistent with the cancer stem cell model [8]. Many cancers have been found to contain cells with properties of stem cells. However, in most cases the existence of cancer stem cells has been documented functionally: the presence of cancer stem cells in the bulk of cancer cells is discerned by their capacity to form tumours after transplantation into an immunocompromised animal host, most commonly a mouse. These assays reveal that only a small fraction of cancer cells are capable of forming new tumours in the host. Importantly, these cells not only can form tumours upon transplantation but also can recapitulate tumour heterogeneity [9]. However, until very recently, the isolation of a cancer stem cell population using molecular signatures, cell surface markers, or mutation profiles has proven to be extremely difficult [7,10,11].

Recently, numerous studies have shown that cancer stem cells can be enriched via different cell surface markers, such as CD133, CD44, CD90, and EpCAM (CD326) (Table 3.6.1) [12–30]. However, although some markers are common to different types of cancer stem cells,

so far no single marker (or combination of markers) has been shown to be able to distinguish these cells across all cancer types. This lack of universal expression of surface markers limits their use. In addition, surface markers should be interpreted carefully, considering the tissue context and functional assessments (e.g. tumorigenic, clonogenic, and sphere formation assays) and co-expression with stemness markers [11]. In spite of these weaknesses, many studies have taken advantage of surface markers to shed light on the biology of putative cancer stem cells. Some markers are common to several malignancies (e.g. CD44, CD133) and, interestingly, some markers are common to normal stem or progenitor cells (e.g. CD133, EpCAM). Indeed, the cell surface expression of the human prominin-1 (CD133) antigen is common to haematopoietic progenitors, and it is among the most frequently studied markers of cancer stem cells [31].

In addition to surface markers, cancer stem cells may share many key properties with embryonic stem cells. These properties include infinite proliferation potential and the capacity to invade tissues and organs and to promote formation of blood vessels for their own oxygenation. Therefore, cancer stem cells may contribute to the heterogeneity of most human cancers [8]. Although important progress has been made in the identification of cancer stem cells, their origin remains obscure. Cancer stem cells are believed to arise in different ways. First, cancer stem cells can be derived from normal tissue-specific stem cells as a result of specific genetic and epigenetic changes that abrogate proliferation control in the normal cells. Second, differentiated cells that normally have a limited lifespan can regain stem cell properties, that is de-differentiate and become cancer stem cells. Third, normal stem cells may fuse with various differentiated cells and the resulting hybrid cells may be cancer-initiating cells with stem cell properties [32]. These hypotheses are not mutually

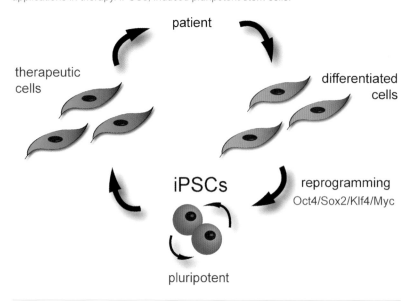

Fig. 3.6.4. Cell reprogramming factors can induce pluripotent stem cells, with potential applications in therapy. iPSCs, induced pluripotent stem cells.

The discovery of stem cell master genes has enabled another, even more insightful branch of research: the transition of differentiated cells into immature pluripotent (stem) cells. This phenotypic reversal or de-differentiation essentially involves enabling specialized cells such as neurons or muscle fibres to regain stem cell properties, which would allow the generation of practically any type of cell. Such a scenario may solve important ethical issues associated with the use of embryos as a source of stem cells, as demonstrated by recent studies [3]. Several laboratories have demonstrated that the introduction of as few as four master genes into either human or murine differentiated cells mediates the emergence of stem cells. This remarkable phenomenon provides support for the argument that differentiated cells can be reprogrammed and that the course of events that normally characterizes differentiation can be reversed. An important implication of these findings is that

exclusive, and the genesis of cancer stem cells may involve more than one mechanism.

cell pool may be rapidly depleted. Depletion of the stem cell pool can impede regeneration and compromise the integrity of normal tissue, leading to degenerative disease [34].

Genomic determination of stem cell identity

Although the features that distinguish stem cells from differentiated cells have been known for many decades, the genetic basis of stem cell identity only began to be understood recently. The development of powerful methodologies in genomics for genome-wide screening enabled the identification of genes and gene networks that maintain stem cells in a special state. With these methods, a limited number of genes have been discovered that are necessary and sufficient to maintain self-renewal and pluripotency – the two distinguishing features of stem cells. These genes have been referred to as "masters of stemness". The genes *Oct4*, *Sox2*, and *Nanog* belong to this exclusive category [33]. These genes encode transcription factors that control the transcription of other genes (Fig. 3.6.4). Such signal transduction pathways maintain stem cell behaviour and identity. When the relevant genes are inactivated or mutated, stem cells may differentiate into specialized cells and the stem

Fig. 3.6.5. Reprogramming can alter any cell of the body so that it may function as a pluripotent stem cell. Shown are human induced pluripotent stem cells derived from dermal fibroblasts. Immunofluorescence analysis with an antibody against Nanog protein (red) is used to indicate that Nanog (a master transcription factor critically involved in stem cells and a widely used marker of the pluripotent state) is expressed and that cells have been successfully reprogrammed.

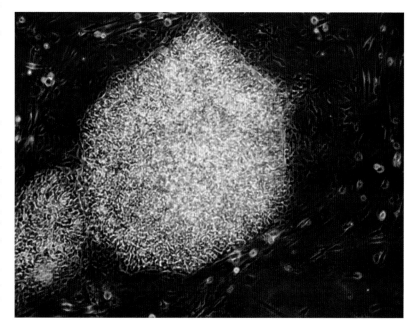

Fig. 3.6.6. Conventional therapies may reduce tumour size by killing mainly differentiated tumour cells. If the putative cancer stem cells are less sensitive to these therapies, then cancer stem cells will remain viable after therapy and re-establish the tumour. By contrast, if therapies can be targeted against cancer stem cells, then they might more effectively kill the cancer stem cells, rendering the tumours unable to maintain themselves or grow. Thus, even if cancer stem cell-directed therapies do not shrink tumours initially, they may eventually lead to cures. CSC, cancer stem cell.

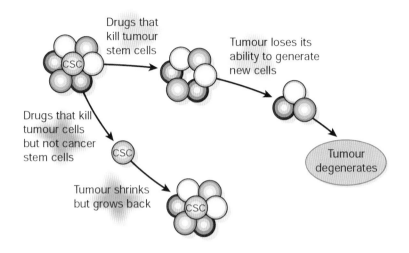

Stem cells and cancer therapy

Much current interest in stem cells and cancer stem cells is predicated on the realization that this tiny, yet critical, population of cancer cells represents an opportunity to devise novel strategies for cancer therapy [35]. Many currently used protocols for cancer therapy are now understood to fail – marked by the reappearance of disease – due to an inability to eradicate cancer stem cells. Classic chemotherapy regimes have been developed to rapidly shrink tumours. However, these changes are often transient and are followed by recurrence (Fig. 3.6.6). Such a clinical course suggests that the therapy used specifically targets rapidly growing tumour cells, whereas more slowly growing cancer stem cells may be spared. Thus, major challenges will be (i) to discover efficient ways to identify and isolate tissue-specific stem cells and cancer stem cells, (ii) to gain insights into the mechanisms of self-renewal and pluripotency of normal stem cells and cancer stem cells, and (iii) to identify genetic and epigenetic events that are critical to cancer-initiating reprogramming and cancer stem cell development (see "Stem cells in cancer: determinants of clinical outcome?").

The ever-increasing research efforts in the field of stem cells have the potential to identify processes that are currently unknown and yet key in cancer development, which will ultimately have a major impact on the development of novel strategies to control and perhaps eliminate cancer.

cancer stem cells may also arise by non-genetic changes that confer certain features on differentiated cells. This hypothesis is supported by the knowledge that all cells, including stem cells, in any given organism share an identical genome.

Experimental evidence from various recent studies suggests a similar conclusion to that just described: cell differentiation is not unidirectional, and different factors may lead to reversal of cell differentiation under either physiological or pathological conditions. In the same way that tumorigenesis may be identified with the acquisition of self-renewal and pluripotency in vivo, manipulation of differentiated cells in vitro may lead to a controlled version of the same process. Conversely, cells with established stemness features may acquire characteristics of partial differentiation. The balance between stemness and a differentiated character appears to be different during critical periods of life, such as embryonic development. An extrapolation of the same idea is evidenced by the increasing interest being accorded to the effects of early-life exposures on the development of later disease. In this sense, early in utero life represents a critical period where pluripotency and differentiation networks interact dynamically and where environmental exposures may have an impact beyond that initially perceived.

References

1. Takahashi K, Yamanaka S (2006). Induction of pluripotent stem cells from mouse embryonic and adult fibroblast cultures by defined factors. *Cell*, 126:663–676. http://dx.doi.org/10.1016/j.cell.2006.07.024 PMID:16904174

2. Yamanaka S (2007). Strategies and new developments in the generation of patient-specific pluripotent stem cells. *Cell Stem Cell*, 1:39–49. http://dx.doi.org/10.1016/j.stem.2007.05.012 PMID:18371333

3. Bellin M, Marchetto MC, Gage FH, Mummery CL (2012). Induced pluripotent stem cells: the new patient? *Nat Rev Mol Cell Biol*, 13:713–726. http://dx.doi.org/10.1038/nrm3448 PMID:23034453

4. Polyak K, Hahn WC (2006). Roots and stems: stem cells in cancer. *Nat Med*, 12:296–300. http://dx.doi.org/10.1038/nm1379 PMID:16520777

5. Baumann M, Krause M, Hill R (2008). Exploring the role of cancer stem cells in radioresistance. *Nat Rev Cancer*, 8:545–554. http://dx.doi.org/10.1038/nrc2419 PMID:18511937

6. Rossi DJ, Jamieson CH, Weissman IL (2008). Stems cells and the pathways to aging and cancer. *Cell*, 132:681–696. http://dx.doi.org/10.1016/j.cell.2008.01.036 PMID:18295583

7. Valent P, Bonnet D, De Maria R et al. (2012). Cancer stem cell definitions and terminology: the devil is in the details. *Nat Rev Cancer*, 12:767–775. http://dx.doi.org/10.1038/nrc3368 PMID:23051844

8. Magee JA, Piskounova E, Morrison SJ (2012). Cancer stem cells: impact, heterogeneity, and uncertainty. *Cancer Cell*, 21:283–296. http://dx.doi.org/10.1016/j.ccr.2012.03.003 PMID:22439924

9. Visvader JE, Lindeman GJ (2008). Cancer stem cells in solid tumours: accumulating evidence and unresolved questions. *Nat Rev Cancer*, 8:755–768. http://dx.doi.org/10.1038/nrc2499 PMID:18784658

10. Tirino V, Desiderio V, Paino F et al. (2011). Human primary bone sarcomas contain CD133⁺ cancer stem cells displaying high tumorigenicity in vivo. *FASEB J*, 25:2022–2030. http://dx.doi.org/10.1096/fj.10-179036 PMID:21385990

11. Tirino V, Desiderio V, Paino F et al. (2013). Cancer stem cells in solid tumors: an overview and new approaches for their isolation and characterization. *FASEB J*, 27:13–24. http://dx.doi.org/10.1096/fj.12-218222 PMID:23024375

12. Lapidot T, Sirard C, Vormoor J et al. (1994). A cell initiating human acute myeloid leukaemia after transplantation into SCID mice. *Nature*, 367:645–648. http://dx.doi.org/10.1038/367645a0 PMID:7509044

13. Al-Hajj M, Wicha MS, Benito-Hernandez A et al. (2003). Prospective identification of tumorigenic breast cancer cells. *Proc Natl Acad Sci U S A*, 100:3983–3988. http://dx.doi.org/10.1073/pnas.0530291100 PMID:12629218

14. Wright MH, Calcagno AM, Salcido CD et al. (2008). *Brca1* breast tumors contain distinct CD44⁺/CD24⁻ and CD133⁺ cells with cancer stem cell characteristics. *Breast Cancer Res*, 10:R10. http://dx.doi.org/10.1186/bcr1855 PMID:18241344

15. Shi C, Tian R, Wang M et al. (2010). CD44⁺CD133⁺ population exhibits cancer stem cell-like characteristics in human gallbladder carcinoma. *Cancer Biol Ther*, 10:1182–1190. http://dx.doi.org/10.4161/cbt.10.11.13664 PMID:20948317

16. Takaishi S, Okumura T, Tu S et al. (2009). Identification of gastric cancer stem cells using the cell surface marker CD44. *Stem Cells*, 27:1006–1020. http://dx.doi.org/10.1002/stem.30 PMID:19415765

17. Singh SK, Clarke ID, Terasaki M et al. (2003). Identification of a cancer stem cell in human brain tumors. *Cancer Res*, 63:5821–5828. PMID:14522905

18. Singh SK, Hawkins C, Clarke ID et al. (2004). Identification of human brain tumour initiating cells. *Nature*, 432:396–401. http://dx.doi.org/10.1038/nature03128 PMID:15549107

19. Prince ME, Sivanandan R, Kaczorowski A et al. (2007). Identification of a subpopulation of cells with cancer stem cell properties in head and neck squamous cell carcinoma. *Proc Natl Acad Sci U S A*, 104:973–978. http://dx.doi.org/10.1073/pnas.0610117104 PMID:17210912

20. Yin S, Li J, Hu C et al. (2007). CD133 positive hepatocellular carcinoma cells possess high capacity for tumorigenicity. *Int J Cancer*, 120:1444–1450. http://dx.doi.org/10.1002/ijc.22476 PMID:17205516

21. Haraguchi N, Ishii H, Mimori K et al. (2010). CD13 is a therapeutic target in human liver cancer stem cells. *J Clin Invest*, 120:3326–3339. http://dx.doi.org/10.1172/JCI42550 PMID:20697159

22. Yang ZF, Ho DW, Ng MN et al. (2008). Significance of CD90⁺ cancer stem cells in human liver cancer. *Cancer Cell*, 13:153–166. http://dx.doi.org/10.1016/j.ccr.2008.01.013 PMID:18242515

23. Yamashita T, Ji J, Budhu A et al. (2009). EpCAM-positive hepatocellular carcinoma cells are tumor-initiating cells with stem/progenitor cell features. *Gastroenterology*, 136:1012–1024, e4. http://dx.doi.org/10.1053/j.gastro.2008.12.004 PMID:19150350

24. Eramo A, Lotti F, Sette G et al. (2008). Identification and expansion of the tumorigenic lung cancer stem cell population. *Cell Death Differ*, 15:504–514. http://dx.doi.org/10.1038/sj.cdd.4402283 PMID:18049477

25. Fang D, Nguyen TK, Leishear K et al. (2005). A tumorigenic subpopulation with stem cell properties in melanomas. *Cancer Res*, 65:9328–9337. http://dx.doi.org/10.1158/0008-5472.CAN-05-1343 PMID:16230395

26. Tang KH, Dai YD, Tong M et al. (2013). A CD90⁺ tumor-initiating cell population with an aggressive signature and metastatic capacity in esophageal cancer. *Cancer Res*, 73:2322–2332. http://dx.doi.org/10.1158/0008-5472.CAN-12-2991 PMID:23382045

27. Zhao JS, Li WJ, Ge D et al. (2011). Tumor initiating cells in esophageal squamous cell carcinomas express high levels of CD44. *PLoS One*, 6:e21419. http://dx.doi.org/10.1371/journal.pone.0021419 PMID:21731740

28. Baba T, Convery PA, Matsumura N et al. (2009). Epigenetic regulation of *CD133* and tumorigenicity of CD133+ ovarian cancer cells. *Oncogene*, 28:209–218. http://dx.doi.org/10.1038/onc.2008.374 PMID:18836486

29. Hermann PC, Huber SL, Herrler T et al. (2007). Distinct populations of cancer stem cells determine tumor growth and metastatic activity in human pancreatic cancer. *Cell Stem Cell*, 1:313–323. http://dx.doi.org/10.1016/j.stem.2007.06.002 PMID:18371365

30. Collins AT, Berry PA, Hyde C et al. (2005). Prospective identification of tumorigenic prostate cancer stem cells. *Cancer Res*, 65:10946–10951. http://dx.doi.org/10.1158/0008-5472.CAN-05-2018 PMID:16322242

31. Yin AH, Miraglia S, Zanjani ED et al. (1997). AC133, a novel marker for human hematopoietic stem and progenitor cells. *Blood*, 90:5002–5012. PMID:9389720

32. Bjerkvig R, Tysnes BB, Aboody KS et al. (2005). The origin of the cancer stem cell: current controversies and new insights. *Nat Rev Cancer*, 5:899–904. http://dx.doi.org/10.1038/nrc1740 PMID:16327766

33. Boiani M, Schöler HR (2005). Regulatory networks in embryo-derived pluripotent stem cells. *Nat Rev Mol Cell Biol*, 6:872–884. http://dx.doi.org/10.1038/nrm1744 PMID:16227977

34. Erlandsson A, Morshead CM (2006). Exploiting the properties of adult stem cells for the treatment of disease. *Curr Opin Mol Ther*, 8:331–337. PMID:16955696

35. Visvader JE, Lindeman GJ (2012). Cancer stem cells: current status and evolving complexities. *Cell Stem Cell*, 10:717–728. http://dx.doi.org/10.1016/j.stem.2012.05.007 PMID:22704512

3.7 Tumour microenvironment

3 BIOLOGY

Robert R. Langley

Chris Paraskeva (reviewer)
Theresa L. Whiteside (reviewer)
Jiri Zavadil (reviewer)

Summary

- The tumour microenvironment refers to the biochemical and cellular composition of the tissue encompassing a tumour and comprises a heterogeneous population of cancer cells, a variety of non-cancer cells, soluble proteins, blood vessels, peritumoural lymphatic vessels, and a supporting structural matrix.

- Bidirectional signalling between cancer cells and stromal cells leads to enhanced cancer cell division, suppressed immune cell function, and resistance to therapeutic intervention, all of which result in poor clinical outcome.

- Cancer-associated inflammation parallels disease progression, and tumours have been characterized as "wounds that do not heal".

- Accumulating evidence suggests that combined therapeutic regimens that both target cancer cells (e.g. chemotherapy) and modify the tumour microenvironment (i.e. anti-angiogenic therapy) are superior to treatments directed against only cancer cells.

Over the past several years, it has become increasingly apparent that the reciprocal signalling that takes place between cancer cells and the cellular and molecular components of the surrounding tissue plays a decisive role in determining tumour growth, metastasis, and responsiveness to therapy. Tumour growth is accompanied by an ever-increasing recruitment and activation of previously quiescent cells, whose cumulative response is one that perpetuates disease progression (Fig. 3.7.1). Treatment efforts are hindered by a unique set of physiological parameters present in the tumour microenvironment. Consequently, much effort is currently directed towards the development of therapeutic strategies that both target cancer cells and modify the tumour microenvironment. Several key aspects of the tumour microenvironment are described in this chapter.

Tumour vasculature

The proximity of a cancer cell to a blood vessel determines its fate; cancer cells located within 75 μm of a blood vessel enter the cell division cycle, whereas cancer cells located farther than 150 μm from a vessel undergo programmed cell death [1]. Tumour growth to a size beyond a few millimetres in diameter leads to hypoxia and nutrient deprivation, which activate the "angiogenic switch" and allow tumours to progress [2]. Cancer cells produce cytokines and growth factors that act in an autocrine manner to promote their own expansion, and in a paracrine fashion to convey information to quiescent adjacent cells. The initial target cells for signal-releasing cancer cells are resident microvascular endothelial cells, which respond by activating programmes that culminate in the formation of new vascular networks (i.e. angiogenesis) (Fig. 3.7.2). Angiogenesis diminishes the metabolic pressures associated with unrestricted cancer cell division and increases the likelihood of cancer cell dissemination. The tumour microenvironment becomes enriched in vascular endothelial growth factor (VEGF), a primary mediator of pathological angiogenesis.

Angiogenesis is most pronounced at the interface between tumour and normal tissue, although the intensity of the neovascularization response varies between different types of tumours (Fig. 3.7.3). Angiogenesis is greatest in glioblastoma and renal cell carcinoma and least in tumours of the prostate and lung [3]. Some cancer cells (e.g. melanoma cells) may forgo angiogenesis altogether and satisfy their metabolic demands by proliferating along the length of pre-existing

Fig. 3.7.1. Illustration depicting the complexity of the interplay between cancer cells and stromal cells. (A) Transforming growth factor β (TGF-β) produced from initiated epithelial cells activates tissue fibroblasts. Activated fibroblasts (myofibroblasts) generate hepatocyte growth factor (HGF), which binds to the MET receptor on epithelial cells. Activation of MET signalling has been shown to stimulate pathways that promote cell division, motility, and anti-apoptotic activity. (B) Cancer cells produce the pro-angiogenic protein vascular endothelial growth factor (VEGF), in response to declining oxygen tension. (C) VEGF is chemotactic for macrophages, which contribute to the pool of pro-angiogenic proteins. (D) Myofibroblast-derived HGF activates invasive and migratory programmes in cancer cells, allowing them to penetrate structurally deficient angiogenic vessels and spread to distal tissues. (E) Interleukin-1 (IL-1) produced by myofibroblasts leads to the recruitment of inflammatory cells. (F) Tumour-associated macrophages generate VEGF-C, which signals for lymphangiogenesis, increasing the likelihood of lymph node metastasis. (G) Macrophages and myofibroblasts secrete matrix metalloproteinases (MMPs), which remodel the extracellular matrix. (H) Cancer cell chemokines including chemokine ligand 2 (CCL2) and CCL5 direct circulating monocytes to the tumour. Macrophage colony-stimulating factor (MCSF) promotes the differentiation of monocytes to macrophages. (I) Cancer cell-derived IL-6 and IL-10 polarize macrophages to an M2 phenotype with pro-angiogenic and immunosuppressive properties.

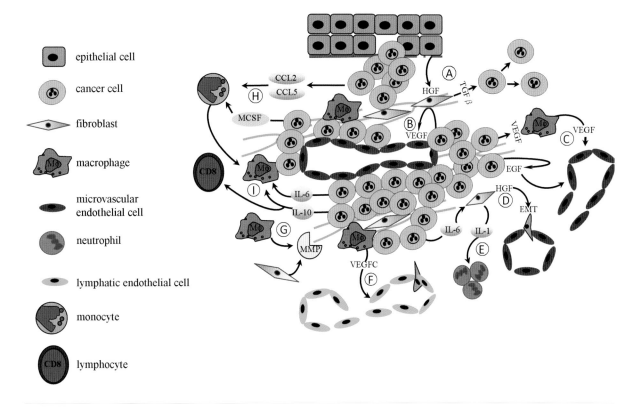

blood vessels in a process referred to as vessel co-option. Cancer cells may co-opt blood vessels when challenged with anti-angiogenic agents.

Pharmacological suppression of angiogenesis as a means to control tumour growth is an area of intense investigation. Several inhibitors of the VEGF signalling pathway are currently in clinical use; these include bevacizumab, a monoclonal antibody that neutralizes VEGF, and small-molecule inhibitors of the tyrosine kinase receptor VEGFR2 (e.g. sorafenib, sunitinib). The addition of bevacizumab to standard therapy was found to increase overall survival in patients with advanced malignancies, including non-small cell lung cancer and metastatic colorectal cancer. However, many tumours are inherently resistant to anti-angiogenic agents, and those tumours that initially respond to treatment eventually become refractory to therapy and recur.

Independent investigations concluded that cancer cells circumvent anti-VEGF therapies by upregulating alternative angiogenic proteins, such as basic fibroblast growth factor and interleukin-8. Recent data suggest that stromal cells also contribute to resistance to anti-VEGF agents. Indeed, preclinical studies using cross-species hybridization of microarrays concluded that most of the gene expression changes associated with acquired resistance of non-small cell lung cancers to bevacizumab occur in stromal cells [4]. The epidermal growth factor receptor (*EGFR*) gene was identified as a network hub activated on stromal cells of bevacizumab-resistant non-small cell lung tumours. Co-localization studies revealed a 10-fold increase in the number of pericytes expressing the activated form of EGFR in experimental bevacizumab-

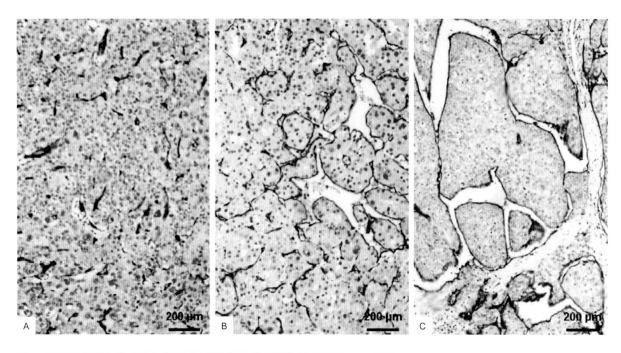

Fig. 3.7.2. Morphological classification of tumour vasculature in hepatocellular carcinoma. Three human hepatocellular carcinomas were stained with anti-CD34 antibody to show their vasculature. The vasculature can be (A) capillary-like microvessels, (B) a mixture of capillary-like and sinusoid-like vasculature, or (C) sinusoid-like vasculature. The prognosis of patients harbouring these three vasculature types differs; capillary-like microvessels correspond to the best prognosis and sinusoid-like tumour vasculature the worst.

resistant tumours compared with control tumours. Dual inhibition of VEGFR and EGFR pathways reduced pericyte coverage of tumour blood vessels and, moreover, delayed emergence of the resistant phenotype [4].

In other animal models of cancer, tumour refractoriness to anti-VEGF therapy was dependent on the tumour's ability to prime and recruit CD11b+Gr1+ granulocyte-macrophage cells [5]. Cancer cells and tumour-associated fibroblasts synthesize and secrete granulocyte-macrophage colony-stimulating factor and stromal cell-derived factor 1, which stimulate myeloid recruitment into the tumour microenvironment. In addition to providing a rich reserve of angiogenic proteins, CD11b+Gr1+ cells also suppress the immune response of CD4+ and CD8+ T cells through several different mechanisms, including upregulation of reactive oxygen species, nitric oxide, and immunosuppressive cytokines.

Physiological parameters of the tumour microenvironment

Tumour blood vessels are distinct from normal vessels in that they are dilated, tortuous, and heterogeneously distributed, and comprise constitutively activated endothelial cells. VEGF renders the tumour vascular bed hyperpermeable to macromolecules, and extravasated proteinaceous fluid accumulates in the tumour matrix due to a lack of functional intratumour lymphatic vessels. Consequently, tumour interstitial colloid osmotic pressures are significantly greater than those of normal tissues and most tumours have grossly elevated interstitial fluid pressures. The elevated interstitial fluid pressure creates a barrier to transcapillary transport, which limits the uptake of therapeutic agents in tumours. Interventions that lower interstitial fluid pressure, such as anti-VEGF therapies, are reported to normalize the tumour vasculature and improve drug uptake.

Chemotherapy and radiotherapy require optimal tumour blood flow to achieve maximal benefit, whereas anti-angiogenic therapies and vascular disrupting agents seek to completely abolish neoplastic blood flow. Blood flow to tumours is heterogeneous, and marked variability exists even in tumours with a similar histological classification growing in the same anatomical region [6]. Elevated interstitial fluid pressure may compress tumour blood vessels and diminish tumour blood flow. Blood flow fluctuations (and vascular stasis) occur frequently in the tumour circulation and are associated with periods of hypoxia. Fluctuations in erythrocyte flux in tumour blood vessels predispose tumour cells to periods of transient hypoxia and reoxygenation.

Estimates indicate that 50–60% of advanced tumours contain heterogeneously distributed hypoxic regions. There are two forms of hypoxia in human tumours. Diffusion-limited hypoxia refers to limitations in the diffusion distance of oxygen from a blood vessel. The diffusion distance of oxygen from tumour blood vessels has been measured and is approximately 120 μm. Perfusion-limited hypoxia results from non-uniform blood flow patterns caused by structural and functional alterations in tumour vessels. For example, a rapidly expanding tumour may impinge on its vasculature and temporarily or permanently block blood flow, thereby creating areas deficient in oxygen. Arteriovenous shunting is also a common feature in tumour circulation; approximately one third of arterial blood can pass through tumours without taking part in the microcirculatory exchange process.

The oxygenation status of tumours has important clinical implications. Radiotherapy and chemotherapy are significantly more effective in an aerobic environment. Aerobic cells are 3 times as sensitive as hypoxic cells to the effects of radiation. Hypoxia acts as a physiological selective pressure for variants with diminished apoptotic potential, enhanced genetic instability, and increased invasive capacity.

Oxygen deprivation is associated with increased metastasis and poor outcomes in patients with head and neck carcinomas and cervical cancer.

Studies evaluating the genetic stability of the stromal compartment have yielded conflicting results. Examinations of formalin-fixed, paraffin-embedded archival tumours reported loss of heterozygosity (LOH) and changes in copy number of certain loci in cancer-associated fibroblasts, whereas studies performed on fresh-frozen tissues failed to detect chromosomal changes in cancer-associated fibroblasts. A recent genome-wide copy number and LOH analysis of fresh-frozen breast and ovarian cancers using array analysis for hundreds of thousands of single-nucleotide polymorphisms reported that LOH and copy number alterations are extremely rare in cancer-associated fibroblasts [7].

There is no debate about the importance of inflammation to carcinogenesis and neoplastic progression (see "Inflammation and cancer" in Chapter 2.4). Epidemiological reports indicate that chronic inflammation in select organs increases the risk for development of cancer and that non-steroidal anti-inflammatory drugs reduce the incidence of, and mortality from, several tumour types [8]. An inflammatory component is also present in the microenvironment of tumours that are not epidemiologically related to inflammation. In general, cancer-associated inflammation parallels disease progression and contributes to cancer cell division and survival, angiogenesis, metastasis, subversion of adaptive immunity, and reduced response to therapy [8].

Tumour-associated macrophages

Macrophages are among the most represented innate immune cells in the tumour microenvironment. A correlation exists between high macrophage content and poor prognosis in many human tumours. Circulating monocytes traffic to tumours in response to chemokines including chemokine ligand 2 (CCL2) and CCL5, growth factors such as VEGF, and vasoactive peptides including endothelins. Cancer cell-derived factors mediate the differentiation and orientation of incoming monocytes. Macrophage colony-stimulating factor promotes the differentiation of monocytes to resident macrophages, whereas interleukin-6 (IL-6) and IL-10 polarize macrophages towards an M2 phenotype [9]. Results from clinical and experimental studies suggest that the functional properties of M2 macrophages favour tumour progression. M2 macrophages possess limited antigen-presenting capacity and suppress Th1 adaptive immunity while actively promoting angiogenesis and tissue remodelling processes.

Tumour-associated macrophages are also a major source of matrix metalloproteinases (MMPs), a family of zinc-containing endopeptidases, which play a critical role in tissue remodelling processes. MMPs are

Fig. 3.7.3. Novel assays for measuring surrogate markers of tumour angiogenesis activity. The complex biology of angiogenesis inhibitors has accentuated the need to develop technologies that can be used to assess the effects of biological markers. A compilation of data from multiple assays, including measuring angiogenic factors in serum, plasma, and urine; tumour biopsy analysis; radiological imaging; and, recently, ex vivo analyses of isolated peripheral blood cells (labelled circulating endothelial cells) may facilitate defining the optimal biological dose for subsequent clinical studies of angiogenesis inhibitors.

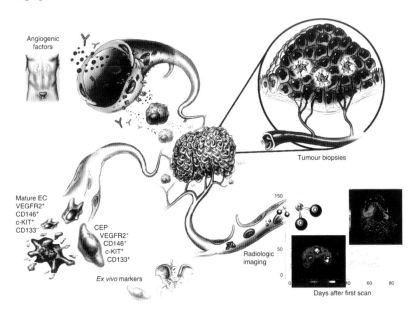

initially expressed as inactive zymogens, and activation requires cleavage of an autoinhibitory pro-domain. MMP-mediated proteolytic destruction of the extracellular matrix results in the release of matrix-embedded bioactive fragments and growth factors that encourage cancer cell division, angiogenesis, and neutrophil recruitment processes. Expression and activity levels of MMPs are up-regulated in most human cancers and correlate with advanced tumour stage, increased invasion and metastasis, and shortened survival [10].

Macrophages express an extensive array of pro-angiogenic proteins sufficient to trigger the angiogenic switch or amplify an ongoing neovascularization response. Conditions that enhance angiogenic activity in macrophages include hypoxia and elevated levels of pyruvate, lactate, and hydrogen ions, all of which are characteristic of the tumour micro-environment. Macrophage-produced VEGF and prostaglandins diminish endothelial cell barrier function by increasing the permeability of tumour vasculature. Macrophage-derived VEGF-C and VEGF-D ligands signal for peritumoural lymphangiogenesis, which may increase the spread of cancer cells to regional lymph nodes.

Microenvironment in metastasis

Most deaths due to cancer result from the progressive growth of metastases that are resistant to conventional therapies. The process of metastasis involves a complex series of interrelated steps that begins when cancer cells detach from the primary mass and invade the surrounding stroma (Fig. 3.7.4). Carcinoma cells at the invasive front adopt morphological features and patterns of gene expression that are characteristic of mesenchymal cells during a process referred to as epithelial–mesenchymal transition (EMT). EMT plays a critical role during embryonic development and contributes to tissue repair processes in the adult. Disseminating carcinoma cells reactivate this developmental programme and re-press epithelial proteins E-cadherin, β-catenin, and cytokeratin and up-regulate mesenchymal-associated proteins N-cadherin, vimentin, and fibronectin. Recent studies suggest that cancer cells undergoing EMT may also acquire stem cell-like properties and become resistant to

Fig. 3.7.4. The process of metastasis consists of sequential, interlinked, and selective steps. Each step of the metastatic process is considered rate-limiting in that failure of a tumour cell to complete any step effectively terminates the process. The formation of clinically relevant metastases represents the survival and growth of a unique subpopulation of cells that pre-exist in primary tumours. See the text for a detailed description of the individual steps of the metastatic process.

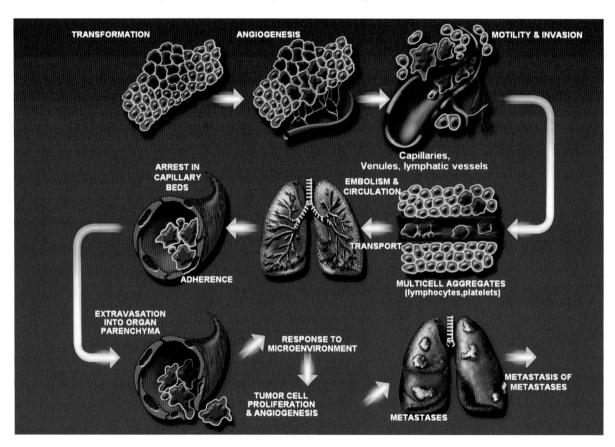

anticancer therapies [11]. Reciprocal signalling between cancer cells and cancer-associated fibroblasts is reported to stimulate EMT in some experimental models. Invading cancer cells gain access to the systemic circulation by penetrating thin-walled blood vessels and lymphatic channels. Circulating cancer cells are retained in target organs by adhering to microvascular endothelial cells or the sub-endothelial basement membrane. Extravasated cancer cells are thought to undergo mesenchymal–epithelial transition in the secondary tissue, by a yet-unknown mechanism. Cancer cells that leave the cell cycle or are unable to trigger the angiogenic switch may enter a period of dormancy or undergo apoptosis.

The process of metastasis is extremely inefficient in that less than 0.1% of circulating tumour cells eventually form metastases. That certain tumours have a tendency to form metastases in specific organs provided the foundation for the "seed and soil" hypothesis, which was proposed well over a century ago. In essence, Paget's hypothesis states that tumour cells ("seed") grow preferentially in the microenvironment of select organs ("soil"). In the concluding sections of this chapter, the discussion focuses on the microenvironment of the brain and bone, two frequent target organs of metastasis.

Brain microenvironment

Estimates indicate that approximately 200 000 cases of brain metastases occur each year in the USA, and that 20–40% of patients with systemic cancers develop brain metastases during the course of their disease. Brain metastasis has several unmet clinical needs; there are few clinically relevant tumour models, no targeted therapies exist that are specific for brain metastases, and the median survival for untreated patients is 5 weeks [12]. Most brain metastases arise from primary tumours that originate in the lung (40–50%), breast (15–20%), or skin (5–10%). Patients tend to present with multiple brain metastases, 80% of which are located in the cerebral hemispheres.

Comparative genome expression analysis was used to study the molecular mechanisms that mediate breast cancer cell arrest and extravasation in the brain. Cyclo-oxygenase 2 (COX-2), heparin-binding EGF-like growth factor (HB-EGF), and α-2,6-sialyltransferase 5 (ST6GALNAC5) were identified as key regulatory molecules that control the passage of breast cancer cells through the blood–brain barrier [13]. ST6GALNAC5 enhances the affinity of breast cancer cells for brain endothelial cells, whereas COX-2 increases the permeability of brain vasculature. Autocrine activation of breast cancer cell EGFR by HB-EGF signals for invasion of the brain parenchyma.

Results from real-time imaging studies suggest that survival of cancer cells in the central nervous system is dependent on their ability to communicate with vascular endothelial cells. Failure to stimulate angiogenesis leads to regression of lung adenocarcinoma cell brain metastases, whereas the inability to locate cerebral vessels for co-option leads to activation of cell death programmes in melanoma brain metastases [14]. Brain endothelial cells also protect brain metastases from the cytotoxic effects of chemotherapy. Unlike endothelial cells from other regional circulations, brain endothelial cells constitutively express the P-glycoprotein transporter on their apical membrane, which mediates the efflux of several chemotherapeutic agents, including vinblastine, methotrexate, vincristine, doxorubicin, and etoposide. P-glycoprotein also limits the central nervous system uptake of several small-molecule targeted therapies, such as erlotinib, gefitinib, and imatinib.

One hallmark of human brain metastases is reactive astrogliosis, the process in which astrocytes alter their patterns of gene expression and undergo changes in cell morphology. Astrogliosis is characterized by upregulation of the intermediate filament protein called glial fibrillary acidic protein, and hypertrophy of astrocyte cellular processes. Astrocytes encircle and infiltrate brain metastases, and the magnitude of astrogliosis parallels tumour growth. The precise mechanism responsible for astrogliosis remains unclear. Results obtained from co-culture systems using astrocytes and human cancer cells demonstrated that astrocytes protect cancer cells from chemotherapeutic agents through gap junction-mediated communication that results in upregulation of GSTA5, BCL2L1, and TWIST1 survival genes in cancer cells [15].

Bone microenvironment

Bone metastasis is also a significant public health concern; it occurs in up to 70% of individuals with advanced cancer of the breast or prostate and in approximately 40% of patients with carcinomas of the lung or kidney. The pathophysiology of bone metastasis involves several different cell populations and a variety of regulatory proteins. Bone metastases are classified as either osteoblastic or osteolytic, depending on whether the pathology involves bone formation or bone destruction. Pathological bone remodelling results in significant skeletal complications, including pain, hypercalcaemia, fractures, spinal cord compression, and immobility.

The highly vascularized metaphyseal bone found at the ends of long bones, ribs, and vertebrae is a target site for bone-homing tumour cells. The bone is enriched in several cytokines and growth factors that act as homing signals for cancer cells. Studies suggest that stromal cell-derived factor 1 and its receptor, CXCR4, may direct the trafficking of a variety of cancer cells to bone. Stromal cell-derived factor 1 is constitutively expressed in the bone microenvironment by fibroblasts, endothelial cells, and osteoblasts. Neutralizing antibodies and synthetic peptide antagonists directed against CXCR4 expressed on prostate and breast cancer cells were found to reduce the number of bone metastases in experimental models. *CXCR4* was identified as one of a small set of genes that mediate breast cancer metastasis to bone. Activation of CXCR4 on cancer cells transduces Src-dependent survival signals and increases their affinity for microvascular endothelial cells.

Several factors have been implicated in the skeletal remodelling that accompanies metastatic bone cancer. One of the most studied mediators of bone metastasis is parathyroid hormone-related peptide (PTHrP). More than 90% of breast cancer bone metastases are PTHrP-positive, whereas only 20% of breast cancers in non-bone metastatic sites express PTHrP. PTHrP produced by breast cancer cells binds to parathyroid hormone receptor 1 on osteoblasts and stimulates upregulation of receptor activator of nuclear factor κB ligand (RANKL). RANKL then binds to its receptor on osteoclasts and promotes cell differentiation and activation. Bone resorption liberates from the bone matrix transforming growth factor β, which then binds to its receptor on cancer cells and activates a positive feedback loop by signalling for increased production of PTHrP from cancer cells. Agents that target RANKL and interfere with osteoclastogenesis decrease the incidence of skeletal complications and are the current standard of care for patients with bone metastasis [16].

Fig. 3.7.5. The role of platelet-derived growth factor receptor β (PDGFR-β) in the pathogenesis of hormone-refractory prostate cancer bone metastasis. (A) Circulating prostate cancer cells ensure their retention in the bone by exploiting their sialyl Lewis[x] antigen to adhere to E-selectin expressed on bone endothelial cells. (B) Extravasating tumour cells express interleukin-6 (IL-6), which is chemotactic for monocytes and imparts M2 functional properties to macrophages. Tumour necrosis factor α (TNFα) produced by macrophages stimulates prostate cancer cells to increase their production of IL-6. (C) TNFα activates osteoclasts and signals for activation of the bone remodelling process. (D) Transforming growth factor β (TGF-β) released from the bone matrix binds to its receptor on prostate cancer cells, where it stimulates production of platelet-derived growth factor (PDGF). (E) PDGF acts in an autocrine manner by binding to PDGFR-β expressed on cancer cells and stimulating cell division. (F) Phosphorylation of PDGFR-β on tumour-associated endothelial cells promotes activation of angiogenic programmes in resident endothelial cells.

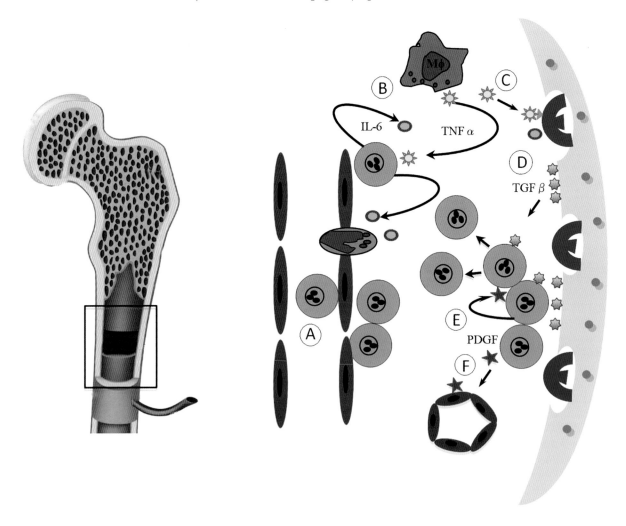

Mortality from prostate cancer usually results from metastasis of hormone-refractory prostate cancer cells. The spread of prostate cancer to the bone is thought to involve both anatomical components (i.e. the Batson venous plexus) and site-specific molecular adhesive interactions between the tetrasaccharide sialyl Lewis[x] antigen on prostate cancer cells and its receptor E-selectin, which is constitutively expressed on bone endothelial cells. Preclinical studies of androgen-independent prostate cancer cells implanted into the bone of mice implicated platelet-derived growth factor receptor β (PDGFR-β) in metastatic progression in that inhibition of PDGFR-β activation with imatinib therapy produced apoptosis of both cancer cells and the tumour-associated blood vessels. PDGFR-β signalling promotes survival of bone endothelial cells, and the receptor is expressed in its phosphorylated form on tumour-associated endothelial cells and cancer cells in clinical bone marrow samples from prostate cancer patients. PDGFR-β was also identified as one of the five genes that predicted recurrence after prostatectomy. The role of PDGFR-β in hormone-refractory prostate cancer bone metastasis is illustrated in Fig. 3.7.5.

Conclusion

Over the past 5 years, the number of investigations into the cellular interactions that take place in the tumour microenvironment has increased dramatically. During this same period, both the United States National Cancer Institute and the European Commission have established major research initiatives focused exclusively on an improved understanding of the cellular communication that takes place between cancer cells and the stromal compartment. One consequence of these efforts has been the realization that therapeutic targeting of both cancer cells and components of the microenvironment leads to improved clinical outcomes. Continued study of the complex cross-talk between cancer cells and the microenvironment of target organs of metastasis is likely to yield new opportunities for therapeutic intervention.

References

1. Fidler IJ, Yano S, Zhang RD et al. (2002). The seed and soil hypothesis: vascularisation and brain metastases. *Lancet Oncol*, 3:53–57. http://dx.doi.org/10.1016/S1470-2045(01)00622-2 PMID:11905606

2. Weis SM, Cheresh DA (2011). Tumor angiogenesis: molecular pathways and therapeutic targets. *Nat Med*, 17:1359–1370. http://dx.doi.org/10.1038/nm.2537 PMID:22064426

3. Eberhard A, Kahlert S, Goede V et al. (2000). Heterogeneity of angiogenesis and blood vessel maturation in human tumors: implications for antiangiogenic tumor therapies. *Cancer Res*, 60:1388–1393. PMID:10728704

4. Cascone T, Herynk MH, Xu L et al. (2011). Upregulated stromal EGFR and vascular remodeling in mouse xenograft models of angiogenesis inhibitor-resistant human lung adenocarcinoma. *J Clin Invest*, 121:1313–1328. http://dx.doi.org/10.1172/JCI42405 PMID:21436589

5. Shojaei F, Wu X, Malik AK et al. (2007). Tumor refractoriness to anti-VEGF treatment is mediated by CD11b+Gr1+ myeloid cells. *Nat Biotechnol*, 25:911–920. http://dx.doi.org/10.1038/nbt1323 PMID:17664940

6. Vaupel P, Kallinowski F, Okunieff P (1989). Blood flow, oxygen and nutrient supply, and metabolic microenvironment of human tumors: a review. *Cancer Res*, 49:6449–6465. PMID:2684393

7. Qiu W, Hu M, Sridhar A et al. (2008). No evidence of clonal somatic genetic alterations in cancer-associated fibroblasts from human breast and ovarian carcinomas. *Nat Genet*, 40:650–655. http://dx.doi.org/10.1038/ng.117 PMID:18408720

8. Colotta F, Allavena P, Sica A et al. (2009). Cancer-related inflammation, the seventh hallmark of cancer: links to genetic instability. *Carcinogenesis*, 30:1073–1081. http://dx.doi.org/10.1093/carcin/bgp127 PMID:19468060

9. Sica A, Allavena P, Mantovani A (2008). Cancer related inflammation: the macrophage connection. *Cancer Lett*, 267:204–215. http://dx.doi.org/10.1016/j.canlet.2008.03.028 PMID:18448242

10. Page-McCaw A, Ewald AJ, Werb Z (2007). Matrix metalloproteinases and the regulation of tissue remodelling. *Nat Rev Mol Cell Biol*, 8:221–233. http://dx.doi.org/10.1038/nrm2125 PMID:17318226

11. Thiery JP, Acloque H, Huang RY, Nieto MA (2009). Epithelial-mesenchymal transitions in development and disease. *Cell*, 139:871–890. http://dx.doi.org/10.1016/j.cell.2009.11.007 PMID:19945376

12. Langley RR, Fidler IJ (2013). The biology of brain metastasis. *Clin Chem*, 59:180–189. http://dx.doi.org/10.1373/clinchem.2012.193342 PMID:23115057

13. Bos PD, Zhang XH, Nadal C et al. (2009). Genes that mediate breast cancer metastasis to the brain. *Nature*, 459:1005–1009. http://dx.doi.org/10.1038/nature08021 PMID:19421193

14. Kienast Y, von Baumgarten L, Fuhrmann M et al. (2010). Real-time imaging reveals the single steps of brain metastasis formation. *Nat Med*, 16:116–122. http://dx.doi.org/10.1038/nm.2072 PMID:20023634

15. Kim SJ, Kim JS, Park ES et al. (2011). Astrocytes upregulate survival genes in tumor cells and induce protection from chemotherapy. *Neoplasia*, 13:286–298. PMID:21390191

16. Weilbaecher KN, Guise TA, McCauley LK (2011). Cancer to bone: a fatal attraction. *Nat Rev Cancer*, 11:411–425. http://dx.doi.org/10.1038/nrc3055 PMID:21593787

Websites

Tumor Microenvironment Network: http://tmen.nci.nih.gov/

MicroEnviMet: Seventh Framework Programme: http://www.microenvimet.eu/

3.8

Signal transduction and targeted therapy

3 BIOLOGY

Fabio Savarese
Martin Holcmann
Maria Sibilia

Zdenko Herceg (reviewer)
Michael P. Brown (contributor)
Nikki Burdett (contributor)

Summary

- Signalling pathways regulate a plethora of biological processes in all cells of complex organisms.

- Consistent with mediating cell survival, proliferation, response of growth factors, and related biological processes, components of such signalling pathways are often variously modified by mutation or epigenetic effects in different types of cancer.

- A range of small-molecule inhibitors and monoclonal antibodies are categorized as targeted therapies because the benefits these agents provide depend upon perturbation of particular signalling pathways in malignant cells.

- One particularly well-studied signalling network is the epidermal growth factor receptor (EGFR) pathway. Due to the role of this pathway in maintaining the transformed phenotype in tumours such as non-small cell lung cancer and squamous cell carcinoma of the head and neck, the EGFR pathway is a prominent target for pharmacological inhibition.

- A major problem with therapies aimed at inhibiting signalling pathways is that tumour cells manifest a wide array of strategies, which render them refractory to drug treatment.

- Modern whole-genome sequencing techniques offer great potential for the provision of optimal targeted therapy on an individual basis, as demonstrated by their initial successful application in the clinic.

Responsiveness to extracellular signals is a fundamental attribute of all living organisms. For instance, bacteria sense nutrition gradients through signalling cascades mediated by transmembrane receptors, which result in bacterial motion towards nutrients [1]. This paradigm of receptor-mediated signal transduction reaches its highest level of complexity in mammals, where hundreds of different cell types communicate with each other – both locally, as involving the paracrine system, and over relatively vast distances, as identified by the endocrine system. Virtually every biological process is at least co-regulated by the integration of extracellular signals from cells and organs. This chapter focuses on the molecular events that mediate signal transduction, how these signalling cascades are dysregulated in cancer, and how targeting these signalling networks may increase the efficiency of anticancer therapy.

Receptor tyrosine kinases – molecular biology and functions

In humans, various signalling cascades with distinct molecular properties play key roles in health and disease. The major signalling pathways perturbed in various tumour types (Table 3.8.1) mediate organ development and homeostasis in normal tissue. The receptor tyrosine kinases identify a specific group of receptor molecules [2]. In humans, 58 different receptor tyrosine kinases have been identified, grouped into 20 subfamilies. Members of the ERBB receptor subfamily, namely ERBB1 (also named epidermal growth factor receptor [EGFR]), ERBB2, ERBB3, and ERBB4, all play important roles in development and homeostasis but are dysregulated in various human tumours and therefore constitute therapeutic targets in the treatment of cancer [3].

Generally, receptor tyrosine kinases function as homodimers and heterodimers, including the ERBB family members. Each monomer consists of an extracellular N-terminal domain, which primarily serves as a binding site for various ligands; a hydrophobic transmembrane domain; and an

Pathway	Molecular features of signal transduction	Examples of associated cancers
RTKs	Receptor tyrosine kinases (RTKs) initiate phosphorylation cascades that involve adaptor proteins and various mitogen-activated protein kinases (MAPKs), ultimately modulating transcription of genes involved in proliferation and differentiation.	Most cancers
PI3K	Activation by RTKs leads to the chemical modification of components of the cell membrane, which through a multistep process leads to increased cell growth and survival.	Ovarian cancer
JAK-STAT	Activation by receptors, like cytokine receptors or the RTK family. Directly activates proteins called signal transducer and activator of transcription (STATs).	Lymphoma
NF-κB	Cytokine receptors activate a complex protein network, which through proteolysis of inhibitory factors ultimately leads to the nuclear translocation and activation of transcription factors belonging to the NF-κB family.	Lymphoma, breast cancer
Notch	Activation of the transmembrane receptor Notch leads to the proteolysis of its intracellular domain, which shuttles to the nucleus and ultimately serves as a transcription factor.	Pancreatic cancer
Hedgehog	Ligand binding to the receptor Patched leads to its inactivation and inhibits the repressive role of Patched on another receptor, Smoothened. Activated Smoothened initiates a signalling cascade that results in changes in gene expression.	Basal cell carcinoma, medulloblastoma
WNT	In a very complex signalling cascade, activation of various receptors by WNT ligands inhibits the activity of an important cytoplasmic kinase, GSK3B, which in turn stabilizes β-catenin protein, which subsequently shuttles to the nucleus and serves as a transcription factor.	Colon cancer
TGF-β	Activation of the TGF-β receptors phosphorylates proteins called SMADs, which subsequently enter the nucleus and regulate expression of genes required for processes such as proliferation or cell motility.	Breast cancer, colon cancer

NF-κB, nuclear factor kappa-light-chain-enhancer of activated B cells; PI3K, phosphatidylinositol 3-kinase; TGF-β, transforming growth factor β.

intracellular C-terminal region containing the catalytic kinase domains (Fig. 3.8.1). Signal transduction is initiated by binding of a ligand to the extracellular domain of a receptor molecule, inducing homodimerization when a second identical receptor molecule is involved, or heterodimerization, which involves a different receptor molecule, usually of the same family, with subsequent conformational changes. Dimerization causes activation of the intracellular kinase domain within the receptor. This leads to phosphorylation (usually in *trans*) of various tyrosine residues, which are located in the C-terminal part of these proteins (Fig. 3.8.1). In biochemical terms, the phosphate group (PO_4) of ATP, the phosphate donor in most biochemical reactions, is covalently linked to a tyrosine residue of the receptor by the catalytic activity of its kinase domain. As is discussed later, these two steps, namely receptor dimerization and ATP catalysis, underpin therapeutic strategies targeting signalling pathways [4].

Once receptor phosphorylation has occurred, multiple proteins ensure that the original signal is amplified and transduced within the cell to different compartments. Adaptor proteins bind to the phosphorylated residues of the receptor tyrosine kinases and propagate the stimulus by protein–protein interactions, many of which result in further phosphorylation events. Particular propagators of the signalling cascade initiated by ERBB receptors are the protein SOS and the small GTPase RAS, which are frequently mutated in various cancers. Cellular processes affected by ERBB signalling include (i) the regulation of gene expression, mediated mainly by mitogen-activated protein kinase (MAPK)-regulated activity of the activator protein 1 (AP1) transcription factors; (ii) AKT-mediated cell survival; and (iii) changes in cell motility, controlled by RHO and RAC proteins. This signalling cascade is kept in a dynamic state as multiple molecular mechanisms mediate the turnover of activated receptor tyrosine kinases. These mechanisms range from the dephosphorylation of the cytoplasmic domains by phosphatases to the internalization and ubiquitin-mediated degradation of receptor complexes, all intended to terminate the activating signal. Mutations in genes that are required for turning off activated receptor tyrosine kinases may contribute to cancer development.

Functions of ErbB signalling in health and disease

Analyses of mice carrying mutated alleles of the genes encoding the various ErbB receptors have greatly contributed to understanding the role of these proteins in various tissues and organs. In general, the genetic inactivation of *ErbB2*, *ErbB3*, or *ErbB4* leads to early embryonic lethality in mice [5]. Likewise, mice lacking Egfr show embryonic lethality or die during the first weeks after birth, depending on the genetic background, with defects in several epithelia and in the brain [6]. Conditional inactivation of the *Egfr* allele has contributed to overcoming this early lethality and therefore to an improved understanding of the function of Egfr signalling in adult tissues [7]. The analysis of animals in which *Egfr* was specifically mutated in distinct cell types has revealed roles in epithelial development and differentiation as well as in liver regeneration and proper brain patterning and function. Egfr signalling in these tissues induces (i) the

Fig. 3.8.1. (A,B) Structural change in the transmembrane protein epidermal growth factor receptor (EGFR) caused by binding of its ligand. (A) EGFR (blue) is a transmembrane receptor with an extracellular ligand-binding domain (the ligand EGF is shown in red), a transmembrane domain (the membrane is drawn in grey), and an intracellular domain. (B) Binding of EGF leads to receptor dimerization and activation of the intracellular kinase domains. (C) Principles of signal transduction via ERBB receptors: (1) ligand binding leads to receptor dimerization and the activation of the intracellular kinase domain; (2) various adaptor proteins and kinases lead to the transduction of the signal into the nucleus; (3) activation of transcription factors results in induction of gene expression.

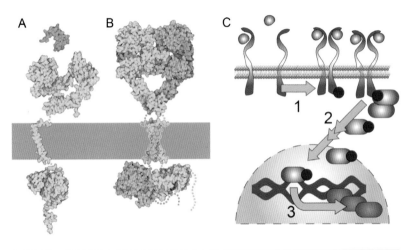

suppression of differentiation at the expense of proliferation and (ii) pro-survival signalling. Increased proliferation and aberrant cell survival contribute to cancer development, and indeed various studies in mice have revealed the role of aberrant Egfr signalling in different models of murine tumorigenesis.

Multiple components of the ERBB signalling network may be mutated in cancer. EGFR stimulates basic cellular functions such as proliferation and cell survival, and mutations that lead to enhanced EGFR signalling are frequently found in tumour cells [8]. Several different mutations may result in pro-tumorigenic signalling through EGFR; the most notable involve (i) overexpression, (ii) activating mutations, (iii) heterodimerization with other ERBB family members, (iv) autocrine ligand production, and (v) reduced downregulation of ERBB signalling (Fig. 3.8.2). Interestingly, different types of mutations are found in different tumours. For example, EGFR overexpression is frequently found in brain, liver, and colon cancers, whereas activating mutations are found in non-small cell

lung cancer (e.g. EGFRL858R) and glioblastomas (e.g. EGFRvIII: deletion of exons 2–7). Mechanistically, overexpression may be caused by higher transcriptional activity of the corresponding genes or by gene amplification. Often, in individual tumours of patients with a particular type of cancer, increased transcriptional activity as well as gene duplication can be observed, alone or together with activating mutations, such as in colorectal cancer or non-small cell lung cancer.

Role of EGFR in distinct types of cancer

EGFR and glioblastoma

Both gene amplification and activating mutations of EGFR can be found in patients with glioblastoma multiforme. Two subtypes of glioblastoma can be distinguished, based on their ontogeny: primary glioblastomas arise de novo, whereas secondary glioblastomas develop from low-grade astrocytoma. Interestingly, 97% of primary glioblastomas are known to contain additional copies of the EGFR gene but show no

mutations in the tumour suppressor p53 protein encoded by TP53. In addition to EGFR amplification, the EGFRvIII mutation is frequently encountered in glioblastoma, and overall more than 60% of all types of glioblastoma show dysregulated EGFR expression or function. In contrast, secondary glioblastomas are associated with frequent mutations in TP53, while EGFR amplifications or mutations are rare. Unfortunately, targeted anti-EGFR therapies have been shown to have very limited success in the treatment of glioblastomas [9].

EGFR, skin cancers, and tumours of the head and neck

Skin cancer is one of the most frequent diseases in humans worldwide. One of its most common forms is squamous cell carcinoma, and EGFR is frequently amplified and EGFR overexpressed in squamous cell carcinoma. In melanoma, a frequently metastatic skin cancer, EGFR is often amplified in late-stage tumours.

In addition to squamous cells in skin tumours, EGFR is also frequently overexpressed in head and neck squamous cell carcinomas (HNSCCs), which arise from mucosal epithelia of the head and neck (lips, oral and nasal cavities, larynx, or pharynx). High EGFR levels are found in 90% of all HNSCCs and indicate a poor prognosis. More than 80% of HNSCC patients with normal EGFR expression survive longer than 5 years, compared with 25% of patients in whom EGFR overexpression has been detected. Currently, the most frequently used therapeutic approach in HNSCC patients is a combination of radiotherapy and targeted anti-EGFR therapies [10].

EGFR and non-small cell lung carcinoma

Non-small cell lung carcinoma refers to any type of epithelial lung cancer other than small cell lung carcinoma. Lung cancers account for about one third of all cancer deaths worldwide, and more than 80% of all lung tumours can be classified as non-small cell lung carcinomas, which are mainly adenocarcinoma and squamous cell carcinoma. The most common genetic mutations found in non-small cell lung carcinoma affect the genes that express EGFR and K-RAS, a signalling protein downstream of receptor tyrosine kinases, demonstrating the role of dysregulated ERBB signalling in this disease. *EGFR* and *K-RAS* mutations are mutually exclusive, indicating that a constitutively active downstream mediator (RAS) of the ERBB cascade does not require increased receptor levels for oncogenicity. Non-small cell lung carcinomas frequently display specific *EGFR* mutations, which are very rarely observed in other cancers, and which result in expression of mutated EGFR protein with constitutively active kinase domains. Anti-EGFR targeted therapies are singularly effective in patients harbouring these mutations, although ultimately hampered by the development of resistance [11].

Therapeutic approaches that target signal transduction

Various molecular strategies aimed at the functional inactivation of oncogenes are currently being developed and tested in numerous clinical trials [3]. At present, however, all types of anticancer drugs that inhibit receptor tyrosine kinases either belong to the class of small-molecule inhibitors or are recombinant antibodies that bind and inhibit the specific receptors (Table 3.8.2). Advances in resolving protein structures have facilitated the design of small molecules targeting oncoproteins specifically. For a protein to be "druggable" by this approach, the protein must have an active domain shaped like a cleft or a pocket that is accessible to water. Small-molecule inhibitors of protein kinases, exemplified by the intracellular domains of the ERBB receptors, primarily affect enzymatic activity by inhibiting ATP catalysis occurring within the kinase domain (Fig. 3.8.3).

Several parameters influence the efficacy of small-molecule inhibitors. Drugs binding irreversibly to their target permanently inhibit kinase function, as opposed to the activity of reversible inhibitors. Irreversible inhibition is more effective but much more toxic. Another parameter is the specificity of the drug – either targeting the ATP-binding domain of a kinase, which usually leads to a highly specific drug, or targeting ATP itself. Recent studies demonstrate frequent interactions of protein kinase inhibitors, previously believed to be specific, with multiple other protein kinases. These off-target effects present a major challenge since they might be the cause of potentially detrimental side-effects. However, in some cases this non-selectiveness can prove beneficial, as in the case of sorafenib [12]. Sorafenib was originally identified as a RAF inhibitor, but the clinical success of this agent is attributable to an inhibitory effect on the kinases of the vascular endothelial growth factor receptor 2 (VEGFR2), platelet-derived growth factor receptor (PDGFR), and fibroblast growth factor receptor (FGFR) types. Similarly, oral multikinase inhibitors such as sunitinib target PDFGRs, VEGFRs,

KIT, RET, CSF1R, and FLT3 and have been successfully used for the cure of renal cell carcinoma and imatinib-resistant gastrointestinal stromal tumours.

As well as small-molecule inhibitors, monoclonal antibodies to the extracellular domain of transmembrane receptors have been successfully established for the treatment of certain types of cancer [13]. An example is the chimeric antibody cetuximab, which inhibits heterodimerization and consequently the activation of the signalling cascade downstream of EGFR (Fig. 3.8.3). In addition, antibodies may act via the induction of an anti-tumour immune response by a process designated antibody-dependent cytotoxicity. The difference in size between the small-molecule inhibitor erlotinib and the antibody cetuximab is illustrated in Fig. 3.8.3.

Clinical application of targeted therapies

In most cases, tumours from patients with non-small cell lung carcinoma exhibit hyperactive EGFR signalling. Hence, when drugs that selectively

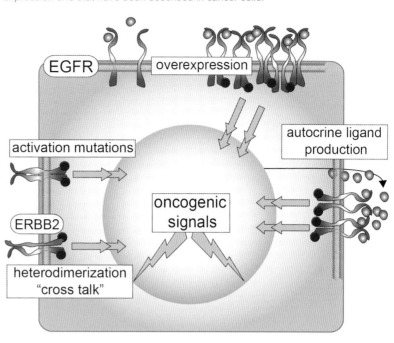

Fig. 3.8.2. Various types of structural change that may result in alterations of ERBB expression and that have been described in cancer cells.

inhibit EGFR, namely the small-molecule inhibitors gefitinib and erlotinib, first became available, efficient treatment of this disease was anticipated. However, from the outset, clinical trials indicated that only a small percentage of patients responded well to treatment [14]. It became apparent that the therapy was beneficial for patients carrying mutations in the kinase domain of EGFR but not for individuals with tumours that overexpress wild-type EGFR. However, secondary EGFR mutations arose, specifically in patients initially responsive to gefitinib and erlotinib, and these mutations rendered the protein resistant to inhibition by these compounds. In preclinical trials, treatment of such gefitinib/erlotinib-resistant tumour cells with other classes of drugs, such as the EGFR/ErbB2 inhibitor lapatinib or the irreversible kinase inhibitor afatinib, overcame resistance towards anti-EGFR therapy. However, due to toxicity, a combinatorial treatment has yet to be adopted clinically.

In HNSCC patients in whom abnormally activated EGFR signalling has been detected, a combination of radiotherapy and the EGFR-targeting antibody cetuximab is widely used at present. Cetuximab is a humanized mouse antibody, and binding of this antibody to the extracellular part of EGFR not only inhibits the activation of the downstream signalling cascade but also inhibits receptor turnover and renders tumour cells more immunogenic, leading to increased levels of antibody-dependent cellular toxicity. However, similarly to non-small cell lung carcinoma patients treated with gefitinib and erlotinib, HNSCC patients quickly develop resistance to cetuximab [15]. In general, the use of EGFR-targeted drugs currently leads to prolonged survival of patients diagnosed with cancer, but not to reduced mortality.

In summary, the use of drugs inhibiting the function of EGFR and

Table 3.8.2. Monoclonal antibodies and small-molecule inhibitors currently in clinical use that target diverse signal transduction pathways

Generic name	Target	EMA-approved indications	FDA-approved indications
Monoclonal antibodies			
Bevacizumab	VEGF	Metastatic colorectal cancer, breast cancer, non-small cell lung cancer, renal cell carcinoma, grade IV glioma; epithelial ovarian, fallopian tube, or primary peritoneal cancer	Metastatic colorectal cancer, non-small cell lung cancer, glioblastoma, metastatic renal cell carcinoma
Cetuximab	EGFR	Head and neck squamous cell carcinoma, EGFR-positive K-RAS wild-type colorectal cancer	Head and neck squamous cell carcinoma, EGFR-positive colorectal cancer
Ipilimumab	CTLA-4	Unresectable or metastatic melanoma	Unresectable or metastatic melanoma
Panitumumab	EGFR	K-RAS wild-type metastatic colorectal cancer (conditional)	K-RAS-negative metastatic colorectal cancer
Pertuzumab	HER2	HER2-positive unresectable or metastatic breast cancer	HER2-positive metastatic breast cancer
Trastuzumab	HER2	HER2-positive breast cancer; HER2-positive gastric or gastro-oesophageal junction adenocarcinoma	HER2-positive breast cancer, HER2-positive gastric or gastro-oesophageal junction cancer
Small-molecule inhibitors			
Afatinib	EGFR, HER2, HER4	Treatment of EGFR tyrosine kinase inhibitor-naive adult patients with locally advanced or metastatic non-small cell lung cancer with activating *EGFR* mutation(s)	First-line treatment of patients with metastatic non-small cell lung cancer whose tumours have *EGFR* exon 19 deletions or exon 21 (L858R) substitution mutations as detected by an FDA-approved test
Axitinib	VEGFR, PDGFR	Advanced renal cell carcinoma	Advanced renal cell carcinoma
Cabozantinib	VEGFR, MET, RET	None	Metastatic medullary thyroid cancer
Crizotinib	ALK, MET	ALK-positive non-small cell lung cancer (conditional)	ALK-positive non-small cell lung cancer
Dabrafenib	V600E BRAF	None	BRAF V600E-positive unresectable or metastatic melanoma
Erlotinib	EGFR	*EGFR* mutation-positive non-small cell lung cancer, pancreatic cancer	Non-small cell lung cancer, pancreatic cancer
Gefitinib	EGFR	Locally advanced or metastatic *EGFR* mutation-positive non-small cell lung cancer	Non-small cell lung cancer

ALK, anaplastic lymphoma kinase; CSF1R, colony-stimulating factor 1 receptor; EGFR, epidermal growth factor receptor; EMA, European Medicines Agency; FDA, United States Food and Drug Administration; GnRH, gonadotropin-releasing hormone; mTOR, mammalian target of rapamycin; PDGFR, platelet-derived growth factor receptor; VEGF, vascular endothelial growth factor; VEGFR, vascular endothelial growth factor receptor.

Generic name	Target	EMA-approved indications	FDA-approved indications
Imatinib	PDGFR, KIT	KIT-positive gastrointestinal stromal tumours, adjuvant or unresectable	KIT-positive gastrointestinal stromal tumours, adjuvant or unresectable
Lapatinib	EGFR, HER2	HER2-positive breast cancer (conditional)	HER2-positive breast cancer
Pazopanib	VEGFR, KIT, PDGFR	Advanced renal cell carcinoma, advanced soft tissue sarcoma (conditional)	Advanced renal cell carcinoma, advanced soft tissue sarcoma
Regorafenib	PDGFR, KIT, RET, VEGFR	None	Metastatic colorectal cancer
Sorafenib	VEGR, PDGFR, CRAF, FLT3	Hepatocellular carcinoma, advanced renal cell carcinoma	Unresectable hepatocellular carcinoma, advanced renal cell carcinoma
Sunitinib	VEGFR, PDGFR, KIT, FLT3, RET, CSF1R	Advanced renal cell carcinoma, unresectable or metastatic malignant gastrointestinal stromal tumours, pancreatic neuroendocrine tumours	Advanced renal cell carcinoma, progressive gastrointestinal stromal tumours, pancreatic neuroendocrine tumours
Trametinib	V600 BRAF	None	BRAF V600-positive unresectable or metastatic melanoma
Vandetanib	VEGFR, EGFR, RET	Medullary thyroid cancer (conditional)	Medullary thyroid cancer
Vemurafenib	V600 BRAF	BRAF V600-positive unresectable or metastatic melanoma	BRAF V600E-positive unresectable or metastatic melanoma
Small-molecule allosteric inhibitors			
Everolimus	mTOR	Advanced renal cell carcinoma; unresectable pancreatic neuroendocrine tumours; hormone-receptor-positive, HER2-negative postmenopausal breast cancer; subependymal giant cell astrocytoma (conditional)	Advanced renal cell carcinoma; unresectable pancreatic neuroendocrine tumours; subependymal giant cell astrocytoma; hormone-receptor-positive, HER2-negative postmenopausal breast cancer
Temsirolimus	mTOR	Advanced renal cell carcinoma	Advanced renal cell carcinoma
Small-molecule Smoothened antagonist			
Vismodegib	Smoothened receptor	None	Metastatic or recurrent basal cell carcinoma
Recombinant decoy receptor			
Ziv-aflibercept	VEGFR	Metastatic colorectal cancer	Metastatic colorectal cancer
Antibody–drug conjugate			
Ado-trastuzumab emtansine	HER2	None	HER2-positive metastatic breast cancer
Hormonal agents			
Abiraterone	Androgen synthesis–CYP17A1 inhibition	Metastatic castration-resistant prostate cancer	Metastatic castration-resistant prostate cancer
Anastrazole	Aromatase	None	Hormone-receptor-positive postmenopausal breast cancer, or hormone-receptor-negative disease after tamoxifen
Bicalutamide	Androgen receptor	None	Metastatic prostate cancer
Degarelix	GnRH receptor	Advanced prostate cancer	Advanced prostate cancer
Enzalutamide	Androgen receptor	None	Metastatic castration-resistant prostate cancer
Exemestane	Aromatase	None	Estrogen-receptor-positive postmenopausal breast cancer, or estrogen-receptor-negative disease after tamoxifen
Flutamide	Androgen receptor	None	Prostate cancer
Goserelin	GnRH receptor	None	Prostate cancer, palliative treatment of premenopausal breast cancer
Letrozole	Aromatase	None	Postmenopausal breast cancer
Leuprorelin acetate	GnRH receptor	None	Palliative treatment of prostate cancer
Tamoxifen	Estrogen receptor	None	Metastatic breast cancer

ALK, anaplastic lymphoma kinase; CSF1R, colony-stimulating factor 1 receptor; EGFR, epidermal growth factor receptor; EMA, European Medicines Agency; FDA, United States Food and Drug Administration; GnRH, gonadotropin-releasing hormone; mTOR, mammalian target of rapamycin; PDGFR, platelet-derived growth factor receptor; VEGF, vascular endothelial growth factor; VEGFR, vascular endothelial growth factor receptor.

Fig. 3.8.3. (A) The action of tyrosine kinase inhibitors (TKIs) and inhibitory antibodies (cetuximab). TKIs inhibit signal transduction by blocking the activation of the receptor through inhibition of the kinase domain. In contrast, cetuximab impairs the dimerization of epidermal growth factor receptor (EGFR). (B) Size comparison between ATP and erlotinib, and between EGFR and cetuximab. Erlotinib is a small-molecule inhibitor and is approximately the same size as ATP, the molecule essential for the phosphorylation of the receptor after dimerization. Cetuximab and EGFR are approximately 400 times bigger, as indicated by the magnifying glass.

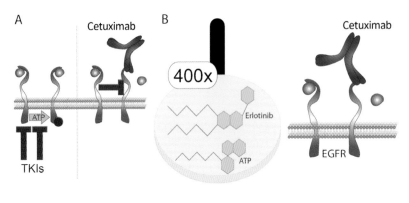

other receptor tyrosine kinases achieves an initial response, but the regrowth of tumours resistant to these drugs is commonly observed; such a scenario is attributable to inherent genetic instability, as evidenced by rapid mutation. Emergence of new mutations under the selective pressure of treatment with receptor tyrosine kinase inhibitors allows tumour cells to continue growth despite drug treatment. Ideally, this scenario is resolved by the identification of secondary mutations and the development of new treatment strategies. Although great progress has been made in developing targeted anticancer drugs to be applied specifically in preselected cancer patients, mechanisms of resistance have yet to be fully elucidated.

A better understanding of resistance mechanisms would lead to the identification of new targets against which new drugs could be designed and developed. Importantly, mechanisms mediating resistance to broad classes of drugs have to be identified and to be distinguished from processes specific to particular agents. The search for biomarkers, which predict the response of certain tumours or patients to therapeutic treatment, has thus become a focus of many pharmaceutical companies and research laboratories [16].

The catch of anticancer therapy: acquired drug resistance

Research addressing mechanisms of resistance to therapy targeted against signalling pathways, including anti-EGFR drugs, has markedly increased in recent years. Currently, recognized resistance mechanisms to anti-EGFR drugs include (i) additional mutations of EGFR; (ii) compensatory signalling via other receptors, such as VEGFR, insulin-like growth factor receptor (IGFR), and AXL; (iii) increased expression of VEGF, which modulates angiogenesis and may reduce localized drug concentration; and (iv) mutations in molecules downstream of EGFR, such as RAS or RAF (Fig. 3.8.4). Such downstream activating mutations render the tumour cells independent of EGFR function and therefore refractory to treatment with drugs against EGFR [17].

Mutations in downstream mediators of EGFR signalling commonly occur in tumours exhibiting neither *EGFR* mutation nor overexpression. An example involves metastatic melanoma, in which an activating mutation in *BRAF*, V600E, is frequently found. Recently, treatment of metastatic melanoma with the BRAF inhibitor vemurafenib yielded promising initial results [18]. In one clinical study, more than 50% of patients receiving vemurafenib experienced prolonged survival compared with untreated patients, and in an independent study more than 80% of treated patients showed partial to complete regression of tumours compared with non-treated individuals. However, tumour regression lasted only 2–18 months, and subsequently vemurafenib-resistant tumours appeared. Furthermore, vemurafenib had severe side-effects, giving rise in some cases to cutaneous squamous cell carcinoma or keratoacanthoma [19].

New insights gained from the genomic revolution

The new millennium has seen the complete sequencing of the human genome and genomes of other important organisms and pathogens. In particular, recent advances in whole-genome sequencing are revolutionizing modern medicine [20]. A pioneering study comparing the whole genomes of tumour and normal cells in a patient with acute myeloid leukaemia led to the discovery of various somatic mutations in malignant cells, one of them affecting the gene encoding the receptor tyrosine kinase FLT3 [21], demonstrating the power of modern genomic techniques. With such powerful tools available, a major goal for cancer therapy comes within reach: the identification of genetic mutations responsible for cancer development as well as those occurring during cancer progression. This would enable treatment strategies to be adapted based on the genetic changes during the course of the disease. In particular, mutations in cellular processes that "drive" tumorigenesis present attractive targets for therapeutic intervention. Notably, more than half of the "tumour driver" gene classes are constituted by components of signalling pathways [22]. Whole-genome sequencing of cancer patients leads to the discovery of sequence variations that can be used to predict whether a patient or an individual tumour can respond to a certain drug, which is referred to as pharmacogenomics [23].

Prospects

Ever-expanding knowledge about signal transduction networks underpins the design of novel agents and improved anticancer strategies. However, greater knowledge also reveals another degree of complexity in relation to contemporary understanding of tumour biology. Consequently, for every drug that successfully targets a specific pathway, multiple resistance mechanisms following from the initial treatment may be anticipated. Such an outlook, if applicable universally, is daunting but may be offset by the following considerations.

First, the expanding repertoire of drugs targeting proteins mediating every step of a signalling cascade will also increase our repertoire for ameliorating secondary and subsequent mutations. Perhaps even more importantly, modern screening techniques of gene expression patterns, or the identification of novel biomarkers of individual tumours, will allow

Fig. 3.8.4. Resistance mechanisms against drugs targeting the ERBB signalling network: (1) activating mutations in downstream effector molecules make the pathway completely independent of receptor function; (2) activating mutations in the kinase domain lead to constitutively active receptors; (3) mutations in the extracellular domain interfere with binding of cetuximab; (4) overproduction of vascular endothelial growth factor (VEGF) leads to altered angiogenesis and reduced exposure to drugs; (5) compensatory signalling via other receptors.

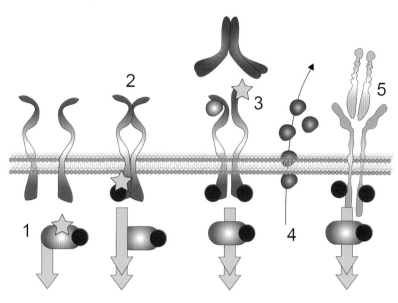

more informed development of combinations of therapeutics that have the highest chance of success in an individual patient. The introduction of massively parallel DNA sequencing technologies will soon provide comprehensive data at low cost. The term "personalized medicine" will no longer connote response to a single agent but will indicate therapy based on the biological characteristics of individual tumours, specified with reference to tumour progression in real time [24].

We thank Thomas Bauer for the artwork and design of the figures.

References

1. Falke JJ, Bass RB, Butler SL *et al.* (1997). The two-component signaling pathway of bacterial chemotaxis: a molecular view of signal transduction by receptors, kinases, and adaptation enzymes. *Annu Rev Cell Dev Biol*, 13:457–512. http://dx.doi.org/10.1146/annurev.cellbio.13.1.457 PMID:9442881

2. Lemmon MA, Schlessinger J (2010). Cell signaling by receptor tyrosine kinases. *Cell*, 141:1117–1134. http://dx.doi.org/10.1016/j.cell.2010.06.011 PMID:20602996

3. Levitzki A, Klein S (2010). Signal transduction therapy of cancer. *Mol Aspects Med*, 31:287–329. http://dx.doi.org/10.1016/j.mam.2010.04.001 PMID:20451549

4. Schlessinger J (2002). Ligand-induced, receptor-mediated dimerization and activation of EGF receptor. *Cell*, 110:669–672. http://dx.doi.org/10.1016/S0092-8674(02)00966-2 PMID:12297041

5. Sibilia M, Kroismayr R, Lichtenberger BM *et al.* (2007). The epidermal growth factor receptor: from development to tumorigenesis. *Differentiation*, 75:770–787. http://dx.doi.org/10.1111/j.1432-0436.2007.00238.x PMID:17999740

6. Sibilia M, Wagner EF (1995). Strain-dependent epithelial defects in mice lacking the EGF receptor. *Science*, 269:234–238. http://dx.doi.org/10.1126/science.7618085 PMID:7618085

7. Wagner B, Natarajan A, Grünaug S *et al.* (2006). Neuronal survival depends on EGFR signaling in cortical but not midbrain astrocytes. *EMBO J*, 25:752–762. http://dx.doi.org/10.1038/sj.emboj.7600988 PMID:16467848

8. Normanno N, De Luca A, Bianco C *et al.* (2006). Epidermal growth factor receptor (EGFR) signaling in cancer. *Gene*, 366:2–16. http://dx.doi.org/10.1016/j.gene.2005.10.018 PMID:16377102

9. Mellinghoff IK, Wang MY, Vivanco I *et al.* (2005). Molecular determinants of the response of glioblastomas to EGFR kinase inhibitors. *N Engl J Med*, 353:2012–2024. http://dx.doi.org/10.1056/NEJMoa051918 PMID:16282176

10. Sundvall M, Karrila A, Nordberg J *et al.* (2010). EGFR targeting drugs in the treatment of head and neck squamous cell carcinoma. *Expert Opin Emerg Drugs*, 15:185–201. http://dx.doi.org/10.1517/14728211003716442 PMID:20415599

11. da Cunha Santos G, Shepherd FA, Tsao MS (2011). EGFR mutations and lung cancer. *Annu Rev Pathol*, 6:49–69. http://dx.doi.org/10.1146/annurev-pathol-011110-130206 PMID:20887192

12. Adnane L, Trail PA, Taylor I, Wilhelm SM (2006). Sorafenib (BAY 43-9006, Nexavar), a dual-action inhibitor that targets RAF/MEK/ERK pathway in tumor cells and tyrosine kinases VEGFR/PDGFR in tumor vasculature. *Methods Enzymol*, 407:597–612. http://dx.doi.org/10.1016/S0076-6879(05)07047-3 PMID:16757355

13. Astsaturov I, Cohen RB, Harari P (2007). EGFR-targeting monoclonal antibodies in head and neck cancer. *Curr Cancer Drug Targets*, 7:650–665. http://dx.doi.org/10.2174/156800907782418365 PMID:18045070

14. Sridhar SS, Seymour L, Shepherd FA (2003). Inhibitors of epidermal-growth-factor receptors: a review of clinical research with a focus on non-small-cell lung cancer. *Lancet Oncol*, 4:397–406. http://dx.doi.org/10.1016/S1470-2045(03)01137-9 PMID:12850190

15. Brand TM, Iida M, Wheeler DL (2011). Molecular mechanisms of resistance to the EGFR monoclonal antibody cetuximab. *Cancer Biol Ther*, 11:777–792. http://dx.doi.org/10.4161/cbt.11.9.15050 PMID:21293176

16. Brooks JD (2012). Translational genomics: the challenge of developing cancer biomarkers. *Genome Res*, 22:183–187. http://dx.doi.org/10.1101/gr.124347.111 PMID:22301132

17. Wheeler DL, Dunn EF, Harari PM (2010). Understanding resistance to EGFR inhibitors – impact on future treatment strategies. *Nat Rev Clin Oncol*, 7:493–507. http://dx.doi.org/10.1038/nrclinonc.2010.97 PMID:20551942

18. Chapman PB, Hauschild A, Robert C *et al.*; BRIM-3 Study Group (2011). Improved survival with vemurafenib in melanoma with *BRAF* V600E mutation. *N Engl J Med*, 364:2507–2516. http://dx.doi.org/10.1056/NEJMoa1103782 PMID:21639808

19. Anforth R, Fernandez-Peñas P, Long GV (2013). Cutaneous toxicities of RAF inhibitors. *Lancet Oncol*, 14:e11–e18. http://dx.doi.org/10.1016/S1470-2045(12)70413-8 PMID:23276366

20. Kilpivaara O, Aaltonen LA (2013). Diagnostic cancer genome sequencing and the contribution of germline variants. *Science*, 339:1559–1562. http://dx.doi.org/10.1126/science.1233899 PMID:23539595

21. Ley TJ, Mardis ER, Ding L *et al.* (2008). DNA sequencing of a cytogenetically normal acute myeloid leukaemia genome. *Nature*, 456:66–72. http://dx.doi.org/10.1038/nature07485 PMID:18987736

22. Vogelstein B, Papadopoulos N, Velculescu VE *et al.* (2013). Cancer genome landscapes. *Science*, 339:1546–1558. http://dx.doi.org/10.1126/science.1235122 PMID:23539594

23. McLeod HL (2013). Cancer pharmacogenomics: early promise, but concerted effort needed. *Science*, 339:1563–1566. http://dx.doi.org/10.1126/science.1234139 PMID:23539596

24. van't Veer LJ, Bernards R (2008). Enabling personalized cancer medicine through analysis of gene-expression patterns. *Nature*, 452:564–570. http://dx.doi.org/10.1038/nature06915 PMID:18385730

3.9 Immunology and immunotherapy

3 BIOLOGY

Giorgio Trinchieri

Jean-Pierre Abastado (reviewer)

Summary

- Inflammation and immunity affect cancer initiation, progression, dissemination, co-morbidities, and response to therapy. Cancer often originates in chronically inflamed tissue, due to infections or other causes. Tumour-elicited inflammation contributes to progression and dissemination. Cancer incidence is reduced by eliminating the causes of inflammation or by prolonged use of non-steroidal anti-inflammatory drugs.

- Anti-tumour immunity is evident in established tumours and may affect progression negatively or positively. Histological evidence of a brisk immune response is correlated with more favourable prognosis. Tumours, however, use various mechanisms to escape the immune response.

- Tumour immunotherapy protocols have used pro-inflammatory therapies, cytokines, antibodies, adoptive T-cell transfer, and a variety of therapeutic vaccines, with mixed success. Antibodies that block immune checkpoints may prevent tumour immune evasion. When successful, immunotherapy provides more durable remissions than cytotoxic
or targeted therapies, suggesting that combined treatment protocols may prove efficacious.

Cancer cells initially maintain altered morphological and functional characteristics of their tissue of origin, representing almost a caricature of it. The organism does not ignore the growing tumour but reacts to it similarly to the response evoked by tissue damage and, as in wound repair, by establishing a symbiotic relationship that favours tumour growth and dissemination. An adaptive immune response reminiscent of that against foreign pathogens is also often present, with variable effects on tumour growth. Inflammation and immunity likely have an instrumental role in cancer initiation, progression, and dissemination and are also responsible for co-morbidities such as anorexia/cachexia [1] (Fig. 3.9.1).

The study of cancer etiopathogenesis and the identification of therapeutic targets were initially focused on intrinsic cancer cell traits that affect the ability of malignant cells to proliferate and invade local or distant tissues [2]. For a tumour to thus establish itself or form metastases, not only are the transformed cells (the "seed") important, but equally so is the tissue that receives them (the "soil") [3]. Hence, the tumour microenvironment is key, not only as a participant in the neoplastic process but also as a possible therapeutic target [2]. The tumour is a complex organized tissue formed by both the transformed clonal cells and stromal cells. The genetic and epigenetic evolution of successful malignant cells is dependent on their fitness to the microenvironment, resulting in optimal access to nutrients and tissue remodelling. The microenvironment of most tumours is infiltrated by innate and adaptive immune inflammatory cells that influence the survival and adaptation of the transformed cells.

Inflammation and cancer

Chronic inflammation related to bacterial, viral, or parasitic infections has been associated with the etiopathogenesis of about one fifth of cancer cases worldwide, particularly in developing or less-developed countries [4]. Particular pathogens such as *Helicobacter pylori*, human papillomaviruses (HPV), Epstein–Barr virus, and hepatitis B and C viruses account for the majority of those cases. Some of these pathogens, for example HPV or Epstein–Barr virus, directly transform the infected cells, whereas others, such as *H. pylori*, induce tissue inflammation that favours cancer initiation and progression (Fig. 3.9.2). However,

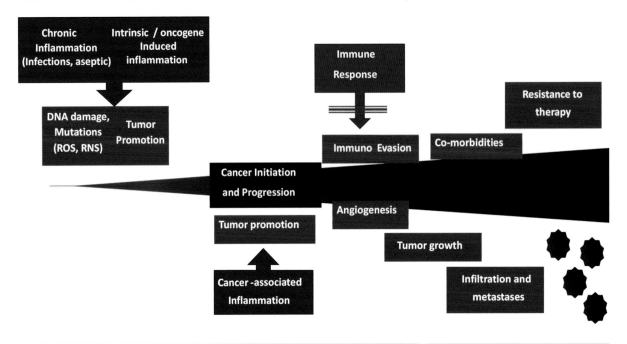

Fig. 3.9.1. The multiple links between inflammation and cancer. With time (left to right), a tumour progresses in size and metastasizes (right). Inflammation (intrinsic in the tissue of tumour origin or induced by the growing tumour, purple) contributes to the mechanisms of tumour induction/progression, co-morbidities, or response to therapy (red). Tumour-specific immune response (blue) generally has an anti-tumour effect, which should be evaded or redirected for the tumour to progress.

the inflammatory response to oncogenic pathogens may also act as a tumour promoter. Cancer resulting from infection can be prevented by prophylactic vaccination, as is the case for HPV and hepatitis B virus, or by antibiotic treatment in the case of *H. pylori*. Early data indicate that HPV vaccines are efficient not only in preventing infections but also in preventing development of precancerous lesions in the cervix and at other anatomical locations [5]. A reduction in the prevalence of *H. pylori* in Caucasian individuals in the USA and other areas of the world has been paralleled by a dramatic decline in stomach cancer incidence, although accompanied by increased incidence of oesophageal adenocarcinoma, which may be associated with concurrent increases in obesity and gastro-oesophageal reflux or with bacterial dysbiosis in the upper digestive tract in the absence of *H. pylori* [6]. The chronic nature of the cancer-inducing infections and the persistence of pathogenic genes in malignant cells suggest the possibility of targeting infection-driven

cancer with post-exposure vaccines to prevent cancer development or with therapeutic vaccine to treat established cancers.

Other cancers, not associated with infection, originate in chronically inflamed tissues injured by chemical or physical agents, such as irradiation or lung-irritating particles, or are dependent on conditions resulting from mutation of digestive enzymes or of inflammatory genes. In the absence of pathogens, altered composition or interaction with the commensal microbiota at the body interfaces may result both locally and systemically in a distorted inflamed state that favours cancer initiation; an example is increased risk of colon cancer in patients with inflammatory bowel diseases characterized by intestinal dysbiosis and chronic inflammation. Intestinal dysbiosis may also mediate increased cancer incidence in obese populations, the pathogenesis of cancer co-morbidities, and chemotherapy side-effects [1].

Infiltrating inflammatory and immune haematopoietic cells charac-

terize inflamed tissue, but epithelial, stromal, and endothelial cells also produce and respond to inflammatory mediators, affecting their proliferation and functions and attracting haematopoietic cells. Activation of oncogenes such as *Ras*, *Myc*, *Ret*, and *Src* is associated with intrinsic inflammation through production of growth factors, cytokines, chemokines, and tissue remodelling enzymes acting on the transformed cells with an autocrine feedback loop, while simultaneously reprogramming the tumour microenvironment and attracting haematopoietic cells and affecting their functional differentiation [7].

Chronic inflammation favours cancer initiation by multiple mechanisms, including genetic and epigenetic instability mediated in part by reactive oxygen species that induce or amplify DNA damage after toxic insults. Inflammation also acts as a tumour promoter by providing growth factors and tissue remodelling factors and by supporting angiogenesis. Once the tumour is established, cancer-induced inflammation, revealed by tumour-

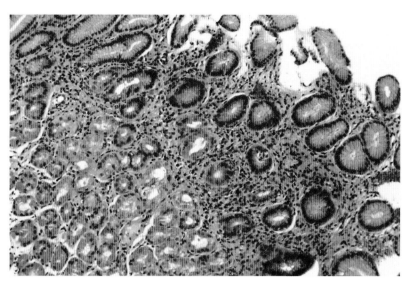

Anti-tumour immunity and immunosurveillance

Tumour cell immunogenicity refers to the ability of tumour cells to express antigens recognized by the immune system. These tumour antigens can be: molecules encoded by cancer-germline genes that tend not to be efficiently presented by central tolerance-inducing medullary thymic epithelial cells; tumour-specific antigenic polypeptides resulting from mutation of key regulatory genes, for example the products of activated oncogenes; oncogenic viral proteins; and molecules selectively overexpressed by tumours, including wild-type p53 [11]. For recognition by T cells, antigenic peptides are presented by major histocompatibility complex (MHC) molecules: class I for CD8 cytotoxic T cells and class II for CD4 helper T cells. Loss of MHC expression prevents tumour immunogenicity, although tumour antigens can be cross-presented by antigen-presenting cells, such as dendritic cells, in the tumour microenvironment. Tumour antigens exposed on the cell surface are recognized by antibodies that may have both anti-tumour and pro-tumour effects (see "Role of the innate and acquired immune systems in mammary development and breast cancer"). Similarly, anti-tumour T-cell-mediated immunity may have variable effects on tumour growth. Certain types of immune response, in particular T helper type 1 (Th1) responses, are generally considered to be anti-tumour, whereas Th2 responses are pro-tumour growth or favourable to metastasis formation [12]. The more recently described Th17 response in different situations may be either pro- or anti-tumour.

Anticancer immunity is evidenced by patients with paraneoplastic neurological degeneration and smouldering tumours in whom neurological disorders are triggered by an antibody response to neuronal antigens expressed on tumour cells [13]. Historically, the presence of lymphocyte infiltrates in tumours has been considered a positive prognostic factor for several tumour types.

associated haematopoietic cells, is a constant in most tumours, including those not known to originate from an inflamed tissue. Tumour-elicited inflammation mediates promotion, facilitates tumour dissemination, and creates an immunosuppressive environment responsible for immune escape [8]. Thus, for example, the oncogene-driven secretion of granulocyte-macrophage colony-stimulating factor (GM-CSF) endows tumour-infiltrating myeloid cells with immunosuppressive activity.

Anti-inflammatory therapies and cancer prevention

Regular use of aspirin or other non-steroidal anti-inflammatory drugs over extended periods decreases cancer incidence and specifically reduces the risk of colorectal cancer or polyp recurrence [9]. Meta-analysis of randomized trials of cardiovascular disease prevention in which patients took aspirin daily for more than 7.5 years indicated that the 20-year risk of cancer death was reduced by 40% for gastrointestinal cancers and by approximately 20% for all solid cancers, including lung, brain, and prostate cancers and melanoma [10]. Non-steroidal anti-inflammatory drugs inhibit the cyclooxygenases COX-1 and COX-2 that catalyse the production of prostaglandins from fatty acids. Drugs like aspirin inhibit both COX-1 and COX-2 and thus are toxic to the stomach and intestinal lining, whereas COX-2 inhibitors do not alter the gastrointestinal homeostasis, although their cardiovascular toxicity has severely limited their use, especially for prophylactic therapies. While cyclooxygenase inhibitors are anti-inflammatory, their preventive effect on cancer may also be due to non-inflammation-related effects of prostaglandins on vasodilation, angiogenesis, DNA mutation rate, epithelial cell adhesion, or apoptosis. At the concentrations used in cardiovascular studies, aspirin inhibits cyclooxygenases but has no effect on major pathways of cancer-related inflammation, such as those downstream of activation of nuclear factor kappa-light-chain-enhancer of activated B cells (NF-κB), which are inhibited only at much higher dosages. The inflammatory pathways hijacked by tumours to promote their own progression are also required for physiological tissue homeostasis, resistance to infections, and response to tissue damage. Targeting these molecular pathways without affecting their physiological roles may be difficult.

Role of the innate and acquired immune systems in mammary development and breast cancer

Zena Werb

The tumour-promoting role of the immune system has long been recognized. Postnatal development of the mammary gland occurs in an immunocompetent environment. In breast cancer, the immune environment is compromised, allowing neoplastic progression and metastasis to proceed. Activation of CD4+ T cells by antigen-presenting cells is evident within the developing mammary gland, and production of interferon-gamma by T helper type 1 (Th1) effector T cells negatively regulates postnatal mammary gland development.

First, the importance of tissue antigen-presenting cells was demonstrated, by depletion of CD11c^high/ MHCII^high mammary antigen-presenting cells in vivo in mice and ex vivo in three-dimensional primary organotypic cultures, which increased ductal invasion and epithelial branching. Second, depletion of α/β T cells, blocking antibodies to MHCII and CD4, and T-cell proliferation assays all suggested that regulation of mammary postnatal organogenesis by antigen-presenting cells and CD4+ T cells is antigen-mediated. The production of interferon-gamma by Th1 effector cells inhibited mammary postnatal organogenesis by acting directly on the mammary luminal epithelial cells. These results suggest a novel regulatory role for the adaptive immune system in normal tissue remodelling, even in the absence of injury or inflammation.

As tumours develop, the inflammatory compartment changes dramatically. Tumour-associated macrophages and antigen-presenting cells and CD11b+Gr1+ cells increase markedly, starting very early before malignant conversion. While the tumour antigen-presenting cells still interact with T cells, the T cells no longer are activated for anti-tumour functions. These myeloid cells also increase in tissues distant from the primary tumour, establishing sites for metastasis. The expansion of inflammatory cells contributes to the events stimulating tumour growth and metastasis. Characterization of the molecular pathways that regulate these populations will lead to identification of pathways and molecules that could be targeted to prevent tumour progression and metastasis.

Reference

Egeblad M et al. (2010). Dev Cell, 18:884–901. http://dx.doi.org/10.1016/j.devcel.2010.05.012 PMID:20627072

In human colon cancer, a particular immune contexture, characterized by a high density of Th1/cytotoxic memory T lymphocytes located both in the centre and at the invasive margin of the primary tumour, is positively correlated with disease-free and overall survival and lower incidence of relapse and metastasis [14], a finding that is being extended to other tumour types. This immunoscore classification distinguishes high- and low-risk patients in both initial and advanced stages of the disease, and it is independent and more informative than conventional staging methods.

The historical concept of immunosurveillance has been more recently defined by studies in experimental animals that have identified major phases of tumour growth regulated by the anti-tumour immune response: elimination of nascent tumours, equilibrium with dormant tumours, editing of progressing tumours, and finally escape and uncontrolled growth [15]. A role for immunosurveillance in humans is indicated by increased cancer incidence in immunosuppressed patients. Such kidney transplant recipients or HIV-infected patients appear to have a strikingly increased risk of tumour types of possible viral etiology. However, epidemiological evidence of an increased risk of other tumour types – such as colon and breast tumours, which have an increased incidence in immunodeficient mice – is less compelling. Immunodeficient mice have increased infections and microbial dysbiosis, and this may compound the effect of lack of immunity on tumour susceptibility. Long-term clinical cancer dormancy is often observed – for example, in survivors of breast cancer and melanoma – and transplantation of organs from these patients into immunosuppressed recipients results in break of dormancy and donor tumour progression. However, the relative contribution of an immune equilibrium compared with the contribution of other homeostatic mechanisms in clinical cancer dormancy remains to be fully defined [16].

Tumour immune escape

Even in the presence of immunity, clinical tumours progress and disseminate; spontaneous regressions are rare. Tumour growth can be attributed in part to the induction of inefficient types of immune response, such as Th2 rather than Th1, and by an immunosuppressive tumour microenvironment. The activity of both effector T and B cells, as well as that of antigen-presenting cells, is depressed in the tumour microenvironment. Tumour immunosuppression is maintained by immunoregulatory cell types, such as regulatory T and B cells, as well as myeloid-derived suppressor cells. Immunosuppressive or anti-inflammatory molecules, such as interleukin-10 (IL-10), vascular endothelial growth factor, transforming growth factor β, IL-4, IL-13, nitric oxide, arginase, and indoleamine

256

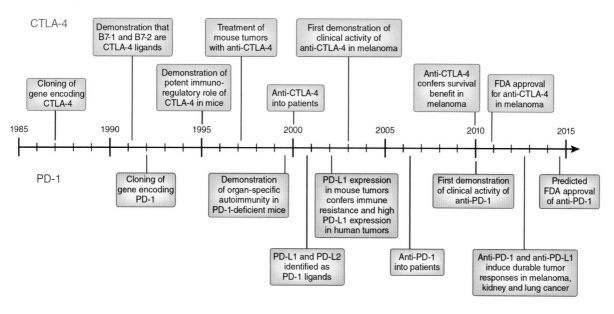

Fig. 3.9.3. Timeline and milestones of the development of therapies involving anti-CTLA-4 and anti-PD-1, from gene discovery to clinical development.

2,3-dioxygenase, are produced in the tumour microenvironment [12].

One of the major mechanisms of tumour escape is the loss or mutation of tumour antigens, as demonstrated experimentally by the immmunoediting of tumour cells in immunocompetent animals, as well as by decreased or lost expression of MHC molecules on the cell surface [15].

Immunity is modulated by a series of co-stimulatory receptor–ligand pairs expressed on antigen-presenting cells and T cells that amplify the T-cell response to antigen–MHC complexes [17]. The CD28/B7 family represents the best example of co-stimulatory molecules. Other members of this family are co-inhibitor molecules – such as, for example, CTLA-4 – that downregulate immune responses when no longer needed. Tumours may escape the immune response by using these receptors and mechanisms involved in the physiological downregulation of the immune response. The programmed cell death 1 (PD1) receptor and its ligand PD-L1 (also called B7-H1) are particularly relevant because PD-L1, unlike B7-1/B7-2, is selectively upregulated on many human tumour cells (Fig. 3.9.3).

Tumour immunotherapy

Since the early attempts of Coley to cure solid tumours with bacterial preparations ("Coley toxin"), investigators have attempted to harness the immune system to reject cancer by stimulating innate resistance or using adaptive immunity for cancer therapy. Various bacterial preparations have been used to induce inflammation and innate resistance, with some positive results, specifically including the use of bacillus Calmette–Guérin (BCG) for the topical treatment of bladder cancer [18]. Granted the role of innate receptors in the inflammatory response to bacterial products, use of Toll-like receptor (TLR) ligands in cancer therapy has been investigated; the TLR7 ligand imiquimod is approved for skin cancer, and the TLR4 ligand monophosphoryl lipid A as an adjuvant in a HPV vaccine.

Many pro-inflammatory cytokines have shown promise in experimental animals but have proven ineffective or highly toxic in clinical trials. Type I interferon and IL-2 are approved as single agents for cancer therapy. Interferon is approved for adjuvant therapy of melanoma and for the treatment of certain haematopoietic malignancies, of Kaposi sarcoma, and, in combination with anti-angiogenic compounds, of renal cancer. With the development of targeted therapies, the use of interferon for melanoma has been declining. IL-2 is approved for advanced melanoma and renal cell carcinoma. Other immunoregulatory cytokines that affect T-cell expansion and activation, such as IL-7, IL-12, and IL-15, are being clinically tested, alone or as part of immune-enhancing therapy. Granulocyte colony-stimulating factor and GM-CSF are approved to shorten the time to neutrophil recovery and reduce the incidence of infections after cancer chemotherapy.

Immunotherapy based on the adoptive transfer of either naturally occurring tumour-infiltrating T cells or T cells engineered to express genes encoding well-defined antitumour T-cell receptors or designed chimeric receptors mediate tumour regression in a large proportion of patients with metastatic cancer, particularly when infused after lymphodepletion [19]. Current efforts are focused on increasing the accuracy of targeting tumour antigens and the associated vasculature, as well as on identification and purification of T-cell subsets that are more efficient in expanding and mediating tumour eradication.

Since the development of monoclonal antibody technology, great effort has been devoted to using antibodies in cancer therapy [20]. Therapeutic antibodies can be directed against surface antigens selectively expressed on tumour cells. These antibodies induce tumour cell death by antibody-dependent cell-mediated cytotoxicity, recruiting effector cells such as natural killer cells and macrophages via binding of the Fc portion of the immunoglobulin G antibodies to Fc receptors expressed on effector cells. The cytotoxic effect can be amplified by conjugating radioisotopes, cytotoxic drugs, or toxins to the antibody. Alternatively, cell-mediated cytotoxicity can be facilitated by chimeric antibodies combining specificity for tumour antigens with specificity for activating receptors on immune cells, thus cross-linking tumour and effector cells while activating cytotoxic mechanisms. Unconjugated anti-CD20 and anti-CD5 antibodies and radioisotope- or ozogamicin-conjugated anti-CD20 and anti-CD33 antibodies are approved for haematopoietic malignancies, and unconjugated anti-HER2 antibodies for breast cancer. Another mechanism of action of antibodies in cancer is the functional inhibition of growth factor receptors or pro-tumour factors. Anti-epithelial growth factor receptor and anti-vascular endothelial growth factor unconjugated antibodies are approved for colorectal cancer and other solid tumours.

Unlike the success of prophylactic vaccines against oncogenic viruses, efficient therapeutic vaccines able to induce an immune response against established tumours have been difficult to develop. Although knowledge of the mechanisms of tumour immunity has been extensively applied in both experimental and clinical trials, clinical responses to tested cancer vaccines have been modest, and T-cell-mediated anti-tumour immunity elicited by vaccines was followed by clinical response in only a minority of patients [19]. Different formulations of antigens and adjuvants, including gene-based vaccination, have been used to harness the immunostimulatory ability of dendritic cells, either by adoptively transferring them after in vitro activation and exposure to tumour antigens or by targeting them in vivo with tumour antigen-conjugated antibodies directed against their surface receptors [21]. Sipuleucel-T, the only approved vaccine for metastatic hormone-independent prostate cancer, has in clinical trials significantly but modestly increased survival by approximately 4 months [19]. Sipuleucel-T is prepared by exposing the patient's dendritic cells to a fusion protein containing GM-CSF and the antigen prostatic acid phosphatase.

The poor efficacy of cancer vaccines is probably due to persistence of an immunosuppressive tumour microenvironment, which prevents the development of the anti-tumour response [18]. Immunosuppression might be reversed by developing better adjuvants or by blocking immunosuppressive factors, such as transforming growth factor β, indoleamine 2,3-dioxygenase, or IL-10. Use of antibodies that block co-inhibitory molecules has

Fig. 3.9.4. Generation and regulation of anti-tumour immunity. Active cancer immunotherapy may target antigen presentation at the level of dendritic cells, promote generation of anticancer T cells, and reverse the immunosuppressive mechanisms of the tumour microenvironment. The dendritic cells that have captured tumour antigens from dead or dying tumour cells (A) migrate to the draining lymph nodes, where they present captured antigenic peptides on major histocompatibility complex (MHC) class II and class I molecules to T cells (B), inducing an anticancer effector T-cell response if immunogenic maturation stimuli are present (C) or alternatively, in their absence, inducing tolerance and immunosuppression (D). Depending on the maturation stimulus, dendritic cells will differentially express co-stimulatory molecules and produce immunoregulatory cytokines, affecting the quality and the class of the T-cell response. Interaction of CD28 or OX40 with B7-1/B7-2 or OX40L favours protective T-cell responses, whereas interaction of CTLA-4 with B7-1/B7-2 or of PD-1 with PD-L1/PD-L2 will suppress T-cell responses. Effector T cells will re-enter the tumour microenvironment (E), where their anticancer ability will be limited by immunosuppressive mechanisms that include upregulation of PD-L1/PD-L2 on the cancer cell surface and release of IL-10, vascular endothelial growth factor, transforming growth factor β, IL-4, IL-13, nitric oxide, arginase, and indoleamine 2,3-dioxygenase. NK, natural killer cell; T$_{reg}$, regulatory T cell.

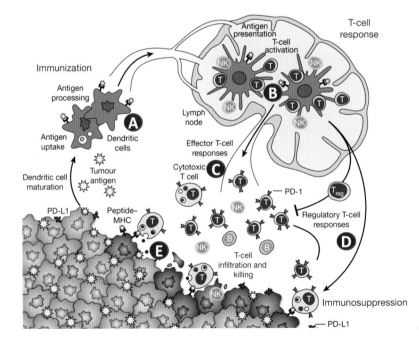

Premortem autophagy and endoplasmic reticulum stress as immunogenic signals in cancer therapy

Guido Kroemer

The ultimate goal of anticancer therapy is the induction of tumour cell death. Physiological cell death, which occurs as a continuous by-product of cellular turnover, is non-immunogenic or even tolerogenic, thereby avoiding autoimmunity. However, cancer cell death elicited by radiotherapy and some chemotherapeutic agents, such as anthracyclines and oxaliplatin, can be immunogenic. Immunogenic death involves changes in the composition of the cell surface, as well as the release of soluble immunogenic signals that occur in a defined temporal sequence. This "key" then operates on a series of receptors expressed by dendritic cells (the "lock") to allow for the presentation of tumour antigens to T cells and for the initiation of a productive immune response. Immunogenic cell death is characterized by the early cell-surface exposure of calreticulin, which determines the uptake of tumour antigens by dendritic cells. The late release of the high-mobility group box 1 protein, which acts on Toll-like receptor 4, is required for the presentation of antigens from dying tumour cells. In addition, the release of ATP from dying cells causes the P2RX7 purinergic receptor-dependent activation of the NLRP3 inflammasome in dendritic cells, thereby allowing them to release interleukin-1β and to polarize tumour antigen-specific CD8 T cells towards a Tc1 cytokine pattern.

It may be hypothesized that the immune system determines the long-term success of anticancer therapies and that this immune response is dictated by immunogenic tumour cell death. Thus, therapeutic failure can result from failure to undergo immunogenic cell death (rather than cell death as such). Agents that fail to induce immunogenic cell death cannot yield a long-term success in cancer therapy. Moreover, tumours that are intrinsically unable to undergo immunogenic cell death are incurable. Importantly, it appears that mitochondrial events determine whether cancer cells die in response to chemotherapy, while an endoplasmic reticulum stress response combined with autophagy determines whether this cell death is perceived as immunogenic. Strategies may be developed to restore the immunogenicity of cell death in the context of deficient autophagy or endoplasmic reticulum stress.

Reference

Senovilla L *et al.* (2012). *Science*, 337: 1678–1684. http://dx.doi.org/10.1126/science. 1224922 PMID:23019653

promise. The monoclonal antibody to CTLA-4 (ipilimumab) is approved for use in patients with metastatic melanoma; increased survival is reasonably attributable to amplification of the endogenous anti-tumour T-cell response (Fig. 3.9.4). In several clinical trials, antibodies against PD1 receptor or its ligand PD-L1 are showing significant responses in patients with melanoma or other solid tumours, such as lung cancer [17]. These new drugs may amplify the anti-tumour immune response elicited by cancer vaccines or the endogenous immune response induced after tumour destruction by certain therapies, resulting in clinical benefit. A downside of any therapy that increases anti-tumour immunity by reversing physiological immune checkpoints is that regulation of self-tolerance and antimicrobial resistance are also affected, with possible autoimmune and inflammatory side-effects.

Combination of chemotherapy, targeted therapy, and immunotherapy

Cytotoxic agents have underpinned cancer therapy. Increasingly, agents that specifically target molecular pathways underlying malignant transformation have been developed (see Chapter 3.8). Both cytotoxic and targeted drugs may adversely affect the anticancer immune response. However, in experimental animals, certain drugs, including some widely used chemotherapy compounds, induce immunogenic cell death, which favours generation of a tumour-specific immune response able to eradicate or delay tumour progression. Immunogenic cell death is characterized by expression of endogenous activators of inflammation – surface exposure of the endoplasmic reticulum protein calreticulin, and release of ATP and high-mobility group box 1 protein – resulting in effective cross-presentation of tumour antigens and protective anticancer immunity [22] (see "Premortem autophagy and endoplasmic reticulum stress as immunogenic signals in cancer therapy"). In addition, certain chemotherapeutic agents induce the intratumour expression of T-cell-attracting chemokines [23].

Combination of non-specific or targeted tumour therapies with immunotherapy approaches may provide successful cancer therapy. Although cytotoxic and targeted therapies are effective, clinical responses are often temporary. Experimental and clinical evidence suggests that immunotherapy, when successful, provides durable responses or even tumour eradication [18]. Immunity may be able to destroy cancer stem cells that are unresponsive to standard or targeted therapies. While cytotoxic or targeted therapy may select tumour cells that became insensitive or had mutations in the targeted genes, strong anticancer immunity may destroy a small proportion of mutated cells present within the antigenic tumours. Anti-tumour immunity not only mediates direct cytotoxicity of antigenic tumour cells but also activates humoral and cellular inflammatory mechanisms that damage tumour cells as well as their microenvironment, stroma, and vasculature by cross-presentation of tumour antigen on stromal antigen-presenting cells. Progress in understanding these mechanisms will define optimal clinical protocols that combine different therapeutic approaches with immunotherapy.

References

1. Trinchieri G (2012). Cancer and inflammation: an old intuition with rapidly evolving new concepts. *Annu Rev Immunol*, 30:677–706. http://dx.doi.org/10.1146/annurev-immunol-020711-075008 PMID:22224761

2. Hanahan D, Weinberg RA (2011). Hallmarks of cancer: the next generation. *Cell*, 144:646–674. http://dx.doi.org/10.1016/j.cell.2011.02.013 PMID:21376230

3. Fidler IJ (2003). The pathogenesis of cancer metastasis: the 'seed and soil' hypothesis revisited. *Nat Rev Cancer*, 3:453–458. http://dx.doi.org/10.1038/nrc1098 PMID:12778135

4. de Martel C, Ferlay J, Franceschi S *et al.* (2012). Global burden of cancers attributable to infections in 2008: a review and synthetic analysis. *Lancet Oncol*, 13:607–615. http://dx.doi.org/10.1016/S1470-2045(12)70137-7 PMID:22575588

5. Lowy DR, Schiller JT (2012). Reducing HPV-associated cancer globally. *Cancer Prev Res (Phila)*, 5:18–23. http://dx.doi.org/10.1158/1940-6207.CAPR-11-0542 PMID:22219162

6. Atherton JC, Blaser MJ (2009). Coadaptation of *Helicobacter pylori* and humans: ancient history, modern implications. *J Clin Invest*, 119:2475–2487. http://dx.doi.org/10.1172/JCI38605 PMID:19729845

7. Mantovani A, Allavena P, Sica A, Balkwill F (2008). Cancer-related inflammation. *Nature*, 454:436–444. http://dx.doi.org/10.1038/nature07205 PMID:18650914

8. Grivennikov SI, Greten FR, Karin M (2010). Immunity, inflammation, and cancer. *Cell*, 140:883–899. http://dx.doi.org/10.1016/j.cell.2010.01.025 PMID:20303878

9. Wang D, Dubois RN (2010). Eicosanoids and cancer. *Nat Rev Cancer*, 10:181–193. http://dx.doi.org/10.1038/nrc2809 PMID:20168319

10. Rothwell PM (2013). Aspirin in prevention of sporadic colorectal cancer: current clinical evidence and overall balance of risks and benefits. *Recent Results Cancer Res*, 191:121–142. http://dx.doi.org/10.1007/978-3-642-30331-9_7 PMID:22893203

11. Blankenstein T, Coulie PG, Gilboa E, Jaffee EM (2012). The determinants of tumour immunogenicity. *Nat Rev Cancer*, 12:307–313. http://dx.doi.org/10.1038/nrc3246 PMID:22378190

12. Coussens LM, Zitvogel L, Palucka AK (2013). Neutralizing tumor-promoting chronic inflammation: a magic bullet? *Science*, 339:286–291. http://dx.doi.org/10.1126/science.1232227 PMID:23329041

13. Albert ML, Darnell RB (2004). Paraneoplastic neurological degenerations: keys to tumour immunity. *Nat Rev Cancer*, 4:36–44. http://dx.doi.org/10.1038/nrc1255 PMID:14708025

14. Fridman WH, Pagès F, Sautès-Fridman C, Galon J (2012). The immune contexture in human tumours: impact on clinical outcome. *Nat Rev Cancer*, 12:298–306. http://dx.doi.org/10.1038/nrc3245 PMID:22419253

15. Schreiber RD, Old LJ, Smyth MJ (2011). Cancer immunoediting: integrating immunity's roles in cancer suppression and promotion. *Science*, 331:1565–1570. http://dx.doi.org/10.1126/science.1203486 PMID:21436444

16. Uhr JW, Pantel K (2011). Controversies in clinical cancer dormancy. *Proc Natl Acad Sci U S A*, 108:12396–12400. http://dx.doi.org/10.1073/pnas.1106613108 PMID:21746894

17. Pardoll DM (2012). Immunology beats cancer: a blueprint for successful translation. *Nat Immunol*, 13:1129–1132. http://dx.doi.org/10.1038/ni.2392 PMID:23160205

18. Mellman I, Coukos G, Dranoff G (2011). Cancer immunotherapy comes of age. *Nature*, 480:480–489. http://dx.doi.org/10.1038/nature10673 PMID:22193102

19. Restifo NP, Dudley ME, Rosenberg SA (2012). Adoptive immunotherapy for cancer: harnessing the T cell response. *Nat Rev Immunol*, 12:269–281. http://dx.doi.org/10.1038/nri3191 PMID:22437939

20. Weiner LM, Surana R, Wang S (2010). Monoclonal antibodies: versatile platforms for cancer immunotherapy. *Nat Rev Immunol*, 10:317–327. http://dx.doi.org/10.1038/nri2744 PMID:20414205

21. Palucka K, Banchereau J (2012). Cancer immunotherapy via dendritic cells. *Nat Rev Cancer*, 12:265–277. http://dx.doi.org/10.1038/nrc3258 PMID:22437871

22. Zitvogel L, Kepp O, Kroemer G (2011). Immune parameters affecting the efficacy of chemotherapeutic regimens. *Nat Rev Clin Oncol*, 8:151–160. http://dx.doi.org/10.1038/nrclinonc.2010.223 PMID:21364688

23. Abastado JP (2012). The next challenge in cancer immunotherapy: controlling T-cell traffic to the tumor. *Cancer Res*, 72:2159–2161. http://dx.doi.org/10.1158/0008-5472.CAN-11-3538 PMID:22549945

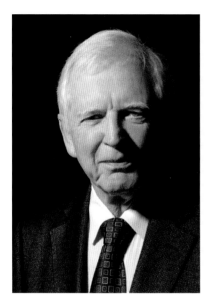

Harald zur Hausen
in collaboration with Ethel-Michele de Villiers

Prenatal infections with subsequent immune tolerance could explain the epidemiology of common childhood cancers

Harald zur Hausen has devoted his scientific life to investigating to what extent infectious agents contribute to human cancer. He was awarded the Nobel Prize in Physiology or Medicine 2008 for his research demonstrating that human papillomavirus (HPV) causes cervical cancer and for the identification of the high-risk types of HPV. His work has resulted in improved screening and treatment of cervical cancer and has paved the way for the development of vaccines against high-risk HPV. Dr zur Hausen studied medicine at the Universities of Bonn, Hamburg, and Düsseldorf. He was a researcher and professor at the University of Würzburg, the University of Erlangen-Nürnberg, and the University of Freiburg, and he served as the scientific director of the German Cancer Research Center (Deutsches Krebsforschungszentrum) from 1983 to 2003. Dr zur Hausen's contributions to the field of virology have informed our understanding of the connections between infections and chronic diseases.

Summary

This Perspective summarizes sets of epidemiological data on early childhood tumours favouring their etiology as a result of interactions between specific host-cell chromosomal modifications and infectious events. This is discussed mainly for acute lymphoblastic leukaemia but also for neuroblastomas and brain tumours. In contrast to the majority of previous publications, this report underlines evidence in support of a prenatal infection, resulting in immune tolerance for the infecting agent. Episomally persisting single-stranded DNA viruses with a circular genome are discussed as potential candidates. Prenatal infections have been documented for torque teno (TT) viruses. They are widespread in all human populations, replicate in cells of bone marrow and the peripheral blood, and respond to interferon treatment. Thus far, in part due to the type heterogeneity of this virus family, no follow-up studies are available demonstrating induction of immune tolerance in cases of prenatal infections.

If we include the approximately 10% of gastric cancers linked to Epstein–Barr virus infections and the increasing percentage of head and neck cancers linked to high-risk human papillomavirus (HPV) infections, then slightly more than 20% of the global cancer incidence can be linked to infectious events [1]. Many of the existing links were originally identified based on epidemiological observations. This poses an interesting question: can we identify malignant disorders where epidemiological data may point to an infectious origin, although no convincing supportive evidence has thus far been obtained by different approaches? Cancers that could be considered from this perspective have been discussed before [2].

Particular childhood malignancies

This Perspective will concentrate on a specific set of childhood malignancies: acute lymphoblastic leukaemia (ALL), neuroblastomas, and central nervous system (CNS) cancers, with some sidestepping to acute myeloid leukaemia (AML) and Hodgkin disease. None of the malignancies discussed here has been consistently connected to infectious disorders, except for Hodgkin disease, where 25–35% of cases in developed countries have been linked to Epstein–Barr virus infections. Since the majority of epidemiological studies have analysed ALL data, this cancer will be specifically emphasized.

At least two events contribute to ALL development, according to prevailing views: chromosomal modifications acquired during the fetal period and an additional postnatal event, commonly discussed as an unspecified infection [3–6]. Specific chromosomal translocations, for example *TEL-AML* and t(11;19)(q23;p13), have been documented for the prenatal period [7] (reviewed in [8]). They occur, however, "at a substantially higher frequency (~100×) before birth than the cumulative incidence or risk of disease, reflecting the requirement for complementary and secondary genetic events that occur postnatally" [8], and they are thus not sufficient to cause leukaemia [9].

This Perspective summarizes sets of epidemiological data favouring the interaction of specific molecular modifications with an infectious event. In contrast to the majority of previous publications, it underlines evidence in support of a prenatal infection, resulting in immune tolerance for the infecting agent.

Infections that mediate protection

During the past decades, several reports have described a protective effect of multiple infections during early childhood for ALL (reviewed in [10], [11]), neuroblastomas [12–14], CNS cancers [15], and Hodgkin disease [16,17]. Only a few studies have failed to confirm these observations for leukaemias (reviewed in [10], [11]). Some publications referred to a higher risk of ALL development after maternal infections during pregnancy (reviewed in [10]). Early immunization against *Haemophilus influenzae* type b seems to reduce the risk of ALL [18,19]. Even human leukocyte antigen (HLA) haplotype may influence ALL susceptibility [20,21]. Interestingly, about 2% of childhood cancers are present at the time of delivery. Neuroblastomas are the most frequent connatal malignancy among the tumours discussed here, followed by CNS tumours and leukaemias (reviewed in [22]).

Attendance at day-care centres, number of siblings, and less breastfeeding during the first year of life have been implicated as surrogate markers for multiple infections and for the likelihood of childhood infection. Breastfeeding for more than 6 months has been repeatedly reported as a protective factor for ALL development (see reviews in [10], [11]). The protective role of communicative contacts is well documented by the lower risk for subsequent siblings compared with the first-born child in a pooled analysis from five states in the USA [13]. In addition, allergies acquired during the first year of life have been identified as protective factors. Most studies to date have reported an inverse association between allergies and childhood leukaemia (reviewed in [23]).

Thus far, protective factors for ALL, and to a more limited degree for neuroblastomas and CNS tumours, have been discussed. Several risk factors can also be clearly identified; they concern, in particular, a high socioeconomic status and a protected environment. The rate of ALL is clearly higher in countries with high standards of living than in poorer societies [24]. As an overriding risk factor, however, were considered molecular changes, specifically chromosomal translocations, occurring during the intrauterine phase of life [4–8,25]. These observations soon led to the conclusion that ALL arises in utero already, although it has quickly been recognized that genetic modifications are not sufficient for leukaemia development [8,9]. It became a common postulate that, as the regular course, first a genetic event occurs during the fetal period, followed by a second one, possibly an infection, during the postnatal phase.

Specific predictions

If infections are involved in the etiology of those childhood cancers discussed here, the occurrence of connatal neuroblastomas, CNS tumours, and ALL would be an indication for prenatal (fetal) infections with a high likelihood of interaction with specific chromosomal

modifications. Prenatal infections with subsequent postnatal persistence will result in acceptance of the respective antigens by the immune system of the carrier, and thus in immune tolerance [26–28]. Anticipating prenatal infections and a resulting immune tolerance of the persisting agent, several predictions can be made:

- The respective tumours should not increase under conditions of immunosuppression (in organ allograft recipients and persons with HIV infection);
- The agent should retain its susceptibility to antiviral cytokines (e.g. interferons);
- Interferon-inducing nonspecific infections should negatively interfere with the suspected infection;
- Interferon-inducing allergic conditions should also negatively interfere with the suspected infection;
- Interferon that is present in breast milk should also have protective properties;
- Conditions that avoid multiple infections in early childhood should increase the risk for these tumours;
- The cancer risk for the first-born child (with a reduced risk for early childhood infections) should be higher than that for subsequent siblings (with a higher risk for communicative infections);
- Prenatal chromosomal modifications have been identified as risk factors but not as sufficient for cancer induction; thus, there should be a syncarcinogenic interaction between these modifications and the respective infection.

Immune tolerance has not yet been proven for antigens in the tumours discussed here. In case it exists for antigens of potentially oncogenic agents, it is anticipated that immunosuppression should not favour an enhanced outgrowth of the respective tumour type. However, antiviral cytokines (e.g. interferon-gamma), whose synthesis is not exclusively controlled by the lymphatic system, should retain a broad function in antiviral defence [29]. Similarly, nonspecific infections leading to interferon synthesis should interact protectively. In this respect it seems to be interesting that enhanced interferon-gamma synthesis has been described for allergic conditions [30–33] and was also demonstrated in human breast milk for extended breastfeeding periods [34–37].

The major risk factors are obviously specific chromosomal translocations and gene modifications, which, as discussed before, clearly emerge as risk factors but are not sufficient to trigger malignant growth. The other major predisposing factor for the tumour types analysed here appears to be the absence of multiple infections during the first year of life, lack of many communicative contacts, and an environment not exposing the infant to conditions of poor hygiene.

If we take prenatal infection and resulting immune tolerance for granted, all these data are readily compatible with a model we proposed in 2005 [38]. It is shown, with some minor modifications, in Fig. P3.1. If "Peri- and postnatal respiratory infections" is replaced by "Interferon-gamma production due to allergic conditions or prolonged breastfeeding", the basic features of the scheme remain unaltered.

Prenatal infections implicated

Do prenatal infections exist that would fit into this picture? Obviously several infections have been identified as occurring during fetal life, among them cytomegalovirus and rubella infections, in part with grave consequences for the developing fetus. If we analyse, however, those infections that would fit into the criteria outlined here, very few of the identified agents would remain. Besides vertical transmission, additional properties should be subsequent development

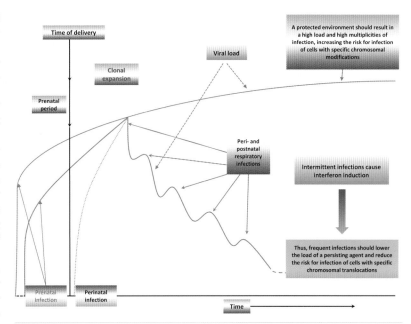

Fig. P3.1. The target cell conditioning model based on prenatal or perinatal torque teno (TT) virus-like infections. Transplacental as well as perinatal infections should lead to virus persistence and an increasing viral load. Multiple intermittent infections with interferon-inducing agents should reduce the viral load substantially and thus decrease the risk for virus-induced chromosomal modifications.

of immune tolerance, replication or effective persistence within the precursor cells of ALL and possibly the other cancers discussed here, and finally responsiveness to interferon. Polyomaviruses and anelloviruses (torque teno [TT] viruses) emerge as potential candidates [11,38].

Particularly anelloviruses seem to represent promising candidates. Vertical transmission of TT virus DNA has been demonstrated by detection in umbilical cord blood [39–41]. These viruses replicate in mononuclear cells of bone marrow and the peripheral blood [42–44] and, as shown by interferon treatment of hepatitis C virus carriers, they respond well to interferon treatment [45–47]. The question of whether these viruses induce immune tolerance after prenatal infections remains open and is

currently difficult to study in view of their remarkable heterogeneity. Their analysis is being complicated by observations of frequent intragenomic rearrangements, resulting in novel open reading frames [48,49]. A synergistic function with specific cellular genetic modifications still requires further investigation.

It would be difficult, if not impossible, to reconcile a chain of mutational events with the published epidemiological data available concerning the etiology of the tumours discussed here. A prenatal infection with resulting immune tolerance, however, acting syncarcinogenically with cellular gene modifications, seems to be in line with all epidemiological observations thus far reported. Virological studies, however, have not yet led to the identification of responsible infectious factors.

References

1. zur Hausen H (2006). *Infections Causing Human Cancer.* Weinheim, Germany: Wiley. http://dx.doi.org/10.1002/3527609318

2. zur Hausen H (2009). The search for infectious causes of human cancers: where and why. *Virology*, 392:1–10. http://dx.doi.org/10.1016/j.virol.2009.06.001 PMID:19720205

3. Greaves MF, Alexander FE (1993). An infectious etiology for common acute lymphoblastic leukemia in childhood? *Leukemia*, 7:349–360. PMID:8445941

4. Greaves M (1999). Molecular genetics, natural history and the demise of childhood leukaemia [Review]. *Eur J Cancer*, 35:1941–1953. http://dx.doi.org/10.1016/S0959-8049(99)00296-8 PMID:10711237

5. Taub JW, Ge Y (2004). The prenatal origin of childhood acute lymphoblastic leukemia. *Leuk Lymphoma*, 45:19–25. http://dx.doi.org/10.1080/1042819031000149403 PMID:15061193

6. Kim AS, Eastmond DA, Preston RJ (2006). Childhood acute lymphocytic leukemia and perspectives on risk assessment of early-life stage exposures. *Mutat Res*, 613:138–160. http://dx.doi.org/10.1016/j.mrrev.2006.09.001 PMID:17049456

7. Mahmoud HH, Ridge SA, Behm FG *et al.* (1995). Intrauterine monoclonal origin of neonatal concordant acute lymphoblastic leukemia in monozygotic twins. *Med Pediatr Oncol*, 24:77–81. http://dx.doi.org/10.1002/mpo.2950240203 PMID:7990767

8. Greaves M (2005). In utero origins of childhood leukaemia. *Early Hum Dev*, 81:123–129. http://dx.doi.org/10.1016/j.earlhumdev.2004.10.004 PMID:15707724

9. Greaves MF, Wiemels J (2003). Origins of chromosome translocations in childhood leukaemia. *Nat Rev Cancer*, 3:639–649. http://dx.doi.org/10.1038/nrc1164 PMID:12951583

10. O'Connor SM, Boneva RS (2007). Infectious etiologies of childhood leukemia: plausibility and challenges to proof. *Environ Health Perspect*, 115:146–150. http://dx.doi.org/10.1289/ehp.9024 PMID:17366835

11. zur Hausen H (2009). Childhood leukemias and other hematopoietic malignancies: interdependence between an infectious event and chromosomal modifications. *Int J Cancer*, 125:1764–1770. http://dx.doi.org/10.1002/ijc.24365 PMID:19330827

12. Menegaux F, Olshan AF, Neglia JP *et al.* (2004). Day care, childhood infections, and risk of neuroblastoma. *Am J Epidemiol*, 159:843–851. http://dx.doi.org/10.1093/aje/kwh111 PMID:15105177

13. Von Behren J, Spector LG, Mueller BA *et al.* (2011). Birth order and risk of childhood cancer: a pooled analysis from five US States. *Int J Cancer*, 128:2709–2716. http://dx.doi.org/10.1002/ijc.25593 PMID:20715170

14. Maule MM, Zuccolo L, Magnani C *et al.* (2006). Bayesian methods for early detection of changes in childhood cancer incidence: trends for acute lymphoblastic leukaemia are consistent with an infectious aetiology. *Eur J Cancer*, 42:78–83. http://dx.doi.org/10.1016/j.ejca.2005.07.028 PMID:16324832

15. Altieri A, Castro F, Bermejo JL, Hemminki K (2006). Association between number of siblings and nervous system tumors suggests an infectious etiology. *Neurology*, 67:1979–1983. http://dx.doi.org/10.1212/01.wnl.0000247036.98444.38 PMID:17159104

16. Paffenbarger RS Jr, Wing AL, Hyde RT (1977). Characteristics in youth indicative of adult-onset Hodgkin's disease. *J Natl Cancer Inst*, 58:1489–1491. PMID:857036

17. Roman E, Ansell P, Bull D (1997). Leukaemia and non-Hodgkin's lymphoma in children and young adults: are prenatal and neonatal factors important determinants of disease? *Br J Cancer*, 76:406–415. http://dx.doi.org/10.1038/bjc.1997.399 PMID:9252212

18. Groves FD, Gridley G, Wacholder S *et al.* (1999). Infant vaccinations and risk of childhood acute lymphoblastic leukaemia in the USA. *Br J Cancer*, 81:175–178. http://dx.doi.org/10.1038/sj.bjc.6690668 PMID:10487630

19. Groves F, Auvinen A, Hakulinen T (2000). *Haemophilus influenzae* type b vaccination and risk of childhood leukemia in a vaccine trial in Finland [Abstract]. *Ann Epidemiol*, 10:474. http://dx.doi.org/10.1016/S1047-2797(00)00110-1 PMID:11018411

20. Dorak MT, Oguz FS, Yalman N *et al.* (2002). A male-specific increase in the HLA-DRB4 (DR53) frequency in high-risk and relapsed childhood ALL. *Leuk Res*, 26:651–656. http://dx.doi.org/10.1016/S0145-2126(01)00189-8 PMID:12008082

21. Taylor GM, Dearden S, Payne N *et al.* (1998). Evidence that an *HLA-DQA1-DQB1* haplotype influences susceptibility to childhood common acute lymphoblastic leukaemia in boys provides further support for an infection-related aetiology. *Br J Cancer*, 78:561–565. http://dx.doi.org/10.1038/bjc.1998.540 PMID:9744491

22. Moore SW, Satgé D, Sasco AJ *et al.* (2003). The epidemiology of neonatal tumours. Report of an international working group. *Pediatr Surg Int*, 19:509–519. http://dx.doi.org/10.1007/s00383-003-1048-8 PMID:14523568

23. Chang JS, Wiemels JL, Buffler PA (2009). Allergies and childhood leukemia. *Blood Cells Mol Dis*, 42:99–104. http://dx.doi.org/10.1016/j.bcmd.2008.10.003 PMID:19049852

24. Pisani P, Parkin DM, Bray F, Ferlay J (1999). Estimates of the worldwide mortality from 25 cancers in 1990. *Int J Cancer*, 83:18–29. http://dx.doi.org/10.1002/(SICI)1097-0215(19990924)83:1<18::AID-IJC5>3.0.CO;2-M PMID:10449602

25. Gruhn B, Taub JW, Ge Y *et al.* (2008). Prenatal origin of childhood acute lymphoblastic leukemia, association with birth weight and hyperdiploidy. *Leukemia*, 22:1692–1697. http://dx.doi.org/10.1038/leu.2008.152 PMID:18548099

26. Jamieson BD, Ahmed R (1988). T-cell tolerance: exposure to virus in utero does not cause a permanent deletion of specific T cells. *Proc Natl Acad Sci U S A*, 85:2265–2268. http://dx.doi.org/10.1073/pnas.85.7.2265 PMID:3258424

27. Dietert RR (2009). Developmental immunotoxicity (DIT), postnatal immune dysfunction and childhood leukemia [Review]. *Blood Cells Mol Dis*, 42:108–112. http://dx.doi.org/10.1016/j.bcmd.2008.10.005 PMID:19019708

28. Malhotra I, Dent A, Mungai P *et al.* (2009). Can prenatal malaria exposure produce an immune tolerant phenotype? A prospective birth cohort study in Kenya. *PLoS Med*, 6:e1000116. http://dx.doi.org/10.1371/journal.pmed.1000116 PMID:19636353

29. Hara T, Ohashi S, Yamashita Y *et al.* (1996). Human V delta 2+ gamma delta T-cell tolerance to foreign antigens of *Toxoplasma gondii*. *Proc Natl Acad Sci U S A*, 93:5136–5140. http://dx.doi.org/10.1073/pnas.93.10.5136 PMID:8643541

30. Smart JM, Horak E, Kemp AS *et al.* (2002). Polyclonal and allergen-induced cytokine responses in adults with asthma: resolution of asthma is associated with normalization of IFN-gamma responses. *J Allergy Clin Immunol*, 110:450–456. http://dx.doi.org/10.1067/mai.2002.127283 PMID:12209093

31. Brown V, Warke TJ, Shields MD, Ennis M (2003). T cell cytokine profiles in childhood asthma. *Thorax*, 58:311–316. http://dx.doi.org/10.1136/thorax.58.4.311 PMID:12668793

32. Friedlander SL, Jackson DJ, Gangnon RE *et al.* (2005). Viral infections, cytokine dysregulation and the origins of childhood asthma and allergic diseases. *Pediatr Infect Dis J*, 24 Suppl:S170–S176, discussion S174–S175. PMID:16378042

33. Simon D, Braathen LR, Simon HU (2007). Increased lipopolysaccharide-induced tumour necrosis factor-alpha, interferon-gamma and interleukin-10 production in atopic dermatitis. *Br J Dermatol*, 157:583–586. http://dx.doi.org/10.1111/j.1365-2133.2007.08050.x PMID:17596153

34. Daniels JL, Olshan AF, Pollock BH *et al.* (2002). Breast-feeding and neuroblastoma, USA and Canada. *Cancer Causes Control*, 13:401–405. http://dx.doi.org/10.1023/A:1015746701922 PMID:12146844

35. Kwan ML, Buffler PA, Abrams B, Kiley VA (2004). Breastfeeding and the risk of childhood leukemia: a meta-analysis. *Public Health Rep*, 119:521–535. http://dx.doi.org/10.1016/j.phr.2004.09.002 PMID:15504444

36. Martin RM, Gunnell D, Owen CG, Smith GD (2005). Breast-feeding and childhood cancer: a systematic review with metaanalysis. *Int J Cancer*, 117:1020–1031. http://dx.doi.org/10.1002/ijc.21274 PMID:15986434

37. Tomicić S, Johansson G, Voor T *et al.* (2010). Breast milk cytokine and IgA composition differ in Estonian and Swedish mothers–relationship to microbial pressure and infant allergy. *Pediatr Res*, 68:330–334. http://dx.doi.org/10.1203/PDR.0b013e3181ee049d PMID:20581738

38. zur Hausen H, de Villiers EM (2005). Virus target cell conditioning model to explain some epidemiologic characteristics of childhood leukemias and lymphomas. *Int J Cancer*, 115:1–5. http://dx.doi.org/10.1002/ijc.20905 PMID:15688417

39. Gerner P, Oettinger R, Gerner W *et al.* (2000). Mother-to-infant transmission of TT virus: prevalence, extent and mechanism of vertical transmission. *Pediatr Infect Dis J*, 19:1074–1077. http://dx.doi.org/10.1097/00006454-200011000-00009 PMID:11099089

40. Goto K, Sugiyama K, Ando T *et al.* (2000). Detection rates of TT virus DNA in serum of umbilical cord blood, breast milk and saliva. *Tohoku J Exp Med*, 191:203–207. http://dx.doi.org/10.1620/tjem.191.203 PMID:11038012

41. Martínez-Guinó L, Kekarainen T, Segalés J (2009). Evidence of Torque teno virus (TTV) vertical transmission in swine. *Theriogenology*, 71:1390–1395. http://dx.doi.org/10.1016/j.theriogenology.2009.01.010 PMID:19249089

42. Okamoto H, Takahashi M, Nishizawa T *et al.* (2000). Replicative forms of TT virus DNA in bone marrow cells. *Biochem Biophys Res Commun*, 270:657–662. http://dx.doi.org/10.1006/bbrc.2000.2481 PMID:10753679

43. Mariscal LF, López-Alcorocho JM, Rodríguez-Iñigo E *et al.* (2002). TT virus replicates in stimulated but not in nonstimulated peripheral blood mononuclear cells. *Virology*, 301:121–129. http://dx.doi.org/10.1006/viro.2002.1545 PMID:12359452

44. Kakkola L, Hedman K, Qiu J *et al.* (2009). Replication of and protein synthesis by TT viruses [Review]. *Curr Top Microbiol Immunol*, 331:53–64. http://dx.doi.org/10.1007/978-3-540-70972-5_4 PMID:19230557

45. Maggi F, Pistello M, Vatteroni M *et al.* (2001). Dynamics of persistent TT virus infection, as determined in patients treated with alpha interferon for concomitant hepatitis C virus infection. *J Virol*, 75:11999–12004. http://dx.doi.org/10.1128/JVI.75.24.11999-12004.2001 PMID:11711590

46. Lai YC, Hu RT, Yang SS, Wu CH (2002). Coinfection of TT virus and response to interferon therapy in patients with chronic hepatitis B or C. *World J Gastroenterol*, 8:567–570. PMID:12046094

47. Moreno J, Moraleda G, Barcena R *et al.* (2004). Response of TT virus to IFN plus ribavirin treatment in patients with chronic hepatitis C. *World J Gastroenterol*, 10:143–146. PMID:14695786

48. de Villiers EM, Kimmel R, Leppik L, Gunst K (2009). Intragenomic rearrangement in TT viruses: a possible role in the pathogenesis of disease. *Curr Top Microbiol Immunol*, 331:91–107. http://dx.doi.org/10.1007/978-3-540-70972-5_6 PMID:19230559

49. de Villiers EM, Borkosky SS, Kimmel R *et al.* (2011). The diversity of torque teno viruses: in vitro replication leads to the formation of additional replication-competent subviral molecules. *J Virol*, 85:7284–7295. http://dx.doi.org/10.1128/JVI.02472-10 PMID:21593173

4

Cancer
prevention

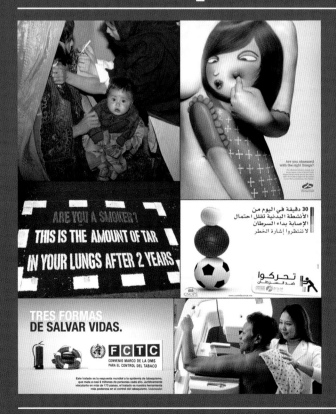

Preventing cancer by avoiding exposure to particular carcinogens follows from knowledge of causation. Priorities for cancer prevention differ on national, and sometimes local, scales. Certain individual lifestyle choices are also identified as key to reducing cancer incidence. Tobacco-related mortality has prompted measures from supporting smoking cessation to adopting an international treaty. In communities where cancers are clearly attributable to alcohol drinking and/or avoidable sunlight exposure, corresponding behaviour change is warranted. Beyond exposure to specific carcinogens, various cancer types are attributable to the joint effect of diet, obesity, and physical inactivity, providing imperatives for prevention of diabetes, heart disease, and cancer, particularly in high-income countries. Primary prevention of some infection-caused cancers is achievable by vaccination, and regulatory measures have been proven to reduce or eliminate cancer caused by workplace or environmental pollutants. Secondary prevention by detecting premalignant or early stages of disease can reduce morbidity and mortality from particular tumours.

4.1 Changing behaviours – tobacco control

4 PREVENTION

Ron Borland
Maria E. Leon

Frank J. Chaloupka (reviewer)
Hana Ross (reviewer)
Melanie Wakefield (reviewer)

Summary

- Tobacco use, particularly cigarette smoking, remains a major cancer control priority as well as being a priority for other areas of disease prevention.

- The WHO Framework Convention on Tobacco Control is at the centre of international efforts to reduce tobacco-related harms.

- Uptake and continuation of tobacco use by individuals is influenced by personal and societal/environmental factors. The practice of tobacco companies to actively market their products is a major influence.

- Government-supported tobacco control policies are necessary to constrain the activities of the tobacco industry, to deter tobacco use, and to encourage existing users to quit.

- A comprehensive tobacco control programme requires policies that adequately regulate the practices of tobacco companies, by eliminating their capacity to promote their products; do all that is possible to reduce the harmfulness and allure of tobacco products; create a disincentive to use these products through high taxes; protect people from involuntary smoking; ensure that the public is adequately informed; and support services to help those unable to quit unassisted.

Cigarette smoking is the most frequent form of tobacco use and a major cause of cancer as well as many other diseases, but stopping use can reverse some of the damage and prevent other risks from continuing to rise [1]. Other forms of tobacco are also harmful. Most of the harms to health are caused by the delivery of carcinogens and additional toxic substances, not by the nicotine, which is the main psychoactive substance in tobacco and the core reason people use and continue to use tobacco. Tobacco use is also partly sustained by beliefs that users hold and by the roles that tobacco use plays in society, both of which are influenced by tobacco industry marketing. Quitting smoking can be facilitated by an environment where non-smoking has become the norm, but this is not sufficient for many smokers. Non-smokers need to be protected from involuntary smoking. The importance of tobacco control to health and the need for coordinated international action has been recognized by the international community through the WHO Framework Convention on Tobacco Control (FCTC) [2].

Prevention of initiation and promotion of cessation are the two main objectives guiding efforts towards reducing smoking. Along with protecting others from involuntary smoking and reducing the

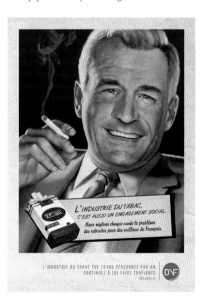

Fig. 4.1.1. Campaign poster from the French association Droits des Non-Fumeurs (Non-Smokers' Rights): "The tobacco industry also has a social commitment. Every year, we solve the problems of thousands of French pensioners. The tobacco industry kills 73 000 people every year. Keep trusting them."

harmfulness of tobacco products, these form the four pillars of a comprehensive approach to tobacco control. The ideal is to prevent uptake, but this is never likely to be universal, so other strategies are needed as well. This chapter focuses on reducing cigarette smoking, although much of the discussion can be generalized to the control of other forms of tobacco use.

Tobacco use: the scope of the challenge

The prevalence of cigarette smoking varies greatly across the world and also varies greatly by sex [3] but remains unacceptably high everywhere. In several countries, more than 50% of men smoke cigarettes; these include China, Indonesia, and the Russian Federation, three of the largest countries. In some African countries, less than 10% of men smoke. Overall, far fewer women than men smoke. In some small countries, more than 40% of women smoke, but the prevalence is less than 5% in many countries, including China. Use of other smoked products, notably bidis, is very high in India and other parts of South Asia. Use of a variety of smokeless tobacco products is most prevalent in South Asia and parts of Africa, where smokeless tobacco products are often the main form of tobacco use among women, and in parts of Scandinavia among men.

Tobacco use is addictive, due to the psychoactive effects of the nicotine. However, the addiction is more to the way in which the nicotine is delivered than to the drug itself. Cigarettes are the most addictive form of nicotine delivery, whereas nicotine provided in transdermal patches to facilitate cessation appears to have no addiction potential. There is evidence that it is easier to quit smokeless tobacco use than cigarette smoking [4]. Hence, the development and maintenance of addiction or dependence is a biopsychosocial phenomenon [5,6]. Rituals associated with tobacco use, sustained in part

by social conventions, become part of what is hard to give up. Tobacco dependence develops as the cumulative effect of tobacco use, usually in adolescence, and becomes a barrier – physiological or/and psychological – to stopping use [7].

The majority of smokers start using tobacco as teenagers, with a younger age of initiation in high-income countries compared with middle- and low-income countries [8]. The stages in the development of the habit in a tobacco user include never-use, trial, experimentation, and established use (with varying degrees of dependence), followed by an often-repeated cycle of quit attempts and relapse, leading to either permanent cessation or continued use [9]. Preventing initial trial or progression of use after initial trial are the most important goals of tobacco control policies, as their achievement effectively eliminates the health risk, but while a population of smokers persists, additional efforts are required.

Tobacco control is grounded in the harms of the behaviour. Smoking behaviour is maintained by two sets of factors: the experienced effects of tobacco use, and the ways in which smoking has become socially useful. As smoking became more prevalent, rituals associated with it became part of the prevailing culture of countries, as illustrated by the offering of cigarettes to others to facilitate socialization and the giving of cigarettes as gifts. These factors not only help sustain use but also provide reasons for use and reasons to oppose efforts to control use. The denormalization of smoking involves eliminating as far as possible these social benefits of tobacco use, leaving only the experienced effects to be overcome for those motivated to quit. Denormalization takes time, and much of it occurs as a side-effect of strong public education campaigns and the introduction of smoke-free places. As smoking becomes less valued socially, policy-makers may more easily enact stronger laws to further

constrain use, thus creating a virtuous cycle of activity. Changing the social conditions or normative context to discourage tobacco use reduces the incentives to take up or continue smoking and should make quitting easier. However, part of the addiction is caused by factors within the individual; thus, normative change, while helping to drive down the prevalence of smoking, is not enough to assist many smokers who remain unable to quit [10].

Measurement and evaluation

Central to any systematic, scientifically grounded approach to reducing the tobacco epidemic is regular monitoring of smoking prevalence and high-quality evaluation of the impacts of control efforts. There are now coordinated international efforts to monitor use [11]. The key instruments are the Global Adult Tobacco Survey [12] and the Global Youth Tobacco Survey [13]. The Global Adult Tobacco Survey is a more recent innovation and has not extended to many countries yet. The use of the Global Youth Tobacco Survey is more widespread (Figure 4.1.2). There are similar pre-existing surveys of both adults and children in most developed countries.

Trends indicated by survey data provide key indicators of progress. Surveys should be sufficiently large as to provide data about important subgroups, for example to indicate whether progress is equivalent across levels of socioeconomic status or by sex. Youth surveys are determinative in monitoring efforts to prevent uptake.

Volume 12 of the IARC Handbooks of Cancer Prevention, on methods for evaluating tobacco control policies, presents an extensive set of measures or variables, collected from multiple surveys, to monitor the natural history of tobacco use [14]. However, cross-sectional repeat surveys, while an excellent method for assessing prevalence and changes in prevalence, lack specificity to reveal the mechanisms by which any observed changes have taken place. Cohort

Fig. 4.1.2. Global Youth Tobacco Survey (GYTS): monitoring of cigarette smoking in (A) boys and (B) girls. Regions: AFR, Africa; AMR, the Americas; EMR, Eastern Mediterranean; EUR, Europe; SEAR, South-East Asia; WPR, Western Pacific.

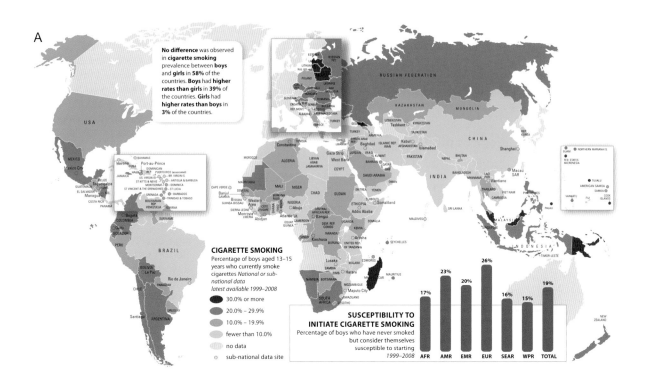

A

No difference was observed in cigarette smoking prevalence between boys and girls in 58% of the countries. Boys had higher rates than girls in 39% of the countries. Girls had higher rates than boys in 3% of the countries.

CIGARETTE SMOKING
Percentage of boys aged 13–15 years who currently smoke cigarettes National or sub-national data latest available 1999–2008

- 30.0% or more
- 20.0% – 29.9%
- 10.0% – 19.9%
- fewer than 10.0%
- no data
- ○ sub-national data site

SUSCEPTIBILITY TO INITIATE CIGARETTE SMOKING
Percentage of boys who have never smoked but consider themselves susceptible to starting 1999–2008

AFR	AMR	EMR	EUR	SEAR	WPR	TOTAL
17%	23%	20%	26%	16%	15%	19%

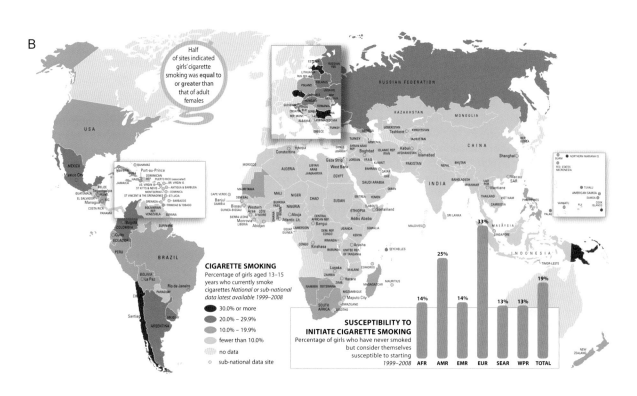

B

Half of sites indicated girls' cigarette smoking was equal to or greater than that of adult females

CIGARETTE SMOKING
Percentage of girls aged 13–15 years who currently smoke cigarettes National or sub-national data latest available 1999–2008

- 30.0% or more
- 20.0% – 29.9%
- 10.0% – 19.9%
- fewer than 10.0%
- no data
- ○ sub-national data site

SUSCEPTIBILITY TO INITIATE CIGARETTE SMOKING
Percentage of girls who have never smoked but consider themselves susceptible to starting 1999–2008

AFR	AMR	EMR	EUR	SEAR	WPR	TOTAL
14%	25%	14%	33%	13%	13%	19%

or panel studies are much more powerful in this regard. A good example of high-quality evaluation is the International Tobacco Control Policy Evaluation project, which not only uses cohorts of smokers within countries but also attempts to measure all of the main theorized mediators of policy effects as well as indicators of policy reach and proximal impact. These data are generated using parallel surveys in different countries, which permit results in a country that implements a policy to be compared with those in control countries that do not, and also allow for exploration of possible differences in policy impact because of cultural traditions or the presence of complementary policies and the history of past efforts. These methods can also help to tease out interactions between multiple policies. This kind of approach is realizing the intention of the WHO FCTC to be an evidence-grounded treaty, by generating valid scientific data that are used to inform policy.

Tobacco control interventions

The two main domains and the key elements of tobacco control that are considered in this section are outlined in Fig. 4.1.3 [14]. The first is tobacco industry control, which is directed at regulating the marketing resources of the industry and targets the product, its price, its availability, and its packaging. The second is tobacco use control, which focuses more directly on users or on individuals vulnerable to become users, and includes restrictions on where people can smoke, educational interventions, and provision of support for cessation. Both types of controls are shown in Table 4.1.1.

Price and taxation

Price is a factor that theoretically acts to reduce consumption independently of whether people believe that use is harmful. Imposition of taxes to increase the retail price of tobacco reduces the prevalence and frequency of tobacco use in

the population. Similarly, decreasing prices are associated with increased use. Taxation is considered the single most effective intervention to change tobacco behaviours [15,16], but this may be because its impact is easy to quantify as it typically occurs immediately after the price changes, whereas other strategies, for example educational interventions, have rather more diffuse and longer-term effects.

Because price increases reduce consumption and smoking prevalence, ensuring that the price is as high as possible is a key tobacco control strategy. A significant proportion of the retail price of a tobacco product involves taxes, and a change in the tax rate is the main way that governments can influence the retail price. Although WHO recommends that excise taxes should account for a minimum of 70% of the retail price of tobacco products, this level has been achieved by only a few countries in the world [17,18] and sometimes only for

some tobacco products. Apart from taxes, other ways that governments can influence retail prices include banning gifts with cigarette purchases, price controls exemplified by minimum price laws, and strong enforcement of penalties for evading tobacco taxes. These options necessitate registration of manufacturers and monitoring of national production as well as efforts to minimize smuggling [16]. There is now a Protocol to the WHO FCTC – the Protocol to Eliminate Illicit Trade in Tobacco Products – that, when implemented, should help international coordination to reduce the illegal trade in tobacco products, which is currently a major problem in some countries [2].

The impact of tobacco taxes on prices can also be lessened by legal responses to the tax increase [16]. For instance, in anticipation of or in response to a tax increase, tobacco companies can limit price increases by reducing profit margins, sometimes targeted at those

Fig. 4.1.3. Schematic overview of tobacco control interventions and how they relate to tobacco products, users, and potential users.

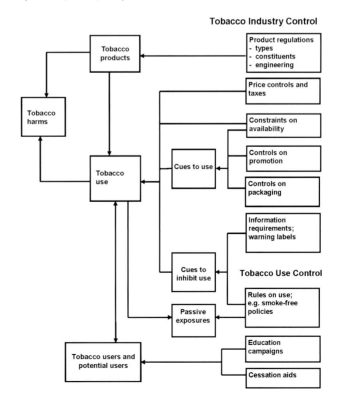

Table 4.1.1. Tobacco control interventions

Intervention	Aims	Examples
Tobacco industry controls – targeted at producers		
Product controls	To reduce use, and to reduce harmfulness of products	Rules preventing the establishment of new products (prohibition of marketing and sales of snus in the European Union, with the exception of Sweden); rules limiting the appeal of products (bans on the use of flavourings or imposing limits on constituents); rules restricting the levels of constituents and emissions (upper limits on tar, nicotine, and carbon monoxide)
Price controls	To reduce use in current users, and to deter use in never-users and former users	Increase in excise taxes passed onto the retail price of tobacco products; price policies that include a minimum price floor to counteract industry's marketing discounts
Promotion controls	To reduce use and appeal of products	Bans on paid advertisement, sponsorship, and place-ment of products, including restrictions on packaging (generic packaging); bans on product price-reducing promotions
Availability controls	To reduce availability of products and discourage use in certain venues	Restrictions on the number and types of outlets; restrictions about to whom products can be sold (age limits and vending machines); ban on sales in bars
Packaging controls	To reduce cues to use, and to make the product less attractive	Rules on descriptors of package content; ban on sales of single cigarettes; establishment of a minimum pack size
Form and content of warnings	To discourage use and inform the public of adverse health effects	Inclusion of facts about the harms of tobacco use or the health benefits of quitting use; information about toxin levels
Provisions to detect compliance with tax directives	To limit tobacco tax avoidance and evasion	Use of tax stamps and of systems for tracking and tracing tobacco products
Tobacco use controls – targeted at users or potential users		
Rules about use	To reduce use, and to protect non-users	Smoke-free policies that protect non-smokers and also have effects on users (reduction in consumption)
Public communication campaigns	To disseminate to as many people as possible the messages of anti-tobacco campaigns	Mass media campaigns to promote programmes designed to inform people while minimizing the risk of awakening the desires of experimenting with tobacco
Programmes to disseminate the availability of tobacco cessation services	To increase the level of information about cessation resources in place to increase their use	Rules regulating cessation medications, availability of services, and existence of subsidies on medications and services (among these: quitlines, "quit to win" campaigns, brief advice from physicians, nurses, and/or other health-care providers)

products most used by young people and/or lower-income smokers. Companies can also turn a sudden tax increase into a series of gradual increases in the hope that consumers will not notice and thus the impact on consumption will be less. Where products are differentially taxed, consumers can shift to products that are taxed less and are thus cheaper.

The demand for tobacco products is inversely related to price. The magnitude of this response is measured by the price elasticity of the demand for tobacco products, usually expressed in terms of the percentage change in use that results from a 10% increase in price. The more price-elastic the demand, the more effective is a tobacco price increase in lowering use. The price elasticity of demand can be estimated by using aggregate data or with household-level or individual-level data, based on surveys. Individual-level data allow the effect of price on consumption to be assessed by sex, age group, socioeconomic status, and other attributes of the population, potentially revealing differences between subgroups in sensitivity to price changes. Aggregate data do not allow the effects on prevalence to be separated, independent of consumption per user.

There is an inverse relationship between cigarette prices and cigarette consumption across all countries. Data from the USA and the United Kingdom, where most studies have been conducted, indicate that the magnitude of the price elasticity of cigarette demand is about −0.4 (range, −0.2 to −0.6); that is, for a 10% increase in price a 4% decrease in consumption is

Fig. 4.1.4. Campaign poster from the Australian Department of Health and Ageing describing the gradual positive effects that quitting tobacco has on the human body.

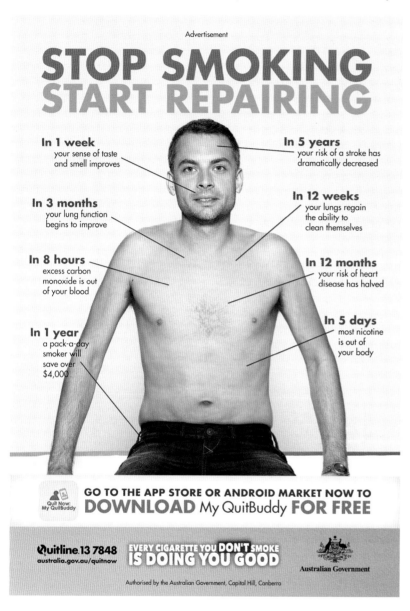

that all other tobacco products are similarly price-elastic. Some studies have documented substitution among these products in response to increases in their relative prices, specifically between cigarettes and smokeless tobacco after increases in taxes on cigarettes, and between cigarettes and cigars after increases in the price of cigarettes [20].

Price elasticity for tobacco products within countries also depends on income levels of potential consumers. Indeed, after considering potential confounders, as aggregate income increases the aggregate demand for tobacco typically increases. The policy implication is that the price of tobacco products must increase at least as fast as income growth to avoid tobacco products becoming more affordable. Younger tobacco users are expected to be more sensitive to increases in prices or taxes than adults because they have less disposable income and a lower level of tobacco dependence [16]. Younger users are also more influenced by peer use and are more concerned with immediate costs than with health outcomes in the long term. These expectations have been confirmed. Both smoking prevalence and intensity among young people diminish in response to cigarette price increases. The magnitude of the overall elasticity in high-income countries, where most studies has been conducted, ranges between −0.50 and −1.2 [16].

Restrictions on tobacco promotion

Many of the techniques now ubiquitous in mass marketing were first used, or first perfected, for selling manufactured cigarettes [21,22]. Advertising and other forms of promotion can be a powerful force for increasing product use. Legislative bans or other agreements to eliminate tobacco advertising are thus a critical aspect of tobacco control efforts (Article 13 of the WHO FCTC) (Table 4.1.2). Advertising involves far more than advertisements on television, on billboards, or in

observed [8]. Elasticity estimates from other high-income countries are more varied. Greater elasticity is often observed in low- and middle-income countries, with estimates between −0.2 and −0.8 [16]. In those environments with elasticity estimates that are very low, cigarettes are very cheap or their affordability has risen significantly over time (due to increased earnings), rendering tax increases less effective.

A smaller number of studies have assessed the effect of increases in cigarette prices on smoking cessation in adults. Higher taxes and prices reduce the duration of smoking, increase quit attempts, and increase the number of smokers who successfully quit [16,19]. About half of the impact of the price increase is on adult prevalence and about half is on the number of cigarettes consumed by adult smokers [16]. Limited evidence indicates

Article	Description
Article 5.3	Designed to restrict the influence of the tobacco industry in decision-making related to implementation of the treaty.
Article 6	Price and tax measures to reduce the demand for tobacco. Guidelines recommend trying to raise taxes so that they account for at least 70% of the retail price.
Article 8	Protection from exposure to tobacco smoke.
Article 9	Regulation of the contents of tobacco products.
Article 10	Regulation of tobacco product disclosures.
Article 11	Packaging and labelling of tobacco products. Mandates health warnings covering at least 30% of both main surfaces of packages. Guidelines suggest graphic warnings covering at least 50% of the package and consideration of plain packaging.
Article 12	Education, communication, training, and public awareness. Requires public education and training of health professionals, and participation of civil society in such activities.
Article 13	Tobacco advertising, promotion, and sponsorship. Requires prohibiting this as far as possible within constitutional limits.
Article 14	Demand reduction measures concerning tobacco dependence and cessation. Mandates developing guidelines and programmes for delivery of effective aids and services to help smokers quit.
Article 15	Illicit trade in tobacco products. Expanded with first Protocol to the treaty, requiring a range of actions to control international trade so as to eliminate illicit trade.
Article 16	Sales to and by minors. Designed to stop sales to minors, and includes suggestions for bans on vending machines and other channels where restrictions on sales may be problematic.
Articles 20–22	Research, which includes surveillance, intervention development, and evaluation to ensure that the WHO Framework Convention on Tobacco Control is evidence-based and progress can be monitored.

newspapers; it also includes posters and the display of the products at point of sale as well as the branding and associated designs on the packaging. Internet advertising should also be recognized, but its control may require international cooperation. A comprehensive policy also requires cigarettes to be kept from view – to eliminate the promotional aspect of large, prominent cigarette displays – and removing as much branding as possible from packaging, ultimately by plain packaging (see "Australia's plain packaging of tobacco products"). Restrictions on advertising need to be reasonably extensive before effects on use can be detected, at least in part due to the capacity of the industry to shift promotion to channels that are still permitted [8].

Availability of products

Tobacco remains one of the most readily available consumer products on the market. Many countries have prohibited sales to minors. A few countries, like France, limit tobacco sales to specialist retailers. In most countries, however, tobacco is still available in places like convenience stores, which, in turn, are often frequented by children. The density of tobacco outlets is related to the prevalence of smoking in the area [23]. An increased focus on restricting where tobacco products can be sold is anticipated in future policy initiatives.

Product regulation

Use of filters is the only viable way of cleaning up tobacco smoke. However, use of filters is severely limited in its efficacy because filters either remove nicotine or create conditions where nicotine cannot be carried as effectively into the lungs, thereby diminishing consumer appeal. While cigarettes and other forms of smoked tobacco continue to be used, it is important to progressively reduce the toxicity of these products as far as possible. It is possible to remove the bulk of toxins from smokeless forms of tobacco, so this is a viable strategy for reducing the harm that smokeless tobacco causes. Low-toxin smokeless tobacco causes far less harm than other forms of tobacco [24], but it does contain carcinogens [25]. These products also contain nicotine, which reinforces future use, thus prolonging the duration of the habit and increasing the cumulative use, thereby increasing the likelihood of damage to health.

The main forms of product regulation have been to set limits on the amount of tar, nicotine, and, often, carbon monoxide produced by cigarettes as determined using a standard machine. This prompted companies to market certain cigarettes as "light" and "mild", implying that these products were less harmful, sometimes by suggesting that they were an alternative to quitting. However, cigarettes that actually delivered low levels of nicotine were not used in the long term by individual consumers. The industry addressed this problem by using filter ventilation: small holes in the paper surrounding the filter, thereby permitting air to mix with the smoke. This allowed cigarettes that, although they were determined by a testing machine to be low in tar and nicotine yield, actually delivered similar amounts of nicotine and the accompanying tar to smokers as did regular cigarettes [26]. Smokers compensated for the dilution effect; they blocked some of the holes and took larger and deeper puffs [27]. The WHO FCTC mandates prohibiting the misleading use of the terms "mild" and "light", and recommends removing misleading yield measures from packaging where

Australia's plain packaging of tobacco products

Simon Chapman

On 1 December 2012, Australia became the first country to require that all tobacco products be sold in standardized "plain" packaging. The Tobacco Plain Packaging Act 2011 mandates an identical standard for all brands for all aspects of packaging [1]. Parallel legislation mandated graphic health warnings, now the world's largest at 75% of the pack's front surface and 90% of the back surface [2]. All brands are now sold in the same dull brown colour; the only differentiation is the brand name and variant, printed in a standard font. All aspects of the new design reflect detailed research with smokers about the options that are the least attractive and cause the most concerns about health [3].

The Australian government introduced the bill following advice from its Preventative Health Task Force, which argued that Australia's tobacco advertising ban failed to address what had long been a major loophole: the role of the pack

as advertising. As with all other industries, internal tobacco industry documents and the tobacco trade press discuss candidly the central role of packs in promoting the attractions of brands and smoking.

Plain packaging is anticipated to have less effect on older, heavily dependent smokers, who tend to be brand-loyal and less image-conscious. However, without branding, future generations will grow up never having seen category A carcinogens packaged in attractive packs. Today's 20-year-olds in Australia have never seen local tobacco advertising, and youth smoking rates are at an all-time low. Plain packs are expected to turbocharge this trend.

A large-scale evaluation of the impact of the packaging commenced well before it was implemented. Early feedback suggests that many smokers believe their cigarettes now taste worse than before, an effect predictable from market research into how

packaging powerfully conditions expectations and consumers' experience of products. Reports are also common that smokers feel that the large health graphic health warnings are disturbing and embarrassing.

The new law has already survived a tobacco industry challenge in the Australian High Court, with only one judge of seven not supporting the government. The industry campaigned vigorously against the policy and is expected to engage in heavy price discounting to try and show the world that the policy failed and should not be adopted elsewhere. The government can counteract this by raising the tobacco tax.

Australia's historic plain cigarette packaging legislation is a weapons-grade public health policy now causing major concern in the international industry because of its potential to have a domino effect on other countries' tobacco control policies. No other product is subject to such complete control, sending a powerful message to the population that tobacco is an exceptionally unhealthy product, deserving exceptional controls.

References

1. Australian Government, Department of Health and Ageing (2012). Tobacco. Plain packaging of tobacco products. Available at http://www.health.gov.au/internet/main/publishing.nsf/content/tobacco-plain.

2. Australian Government, Department of Health and Ageing (2012). Tobacco. Health warnings. Available at http://www.health.gov.au/internet/main/publishing.nsf/content/tobacco-warn.

3. Australian Government, Department of Health and Ageing (2012). Market Research Reports on tobacco plain packaging and graphic health warnings. Available at http://www.health.gov.au/internet/yourhealth/publishing.nsf/Content/mr-plainpack#.UOpDL7ZhNT4.

Fig. B4.1.1. Health warning statements on tobacco packages have evolved significantly in Australia, from text-only health warnings (left) until the introduction of graphic health warnings on 1 March 2006, to the introduction of the new plain packaging (right) on 1 December 2012.

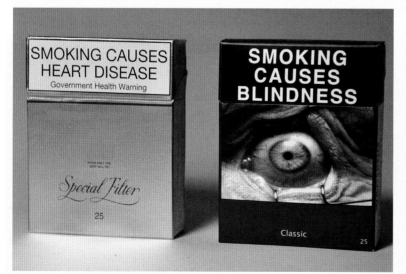

Fig. 4.1.5. Campaign material from the Vietnamese Ministry of Health: "Tobacco has ravaging effects on your body and your baby's. Quit today. From 01/01/2010, make sure to strictly implement the provisions of the government smoking ban in public places and workplaces."

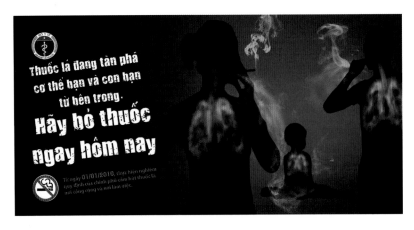

smoke-free environments, including mass anti-tobacco campaigns and dissemination of information about the availability of cessation services or medications.

Globally, exposure to second-hand smoke varies significantly across countries, and a large part of the world's population continues to be exposed to the health hazards of involuntary smoking both at work and at home. For example, 63% of Chinese workers report being exposed to smoke in their workplace (see "Tobacco and China"). The proportion of adolescents living in homes where others smoke in their presence can be high even in high-income countries.

they had been mandated. These bans have had a limited impact [28]. Consumers experience these cigarettes as slightly less harsh and interpret this reduced averseness as reduced harmfulness [29]. The core problem of filter ventilation has not been addressed, and remains [27].

Reducing product toxicity is one aim of Articles 9 and 10 of the WHO FCTC (Table 4.1.2). Product regulation also needs to consider both the addictiveness and the related attractiveness of tobacco products that continue to be harmful. Several countries, including Canada and Brazil, now ban all or nearly all additives to cigarettes that are designed to affect flavour. Products containing high levels of toxins still dominate the market in many countries.

One recent product development that has evoked interest as a harm reduction option is electronic cigarettes (e-cigarettes), also referred to as electronic nicotine delivery systems (ENDS). This product is designed to deliver nicotine to the lungs without combustion. Several groups of ex-smokers use and promote e-cigarettes as low-harm alternatives to smoking. The safety and efficacy of this product as a cessation aid is under study. Like smokeless tobacco, the potential role of e-cigarettes in reducing smoking is unclear [30], but

evidence is emerging that e-cigarettes will be a much easier product to switch to and that they may be effective cessation aids [31].

Smoke-free laws

Smoke-free legislation is primarily designed to protect non-smokers. Comprehensive laws that are well complied with greatly reduce involuntary smoking. Smoke-free policies also contribute to a reduction in the level of daily cigarette consumption by smokers, to a drop in the prevalence of smoking, and to deter smoking initiation among young people [32,33]. Bans on workplace smoking reduce daily cigarette consumption by an average of 2–4 cigarettes. One large United States study found that after controlling for potential confounders, the percentage of a state's population that was covered by smoke-free air laws was correlated with a decreased odds of susceptibility to smoking, current smoking, and established smoking in young people [33]. Comprehensive smoke-free policies create strong anti-smoking norms that lead to voluntary interventions such as smoking bans in private homes, which reduce exposure of children to second-hand smoke, with resulting effects in reducing adult smoking. Regular efforts are needed to remind the population of the health benefits of

Educational efforts

The knowledge that tobacco use is harmful is central to any efforts to control its use, although sometimes the pervasiveness of this knowledge makes demonstrating effects from specific interventions difficult. The two main ways of informing the public are through mass media, increasingly via the Internet, and by provision of warning material on tobacco packaging. For young people, school-based education is another source of information, although it has only modest effects on preventing uptake unless complemented with other strategies [34]. Warning labels on packaging can improve knowledge and generate concerns about smoking, and thereby stimulate increased quitting [35], although their net effect on cessation is probably small. Large graphic warnings are the most effective. The mass media are the main source of health information for most people and, even taking the Internet into account, remain the main source of unsolicited information. The mass media convey new information and remind people about knowledge they already possess but have forgotten or are ignoring (see also Chapter 4.3). The more attention is paid to tobacco in the mass media, the more quitting-related activity occurs [36].

Tobacco and China

Judith Mackay

The epidemic

The Chinese government owns the world's largest tobacco company. China is the largest producer and consumer of tobacco, with about 350 million smokers, mostly male. One third of all cigarettes smoked in the world are smoked in China. In 2010 it was estimated that 53% of the male population and 2.4% of the female population in China were smokers [1]. Tobacco currently causes 1.2 million deaths annually in China (equal to 3000 deaths every day), the highest number for any one country – and this figure is predicted to rise to more than 3 million by 2030 [2]. More than 70% of the population are regularly exposed to second-hand smoke. Only recently have small numbers of smokers attempted to quit.

Economic costs

Smoking puts great pressures on economic development. Between 2000 and 2008, the attributable costs of tobacco use in China quadrupled, from US$ 7.2 billion to US$ 28.9 billion, or 0.7% of the gross domestic product [3].

Tobacco control action

In 1979, the Ministries of Health, Finance, and Agriculture jointly issued the Circular of Publicity on the Harm of Smoking and Control on Smoking. Since the 1980s, central and local governments have passed and expanded laws for the control of smoking in public places, protection of minors, and bans on tobacco promotion, and have issued many circulars. In 1997, Beijing hosted the 10th World Conference on Tobacco or Health, opened by President Jiang Zemin, which brought considerable attention to the issue of smoking. China ratified the WHO Framework Convention on Tobacco Control (FCTC) in 2005 and was the second country to sign the Protocol to Eliminate Illicit Trade in Tobacco Products in 2013. China is one of only four countries where tobacco control is included in both the National Development Plan and the United Nations Development Assistance Frameworks.

Obstacles and challenges

The obstacles and challenges are common to most countries, and include a focus on curative, not preventive, medicine. The state tobacco monopoly has jurisdiction over most tobacco control in China – a clear conflict of interest. The public still lacks accurate awareness of the harms of smoking and second-hand smoke. There is no national ban on smoking in public places and the workplace, where smoking is still very common. City-level smoke-free initiatives are neither comprehensive nor well-enforced. China has weak text-only package warnings and no graphic warnings. Very cheap brands discourage smokers from attempting to quit. Despite some bans on direct tobacco advertising, there is heavy exposure to tobacco promotion through event sponsorships, outdoor displays, and entertainment media [2].

The future

As part of comprehensive tobacco control action, the responsibility for tobacco control legislation and the WHO FCTC should be removed from the dominion of the state tobacco monopoly, coupled with an effective taxation policy.

References

1. Centers for Disease Control and Prevention (2010). Global Adult Tobacco Survey (GATS) Fact Sheet China: 2010. Available at http://apps.nccd.cdc.gov/gtssdata/Ancillary/DataReports.aspx?CAID=1.

2. International Tobacco Control Policy Evaluation Project (2012). *ITC China Project Report. Findings from the Wave 1 to 3 Surveys (2006–2009)*. Waterloo, Ontario, Canada: University of Waterloo; Beijing, China: Office of Tobacco Control, Chinese Center for Disease Control and Prevention. Available at http://www.itcproject.org/documents/keyfindings/itcchinanrenglishwebdec142012finalpdf.

3. Yang L, Sung H-Y, Mao Z et al. (2011). *Tob Control*, 20:266–272. http://dx.doi.org/10.1136/tc.2010.042028 PMID:21339491

Well-constructed advertisements about the harms of smoking raise the profile of the issue and make the harms more personally relevant, thus encouraging smokers to quit and others not to start or resume smoking [37,38]. Part of the preventive effect seems to stem from disgust associated with the unattractive and disfiguring aspects of disease linked to smoking, rather than from anxiety about future harms. Anti-smoking advertisements appear to have their effects by essentially the same mechanisms as health warnings on packs. Television advertisements can convey a much more engaging message than comparable pack warnings, but smokers are exposed to them far less often. Although advertising is expensive, it can reach large numbers of people quite cheaply per person influenced, so it is very cost-effective.

The mass media are effective in reaching smokers in lower socio-economic groups, especially when the advertising is both designed to be seen as relevant and shown in programmes that these groups tend to view, and is at least as effective in influencing these groups as in influencing smokers in more socio-economically advantaged groups. Smokers in less-advantaged socio-economic groups may also require more intensive assistance if they are to quit successfully. Having the issue of smoking prominent in the mass media can also motivate health professionals by making them more aware and also more

Fig. 4.1.6. A WHO poster for World No Tobacco Day 2013 calls for legislative bans on tobacco advertising, promotion, and sponsorship.

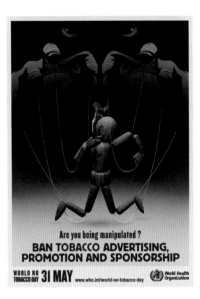

A wide range of behavioural interventions, including structured self-help manuals, tailored self-help resources, quitlines, and face-to-face individual or group programmes, all help smokers to quit, and the success rates increase with increased involvement, up to several sessions [40,42]. The effectiveness of such interventions is directly related to their intensity, typically measured by the amount of support, at least up to about four substantial sessions, but beyond that, there is little evidence that even more intensive interventions are effective. Intensive advice-based programmes are increasingly delivered via the telephone rather than face-to-face. Use of automated advice programmes, consisting of tailored personalized advice on the Internet and/or short, frequent advice messages to mobile phones, is markedly increasing. Both forms of automated intelligent programmes are effective. Combining advice-based programmes with medication gives the best results as the two seem to have largely independent effects [40]. There is no evidence of reduced relapse associated with any intervention after it ceases [43].

Factors that influence smokers to try to quit are somewhat different to those that influence success in quitting [44]. Evidence is also beginning to emerge that determinants of short-term success may differ from those for long-term maintenance [10]. If so, different strategies are needed to help those who survive the difficult early weeks to maintain cessation in the long term, which is the ultimate challenge. Although this aspect is rarely subject to specific investigation, population-based studies indicate that a small percentage of ex-smokers continue to use nicotine replacement therapy in the long term. E-cigarettes currently hold the most promise of being viable substitutes for the largest number of smokers, but research is needed to document or confirm both safety and effectiveness as a cessation aid.

The outcome of interventions is not only a matter of how effective those interventions are when used but also a function of what proportion of smokers are prepared to use them in their quit attempts. As noted above, reference to smoking behaviour in the media drives people to seek help, as does product-specific advertising. To achieve the highest cessation rates requires a population of smokers who are motivated to quit, who are prepared to use the best possible help, and who are able to access aids that will maximize success. Uptake of help, particularly advice-based help, remains low, even when services are subsidized or free. This is probably due to a combination of beliefs that "I should be able to do this by myself" and deep ambivalence about change in relation to tobacco use and other dependencies. Use of services is also influenced by the way the services are provided. For example, in the United Kingdom, there is much greater use of face-to-face services than there is of a well-organized and readily available network of other services. However, in most other countries that have systems to provide help, telephone-based quitlines are generally preferred to face-to-face services, at least in part due to the convenience.

Comprehensive efforts

As recognized by the WHO FCTC, efforts on multiple fronts are required if significant progress is to be made in tobacco control [2]. There are huge challenges. In low- and middle-income countries, governments may have other priorities and sometimes lack the infrastructure to support policy. In high-income countries, smoking is increasingly concentrated among less-advantaged socioeconomic groups, further exacerbating inequalities. Much remains to be done, but progress is being made.

likely to raise the issue with their clients. The new social media, which includes the Internet and mobile telephony, provides both huge challenges and opportunities for tobacco control. The challenges come from the difficulty of regulating any pro-smoking activity. The opportunities arise from the potential of social media to provide more genuine personal engagement and the opportunity for well-informed members of the community to become active in communicating the messages.

Cessation aids

There is now a range of effective medications for smoking cessation when used for periods of about 6–12 weeks [39–41]. These medications, which include nicotine itself (as nicotine replacement therapy) plus three other drugs (bupropion, varenicline, and cytisine, which impinge on different aspects of the brain's reward system), are all demonstrably effective. There is evidence that using medication for an extended period can at least delay relapse, but only for the period during which the drug is being used.

References

1. IARC (2007). IARC Handbooks of Cancer Prevention, Vol. 11: *Tobacco Control: Reversal of Risk After Quitting Smoking.* Lyon: IARC.

2. WHO (2003). *WHO Framework Convention on Tobacco Control.* Geneva: WHO. Available at http://www.who.int/fctc/en/index.html.

3. Eriksen M, Mackay J, Ross H (2012). *The Tobacco Atlas,* 4th ed. Atlanta, GA: American Cancer Society, World Lung Foundation. Available at http://www.tobaccoatlas.org.

4. Fagerström K, Eissenberg T (2012). Dependence on tobacco and nicotine products: a case for product-specific assessment. *Nicotine Tob Res,* 14:1382–1390. http://dx.doi.org/10.1093/ntr/nts007 PMID:22459798

5. West R, Brown J (2013). *Theory of Addiction,* 2nd ed. Oxford: Wiley.

6. Henningfield JE, Benowitz NL (2010). Pharmacology of tobacco addiction. In: Boyle P, Gray N, Henningfield J et al., eds. *Tobacco: Science, Policy, and Public Health,* 2nd ed. Oxford: Oxford University Press, pp. 155–170.

7. DiFranza JR, Savageau JA, Fletcher K et al. (2002). Measuring the loss of autonomy over nicotine use in adolescents: the DANDY (Development and Assessment of Nicotine Dependence in Youths) study. *Arch Pediatr Adolesc Med,* 156:397–403. http://dx.doi.org/10.1001/archpedi.156.4.397 PMID:11929376

8. Jha P, Chaloupka FJ, eds (1999). *Curbing the Epidemic: Governments and the Economics of Tobacco Control.* Washington, DC: World Bank.

9. Partos TR, Borland R, Yong HH et al. (2013). The quitting rollercoaster: how recent quitting history affects future cessation outcomes (data from the International Tobacco Control 4-country cohort study). *Nicotine Tob Res,* 15:1578–1587. http://dx.doi.org/10.1093/ntr/ntt025 PMID:23493370

10. Borland R. (2014). *Understanding Hard to Maintain Behaviour Change: A Dual Process Approach.* Oxford: Wiley.

11. Global Tobacco Surveillance System Collaborating Group (2005). Global Tobacco Surveillance System (GTSS): purpose, production, and potential. *J Sch Health,* 75:15–24. http://dx.doi.org/10.1111/j.1746-1561.2005.tb00004.x PMID:15779140

12. WHO (2012). Global Adult Tobacco Survey. Available at http://www.who.int/tobacco/surveillance/gats/en.

13. WHO (2012). Global Youth Tobacco Survey. Available at http://www.who.int/tobacco/surveillance/gyts/en/.

14. IARC (2008). IARC Handbooks of Cancer Prevention, Vol. 12: *Tobacco Control: Methods for Evaluating Tobacco Control Policies.* Lyon: IARC.

15. WHO (2008). *WHO Report on the Global Tobacco Epidemic, 2008: The MPOWER Package.* Geneva: WHO.

16. IARC (2011). IARC Handbooks of Cancer Prevention, Vol. 14: *Tobacco Control: Effectiveness of Tax and Price Policies for Tobacco Control.* Lyon: IARC.

17. WHO (2013). *WHO Report on the Global Tobacco Epidemic, 2013: Enforcing Bans on Tobacco Advertising, Promotion and Sponsorship.* Geneva: WHO. Available at http://apps.who.int/iris/bitstream/10665/85380/1/9789241505871_eng.pdf.

18. WHO (2010). WHO *Technical Manual on Tobacco Tax Administration.* Geneva: WHO. Available at http://www.who.int/tobacco/publications/tax_administration/en/.

19. Franz GA (2008). Price effects on the smoking behaviour of adult age groups. *Public Health,* 122:1343–1348. http://dx.doi.org/10.1016/j.puhe.2008.05.019 PMID:18951594

20. Delnevo CD, Hrywna M, Foulds J, Steinberg MB (2004). Cigar use before and after a cigarette excise tax increase in New Jersey. *Addict Behav,* 29:1799–1807. http://dx.doi.org/10.1016/j.addbeh.2004.04.024 PMID:15530722

21. Brandt AM (2007). *The Cigarette Century: The Rise, Fall, and Deadly Persistence of the Product That Defined America.* New York: Basic Books.

22. Proctor RN (2012). *Golden Holocaust: Origins of the Cigarette Catastrophe and the Case for Abolition.* Berkeley, CA: University of California Press.

23. Chuang Y-C, Cubbin C, Ahn D, Winkleby MA (2005). Effects of neighbourhood socioeconomic status and convenience store concentration on individual level smoking. *J Epidemiol Community Health,* 59:568–573. http://dx.doi.org/10.1136/jech.2004.029041 PMID:15965140

24. Royal College of Physicians (2007). *Harm Reduction in Nicotine Addiction: Helping People Who Can't Quit.* A report by the Tobacco Advisory Group of the Royal College of Physicians. London: Royal College of Physicians.

25. IARC (2012). Personal habits and indoor combustions. *IARC Monogr Eval Carcinog Risks Hum,* 100E:1–575. PMID:23193840

26. Kozlowski LT, Frecker RC, Khouw V, Pope MA (1980). The misuse of 'less-hazardous' cigarettes and its detection: hole-blocking of ventilated filters. *Am J Public Health,* 70:1202–1203. http://dx.doi.org/10.2105/AJPH.70.11.1202 PMID:7425194

27. Kozlowski LT, O'Connor RJ (2002). Cigarette filter ventilation is a defective design because of misleading taste, bigger puffs, and blocked vents. *Tob Control,* 11 Suppl 1:I40–I50. http://dx.doi.org/10.1136/tc.11.suppl_1.i40 PMID:11893814

28. Yong HH, Borland R, Cummings KM et al. (2011). Impact of the removal of misleading terms on cigarette pack on smokers' beliefs about 'light/mild' cigarettes: cross-country comparisons. *Addiction,* 106:2204–2213. http://dx.doi.org/10.1111/j.1360-0443.2011.03533.x PMID:21658140

29. Shiffman S, Pillitteri JL, Burton SL et al. (2001). Smokers' beliefs about "light" and "ultra light" cigarettes. *Tob Control,* 10 Suppl 1:i17–i23. PMID:11740040

30. Etter J-F, Bullen C, Flouris AD et al. (2011). Electronic nicotine delivery systems: a research agenda. *Tob Control,* 20:243–248. http://dx.doi.org/10.1136/tc.2010.042168 PMID:21415064

31. Bullen C, Howe C, Laugesen M et al. (2013). Electronic cigarettes for smoking cessation: a randomised controlled trial. *Lancet,* 382:1629–1637. http://dx.doi.org/10.1016/S0140-6736(13)61842-5 PMID:24029165

32. IARC (2009). IARC Handbooks of Cancer Prevention, Vol. 13: *Tobacco Control: Evaluating the Effectiveness of Smoke-free Policies.* Lyon: IARC.

33. Farrelly MC, Loomis BR, Han B et al. (2013). A comprehensive examination of the influence of state tobacco control programs and policies on youth smoking. *Am J Public Health,* 103:549–555. http://dx.doi.org/10.2105/AJPH.2012.300948 PMID:23327252

34. Pierce JP, Distefan JM, Hill D (2010). Adolescent smoking. In: Boyle P, Gray N, Henningfield J et al., eds. *Tobacco: Science, Policy, and Public Health,* 2nd ed. Oxford: Oxford University Press, pp. 313–322.

35. Borland R, Yong H-H, Wilson N et al. (2009). How reactions to cigarette packet health warnings influence quitting: findings from the ITC Four-Country survey. *Addiction,* 104:669–675. http://dx.doi.org/10.1111/j.1360-0443.2009.02508.x PMID:19215595

36. Pierce JP, Gilpin EA (2001). News media coverage of smoking and health is associated with changes in population rates of smoking cessation but not initiation. *Tob Control*, 10:145–153. http://dx.doi.org/10.1136/tc.10.2.145 PMID:11387535

37. Durkin S, Brennan E, Wakefield M (2012). Mass media campaigns to promote smoking cessation among adults: an integrative review. *Tob Control*, 21:127–138. http://dx.doi.org/10.1136/tobaccocontrol-2011-050345 PMID:22345235

38. Wakefield MA, Loken B, Hornik RC (2010). Use of mass media campaigns to change health behaviour. *Lancet*, 376:1261–1271. http://dx.doi.org/10.1016/S0140-6736(10)60809-4 PMID:20933263

39. Cahill K, Stevens S, Perera R, Lancaster T (2013). Pharmacological interventions for smoking cessation: an overview and network meta-analysis. *Cochrane Database Syst Rev*, 5:CD009329. http://dx.doi.org/10.1002/14651858.CD009329.pub2 PMID:23728690

40. Treatobacco (2012). Available at www.treatobacco.net.

41. Hartmann-Boyce J, Stead LF, Cahill K, Lancaster T (2013). Efficacy of interventions to combat tobacco addiction: Cochrane update of 2012 reviews. *Addiction*, 108:1711–1721. http://dx.doi.org/10.1111/add.12291 PMID:23834141

42. The Cochrane Library (2012). Tobacco. Available at www.thecochranelibrary.com/view/0/index.html#http://www.thecochranelibrary.com/view/0/browse.html.

43. Hajek P, Stead LF, West R *et al.* (2009). Relapse prevention interventions for smoking cessation. *Cochrane Database Syst Rev*, 8:CD003999. http://dx.doi.org/10.1002/14651858.CD003999.pub4 PMID:23963584

44. Vangeli E, Stapleton J, Smit ES *et al.* (2011). Predictors of attempts to stop smoking and their success in adult general population samples: a systematic review. *Addiction*, 106:2110–2121. http://dx.doi.org/10.1111/j.1360-0443.2011.03565.x PMID:21752135

Websites

Global Adult Tobacco Survey (GATS):
http://www.who.int/tobacco/surveillance/gats/en/

Global Youth Tobacco Survey (GYTS):
http://www.who.int/tobacco/surveillance/gyts/en/

Global Youth Tobacco Survey Results:
www.cdc.gov/tobacco/global/gtss/tobacco_atlas/pdfs/part3.pdf

The International Tobacco Control Policy Evaluation Project: http://www.itcproject.org

The Tobacco Atlas:
http://www.tobaccoatlas.org

WHO Framework Convention on Tobacco Control:
http://www.who.int/fctc/en/index.html

4.2

Changing behaviours – physical activity and weight control

4 PREVENTION

Rena R. Wing
Kathryn R. Middleton

Christine M. Friedenreich (reviewer)
Isabelle Romieu (reviewer)

Summary

- In trials, weight loss and increased physical activity have reduced the risk of diabetes among participants.

- Behavioural weight management programmes typically produce weight losses of about 7–10% of initial body weight after 6–12 months of treatment, and increasingly include extended-care sessions.

- Typical goals in behavioural weight loss programmes include reducing caloric intake by approximately 500–1000 kcal (2000–4000 kJ) per day and increasing participation in moderate-intensity physical activity to 250 minutes or more per week.

- Behavioural weight management programmes focus on using self-monitoring, problem-solving, and goal setting to enact changes to the antecedents and consequences of behaviour.

- Benefits of adhering to weight loss, physical activity, and related guidelines are being evaluated in relation to reduced cancer incidence in relevant trials.

Earlier chapters in this Report (see Chapter 2.6 and Chapter 3.5) present strong observational evidence that obesity and physical inactivity may be related to the development of some forms of cancer (see "Energy restriction, age, and cancer risk") and suggest plausible biological pathways for this association. Indeed, epidemiological studies suggest that physical activity and weight loss can lower breast cancer risk and improve survival, evidence that researchers have suggested warrants further clinical trials investigating the impact of behavioural weight management on preventing cancer and improving survival [1]. To develop such studies, it is important to understand the basic strategies that might be used to help individuals change their weight and/or their physical activity, and the type of results that can be achieved.

Outcomes of behavioural weight loss programmes

Behavioural programmes typically produce weight losses of about 7–10% of initial body weight after 6–12 months of treatment. These weight losses have been shown to have clinically significant health benefits. The strongest evidence comes from the Diabetes Prevention Program, a multicentre randomized controlled trial, which demonstrated that behavioural weight loss led to significantly larger reductions in diabetes incidence than did treatment with metformin [2]. In that study, more than 3000 overweight or obese individuals with impaired glucose tolerance were randomly assigned to receive lifestyle intervention, metformin (a drug usually used to treat diabetes), or placebo. The goals of the lifestyle intervention included weight loss of at least 7% of initial body weight (by decreasing dietary fat intake, reducing total caloric intake, and increasing physical activity) and increasing participation in moderate-intensity physical activity to 150 minutes per week. To reach these goals, a 16-session core curriculum was delivered to participants individually over the first 6 months of the study, with continuing contact (at least once every 2 months) during the remainder of the trial. The Diabetes Prevention Program trial was stopped early (after an average of 3.2 years of follow-up) because of the positive effects of lifestyle intervention on diabetes incidence.

The lifestyle intervention resulted in an average weight loss of 6.5 kg at the end of the core curriculum and a weight loss of 4.5 kg at 3 years. Of participants in this arm, 49% achieved the 7% weight loss goal at 6 months and 37% at the final visit. On average, physical activity increased to 224 minutes per week

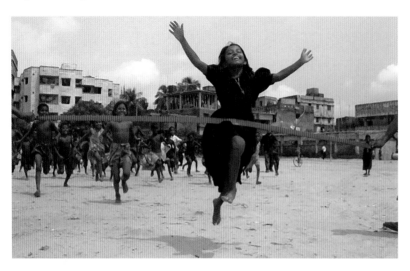

at the end of the core curriculum and 227 minutes at the end of the trial. The exercise goal was achieved by 74% of participants at week 24 and 67% at the final visit.

Although they are relatively modest, these weight losses and increases in physical activity produced dramatic effects on diabetes incidence. The lifestyle intervention reduced the risk of developing diabetes by 58% relative to placebo. Weight loss was the dominant predictor of the reduced incidence of diabetes. Moreover, when participants were followed up for 10 years, the benefits of lifestyle intervention for preventing diabetes were still apparent, although there were no longer any differences in weight loss between the three arms. As diabetes has been demonstrated to be an independent predictor of cancer mortality (beyond body mass index) [3], the impact of intervention on diabetes incidence suggests that these trials may be beneficial for lowering cancer mortality.

The findings from the Diabetes Prevention Program, indicating that modest weight losses and increases in physical activity can be achieved and can have important health benefits, have been confirmed recently in another clinical trial, called Look AHEAD. The Look AHEAD study involved more than 5000 overweight or obese individuals with type 2 diabetes, who were assigned to an intensive lifestyle intervention or the control group [4]. The lifestyle intervention was similar to that used in the Diabetes Prevention Program, but participants were given a higher physical activity goal of 175 minutes per week and encouraged to lose 10% of their initial body weight, and meal replacement products were provided to increase adherence to the dietary prescription. The intervention was delivered in group format with periodic individual sessions; participants were seen weekly for the first 6 months, seen 3 times per month for months 7–12, and then seen or contacted by phone or e-mail at least twice a month. Participants in the lifestyle intervention arm had lost an average of 8.6% of their body weight at 1 year (vs 0.7% in the control group). At 4 years, participants in the intensive lifestyle intervention group had maintained on average a loss of 4.7% of their initial body weight, whereas the control group had maintained a loss of 1.1%. Fitness levels also improved markedly in the lifestyle intervention group relative to the control group at both 1 year and 4 years. Improvements in glycaemic control and in several important cardiovascular risk factors were greater in the intensive lifestyle intervention group than in the control group throughout the 4 years [5]. The long-term results of the Look AHEAD trial, which indicate many health benefits of intensive lifestyle intervention but a lack of benefit for cardiovascular morbidity and mortality, will be described in future publications.

Indications of possible cancer-related benefits of behavioural weight loss programmes have been evident for more than a decade. Thus, a randomized trial of a physical-activity-based weight management programme in breast cancer survivors ($n = 68$) demonstrated larger weight losses in the treatment group compared with the control group (5.7 kg vs 0.2 kg) and favourable changes in levels of inflammatory cytokines for intervention participants but not for control participants [6]. Furthermore, within participants assigned to the treatment group, participation in physical activity was significantly associated with favourable changes in interleukin-6 levels.

Theoretical premise of behavioural weight loss programmes

Behaviour-based weight loss programmes, such as those used in the Diabetes Prevention Program and Look AHEAD trials, are based primarily on social learning theory [7]. These programmes focus on helping individuals make long-term changes in both their eating and exercise behaviours to produce weight loss and maintenance. This approach assumes that providing information about diet and activity may be important and helpful to individuals but is not sufficient. Rather, it is important to help people understand their current eating and exercise behaviours and the variables that are influencing these behaviours (e.g. to appreciate the learned connection between going to the movies and eating popcorn). Behavioural treatment programmes then focus on teaching participants strategies for changing the variables that are

Energy restriction, age, and cancer risk

Piet van den Brandt

Caloric restriction (CR) – reduced energy intake without malnutrition – is the most robust nutritional intervention known to date that increases lifespan in many species, such as yeast, nematodes, fruit flies, and mammals [1]. In rodents exposed to young-onset CR (age, 1–3 months), CR inhibits spontaneous and induced tumours in various organs. Effects of middle-age-onset CR on cancer risk are less clear, although beneficial effects are seen on age-related processes. In mice, a CR of 15–53% below usual ad libitum intake resulted in a proportionate linear reduction of 20–62% in tumour incidence. Effects of CR seem larger on spontaneous tumours: a meta-analysis showed 55% fewer spontaneous mammary tumours, with no heterogeneity according to study characteristics such as age, duration and degree of CR, and nutrient type.

Two 20-year-long randomized trials in nonhuman primates have evaluated the effects of long-term CR on mortality and cancer risk in rhesus monkeys. In the Wisconsin National Primate Research Center (WNPRC) trial, an adult-onset CR of 30% non-significantly reduced overall mortality; incidence of cancer (gastrointestinal adenocarcinoma) was reduced by 50% compared with apes fed ad libitum. The National Institute on Aging (NIA) trial investigated moderate CR in young and old monkeys and found no differences in survival. Nevertheless, cancer incidence was significantly reduced in monkeys with young-onset CR compared with controls [2]. Several differences between these two trials limit the ability to draw conclusions, including less CR, a healthier control diet, and no ad libitum controls in the NIA trial.

Indications that energy restriction may be important for cancer in humans stem from observational research. Overweight, as an indicator of a positive energy balance, is positively related to risk of various cancers. With respect to CR, Dutch and Norwegian cohort studies of individuals who experienced 50–70% reduced food rationing (for < 1 year) in early life during the Second World War showed subsequently decreased risk of colorectal cancer [3] and (less consistently) of breast cancer, which may be due partly to confounding and malnutrition.

Ecological evidence on CR without malnutrition comes from Okinawans, who consume 15% fewer calories than mainland Japanese and have markedly lower cancer mortality rates. One randomized controlled trial is currently under way on effects of short-term CR (20–25% reduction for 6–12 months) in overweight subjects. Risk factors for coronary heart disease and cancer improved, but CR adherence was low in the longer-term group. However, applying CR to subjects of normal weight to achieve a low-normal body mass index of < 21 kg/m^2 (as in nonhuman studies) differs from applying CR to overweight or obese individuals when studying health effects [1].

Possible mechanisms underlying beneficial effects of CR involve metabolic adaptations to CR, effects of CR on tumorigenic processes, for example upregulated DNA repair and downregulated insulin/IGF-1/mTOR pathways [1], and epigenetic influences [3]. In summary, CR has beneficial effects on longevity and cancer incidence in different species; effects seem clearer with young-onset CR. Effects in humans remain promising but uncertain due to the relatively few randomized controlled trials that have concluded.

References

1. Omodei D, Fontana L (2011). FEBS Lett, 585:1537–1542. http://dx.doi.org/10.1016/j.febslet.2011.03.015 PMID:21402069

2. Mattison JA et al. (2012). Nature, 489:318–321. http://dx.doi.org/10.1038/nature11432 PMID:22932268

3. Hughes LAE et al. (2009). PLoS One, 4:e7951. http://dx.doi.org/10.1371/journal.pone.0007951 PMID:19956740

leading to inappropriate eating and sedentary behaviour as well as ways to evaluate the effect of the changes on their eating and exercise habits and ultimately their body weight.

Format of behavioural weight loss programmes

Typically, behavioural weight loss programmes are offered in group settings, with about 10–20 participants treated together. Groups are often closed-format; participants all start at the same time and remain in the same group. Meetings (typically 60 minutes long) are held weekly for 6 months, every 2 weeks for the next 6 months, and then monthly for the following 6 months. This extended schedule of treatment contact has been shown to improve long-term outcomes [8]. Groups are typically led by a multidisciplinary team of nutritionists, exercise physiologists, and behavioural therapists. The protocols for the lifestyle intervention used in the Diabetes Prevention Program and Look AHEAD trials are available online.

Energy balance

Change in body weight is influenced by the balance of caloric intake relative to caloric expenditure. Thus, behavioural interventions typically focus on lowering caloric intake – typically by approximately 500–1000 kcal (2000–4000 kJ) per day – while increasing physical activity. The dietary and physical activity components of the energy balance are reviewed below, and recommendations are offered.

Diet

Calorie goals given to participants typically vary by baseline body weight [9]. Individuals who weigh 200 pounds (90 kg) or less at baseline are given calorie goals of approximately 1200 kcal (5000 kJ) per day, whereas those who weigh more than 200 pounds (90 kg) are given goals of 1500–1800 kcal (6250–7500 kJ) per day. These goals should lead to caloric intake deficits of approximately 500–1000 kcal (2000–4000 kJ) per day, which are associated with a weight loss of 1–2 pounds (0.5–1 kg) per week. In addition, participants are recommended to decrease their fat intake, typically by consuming less than 25% of caloric intake from fat. Furthermore, participants are encouraged to increase intake of fruits and vegetables while decreasing intake of foods that observational studies suggest may be associated with obesity, such as sugar-sweetened beverages and high-fat snack foods [10].

Physical activity

Participants in behavioural weight loss programmes are encouraged not only to decrease their caloric intake but also to increase their level of participation in physical activity. This is often approached in two ways: (i) by increasing participation in moderate-intensity physical activity and (ii) by increasing overall lifestyle physical activity. The American College of Sports Medicine [11] recommends 150–200 minutes per week of moderate-intensity activity (such as brisk walking) for individuals trying to maintain weight, and more than 250 minutes per week for those trying to lose weight. Participants are encouraged to work up to these goals by gradually adding 10 minutes per week above baseline. In addition, participants typically track unstructured, lifestyle physical activity using pedometers or accelerometers and aim to gradually increase their activity to reach a goal of 10 000 steps per day.

Key components of weight management programmes

In addition to providing information about diet and physical activity, other key components of weight management programmes focus on improving self-regulatory skills and changing the antecedents and consequences of dietary and physical activity behaviours. These key components are discussed below.

Goal setting

Self-regulation is generally viewed as an internal process that involves goal setting, self-monitoring, and evaluation of success or failure of goal achievement. Setting clear goals for caloric intake and physical activity provides structure and direction. Individuals are encouraged to set goals that are short-term (typically a weekly weight loss goal vs a "goal weight"), measurable (e.g. eating an apple as a snack on three days during the week vs "eating more fruit"), and attainable (e.g. setting a starting activity goal to walk for 15 minutes three days per week vs running for an hour every day).

Self-monitoring

Self-monitoring, a key step in evaluating progress towards goal achievement, may involve keeping records of body weight, caloric intake (as indicated by food consumed), and physical activity (by using a pedometer or accelerometer). Self-monitoring allows individuals to assess their progress towards goals and to receive feedback on the adequacy of their goal-directed behaviours. Adherence to self-monitoring has been demonstrated to be significantly associated with success in both weight loss and long-term maintenance of weight loss [12].

Problem-solving skills

Problem-solving is a process by which individuals can address barriers to behaviour change [13]. Typically, problem-solving includes five distinct steps (Box 4.2.1). An example of a problem-solving participant worksheet is shown in Fig. 4.2.2. The five-step problem-solving model is generally viewed as an iterative process, and if the chosen solution does not adequately address the barrier, individuals are encouraged to cycle back to steps 3 and 4 to try alternative solutions.

Changing behavioural antecedents

Behaviour is affected both by antecedents – events that happen before the given behaviour – and by consequences, which are both positive or negative events that occur after the behaviour (Fig. 4.2.3). For example, an individual's choice of lunch can

Box 4.2.1. Problem-solving skills training: the five-step problem-solving model.

Step 1.
Positive problem orientation.
The view that problems are a normal part of behaviour change versus evidence of overall failure.

Step 2.
Problem definition.
Individuals clearly describe the barrier to change in objective, concrete terms.

Step 3.
Generation of alternatives.
Individuals brainstorm potential solutions, seeking quantity of ideas over quality.

Step 4.
Decision-making.
Participants evaluate decisions to decide which would be the best solution to the given problem.

Step 5.
Solution implementation and verification.
Participants implement the chosen solution and evaluate (through self-monitoring) whether this solution works.

Problem-Solving Skills Worksheet

What is the problem?_____

What are potential solutions?

_____
_____
_____

Choose one solution!

I will: _____ When? _____

Roadblocks that may come up: I will handle them by:

_____   _____

_____   _____

I will do this to make success more likely:

_____

be affected by their environment, and specifically the availability of nearby restaurants, and by thoughts and feelings (such as cravings, or feeling stressed or upset). These antecedents can often be manipulated by participants to assist with health behaviour change, as discussed below.

Stimulus control

Environmental factors have been demonstrated to affect both eating behaviours and physical activity. For example, the easy availability of high-calorie, highly palatable "junk food" can increase caloric intake, and lack of recreation facilities, safe walking areas, or sidewalks can decrease participation in physical activity. Individuals have some control over their environments and can often enact positive environmental change at home and work.

Changing cognitions

Thoughts and feelings can also represent the antecedents in Fig. 4.2.3. According to the cognitive behavioural model of behaviour, an individual's thoughts affect their feelings, which can then affect behaviour. Thus, a person having the thought "I'll never be able to lose weight" is likely to feel upset, frustrated, or angry, which may lead to the behaviour

of overeating or avoiding planned exercise. The process of cognitive restructuring involves identifying maladaptive thoughts, labelling these thoughts, and replacing them with more rational thoughts. For example, the thought "I'll never be able to lose weight" can be replaced with the thought "I may have had a challenging week, but I've lost 15 pounds so far and can recover from this slip."

Changing behavioural consequences

In addition to changing behavioural antecedents, the consequences of behaviour can be modified to affect future behaviour. Individuals will be more likely to engage in a behaviour

if it is tied in with a reward versus a punishment. Thus, manipulating the consequences of behaviour can lead to positive behaviour change. In general, individuals are encouraged to use non-food rewards, such as stickers, positive notes, buying new clothing, and so on. Increasing social support for behaviour change and use of programmatic incentives have also been demonstrated to lead to positive behaviour change.

Social support

A group format for lifestyle weight management interventions has been used to invoke social support for individual behaviour change. Group cohesion has been shown to enhance the effectiveness of weight management treatment, even for people who indicate before intervention that they would prefer individual treatment. Sharing success at behaviour change with the group can elicit positive support, acting as a social reward for the individual.

Incentives

The use of incentives in weight management stems from literature in behavioural economics, which has demonstrated that people tend to discount long-term rewards in favour of short-term gains. This applies to weight management in that long-term benefits of improved dietary and activity behaviours, including weight loss and improvements in metabolic risk factors, can be less motivating than short-term benefits such as the pleasure of eating or being

Fig. 4.2.3. The A-B-C model of behaviour.

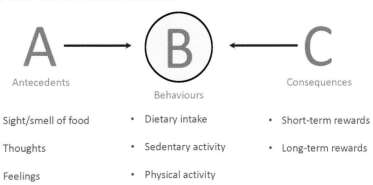

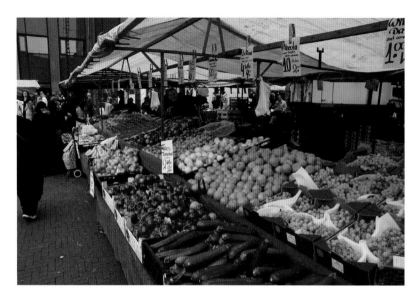

successful at maintaining weight loss tend to continue to consume a low-calorie, low-fat diet, eat breakfast, regularly self-monitor body weight and food intake, and engage in high levels of physical activity [18].

Dissemination and novel interventions

While behavioural weight management programmes have demonstrated efficacy and effectiveness, dissemination remains a barrier to wide access to treatment. Cost and availability of trained staff often limit the reach of these programmes, especially the high-intensity programmes most often delivered in research settings: typically 3–6 months of weekly groups, followed by several months of extended-care groups, meeting every 2 weeks and then monthly. Thus, increasing research has focused on lower-cost delivery of these programmes, including stepped-care, phone-based, and Internet-based programmes. Interventions using newer self-monitoring technologies, including activity monitors and smartphone applications that allow individuals to track their weight, food intake, and activity, hold promise as access to computers and smartphones across the population has been increasing substantially.

sedentary. Incentives for behaviour change and weight loss can provide additional reinforcement to the consequence end of the model shown in Fig. 4.2.3. Monetary incentives or deposit contracts, where participants deposit money that is returned only if they meet programme goals, have been shown to improve initial treatment results, but their long-term effects are still unclear [14].

Maintenance of weight loss

Long-term maintenance of weight loss has remained a substantial challenge [15,16]. After an intervention ends, individuals tend to regain lost weight, typically regaining one third to one half within 1 year of the end of treatment and returning to baseline weight within 3–5 years after treatment [17]. Research has focused on identifying factors that improve the long-term maintenance of weight loss; to date, one of the most successful factors has been the provision of extended care. A recent review of the literature on maintenance of weight loss suggested that the provision of extended care leads to the maintenance of an additional 3.2 kg of weight loss over 17.6 months after the intervention

compared with the control group [8]. Researchers are currently working to develop additional approaches to improving long-term maintenance of weight loss.

In addition, individual factors that promote long-term maintenance have been investigated. Using a national registry of people who have been successful in losing at least 13.6 kg and maintaining this loss for at least 1 year, researchers have found that people who are

Fig. 4.2.5. The National Health Service in the United Kingdom has a website on healthy living, called Change4Life. The "Eat well" section of the website enables people to plan healthy meals.

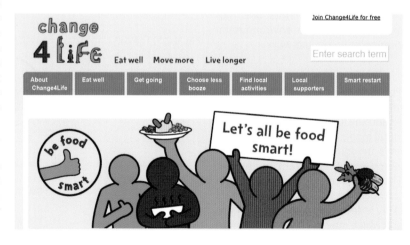

EPIC as a model study vehicle

Elio Riboli

The European Prospective Investigation into Cancer and Nutrition (EPIC) was developed at IARC, in close collaboration with several major national research institutions, as a long-term multicentre prospective cohort study in western Europe designed specifically to investigate the relationship between lifestyle, diet, and cancer. Enrolment of EPIC participants began in 1992, with the invitation of mainly healthy subjects aged 35–70 years from the general population in certain geographical areas. By the end of the recruitment phase, in 2000, EPIC was the largest prospective cohort study with a baseline biorepository aimed at investigating cancer etiology, with 521 330 participants from 23 study centres in 10 European countries.

Participants completed questionnaires on diet and lifestyle factors, including physical activity, and underwent measurements of anthropometric characteristics (e.g. weight, height, waist and hip circumferences), blood pressure, and pulse rate. Anonymized data are stored in a central secured database at IARC. EPIC was the first prospective study to collect and store blood from such a large number of participants: 388 467 blood samples of 30 ml each were collected and aliquoted into 28 plastic straws stored in liquid nitrogen, with aliquots divided between the central biorepository at IARC and each national centre. Since initial baseline collection, EPIC participants have been followed up to monitor changes in major dietary and lifestyle factors. Follow-up aimed at identifying cancer cases and dates and causes of death occurring among the EPIC cohort is principally based on record linkage with data from population cancer registries and regional or national death registries [1].

The design of the EPIC cohort is key to facilitating studies of cancer etiology. It was the first prospective study with a bespoke biorepository of its size in the world. Wide geographical coverage also means that EPIC includes populations with varying dietary and lifestyle habits and different underlying cancer incidence rates; this strategy was conceived to increase the overall statistical power to identify diet–disease relationships. The range of data as well as biological samples that were collected before diagnosis from the same population enables integrated analyses of cancer risk factors. Finally, through long-term follow-up spanning almost two decades, more than 60 000 newly incident cancer cases have been reported, giving scope for well-powered studies.

EPIC has proven to be a powerful resource to investigate the association between complex nutritional, metabolic, and genetic characteristics and cancer risk. An example is the identification using EPIC of links between metabolic syndrome and cancer risk. Metabolic syndrome is a cluster of metabolic abnormalities, including abdominal obesity, elevated blood pressure, abnormal glucose metabolism, and dyslipidaemia. It was shown that individual components of metabolic syndrome, such as insulin resistance (as measured by serum C-peptide levels) and central obesity, are associated with increased risk of several types of cancer [2]. While metabolic syndrome was associated with colorectal cancer risk, this could be accounted for by individual components of the syndrome, namely abnormal glucose

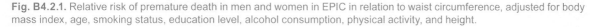

Fig. B4.2.1. Relative risk of premature death in men and women in EPIC in relation to waist circumference, adjusted for body mass index, age, smoking status, education level, alcohol consumption, physical activity, and height.

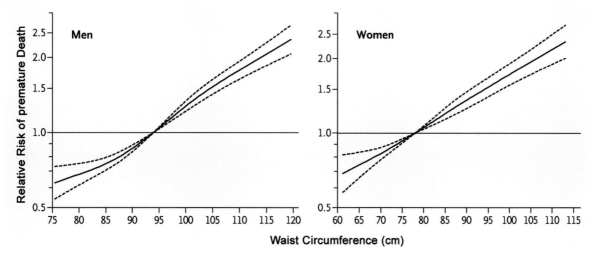

metabolism and central obesity, indicating that complex definitions of metabolic syndrome may not be of additional clinical utility in identifying individuals at increased risk of colorectal cancer.

Concerning central obesity, EPIC data allowed clarification of the apparent paradox by which being very slim (body mass index [BMI], 20–23 kg/m²) and being overweight (BMI, 26–30 kg/m²) appeared to be associated with similarly higher risk of all-cause mortality in adult life, compared with having a medium BMI (about 24–25 kg/m²). This paradox was often described as a J-shaped risk function of BMI versus mortality rates. EPIC showed that waist circumference adjusted for BMI is linearly related to the risk of premature death, that having a slim waist is associated with the lowest mortality, and that the apparent excess is due to individuals with low BMI but with low muscular mass and excess abdominal adiposity (Fig. B4.2.1) [3].

References

1. Bingham S, Riboli E (2004). *Nat Rev Cancer*, 4:206–215. http://dx.doi.org/10.1038/nrc1298 PMID:14993902

2. Jenab M *et al.* (2007). *Int J Cancer*, 121:368–376. http://dx.doi.org/10.1002/ijc.22697 PMID:17372899

3. Pischon T *et al.* (2008). *N Engl J Med*, 359:2105–2120. http://dx.doi.org/10.1056/NEJMoa0801891 PMID:19005195

Given the evidence that excess body weight and low levels of physical activity are associated with cancer risk and poorer survival outcomes (see "EPIC as a model study vehicle"), there is a need to conduct clinical trials to determine whether behavioural weight loss interventions can improve survival and/or help to prevent cancer [1]. Behavioural weight loss programmes are effective in helping participants lose 7–10% of their initial body weight; these weight losses produce numerous health benefits and should be evaluated further for cancer prevention and survival. A current randomized controlled trial, including 962 patients in 40 centres, is investigating the impact of physical activity on disease outcome in colon cancer survivors [19].

Data relating to cancer outcomes affected by adherence to weight control and/or physical activity guidelines are becoming available. Consequences of adherence to World Cancer Research Fund recommendations were monitored among approximately 30 000 postmenopausal women aged 50–76 years at baseline in 2000–2002

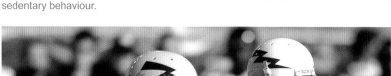

Fig. 4.2.6. Paradoxically, sport shown on television may play a role in determining sedentary behaviour.

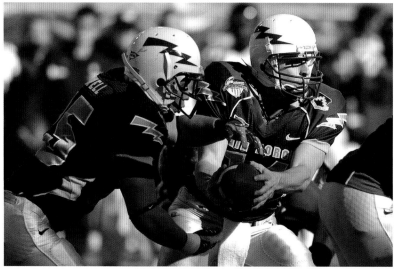

with no history of breast cancer. Meeting these cancer prevention recommendations, specifically those related to alcohol, body fatness, and intake of plant foods, was associated with reduced breast cancer incidence [20]. Benefits to cancer survivors have also been observed [21]. Cancer prevention through promotion of physical activity and dietary change in cancer screening settings is also being explored [22]. Future trials will investigate the role of weight loss and/or increased physical activity in primary prevention of various tumour types.

References

1. Ballard-Barbash R, Hunsberger S, Alciati MH et al. (2009). Physical activity, weight control, and breast cancer risk and survival: clinical trial rationale and design considerations. J Natl Cancer Inst, 101:630–643. http://dx.doi.org/10.1093/jnci/djp068 PMID:19401543

2. Knowler WC, Barrett-Connor E, Fowler SE et al.; Diabetes Prevention Program Research Group (2002). Reduction in the incidence of type 2 diabetes with lifestyle intervention or metformin. N Engl J Med, 346:393–403. http://dx.doi.org/10.1056/NEJMoa012512 PMID:11832527

3. Coughlin SS, Calle EE, Teras LR et al. (2004). Diabetes mellitus as a predictor of cancer mortality in a large cohort of US adults. Am J Epidemiol, 159:1160–1167. http://dx.doi.org/10.1093/aje/kwh161 PMID:15191933

4. Wadden TA, Neiberg RH, Wing RR et al.; Look AHEAD Research Group (2011). Four-year weight losses in the Look AHEAD study: factors associated with long-term success. Obesity (Silver Spring), 19:1987–1998. http://dx.doi.org/10.1038/oby.2011.230 PMID:21779086

5. Jakicic JM, Egan CM, Fabricatore AN et al. (2013). Four-year change in cardiorespiratory fitness and influence on glycemic control in adults with type 2 diabetes in a randomized trial: the Look AHEAD trial. Diabetes Care, 36:1297–1303. http://dx.doi.org/10.2337/dc12-0712 PMID:23223405

6. Pakiz B, Flatt SW, Bardwell WA et al. (2001). Effects of a weight loss intervention on body mass, fitness, and inflammatory biomarkers in overweight or obese breast cancer survivors. Int J Behav Med, 18:333–341. http://dx.doi.org/10.1007/s12529-010-9079-8 PMID:21336679

7. Bandura A (1986). Social Foundations of Thought and Action: A Social Cognitive Theory. Englewood Cliffs, NJ: Prentice-Hall.

8. Ross Middleton KM, Patidar SA, Perri MG (2012). The impact of extended care on the long-term maintenance of weight loss: a systematic review and meta-analysis. Obes Rev, 13:509–517. http://dx.doi.org/10.1111/j.1467-789X.2011.00972.x PMID:22212682

9. Wing RR (2008). Behavioral approaches to the treatment of obesity. In: Bray GA, Bouchard C, eds. Handbook of Obesity: Clinical Applications, 3rd ed. New York: Informa Healthcare, pp. 227–248.

10. Mozaffarian D, Hao T, Rimm EB et al. (2011). Changes in diet and lifestyle and long-term weight gain in women and men. N Engl J Med, 364:2392–2404. http://dx.doi.org/10.1056/NEJMoa1014296 PMID:21696306

11. Donnelly JE, Blair SN, Jakicic JM et al.; American College of Sports Medicine (2009). American College of Sports Medicine Position Stand. Appropriate physical activity intervention strategies for weight loss and prevention of weight regain for adults. Med Sci Sports Exerc, 41:459–471. http://dx.doi.org/10.1249/MSS.0b013e3181949333 PMID:19127177

12. Burke LE, Wang J, Sevick MA (2011). Self-monitoring in weight loss: a systematic review of the literature. J Am Diet Assoc, 111:92–102. http://dx.doi.org/10.1016/j.jada.2010.10.008 PMID:21185970

13. D'Zurilla T, Nezu AM (2006). Problem-Solving Therapy: A Positive Approach to Clinical Intervention, 3rd ed. New York: Springer.

14. Burns RJ, Donovan AS, Ackermann RT et al. (2012). A theoretically grounded systematic review of material incentives for weight loss: implications for interventions. Ann Behav Med, 44:375–388. http://dx.doi.org/10.1007/s12160-012-9403-4 PMID:22907712

15. Jeffery RW, Drewnowski A, Epstein LH et al. (2000). Long-term maintenance of weight loss: current status. Health Psychol, 19 Suppl: 5–16. http://dx.doi.org/10.1037/0278-6133.19.Suppl1.5 PMID:10709944

16. Perri MG, Foreyt JP, Anton SD (2008). Preventing weight regain after loss. In: Bray GA, Bouchard C, eds. Handbook of Obesity: Clinical Applications, 3rd ed. New York: Informa Healthcare, pp. 249–268.

17. Thomas PR, Stern JS (1995). Weighing the Options: Criteria for Evaluating Weight-Management Programs. Washington, DC: National Academy Press.

18. Wing RR, Hill JO (2001). Successful weight loss maintenance. Annu Rev Nutr, 21:323–341. http://dx.doi.org/10.1146/annurev.nutr.21.1.323 PMID:11375440

19. Courneya KS, Booth CM, Gill S et al. (2008). The Colon Health and Life-Long Exercise Change trial: a randomized trial of the National Cancer Institute of Canada Clinical Trials Group. Curr Oncol, 15:279–285. http://dx.doi.org/10.3747/co.v15i6.378 PMID:19079628

20. Hastert TA, Beresford SAA, Patterson RE et al. (2013). Adherence to WCRF/AICR cancer prevention recommendations and risk of postmenopausal breast cancer. Cancer Epidemiol Biomarkers Prev, 22:1498–1508. http://dx.doi.org/10.1158/1055-9965.EPI-13-0210 PMID:23780838

21. Inoue-Choi M, Lazovich D, Prizment AE, Robien K (2013). Adherence to the World Cancer Research Fund/American Institute for Cancer Research recommendations for cancer prevention is associated with better health-related quality of life among elderly female cancer survivors. J Clin Oncol, 31:1758–1766. http://dx.doi.org/10.1200/JCO.2012.45.4462 PMID:23569318

22. Anderson AS, Mackison D, Boath C, Steele R (2013). Promoting changes in diet and physical activity in breast and colorectal cancer screening settings: an unexplored opportunity for endorsing healthy behaviors. Cancer Prev Res (Phila), 6:165–172. http://dx.doi.org/10.1158/1940-6207.CAPR-12-0385 PMID:23324132

Websites

Diabetes Prevention Program Study Documents Web Site:
http://www.bsc.gwu.edu/DPP/index.htmlvdoc

Look AHEAD: Action for Health in Diabetes:
https://www.lookaheadtrial.org/

4.3

Designing and evaluating population-wide campaigns

4 PREVENTION

David Hill
Melanie Wakefield

Joakim Dillner (reviewer)
Surendra S. Shastri (reviewer)

Summary

- Population-wide campaigns can be an effective and efficient way to modify cancer risk in populations where more immediate channels of personal communication and influence are not feasible.

- In the design and evaluation of campaigns, a balance should be struck between influencing the environment and context in which individual cancer-related behaviours take place, and the intrapersonal determinants of those behaviours.

- Hypothesized causal pathways for change in individuals should be specified in advance, as this will help focus the interventions that make up the campaign as well as defining measures of outcome that will demonstrate and explain effects.

- Campaign messages need to take into account psychological factors that oppose, and facilitate, change in cancer-related behaviour.

- All campaigns should be subject to evaluation using specified criteria, particularly with reference to novel elements.

- While campaigns should be sensitive to local cultural factors, there is evidence that many campaigns can be successfully re-used or adapted for use in different countries.

When is a campaign the right approach?

Population-wide campaigns for primary or secondary prevention of cancer should be considered when the risk or risk factors for a prevalent cancer are spread widely through a population. Such campaigns invariably make use of mass media, often through carefully planned paid advertising, as well as other simultaneous communication and policy interventions. Campaigns would not normally be considered for rare tumours or those concentrated in subpopulations, such as in certain occupations or locations, or for influencing risk behaviours in small demographic subgroups. There are almost certainly other more effective and efficient alternative ways to directly communicate and influence risk in such cases, for instance by communicating at antenatal clinics where pregnant smokers are concentrated, or by using broadcast or print media in the preferred language of a targeted population subgroup.

Campaigns in cancer prevention are often conceived and funded by public health authorities as time-limited operations, whereas in reality their objectives can rarely be achieved or maintained without long-term investment of time, effort, and money. A cancer prevention campaign is better thought of as a health service for which the need is continuous (such as palliative care or ambulances) than as a "project" that has a defined end.

This chapter considers campaigns where the objective is to change a defined cancer-related *behaviour* in members of a defined population. It is not concerned with cancer "awareness-raising" campaigns. Indeed, such campaigns are of questionable public health value. Sometimes awareness-raising campaigns can do harm, as when prostate cancer awareness leads to inappropriate screening for the disease and to harms that at least arguably outweigh any benefits [1,2]. Neither should campaigns be undertaken as a substitute for potentially effective public health policy and regulation. Rather, they should build on good policy and generate public acceptance of the need for regulations that facilitate change in behaviours known to increase cancer risk.

Campaigns can be implemented for primary or secondary prevention, but their use in secondary prevention is more limited. Since secondary prevention depends principally on there being a means of detecting cancer early enough for treatment to be more effective than otherwise, health services (for screening, diagnosis, and treatment) need to be in place before the appropriate target group is invited or persuaded to attend. Contacting individuals directly with invitation letters is far more effective than public advertising of a service alone [3], so a campaign is not likely to be a major element in secondary prevention. In addition, unless the relevant health services are equally available to all members of a target population, population-wide campaigns would generate demand that could not be met. Thus, when screening services are introduced into a population in stages, it makes little sense to use mass media to communicate. However, assuming that all required services are ready, there may be a limited role in the early stages for mass communication to engender a level of awareness and public understanding to prime acceptance of personal invitations when they arrive. Later in the programme's life, there may also be a role for mass media in refreshing public interest should participation rates start to fall [4]. Overall, mass media campaigns alone are unlikely to achieve desired participation rates for secondary prevention programmes.

Habitual and non-habitual behaviours

There is a fundamental distinction to be made between strategies designed to change risky *habitual behaviours* such as tobacco use, over-nutrition, under-exercising, and alcohol consumption, and strategies aimed to prompt an individual to *act only once or twice* – such as human papillomavirus (HPV) or hepatitis B virus (HBV) vaccination – or *intermittently*, as is required for effective screening. Campaigns to change habitual behaviours are far more difficult to implement successfully.

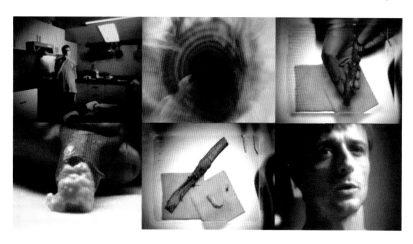

Fig. 4.3.1. Series of images from a video used by Australia's National Tobacco Campaign in 1997–2001. This particular advertisement highlighted how smoking causes arteries to become blocked, graphically emphasizing that "every cigarette is doing you damage".

The norm is for incremental change, at best, in population rates of a habitual target behaviour, whereas participation rates approaching 50% may rapidly follow the introduction of a screening or vaccination service that was supported by direct invitations and media publicity [5,6].

Habits are the result of a person's lifelong operant learning history, and are likely to be highly resistant to change. In the case of tobacco at least, the difficulties of reversing a habit are further complicated by the addictive qualities of nicotine. Nevertheless, campaigns have been shown to be effective in changing population risk behaviours, including tobacco use, albeit at incremental levels. It is noteworthy that small percentage changes in risk factor behaviours equate to large numbers of people when a risk factor is common, and that where relative risks are large, the potential for reducing early death is substantial. Furthermore, small percentage changes that are sustained over several years add up to big effects. As well as initiating trends, campaigns play a vital role in sustaining them [7,8].

Types of campaign message

Formulating the campaign message – what the communication actually says to the target individual and how

it is said – is at the core of campaign planning. Judicious application of psychological knowledge is helpful, if not essential. It is important that campaign planners are explicit about the way in which their message is expected to influence the receiver, because this sharpens the focus of the intervention and assists in formulating measures to evaluate whether the campaign is "working". Many laboratory studies have investigated the underlying nature of effective health messages – for instance, the relative merits of gain- or loss-framed wording [9] – but the applicability of results obtained to population-wide communications is uncertain. A smaller number of studies have explored message characteristics as they apply to broadcast cancer prevention campaigns [10].

A common issue is when, and when not, to use confronting, shocking, or "scary" message content [11]. One would hesitate to use such messages to promote participation in cancer screening. This is because people contemplating a screening offer are likely in a psychologically conflicted "approach–avoidance" state of mind, in which they are attracted by the possibility that they will get a reassuring all-clear report but at the same time are fearful of (and wishing to avoid) the possibility of a cancer diagnosis. Hence, a message

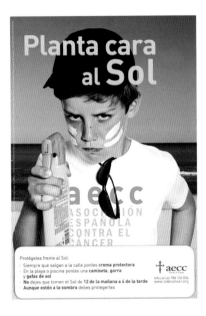

Fig. 4.3.2. Poster from the Spanish Association against Cancer (AECC) campaign for skin cancer prevention: "Stand up to the sun. Protect yourself against the sun. Whenever outside, put sunscreen on. At the beach or swimming pool, wear a shirt, a hat, and sunglasses. Don't let them go into the sun between 12 and 4 pm. Even in the shade, you have to protect yourself."

emphasizing how bad cancer can be might simply amplify avoidance without influencing approach tendencies. Positive portrayals of the reassurance offered by a favourable test result might be more effective. In contrast, scary messages are appropriate for a person contemplating quitting smoking, who has an "avoidance–avoidance" conflict between wanting to avoid lung cancer and wanting to avoid withdrawal symptoms. Messages that increase the desire to avoid lung cancer – by using vivid imagery, or eliciting powerful negative emotions through the use of personal testimonials or by dramatizing someone confronting a situation in which members of the target audience could envision themselves – might well tip the balance in favour of behaviour change in the smoker, who may then be more willing to tolerate withdrawal symptoms to avoid the feared health consequences.

In recent years, there has been a body of work on the efficacy of specific cancer prevention messages in different populations around the world, and certain principles stand out. At least in tobacco control, messages that communicate the serious health harms of smoking by eliciting emotional discomfort in viewers elicit similar responses in smokers in many countries of the world, suggesting great potential for sharing and recycling of advertisements across jurisdictions. These kinds of messages have high memorability, elicit early responses predictive of smoking behaviour change across many population subgroups within and between countries, and are more likely to generate cessation attempts in response to campaign exposure. This suggests that they are likely to be effective messages for wide dissemination [12–16]. Overall, this research supports the assumption on which many campaigns have been based: that an underlying dynamic of health behaviour change arises from a desire to reduce psychological discomfort felt when continuing to engage in the risk behaviour.

Campaign formulation

Prevention campaigns are usually created and implemented by teams of professionals from varying backgrounds, who all contribute according to their skills. The teams may include behavioural scientists, medical experts, health promotion specialists, copywriters, graphic designers, filmmakers, media specialists, journalists, and so on. Consistent messaging therefore needs to be built on a shared understanding of the way in which the communications are expected to influence the behaviour of people who are the targets of the campaign. Ideally, a small group, which includes a behavioural scientist experienced in such campaigns, would develop a behavioural model tailored to this campaign. Useful models can be found in the literature (Box 4.3.1) [17,18].

Models are based on principles derived from basic research in the behavioural sciences, for instance, in the fields of cognition, social learning, operant conditioning (positive and negative reinforcement), memory, modelling, motivation, and self-efficacy. By their nature, models in the theoretical literature are comprehensive and it is not always useful to try to apply them entirely in formulating a campaign. Rather, the planning group should take inspiration from them and then create and articulate a model suited to the intended campaign. The model becomes the reference point for all those who apply their creative talents to developing the campaign [19].

Box 4.3.1. "Big Five" principles of behaviour change

Hill and Dixon [18] proposed a set of principles they call the "Big Five", which encapsulate a large body of psychological and behavioural research on determinants of human behaviour.

Few, if any, cancer-related behaviours are the result of a single influence, so it follows that the more determinants a campaign can activate simultaneously, the more likely it is that change will occur.

Change in behaviour is likely to occur to the extent that a person:

1. Wants to do it (motivation)
2. Sees others doing it (modelling)
3. Has the capacity to do it (resources and self-efficacy beliefs)
4. Remembers to do it (memory)
5. Is reinforced for doing it, or suffers for not doing it (positive and negative reinforcement).

The "Big Five" principles can be used in campaign planning as a checklist to maximize forces for population behaviour change.

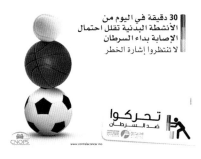

As well as making explicit the intended pathways of influence of campaign communications, the elements of a behavioural model enrich the campaign by providing a checklist of opportunities to intervene. Most behaviours, and certainly those behaviours involved in cancer prevention, have multiple "causes". It therefore follows that the more of these causes can be influenced by the campaign, the more likely it is that behaviour change will occur. For instance, a campaign that not only *modelled the desired behaviour* in a respected person but also *strengthened motivation* by communicating a fresh reason to change and promised *positive reinforcement* would more likely be effective than one that relied solely on modelling.

Market segmentation
Commercial marketing assumes a product or products that can be rendered relatively more attractive to a consumer. Different products can be created, varied, and packaged for population segments in ways that recommended health behaviours cannot. But even assuming that a behaviour can be equated to a product, one cannot create variants of the behaviour simply to suit the tastes of population segments.

Experience with primary prevention campaigns generally suggests that at any given time only a certain proportion of those at risk are ready to consider behaviour change. This is the segment that mass communications are most likely to activate. This is also a reason why campaigns need to extend over long periods: so that they will influence new segments or "waves" of people as they become ready to change.

That good health and avoiding disease is a universal (i.e. "unsegmented") human aspiration probably explains the fortunate finding that anti-smoking television advertisements made in high-income countries can readily be adapted for effective use in campaigns in low- and middle-income countries [12,16,20].

Channels of communication
The choice of channels to reach a target audience should be based on analysis of that population group's exposure to various communication channels. Such data are usually available commercially in low- and middle-income countries as well as high-income countries. This analysis will underpin media planning decisions about relative balance of effort and expenditure between television, radio, print, outdoor, transit, direct mail, and so on.

Although social media such as Facebook and Twitter are likely to be a means to achieve advocacy goals and strengthen the impact of broadcast campaigns to change cancer-related behaviour, the evidence base remains small [21]. However, promising results have been reported for pioneering work in low- and middle-income countries, including Viet Nam and Egypt [22,23].

Evaluation
It is helpful to think of a campaign as a hypothesis (or set of hypotheses) to be tested. Whether the campaign will "work" can never be known in advance, no matter how well grounded it is in prior research. Every new campaign will have novel elements, if only because it should be formulated to resonate with the specific culture in which it is implemented. Those implementing campaigns should pay as much attention to evaluation as to implementation, since that is the path to continuous improvement.

Careful pre-testing of campaign elements can lead to final improvements in communications before the campaign is launched. It may give useful insights into how the campaign will be received and how to manage misunderstandings or other difficulties that may arise [23]. Most campaigns rely heavily on self-reports from individuals, so it is important to use forms of questioning that minimize response bias [24] and that preferably have been validated objectively (e.g. biochemical validation of smoking status, or unobtrusive observation).

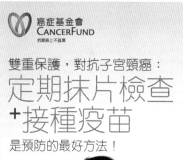
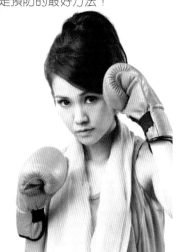

Fig. 4.3.5. A campaign for breast cancer prevention in Singapore: "Are you obsessed with the right things? The difference between a pimple and breast cancer is that of life and death. Regular breast checks are the best way to fight cancer. Show support for the women in your life by purchasing a Pink Ribbon."

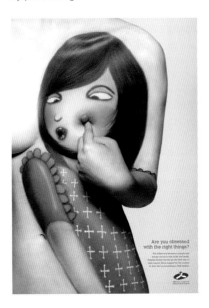

It is when measures of campaign effectiveness are being considered that the investment in clear articulation of hypothesized pathways of influence, as mentioned above, becomes apparent. The campaign evaluation should aim to quantify change at as many points as possible in the pathway, not merely the targeted risk behaviour itself. For instance, a campaign aiming to get smokers to make a cessation attempt by broadcasting new messages about macular degeneration should use representative sample surveys to assess population changes in knowledge about macular degeneration and to test whether such knowledge was associated with intentions to quit, as well as to assess changes over time in quitting behaviour itself.

As well as being effective, campaigns should be cost-effective – meaning they should achieve prevention outcomes at a lower per capita cost than alternative approaches. For example, there is good evidence that anti-tobacco

campaigns and skin cancer prevention campaigns are cost-effective [25,26]. Unsurprisingly, tobacco control campaigns (together with rigorous evaluations) have been the most common, leading to a substantial knowledge base, some of which has relevance for campaigns on other cancer risk behaviours.

Examples of successful campaigns

Anti-tobacco
An early, landmark campaign was the New South Wales "Quit. For Life" campaign (starting in 1983), which used a powerful image of tar being squeezed from a sponge to convey the build-up of carcinogenic particulate matter in lungs from tobacco smoke. The campaign resulted in an estimated short-term reduction in smoking prevalence of 2.8% [27]. This effect was replicated with the onset of the campaign in the adjoining state of Victoria the following year [28].

California conducted a well-funded and long-term campaign and showed reductions in smoking prevalence, resulting in a 4% difference between California and the rest of the USA in 1995, although momentum later waned, probably as a result of decreased government funding and increased pro-tobacco advertising [29].

New York State used strong graphic and emotional content in a televised mass media campaign supplemented by advertisements to build confidence in the ability to quit smoking, and between 2003 and 2009 reported a fall in prevalence of 18%, compared with a fall of only 5% nationally [30].

In Massachusetts, after the introduction of a comprehensive campaign that included significant price (tax) increases in 1993, the prevalence of smoking fell at an average annual rate of 4% until 1999, in contrast to little or no change in the rest of the USA, excluding California [31].

A national television and radio campaign to warn of the hazards of smokeless tobacco use in India

was shown to produce effects on precursors of behaviour change, including intentions to modify smokeless tobacco use, in the target population [32].

Sun protection
The commencement of the SunSmart campaign in Victoria, Australia, in 1989 was followed by a significant improvement in sun-related beliefs and behaviours and a reduction in prevalence of sunburn (assumed to be an intermediate marker of carcinogenic risk), after adjusting for ambient levels of ultraviolet radiation at the time observations were made [33], and long-term follow-up showed a continuing effect [34].

Diet/nutrition
The "1% or Less" campaign was an intensive 6-week mass media campaign to promote the use of low-fat milk in Wheeling, West Virginia, in the USA. After the campaign, 34% of milk drinkers indicated that they had changed to low-fat milk, compared with 3.6% in the control community [35]. Also, sales of low-fat milk increased from 29% to 46% in the intervention community.

Physical activity
The VERB campaign (Fig. 4.3.6), which was implemented nationally in the USA from 2002 to 2006, used commercial advertising and marketing techniques to increase physical activity levels in children. Changes that suggested an effect of the campaign were reported in attitudes and behaviour [36].

Campaign principles applied to subpopulations
Using Vietnamese-language media, a campaign to promote colorectal cancer screening among Vietnamese Americans in Alameda and Santa Clara counties in California in 2004–2006 resulted in greater screening participation than in comparison communities that did not receive the campaign [37].

Also using Vietnamese-language media, a campaign in Houston,

Texas, to promote the receipt of three hepatitis B virus vaccinations for Vietnamese American children aged 3–18 years resulted in increased knowledge among parents about such vaccinations and a significantly higher increase in the rate of vaccinations compared with a control community [38].

The cancer prevention environment

All behaviour is a product both of intra-individual factors and of the environments in which behaviours take place. Campaigns take place in, and can be affected both positively and negatively by, the prevailing social, policy, and regulatory environments. So the best campaigns not only rely on a conducive environment; successful prevention campaigns help to create such environments.

Ideally, to make a public health impact, the social and regulatory environments will need to move in concert with successive phases of public communication campaigns.

Fig. 4.3.6. One of many posters used for the VERB campaign in the USA. The 2002–2006 campaign was aimed at increasing and maintaining physical activity among tweens (ages 9–13).

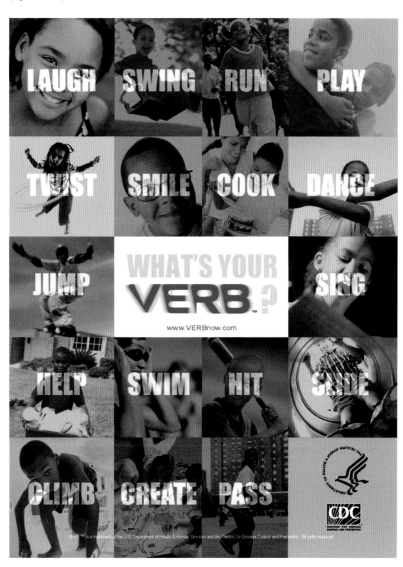

References

1. Chapman S, Barratt A, Stockler M (2010). *Let Sleeping Dogs Lie? What Men Should Know before Getting Tested for Prostate Cancer.* Sydney, Australia: Sydney University Press.

2. Schröder FH, Hugosson J, Roobol MJ *et al.*; ERSPC Investigators (2009). Screening and prostate-cancer mortality in a randomized European study. *N Engl J Med*, 360:1320–1328. http://dx.doi.org/10.1056/NEJMoa0810084 PMID:19297566

3. Ferroni E, Camilloni L, Jimenez B *et al.*; Methods to Increase Participation Working Group (2012). How to increase uptake in oncologic screening: a systematic review of studies comparing population-based screening programs and spontaneous access. *Prev Med*, 55:587–596. http://dx.doi.org/10.1016/j.ypmed.2012.10.007 PMID:23064024

4. Mullins R, Wakefield M, Broun K (2008). Encouraging the right women to attend for cervical cancer screening: results from a targeted television campaign in Victoria, Australia. *Health Educ Res*, 23:477–486. http://dx.doi.org/10.1093/her/cym021 PMID:17615181

5. Ladner J, Besson MH, Hampshire R *et al.* (2012). Assessment of eight HPV vaccination programs implemented in lowest income countries. *BMC Public Health*, 12:370. http://dx.doi.org/10.1186/1471-2458-12-370 PMID:22621342

6. Brotherton J, Gertig D, Chappell G *et al.* (2011). Catching up with the catch-up: HPV vaccination coverage data for Australian women aged 18–26 years from the National HPV Vaccination Program Register. *Commun Dis Intell Q Rep*, 35:197–201. PMID:22010515

7. Wakefield MA, Bowe SJ, Durkin SJ *et al.* (2013). Does tobacco-control mass media campaign exposure prevent relapse among recent quitters? *Nicotine Tob Res*, 15:385–392. http://dx.doi.org/10.1093/ntr/nts134 PMID:22949574

8. Niederdeppe J, Farrelly MC, Hersey JC, Davis KC (2008). Consequences of dramatic reductions in state tobacco control funds: Florida, 1998–2000. *Tob Control*, 17:205–210. http://dx.doi.org/10.1136/tc.2007.024331 PMID:18390911

9. Gallagher KM, Updegraff JA (2012). Health message framing effects on attitudes, intentions, and behavior: a meta-analytic review. *Ann Behav Med*, 43:101–116. http://dx.doi.org/10.1007/s12160-011-9308-7 PMID:21993844

10. Durkin S, Brennan E, Wakefield M (2012). Mass media campaigns to promote smoking cessation among adults: an integrative review. *Tob Control*, 21:127–138. http://dx.doi.org/10.1136/tobaccocontrol-2011-050345 PMID:22345235

11. Hill D, Chapman S, Donovan R (1998). The return of scare tactics. *Tob Control*, 7:5–8. http://dx.doi.org/10.1136/tc.7.1.5 PMID:9706747

12. Wakefield M, Durrant R, Terry-McElrath Y *et al.* (2003). Appraisal of anti-smoking advertising by youth at risk for regular smoking: a comparative study in the United States, Australia, and Britain. *Tob Control*, 12 Suppl 2:ii82–ii86. http://dx.doi.org/10.1136/tc.12.suppl_2.ii82 PMID:12878778

13. Durkin SJ, Biener L, Wakefield MA (2009). Effects of different types of antismoking ads on reducing disparities in smoking cessation among socioeconomic subgroups. *Am J Public Health*, 99:2217–2223. http://dx.doi.org/10.2105/AJPH.2009.161638 PMID:19833980

14. Farrelly MC, Duke JC, Davis KC *et al.* (2012). Promotion of smoking cessation with emotional and/or graphic antismoking advertising. *Am J Prev Med*, 43:475–482. http://dx.doi.org/10.1016/j.amepre.2012.07.023 PMID:23079169

15. Davis KC, Nonnemaker J, Duke J *et al.* (2013). Perceived effectiveness of cessation advertisements: the importance of audience reactions and practical implications for media campaign planning. *Health Commun*, 28:461–72. http://dx.doi.org/10.1080/10410236.2012.696535 PMID:22812702

16. Wakefield M, Bayly M, Durkin S *et al.*; International Anti-Tobacco Advertisement Rating Study Team (2013). Smokers' responses to television advertisements about the serious harms of tobacco use: pre-testing results from 10 low- to middle-income countries. *Tob Control*, 22:24–31. http://dx.doi.org/10.1136/tobaccocontrol-2011-050171 PMID:21994276

17. Hornik R, Yanovitzky I (2003). Using theory to design evaluations of communication campaigns: the case of the national youth anti-drug media campaign. *Commun Theory*, 13:204–224. http://dx.doi.org/10.1111/j.1468-2885.2003.tb00289.x

18. Hill D, Dixon H (2010). Achieving behavioural changes in individuals and populations. In: Elwood JM, Sutcliffe SB, eds. *Cancer Control.* Oxford: Oxford University Press, pp. 43–61.

19. Hill D, Carroll T (2003). Australia's National Tobacco Campaign. *Tob Control*, 12 Suppl 2:ii9–ii14. http://dx.doi.org/10.1136/tc.12.suppl_2.ii9 PMID:12878768

20. Cotter T, Perez D, Dunlop S *et al.* (2010). The case for recycling and adapting anti-tobacco mass media campaigns. *Tob Control*, 19:514–517. http://dx.doi.org/10.1136/tc.2009.035022 PMID:20852321

21. Chou WY, Prestin A, Lyons C, Wen KY (2013). Web 2.0 for health promotion: reviewing the current evidence. *Am J Public Health*, 103:e9–e18. http://dx.doi.org/10.2105/AJPH.2012.301071 PMID:23153164

22. Hefler M, Freeman B, Chapman S (2012). Tobacco control advocacy in the age of social media: using Facebook, Twitter and Change. *Tob Control*, 22:210–214. http://dx.doi.org/10.1136/tobaccocontrol-2012-050721 PMID:23047890

23. World Lung Foundation Tobacco Control Mass Media Resource. 360 Mass Media Process. Available at http://67.199.72.89/mmr/english/360formativeResearch.html.

24. Dillman DA (1978). *Mail and Telephone Surveys: The Total Design Method.* New York: Wiley.

25. Hurley SF, Matthews JP (2008). Cost-effectiveness of the Australian National Tobacco Campaign. *Tob Control*, 17:379–384. http://dx.doi.org/10.1136/tc.2008.025213 PMID:18719075

26. Carter R, Marks R, Hill D (1999). Could a national skin cancer primary prevention campaign in Australia be worthwhile? An economic perspective. *Health Promot Int*, 14:73–82. http://dx.doi.org/10.1093/heapro/14.1.73

27. Dwyer T, Pierce JP, Hannam CD, Burke N (1986). Evaluation of the Sydney "Quit. For Life" anti-smoking campaign. Part 2. Changes in smoking prevalence. *Med J Aust*, 144:344–347. PMID:3485760

28. Pierce JP, Macaskill P, Hill D (1990). Long-term effectiveness of mass media led antismoking campaigns in Australia. *Am J Public Health*, 80:565–569. http://dx.doi.org/10.2105/AJPH.80.5.565 PMID:2327533

29. Pierce JP, Gilpin EA, Emery SL *et al.* (1998). Has the California tobacco control program reduced smoking? *JAMA*, 280:893–899. http://dx.doi.org/10.1001/jama.280.10.893 PMID:9739973

30. Davis KC, Farrelly MC, Duke J *et al.* (2012). Antismoking media campaign and smoking cessation outcomes, New York State, 2003–2009. *Prev Chronic Dis*, 9:E40. http://dx.doi.org/10.5888/pcd9.110102 PMID:22261250

31. Biener L, Harris JE, Hamilton W (2000). Impact of the Massachusetts tobacco control programme: population based trend analysis. *BMJ*, 321:351–354. http://dx.doi.org/10.1136/bmj.321.7257.351 PMID:10926595

32. Murukutla N, Turk T, Prasad CV *et al.* (2012). Results of a national mass media campaign in India to warn against the dangers of smokeless tobacco consumption. *Tob Control*, 21:12–17. http://dx.doi.org/10.1136/tc.2010.039438 PMID:21508418

33. Hill D, White V, Marks R, Borland R (1993). Changes in sun-related attitudes and behaviours, and reduced sunburn prevalence in a population at high risk of melanoma. *Eur J Cancer Prev*, 2:447–456. http://dx.doi.org/10.1097/00008469-199311000-00003 PMID:8287008

34. Dobbinson SJ, Wakefield MA, Jamsen KM *et al.* (2008). Weekend sun protection and sunburn in Australia: trends (1987–2002) and association with SunSmart television advertising. *Am J Prev Med*, 34:94–101. http://dx.doi.org/10.1016/j.amepre.2007.09.024 PMID:18201638

35. Reger B, Wootan MG, Booth-Butterfield S (1999). Using mass media to promote healthy eating: a community-based demonstration project. *Prev Med*, 29:414–421. http://dx.doi.org/10.1006/pmed.1998.0570 PMID:10564633

36. Huhman ME, Potter LD, Duke JC *et al.* (2007). Evaluation of a national physical activity intervention for children: VERB campaign, 2002–2004. *Am J Prev Med*, 32:38–43. http://dx.doi.org/10.1016/j.amepre.2006.08.030 PMID:17218189

37. Nguyen BH, McPhee SJ, Stewart SL, Doan HT (2010). Effectiveness of a controlled trial to promote colorectal cancer screening in Vietnamese Americans. *Am J Public Health*, 100:870–876. http://dx.doi.org/10.2105/AJPH.2009.166231 PMID:20299659

38. McPhee SJ, Nguyen T, Euler GL *et al.* (2003). Successful promotion of hepatitis B vaccinations among Vietnamese-American children ages 3 to 18: results of a controlled trial. *Pediatrics*, 111:1278–1288. http://dx.doi.org/10.1542/peds.111.6.1278 PMID:12777542

4.4

Prevention strategies common to noncommunicable diseases

Pekka Puska

Thiravud Khuhaprema (reviewer)
Richard Muwonge (reviewer)

Summary

- Extensive research during the past few decades has provided strong evidence for prevention of cancer and other major noncommunicable diseases. Although preventive actions among people at high risk are important and there are multiple tumour-specific measures, the greatest potential for cancer prevention in the general population is through integrated health promotion and policies that target certain lifestyle-related risk factors to prevent noncommunicable diseases.

- The WHO Global Strategy for the Prevention and Control of Noncommunicable Diseases targets four behavioural risk factors – tobacco, unhealthy diet, physical inactivity, and harmful use of alcohol – with specific strategies.

- The WHO Framework Convention on Tobacco Control describes the most effective measures, especially for demand reduction, and is binding for the countries that have ratified it.

- The WHO Global Strategy on Diet, Physical Activity, and Health includes a range of evidence-based interventions to influence diet and physical activity in the general population. Emphasis is placed on measures to promote production, availability, and marketing of healthier food stuffs.

- The WHO Global Strategy to Reduce the Harmful Use of Alcohol describes initiatives to reduce the harmful use of alcohol, with emphasis on alcohol policy.

- The major challenge to framing preventive measures for noncommunicable diseases is the gap between the scientific knowledge of risk and its extrapolation to achieve reduced incidence.

During the past two decades, the globalization of public health priorities has proceeded rapidly. Studies of the burden of disease worldwide have established that noncommunicable diseases (NCDs) are now the main causes of death, not only in developed countries but also in developing countries [1]. A landmark publication was *The World Health Report 2002*, which documented both the change in the burden of disease and the impact of the main risk factors [2].

As a consequence of the emerging NCD epidemic, the WHO Global Strategy for the Prevention and Control of Noncommunicable Diseases was approved by the World Health Assembly in 2000 [3]. It was based on the global increase of NCDs, the causal role of certain behaviour-linked risk factors, the accumulated scientific evidence indicating possibilities for NCD prevention, and the experience in several countries.

The potential of NCD prevention

The WHO Global Strategy for the Prevention and Control of Noncommunicable Diseases [3] acknowledged for the first time that NCDs are a priority area for WHO. The strategy focused on the four main groups of NCDs: cardiovascular disease, cancer, diabetes, and chronic pulmonary disease. It included comprehensive NCD control activities but emphasized prevention as the key public health approach.

Although the causal role of the main risk factors for NCDs was established beyond any reasonable doubt before 2000, the understanding of the great potential of NCD prevention has grown most rapidly since then. In Finland, large reductions in the age-specific rates of cardiovascular disease and cancer have occurred as a result of the preventive work begun in the 1970s [4].

In the early years of NCD prevention, emphasis was placed on early detection, individual treatment, and education about causative agents. This is commonly known as the "high-risk" approach. However, both epidemiological and behavioural/social considerations emphasize "population-based" prevention as the most effective public health approach [5,6].

The WHO Global Strategy for the Prevention and Control of Noncommunicable Diseases introduced the concept of integrated prevention. It was recognized that although specific activities related to different diseases are needed, the most effective public health approach requires intervention to reduce the impact on the entire population of risk factors that are common to several major NCDs. The WHO strategy specifically addresses tobacco use, unhealthy diet, physical inactivity, and harmful use of alcohol.

This chapter discusses cancer prevention in the general population through this integrated NCD prevention perspective. This is the most cost-effective and sustainable public health approach to achieving a major reduction of the cancer burden in general populations. However, it should be recognized that several other measures, discussed elsewhere in this Report, can substantially contribute to cancer prevention. These include various screening programmes, measures to control certain infectious diseases, and action to prevent skin cancers by restricting exposure to ultraviolet radiation and to prevent lung cancer by addressing outdoor and indoor air pollution, specifically including clean stove programmes in relevant countries.

Population-based integrated NCD prevention targets risk-related behaviours or lifestyles in the community as a whole and requires emphasis on the built and social environments as determining lifestyle, and on broad health promotion and policy interventions. This has also led to

consideration of the social determinants of particular lifestyles, and possibilities to influence them [7]. The early approaches to health education have, more recently, been supplemented by attempts to influence environments – physical and social. Such an "ecological" approach calls for comprehensive activities by different authorities, which may be equated to multisectoral actions, among which are policy measures by different sectors of the government, such as the Finnish initiative Health in All Policies [8].

Since the 2000 WHO strategy on NCDs, WHO has developed several major methodologies and tools for national interventions directed towards four behavioural risk factors: tobacco use, unhealthy diet, physical inactivity, and harmful use of alcohol.

WHO Framework Convention on Tobacco Control

The WHO Framework Convention on Tobacco Control (FCTC) was adopted in 2003 [9]. As of September 2013, 177 countries have ratified it. This is first time that international law has been used in the field of public health. The WHO FCTC specifies evidence-based elements of successful tobacco control; most initiatives are directed towards reducing demand for tobacco products. Demand may be reduced through education and communication (Fig. 4.4.1). Comprehensive educational, public awareness, and training programmes on tobacco control are directed towards health workers, other professionals, community groups, and decision-makers. Reducing tobacco use is difficult because of the strong addictive effects of nicotine and also because of the social dependence. Both pharmacological and non-pharmacological methods, the latter involving psychological and educational approaches, have been developed to effectively help tobacco users to quit. Tobacco control policies should include measures to provide cessation services [10].

The global tobacco epidemic is an immediate outcome of the

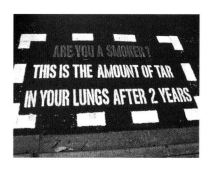

Fig. 4.4.1. An anti-smoking message painted on a pedestrian crossing in the Orchard Road area of Singapore.

powerful leverage of the multinational tobacco industry, exercised through advertising, promotion, sponsorship, and lobbying. Thus, an important component of tobacco control is a comprehensive ban on advertising, promotion, and sponsorship. In relation to this challenge, an international agreement is especially important because of the cross-border spread of advertising material.

Price and tax measures are effective and important means of reducing tobacco consumption, particularly among young people (see Chapter 4.1). Although there are no safe tobacco products, national or other relevant authorities can introduce regulations on testing and measuring tobacco products, and on levels of particular components in, and emissions from, these products.

Exposure to second-hand tobacco smoke, especially indoors, is recognized as causing multiple NCDs [11] and adversely affects vulnerable groups within the population, such as children. Smoke-free environments discourage people from initiating smoking and continuing to smoke. Thus, any tobacco control policy should include prohibition of smoking in indoor workplaces, on public transportation, in other indoor settings, and in public places such as stadiums.

Packaging for tobacco products should not promote the product by presenting misleading messages. Such misleading messages may include terms like "low tar", "light", "ultralight", or "mild". Tobacco packages

Fig. 4.4.2. New graphics and warnings on cigarette packaging are being implemented in several countries. This example from Brazil includes "Horror, Danger, Gangrene, Impotence, Pain, Death". Although community awareness of smoking as a cause of lung cancer predominates, morbidity and mortality due to smoking include the consequences of respiratory, cardiovascular, and other diseases.

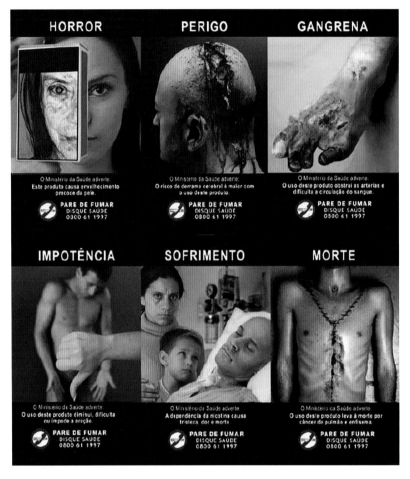

should carry large and clear health warnings in text or in the form of pictures, and/or be generic (Fig. 4.4.2). Australia was the first country to adopt the plain packaging of cigarettes [12].

The WHO FCTC specifies a range of measures to reduce supply. The sale of tobacco to minors should be prohibited, and this legislation should be comprehensively enforced. Vending machines should be placed so that children cannot obtain access. Surprisingly, a nontrivial percentage of the tobacco used worldwide is smuggled, manufactured illicitly, or counterfeited. Therefore, elimination of illicit trade in tobacco products is an issue requiring international collaboration by relevant authorities.

Although the scientific basis for tobacco control is very strong, further research is needed in several areas, including, for example, the vulnerability of particular populations. It is important for every country to identify its own research needs in the light of local circumstances. Monitoring trends in tobacco use in the general population and in subgroups is crucial. It is also important to monitor determinants and patterns of tobacco use, as well as the impact of activities related to tobacco control.

In 2009, the WHO FCTC Secretariat published a report on the global implementation of the convention [13]. The report concluded that the implementation varies substantially. Overall, most countries report high implementation rates for measures on packaging and labelling, sales to minors, and education and training. In general, implementation rates for programmes directed towards cessation remain low.

Promoting healthy diet and physical activity

Diet and physical activity are different from tobacco smoking in many fundamental respects [14]. Tobacco smoking is a very harmful practice and, in principle, not needed at all. Diet and physical activity are part of everyday life. Physical activity and eating a healthy diet are positive behaviours to be promoted [15]. Also, the health implications of diet are multiple and complicated. Furthermore, although there are general recommendations, the relationships of different nutrients and foods to different NCDs vary.

In 2004, WHO adopted a Global Strategy on Diet, Physical Activity, and Health [16]. This strategy provides countries with a comprehensive range of options to influence dietary practices and physical activity in their populations (Fig. 4.4.3). As background for this strategy, WHO, in collaboration with FAO, published the report *Diet, Nutrition and Prevention of Chronic Diseases* [17]. Based on expert advice, the report reviewed the evidence relating to nutrition as a means of preventing cardiovascular disease, cancer, diabetes, obesity, osteoporosis, and dental caries.

The WHO strategy's recommendations concerning diet for populations and individuals were the following:

- Achieve energy balance and a healthy weight.
- Limit energy intake from total fats, and shift fat consumption away from saturated fats to unsaturated fats; eliminate the intake of transfatty acids (also called trans fats).

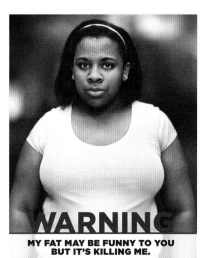

Fig. 4.4.3. Poster from the Strong4Life campaign to prevent childhood obesity, in Atlanta, USA. Obesity increases the risk of diabetes, cardiovascular disease, and certain cancers – the major noncommunicable diseases – worldwide.

- Increase consumption of fruits and vegetables, legumes, whole grains, and nuts.
- Limit the intake of free sugars.
- Limit salt (sodium) consumption.

Individuals were encouraged to engage in optimal levels of physical activity throughout their lives. Different types and amounts of physical activity are required to achieve different health outcomes; at least 30 minutes of regular, moderate-intensity physical activity on most days reduces the risk of cardiovascular disease, diabetes (Fig. 4.4.4), colon cancer, and probably breast cancer.

The strategies – both policies and necessary actions to achieve them – must be adopted comprehensively, taking a long-term perspective and engaging all sectors of society. The complex interactions between personal choices, social norms, and economic and environmental factors must be recognized. A life-course perspective is essential, and the strategies should be part of broad public health programmes. Priority should be

accorded to activities targeting the lowest-income population groups and communities.

Governments

Governments have a primary steering role and are encouraged to act within the context of comprehensive NCD prevention and health promotion. National strategies should identify the required measures and should include specific goals, objectives, and actions. Governments should take action in the following areas:
- Education, communication, and public awareness.
- Marketing, advertising, sponsorship, and promotion.
- Labelling of food products.
- Health claims.

School policies and programmes should support the adoption of healthy diets and physical activity of children, and health services should target the habits of patients and the general population. Governments should also invest in research and evaluation of nutrition and physical activity in the general population. National institutions for public health, nutrition, and physical activity have an important role to play in the implementation of programmes and in monitoring and evaluation.

Private sector and civil society

The private sector can also influence dietary practices and physical activity [18]. The food industry, retailers, catering organizations (including those responsible for meals at schools or workplaces), sporting-goods manufacturers, advertising and recreation businesses, and the media may all contribute to the adoption of good health practices. Moreover, commentaries note that food systems are rarely driven to deliver optimal human diets but predominantly to maximize profits, with increased obesity as the immediate outcome [19].

Recommendations to the food processing industry may include the following:

- Limit the levels of saturated fats, trans fats, sugars, and salt in products.
- Continue to develop and provide affordable, healthy, and nutritious choices to consumers.
- Introduce new products with better nutritional value than was previously available.
- Provide consumers with adequate and understandable product and nutritional information.
- Practise responsible marketing.
- Provide simple, clear, and consistent food labels and evidence-based health claims.
- Assist in the development and implementation of physical activity programmes.

Workplaces provide settings for health promotion and disease prevention, and should make provision for healthy food choices and encouragement of physical activity.

Civil society and nongovernmental organizations can advocate for healthy lifestyles and influence the food industry to provide healthy products. Such organizations can mobilize community sentiment and influence the public agenda. Nongovernmental and civic groups can support the dissemination of information on healthy diets and physical activity.

Alcohol control

Alcohol consumption is among the top 10 causes of mortality worldwide,

Fig. 4.4.4. Testing of blood glucose with a blood glucose meter, used to help manage diabetes. Reduced incidence of diabetes, cardiovascular disease, and certain tumour types may be identified as benefits from reduced obesity, an outcome sought through adoption of better dietary practices and increased physical activity.

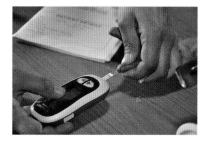

The global economics of chronic and noncommunicable diseases

Felicia Marie Knaul and Andrew Marx

Chronic and noncommunicable diseases (CNCDs) have massive ramifications for global poverty, financial security, and equity [1,2]. The World Economic Forum's *Global Risks 2010* report ranked chronic disease among the three most likely and severe risks facing the planet, with potential economic losses of more than US$ 1 trillion [1].

Between 2005 and 2015, income losses of US$ 558 billion in China and US$ 237 billion in India are predicted due to stroke, heart disease, and diabetes alone [3]. And the economic impact of CNCDs on low- and middle-income countries (LMICs) will become more severe over time, particularly affecting working-age populations. Although the predicted proportion of deaths from NCDs among those aged 15–59 years will fall globally by 2030, it will increase in LMICs [2].

Tobacco is a huge economic risk for LMICs. Tobacco's estimated annual burden of US$ 500 billion exceeds the total yearly health expenditure of all LMICs combined. Tobacco consumption is estimated to reduce global economic gross domestic product by 3.6% per year. If consumption continues to rise, the global annual economic cost of tobacco may reach US$ 1 trillion between 2020 and 2030 [4].

The estimated annual cost of scaling up interventions to reduce risk factors such as tobacco use and harmful alcohol consumption is only US$ 2 billion for all LMICs – less than US$ 0.40 per person. After including additional interventions

such as vaccinations against hepatitis B virus to prevent liver cancer and against human papillomavirus to prevent cervical cancer, the annual cost increases to US$ 9.4 billion: an annual per capita investment of less than US$ 1 for low-income countries, US$ 1.50 for lower-middle-income countries, and US$ 3 for upper-middle-income countries [3].

A 50% rise in chronic disease incidence and mortality, such as that projected for Latin America from 2002 to 2030, could slow annual economic growth by more than 2%, widening disparities between high-income countries and LMICs [5]. This projected economic burden exceeds any to date, including those from malaria and HIV/AIDS [3].

CNCDs also have a tremendous negative impact on the economic well-being of families. CNCDs, especially cancer, increase the risk of catastrophic health expenditure, impairing the ability of families to invest in education and nutrition. In South Asia, for example, the chances of catastrophic expenditures from hospitalizations are 160% higher for cancer than for infectious disease [6]. As typified by data from Egypt, people with NCDs have a 25% lower probability of being employed [7]. Furthermore, the burden of caregiving generally falls heavily on women and girls, exacerbating gender inequities by reducing their labour force participation and access to educational opportunities [2].

Inadequately investing in prevention and treatment of CNCDs is recognized as short-sighted

and misguided [1]. In the face of resource constraints, a short-term view would encourage LMICs to focus only on achieving the United Nations Millennium Development Goals. Yet, ignoring CNCDs places many countries at risk of not meeting many of the Millennium Development Goals because of escalating health costs and the health risks to mothers, infants, and young children [3]. Failure to protect populations from preventable health risks will inevitably and severely detract from both economic development and social well-being [3].

References

1. Global Risk Network of the World Economic Forum (2010). *Global Risks 2010: A Global Risk Network Report.* Geneva: World Economic Forum.

2. Nikolic IA *et al.* (2011). *Chronic Emergency: Why NCDs Matter.* Health, Nutrition and Population (HNP) Discussion Paper. Washington, DC: World Bank.

3. WHO (2011). *Global Status Report on Noncommunicable Diseases 2010.* Geneva: WHO.

4. Shafey O, Eriksen M, Ross H, Mackay J (2009). *The Tobacco Atlas*, 3rd ed. Atlanta, GA: American Cancer Society.

5. Stuckler D (2008). *Milbank Q*, 86:273–326. http://dx.doi.org/10.1111/j.1468-0009.2008.00522.x PMID:18522614

6. Engelgau MM *et al.* (2011). *Capitalizing on the Demographic Transition: Tackling Noncommunicable Diseases in South Asia.* Washington, DC: World Bank.

7. Rocco L *et al.* (2011). *Chronic Diseases and Labor Market Outcomes in Egypt.* Policy Research Working Paper 5575. Washington, DC: World Bank.

responsible for 2–3 million deaths per year [20]. NCDs are among the adverse health outcomes of alcohol consumption, which extend from the acute effects of intoxication, which contributes to accidents and anti-social behaviour, to chronic injury, including liver disease, certain

cancers (Fig. 4.4.5), and cardiovascular disease.

A special aspect of alcohol consumption is its addictive nature. Thus, alcohol is "no ordinary commodity" [21]. While certain adverse health consequences of drinking, including road accidents and criminal assault,

are usually a result of "harmful use", the prevalence of harmful use is closely related to the level of alcohol consumption in the general population. Accordingly, interventions should not be confined to "high-risk interventions" among problem users, but should address general alcohol policy and

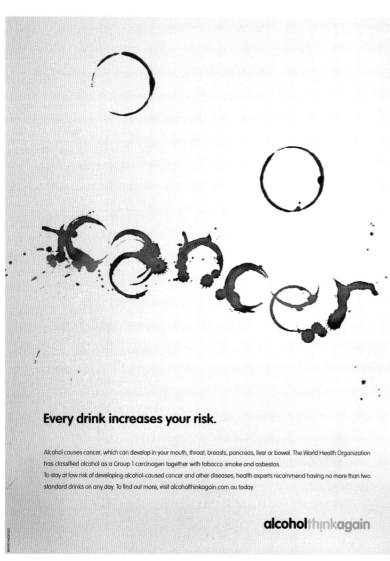

Every drink increases your risk.

Alcohol causes cancer, which can develop in your mouth, throat, breasts, pancreas, liver or bowel. The World Health Organization has classified alcohol as a Group 1 carcinogen together with tobacco smoke and asbestos.

To stay at low risk of developing alcohol-caused cancer and other diseases, health experts recommend having no more than two standard drinks on any day. To find out more, visit alcoholthinkagain.com.au today.

alcoholthinkagain

be population-based interventions. There is consensus about effective interventions to reduce alcohol consumption [21]. Price and availability are the most effective matters for interventions. Among other interventions are measures to limit drinking and driving, and mini-interventions in health services. Information campaigns alone seem to have no direct impact.

In 2010, WHO adopted the Global Strategy to Reduce the Harmful Use of Alcohol [22]. This strategy includes evidence-based policies and measures concerning pricing, availability, and marketing. *Pricing* policies are important because consumers are sensitive to changes in the price of alcohol. Policy options include: taxation, especially taking account of the alcohol content of particular beverages; restricting the use of price reductions for promoting sales; establishing minimum prices; and price concessions for non-alcoholic beverages. Pricing policies should take account of inflation and variation in incomes over time. Strategies that regulate the *availability* of alcohol through regulation, policies and programmes include: appropriate systems to regulate production, wholesaling, and serving (regulations may include government monopolies, regulating hours or days of sale, or sales in certain places or during certain events); minimum age for youth being permitted to purchase these products; and policies to reduce illicit production or smuggling. *Marketing* policies should be aimed at reducing the impact of advertising and other marketing, particularly as these matters affect young people. Frameworks should be established to regulate the nature of, and amount of expenditure on, marketing and sponsorship.

Health services are central to mitigating harm at the individual level among those with conditions caused by alcohol. Health services should address prevention through initiatives to reduce consumption and through treatment interventions for individuals and their families. Mini-interventions, in the form of identification of persons at risk and brief interventions, have proven to be cost-effective.

Conclusion

A range of evidence-based interventions have been identified to reduce the deleterious effects of major lifestyle-related risk factors common to cancer and other NCDs. This approach was recognized in recent global political developments that culminated in the United Nations High-Level Meeting on the Prevention and Control of Noncommunicable Diseases that took place in 2011 in New York [23]. Influencing the behavioural risk factors common to several major NCDs in the general population is a cost-effective and sustainable public health approach immediately relevant to cancer prevention. Although effective treatment of cancer patients is a necessity, it is generally recognized that more should be done to prevent the otherwise increasing burden of malignant disease.

References

1. WHO (2008). *The Global Burden of Disease: 2004 Update*. Geneva: WHO.

2. WHO (2002). *The World Health Report 2002: Reducing Risks, Promoting Healthy Life*. Geneva: WHO.

3. WHO (2000). *Global Strategy for the Prevention and Control of Noncommunicable Diseases (WHAA53/14)*. Geneva: WHO.

4. Puska P, Vartiainen E, Laatikainen T *et al.*, eds (2009). *The North Karelia Project: From North Karelia to National Action*. Helsinki: National Institute for Health and Welfare.

5. Rose G (1992). *The Strategy of Preventive Medicine*. Oxford: Oxford University Press.

6. Puska P (2005). Community change and the role of public health. In: Marmot M, Elliott P, eds. *Coronary Heart Disease Epidemiology: From Aetiology to Public Health*. New York: Oxford University Press, pp. 893–907.

7. WHO (2008). *Closing the Gap in a Generation: Health Equity through Action on the Social Determinants of Health. Final Report of the Commission on Social Determinants of Health*. Geneva: WHO.

8. Puska P, Ståhl T (2010). Health in All Policies – the Finnish initiative: background, principles, and current issues. *Annu Rev Public Health*, 31:315–328. http://dx.doi.org/10.1146/annurev.publhealth.012809.103658 PMID:20070201

9. WHO (2003). *WHO Framework Convention on Tobacco Control*. Geneva: WHO.

10. Pirie K, Peto R, Reeves GK *et al.*; Million Women Study Collaborators (2013). The 21st century hazards of smoking and benefits of stopping: a prospective study of one million women in the UK. *Lancet*, 381:133–141. http://dx.doi.org/10.1016/S0140-6736(12)61720-6 PMID:23107252

11. Oberg M, Jaakkola MS, Woodward A *et al.* (2010). Worldwide burden of disease from exposure to second-hand smoke: a retrospective analysis of data from 192 countries. *Lancet*, 377:139–146. http://dx.doi.org/10.1016/S0140-6736(10)61388-8 PMID:21112082

12. Wakefield MA, Hayes L, Durkin S, Borland R (2013). Introduction effects of the Australian plain packaging policy on adult smokers: a cross-sectional study. *BMJ Open*, 3:e003175. http://dx.doi.org/10.1136/bmjopen-2013-003175 PMID:23878174

13. WHO (2009). *2009 Summary Report on Global Progress in Implementation of the WHO Framework Convention on Tobacco Control*. Geneva: WHO.

14. Friel S, Labonte R, Sanders D (2013). Measuring progress on diet-related NCDs: the need to address the causes of the causes. *Lancet*, 381:903–904. http://dx.doi.org/10.1016/S0140-6736(13)60669-8 PMID:23499037

15. Lee I-M, Shiroma EJ, Lobelo F *et al.*; Lancet Physical Activity Series Working Group (2012). Effect of physical inactivity on major non-communicable diseases worldwide: an analysis of burden of disease and life expectancy. *Lancet*, 380:219–229. http://dx.doi.org/10.1016/S0140-6736(12)61031-9 PMID:22818936

16. WHO (2004). *Global Strategy on Diet, Physical Activity and Health*. Geneva: WHO.

17. Joint WHO/FAO Expert Consultation on Diet, Nutrition and the Prevention of Chronic Diseases (2003). *Diet, Nutrition and the Prevention of Chronic Diseases: Report of a Joint FAO/WHO Expert Consultation*. Geneva: WHO (WHO Technical Report No. 916).

18. Hancock C, Kingo L, Raynaud O (2011). The private sector, international development and NCDs. *Global Health*, 7:23. http://dx.doi.org/10.1186/1744-8603-7-23 PMID:21798001

19. Stuckler D, Nestle M (2012). Big food, food systems, and global health. *PLoS Med*, 9:e1001242. http://dx.doi.org/10.1371/journal.pmed.1001242 PMID:22723746

20. WHO (2009). *Global Health Risks: Mortality and Burden of Disease Attributable to Selected Major Risk Factors*. Geneva: WHO.

21. Babor T, Caetano R, Casswell S *et al.* (2010). *Alcohol: No Ordinary Commodity. Research and Public Policy*, 2nd ed. Oxford: Oxford University Press.

22. WHO (2010). *Global Strategy to Reduce the Harmful Use of Alcohol*. Geneva: WHO.

23. United Nations (2011). Political Declaration of the High-Level Meeting of the General Assembly on the Prevention and Control of Non-communicable Diseases. New York: United Nations. Available at www.who.int/nmh/events/un_ncd_summit2011/political_declaration_en.pdf.

Legislative and regulatory initiatives

4 PREVENTION

Bernard W. Stewart
Robert A. Baan

Vincent Cogliano (reviewer)
Jonathan Liberman (reviewer)
Christopher J. Portier (reviewer)

Summary

- A range of legislative measures, and corresponding regulations, affect exposure to carcinogens, although very few are specifically framed in that context.

- Certain behaviours determine personal exposure to carcinogens, primarily involving tobacco smoking, alcohol consumption, or deliberate sun exposure. Such exposures may be affected by legislative measures, which reflect societal attitudes and concerns and are thus not necessarily framed with specific reference to a carcinogenic risk.

- Beyond national or subnational initiatives, the international WHO Framework Convention on Tobacco Control establishes treaty obligations on Parties to adopt relevant legislation, among other measures.

- Prevention of occupational cancer underpins the banning of a limited number of agents, including asbestos, and the specification of workplace exposure limits for many other carcinogenic substances. However, work-related carcinogenic risks that are not identified with specific

agents are not amenable to such action.

- The incidence of cancer attributable to atmospheric, waterborne, or foodborne contaminants may be reduced by regulatory intervention that results in decreased exposure to pollutants. In certain instances, health benefits have been established.

- Community awareness of regulations to prevent or limit carcinogen exposure is often focused on particular circumstances of involuntary exposure, rather than on measures that reduce such exposure by affecting behaviour.

Scope

A range of legal processes, including international treaties, national and subnational legislation, and associated regulatory measures, are directed at, or relevant to, cancer control. Such measures rely on the outcomes of medical and scientific research, including behavioural research, and are discussed in that context in this chapter. This approach represents a very limited perspective. A comprehensive consideration of legal processes relevant to cancer control would involve describing not only relevant measures but also their

implementation as reflected in monitoring and inspection, their interpretation as indicated by litigation and consequential judicial determinations (see Chapter 6.6), and their impact as indicated, for example, by research to establish the efficacy of a particular measure in reducing exposure, and ultimately in reducing any related burden of disease.

Regulatory measures adopted under legislation to address the risk presented by exposure to carcinogens are almost invariably specific to particular classes of agents or circumstances of exposure. There are controls on occupational, environmental, pesticide, pharmaceutical, and foodborne exposures. One of the most developed regulatory frameworks can be seen in the USA. In that country, relevant legislation includes the Clean Air Act, the Clean Water Act, the Toxic Substances Control Act, the Food Quality Protection Act, the Comprehensive Environmental Response, Compensation, and Liability Act (commonly known as the Superfund law), the Occupational Safety and Health Act, and the Food, Drug and Cosmetic Act. In common with similar legislation in other countries, regulations adopted under such measures serve to limit exposure to carcinogens. Rarely, if ever, is legislation oriented towards cancer prevention; the Delaney Clause (1958),

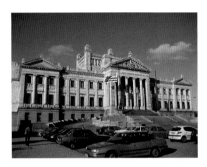

Fig. 4.5.1. The Legislative Palace in Montevideo, Uruguay, is the site where the Uruguayan parliament meets. Governments worldwide have adopted legislation establishing a range of statutory authorities to regulate, for example, exposure to carcinogens through the use of certain categories of consumer and other products.

an amendment (now repealed) to the United States Food, Drug and Cosmetic Act, is an exception [1]. However, as a means of limiting or preventing exposure to carcinogens, regulatory processes and the corresponding enabling legislation play a crucial role. The range of matters relevant to cancer control and appropriately subject to legislation and/or regulation expands in parallel with the understanding of the term "environment" (see "Environmental pollution: old and new").

Apart from limiting exposure to carcinogens, cancer control may be furthered by legislation covering a broad scope. The health-care budget is a major aspect of many national economies and is likely to specify expenditure for cancer control, particularly involving diagnosis of, treatment of, recovery from, and palliation of malignant disease. Lesser funding, but possibly with wider ramifications, may involve services relating to population-based cancer screening or the instigation of vaccination programmes. Statutory action underpins the operation of population-based cancer registries. The entire health-care workforce is dependent on education and training, which is supported by legislation. Against such a broad background, this chapter is limited to measures to prevent or reduce the

likelihood of exposure to carcinogens in various contexts.

In discussions of conditions under which exposure to carcinogens may occur, a distinction is often made between behaviours and unavoidable situations or involuntary circumstances [2]. Rarely are recognized or suspected carcinogens summarily subjected to regulatory control by the imposition of a ban. To address behavioural exposures to carcinogens, banning particular products or agents is often not practicable, even if that option is mentioned to emphasize a particular cause-and-effect relationship. In relation to behavioural exposures, legislative measures short of bans may have a marked and demonstrable effect on the likelihood of exposure to carcinogens.

Minimizing behaviour-related exposures

The circumstances of behaviour-related carcinogenic risk were first identified largely in high-income countries but are now recognized in many instances as occurring worldwide. Such behaviour-related exposures include tobacco smoking, alcohol consumption, and excessive

food intake, as well as unnecessary sun exposure, which is particular to fair-skinned populations. For these factors, although cancer is just one of the adverse health outcomes, it is often the focus of community awareness because it is generally acknowledged as the most feared disease. Accordingly, advocacy directed towards the adoption of relevant measures may be framed primarily with reference to cancer. The benefits of adopting measures to reduce exposure to behaviour-related carcinogens may extend beyond reducing the incidence of cancer.

Tobacco smoking

The WHO Framework Convention on Tobacco Control (FCTC), the first-ever international treaty on health under the auspices of WHO, marks a peak in statutory measures calculated to reduce the burden of disease [3]. The WHO FCTC is one of the fruits of medical and biological evidence that tobacco smoking causes a broad spectrum of diseases, specifically including cancer. Certain legislative measures that may be adopted to reduce tobacco consumption have also been established by research and hence can be adopted

Fig. 4.5.2. A poster illustrating the WHO Framework Convention on Tobacco Control as the theme of World No Tobacco Day 2011.

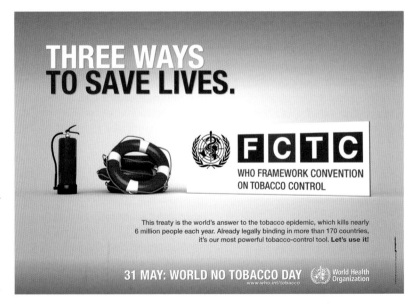

Environmental pollution: old and new

Rodolfo Saracci

"Environmental pollution" is a term collectively denoting all agents noxious to health that contaminate the human environment. In the broad sense, "the environment" includes everything outside the genetic endowment of an individual. Hence, blood represents the body's internal environment, and food, cosmetics, and tobacco smoke are elements of the personal environment, while air, soil, and water as they occur in the home, in buildings, at workplaces, and outdoors constitute the environment in the stricter and more usual sense of the word.

Noxious pollutants of the environment (in the stricter sense) have been a scourge since time immemorial. For centuries, inadequate sanitation of water polluted with sewage caused a heavy burden of infectious disease and death. Early industrial development added urban overcrowding, facilitating the transmission of pathogenic microorganisms, and a massive increase

in the volume of waste and in toxic chemicals from industrial sources. The same still occurs today, particularly in low-income areas of contemporary megacities, exposing large populations to the combined risks of "old" infectious diseases, most often acute, and of "new", pollutant-induced ailments like chronic respiratory diseases and a variety of cancers, which develop slowly over years or decades after the beginning of the exposures.

The occurrence of cancers induced by environmental contaminants depends on several circumstances. Pollutants may be present at low concentrations, producing weak effects, in places where effective hygiene facilities and regulations are available, as in high-income countries. Instead, an increase in cancer risk may derive from the fact that several carcinogenic pollutants are often jointly present and active within the same medium, for example polycyclic aromatic

hydrocarbons, benzene, arsenic, and other inorganic chemicals in urban air or chlorination by-products in drinking-water. Time of exposure plays a role; for instance, exposure during the perinatal period or in early life might predispose to onset of cancers both in childhood and in adult life. Whereas pollutants are often present at relatively low concentrations in the general environment, high concentrations can occur locally around point sources, typically industrial discharges of fumes in air or disposal of waste in waters and soils. Given the variety of exposure circumstances, the proportion of all cancers attributable to carcinogenic pollutants varies from place to place and with time. However, "overall" estimates applicable to whole countries or regions have been attempted, with attributable fractions ranging from 1% (or even less) to 5–10%.

as specific measures recognized in the WHO FCTC. Parties to the WHO FCTC undertake to increase tobacco taxes; protect citizens from exposure to tobacco smoke at work and in other places; ban tobacco advertising, promotion, and sponsorship, and apply restrictions to advertising where constitutional constraints preclude a complete ban; prohibit the use of deceptive terms such as "light" and "mild"; regulate the packaging and labelling of tobacco products, including adoption of health warnings; regulate the testing of emissions from tobacco products; promote public awareness of tobacco control issues; implement programmes to provide for cessation of tobacco use; adopt measures to combat illicit trade in tobacco; prohibit the sale of tobacco products to minors; and implement policies to support alternative sources of income for tobacco workers, growers, and individual sellers.

Some of these provisions, such as those related to cessation programmes, are not immediately addressed by and through legislation. Otherwise, many of the policies may be wholly or largely achieved through legislation to reduce the use of tobacco products. Banning the production and sale of tobacco products is not envisaged under the WHO FCTC and is not considered to be an option in most countries. However, legislative measures to control or discourage practices that contribute to ill health have the potential to contribute markedly to cancer control as well.

The measures adopted by particular countries, or by countries in partnership, to implement tobacco control legislation vary both in the terms of their design and in the time frame for their implementation. In some instances, the prerogative may lie with state or provincial governments to adopt particular legislation. Both the attributable risk of smoking

Fig. 4.5.3. The Tobacco Legislation Amendment Bill 2012, passed by the Legislative Assembly of New South Wales, Australia, provides a basis for regulations to limit smoking in public places.

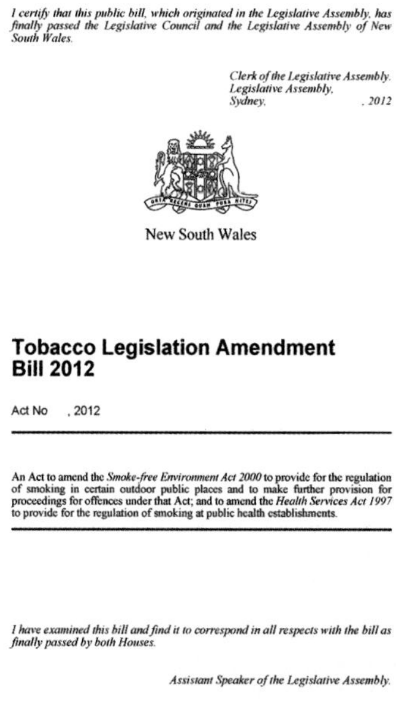

I certify that this public bill, which originated in the Legislative Assembly, has finally passed the Legislative Council and the Legislative Assembly of New South Wales.

*Clerk of the Legislative Assembly.
Legislative Assembly,
Sydney,   . 2012*

New South Wales

Tobacco Legislation Amendment Bill 2012

Act No   . 2012

An Act to amend the *Smoke-free Environment Act 2000* to provide for the regulation of smoking in certain outdoor public places and to make further provision for proceedings for offences under that Act; and to amend the *Health Services Act 1997* to provide for the regulation of smoking at public health establishments.

I have examined this bill and find it to correspond in all respects with the bill as finally passed by both Houses.

Assistant Speaker of the Legislative Assembly.

for lung cancer and the relative risk are so large that the effect of particular measures to discourage smoking may be readily evident in terms of case numbers – a scenario that does not apply to many cancer prevention initiatives. Thus, lung cancer rates in California during 1988–1997 could be distinguished from those in the rest of the USA, an outcome correlated with legislative measures against tobacco use adopted in California [4].

Legislation to control tobacco use is particularly relevant to developing countries, in many of which tobacco consumption has risen dramatically. This challenge is being addressed. In India, for example, beginning with the Cigarettes Act of 1975, several legislative strategies and programmes to curb tobacco use have been implemented, with limited success; currently, the Cigarettes and Other Tobacco Products Act of 2003 is designed to curb the use of tobacco, to protect and promote public health [5]. Tobacco control initiatives are also being undertaken in China [6].

Alcohol consumption

In countries where consumption of alcoholic beverages is legal, the harm attributable to alcohol consumption may be limited by encouraging personal responsibility for drinking behaviour and by adopting a range

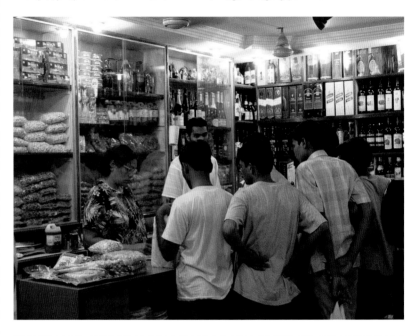

Fig. 4.5.4. Young men buy alcohol from a vendor at a local market in India. In countries where the sale of alcoholic beverages is permitted, consumption is primarily a matter of personal choice. However, the community may regulate availability by specifying that, for example, people must be of a certain minimum age to legally purchase alcohol.

of regulatory options. In contrast to tobacco use, the immediate focus on harm induced by irresponsible alcohol consumption involves, for example, traffic accidents and violent assaults. A longer-term view is that alcohol consumption contributes to chronic disease, including cancer. WHO has adopted a Global Strategy to Reduce the Harmful Use of Alcohol, which addresses the affordability, availability, and promotion of alcohol – all matters that are subject to statutory regulation. Commentary on this WHO initiative refers specifically to the prospect of expansion of the alcohol market in low- and middle-income countries. For example, in Thailand, alcohol consumption was once low, but the adult per capita consumption rose from 0.26 l in 1961 to 8.47 l in 2001 [7].

During the past decade, legislative progress in the European Commission and in Australia and New Zealand to reduce alcohol-related cancers, among other harms, has been modest at best, and there are differences between countries in the involvement of the alcohol industry in developing relevant measures [8]. In Canada, as in many similar countries, the minimum legal drinking age, service to minors, and drinking and driving are subject to regulation, and there are measures addressing the price of alcohol, density of outlets, server intervention, control systems, and community interventions [9].

Table 4.5.1. Text of alcohol warning labels from eight countries

Country	Text of label
Brazil	"Avoid the risks of excessive alcohol consumption"
Ecuador	"Warning. The excessive consumption of alcohol restricts your capacity to drive and operate machinery, may cause damage to your health, and adversely affects your family"
Mexico	"Excessive consumption of this product is hazardous to health"
Portugal	"Drink alcohol in moderation"
Republic of Korea	One of three messages, including: "Warning: Excessive consumption of alcohol may cause liver cirrhosis or liver cancer and, especially, women who drink while they are pregnant increase the risk of congenital anomalies"
Thailand	"Warning: Drinking liquor reduces driving ability" and "Forbidden to be sold to children under 18 years old"
USA	"GOVERNMENT WARNING:" "According to the Surgeon General, women should not drink alcoholic beverages during pregnancy because of the risk of birth defects" or "Consumption of alcohol impairs your ability to drive a car or operate machinery, and may cause health problems"
Zimbabwe	"Alcohol may be hazardous to health if consumed to excess" or "Operation of machinery or driving after the consumption of alcohol is not advisable"

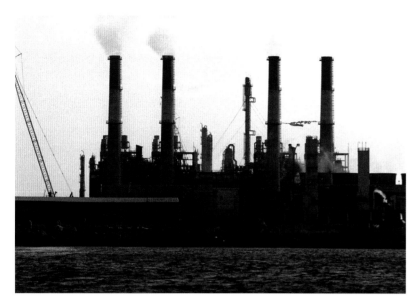

Fig. 4.5.5. A polyvinyl chloride production plant in Turkey. Occupational exposure to specific carcinogens such as vinyl chloride can be readily controlled through regulation of relevant concentrations in the workplace; control of occupational exposure to non-specific waste products, or their impact on the wider community, is more difficult to address.

At least 15 countries have adopted warning labels for alcoholic beverages, and the health effects mentioned include effects on the unborn in some countries; some of these warnings are shown in Table 4.5.1. Cancer is rarely addressed in this context, although reduced consumption of alcohol will contribute to lower incidences of cancers of the oral cavity, oesophagus, liver, female breast, and some other sites.

Exposure to ultraviolet radiation

Unlike virtually all other carcinogens, ultraviolet radiation, primarily from the sun, presents a risk to a particular racial group, namely fair-skinned people. Among such people, the extent of avoidable sun exposure is determined by behaviour and by circumstances. For children, there is a recognized need to address sun protection policies under broad strictures concerning safety [10]. Regulatory measures that specify requirements for childcare centres have been adopted in particular jurisdictions, as exemplified by requirements in Germany [11].

The initial focus of calls to limit provision of commercial indoor tanning operations was the protection of adolescents and young adults. Unequivocal evidence of increased melanoma risk caused by use of ultraviolet-emitting tanning devices, as specified in IARC Monographs Volume 100D, has resulted in access to indoor tanning becoming increasingly restricted around the world [12]. Commercial tanning services are set to be banned in most Australian states in the next few years, and other countries may follow.

For people who work outdoors, appropriate sun protection may involve adoption of particular behaviours, complemented by provision of protective clothing, which may be subject to regulation. It is arguably the task of health education to improve the recognition by adults of the hazard presented by recreational sun exposure. However, the limited progress that has been made in encouraging young people to be "sunsmart" – a term used in Australian campaigns – is prompting consideration of other options, possibly including regulation [13].

Diet

Regulatory measures to reduce obesity are relevant to cancer control but are adopted in the broad context of controlling diabetes and cardiovascular disease. Measures to encourage good nutrition are available and are being further developed (See "Taxing sugar-sweetened beverages: the Brazilian case"), but these are not aimed at reducing exposure to agents generally recognized as carcinogens. In terms of involuntary exposure to carcinogens via food, most attention has been focused on aflatoxin contamination [14]. A singular focus on cancer resulting from food contamination underpinned historic United States legislation – the Delaney Clause mentioned

Table 4.5.2. International limit values (2007) for *ortho*-toluidine

Country	Limit value (8 hours)		Limit value (short-term)	
	ppm	**mg/m³**	**ppm**	**mg/m³**
Belgium	2	8.9		
Canada, Québec	2	8.8		
Denmark	2	9	4	18
France	2	9		
Hungary				0.5
Poland		3		9
Spain	0.2 (skin)	0.89 (skin)		
Switzerland	0.1	0.5		
USA, OSHA	5	22		
United Kingdom	0.2	0.89		

OSHA, United States Occupational Safety and Health Administration.

above – but any such risk is now considered to be best addressed in the context of general food safety legislation [15].

Preventing involuntary exposures

Protecting people from injury caused by exposures over which individuals have little or no control is a particular responsibility of government. Within that broad scope, the prospect or proof of cancer causation has prompted a range of legislative measures, depending on the context in which relevant exposures may occur.

Occupational exposures

Prevention of occupational cancer can be seen in the broader context of avoiding adverse workplace-related health effects due to a broad spectrum of agents. Occupational cancer is wholly preventable by regulatory controls when causation is attributable to a specific chemical or chemicals, as distinct from when increased risk is identified among people engaged in a particular type of work. The adoption of occupational exposure limits for carcinogens is a fundamental regulatory approach and generally involves national standards [16]. In Europe, Registration, Evaluation, Authorisation and Restriction of Chemicals (REACH) regulations are being implemented [17].

Compared with high-income countries, higher levels of exposure to many occupational carcinogens may occur in low- and middle-income countries. The statutory determination of limits for occupational exposure to toxic compounds is being adopted worldwide, as exemplified by initiatives in China [18]. Specific information may be gained from the respective regulatory standards themselves. For carcinogens, international standards for industrial chemicals are systematically summarized in the relevant IARC Monographs. As an example, for the industrial chemical *ortho*-toluidine, which is categorized by IARC as Group 1 (carcinogenic to humans) on

the basis of *sufficient* evidence for causation of bladder cancer in certain workers, exposure limits have been adopted by various countries (Table 4.5.2).

From carcinogenicity data to regulatory control

Measures to prevent occupational cancer or other cancers have often been implemented years, if not decades, after unequivocal evidence of carcinogenic risk was available. Many statutory authorities evaluate evidence of carcinogenicity, and international collaboration in this field is epitomized by the IARC Monographs. Initially, from the early 1970s, IARC Monographs Programme evaluations were based on epidemiological evidence, when available, together with animal bioassay data. The evaluation process was expanded to include mechanistic data, allowing due recognition of

the likely human hazard from, for example, agents that are carcinogenic in experimental animals but for which epidemiological evidence may be scant. Conversely, bioassay findings may be qualified by biological data that suggest differences between mechanisms of tumour induction in certain rodents and those in humans.

This consideration of the overall weight of evidence – including that from mechanistic studies – has resulted in IARC evaluations in Group 1 (carcinogenic to humans) or Group 2A (probably carcinogenic to humans) that would previously not have occurred in view of insufficient epidemiological information. As a result, an imperative may be evident to regulatory authorities without the need to await more definitive epidemiology data. Analysing progress and limitations with respect to the next step – from the categorization

Table 4.5.3. Evidence, IARC evaluations, and United States regulations concerning beryllium

Year	Event
1930s	First industrial uses of beryllium and first reported cases of beryllium-related pneumonitis
1946	Chronic beryllium disease reported for the first time
1949	AEC adopts a 2.0 µg/m³ exposure limit for weapons workers
1970	High lung cancer rates reported among beryllium workers with prior respiratory illness
1971	OSHA adopts a 2.0 µg/m³ exposure limit
1972	IARC Monographs Volume 1: inadequate evidence in humans; sufficient evidence in animals
1979	IARC Monographs Supplement 1: Group 2B (possibly carcinogenic to humans)
1980	Increased lung cancer incidence reported in three studies of beryllium workers
1980	IARC Monographs Volume 23: limited evidence in humans; Group 2A (probably carcinogenic to humans)
1987	IARC Monographs Supplement 7: limited evidence in humans confirmed
1989	DOE proposes a 0.5 µg/m³ exposure limit for DOE weapons and clean-up workers
1993	IARC Monographs Volume 58: sufficient evidence in humans; Group 1 (carcinogenic to humans)
1999	DOE issues a 0.2 µg/m³ exposure limit for DOE weapons and clean-up workers
2006	California OSHSB adopts a 0.2 µg/m³ exposure limit (8-hour TWA)
2009	ACGIH recommends a 0.05 µg/m³ exposure limit (8-hour TWA)
2012	OSHA exposure limit, 2.0 µg/m³; NIOSH recommended exposure limit, 0.5 µg/m³; EPA ambient air limit, 0.01 µg/m³ (30-day TWA)

ACGIH, American Conference of Governmental Industrial Hygienists; AEC, United States Atomic Energy Commission; DOE, United States Department of Energy; EPA, United States Environmental Protection Agency; NIOSH, United States National Institute for Occupational Safety and Health; OSHA, United States Occupational Safety and Health Administration; OSHSB, Occupational Safety and Health Standards Board; TWA, time-weighted average.

Taxing sugar-sweetened beverages: the Brazilian case

Rafael Moreira Claro

Progressively more governments around the world are focusing on ways to use fiscal policies to rectify decades of subsidies for a variety of foods and other goods linked with poor health [1]. WHO has recommended such policies for more than a decade as a way to influence food prices and encourage healthy eating. Evidence based on the Brazilian market indicates that taxing sugar-sweetened beverages would be an effective way to control and reduce the consumption of these products [2].

Trends of prices and consumption of sugar-sweetened beverages, between 1986 and 2003, obtained in three household budget surveys representative of the 11 major metropolitan areas of Brazil, clearly demonstrate how changes in price can affect the consumption of these products (Fig. B4.5.1). As the price of sugar-sweetened beverages decreased from R$ 5.7 per 1000 kcal to

R$ 3.6 per 1000 kcal, their consumption increased significantly from 0.8% to 2.2% of the total calories acquired for household consumption. Since the prices of all other foods and beverages remained stable during this period, the reduction in the price of sugar-sweetened beverages was likely to be even more evident to the population.

The likely impact of taxing sugar-sweetened beverages in Brazil was assessed using national representative data from the early 2000s [2]. A statistically significant reduction in the consumption of these products is expected as a result of increases in price: every 1% increase in price would lead to a 0.84% reduction in consumption in the Brazilian population.

Given that sugar-sweetened beverages are a health hazard regardless of their type, initially no caloric sweetened beverage should be exempted from taxation, to avoid

substitution between types of sugar-sweetened beverages [1]. In addition, effective taxation would have to affect the price of these beverages on all occasions where they are consumed, in the household or away from it.

Even though taxing of sugar-sweetened beverages has the potential to improve health regardless of how the revenue is used, the popularity of such an initiative is likely to increase if the revenues are used to support programmes or policies that promote a healthy lifestyle (such as healthy eating initiatives in schools) [3]. Data from the most recent national food intake survey, conducted in 2008–2009, show that approximately 6.8 billion litres of sugar-sweetened beverages were consumed by the Brazilian population during the study period of 1 year (about 750 ml/person/week); thus, an excise tax of 30% per litre (an average increase of R$ 0.3 in the price per litre) would be high enough to reduce consumption significantly and also generate a revenue of R$ 2.2 billion, or almost US$ 1 billion, an amount sufficient to fund investments in promoting a healthy lifestyle or subsidizing healthy foods.

References

1. Brownell KD *et al.* (2009). *N Engl J Med*, 361:1599–1605. http://dx.doi.org/10.1056/NEJMhpr0905723 PMID:19759377

2. Claro RM *et al.* (2012). *Am J Public Health*, 102:178–183. http://dx.doi.org/10.2105/AJPH.2011.300313 PMID:22095333

3. Caraher M, Cowburn G (2005). *Public Health Nutr*, 8:1242–1249. http://dx.doi.org/10.1079/PHN2005755 PMID:16372919

Fig. B4.5.1. Trends in food prices and consumption of sugar-sweetened beverages in major metropolitan areas of Brazil in 1986–1987, 1995–1996, and 2002–2003. Food prices were adjusted for inflation to represent January 2009 values. Consumption of sugar-sweetened beverages is shown as a percentage of the total calories acquired for household consumption.

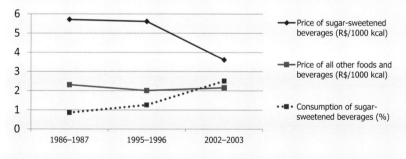

of carcinogenicity to the implementation of regulatory controls – is inherently complicated because it largely identifies national or multinational prerogatives. Progress, or lack of it, is readily evident by considering specific agents.

An international ban on asbestos is in prospect [19], but progress to

this point has taken decades. The categorization of asbestos as carcinogenic to humans readily followed unequivocal epidemiological findings. The first IARC Monograph on asbestos, in 1973, referred to associations between asbestosis and lung cancer that had been reported in 1935, and specified "epidemiological

proof" of the link between exposure to asbestos and increased risks of bronchial carcinoma and mesothelioma. Yet, despite more documentation of attributable injury over half a century, regulatory action was precipitated not by specific research findings, nor by authoritative evaluation of the available data overall, but by the prospect of litigation involving causation being recognized and compensation being required [20].

Soon after the introduction of beryllium in industrial processes in the 1930s, the first reports of related pneumonitis and chronic beryllium disease were published. Some decades later, the carcinogenicity of beryllium became evident: high lung cancer rates were recorded, in particular among beryllium workers with prior respiratory illness. IARC Monograph evaluations of beryllium over four decades have shown a progression, with unequivocal animal data being complemented by successively more definitive epidemiological findings, culminating in a Group 1 evaluation by 1993 (Table 4.5.3). This path has been paralleled by increasingly stringent restrictions – years, and occasionally decades, after the relevant scientific findings. In some instances, beryllium-induced toxic injury apart from cancer, namely multiple types of respiratory disease, has motivated regulatory action.

Pollution

As discussed in Chapter 2.9, air pollution causes a minor fraction of lung cancer in high-income countries. Typically, such pollution, which may include carcinogens such as benzene, formaldehyde, and 1,3-butadiene, is subject to statutory control, as exemplified by the United States Clean Air Act legislation [21]. In many jurisdictions, there are regulatory controls on vehicle emissions [22,23]. The efficacy of regulatory measures to reduce adverse health effects of atmospheric pollution is being progressively established [24].

While such progress in the USA and similar high-income countries is encouraging, this outcome must be set against the knowledge that two thirds of the global burden of disease attributable to air pollution occurs in the low- and middle-income countries of South-East Asia [25]. The relative lack of regulatory control of atmospheric pollution for much of the world's population is indicated by the general lack of relevant measurement data outside North America and the European Union. Between 1990 and 2005, a 6% increase in global population-weighted average ambient concentration of fine particles in the atmosphere occurred, highlighted by increased concentrations in East, South, and South-East Asia and decreases in North America and Europe.

The maximum permissible levels of particular water contaminants are specified by regulation in many countries. In relation to cancer control, the immediate and overwhelming concern is arsenic. Other carcinogens recognized as water contaminants include benzene, trichloroethylene, and chromium VI. In 1942, a United States standard of 50 µg/l for arsenic was set; in 2001, it was reduced to 10 µg/l, the level that had been adopted by WHO as a guideline for drinking-water in 1992. However, introducing the appropriate regulatory response in developing countries where large populations have much higher concentrations of arsenic in drinking-water, often exceeding 100 µg/l, is complex [26].

Statutory authorities and consumer protection

Adverse effects caused by the availability or use of particular commercial products are often the responsibility of statutory authorities that have power in relation to, for example, pesticide licensing or consumer products, including cosmetics. Provisions to protect consumers were invoked in several countries to ban the use of the flame retardant tris(2,3-dibromopropyl) phosphate in children's sleepwear [27]. In some countries, provisions against misleading advertising have served to prevent the marketing of cigarettes using terms such as "light" or "mild", because of the perception, albeit invalid, that such products present a reduced health risk compared with others on the market [28]. Brazil and the European Union were among the first jurisdictions to act [29].

Typically, the responsibility of statutory authorities, or the outcome of consumer protection legislation, does not involve specification of cancer control. However, public outrage at perceived inadequate protection against exposures to carcinogens means that the media often tends to focus on involuntary exposures and regulatory inactivity. Accordingly, the community readily recognizes a need for regulatory intervention to prevent or reduce exposure to carcinogens when such measures address involuntary exposures, exemplified by those occurring in the workplace or as a result of pollution. However, regulatory measures to influence behaviour may well have the greatest impact on cancer incidence and mortality.

References

1. Appel A (1995). Delaney Clause heads for the history books. *Nature*, 376:109. http://dx.doi.org/10.1038/376109a0 PMID:7603551

2. Stewart BW (2012). Priorities for cancer prevention: lifestyle choices versus unavoidable exposures. *Lancet Oncol*, 13:e126–e133. http://dx.doi.org/10.1016/S1470-2045(11)70221-2 PMID:22381935

3. Fong GT, Cummings KM, Borland R et al. (2006). The conceptual framework of the International Tobacco Control (ITC) Policy Evaluation Project. *Tob Control*, 15 Suppl 3:iii3–iii11. http://dx.doi.org/10.1136/tc.2005.015438 PMID:16754944

4. Jemal A, Thun MJ, Ries LA et al. (2008). Annual report to the nation on the status of cancer, 1975–2005, featuring trends in lung cancer, tobacco use, and tobacco control. *J Natl Cancer Inst*, 100:1672–1694. http://dx.doi.org/10.1093/jnci/djn389 PMID:19033571

5. Mehrotra R, Mehrotra V, Jandoo T (2010). Tobacco control legislation in India: past and present. *Indian J Cancer*, 47 Suppl 1:75–80. http://dx.doi.org/10.4103/0019-509X.63870 PMID:20622419

6. Huang J, Zheng R, Emery S (2013). Assessing the impact of the national smoking ban in indoor public places in China: evidence from quit smoking related online searches. *PLoS One*, 8:e65577. http://dx.doi.org/10.1371/journal.pone.0065577 PMID:23776504

7. Casswell S, Thamarangsi T (2009). Reducing harm from alcohol: call to action. *Lancet*, 373:2247–2257. http://dx.doi.org/10.1016/S0140-6736(09)60745-5 PMID:19560606

8. Davoren SL (2011). Legal interventions to reduce alcohol-related cancers. *Public Health*, 125:882–888. http://dx.doi.org/10.1016/j.puhe.2011.09.024 PMID:22036194

9. Giesbrecht N, Stockwell T, Kendall P et al. (2011). Alcohol in Canada: reducing the toll through focused interventions and public health policies. *CMAJ*, 183:450–455. http://dx.doi.org/10.1503/cmaj.100825 PMID:21324848

10. Buller DB, Geller AC, Cantor M et al. (2002). Sun protection policies and environmental features in US elementary schools. *Arch Dermatol*, 138:771–774. http://dx.doi.org/10.1001/archderm.138.6.771 PMID:12056958

11. Aulbert W, Parpart C, Schulz-Hornbostel R et al. (2009). Certification of sun protection practices in a German child daycare centre improves children's sun protection – the 'SunPass' pilot study. *Br J Dermatol*, 161 Suppl 3:5–12. http://dx.doi.org/10.1111/j.1365-2133.2009.09443.x PMID:19775351

12. Pawlak MT, Bui M, Amir M et al. (2012). Legislation restricting access to indoor tanning throughout the world. *Arch Dermatol*, 148:1006–1012. http://dx.doi.org/10.1001/archdermatol.2012.2080 PMID:22801924

13. Goulart JM, Wang SQ (2010). Knowledge, motivation, and behavior patterns of the general public towards sun protection. *Photochem Photobiol Sci*, 9:432–438. http://dx.doi.org/10.1039/b9pp00122k PMID:20354635

14. Pitt JI, Wild CP, Baan RA et al., eds (2012). *Improving Public Health through Mycotoxin Control*. Lyon: IARC (IARC Scientific Publications Series, No. 158).

15. Merrill RA (1997). Food safety regulation: reforming the Delaney Clause. *Annu Rev Public Health*, 18:313–340. http://dx.doi.org/10.1146/annurev.publhealth.18.1.313 PMID:9143722

16. Bolt HM, Huici-Montagud A (2008). Strategy of the scientific committee on occupational exposure limits (SCOEL) in the derivation of occupational exposure limits for carcinogens and mutagens. *Arch Toxicol*, 82:61–64. http://dx.doi.org/10.1007/s00204-007-0260-z PMID:18008062

17. Milan C, Schifanella O, Roncaglioni A, Benfenati E (2011). Comparison and possible use of in silico tools for carcinogenicity within REACH legislation. *J Environ Sci Health C Environ Carcinog Ecotoxicol Rev*, 29:300–323. http://dx.doi.org/10.1080/10590501.2011.629973 PMID:22107165

18. Liang Y, Wong O, Yang L et al. (2006). The development and regulation of occupational exposure limits in China. *Regul Toxicol Pharmacol*, 46:107–113. http://dx.doi.org/10.1016/j.yrtph.2006.02.007 PMID:16624464

19. Sim MR (2013). A worldwide ban on asbestos production and use: some recent progress, but more still to be done. *Occup Environ Med*, 70:1–2. http://dx.doi.org/10.1136/oemed-2012-101290 PMID:23248187

20. Gee D, Greenberg M (2001). Asbestos: from 'magic' to malevolent mineral. In: Harremoës P, Gee D, MacGarvin M et al., eds. *Late Lessons from Early Warnings: The Precautionary Principle 1896–2000*. Copenhagen: European Environmental Agency, pp. 52–63.

21. Woodruff TJ, Axelrad DA, Caldwell J et al. (1998). Public health implications of 1990 air toxics concentrations across the United States. *Environ Health Perspect*, 106:245–251. http://dx.doi.org/10.1289/ehp.98106245 PMID:9518474

22. Bahadur R, Feng Y, Russell LM, Ramanathan V (2011). Impact of California's air pollution laws on black carbon and their implications for direct radiative forcing. *Atmos Environ*, 45:1162–1167. http://dx.doi.org/10.1016/j.atmosenv.2010.10.054

23. Zhou Y, Wu Y, Yang L et al. (2010). The impact of transportation control measures on emission reductions during the 2008 Olympic Games in Beijing, China. *Atmos Environ*, 44:285–293. http://dx.doi.org/10.1016/j.atmosenv.2009.10.040

24. Lioy PJ, Georgopoulos PG (2011). New Jersey: a case study of the reduction in urban and suburban air pollution from the 1950s to 2010. *Environ Health Perspect*, 119:1351–1355. http://dx.doi.org/10.1289/ehp.1103540 PMID:21622086

25. Brauer M, Amann M, Burnett RT et al. (2012). Exposure assessment for estimation of the global burden of disease attributable to outdoor air pollution. *Environ Sci Technol*, 46:652–660. http://dx.doi.org/10.1021/es2025752 PMID:22148428

26. Smith AH, Smith MM (2004). Arsenic drinking water regulations in developing countries with extensive exposure. *Toxicology*, 198:39–44. http://dx.doi.org/10.1016/j.tox.2004.02.024 PMID:15138028

27. de Boer JG, Mirsalis JC, Provost GS et al. (1996). Spectrum of mutations in kidney, stomach, and liver from lacI transgenic mice recovered after treatment with tris(2,3-dibromopropyl)phosphate. *Environ Mol Mutagen*, 28:418–423. http://dx.doi.org/10.1002/(SICI)1098-2280(1996)28:4<418::AID-EM17>3.0.CO;2-I PMID:8991072

28. Anderson SJ, Ling PM, Glantz SA (2007). Implications of the federal court order banning the terms "light" and "mild": what difference could it make? *Tob Control*, 16:275–279. http://dx.doi.org/10.1136/tc.2006.019349 PMID:17652244

29. Borland R, Fong GT, Yong HH et al. (2008). What happened to smokers' beliefs about light cigarettes when "light/mild" brand descriptors were banned in the UK? Findings from the International Tobacco Control (ITC) Four Country Survey. *Tob Control*, 17:256–262. http://dx.doi.org/10.1136/tc.2007.023812 PMID:18426868

4 PREVENTION CHAPTER 4.5

4.6 Vaccination

4 PREVENTION

Rolando Herrero
Silvia Franceschi

Andrew J. Hall (reviewer)
Eduardo Lazcano Ponce (reviewer)
Mark Schiffman (reviewer)

Summary

- Hepatitis B virus (HBV), which causes chronic hepatitis, cirrhosis, and a large fraction of liver cancer cases, is a very common infection in some areas of the world.

- Highly effective vaccines against HBV and liver cancer have been available since 1982, and most countries include HBV vaccination in their childhood immunization programmes.

- A group of about 12 human papillomaviruses (HPVs), particularly HPV types 16 and 18, cause most cervical and anal cancers and an important fraction of vulvar, vaginal, penile, and oropharyngeal cancers.

- Two prophylactic vaccines consisting of empty viral capsids of HPV types 16 and 18 were recently developed. The vaccines are safe and prevent almost 100% of anogenital infections and precancerous lesions among previously unexposed individuals, with enormous potential for cancer control worldwide.

- HPV vaccination of adolescent girls is now recommended and is slowly being implemented in low- and middle-income countries, where more than 80% of cervical cancer cases worldwide occur.

A notable fraction of human cancers (16%) are caused by infections and are largely amenable to effective preventive interventions [1]. Among the most important infections associated with cancers are hepatitis B virus (HBV), hepatitis C virus, human papillomavirus (HPV), and *Helicobacter pylori* (see Chapter 2.4).

Chronic infection with HBV is one of the most important causes of liver cancer (hepatocellular carcinoma) worldwide, particularly in highly endemic areas like sub-Saharan Africa, the Amazon basin, China, the Republic of Korea, and countries in South-East Asia [2]. Vaccines against HBV have been available for several decades and are part of childhood vaccination programmes around the world. The efficacy of the vaccine in preventing chronic HBV infection and liver cancer has now been clearly demonstrated among children and adolescents, and it is expected to reduce incidence of adult hepatocellular carcinoma in many areas when vaccinated populations reach adulthood.

HPV is a very common sexually transmitted virus that causes

Fig. 4.6.1. View from the Chiang Kai-shek Memorial Hall, in Taipei. Taiwan, China, launched a nationwide hepatitis B virus vaccination programme for newborn infants in July 1984.

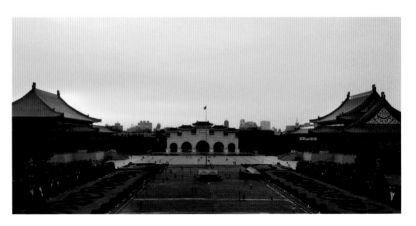

cancers of the cervix, anus, vulva, vagina, penis, and oropharynx among individuals in whom HPV infection is not cleared. Recently, highly effective vaccines have become available to prevent infection by HPV16 and 18, the types responsible for most HPV-related cancers. Vaccine efficacy and cost-effectiveness are maximal among previously unexposed women, and HPV vaccination is being implemented progressively among adolescent girls in developed and developing countries. The vaccines are efficacious to prevent infections and lesions at all the anatomical sites where they have been investigated, and mass vaccination programmes are expected to reduce incidence and mortality from cancers associated with these viruses in the next few decades [3]. This chapter summarizes some of the epidemiological features of HBV and HPV infections and their associated cancers and discusses the characteristics and performance of vaccines against them.

Hepatitis B virus

Hepatitis B virus and liver cancer

HBV is a highly contagious DNA virus transmitted by exposure to infected blood and other body fluids, including semen and vaginal fluids. The virus is transmitted from mother to infant and from child to child, as well as by unsafe injections, sexual contact, and blood transfusions. Perinatal transmission from infected mothers to their newborn infants or from one child to another is very common in highly endemic areas, and the virus can also be transmitted by fomites [4].

HBV infection is a major global health problem. Worldwide, an estimated 2 billion people have been infected with HBV, and more than 360 million have chronic liver infections. HBV causes a life-threatening liver infection, namely hepatitis B, which often leads to chronic liver disease. The occurrence of chronic infection is inversely related to the age of acquisition, from 90% among

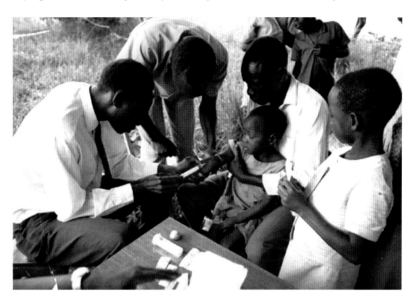

Fig. 4.6.2. A child getting vaccinated in The Gambia. Hepatitis B virus vaccination trials in progress in the country are expected to yield results in the next few years.

people infected perinatally to less than 5% among otherwise healthy adults [5]. HBV-driven persistent inflammation, liver necrosis, and regenerative proliferation lead to cirrhosis and hepatocellular carcinoma. Among people chronically infected, it is estimated that 25% will die from liver disease, including cancer. HBV is responsible for 50–90% of liver cancer cases in high-risk areas [6]. These cancers can also develop without fibrosis because HBV may have a direct carcinogenic effect [4].

Hepatitis B virus vaccine

A vaccine against HBV has been available since 1982. The current vaccine is a recombinant HBV surface antigen produced in yeast or mammalian cells into which the HBV surface antigen gene has been inserted using plasmids. The expressed HBV surface antigen self-assembles into spherical particles that expose the highly immunogenic "a" determinant. Alum (aluminium phosphate) is generally used as an adjuvant. HBV vaccine, of which the initial dose (of a total of three recommended doses) is given within the first 24 hours after birth, is 95% effective in preventing HBV infection and its chronic consequences, even when antibody levels become

undetectable, and was the first vaccine against a major human cancer [7]. The vaccine has an outstanding record of safety and effectiveness. Since 1982, more than 1 billion doses of HBV vaccine have been used worldwide. In many countries where 8–15% of children previously became chronically infected with HBV, vaccination has reduced the rate of chronic infection to less than 1% among immunized children.

Prevention of liver cancer has been demonstrated in children and adolescents in the early vaccinated cohorts in Taiwan, China, where a nationwide HBV immunization programme for newborn infants was initiated in July 1984 [8,9]. Immunization has lowered the prevalence of chronic HBV carriers, incidence of hepatocellular carcinoma, and mortality from fulminant hepatitis [10]; these effects are evident in the birth cohort born in 1981–1984, which received HBV vaccines at preschool ages instead of in infancy. The Republic of Korea also initiated mass HBV vaccination in the early 1980s [11].

A high incidence of liver cancer in Qidong City, China, was attributable to endemic HBV infection and dietary exposure to aflatoxin,

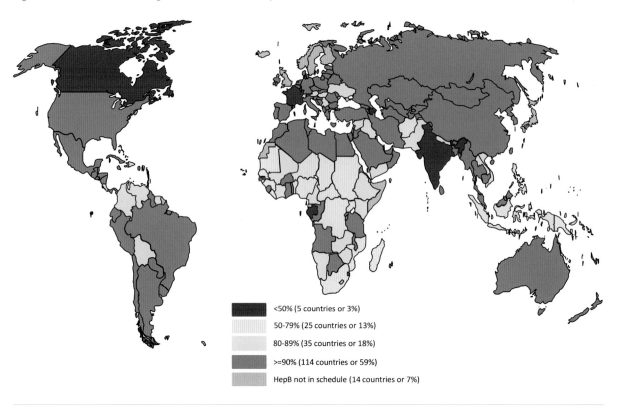

<50% (5 countries or 3%)

50-79% (25 countries or 13%)

80-89% (35 countries or 18%)

>=90% (114 countries or 59%)

HepB not in schedule (14 countries or 7%)

prompting dietary interventions and the initiation of neonatal HBV vaccination. As recently reported, liver cancer incidence has fallen dramatically: compared with 1980–1983, age-specific liver cancer incidence rates in 2005–2008 had significantly decreased by 14-fold at ages 20–24 years, and consistent data were reported for other cohorts [12].

In 2010, 179 countries reported inclusion of the HBV vaccine in their national infant immunization programmes. This is a major increase compared with 31 countries in 1992, the year that the World Health Assembly passed a resolution to recommend global vaccination against HBV. Nearly 70% of children born worldwide received three doses of the HBV vaccine (Fig. 4.6.3).

Human papillomaviruses

Human papillomaviruses and cancer

HPV is considered a necessary cause of cervical cancer, with an attributable fraction of nearly 100%. Multiple epidemiological studies over the past three decades have confirmed the etiological role of about 13 HPV types in cervical cancer; HPV16 and 18 are detectable in about 70% of tumours. The natural history and molecular mechanisms involved in cervical carcinogenesis are well understood [13].

In the cervix, HPV is a sexually transmitted infection acquired by most women shortly after initiation of sexual activity. The most common morphological manifestation of HPV infection consists of minor epithelial abnormalities (equivocal and low-grade cellular changes). The initial infection regresses spontaneously in the majority of women, but among those women where the infection becomes persistent, precancerous lesions (advanced intraepithelial neoplasia) can develop. If not treated, these lesions can lead to cervical cancer after several years. HPVs have well-identified oncogenes whose products interact with tumour

suppressor gene proteins of the host to induce malignant transformation [14]. Prevention of a necessary cause of disease, by definition, should prevent the disease.

An important fraction of other anogenital cancers, including cancers of the anus, vulva, vagina, and penis, are also HPV-related, and in these tumours HPV16 is the strongly predominant type. Although molecular mechanisms similar to those observed in the cervix are probably involved, there is limited knowledge of the natural history of these tumours [13]. Importantly, and similarly to the cervix, most of these tumours show an important increase among immunodeficient individuals. Apart from the lesions in the anogenital tract of both men and women, HPV is implicated in a geographically variable and pathologically distinct fraction of cancers of the oropharynx [15], and the incidence of this cancer has recently tended to increase in several developed countries. In fact, in the USA, where the increase in incidence

Early implementation and monitoring of HPV vaccination in Bhutan

Tandin Dorji and Ugyen Tshomo

Bhutan was the first low-income country to introduce vaccination against human papillomavirus (HPV), the necessary cause of cervical cancer. Cervical cancer is the most common cancer in Bhutanese women. To help prevent the disease, the Ministry of Health developed a national vaccination programme. The Ministry's considerations included disease incidence, the limited reach of screening, the poor outcomes associated with late diagnosis of disease, and the feasibility of a HPV vaccination programme. For national introduction of HPV vaccination, the Ministry recommended immunization with quadrivalent (HPV6, 11, 16, and 18) vaccine for 12-year-old girls and a "catch-up" campaign for girls aged 13–18 years in the first year of the programme. In 2010, a pharmaceutical company provided free quadrivalent HPV vaccine for all girls aged 12–18 years, and for the next 5 years the Australian Cervical Cancer Foundation funded the vaccine for 12-year-old girls. Health workers administered the vaccine in schools; girls not at school received the vaccine at health facilities. In 2010, more than 130 000 doses of quadrivalent HPV vaccine were administered, with a three-dose vaccination coverage rate of 92%. There were no serious adverse events, and the vaccine was well tolerated. The rapid implementation, acceptability, and success of this national HPV vaccination catch-up programme are attributed to strong political commitment and a well-functioning primary health-care system. Bhutan's experience provides an example for other low-income countries considering the introduction of HPV vaccination.

Monitoring of HPV vaccination is challenging: it will take two or three decades before its impact on the onset of cervical cancer will become manifest in cancer registry data. In the near term, the most feasible and informative outcome of vaccination is the decrease in the prevalence of HPV infection and, most notably, the variation in the ratio between HPV types prevented by the current vaccines and other HPV types in sentinel populations of sexually active adolescents and young women. A timely demonstration of the effectiveness in Bhutan will sustain the willingness of other low-income countries to continue their efforts. Therefore, in 2012 the Ministry of Health of Bhutan, in collaboration with Jigme Dorji Wangchuck National Referral Hospital and IARC, started a study that will regularly evaluate HPV prevalence in cervical cells and urine samples of women aged 18 years or older. By 2016, the early impact of vaccination will start to be detectable in women aged 25 years or younger. An expansion of cervical screening and a shift from the current cytology-based screening to HPV-based screening in the country is also being considered in the framework of the same project. This investment will improve cervical cancer prevention in older women and could ultimately serve as the basis for long-term vaccination monitoring.

Fig. B4.6.1. Staff of the Jigme Dorji Wangchuck National Referral Hospital in Thimphu, Bhutan.

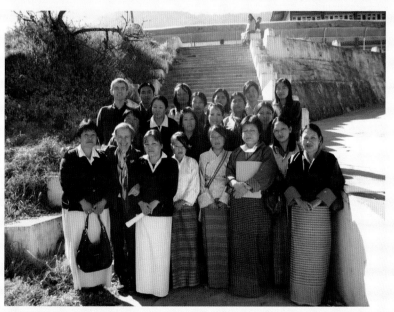

Reference

Ladner J et al. (2012). BMC Public Health, 12:370. http://dx.doi.org/10.1186/1471-2458-12-370 PMID:22621342

of oropharyngeal cancer is observed mainly among men, the number of HPV-related cancers is expected to be higher in men than in women in the next few decades, attributable in part to the consideration that screening has greatly lowered rates of cervical cancer in that country [16]. HPV16 is responsible for about 60% of cervical cancer tumours, but in HPV-associated tumours of other anogenital sites and the oropharynx this viral type is more predominant, responsible for about 90% of the HPV-positive cases.

Introduction and monitoring of a national HPV vaccination programme in Rwanda

Agnès Binagwaho, Maurice Gatera, and Fidele Ngabo

Cervical cancer is the most common cancer among women in Rwanda, where, before 2011, neither cervical cancer screening nor human papillomavirus (HPV) vaccination were available in public health facilities. In 2010, however, the Rwandan Ministry of Health developed a National Strategic Plan for the Prevention, Control, and Management of Cervical Lesions and Cancer. A multidisciplinary

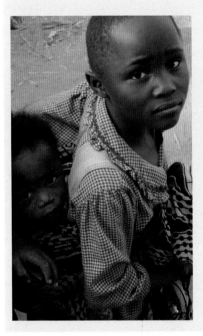

Fig. B4.6.2. A young Rwandan mother and her child.

committee devised a strategic plan for the preparation, implementation, and evaluation of a national HPV vaccination programme, of which the key aspects included: (i) a public–private partnership with a pharmaceutical company to provide free vaccine for 3 years of HPV vaccinations and offer reduced prices for future doses; (ii) a delivery approach based on school grade; (iii) a strong community involvement in identifying and vaccinating girls absent from, or not enrolled in, school; and (iv) a nationwide sensitization campaign preceding the delivery of the first dose.

Since 2011, girls enrolled in primary grade six have been receiving the full three-dose course of HPV vaccine, with additional outreach to the small number of 12-year-old girls not at school. During the programme's second and third years (2012 and 2013), a "catch-up" phase targeting girls in the third year of secondary school has ensured complete coverage of all pre-adolescent and adolescent girls. In 2014 and beyond, only girls in primary grade six will be vaccinated.

In its first year, Rwanda's HPV vaccination programme achieved a three-dose vaccination coverage of 93.2% among an estimated 98 762 eligible girls in grade six. Rwanda is the first example of a successful

nationwide delivery of HPV vaccine in a country eligible for support from the GAVI Alliance, and should motivate other countries to expand their vaccination programmes to include the HPV vaccine, with due customization according to their epidemiological, economic, political, and health system contexts. This is especially timely now that the GAVI Alliance has included the vaccine in its immunization package and the price has been lowered to US$ 5 per vaccine dose for GAVI Alliance-eligible countries.

Rwanda's HPV vaccination programme is expected to have an important impact on the future burden of cervical cancer in Rwanda. In the short term, however, reliable evidence of the effectiveness of the vaccination programme is crucial to help national planners sustain investment in the programme. Thus, a collaboration with IARC is under way to provide timely high-quality data on the impact of the vaccination programme on the prevalence of HPV infection. Such evidence of vaccine effectiveness should also facilitate the introduction of successful programmes into other low- and middle-income countries.

Reference

Binagwaho A et al. (2012). Bull World Health Organ, 90:623–628. http://dx.doi.org/10.2471/BLT.11.097253 PMID:22893746

Human papillomavirus vaccines

Two non-infectious subunit vaccines against HPV have been developed, both composed primarily of virus-like particles and produced by expression of the HPV L1 gene in insect cells (bivalent vaccine) or yeast (quadrivalent vaccine). The L1 gene codes for most of the viral capsid, and after producing the L1 protein, it self-assembles as virus-like particles, which are highly antigenic. They produce a strong antibody

response that prevents infection by neutralizing infectious virus in the mucosa at the time of contagion. A comprehensive review has recently been published [3].

The bivalent vaccine includes HPV16 and HPV18 virus-like particles and is produced with a complex adjuvant system (ASO4) consisting of monophosphoryl lipid A and alum. The quadrivalent vaccine, produced with alum adjuvant, includes HPV16 and HPV18 virus-like particles and, in addition, HPV6 and HPV11 virus-

like particles, the viral types responsible for most benign genital warts.

Both vaccines are almost 100% effective in preventing cervical HPV infections and precancerous lesions associated with the oncogenic viruses included in the vaccine formulations (HPV16 and 18) among women not previously infected, and the vaccines are therefore mainly recommended for adolescent girls before initiation of sexual activity. A summary of demonstrated efficacy of the two cervical cancer

Table 4.6.1. Key findings from clinical trials of HPV VLP vaccines

Study group	Outcome	Quadrivalent vaccine	Bivalent vaccine
Young women	Infection efficacy	Proven	Proven
	CIN2+ efficacy	Proven	Proven
	CIN3 efficacy	Proven	Proven
	VIN/VaIN 2/3 efficacy	Proven	Proven[a]
	Genital warts efficacy	Proven	Not a target
	Anal infection efficacy	Not proven[b]	Proven
	Partial cross-protection infection	Proven	Proven
	Partial cross-protection CIN2+	Proven	Proven
	Therapeutic efficacy	None	None
	Safety	No concerns	No concerns
Mid-adult women[c]	Infection efficacy	Proven	Proven[a]
	CIN2+ efficacy	Proven	Not proven
	Immunogenicity	Proven	Proven
	Safety	No concerns	No concerns
Young men	Infection efficacy	Proven	Not proven
	Genital warts efficacy	Proven	Not a target
	Anal infection efficacy	Proven	Not proven
	AIN2+ efficacy	Proven	Not proven
	Safety	No concerns	No concerns
Children	Infection efficacy	Not proven	Not proven
	Disease efficacy	Not proven	Not proven
	Immunogenicity	Proven	Proven
	Safety	No concerns	No concerns

AIN2+, anal intraepithelial neoplasia, grade 2 or worse; CIN, cervical intraepithelial neoplasia; HPV, human papillomavirus; VaIN, vaginal intraepithelial neoplasia; VIN, vulvar intraepithelial neoplasia; VLP, virus-like particle.
[a] Meeting abstract, not yet published.
[b] "Not proven" indicates that no data have been reported.
[c] See comments in the text on cost-effectiveness for this group.

vaccines is presented in Table 4.6.1 [3]. Although there is evidence of protection by both vaccines against HPV infection and disease among women older than 25 years, the benefit–cost ratio is reduced, in part because of the lower incidence of lesions among women infected by HPV later in life [17].

The vaccines also afford limited protection against HPV types phylogenetically related to HPV16 and 18. Cross-protection against persistent infection of 6 months or more has been reported against HPV31 for the quadrivalent vaccine and against HPV31, 33, 52, 45, and 51 for the bivalent vaccine. However, the significance of early protection against these additional types is not clear

and needs to be monitored over the long term and against cervical disease. Neither of the vaccines is effective against established infections [18].

The quadrivalent vaccine has been shown to also prevent the majority of vulvar and vaginal HPV infections and lesions associated with HPV16 and 18, as well as genital warts (caused by HPV6 and 11). The bivalent vaccine has been shown to prevent anal HPV16 and 18 infections in young women (Table 4.6.1). Based on cross-sectional studies of women aged 18–24 years who received Pap screening in family planning clinics throughout Australia, there was a decrease of 77% in prevalence of HPV types targeted by the quadrivalent

vaccine from the period before (2005–2007) to the period after (2009–2010) the vaccine was widely implemented (Fig. 4.6.4) [19]. Among men, the quadrivalent vaccine has been shown to effectively prevent external genital lesions, including genital warts and penile, perianal, or perineal intraepithelial lesions, and among men who have sex with men it has been demonstrated to prevent anal intraepithelial neoplasia.

Trials of the bivalent and quadrivalent vaccines in terms of infection and lesional end-points have been reviewed [20]. Among HPV-negative women, both vaccines have demonstrated high efficacies against persistent HPV infections and cervical cancer precursors. The quadrivalent

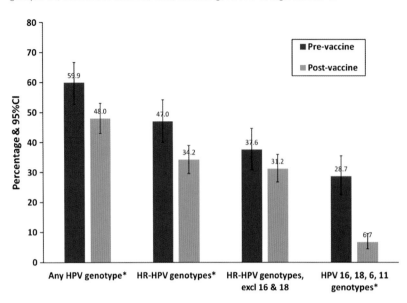

HPV vaccination in Bhutan" and "Introduction and monitoring of a national HPV vaccination programme in Rwanda"). Vaccination of boys to prevent certain cancers in men and to prevent transmission of infection to women is under way in some developed countries. Some areas have implemented vaccination programmes with alternative schedules, including the application of only two doses, based on immunogenicity data showing very similar antibody responses, particularly among young girls. In addition, data from a clinical trial in Costa Rica indicated evidence of protection from fewer than three doses of the bivalent vaccine against persistent infections with relevant viral types [23]. In the same trial, reduced prevalence of oral HPV infection was evident 4 years after vaccination – a result that has implications for the prevention of HPV-associated oropharyngeal cancer, which is increasingly common [24].

New vaccines are being developed that could overcome some of the limitations of current HPV vaccines. In particular, additional protection against other HPV types could eventually eliminate the need for screening. In the meantime, modified screening alternatives will have to be implemented in vaccinated populations, and screening activities will need to continue for the majority of adult women currently alive, who will not benefit from this extraordinary preventive tool.

vaccine is efficacious (> 75% vaccine efficacy) against any of the more severe precursors of vulvar, vaginal, and anal cancers.

Both vaccines have demonstrated an excellent safety record in the several years since they were licensed and have now been incorporated into vaccination programmes in most developed countries. They are recommended for girls before initiation of sexual activity, with additional "catch-up" programmes for young women in some countries. Although the efficacy has not been shown for younger children, immunogenicity bridging studies have shown that the level of the antibody response to the vaccine is stronger in adolescent boys and girls than in young adult women [21]. In general, among women and men of all ages, the vaccines induce a strong immune response to both antigens that persists for at least 8 years, without evidence of declining efficacy so far.

More than 40 countries have already introduced HPV vaccination, mainly among women [22], with a high uptake in some regions but not in others. It will probably only be possible to determine the extent of attributable reduction in cervical cancer incidence after several decades, particularly because vaccination programmes have only recently been initiated in developing countries (see "Early implementation and monitoring of

References

1. de Martel C, Ferlay J, Franceschi S *et al.* (2012). Global burden of cancers attributable to infections in 2008: a review and synthetic analysis. *Lancet Oncol*, 13:607–615. http://dx.doi.org/10.1016/S1470-2045(12)70137-7 PMID:22575588

2. WHO (2006). WHO/UNICEF coverage estimates 1980–2005. Countries having introduced HepB vaccine and infant HepB3 coverage, 2005. Geneva: WHO.

3. Schiller JT, Castellsagué X, Garland SM (2012). A review of clinical trials of human papillomavirus prophylactic vaccines. *Vaccine*, 30 Suppl 5:F123–F138. http://dx.doi.org/10.1016/j.vaccine.2012.04.108 PMID:23199956

4. IARC (2012). Biological agents. *IARC Monogr Eval Carcinog Risks Hum*, 100B: 1–441. PMID:23189750

5. Hyams KC (1995). Risks of chronicity following acute hepatitis B virus infection: a review. *Clin Infect Dis*, 20:992–1000. http://dx.doi.org/10.1093/clinids/20.4.992 PMID:7795104

6. Chen CJ, Yu MW, Liaw YF (1997). Epidemiological characteristics and risk factors of hepatocellular carcinoma. *J Gastroenterol Hepatol*, 12:S294–S308. http://dx.doi.org/10.1111/j.1440-1746.1997.tb00513.x PMID:9407350

7. WHO (2009). Hepatitis B vaccines. *Wkly Epidemiol Rec*, 84:405–419. http://www.who.int/wer/2009/wer8440.pdf PMID:19817017

8. Chang MH, Chen CJ, Lai MS *et al.*; Taiwan Childhood Hepatoma Study Group (1997). Universal hepatitis B vaccination in Taiwan and the incidence of hepatocellular carcinoma in children. *N Engl J Med*, 336:1855–1859. http://dx.doi.org/10.1056/NEJM199706263362602 PMID:9197213

9. Chang MH, Shau WY, Chen CJ *et al.*; Taiwan Childhood Hepatoma Study Group (2000). Hepatitis B vaccination and hepatocellular carcinoma rates in boys and girls. *JAMA*, 284:3040–3042. http://dx.doi.org/10.1001/jama.284.23.3040 PMID:11122592

10. Chiang CJ, Yang YW, You SL *et al.* (2013). Thirty-year outcomes of the national hepatitis B immunization program in Taiwan. *JAMA*, 310:974–976. http://dx.doi.org/10.1001/jama.2013.276701 PMID:24002285

11. Chen TW (2013). Paths towards hepatitis B immunization in Republic of Korea and Taiwan, China. *Clin Exp Vaccine Res*, 2:76–82. http://dx.doi.org/10.7774/cevr.2013.2.2.76 PMID:23858397

12. Sun Z, Chen T, Thorgeirsson SS *et al.* (2013). Dramatic reduction of liver cancer incidence in young adults: 28 year follow-up of etiological interventions in an endemic area of China. *Carcinogenesis*, 34:1800–1805. http://dx.doi.org/10.1093/carcin/bgt007 PMID:23322152

13. Moscicki AB, Schiffman M, Burchell A *et al.* (2012). Updating the natural history of human papillomavirus and anogenital cancers. *Vaccine*, 30 Suppl 5:F24–F33. http://dx.doi.org/10.1016/j.vaccine.2012.05.089 PMID:23199964

14. Doorbar J, Quint W, Banks L *et al.* (2012). The biology and life-cycle of human papillomaviruses. *Vaccine*, 30 Suppl 5:F55–F70. http://dx.doi.org/10.1016/j.vaccine.2012.06.083 PMID:23199966

15. Gillison ML, Alemany L, Snijders PJ *et al.* (2012). Human papillomavirus and diseases of the upper airway: head and neck cancer and respiratory papillomatosis. *Vaccine*, 30 Suppl 5:F34–F54. http://dx.doi.org/10.1016/j.vaccine.2012.05.070 PMID:23199965

16. Chaturvedi AK, Engels EA, Pfeiffer RM *et al.* (2011). Human papillomavirus and rising oropharyngeal cancer incidence in the United States. *J Clin Oncol*, 29:4294–4301. http://dx.doi.org/10.1200/JCO.2011.36.4596 PMID:21969503

17. Westra TA, Rozenbaum MH, Rogoza RM *et al.* (2011). Until which age should women be vaccinated against HPV infection? Recommendation based on cost-effectiveness analyses. *J Infect Dis*, 204:377–384. http://dx.doi.org/10.1093/infdis/jir281 PMID:21742836

18. Hildesheim A, Herrero R, Wacholder S *et al.*; Costa Rican HPV Vaccine Trial Group (2007). Effect of human papillomavirus 16/18 L1 viruslike particle vaccine among young women with preexisting infection: a randomized trial. *JAMA*, 298:743–753. http://dx.doi.org/10.1001/jama.298.7.743 PMID:17699008

19. Tabrizi SN, Brotherton JM, Kaldor JM *et al.* (2012). Fall in human papillomavirus prevalence following a national vaccination program. *J Infect Dis*, 206:1645–1651. http://dx.doi.org/10.1093/infdis/jis590 PMID:23087430

20. Lehtinen M, Dillner J (2013). Clinical trials of human papillomavirus vaccines and beyond. *Nat Rev Clin Oncol*, 10:400–410. http://dx.doi.org/10.1038/nrclinonc.2013.84 PMID:23736648

21. Block SL, Nolan T, Sattler C *et al.*; Protocol 016 Study Group (2006). Comparison of the immunogenicity and reactogenicity of a prophylactic quadrivalent human papillomavirus (types 6, 11, 16, and 18) L1 virus-like particle vaccine in male and female adolescents and young adult women. *Pediatrics*, 118:2135–2145. http://dx.doi.org/10.1542/peds.2006-0461 PMID:17079588

22. Markowitz LE, Tsu V, Deeks SL *et al.* (2012). Human papillomavirus vaccine introduction – the first five years. *Vaccine*, 30 Suppl 5:F139–F148. http://dx.doi.org/10.1016/j.vaccine.2012.05.039 PMID:23199957

23. Kreimer AR, Rodriguez AC, Hildesheim A *et al.*; CVT Vaccine Group (2011). Proof-of-principle evaluation of the efficacy of fewer than three doses of a bivalent HPV16/18 vaccine. *J Natl Cancer Inst*, 103:1444–1451. http://dx.doi.org/10.1093/jnci/djr319 PMID:21908768

24. Herrero R, Quint W, Hildesheim A *et al.*; CVT Vaccine Group (2013). Reduced prevalence of oral human papillomavirus (HPV) 4 years after bivalent HPV vaccination in a randomized clinical trial in Costa Rica. *PLoS One*, 8:e68329. http://dx.doi.org/10.1371/journal.pone.0068329 PMID:23873171

4.7

Screening – principles

4 PREVENTION

Lawrence von Karsa
Peter B. Dean
Silvina Arrossi
Rengaswamy Sankaranarayanan

Ahti Anttila (reviewer)
Anthony B. Miller (reviewer)

Summary

- Early detection and treatment of cancer requires accessible, high-quality health services with adequate human, financial, and technical resources.

- Population-based screening programmes of appropriate quality can reduce morbidity and mortality from breast, cervical, and colorectal cancers. Provided evidence-based methods are used that have been tested under local conditions, these programmes can offer a more effective alternative to early symptomatic detection of disease.

- Cervical cancer screening may involve visual inspection of the cervix, cervical sampling for cytology, or testing for human papillomavirus infection.

- Screening tests for colorectal cancer include faecal occult blood testing and faecal immunochemical testing. Flexible sigmoidoscopy and colonoscopy are also used.

- Screening with mammography permits detection of early-stage breast cancers.

- To maximize the benefit and minimize harm, screening should be implemented only in organized, population-based programmes with adequate resources for planning and training, identification and invitation of the target population, and quality assurance, including monitoring and evaluation.

- Lack of governmental commitment to provide the requisite sustainable resources can be a serious barrier to successful implementation of cancer screening programmes.

Detection of cancer in its early stages and the provision of prompt appropriate treatment are important elements in cancer control. The aim of early detection is to reduce mortality and other serious consequences of advanced disease. This goal may be accomplished if earlier treatment improves life expectancy, locoregional control of disease, and quality of life, and/or permits equally effective therapy with fewer side-effects (Fig. 4.7.1). Key to achieving the potential impact of early detection of cancer is universal access to prompt and effective diagnostic and treatment services. Comprehensive, multidisciplinary quality assurance is essential to maintain an appropriate balance between overall benefit and inherent risk. The concept of early detection of cancer has evolved since the landmark publication by Wilson and Jungner in 1968 [1]. In recent decades the principles established in that publication have been extended through experience gained from implementation of population-based cancer screening programmes [2]. Due to the complexity of the issues that have impacts on the effectiveness and appropriateness of early detection of cancer, this chapter provides an overview of key concepts and sources of information and calls attention to not only the opportunities but also the limitations of cancer screening.

Early detection

Early detection of symptomatic cases

Early diagnosis is particularly relevant for cancers of the breast, cervix, mouth, larynx, colon, rectum, and skin. Before evidence-based screening methods became available, early detection was achieved by improving diagnostic and therapeutic methods and by the education of health-care professionals and the general public to promote early recognition of symptomatic disease. Some early signs of cancer include lumps, sores that fail to heal, abnormal bleeding, persistent indigestion,

Early detection of selected cancers through symptoms or by screening

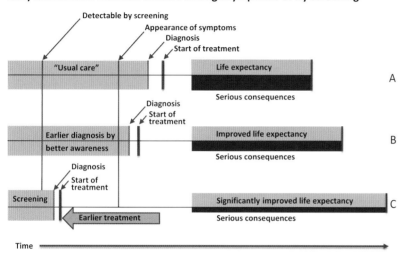

and chronic hoarseness. Increased awareness of cancer warning signs can have a significant impact on the burden of disease, particularly in those health-care systems in low- and middle-income countries in which most patients are currently diagnosed with very-late-stage malignancy [3]. Universal access to adequate diagnosis and treatment is still lacking in many countries and is a serious barrier to the control of symptomatic disease.

Early detection of asymptomatic cancer

In high-income countries, population-based screening has been shown to be effective in reducing cancer-specific mortality, complementing early symptomatic detection of breast, cervical, and colorectal cancers [4–6]. The main objective of screening is to discover latent disease among those who are predominantly asymptomatic and to enable adequate treatment before

the cancer poses a more serious threat to the individual and places an additional burden on the community [1]. Early treatment of invasive lesions, including surgical removal of early invasive breast cancer or endoscopic resection of early colorectal cancer, can be less detrimental than treatment of symptomatic disease [7,8]. Moreover, detection of premalignant

lesions followed by treatment with cryotherapy or the loop electrosurgical excision procedure for intra-epithelial cervical neoplasia, or by endoscopic excision of colorectal adenomas, prevents progression to cervical and colorectal cancer, respectively [5,8,9]. Randomized trials among people at average risk invited to participate in population-based screening have shown a reduction in cervical and colorectal cancer incidence and mortality [6,9].

For cervical cancer, the impact of screening is evident when trends in incidence over decades are compared across 38 countries [10]. Strong downward trends occurred in the highest-income countries, whereas no clear changes, including some increases, were recorded in lower-income settings (Fig. 4.7.2). Due to improvements in survival, the full benefit of mammography screening in terms of the number of breast cancer deaths prevented becomes evident only after a follow-up period of more than two decades. In a large randomized trial, follow-up of 133 065 participants over 29 years showed a 31% reduction in breast cancer mortality in the group assigned to screening compared with the control group; furthermore, most of the deaths prevented by screening would have occurred after a follow-up period of more than 10 years [11]. Two recent studies have also provided insight into long-term effects of colorectal cancer screening [12]. One report estimated that screening colonoscopy

Fig. 4.7.2. Comparison of age-standardized incidence trends of cervical cancer, for ages 30–74 years, between countries of northern Europe and countries of Asia/Africa.

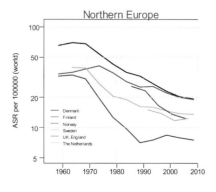

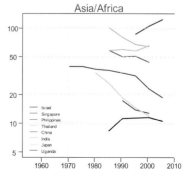

Table 4.7.1. Evidence-based screening methods currently used in national or regional cancer screening programmes

Target cancer	Screening method
Breast	Mammography
Cervical	Cytology (conventional and liquid-based)
	Human papillomavirus testing
	Visual inspection of the cervix with acetic acid
Colorectal	Faecal occult blood testing or faecal immunochemical testing
	Flexible sigmoidoscopy
	Colonoscopy

would have prevented 40% of colorectal cancers over a 22-year period in 88 902 individuals, while the other found that annual faecal occult blood testing reduced mortality by 32% in a 30-year follow-up of 46 551 participants.

A considerably shorter time period was sufficient to demonstrate the efficacy of colorectal cancer screening using once-only flexible sigmoidoscopy between the ages of 55 and 64 years. After 11.2 years of follow-up of 170 038 participants in a randomized controlled study, colorectal cancer incidence and mortality were reduced by 23% and 31%, respectively, in the screening group compared with the control group [13].

A population-based screening programme for detection of asymptomatic disease will also detect cases that are symptomatic, but the detection, on average, will result in earlier treatment for the asymptomatic cases than for the cases of symptomatic disease. It is therefore anticipated that the numbers of detected cancers with a favourable prognosis will be higher in a population-based screening programme of appropriate quality, and over time the effective diagnosis and treatment of these cases will result in a greater decrease in disease-specific mortality than can be achieved by early detection of symptomatic cancer alone. However, early detection may also lead to diagnosis or prolongation of illness without improving a patient's prognosis. Randomized controlled trials are therefore used to eliminate lead-time, length, and selection bias in the evaluation of the effect of cancer screening [4].

The evidence-based screening methods currently used in population-based cancer screening programmes are shown in Table 4.7.1. Suitable screening tests for cervical cancer include cervical sampling for conventional cytology (Pap smear; Fig. 4.7.3) or liquid-based cytology; testing for human papillomavirus (HPV) infection; and visual inspection of the cervix with acetic acid (Fig. 4.7.4). Screening for breast cancer by mammography (Fig. 4.7.5) permits early detection of small breast cancers, most of which have not yet metastasized and can be successfully treated, although some of these might never have presented clinically in the subject's lifetime (overdiagnosis). Bowel cancer screening using faecal occult blood testing, flexible sigmoidoscopy, or colonoscopy may lead to the diagnosis of colorectal polyps (Fig. 4.7.6), removal of which during colonoscopy may prevent their progression to colorectal cancer. Early colorectal cancer that can be effectively treated by endoscopic removal or surgical excision may also be detected. Evidence-based programmes for population-based screening of other major cancers, such as cancers of the ovary, liver, oesophagus, lung, and prostate, have not yet been established.

For high-risk groups, visual screening (Fig. 4.7.7) has been shown to be efficacious in early detection and prevention of deaths from oral cancer [14]. Results of a large randomized controlled trial in the USA showed that screening people at high risk of lung cancer based on age and smoking history with low-dose computed tomography can reduce the number of deaths due to lung cancer [15]. The United States Preventive Services Task Force recently announced a draft

Fig. 4.7.3. Pap smear suggestive of high-grade precancerous lesion: cervical intraepithelial neoplasia grade 3 (CIN3). Inflammatory smear contains many parabasal cells with enlarged nuclei with irregular chromatin (black arrow) and some cells with eosinophilic cytoplasm (purple arrow).

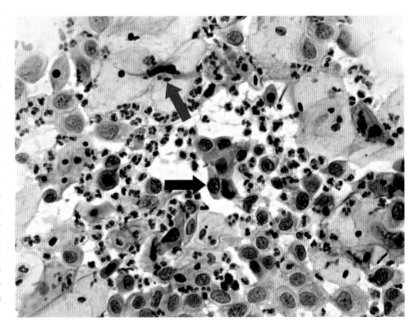

Fig. 4.7.4. Outcomes of visual inspection of the cervix with acetic acid: (A) negative, (B) positive. The circumorificial acetowhite lesion on the right (B) is suggestive of cervical intraepithelial neoplasia.

Fig. 4.7.4. Outcomes of visual inspection of the cervix with acetic acid: (A) negative, (B) positive. The circumorificial acetowhite lesion on the right (B) is suggestive of cervical intraepithelial neoplasia.

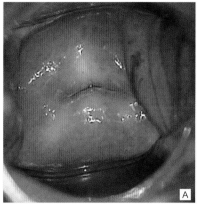
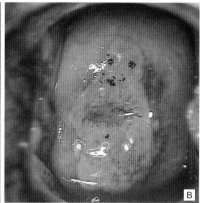

recommendation for annual screening for lung cancer using this procedure in people at high risk [16].

Determinants of harm and benefit

Screening should be conducted only after careful consideration of both harms and benefits. Knowledge has developed about health economic and cost–benefit analysis predicated on the potential health benefits and risks in addition to the financial costs of cancer screening for the people affected [17–19]. Before screening programmes are launched, an analysis of the expected costs and the benefit should be performed using data collected in feasibility and pilot studies in the relevant health-care environment. These analyses should be repeated at intervals in established programmes, typically every 10 years, and before adopting major modifications of existing protocols. The methods applied in cost–benefit analysis are complex, and in interpreting the results, the underlying assumptions as well as the balance between the main benefits and harms of screening should be kept in mind.

Despite the considerable potential of cervical and colorectal cancer screening to prevent invasive cancer through detection and treatment of precancerous lesions, the key

measure of benefit for any such screening programme is mortality reduction, rather than increased detection of early-stage disease. A secondary benefit of earlier diagnosis arises because smaller cancers can often be treated with less debilitating procedures and medications.

The primary harm from screening is morbidity and mortality from the procedures for detection and diagnosis, and the side-effects of treatment

prompted by screening. Exposure to these risks in the absence of any direct health benefit is of particular concern. Such a situation may arise due to false-positive tests or procedures, or from overdiagnosis, i.e. diagnosis through screening of cancers that would not have been detected symptomatically during the lifetime of an individual. Unfortunately, overdiagnosed cancers cannot be individually identified; the likely number of such cases may be estimated after many years of follow-up in a randomized screening trial where screening was never offered to the relevant controls. A related potential harm of screening is overtreatment, which is not limited to those cases that are overdiagnosed. Overtreatment may occur if less-intensive treatment protocols appropriate to early-stage lesions are not available or are not followed.

Quality assurance plays an important role in keeping overdiagnosis and overtreatment in an appropriate range. Studies in Europe addressing overtreatment in breast cancer screening have demonstrated that mastectomy rates decreased markedly after the introduction of population-based mammography screening

Fig. 4.7.5. (A) A normal oblique view mammogram of the left breast of an asymptomatic 57-year-old woman. (B) A small invasive cancer detected at screening 2 years later. This cancer could not be detected with palpation even after it had been detected with mammography.

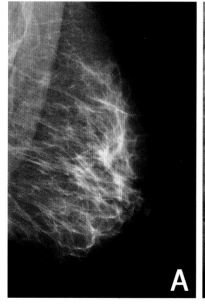
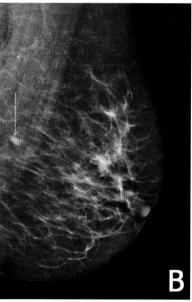

Fig. 4.7.6. A colonoscopy performed as part of the Lampang Province colorectal cancer screening programme in Thailand. Inset at lower right shows a large bowel polyp being removed during the colonoscopy.

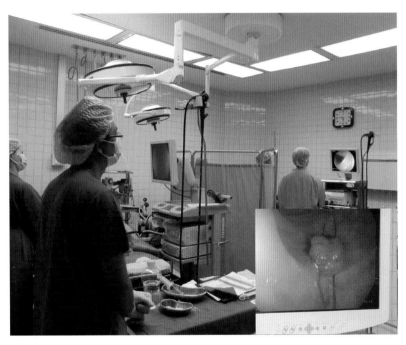

[20,21]. Two recent reviews estimated that for every one or two overdiagnosed cases, at least one death due to breast cancer was avoided, a balance between benefit and harm considered to be appropriate [22,23].

The potential for overdiagnosis is substantial when screening for prostate cancer by determining serum prostate-specific antigen levels [24]. Whereas data from the Prostate, Lung, Colorectal, and Ovarian Cancer Screening Trial in the USA [25], unlike results from the European Randomized Study of Screening for Prostate Cancer [26], have not indicated a disease-specific mortality reduction, both trials suggest that systematic screening would result in significant levels of overdiagnosis. Due to uncertainties about the benefits and the risks, population-based prostate cancer screening is not supported by currently available evidence.

Since estimation of overdiagnosis requires the application of complex statistical methods,all such estimates are subject to uncertainty. Whereas cancer-registry-based studies tend to be imprecise and underestimate the benefits of screening, calculations of the mortality benefit based on precise individual data tend to be highly accurate. Although many people consider the benefit of an averted cancer death to greatly outweigh the risks of overdiagnosis and overtreatment, strict quality assurance practices must be maintained to minimize all risks associated with screening.

Organization of screening

People eligible for population-based screening are defined by age and/or gender, as well as the cancer burden for the relevant tumour type. In most countries breast cancer screening is offered to normal-risk women from the age of 40–50 years and extending to the age of 70–75 years, typically at 2-year intervals. Cervical cancer screening is generally offered to women from the age of 25–30 years and extending to the age of 60–65 years. The recommended interval commonly varies between 3 and 5 years. In low- and middle- income countries, cervical screening may be provided in a narrower age range or only once or a few times in a lifetime. Colorectal cancer screening is generally offered to women and men from the age of 50 years and extending to the age of 74 years. Depending on the screening protocol, which may use faecal occult blood testing, faecal immunochemical testing, flexible sigmoidoscopy, or colonoscopy, the recommended interval commonly varies between 2 and 10 years, and endoscopic screening may be performed only once in a lifetime [27,28].

Screening of high-risk groups is generally not considered a population-based strategy since only a small portion of the total population is affected [3]. For evidence-based screening of high-risk groups, a programmatic approach can be recommended, provided the quality and the cost-effectiveness of the screening process are assured.

Organized programmes

For a programme to be considered an organized screening programme, a public cancer screening policy documented in a law, or an official regulation, decision, directive, or recommendation is required. The policy should define, as a minimum, the screening protocol and repeat interval, and determinants of eligibility for screening. The screening examinations should be financed by public sources (apart from a possible co-payment in high-income countries). Provision of screening in organized programmes is recommended because these include an administrative structure responsible for service delivery, quality assurance, and evaluation [29].

The rules and regulations applicable to an organized programme generally provide for a team at the national or regional level that is responsible for implementation, i.e. for coordinating the delivery of the screening services, maintaining the requisite quality, and reporting on performance and results. Such organizational and managerial elements generally

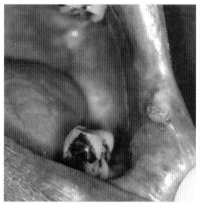 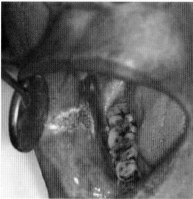

provide for supervision and monitoring of most steps in the screening process, as well as comprehensive guidelines and rules defining standard operating procedures. In addition, a quality assurance structure is required, and a means of ascertaining the population burden of the disease must be available so that the programme can be evaluated [4].

Population-based programmes

Population-based screening programmes identify and individually invite each person in the eligible population to attend each round of screening. Individual invitations aim to give each person in the eligible population an equal chance of benefiting from screening and to thereby reduce health-care inequalities [29]. The invitations should be supported by effective communication for groups with limited access to screening, such as less-advantaged socioeconomic groups. This communication, in turn, should support an informed decision about participation, based on information about the risks and benefits of screening [30,31]. Invitations indicating a date, time, and place for the screening examination have been most effective in high-resource settings. These invitations have usually been sent by letter, often followed up with reminders to non-responders. Recent experience with call centres and electronic messaging

via mobile phones suggests that such methods of communication warrant further investigation [30].

Opportunistic programmes

"Opportunistic" screening is a less cost-effective form of screening and is less amenable to quality assurance than is population-based screening. Such screening relies on a health-care provider taking the initiative to offer screening or to encourage individuals to participate in a screening programme, or to undertake screening outside the context of any programme (so-called wild screening). In high-resource settings, opportunistic screening has been associated with lower overall impact of screening and lower participation rates [32]. In addition, the total volume of resources consumed tends to be significantly higher with opportunistic screening. This leads to overuse of screening resources by part of the target population and underuse by, or lack of coverage of, the rest of the population [33,34].

Importance of quality assurance

The importance of quality assurance in cancer screening goes beyond the need to ensure that any medical intervention is performed adequately, efficiently, and with minimum risk and maximum benefit. At any given time, only a small number of people invited to attend population-based screening

(usually < 1%) will have undetected cancer or precancerous lesions that can be treated effectively. Therefore, only a small number of people can derive a direct health benefit from attending screening. However, all participants are exposed to the risks of screening, and although these are slight, the risks add up. To achieve the benefit of cancer screening, quality must be optimal at every step in the screening process, including identification and personal invitation of each eligible individual; performance of the screening test, examination, or procedure; diagnostic work-up of people with detected abnormalities; and, when necessary, treatment, surveillance, and aftercare (Fig. 4.7.8) [6]. In practice, the process of screening is much more complex than the schematic diagram in Fig. 4.7.8 suggests. For example, in a quality-assured colorectal cancer screening programme using a faecal occult blood testing kit, receipt of the test result indicating whether diagnostic work-up is warranted involves at least five different activities. Diagnostic work-up and clinical management of the lesions detected in screening require multidisciplinary teamwork and can be complicated. That is why organized, quality-assured screening programmes follow comprehensive quality assurance guidelines with evidence-based standards, procedures, and protocols of best practice that are continuously being improved [6,7,35].

Evaluation of the impact of a screening programme on cancer mortality is a long-term objective of quality assurance. The actual effect cannot be exactly quantified because mortality in the screened population would have to be compared with mortality in the same population in the absence of screening. To estimate the effect, various study designs have been used, such as comparing screened and matched unscreened populations, time trends in mortality, case–control studies, and modelling studies. However, changes attributable to improved awareness and treatments cannot be completely

Fig. 4.7.8. The cancer screening process.

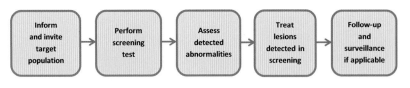

| Inform and invite target population | → | Perform screening test | → | Assess detected abnormalities | → | Treat lesions detected in screening | → | Follow-up and surveillance if applicable |

disentangled from the outcomes of screening programmes. Evidence on the effectiveness of population-based cancer screening is predominantly available from programmes in high-income countries.

To fully evaluate the impact of a screening programme, the potential harms mentioned above must also be determined, such as those due to false-positive tests and overdiagnosis. Since the full impact of a screening programme will not be known for many years after its initiation, it is also necessary to proactively monitor and continuously improve performance of all activities in the screening process from the outset, i.e. long before the impact is actually discernible. That will permit the timely recognition of steps that must be taken to continuously improve communication, organization, professional performance, and equipment.

Low coverage of the target population substantially limits the effectiveness and the cost-effectiveness of any programme. Health-care professionals, responsible authorities, and governments should also be aware of this and other constraints that may limit the achievable impact of cancer screening programmes. A common pitfall is the adoption of non-validated working models and methods. Of prime importance is the availability and sustainability of adequate human, financial, and technical resources to ensure that the programme achieves an appropriate balance between benefit and harm.

Outlook

It may take several years to implement a population-based cancer screening programme, from the beginning of planning to completion of roll-out across an entire country or region. Determinants of successful implementation of population-based cancer screening programmes have been developed for application to screening for any target cancer. Insights into the implementation of such programmes are provided in Chapter 4.8, which illustrates the need for comprehensive quality assurance in the establishment and delivery of multidisciplinary screening services at all resource levels. It also shows the importance of universal access to prompt and effective diagnostic and treatment services, which is a common goal in all attempts to improve cancer control through early detection.

References

1. Wilson JMG, Jungner G (1968). *Principles and Practice of Screening for Disease*. Geneva: WHO. Available at http://whqlibdoc.who.int/php/WHO_PHP_34.pdf/.

2. Lansdorp-Vogelaar I, von Karsa L (2012). European guidelines for quality assurance in colorectal cancer screening and diagnosis. First edition - Introduction. *Endoscopy*, 44 Suppl 3:SE15–SE30. http://dx.doi.org/10.1055/s-0032-1308898 PMID:23012118

3. WHO (2007). *Cancer Control: Knowledge into Action. WHO Guide for Effective Programmes*. Module 3: Early Detection. Geneva: WHO. Available at http://www.who.int/cancer/publications/cancer_control_detection/en/index.html.

4. IARC (2002). IARC Handbooks of Cancer Prevention, Vol. 7: *Breast Cancer Screening*. Lyon: IARC.

5. IARC (2005). IARC Handbooks of Cancer Prevention, Vol. 10: *Cervix Cancer Screening*. Lyon: IARC.

6. von Karsa L, Patnick J, Segnan N *et al.*; European Colorectal Cancer Screening Guidelines Working Group (2013). European guidelines for quality assurance in colorectal cancer screening and diagnosis: overview and introduction to the full supplement publication. *Endoscopy*, 45:51–59. http://dx.doi.org/10.1055/s-0032-1325997 PMID:23212726

7. Perry N, Broeders M, de Wolf C *et al.* (2008). European guidelines for quality assurance in breast cancer screening and diagnosis. Fourth edition - Summary document. *Ann Oncol*, 19:614–622. http://dx.doi.org/10.1093/annonc/mdm481 PMID:18024988

8. Segnan N, Patnick J, von Karsa L, eds (2010). *European Guidelines for Quality Assurance in Colorectal Cancer Screening and Diagnosis - First Edition*. Luxembourg: European Commission, Publications Office of the European Union.

9. Sankaranarayanan R, Nene BM, Shastri SS *et al.* (2009). HPV screening for cervical cancer in rural India. *N Engl J Med*, 360:1385–1394. http://dx.doi.org/10.1056/NEJMoa0808516 PMID:19339719

10. Vaccarella S, Lortet-Tieulent J, Plummer M *et al.* (2013). Worldwide trends in cervical cancer incidence: Impact of screening against changes in disease risk factors. *Eur J Cancer*, 49:3262–3273. http://dx.doi.org/10.1016/j.ejca.2013.04.024 PMID:23751569

11. Tabar L, Vitak B, Chen TH *et al.* (2011). Swedish two-county trial: impact of mammographic screening on breast cancer mortality during 3 decades. *Radiology*, 260:658–663. http://dx.doi.org/10.1148/radiol.11110469 PMID:21712474

12. Levin TR, Corley DA (2013). Colorectal-cancer screening – coming of age. *N Engl J Med*, 369:1164–1166. http://dx.doi.org/10.1056/NEJMe1308253 PMID:24047066

13. Atkin WS, Edwards R, Kralj-Hans I *et al.* (2010). Once-only flexible sigmoidoscopy screening in prevention of colorectal cancer: a multicentre randomised controlled trial. *Lancet*, 375:1624–1633. http://dx.doi.org/10.1016/S0140-6736(10)60551-X PMID:20430429

14. Sankaranarayanan R, Ramadas K, Somanathan T *et al.* (2013). Long term effect of visual screening on oral cancer incidence and mortality in a randomized trial in Kerala, India. *Oral Oncol*, 49:314–321. http://dx.doi.org/10.1016/j.oraloncology.2012.11.004 PMID:23265945

15. Church TR, Black WC, Aberle DR *et al.*; National Lung Screening Trial Research Team (2013). Results of initial low-dose computed tomographic screening for lung cancer. *N Engl J Med*, 368:1980–1991. http://dx.doi.org/10.1056/NEJMoa1209120 PMID:23697514

16. U.S. Preventive Services Task Force (2013). Screening for Lung Cancer: Draft Recommendation Statement. AHRQ Publication No. 13-05196-EF-3. Available at http://www.uspreventiveservicestaskforce.org/uspstf13/lungcan/lungcandraftrec.htm.

17. Wilschut JA, Habbema JD, van Leerdam ME *et al.* (2011). Fecal occult blood testing when colonoscopy capacity is limited. *J Natl Cancer Inst*, 103:1741–1751. http://dx.doi.org/10.1093/jnci/djr385 PMID:22076285

18. de Kok IM, van Rosmalen J, Dillner J *et al.* (2012). Primary screening for human papillomavirus compared with cytology screening for cervical cancer in European settings: cost effectiveness analysis based on a Dutch microsimulation model. *BMJ*, 344:e670. http://dx.doi.org/10.1136/bmj.e670 PMID:22391612

19. Heijnsdijk EA, Wever EM, Auvinen A *et al.* (2012). Quality-of-life effects of prostate-specific antigen screening. *N Engl J Med*, 367:595–605. http://dx.doi.org/10.1056/NEJMoa1201637 PMID:22894572

20. Paci E, Duffy SW, Giorgi D *et al.* (2002). Are breast cancer screening programmes increasing rates of mastectomy? Observational study. *BMJ*, 325:418. http://dx.doi.org/10.1136/bmj.325.7361.418 PMID:12193357

21. Lawrence G, Kearins O, Lagord C *et al.* (2011). *The Second All Breast Cancer Report*. London: National Cancer Intelligence Network. Available at http://www.ncin.org.uk/view.aspx?rid=612

22. Paci E; EUROSCREEN Working Group (2012). Summary of the evidence of breast cancer service screening outcomes in Europe and first estimate of the benefit and harm balance sheet. *J Med Screen*, 19 Suppl 1:5–13. http://dx.doi.org/10.1258/jms.2012.012077 PMID:22972806

23. Marmot MG, Altman D, Cameron D *et al.*; Independent UK Panel on Breast Cancer Screening (2012). *The Benefits and Harms of Breast Cancer Screening: An Independent Review*. Cancer Research UK and the Department of Health (England). Available at www.cruk.org/breastscreeningreview.

24. Draisma G, Etzioni R, Tsodikov A *et al.* (2009). Lead time and overdiagnosis in prostate-specific antigen screening: importance of methods and context. *J Natl Cancer Inst*, 101:374–383. http://dx.doi.org/10.1093/jnci/djp001 PMID:19276453

25. Andriole GL, Crawford ED, Grubb RL 3rd *et al.*; PLCO Project Team (2012). Prostate cancer screening in the randomized Prostate, Lung, Colorectal, and Ovarian Cancer Screening Trial: mortality results after 13 years of follow-up. *J Natl Cancer Inst*, 104:125–132. http://dx.doi.org/10.1093/jnci/djr500 PMID:22228146

26. Schröder FH, Hugosson J, Carlsson S *et al.* (2012). Screening for prostate cancer decreases the risk of developing metastatic disease: findings from the European Randomized Study of Screening for Prostate Cancer (ERSPC). *Eur Urol*, 62:745–752. http://dx.doi.org/10.1016/j.eururo.2012.05.068 PMID:22704366

27. von Karsa L, Anttila A, Ronco G *et al.* (2008). *Cancer Screening in the European Union: Report on the Implementation of the Council Recommendation on Cancer Screening - First Report*. Luxembourg: European Communities. Available at http://ec.europa.eu/health/ph_determinants/genetics/documents/cancer_screening.pdf.

28. International Cancer Screening Network (2013). Cancer Sites. National Cancer Institute. Available at http://appliedresearch.cancer.gov/icsn/sites.html.

29. Karsa LV, Lignini TA, Patnick J *et al.* (2010). The dimensions of the CRC problem. *Best Pract Res Clin Gastroenterol*, 24:381–396. http://dx.doi.org/10.1016/j.bpg.2010.06.004 PMID:20833343

30. Austoker J, Giordano L, Hewitson P *et al.* (2012). European guidelines for quality assurance in colorectal cancer screening and diagnosis. First edition - Communication. *Endoscopy*, 44 Suppl 3:SE164–SE185. http://dx.doi.org/10.1055/s-0032-1309809 PMID:23012120

31. von Karsa L (1995). Mammography screening – comprehensive, population-based quality assurance is required! [in German] *Z Allgemeinmed*, 71:1863–1867.

32. Malila N, Senore C, Armaroli P (2012). European guidelines for quality assurance in colorectal cancer screening and diagnosis. First edition - Organisation. *Endoscopy*, 44 Suppl 3:SE31–SE48. http://dx.doi.org/10.1055/s-0032-1309783 PMID:23012121

33. Arbyn M, Anttila A, Jordan J *et al.* (2010). European guidelines for quality assurance in cervical cancer screening. Second edition - Summary document. *Ann Oncol*, 21:448–458. http://dx.doi.org/10.1093/annonc/mdp471 PMID:20176693

34. Anttila A, von Karsa L, Aasmaa A *et al.* (2009). Cervical cancer screening policies and coverage in Europe. *Eur J Cancer*, 45:2649–2658. http://dx.doi.org/10.1016/j.ejca.2009.07.020 PMID:19699081

35. Cancer Care Ontario (2012). Colorectal cancer screening. Surveillance guidelines. Available at https://www.cancercare.on.ca/pcs/screening/coloscreening/cccstandardsguidelines/.

Websites

International Cancer Screening Network: http://appliedresearch.cancer.gov/icsn/

Screening Group, Section of Early Detection and Prevention, IARC: http://www.iarc.fr/en/research-groups/SCR/index.php

4.8

Screening – implementation

4 PREVENTION

Lawrence von Karsa
You-Lin Qiao
Kunnambath Ramadas
Namory Keita
Silvina Arrossi
Peter B. Dean
Nada Al Alwan
Rengaswamy Sankaranarayanan

Ahti Anttila (reviewer)
Anthony B. Miller (reviewer)

Summary

- Global implementation of population-based cancer screening reveals heterogeneity, and broad knowledge is restricted to three cancer types: breast, cervical, and colorectal cancer.

- In many high-income countries and some middle-income countries, population-based screening programmes for breast and cervical cancer have been established for decades, or shorter periods, and some have achieved significant reductions in cancer-specific mortality. Colorectal cancer screening programmes have been introduced more recently.

- There are few population-based screening programmes in low- and middle-income countries.

- Screening programmes require political commitment, engagement of civil society, competent oversight, and adequate, sustainable resources.

- Programme management should have the authority to coordinate all activities essential for provision of screening services, including training, documentation, monitoring, and other aspects of quality assurance.

- Programmes should be implemented gradually, tailoring expansion of the screening service to the capacity of the health-care system and with optimal accessibility for less-advantaged groups in the target population.

Implementation of quality-assured population-based cancer screening programmes affects very large numbers of people in the eligible age range (see Chapter 4.7). The process requires many years, beginning with the development and testing of a comprehensive quality assurance system to ensure the provision of cost-effective, affordable, and acceptable services for the entire target population. Carefully planned, long-term investment of time and financial resources is justified because the impact of a population-based programme goes far beyond the services provided. Screening can stimulate health systems development and raises the level of awareness of cancer symptoms among health-care professionals and the general public. A quality-assured population-based screening programme raises the standards of cancer diagnosis and treatment throughout the medical community. Professionals trained to meet the standards of the screening programme may also care for

patients outside the programme. These factors, in combination, lead to an overall improvement in the level of cancer care [1].

Criteria for successful implementation of screening

Successful implementation of population-based cancer screening programmes requires expertise in areas relevant to other prevention activities, such as motivation, communication, and reinforcement of efforts designed to prevent cancer [2]. The ability to mobilize large numbers of health-care professionals, other stakeholders, and the target population itself in collective actions focused on a common goal is crucial to the success of any screening programme [3].

Programme implementation begins with a planning and feasibility phase, which includes large-scale pilot studies to evaluate whether screening conducted as planned fulfils the key performance targets and is likely to be cost-effective. It may take several years to collect sufficient data for valid conclusions to be drawn about routine implementation and to make any necessary adjustments to the screening protocol warranted by the pilot results. Pilot studies are also needed to provide information on the cost-effectiveness of screening in the context of

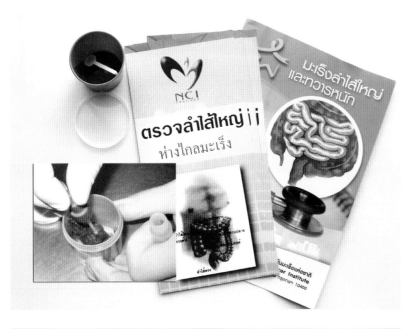

an individual country. After successful pilot studies, gradual, quality-controlled roll-out of the programme across the country begins, with the health-care system controlling the pace of programme expansion, with particular reference to specialized training of staff and investment in infrastructure. The entire process of programme implementation rarely takes less than 10 years [1].

Certain conditions are essential to assure quality in population-based screening programmes. These include long-term political commitment and competent oversight, adequate and sustainable resources, engagement of the community, international collaboration, and autonomous programme management with effective coordination of all activities, particularly communication and training, organizational development, and control of programme resources [4]. Programme resources include a dedicated budget and staff, computerized information systems, and registries for cancer, population, and screening, all based on individual data [5]. Successful implementation of effective screening programmes

requires national investment [6]. In a fully established programme, the proportion of the expenditure devoted to quality assurance in a high-resource setting should be no less than 10–20% [7]. A substantial proportion of these resources are required for well-organized information systems, such as those used by cancer and screening registries, to provide reports on test results for participants and health professionals, to confirm that appropriate action follows a positive screening test, and to monitor performance and evaluate the impact of any screening programme [4].

Setting priorities in implementing screening programmes

Given the substantial resources required for successful implementation of population-based cancer screening programmes, efforts to improve early detection of cancer should be integrated into national comprehensive cancer control plans that establish overall priorities in the health-care agenda and take into account all relevant activities, such as

national or regional programmes for reproductive health [8,9].

In most high-income countries, the burden of cancer has resulted in coordinated efforts to implement population-based screening for all of the tumour types for which evidence-based methods are currently established (breast, cervical, and colorectal cancer). In other countries, due to the comparatively long period required to successfully establish population-based screening programmes, time trends in cancer incidence and mortality should be taken into account when prioritizing potential target cancers for screening [1]. On this basis, cancers currently suitable for screening in low- and middle-income countries include, for example, cervical cancer in sub-Saharan Africa, India, and Latin America; breast cancer in Latin America, the Middle East, and some countries in Asia; and colorectal cancer in countries in transition, such as Brazil and China. Before a commitment is made to the roll-out of a screening programme, the potential cost-effectiveness of the programme in the country should be taken into account. If pilot studies indicate that the cost per year of life saved by a given intervention is less than the per capita gross national product, a screening programme can be considered to be highly cost-effective in that setting [10].

The same principles of quality assurance for population-based screening apply to screening of high-risk groups or to early detection and treatment of symptomatic disease where significant proportions and numbers of patients are diagnosed with very-late-stage disease. Priority should be given to providing adequate resources for diagnosis and treatment of currently increasing levels of symptomatic disease, for example through training of competent staff. When access to prompt diagnosis and treatment is available, alternative strategies of early detection can be considered in countries where low incidence rates do not yet justify population-based screening programmes for asymptomatic

Fig. 4.8.2. Women lining up at Kanungu Health Centre IV in Uganda to receive HIV counselling and cervical cancer screening, and to learn more about available family planning services.

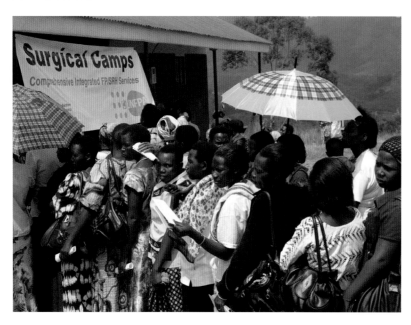

people. In Iraq, for example, recent surveys show significant knowledge gaps in the educated population about the relative importance of breast cancer in the Iraqi population and the performance of breast self-examination, suggesting a potential to increase early detection of breast cancer through better awareness [11]. Morocco is currently establishing universal access to comprehensive cancer diagnosis, treatment, and palliative care according to the 2010–2019 national cancer control plan. This includes a nationwide early detection programme for clinically detectable breast cancer [12].

Screening programmes in high-income countries

The first population-based cancer screening programmes were launched in middle- and high-income countries in the 1960s to 1980s, for cervical cancer screening. These programmes were based on conventional cytology, and many led to reductions of 50–80% in cervical cancer mortality within two to three decades of implementation [13]. In recent years, primary cervical cancer

screening by human papillomavirus (HPV) testing has been established as more accurate and effective. HPV testing is therefore expected to become the preferred screening test for cervical cancer in the medium and long term [14,15].

The first population-based breast screening programmes based on mammography were initiated in Europe, Canada, and Australia in the late 1980s after randomized controlled trials showed the efficacy of screening [16,17]. By 2012, population-based breast screening programmes were running or being established in 24 countries in the European Union and in several countries in Asia and the Americas. Screen-film mammography is being increasingly replaced by digital mammography [18]. Now that screening has been performed for more than two decades in several population-based programmes in Europe, methodologies used to estimate the impact of screening and the level of overdiagnosis have been evaluated using data from service screening programmes [19]. Registry studies analysing population breast cancer mortality rates

over time underestimate the impact of screening on breast cancer mortality because of their inability to exclude deaths in women with breast cancer diagnosed before invitation to screening, and due to the inability to discriminate between data of screened and unscreened women during the gradual implementation of a screening programme in a country or region [20].

Estimates of the impact of service screening in Europe have recently been obtained from a review of all available observational studies from which sufficient longitudinal individual data were available, directly linking a woman's screening history to her cause of death. The authors considered that the most reliable estimates of reduction in breast cancer mortality were 25–31% for women invited for screening and 38–48% for women actually screened [21].

Reviews of all randomized clinical trials that evaluated annual or biennial guaiac-based faecal occult blood testing indicate that trial participants allocated to screening had a 16% lower relative risk of colorectal cancer mortality [22]. Population-based colorectal cancer screening programmes in developed countries are recent, and are still evolving in most countries. Acceptable and desirable levels of performance have recently been developed for the population-based programmes in Europe based on results achieved in randomized trials

Fig. 4.8.3. Augusta Victoria Hospital in Jerusalem operates this mobile mammography unit, which strives to identify women with breast cancer at an early stage so that they may be referred to the hospital for treatment, with better outcomes.

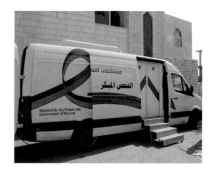

and routine programmes [23]. Efforts are under way to improve programme performance in many countries [24].

Screening programmes in upper-middle-income countries

Opportunistic, large-scale cervical cancer screening has been conducted in some upper-middle-income countries for several years. The resulting impact on cervical cancer incidence and mortality has been limited, due to poor coverage and lack of quality assurance in cytology screening, suboptimal adherence by screen-positive women to further diagnosis and treatment, and lack of information systems to monitor progress and assess impact. In Latin America, this has led to initiatives to reassess the approaches to cervical cancer control, taking into account opportunities to improve organization and quality assurance, as well as the introduction of HPV testing for cervical cancer screening, and HPV vaccination [25]. Self-sampling has also been investigated and shows potential to increase cervical screening effectiveness by increasing participation, especially in women who are difficult to reach or who do not regularly attend cervical cancer screening [26]. In recent years, many of these programmes have been reorganized, and HPV testing is being integrated into routine screening in a phased manner in countries such as Argentina and Mexico. Sporadic and opportunistic mammography screening is widespread, but population-based breast cancer screening programmes have yet to evolve in many upper-middle-income countries. Colorectal cancer screening is less widespread; a national programme exists in Uruguay.

Screening programmes in lower-middle-income and low-income countries

Cancer screening programmes are operational in very few lower-middle-income and low-income countries in Africa, Asia, Central America, and the Caribbean, despite the high risk

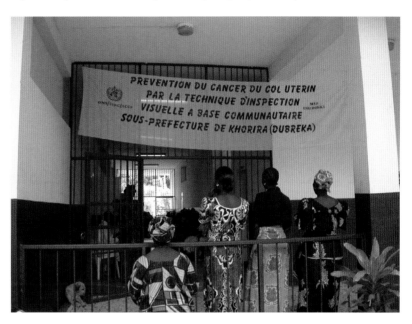

Fig. 4.8.4. Women waiting to be screened during a cervical cancer prevention campaign organized by IARC and Conakry University Hospital, in the Republic of Guinea.

of cervical cancer and the increasing incidence of breast cancer in these regions. Limited resources and inadequate development of health services currently preclude introducing screening programmes in most of these countries. The challenges to introducing cytology screening and to improving treatment of screen-positive women, as well as the limited impact of Pap smear screening in upper-middle-income countries, have prompted the search for alternative screening methods and algorithms for cervical cancer control in low-resource settings. HPV testing and visual inspection of the cervix with acetic acid have been evaluated as alternative methods, and single-visit approaches, involving diagnosis and treatment of screen-positive women in the same sitting as screening, have been explored to improve compliance with treatment. Recent results from such studies have prompted the introduction of visual inspection of the cervix with acetic acid screening programmes in Bangladesh [27], Tamil Nadu state in India, Thailand [28], and Zambia [29], as well as demonstration programmes in 43 counties of 31

provincial administrative areas in China and in several countries in sub-Saharan Africa (Fig. 4.8.4) and Central America. Implementation of acetic acid-based screening may improve development of screening infrastructure, which may, in turn, facilitate the introduction of HPV screening when simple and affordable viral tests become widely available.

Limited resources and inadequate development of health services preclude introducing mammography screening programmes in most lower-middle-income and low-income countries. Improving breast awareness may facilitate earlier clinical diagnosis among symptomatic women in such settings, but these efforts may be counterproductive if the women cannot obtain timely diagnostic and therapeutic services. For the same reason, systematic approaches to early detection based on breast examination and imaging methods are required in countries that have an increasing burden of breast cancer but that currently lack adequate diagnostic and therapeutic services [30,31]. Population-based colorectal cancer screening does not exist in any low-income or lower-middle-income country, with the exception of Thailand, where a pilot colorectal cancer screening programme has been introduced as a forerunner to the phased national expansion.

Outlook

Breast, cervical, and colorectal cancer screening programmes have been improved globally through research in terms of quality inputs, efficiency, and effectiveness. New research findings have catalysed the planning and organization of new screening programmes in some countries [32]. In the foreseeable future, HPV vaccination programmes seem likely to reduce the prevalence of this viral infection and related precancerous lesions, necessitating more sensitive and objective screening tests [33]. Research has indicated the efficacy of mammography and faecal occult blood screening and paved the way for population-based screening programmes. Screening approaches for other tumour types, such as lung, ovarian, oesophageal, stomach, and prostate cancer, are currently being investigated in research settings (Fig. 4.8.5), and in the case of gastric cancer also in the context of a population-based cancer screening programme in the Republic of Korea [34]. Unless these initiatives prove their efficacy, feasibility, and cost-effectiveness in those settings, population-based programmes are unlikely to be established and widely implemented.

Population-based screening programmes for breast, cervical, and colorectal cancer have been introduced as part of cancer control in many high-income countries. Population-based cancer screening programmes do not exist in most

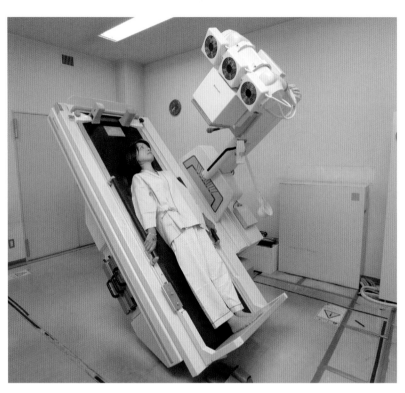

Fig. 4.8.5. A woman being screened for stomach cancer at the Osaka Cancer Prevention and Detection Center, in Japan, in research directed towards the development of a population-based protocol for this tumour type.

low- and middle-income countries, where cancers are mainly detected through very-late-stage symptoms and many are not reported. Recent research may lead to new approaches to early detection and treatment using improved awareness of symptomatic disease and population-based screening of asymptomatic people.

Success in decreasing the burden of cancer will depend on the acceptance by the population of a screening programme that is anchored in a comprehensive and well-structured cancer control programme, and on the capacity of the health-care system to make efficient

and appropriate diagnostic and therapeutic services universally available for the cases detected early. Provision of adequate resources will be decisive.

International cooperation can enable countries to avoid common pitfalls in the implementation of screening programmes and other early detection programmes, and to share knowledge about successful methods and approaches. Sharing of expertise may enable a country to implement programmes more successfully and to avoid unnecessary expenditure and delay.

References

1. Karsa LV, Lignini TA, Patnick J et al. (2010). The dimensions of the CRC problem. *Best Pract Res Clin Gastroenterol*, 24:381–396. http://dx.doi.org/10.1016/j.bpg.2010.06.004 PMID:20833343

2. Hill D, Dixon H (2010). Achieving behavioural changes in individuals and populations. In: Elwood JM, Sutcliffe SB, eds. *Cancer Control*. Oxford: Oxford University Press, pp. 43–61.

3. Hanleybrown F, Kania J, Kramer M (2012). Channeling change: making collective impact work. *Stanford Social Innovation Review*, 1–8. Available at http://www.ssireview.org/blog/entry/channeling_change_making_collective_impact_work/.

4. Lynge E, Törnberg S, von Karsa L et al. (2012). Determinants of successful implementation of population-based cancer screening programmes. *Eur J Cancer*, 48:743–748. http://dx.doi.org/10.1016/j.ejca.2011.06.051 PMID:21788130

5. von Karsa L, Arrossi S (2013). Development and implementation of guidelines for quality assurance in breast cancer screening: the European experience. *Salud Publica Mex*, 55:318–328. PMID:23912545

6. National Colorectal Screening Programme (2011). *International Peer Review Panel Report of Quality Assurance Standards, 10–11 March 2011*. NCSS/PUB/Q-3 Rev 2. Dublin, Ireland: National Cancer Screening Service. Available at http://www.cancerscreening.ie/publications/Colorectal_Peer_Review_Report_Rev_2.pdf.

7. von Karsa L, Suonio E, Lignini TA et al., eds (2012). *Current Status and Future Directions of Breast and Cervical Cancer Prevention and Early Detection in Belarus*. Cancer Control Assessment and Advice Requested by the Belarus Ministry of Health. Report of Expert Mission to Minsk, Belarus, 15–18 February 2011. Lyon: IARC. Available at http://www.iarc.fr/en/publications/pdfs-online/wrk/wrk6/Belarus_Report.pdf.

8. WHO (2006). *Cancer Control: Knowledge into Action. WHO Guide for Effective Programmes*. Module 1: Planning. Geneva: WHO. Available at http://www.who.int/cancer/publications/cancer_control_planning/en/index.html.

9. WHO (2007). *Cancer Control: Knowledge into Action. WHO Guide for Effective Programmes*. Module 3: Early Detection. Geneva: WHO. Available at http://www.who.int/cancer/publications/cancer_control_detection/en/index.html.

10. Ginsberg GM, Lauer JA, Zelle S et al. (2012). Cost effectiveness of strategies to combat breast, cervical, and colorectal cancer in sub-Saharan Africa and South East Asia: mathematical modelling study. *BMJ*, 344:e614. http://dx.doi.org/10.1136/bmj.e614 PMID:22389347

11. Alwan NA, Al-Attar WM, Eliessa RA et al. (2012). Knowledge, attitude and practice regarding breast cancer and breast self-examination among a sample of the educated population in Iraq. *East Mediterr Health J*, 18:337–345. PMID:22768695

12. Lalla Salma Association Against Cancer (2009). *National Cancer Prevention and Control Plan, 2010–2019: Strategic axes and measures*. Available at http://www.nccp-uicc.org/sites/default/files/plans/Morocco%20National-Cancer-Axes-and-Measures.pdf.

13. Hakama M, Chamberlain J, Day NE et al. (1985). Evaluation of screening programmes for gynaecological cancer. *Br J Cancer*, 52:669–673. http://dx.doi.org/10.1038/bjc.1985.241 PMID:4063143

14. Arbyn M, Ronco G, Anttila A et al. (2012). Evidence regarding human papillomavirus testing in secondary prevention of cervical cancer. *Vaccine*, 30 Suppl 5:F88–F99. http://dx.doi.org/10.1016/j.vaccine.2012.06.095 PMID:23199969

15. Cuzick J, Bergeron C, von Knebel Doeberitz M et al. (2012). New technologies and procedures for cervical cancer screening. *Vaccine*, 30 Suppl 5:F107–F116. http://dx.doi.org/10.1016/j.vaccine.2012.05.088 PMID:23199953

16. Shapiro S, Strax P, Venet L (1971). Periodic breast cancer screening in reducing mortality from breast cancer. *JAMA*, 215:1777–1785. http://dx.doi.org/10.1001/jama.1971.03180240027005 PMID:5107709

17. Tabár L, Fagerberg CJ, Gad A et al. (1985). Reduction in mortality from breast cancer after mass screening with mammography. Randomised trial from the Breast Cancer Screening Working Group of the Swedish National Board of Health and Welfare. *Lancet*, 1:829–832. http://dx.doi.org/10.1016/S0140-6736(85)92204-4 PMID:2858707

18. Timmers JM, den Heeten GJ, Adang EM et al. (2012). Dutch digital breast cancer screening: implications for breast cancer care. *Eur J Public Health*, 22:925–929. http://dx.doi.org/10.1093/eurpub/ckr170 PMID:22158996

19. Paci E; EUROSCREEN Working Group (2012). Summary of the evidence of breast cancer service screening outcomes in Europe and first estimate of the benefit and harm balance sheet. *J Med Screen*, 19 Suppl 1:5–13. http://dx.doi.org/10.1258/jms.2012.012077 PMID:22972806

20. Moss SM, Nyström L, Jonsson H et al.; Euroscreen Working Group (2012). The impact of mammographic screening on breast cancer mortality in Europe: a review of trend studies. *J Med Screen*, 19 Suppl 1:26–32. http://dx.doi.org/10.1258/jms.2012.012079 PMID:22972808

21. Broeders M, Moss S, Nyström L et al.; EUROSCREEN Working Group (2012). The impact of mammographic screening on breast cancer mortality in Europe: a review of observational studies. *J Med Screen*, 19 Suppl 1:14–25. http://dx.doi.org/10.1258/jms.2012.012078 PMID:22972807

22. Hewitson P, Glasziou P, Watson E et al. (2008). Cochrane systematic review of colorectal cancer screening using the fecal occult blood test (hemoccult): an update. *Am J Gastroenterol*, 103:1541–1549. http://dx.doi.org/10.1111/j.1572-0241.2008.01875.x PMID:18479499

23. von Karsa L, Patnick J, Segnan N (2012). European guidelines for quality assurance in colorectal cancer screening and diagnosis. First edition - Executive summary. *Endoscopy*, 44 Suppl 3:SE1–SE8. http://dx.doi.org/10.1055/s-0032-1309822 PMID:23012113

24. Benson VS, Atkin WS, Green J et al.; International Colorectal Cancer Screening Network (2012). Toward standardizing and reporting colorectal cancer screening indicators on an international level: The International Colorectal Cancer Screening Network. *Int J Cancer*, 130:2961–2973. http://dx.doi.org/10.1002/ijc.26310 PMID:21792895

25. Herrero R (2012). A new era begins for cervical cancer control. *HPV Today. Latin America Special Issue*, 27:2. Available at www.g-o-c.org/uploads/12nov_hpvtoday.pdf.

26. Hernández-Ávila M, Lazcano-Ponce E, Cruz-Valdés A et al. (2012). Self-sampled vaginal testing to determine HPV DNA: appropriate technology for women who do not regularly attend cervical screening. *HPV Today. Latin America Special Issue*, 27:7. Available at www.g-o-c.org/uploads/12nov_hpvtoday.pdf.

27. Nessa A, Hussain MA, Rahman JN et al. (2010). Screening for cervical neoplasia in Bangladesh using visual inspection with acetic acid. *Int J Gynaecol Obstet*, 111:115–118. http://dx.doi.org/10.1016/j.ijgo.2010.06.004 PMID:20674919

28. Chumworathayi B, Blumenthal PD, Limpaphayom KK et al. (2010). Effect of single-visit VIA and cryotherapy cervical cancer prevention program in Roi Et, Thailand: a preliminary report. *J Obstet Gynaecol Res*, 36:79–85. http://dx.doi.org/10.1111/j.1447-0756.2009.01089.x PMID:20178531

29. Pfaendler KS, Mwanahamuntu MH, Sahasrabuddhe VV et al. (2008). Management of cryotherapy-ineligible women in a "screen-and-treat" cervical cancer prevention program targeting HIV-infected women in Zambia: lessons from the field. *Gynecol Oncol*, 110:402–407. http://dx.doi.org/10.1016/j.ygyno.2008.04.031 PMID:18556050

30. Mittra I, Mishra GA, Singh S *et al.* (2010). A cluster randomized, controlled trial of breast and cervix cancer screening in Mumbai, India: methodology and interim results after three rounds of screening. *Int J Cancer*, 126:976–984. http://dx.doi.org/10.1002/ijc.24840 PMID:19697326

31. Sankaranarayanan R, Ramadas K, Thara S *et al.* (2011). Clinical breast examination: preliminary results from a cluster randomized controlled trial in India. *J Natl Cancer Inst*, 103:1476–1480. http://dx.doi.org/10.1093/jnci/djr304 PMID:21862730

32. Sankaranarayanan R, Sauvaget C, Ramadas K *et al.* (2011). Clinical trials of cancer screening in the developing world and their impact on cancer health-care. *Ann Oncol*, 22 Suppl 7:vii20–vii28. http://dx.doi.org/10.1093/annonc/mdr422 PMID:22039141

33. Sankaranarayanan R, Nene BM, Shastri SS *et al.* (2009). HPV screening for cervical cancer in rural India. *N Engl J Med*, 360:1385–1394. http://dx.doi.org/10.1056/NEJMoa0808516 PMID:19339719

34. Kim Y, Jun JK, Choi KS *et al.* (2011). Overview of the national cancer screening programme and the cancer screening status in Korea. *Asian Pac J Cancer Prev*, 12:725–730. PMID:21627372

Mel Greaves

An evolutionary foundation for cancer control

Melvyn "Mel" Greaves is a professor of cell biology at the Institute of Cancer Research in London; he established the Leukaemia Research Fund Centre there in 1984. Professor Greaves trained in zoology and obtained his Ph.D. in immunology at University College London, before focusing his research on cancer and leukaemia. His pioneering work includes developing new methods for biological classification of leukaemias, identifying that acute lymphoblastic leukaemia (ALL) develops in the womb, and identifying cancer stem cells that cause ALL. His research has greatly contributed to the dramatic reduction in mortality from childhood leukaemia in the past 30 years. His major research goals include confirming the role that common childhood infections play in the development of leukaemia and identifying the major causal factors of the disease. Professor Greaves is also a successful popular science writer and encourages science writing that is aimed at both scientists and the general public.

"Nothing in biology makes sense except in the light of evolution"
— T. Dobzhansky (1973)

Summary

Epidemiologists, cell and molecular biologists, geneticists and genomics experts, and oncologists can all lay claim to significant contributions towards the advancement of our understanding of cancer and its causation and treatment. But the stark fact remains that the worldwide burden of cancer remains huge and is escalating, and advanced or metastatic disease is mostly intransigent to treatment. Billions of dollars are riding on the premise that personalized medicine and targeted therapy will come to the rescue. But do we really have an adequate grasp of the underlying biology? Do we have a coherent framework for accommodating and rationalizing all the multilayered complexity that exists? Here, I advance the argument that cancer is a complex adaptive system and that its causation, stepwise emergence, and therapeutic resistance all follow an evolutionary biology logic. The implications of this perspective for cancer control are considerable.

Darwinian evolution by natural selection is the fundamental law of biology and provides the framework for an understanding of the totality of the living world, from extremophilic species to human diversity. Modern genomics provides a striking validation of evolutionary

Fig. P4.1. Speciation of living organisms: the ancestral tree. Charles Darwin's speciation "tree" from his notebook B, 1837. Founder 1 gives rise, via a branching architecture, to variants A, B, C, and D.

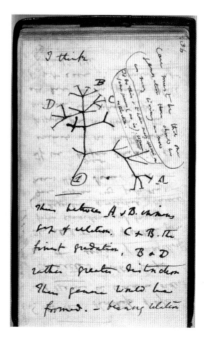

Table P4.1. Evolutionary determinants of vulnerability to cancer

Principle	Liability	Impact in cancer
Principle 1. Evolution just selects from the best available variants.	Limitations or imperfections of design, function, and specificity.	Error-prone replication. Error-prone DNA repair. Stem cells have inherent malignant potential: extensive, replicative, potential migratory phenotype, and quiescence option. Beneficial adaptive responses: inflammation, wound healing, and angiogenesis facilitate cancer promotion. Intrinsically mutagenic enzymes with off-target substrates: RAGs (lymphoid cancers), APOBECs/AID (multiple cancers/lymphoid cancer).
Principle 2. Evolution has "no eyes to the future"; it just selects what fits best, now.	When environmental circumstances change, previously beneficial phenotypes become *mismatched* with our genetic heritage.	Contemporary lifestyles, especially in affluent or "developed" societies, are mismatched with human adaptation to more ancient environments: High UVB exposure versus under-melanized skin: *skin cancers.* Delayed first pregnancy, minimal breast feeding, estrogen-fuelling diets versus non-seasonal estrus: *breast cancer, ovarian cancer.* Diminished infection in infancy versus programmed anticipation of infection in the immune system: *childhood acute lymphoblastic leukaemia.*
Principle 3. Natural selection can only operate on phenotypes that have impacts on survival *and* reproduction.	There is little or no evolutionary resilience for deleterious phenotypes in the post-reproductive period. Adaptive features that are beneficial for reproductive life can later impose a trade-off or penalty (= antagonistic pleiotropy).	Our adaptive phenotypes are optimized for reproductive life versus extensive (decades) post-reproductive longevity: time for accidents to happen (via liabilities 1 and 2 above) (= age-associated cancer incidence).
Principle 4. Natural selection will always happen when replicating units have diversity and there is competition for resources and selective pressures that influence fitness for reproduction and that vary in space and time.	Clonal escape.	Progressive selection of more robust or resilient clonal variants, metastasis, and drug resistance.

AID, activation-induced deaminase; APOBEC, apolipoprotein B mRNA editing enzyme, catalytic polypeptide-like; RAGs, recombination activating genes; UVB, ultraviolet B.

principles, by revealing phylogenetic relationships of species and signatures of prior, positive selection. How odd, then, that medical practice, which deals with dysfunctional biology, should have, until very recently, remained impervious to this principle [1]. How can we understand emergent infectious diseases, antibiotic resistance, modern chronic diseases, drug resistance in cancer, and our vulnerability to cancer without reference to how our biology has been sculpted by evolutionary processes? In this Perspective, I summarize the argument that evolutionary biology provides a coherent framework that recognizes and rationalizes the inherent, multilayered complexity of cancer. Proximate causes and a gene-centric view of cancer can be placed in context. Our apparent vulnerability to cancer and our limited success in treating advanced disease can be seen in a different light. And, critically, an evolutionary biology paradigm can contribute novel ideas to the challenge of how we might best control cancer.

For the historical context of these ideas and more detailed data and argument, see [2–8].

Evolutionary determinants of vulnerability to cancer

Evolution operates by stochastic, or random, genetic variation that provides the substrate for selection in the context of environmental selective pressures. Winners who survive and reproduce have the best adaptive phenotypes or fitness in relation to the prevailing selective forces. This is very different from intelligent design in that evolution can only select from random variation in prior forms, or from the best of what's available. This is a short-term fix strategy with "no eyes to the future" [9]. What is much less appreciated is the baggage, liabilities, and limitations that this inevitably entails (Table P4.1). These considerations can help rationalize the counterintuitive or paradoxical role of endogenous processes in cancer, the ubiquity of mutant clones and premalignant lesions, and the

Fig. P4.2. Speciation of a cancer clone. Diagram showing the phylogenetic tree or evolutionary relationships of seven genetically diverse subclones of acute lymphoblastic leukaemia (ALL), all derived from a single common ancestral cell. All cells have been interrogated for the eight mutations listed on the left. Those mutations were determined by exome sequencing and single-nucleotide polymorphism arrays on whole leukaemic sample B1 (7.1%) normal cells. (Data from [23] using microfluidic-based multiplex quantitative polymerase chain reaction for single-cell genetic analysis.) 0C, loss of both copies; 1C, loss of one copy; het, heterozygous; homo, homozygous.

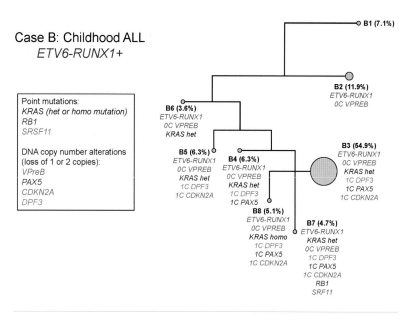

Case B: Childhood ALL
ETV6-RUNX1+

some of which are both consistent with and deleterious to the host – metastasis and drug resistance in particular. Cellular adaptability derives from two principal sources: genetic or mutational diversity, and epigenetic or phenotypic plasticity. Both are critical in cancer.

For the past 3 billion years, whenever replicating entities – molecules, cells, or individuals – have diversified and were confronted with a challenging or competitive environment, evolution by natural selection has occurred (principle 4 in Table P4.1) [17]. This is a, or even *the*, hallmark feature of cancer, at the somatic cell level – although curiously not listed as such [18]. Those 10 cellular features that are considered cancer hallmarks, including angiogenesis, evading cell death, and immune evasion [18], all enhance fitness for survival and/or reproduction – the ultimate register of evolutionary success. The idea that cancer involves sequential genetic changes in cells was evident from chromosome studies for many years [19,20] but was first clearly posited as the clonal evolution paradigm by Peter Nowell in 1976 [2]. Since then, technical advances in genetics, genomics, cell sorting, microscopy, and polymerase chain reaction (PCR)-based assays, culminating in single-cell genomics [21–23], have validated this concept and revealed the extensive and dynamic intraclonal genetic diversity that exists in cancer [7]. The parallels with Darwinian evolutionary speciation in ecosystems, missing from the original vision [2], are now explicitly recognized [7].

Every patient's cancer has a unique evolutionary trajectory or phylogenetic tree, with a branching

high frequency of cancer in ageing humans in modern societies.

Evolutionary considerations may also help us to understand why inherent susceptibility to particular cancers, for example breast or prostate cancer, is highly variable within human populations. Recent genome-wide association studies have provided an audit of inherited gene variants that increase risk [10]. Highly penetrant mutant alleles, such as *BRCA1* and *BRCA2,* exist at relatively high frequencies in certain populations. This is best rationalized not by any historical, adaptive benefit they endowed but from founder effects, i.e. an origin in an individual (2000–3000 years ago for *BRCA1*) who survived a population bottleneck [11]. More common allelic variants are associated with much lower risk levels (odds ratios, 1.01–1.3) [10]. But why should such deleterious variants be common? A significant fraction of the variants that affect breast and prostate cancer are in genes that encode proteins in estrogen or androgen

metabolism and signalling and response pathways [12–14]. One possibility is that the relatively high frequency of these alleles reflects prior positive selection because of a beneficial effect on enhancing fertility [15]. Genomic signatures can reveal whether genes have been subject to positive, adaptive selection during human evolution and the approximate time frames involved [16].

Clonal evolution and cellular adaptability
Cancer is a complex adaptive system with emergent properties,

Table P4.2. Cancer cells' evolutionary resilience and routes to therapeutic escape

Component	Basis of resistance/adaptability [source]
Genetic diversity	Drug (or immunological) targets or components of cellular response mutate [61]. Drug target (e.g. mutant protein) is segregated in subclone.[a]
Epigenetic plasticity	Cells bypass redundant signalling pathways blocked by drugs [45]. Stem cells adopt quiescent "resistant" state [62,63].

[a] Suggested by clonal variegation of mutations [24,25].

clonal architecture, as long recognized in ecological speciation (Figs P4.1, P4.2). Some mutations are consistently present in all cells at the base or trunk of the phylogenetic tree, suggesting that they may be founder or initiating lesions, for example *ETV6-RUNX1* mutations in acute lymphoblastic leukaemia (ALL) [23,24] and von Hippel–Lindau (*VHL*) gene mutations in renal carcinomas [25]. Genetically distinct subclones of cancer frequently exist in distinctive, topographically different regions of tissues [25,26]. This is anticipated from evolutionary principles (consider Galapagos Islands finches) and poses considerable problems for traditional approaches to biopsy-based sampling and prognostics, as well as for biopsy-based genomics [27]. Although only a few studies have integrated serial samples from primary tumours, metastases, and post-therapeutic relapses or recurrences [8,24,28], the patterns that emerge are of dynamic shifts in clonal architecture, with minor subclones emerging after selective sweeps (Fig. P4.2). Dominant clones in relapse [29], drug-resistant recurrence [30,31], or metastasis [28] emerge from previously minor subclones whose existence can be traced back to primary samples.

The evolutionary dynamics of cancer are extremely variable, with intervals between initiation and diagnosis of 1–50 years. The pace of evolution is often characterized by long periods of stasis or slow change, with occasional abrupt or catastrophic changes [8,32], paralleling punctuated equilibrium in ecological evolution [33]. Oncogenic mutations are extremely common in all of us; premalignant lesions are probably ubiquitous, but only a fraction of them evolve to fully fledged malignancy [34]. The implication of this modest evolutionary penetration is that restraints are largely effective and promotional factors are likely critical. The challenge for epidemiologists is taking this protracted and "sluggish" natural history into account, especially with respect to the timing of causative exposures. For

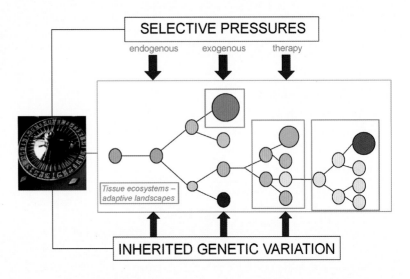

Fig. P4.3. Components of cancer clone evolution. The different colours represent genetically distinct subclones. The roulette wheel symbolizes the role of chance in all components. Endogenous selective pressures include inflammation, anoxia, and metabolic stress [57].

those interested in causation, cancer genomics may provide some vital clues. Although mutations are stochastic in origin, sequencing reveals mutational signatures that are indicative of underlying mechanisms of mutation and, in some cases, reflect the nature of genotoxic exposures [35–37].

Clonal evolution, as with speciation in ecology, is contingent upon ecosystem (tissue-derived or filtered) selective pressures, modulated by inherited susceptibility and chance (Fig. P4.3). Chance is all-pervasive in evolutionary biology and cancer because mutations are stochastic with respect to the functions encoded by genes [3]. The emergence of subclones with

particular putative "driver" mutations can be viewed as an adaptive response to selective pressures, of which environmental and therapeutic exposures are clear examples. Intense therapeutic selective pressure often has the exact opposite effect to that desired: the positive selection of previously silent and innocuous subclones. Metastases are likely to require adaptation to ectopic tissue, fermenting further evolution. Adaptation of cancer cells via beneficial mutations involves both gain-of-function mutants (activating oncogenes) and loss-of-function mutants (deleted tumour suppressor genes), similar to bacteria adapting to adverse conditions [38]. The complex mutation profiles of individual

Table P4.3. Evolutionary parameters are predictive of cancer progression and clinical outcome

Evolutionary parameter	Clinical outcome [source]
Measures of intraclonal genetic diversity (substrate for selection)	Progression of Barrett oesophagus [64] and chronic lymphocytic leukaemia [65]. Survival in head and neck cancer [66].
Burden of stem cells (units of selection)	Progression and outcome in multiple cancers ([67] and references therein; [68]).
Ecosystem diversity (selective pressures)	Survival in breast cancer [69]. Mathematical modelling [70].

Fig. P4.4. Epigenetic plasticity of cancer cells. (A) Illustration of the variation of phenotype within a single subclone. C, cell; D+, differentiating cells; Q, quiescent (out-of-cycle) cells. (B) Depiction of the complex and dynamic signalling networks of an individual cell [43]. Dense coloured regions indicate critical signalling routes. Pathways involved are indicated around the outside of the cell. These data derive from genetic (mutational) analysis of gene interactions in yeast cells. We currently have no such wiring diagram for human cells. The figure underestimates complexity by showing interaction networks under single, steady-state conditions. The reality is considerably more dynamic and complex.

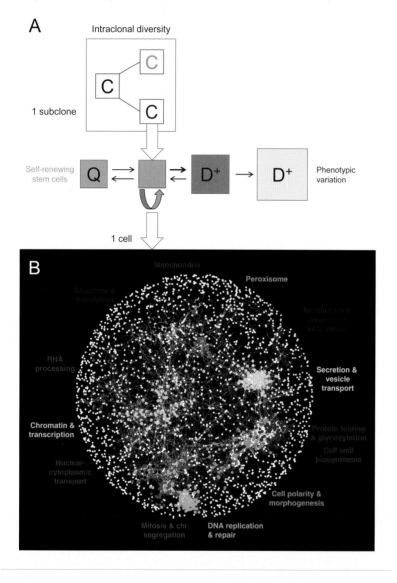

cancer cells reflect combinatorial impacts on cellular fitness and, in some cases, epistatic interactions of mutations, which occur in evolution in general [39]. Genetic instability and chromosomal aneuploidy, common features in cancer, are other adaptive tactics that accelerate the pace of diversification and increase the probability of beneficial mutations arising. Bacteria use the same evolutionary trick under challenging conditions: blind, but more frequent, spinning of the roulette wheel (Fig. P4.3).

Epigenetic plasticity

The adaptive resilience of cancer cells is not solely dependent on mutation. Cells within individual genetically homogeneous clones have epigenetic plasticity and diverse alternative phenotypes that are spatiotemporally expressed (Fig. P4.4A) [40–42]. This facilitates evasion of a therapeutic challenge (Table P4.2). The adaptability of cells is further evidenced at the single-cell level. Each cell has an extensive, complex signalling network that is highly dynamic, robust, and adaptable (Fig. P4.4B) [43]. In cancer, all functionally relevant mutations [44] effectively corrupt these networks, resulting in dysregulation or resetting to a new steady state (e.g. "on" for proliferation). The critical nodes in the signalling networks of normal cells, as well as cancer cells, have built-in redundancy, which provides yet another adaptive route to clonal escape in cancer, for example from targeted therapy (Table P4.2) [45]. The intrinsic adaptability or epigenetic plasticity of cells is itself an ancient evolutionary legacy reflecting built-in safeguards to combat adverse circumstances, particularly for stem cells in more complex long-lived organisms. Cancer stem cells "hunker down" or adopt a dormancy (or quiescent) status under chemotherapeutic challenge [46], an adaptive tactic of considerable evolutionary antiquity [47]. Those cells within subclones that have self-renewal or stem cell competence [48] are crucial to both clonal progression and adaptability as they are, in evolutionary terms, the "units of selection" [49] by virtue of their capacity for extensive or unlimited self-renewal and proliferation [50]. In accordance with a status of "units of selection", cancer stem cells within individual patients are genetically diverse [24] as well as phenotypically plastic [41].

Can we predict and thwart the evolutionary resilience of cancer?

Despite the enthusiasm and some successes for genome-guided personalized medicine and targeted therapeutics in cancer, it is evident

Fig. P4.5. How can we thwart cancer's evolutionary resilience? Numbers on the left indicate the percentage of cancers that might be prevented or controlled by implementing these three approaches. The proportion of 75% for prevention is based on original estimates by Doll and Peto [71]. (1) Vaccines for infection-associated cancers: human papillomavirus, Epstein–Barr virus, hepatitis B virus, hepatitis C virus, *Helicobacter pylori*, etc. (2) Smoking, chronic or intermittent, and exposure to intensive ultraviolet B radiation. (3) Diet and exercise. (4) Surgery for some premalignant lesions (skin, colon, cervix); non-steroidal anti-inflammatory drugs (e.g. aspirin) for premalignant lesions of the gastrointestinal tract and others [72]. (5) As for HIV [52], but applied to cancer [73,74]. (6) See [75]. (7) Molecules that cancer cells invariably depend upon or are addicted to, for example activated MYC, heat shock proteins, self-renewal signalling. (8) Founder lesion in base or trunk of phylogenetic tree [24,25,76]. Target in every cancer cell, for example ABL kinase targeting with imatinib in chronic myeloid leukaemia [77]. (9) Targeting features of self-renewal signatures of cancer stem cells that are different from those of normal stem cells [63,78,79]. (10) Anti-angiogenesis, anti-inflammatories, modest-dose cytostatic versus intensive cytotoxic therapy; see [58–60].

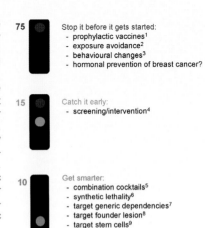

75 **Stop it before it gets started:**
- prophylactic vaccines[1]
- exposure avoidance[2]
- behavioural changes[3]
- hormonal prevention of breast cancer?

15 **Catch it early:**
- screening/intervention[4]

10 **Get smarter:**
- combination cocktails[5]
- synthetic lethality[6]
- target generic dependencies[7]
- target founder lesion[8]
- target stem cells[9]

- the "green" agenda: "evolutionary" tactics, target ecosystem[10]

that the adaptive resilience of cancer cells usually wins out, a pyrrhic victory for the genetic and epigenetic adaptability of cells (Table P4.2). Evolutionary principles of natural selection suggest that the likelihood of therapeutic failure should be predictable by quantitative measures of the major drivers of clonal diversity and selection. In strains of microbial species, mutation rates are predictive of the probability of drug-resistant mutants [51]. The same has long been anticipated for cancer, but here mutation rates are difficult to measure because of dynamic changes and topography of subclones. However, other evolutionary parameters that should be predictive of the likelihood of mutation-based drug resistance can be assayed and quantified: genetic diversity within the clone, the size of the selectable stem cell compartment, and the diversity of the ecosystem. Recent data confirm these expectations (Table P4.3), with considerable implications for instigation of tests that can predict cancer progression of early lesions or therapeutic resistance. The implications for treatment itself are major.

We are pollarding (or pruning) the major branches of the cancer clone phylogenetic tree, largely in ignorance of its architecture and intrinsic resilience. The common consequence, post-therapeutically, is the illusory success of transient tumour shrinkage, followed by florid regeneration as residual minor clones adapt to the new circumstances.

Given the extraordinary adaptability of cells, the sheer number of proliferative cycles (10^{11} per day in the small intestine and bone marrow), and the inherent risk of mutation and the ubiquity of covert tumours [49], it is perhaps surprising that we don't all have malignant cancer at an early age [52]. The reason is that the success of multicellularity as an evolutionary innovation some 600 million years ago required securing the maintenance of tissue integrity with multiple restraints on clonal expansion. This included the innovation of gene functions that can also operate as tumour suppressors [52–54]. And, despite the indulgences of human behaviour, these restraints remain largely successful up to and during our evolutionarily "useful" reproductive lifetime. But the

challenging reality is that approximately one in three individuals will receive a diagnosis of life-threatening cancer. From an evolutionary perspective, the question that needs to be posed is: "How can we best thwart the evolutionary resilience of cancer?" The same issue is central to the control of drug-resistant tuberculosis, malaria, and HIV [55]. Generally, we already know what to do for cancer (Fig. P4.5). The problem is where to put our efforts and resources, and what particular tactics to adopt. The best way to stop evolution is clearly to prevent it starting in the first place. But once it's up and running, there are strategies available that are distinct from current or conventional practice, some of which exploit cancer's evolutionary features and ecological dependencies (Fig. P4.5) [56–60]. To do this effectively would require considerable refocusing of current cancer research and therapeutic priorities. And a recognition of cancer's indelible, evolutionary character.

This Perspective is dedicated to the memory of Professor Pat Buffler.

References

1. Stearns SC, Nesse RM, Govindaraju DR, Ellison PT (2010). Evolution in health and medicine Sackler colloquium: evolutionary perspectives on health and medicine. *Proc Natl Acad Sci U S A*, 107 Suppl 1:1691–1695. http://dx.doi.org/10.1073/pnas.0914475107 PMID:20133821

2. Nowell PC (1976). The clonal evolution of tumor cell populations. *Science*, 194:23–28. http://dx.doi.org/10.1126/science.959840 PMID:959840

3. Greaves M (2000). *Cancer: The Evolutionary Legacy*. Oxford: Oxford University Press.

4. Crespi B, Summers K (2005). Evolutionary biology of cancer. *Trends Ecol Evol*, 20:545–552. http://dx.doi.org/10.1016/j.tree.2005.07.007 PMID:16701433

5. Merlo LMF, Pepper JW, Reid BJ, Maley CC (2006). Cancer as an evolutionary and ecological process. *Nat Rev Cancer*, 6:924–935. http://dx.doi.org/10.1038/nrc2013 PMID:17109012

6. Greaves M (2007). Darwinian medicine: a case for cancer. *Nat Rev Cancer*, 7:213–221. http://dx.doi.org/10.1038/nrc2071 PMID:17301845

7. Greaves M, Maley CC (2012). Clonal evolution in cancer. *Nature*, 481:306–313. http://dx.doi.org/10.1038/nature10762 PMID:22258609

8. Yates LR, Campbell PJ (2012). Evolution of the cancer genome. *Nat Rev Genet*, 13:795–806. http://dx.doi.org/10.1038/nrg3317 PMID:23044827

9. Williams GC (1966). *Adaptation and Natural Selection*. Princeton, NJ: Princeton University Press.

10. Fletcher O, Houlston RS (2010). Architecture of inherited susceptibility to common cancer. *Nat Rev Cancer*, 10:353–361. http://dx.doi.org/10.1038/nrc2840 PMID:20414203

11. Szabo CI, King M-C (1997). Population genetics of BRCA1 and BRCA2. *Am J Hum Genet*, 60:1013–1020. PMID:9150148

12. Low YL, Li Y, Humphreys K *et al.* (2010). Multi-variant pathway association analysis reveals the importance of genetic determinants of estrogen metabolism in breast and endometrial cancer susceptibility. *PLoS Genet*, 6:e1001012. http://dx.doi.org/10.1371/journal.pgen.1001012 PMID:20617168

13. Eeles RA, Kote-Jarai Z, Giles GG *et al.*; UK Genetic Prostate Cancer Study Collaborators; British Association of Urological Surgeons' Section of Oncology; UK ProtecT Study Collaborators (2008). Multiple newly identified loci associated with prostate cancer susceptibility. Nat Genet, 40:316–321. http://dx.doi.org/10.1038/ng.90 PMID:18264097

14. Ghoussaini M, Fletcher O, Michailidou K *et al.*; Netherlands Collaborative Group on Hereditary Breast and Ovarian Cancer (HEBON); Familial Breast Cancer Study (FBCS); Gene Environment Interaction of Breast Cancer in Germany (GENICA) Network; kConFab Investigators; Australian Ovarian Cancer Study Group (2012). Genome-wide association analysis identifies three new breast cancer susceptibility loci. *Nat Genet*, 44:312–318. http://dx.doi.org/10.1038/ng.1049 PMID:22267197

15. Greaves M (2002). Cancer causation: the Darwinian downside of past success? *Lancet Oncol*, 3:244–251. http://dx.doi.org/10.1016/S1470-2045(02)00716-7 PMID:12067687

16. Harris EE, Meyer D (2006). The molecular signature of selection underlying human adaptations. *Am J Phys Anthropol*, 131 Suppl 43:89–130. http://dx.doi.org/10.1002/ajpa.20518 PMID:17103426

17. Buss LW (1987). *The Evolution of Individuality*. Princeton, NJ: Princeton University Press.

18. Hanahan D, Weinberg RA (2011). Hallmarks of cancer: the next generation. *Cell*, 144:646–674. http://dx.doi.org/10.1016/j.cell.2011.02.013 PMID:21376230

19. Boveri T (1929). *The Origin of Malignant Tumors*. London: Baillière, Tindall & Cox.

20. Sandberg AA, Hossfeld DK (1970). Chromosomal abnormalities in human neoplasia. *Annu Rev Med*, 21:379–408. http://dx.doi.org/10.1146/annurev.me.21.020170.002115 PMID:4247449

21. Zong C, Lu S, Chapman AR, Xie XS (2012). Genome-wide detection of single-nucleotide and copy-number variations of a single human cell. *Science*, 338:1622–1626. http://dx.doi.org/10.1126/science.1229164 PMID:23258894

22. Baslan T, Kendall J, Rodgers L *et al.* (2012). Genome-wide copy number analysis of single cells. *Nat Protoc*, 7:1024–1041. http://dx.doi.org/10.1038/nprot.2012.039 PMID:22555242

23. Potter NE, Ermini L, Papaemmanuil E *et al.* (2013). Single cell mutational profiling and clonal phylogeny in cancer. *Genome Res*, [epub ahead of print]. http://dx.doi.org/10.1101/gr.159913.113 PMID:24056532

24. Anderson K, Lutz C, van Delft FW *et al.* (2011). Genetic variegation of clonal architecture and propagating cells in leukaemia. *Nature*, 469:356–361. http://dx.doi.org/10.1038/nature09650 PMID:21160474

25. Gerlinger M, Rowan AJ, Horswell S *et al.* (2012). Intratumor heterogeneity and branched evolution revealed by multiregion sequencing. *N Engl J Med*, 366:883–892. http://dx.doi.org/10.1056/NEJMoa1113205 PMID:22397650

26. Sottoriva A, Spiteri I, Piccirillo SGM *et al.* (2013). Intratumor heterogeneity in human glioblastoma reflects cancer evolutionary dynamics. *Proc Natl Acad Sci U S A*, 110:4009–4014. http://dx.doi.org/10.1073/pnas.1219747110 PMID:23412337

27. Swanton C (2012). Intratumor heterogeneity: evolution through space and time. *Cancer Res*, 72:4875–4882. http://dx.doi.org/10.1158/0008-5472.CAN-12-2217 PMID:23002210

28. Yachida S, Jones S, Bozic I *et al.* (2010). Distant metastasis occurs late during the genetic evolution of pancreatic cancer. *Nature*, 467:1114–1117. http://dx.doi.org/10.1038/nature09515 PMID:20981102

29. Mullighan CG, Phillips LA, Su X *et al.* (2008). Genomic analysis of the clonal origins of relapsed acute lymphoblastic leukemia. *Science*, 322:1377–1380. http://dx.doi.org/10.1126/science.1164266 PMID:19039135

30. Meyer JA, Wang J, Hogan LE *et al.* (2013). Relapse-specific mutations in NT5C2 in childhood acute lymphoblastic leukemia. *Nat Genet*, 45:290–294. http://dx.doi.org/10.1038/ng.2558 PMID:23377183

31. Diaz LA Jr, Williams RT, Wu J *et al.* (2012). The molecular evolution of acquired resistance to targeted EGFR blockade in colorectal cancers. *Nature*, 486:537–540. http://dx.doi.org/10.1038/nature11219 PMID:22722843

32. Baca SC, Prandi D, Lawrence MS *et al.* (2013). Punctuated evolution of prostate cancer genomes. *Cell*, 153:666–677. http://dx.doi.org/10.1016/j.cell.2013.03.021 PMID:23622249

33. Gould SJ, Eldredge N (1993). Punctuated equilibrium comes of age. *Nature*, 366:223–227. http://dx.doi.org/10.1038/366223a0 PMID:8232582

34. Greaves M (2013). Does everyone develop covert cancer? *Nat Rev Cancer*, (in press).

35. Alexandrov LB, Nik-Zainal S, Wedge DC *et al.*; Australian Pancreatic Cancer Genome Initiative; ICGC Breast Cancer Consortium; ICGC MMML-Seq Consortium; ICGC PedBrain (2013). Signatures of mutational processes in human cancer. *Nature*, 500:415–421. http://dx.doi.org/10.1038/nature12477 PMID:23945592

36. Poon SL, Pang S-T, McPherson JR *et al.* (2013). Genome-wide mutational signatures of aristolochic acid and its application as a screening tool. *Sci Transl Med*, 5:ra101. http://dx.doi.org/10.1126/scitranslmed.3006086 PMID:23926199

37. Pfeifer GP (2010). Environmental exposures and mutational patterns of cancer genomes. *Genome Med*, 2:54. http://dx.doi.org/10.1186/gm175 PMID:20707934

38. Hottes AK, Freddolino PL, Khare A *et al.* (2013). Bacterial adaptation through loss of function. *PLoS Genet*, 9:e1003617. http://dx.doi.org/10.1371/journal.pgen.1003617 PMID:23874220

39. Breen MS, Kemena C, Vlasov PK *et al.* (2012). Epistasis as the primary factor in molecular evolution. *Nature*, 490:535–538. http://dx.doi.org/10.1038/nature11510 PMID:23064225

40. Friedl P, Alexander S (2011). Cancer invasion and the microenvironment: plasticity and reciprocity. *Cell*, 147:992–1009. http://dx.doi.org/10.1016/j.cell.2011.11.016 PMID:22118458

41. Kreso A, O'Brien CA, van Galen P *et al.* (2013). Variable clonal repopulation dynamics influence chemotherapy response in colorectal cancer. *Science*, 339:543–548. http://dx.doi.org/10.1126/science.1227670 PMID:23239622

42. Biddle A, Liang X, Gammon L *et al.* (2011). Cancer stem cells in squamous cell carcinoma switch between two distinct phenotypes that are preferentially migratory or proliferative. *Cancer Res*, 71:5317–5326. http://dx.doi.org/10.1158/0008-5472.CAN-11-1059 PMID:21685475

43. Costanzo M, Baryshnikova A, Bellay J *et al.* (2010). The genetic landscape of a cell. *Science*, 327:425–431. http://dx.doi.org/10.1126/science.1180823 PMID:20093466

44. Vogelstein B, Papadopoulos N, Velculescu VE *et al.* (2013). Cancer genome landscapes. *Science*, 339:1546–1558. http://dx.doi.org/10.1126/science.1235122 PMID:23539594

45. Wilson TR, Fridlyand J, Yan Y *et al.* (2012). Widespread potential for growth-factor-driven resistance to anticancer kinase inhibitors. *Nature*, 487:505–509. http://dx.doi.org/10.1038/nature11249 PMID:22763448

46. Frank NY, Schatton T, Frank MH (2010). The therapeutic promise of the cancer stem cell concept. *J Clin Invest*, 120:41–50. http://dx.doi.org/10.1172/JCI41004 PMID:20051635

47. Lewis K (2007). Persister cells, dormancy and infectious disease. *Nat Rev Microbiol*, 5:48–56. http://dx.doi.org/10.1038/nrmicro1557 PMID:17143318

48. Dick JE (2008). Stem cell concepts renew cancer research. *Blood*, 112:4793–4807. http://dx.doi.org/10.1182/blood-2008-08-077941 PMID:19064739

49. Greaves M (2013). Cancer stem cells as 'units of selection'. *Evol Appl*, 6:102–108. http://dx.doi.org/10.1111/eva.12017 PMID:23396760

50. O'Brien CA, Kreso A, Jamieson CHM (2010). Cancer stem cells and self-renewal. *Clin Cancer Res*, 16:3113–3120. http://dx.doi.org/10.1158/1078-0432.CCR-09-2824 PMID:20530701

51. Ford CB, Shah RR, Maeda MK *et al.* (2013). Mycobacterium tuberculosis mutation rate estimates from different lineages predict substantial differences in the emergence of drug-resistant tuberculosis. *Nat Genet*, 45:784–790. http://dx.doi.org/10.1038/ng.2656 PMID:23749189

52. Bissell MJ, Hines WC (2011). Why don't we get more cancer? A proposed role of the microenvironment in restraining cancer progression. *Nat Med*, 17:320–329. http://dx.doi.org/10.1038/nm.2328 PMID:21383745

53. Nakajima Y, Meyer EJ, Kroesen A *et al.* (2013). Epithelial junctions maintain tissue architecture by directing planar spindle orientation. *Nature*, 500:359–362. http://dx.doi.org/10.1038/nature12335 PMID:23873041

54. Domazet-Loso T, Tautz D (2010). Phylostratigraphic tracking of cancer genes suggests a link to the emergence of multicellularity in metazoa. *BMC Biol*, 8:66. http://dx.doi.org/10.1186/1741-7007-8-66 PMID:20492640

55. Goldberg DE, Siliciano RF, Jacobs WR Jr (2012). Outwitting evolution: fighting drug-resistant TB, malaria, and HIV. *Cell*, 148:1271–1283. http://dx.doi.org/10.1016/j.cell.2012.02.021 PMID:22424234

56. Pienta KJ, McGregor N, Axelrod R, Axelrod DE (2008). Ecological therapy for cancer: defining tumors using an ecosystem paradigm suggests new opportunities for novel cancer treatments. *Transl Oncol*, 1:158–164. PMID:19043526

57. Gillies RJ, Verduzco D, Gatenby RA (2012). Evolutionary dynamics of carcinogenesis and why targeted therapy does not work. *Nat Rev Cancer*, 12:487–493. http://dx.doi.org/10.1038/nrc3298 PMID:22695393

58. Silva AS, Kam Y, Khin ZP *et al.* (2012). Evolutionary approaches to prolong progression-free survival in breast cancer. *Cancer Res*, 72:6362–6370. http://dx.doi.org/10.1158/0008-5472.CAN-12-2235 PMID:23066036

59. Gatenby RA, Brown J, Vincent T (2009). Lessons from applied ecology: cancer control using an evolutionary double bind. *Cancer Res*, 69:7499–7502. http://dx.doi.org/10.1158/0008-5472.CAN-09-1354 PMID:19752088

60. Gatenby RA, Silva AS, Gillies RJ, Frieden BR (2009). Adaptive therapy. *Cancer Res*, 69:4894–4903. http://dx.doi.org/10.1158/0008-5472.CAN-08-3658 PMID:19487300

61. Redmond KM, Wilson TR, Johnston PG, Longley DB (2008). Resistance mechanisms to cancer chemotherapy. *Front Biosci*, 13:5138–5154. http://dx.doi.org/10.2741/3070 PMID:18508576

62. Ishikawa F, Yoshida S, Saito Y *et al.* (2007). Chemotherapy-resistant human AML stem cells home to and engraft within the bone-marrow endosteal region. *Nat Biotechnol*, 25:1315–1321. http://dx.doi.org/10.1038/nbt1350 PMID:17952057

63. Saito Y, Uchida N, Tanaka S *et al.* (2010). Induction of cell cycle entry eliminates human leukemia stem cells in a mouse model of AML. *Nat Biotechnol*, 28:275–280. http://dx.doi.org/10.1038/nbt.1607 PMID:20160717

64. Maley CC, Galipeau PC, Finley JC *et al.* (2006). Genetic clonal diversity predicts progression to esophageal adenocarcinoma. *Nat Genet*, 38:468–473. http://dx.doi.org/10.1038/ng1768 PMID:16565718

65. Landau DA, Carter SL, Stojanov P *et al.* (2013). Evolution and impact of subclonal mutations in chronic lymphocytic leukemia. *Cell*, 152:714–726. http://dx.doi.org/10.1016/j.cell.2013.01.019 PMID:23415222

66. Mroz EA, Tward AD, Pickering CR *et al.* (2013). High intratumor genetic heterogeneity is related to worse outcome in patients with head and neck squamous cell carcinoma. *Cancer*, 119:3034–3042. http://dx.doi.org/10.1002/cncr.28150 PMID:23696076

67. Greaves M (2011). Cancer stem cells renew their impact. *Nat Med*, 17:1046–1048. http://dx.doi.org/10.1038/nm.2458 PMID:21900918

68. Lapouge G, Beck B, Nassar D *et al.* (2012). Skin squamous cell carcinoma propagating cells increase with tumour progression and invasiveness. *EMBO J*, 31:4563–4575. http://dx.doi.org/10.1038/emboj.2012.312 PMID:23188079

69. Yuan Y, Failmezger H, Rueda OM *et al.* (2012). Quantitative image analysis of cellular heterogeneity in breast tumors complements genomic profiling. *Sci Transl Med*, 4:ra143. http://dx.doi.org/10.1126/scitranslmed.3004330 PMID:23100629

70. Anderson ARA, Weaver AM, Cummings PT, Quaranta V (2006). Tumor morphology and phenotypic evolution driven by selective pressure from the microenvironment. *Cell*, 127:905–915. http://dx.doi.org/10.1016/j.cell.2006.09.042 PMID:17129778

71. Doll R, Peto R (1981). *The Causes of Cancer*. Oxford: Oxford University Press.

72. Rothwell PM, Fowkes FGR, Belch JFF *et al.* (2011). Effect of daily aspirin on long-term risk of death due to cancer: analysis of individual patient data from randomised trials. *Lancet*, 377:31–41. http://dx.doi.org/10.1016/S0140-6736(10)62110-1 PMID:21144578

73. Al-Lazikani B, Banerji U, Workman P (2012). Combinatorial drug therapy for cancer in the post-genomic era. *Nat Biotechnol*, 30:679–692. http://dx.doi.org/10.1038/nbt.2284 PMID:22781697

74. Sullivan RJ, Lorusso PM, Flaherty KT (2013). The intersection of immune-directed and molecularly targeted therapy in advanced melanoma: where we have been, are, and will be. *Clin Cancer Res*, 19:5283–5291. http://dx.doi.org/10.1158/1078-0432.CCR-13-2151 PMID:24089441

75. Ashworth A, Lord CJ, Reis-Filho JS (2011). Genetic interactions in cancer progression and treatment. *Cell*, 145:30–38. http://dx.doi.org/10.1016/j.cell.2011.03.020 PMID:21458666

76. Yap TA, Gerlinger M, Futreal PA *et al.* (2012). Intratumor heterogeneity: seeing the wood for the trees. *Sci Transl Med*, 4:27ps10. http://dx.doi.org/10.1126/scitranslmed.3003854 PMID:22461637

77. Druker BJ (2008). Translation of the Philadelphia chromosome into therapy for CML. *Blood*, 112:4808–4817. http://dx.doi.org/10.1182/blood-2008-07-077958 PMID:19064740

78. Gupta PB, Onder TT, Jiang G *et al.* (2009). Identification of selective inhibitors of cancer stem cells by high-throughput screening. *Cell*, 138:645–659. http://dx.doi.org/10.1016/j.cell.2009.06.034 PMID:19682730

79. Abrahamsson AE, Geron I, Gotlib J *et al.* (2009). Glycogen synthase kinase 3beta missplicing contributes to leukemia stem cell generation. *Proc Natl Acad Sci U S A*, 106:3925–3929. http://dx.doi.org/10.1073/pnas.0900189106 PMID:19237556

5

Cancer by organ site

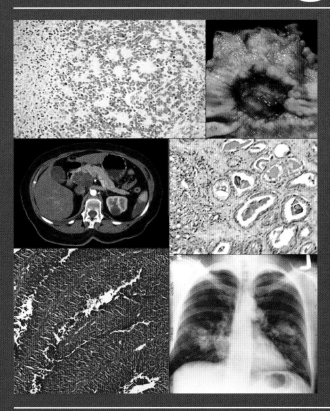

Different tumour types may be characterized with reference to epidemiology, etiology, pathology, genetics, and prevention. Current knowledge in these fields is the culmination of decades, if not centuries, of research, but progress has not been uniform. Notably, remarkable advances have accrued through a particular approach during a relatively short period. This edition of *World Cancer Report* corresponds to a new dimension in characterization of cancer as a genetic disease. Investigation of single genes – epitomized by oncogenes and tumour suppressor genes – has been eclipsed by sequencing of the whole genome, transcriptome, epigenome, or comparable entity for each of the major tumour types, typically involving multi-institutional collaborations based on hundreds of specimens. The benefits – definition of susceptibility, improved means of diagnosis, and development of targeted therapies – vary markedly between tumour types. It is clear that cancer is not a single disease but a multiplicity of different diseases. Identification of exogenous causes, screening methods, high-risk groups, means of diagnosis, and effective therapy vary across tumour types; in most cases the spectrum extends from comprehensive understanding to, as yet, no meaningful impact. Accordingly, knowledge about cancer must be specified with respect to each tumour type.

A guide to the epidemiology data in *World Cancer Report*

Incidence

Incidence is defined as the number of new cases of a disease arising in a given period in a specified population. It can be expressed as an absolute number of cases per year or as a rate per 100 000 persons (or some other denominator) per year. The rate provides an approximation of the average risk of developing a cancer.

Mortality

Mortality is defined as the number of deaths due to a specific underlying cause occurring in a given period in a specified population. It can be expressed as an absolute number of deaths per year or as a rate per 100 000 persons (or some other denominator) per year.

Age standardization

In this Report, all incidence and mortality rates are age-standardized. An age-standardized rate (ASR) is a summary measure of the rate that a population would have if it had a standard age structure. Standardization is necessary when comparing several populations (or the same population at different time points); age has a powerful influence on the risk of cancer, and populations differ with respect to their age distribution. Here, the ASR uses the World Standard Population (of Segi [1], as modified by Doll *et al.* [2]). The calculated incidence or mortality rate is then called the age-standardized incidence or mortality rate (World) and is conventionally expressed per 100 000 persons.

Graphics

Maps, bar charts, pie charts, and time trend figures are shown in the global cancer burden overview (in Section 1) and in site-specific chapters (in Section 5). In the chapters in Section 5, maps, pie charts, and time trend figures are provided for both incidence and mortality where important differences are in evidence (e.g. for breast cancer and colorectal cancer). For cancer sites where survival is relatively low and has changed relatively little, the figures focus on incidence (e.g. for lung cancer and pancreatic cancer). The figures are generally displayed for men and women separately, although for certain sites, a choice has been made to select patterns and trends in either men or women where they are reasonably comparable (e.g. for leukaemia) or where certain sex-specific features can be highlighted (e.g. for thyroid cancer).

Data sources

The graphics are built on three data sources. First, the maps and the pie charts are based on national incidence and mortality *estimates* from GLOBOCAN 2012 [3]. This provides incidence, mortality, and prevalence estimates for 27 site-specific cancers and for all sites combined in 184 countries worldwide. The underlying principle in the estimation process is a reliance on the best available data on cancer incidence and/or mortality within a country to build up the global picture. The results are more accurate or less accurate for different countries, depending on the extent and accuracy of locally available data. Second, the incidence time trends and bar charts are based on *observed* data series from regional or national population-based cancer registries, extracted from *Cancer Incidence in Five Continents* (CI5) Volumes I to X [4,5] and completed with more recent data available from corresponding cancer registry websites. Third, the mortality data for the time trends and bar charts originate from the WHO Mortality Database [6] (or the Centers for Disease Control and Prevention [7] for the USA) and, except for China, are available only at the national level.

Maps

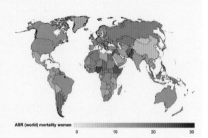

ASR (world) mortality women

The maps provide a global picture of the burden of a cancer site, by sex.

Pie charts

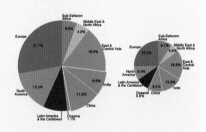

When both incidence and mortality pie charts are presented, the area of the mortality pie is proportional to the number of deaths relative to the number of new cases.

Bar charts

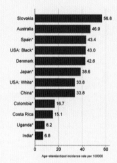

Bar charts of incidence and mortality by cancer, and of incidence and mortality by registry/country for all sites combined, are shown in Chapter 1.1.

Time trends

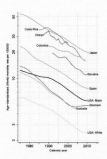

To highlight recent temporal developments, time trends are described from about 1975 onwards. For all cancer sites, data were selected that cover the same set of 11 countries for incidence and 9 countries for mortality (no mortality data were available for Uganda or India, and mortality data for China were available only for specific cancer sites). For the USA, incidence and mortality data are shown separately for Black and White populations. A logarithmic scale is used for the age-standardized rates to show the variety of patterns between populations.

Locally weighted regression curves were fitted to provide smoothed lines through the scatter plot of ASR by calendar year. A bandwidth of 0.3 was used, i.e. 30% of the data were used in smoothing each point. A bandwidth

of 0.5 was used for seven specific cancer sites (oesophagus, liver, pancreas, kidney, testis, thyroid, and nervous system) due to the small number of cases. As annual data for Uganda were not available, natural cubic spline interpolation was used to predict the values for the missing years. Care should be taken when comparing incidence graphs (time trends or bar charts) as the scales used on the vertical axes may differ.

Notes for bar charts

Average annual mortality rates for China are for 1996–2000. Average annual mortality rates for Australia are for 2000–2004.

Notes for time trends and bar charts

Countries represented by regional registries are marked with *; otherwise, registries are national.

Countries represented by one or more than one regional registry: China (Hong Kong Special Administrative Region and Shanghai), Colombia (Cali), India (Chennai and Mumbai), Japan (Miyagi, Nagasaki, and Osaka Prefectures), Spain (Granada, Murcia, Navarra, and Tarragona), Uganda (Kampala), and USA (the Surveillance, Epidemiology

and End Results [SEER] 9 registries: states of Connecticut, Hawaii, Iowa, New Mexico, and Utah and metropolitan areas of San Francisco–Oakland, California; Detroit, Michigan; Seattle–Puget Sound, Washington; and Atlanta, Georgia).

References

1. Segi M (1960). *Cancer Mortality for Selected Sites in 24 Countries* (1950–57). Department of Public Health, Tohoku University of Medicine, Sendai, Japan.

2. Doll R, Payne P, Waterhouse JAH, eds (1966). *Cancer Incidence in Five Continents*, Vol. I. Geneva: International Union Against Cancer.

3. Ferlay J, Soerjomataram I, Ervik M *et al.* (2013). GLOBOCAN 2012 v1.0, Cancer Incidence and Mortality Worldwide: IARC CancerBase No. 11 [Internet]. Lyon: IARC. Available at http://globocan.iarc.fr.

4. Ferlay J, Parkin DM, Curado MP *et al.* (2010). *Cancer Incidence in Five Continents*, Volumes I to IX: IARC CancerBase No. 9 [Internet]. Lyon: IARC. Available at http://ci5.iarc.fr.

5. Forman D, Bray F, Brewster DH *et al.*, eds (2013). *Cancer Incidence in Five Continents*, Vol. X. Available at http://ci5.iarc.fr.

6. WHO Mortality Database. Available at http://www.who.int/healthinfo/statistics/mortality_rawdata/en/index.html.

7. National Center for Health Statistics, U.S. Centers for Disease Control and Prevention. Available at http://www.cdc.gov/nchs/.

5.1 | Lung cancer

Elisabeth Brambilla
William D. Travis

Paul Brennan (reviewer)
Curtis C. Harris (reviewer)
José Rogelio Pérez Padilla (reviewer)

Summary

- Lung cancer is the most common cancer in men and the third most common in women.

- Tobacco smoking, including second-hand smoke, is the predominant cause of lung cancer worldwide. Other causes of lung cancer include radon, occupational exposure to polycyclic aromatic hydrocarbons, certain metals, asbestos, and crystalline silica, as well as exposure circumstances relevant to certain categories of work, and exposure to outdoor air pollution, and specifically to particulate matter and diesel engine exhaust, and to indoor air pollution, including second-hand tobacco smoke and emissions from household combustion of coal.

- Historically, small cell lung carcinoma has been distinguished from non-small cell lung carcinoma, which includes the histological types of adenocarcinoma, squamous cell carcinoma, and large cell carcinoma. Further subtyping is increasingly done on a molecular basis.

- Adenocarcinomas have driver mutations, most commonly involving *EGFR* and *KRAS* mutations as well as *ALK* fusions; squamous cell carcinomas have molecular alterations involving *SOX2*, *TP63*, *FGFR1*, and *DDR2*, and most small cell carcinomas express neuroendocrine markers and have *TP53* and *RB1* mutations. Lung cancers from smokers exhibit up to 10 times as many mutations as tumours from never-smokers.

- Screening for lung cancer is under development.

- Lung cancer is one of the most aggressive human cancers, with a 5-year overall survival of 10–15%.

There are four major histological types of lung cancer: adenocarcinoma, squamous cell carcinoma, small cell carcinoma, and large cell carcinoma. These tumours are defined primarily by morphology; however, in the past 10 years these tumours have started to be classified according to immunohistochemical and genetic characteristics as well.

Etiology

The most common cause of lung cancer is cigarette smoking; tobacco smoke is the most intensively investigated of all known carcinogens [1].

Local forms of tobacco smoking, such as bidis in India (Fig. 5.1.1), are also important. Risk is often related to the product of smoking rate and duration of smoking ("pack-years"), but more precise specification is possible. The lung cancer incidence rate is proportional to the fourth power of age in never-smokers, and the excess in smokers is proportional to the fourth power of smoking duration multiplied by the number of cigarettes smoked per day [2]. Recent analysis based on European and Canadian cases indicated that adenocarcinoma was the most prevalent lung cancer subtype in never-smokers and in women; squamous cell carcinoma predominated in male smokers. Smoking exerted a steeper risk gradient on squamous cell carcinoma and small cell lung cancer than on adenocarcinoma [3]. Diverse indicators of injury to respiratory tissue likely related to tumorigenesis are evident before the onset of clinical disease (see "Earliest molecular evidence of tobacco-induced injury in the airway"). Smoking cessation efforts have resulted in a growing percentage of lung cancers among nonsmokers, particularly those with adenocarcinoma histology.

Although smoking is estimated to account for about 90% of lung cancer cases in high-income countries, a wide range of agents are

Epidemiology

Lung cancer

- Lung cancer remains the most frequent cancer worldwide. There were more than 1.8 million new cases (13% of total cancer incidence) and almost 1.6 million deaths (20% of total cancer mortality), as estimated in 2012. More than one third of all newly diagnosed cases occurred in China.

- Lung cancer is the leading cause of cancer death in men in 87 countries and in women in 26 countries. Age-standardized rates vary 80-fold internationally, are highest in North America, Europe, and East Asia, and tend to still be relatively low in many African countries and some Asian countries.

- Due to a high and rather stable case fatality rate, patterns and trends for mortality rates are similar to those for incidence rates, irrespective of level of resource within a given country.

- Recent trends in lung cancer reflect the evolution of the smoking epidemic. In men, incidence rates have peaked in a number of highly developed countries at a late stage of the tobacco epidemic, while rates continue to rise among women.

- Only in a few countries (Australia and the USA), where the tobacco epidemic is most advanced and smoking prevalence has been declining for several decades, are there recent downward incidence trends among women.

Map 5.1.1. Global distribution of estimated age-standardized (World) incidence rates (ASR) per 100 000, for lung cancer in men, 2012.

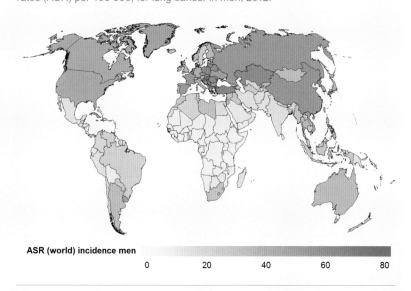

ASR (world) incidence men

0   20   40   60   80

Map 5.1.2. Global distribution of estimated age-standardized (World) incidence rates (ASR) per 100 000, for lung cancer in women, 2012.

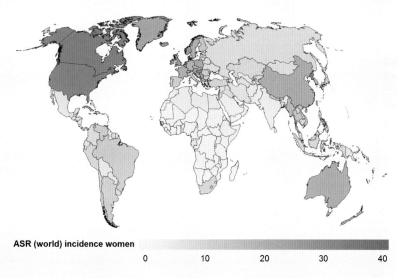

ASR (world) incidence women

0   10   20   30   40

For more details about the maps and charts presented in this chapter, see "A guide to the epidemiology data in *World Cancer Report*".

recognized to cause lung cancer, and for others the evidence is less than definitive. A review of IARC Group 1 carcinogens encountered at highest concentrations in an occupational context predominantly involved causation of lung cancer as covered in, although not restricted to, two volumes of the IARC Monographs. One volume considered arsenic, metals, fibres, and dusts [4]. The other considered mainly organic compounds [5], not only specific chemicals but also certain categories of employment, including work as a painter and work in the rubber industry. In an analysis of the burden of occupational lung cancer in the United Kingdom, asbestos exposure contributed by far the largest number of cases [6]. Radon is also identified as a risk factor for lung cancer [7].

An editorial, prompted by publication of a meta-analysis based on 17 cohorts in nine European studies, specified that air pollution may be recognized as a cause of lung cancer.

Chart 5.1.1. Estimated global number of new cases and deaths with proportions by major world regions, for lung cancer in both sexes combined, 2012

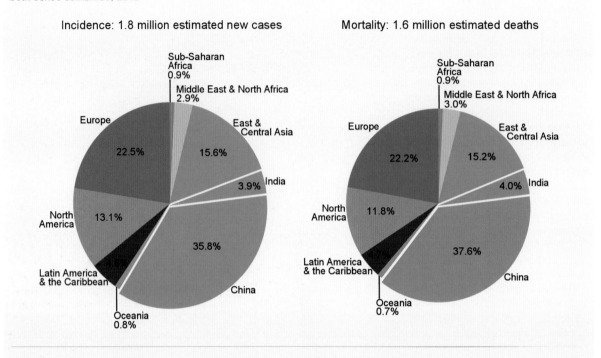

Incidence: 1.8 million estimated new cases

Mortality: 1.6 million estimated deaths

Chart 5.1.2. Age-standardized (World) incidence rates per 100 000 by year in selected populations, for lung cancer in men, circa 1975–2012.

Chart 5.1.3. Age-standardized (World) incidence rates per 100 000 by year in selected populations, for lung cancer in women, circa 1975–2012.

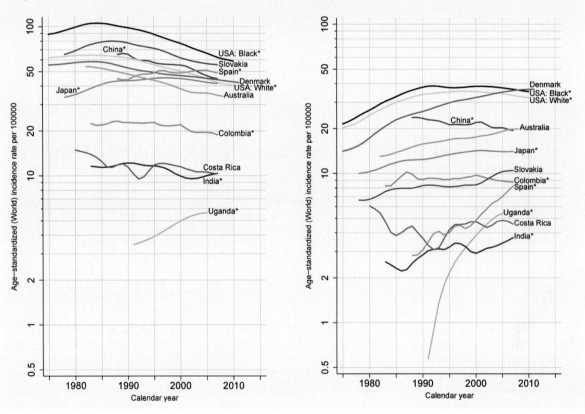

The data included a statistically significant association between risk of lung cancer and particulate matter with a diameter less than 10 μm (PM$_{10}$) (hazard ratio, 1.22; confidence interval, 1.03–1.45) [8]. IARC recently concluded that long-term exposure to outdoor air pollution, and specifically particulate matter in outdoor air, causes lung cancer [9]. Such findings involve outdoor air pollution (see "Biomarkers of air pollution"). Categories of air pollution recognized to cause lung cancer also include exposure to second-hand tobacco smoke and to emissions from household combustion of coal [10,11].

Using defined terminology, the World Cancer Research Fund reported convincing evidence for causation of lung cancer by arsenic in drinking-water and by β-carotene supplements, as well as probable evidence of decreased risk consequent upon consumption of fruits and of foods containing carotenoids [12]. Rare familial cases occur, and compared with nonfamilial cases these patients present with earlier pathological stage and more cancers with adenocarcinoma subtype [13].

Pathology and genetics

Historically, small cell lung carcinoma has been distinguished from non-small cell lung carcinoma (NSCLC), which includes the histological types of adenocarcinoma, squamous cell carcinoma, and large cell carcinoma. However, in the past decade, the distinction between adenocarcinoma and squamous cell carcinoma has been increasingly recognized because of major differences in genetics and also in responses to specific therapies [14]. Therefore, lung cancers are increasingly classified according to molecular subtypes, predicated on particular genetic alterations that drive and maintain lung tumorigenesis. Such driver mutations, and the associated constitutively active mutant signalling proteins, are critical to tumour cell survival, leading to the development of novel targeted therapies. These driver mutations are best established for adenocarcinoma, and more recently a list of oncogenic drivers for squamous cell carcinoma has been discerned, allowing the identification of potential targeted therapies. Nevertheless, for the majority of lung cancers, there is as yet no clear first-line chemotherapy targeting a driver signature.

A genetic basis of susceptibility to lung cancer generally, as distinct from susceptibility to particular tumour types, has been extensively investigated. Large, collaborative genome-wide association studies have identified three separate loci that are associated with lung cancer (5p15, 6p21, and 15q25) and that include genes regulating nicotinic acetylcholine receptors and telomerase production. However, much about genetic risk remains to be discovered, and rarer gene variants, such as those of the *CHEK2* gene, likely account for most of the remaining genetic susceptibility [15]. Studies of single-nucleotide polymorphisms, based on carcinogen metabolism and DNA repair mediating susceptibility to tobacco smoke-induced carcinogenesis, have provided limited insight.

Lung adenocarcinoma

Adenocarcinomas represent 40% of all lung cancers in the USA [16]. Most lung adenocarcinomas are diagnosed in the periphery of the lung (Fig. 5.1.2). Major changes to the 2004 WHO classification are recommended in light of the 2011 International Association for the Study of Lung Cancer, American Thoracic Society, and European Respiratory Society classification of lung adenocarcinoma [17]. The term "bronchioloalveolar carcinoma" is no longer used.

In small biopsies or cytology specimens, a tumour is classified as adenocarcinoma if it shows clear glandular morphology such as acinar, papillary, lepidic, or solid with mucin patterns. In tumours that lack any clear adenocarcinoma or squamous cell carcinoma morphology, the tumour requires further evaluation with immunohistochemistry through a limited work-up using a single adenocarcinoma marker (i.e. TTF-1) and squamous marker (i.e. p63 or p40). If a tumour is positive for TTF-1 but negative for a squamous marker, it is classified as "NSCLC, favour adenocarcinoma" [17]. However, if no adenocarcinoma or squamous differentiation is

Fig. 5.1.1. Older men smoking tobacco in India. Bidis, made of coarse and uncured tobacco, account for about 60% of smoked tobacco products in India, whereas cigarettes account for 20%.

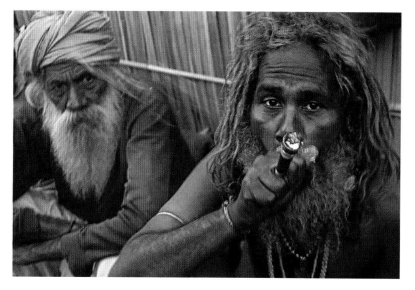

Earliest molecular evidence of tobacco-induced injury in the airway

Avrum Spira

Cigarette smoke creates a molecular "field of injury" in all airway epithelial cells exposed to the toxins associated with that exposure (Fig. B5.1.1). It has been known from early autopsy observations of cellular atypia throughout the airways of smokers that the cellular injury produced by smoking involves the whole respiratory tract. Several studies have shown that bronchial airway epithelial cells of current and former smokers with and without lung cancer display allelic loss, *TP53* mutations, and changes in promoter methylation and in telomerase activity of non-cancerous bronchial epithelial cells [1]. More recently, multiple groups have demonstrated that genome-wide gene expression profiling of bronchial airway epithelial cells collected by brushing at the time of bronchoscopy reflects the physiological response to and damage from exposure to cigarette smoke. The smoking-related changes in the airway transcriptome may be regulated, in part, by changes in DNA methylation and microRNA expression in response to the toxic exposure. While most of these genomic alterations (including those involved in xenobiotic metabolism and oxidative stress) reverse within months of smoking cessation, a subset of these transcriptomic changes are irreversible among former smokers (including those who have stopped smoking for > 10 years) and may be associated with the increased risk of smoking-related lung disease in former smokers.

Based on the heterogeneity in the bronchial airway genomic response to smoking, gene expression biomarkers in the cytologically normal bronchial airway epithelium have been developed for the early detection of lung cancer in current or former smokers being evaluated for clinical suspicion of disease [2]. These gene expression alterations in the airway have also been shown to reflect activation of oncogenic signalling pathways among high-risk smokers that can be reversed with chemopreventive agents that target these pathways. Furthermore, methylation changes in the promoter region of cancer-related genes measured in sputum have been shown to be associated with lung cancer risk among smokers. This molecular field of injury has recently been extended to chronic obstructive pulmonary disease, where gene expression alterations in the bronchial airway have been found among smokers with obstructive airway disease.

These observations suggest that the entire respiratory tree is affected by cigarette smoke, and that easily obtainable upper airway cells might provide insight into the types and degree of epithelial cell injury that have occurred in an individual smoker. Recent studies have indicated that the gene expression responses to smoking in the bronchial airway also occur in the extrathoracic airway epithelium that lines the mouth and nose [3]. This has led to the promise of genomic biomarkers of tobacco exposure and disease risk that can be developed in these non-invasive biosamples and can be applied to large-scale population-based studies.

Fig. B5.1.1. The molecular field of injury that is induced among airway epithelial cells throughout the respiratory tract. miRNA, microRNA; mRNA, messenger RNA; SNPs, single-nucleotide polymorphisms.

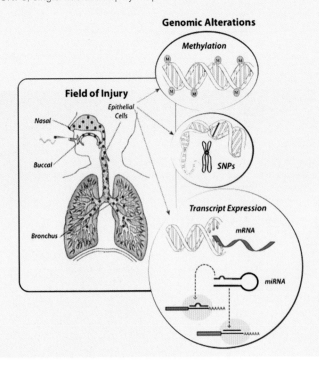

References

1. Steiling K *et al.* (2008). *Cancer Prev Res (Phila)*, 1:396–403. http://dx.doi.org/10.1158/1940-6207.CAPR-08-0174 PMID:19138985

2. Spira A *et al.* (2007). *Nat Med*, 13:361–366. http://dx.doi.org/10.1038/nm1556 PMID:17334370

3. Zhang X *et al.* (2010). *Physiol Genomics*, 41:1–8. http://dx.doi.org/10.1152/physiolgenomics.00167.2009 PMID:19952278

Fig. 5.1.2. Gross appearance of lung adenocarcinoma. The tumour is situated in the periphery of the lung, involving the subpleural tissue with a tan grey cut surface.

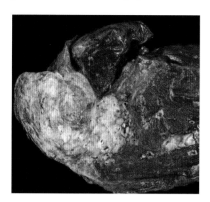

identified by morphology or immunohistochemical staining, the tumour is classified as "NSCLC - not otherwise specified". This is necessary to preserve as much tissue as possible for molecular testing.

Adenocarcinoma in situ is an adenocarcinoma of pure lepidic growth without invasion that measures 3 cm or less. Minimally invasive adenocarcinoma is a lepidic-predominant adenocarcinoma measuring 3 cm or less that has 5 mm or less of an invasive component [17]. Invasive adenocarcinomas are now classified according to the predominant subtype. This classification is based on comprehensive histological subtyping by estimating different histological patterns in a semi-quantitative manner in 5–10% increments (Fig. 5.1.3).

Multiple studies have demonstrated consistent correlations of survival with the predominant subtypes, with very favourable (adenocarcinoma in situ, minimally invasive adenocarcinoma, lepidic), intermediate (acinar, papillary), and poor (solid, micropapillary) prognostic categories. As expected, so far all cases reported as adenocarcinoma in situ and minimally invasive adenocarcinoma have demonstrated 5-year disease-free survival of 100% [14].

The majority of lung adenocarcinomas from never-smokers harbour a mutation in either *EGFR* or *HER2* (*ERBB2*) or a fusion involving *ALK* or *ROS1* [18]. Driver mutations in adenocarcinoma occur in the *EGFR*, *HER2* (*ERBB2*), *KRAS*, *ALK*, *BRAF*, *PIK3CA*, and *ROS1* genes (Fig. 5.1.4A). Mutations in *KRAS* and *EGFR* are mutually exclusive, as are most of the kinase domain mutations listed above, except for *PIK3CA* [19,20]. Several of these genes may have increased gene copy number or amplification, mostly of the mutant allele. *EGFR* (20%), *HER2* (2%), and *MET* (1%) may be amplified preferentially on the mutant allele. *MET* amplification occurs more frequently in resistant disease and is associated with EGFR tyrosine kinase inhibition. All of these mutations offer the possibility of targeted therapy, although only three (*EGFR* mutation, *ALK* and *ROS1* fusion) are subject to targeted treatment with currently approved drugs: gefitinib or erlotinib for *EGFR* mutation and crizotinib for *ALK* and *ROS1* fusion. Agents targeting the others are in development in phase 2 or phase 3 (Table 5.1.1).

Whole-exome and whole-genome sequencing of DNA from 183 pairs of lung adenocarcinoma tumours and matched normal tissues

Fig. 5.1.3. Adenocarcinoma histology. (A) Lepidic pattern: atypical pneumocytes line the alveolar walls with no invasive component. (B) Acinar pattern: cytologically malignant tumour cells form round to oval-shaped glands. (C) Papillary pattern: malignant glandular cells grow along the surface of fibrovascular cores. (D) Micropapillary pattern: these tumour cells form papillae lacking fibrovascular cores. (E) Solid pattern: these malignant cells are growing in sheets with hyperchromatic nuclei. (F) Invasive mucinous adenocarcinoma: malignant cells grow in acinar and lepidic patterns. The tumour cells have abundant apical mucin and small, basally oriented nuclei.

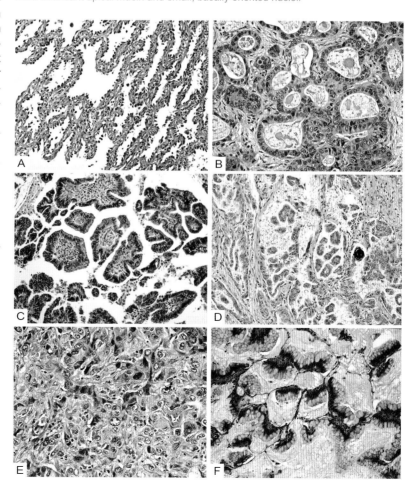

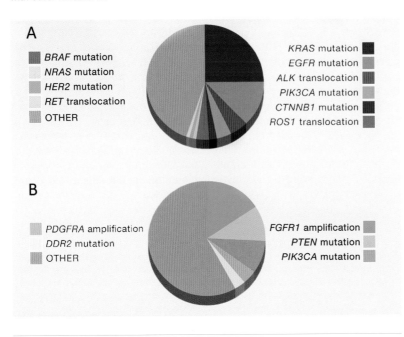

Fig. 5.1.4. (A) Mutation spectrum in adenocarcinoma. Mutations in *TP53* and *STK11/LKB1* are common occurrences, not included in the pie chart due to high overlap with other mutations. (B) Mutation spectrum in squamous cell carcinoma. Mutations in *TP53* are a common occurrence, not included in the pie chart due to high overlap with other mutations.

A
- BRAF mutation
- NRAS mutation
- HER2 mutation
- RET translocation
- OTHER
- KRAS mutation
- EGFR mutation
- ALK translocation
- PIK3CA mutation
- CTNNB1 mutation
- ROS1 translocation

B
- PDGFRA amplification
- DDR2 mutation
- OTHER
- FGFR1 amplification
- PTEN mutation
- PIK3CA mutation

identified, among many other findings, statistically recurrent somatic mutations in the splicing factor gene *U2AF1* and truncating mutations affecting *RBM10* and *ARID1A* [21].

Adenocarcinomas from never-smokers have a higher frequency of *EGFR* mutations (38% vs 14%) and *ALK* rearrangements (12% vs 2%) compared with tumours from former or current smokers [22]. Such a comparison in respect of NSCLC and adjacent normal tissue from 17 patients identified 3726 point mutations and more than 90 insertions or deletions in the coding sequence, with an average mutation frequency more than 10 times higher in smokers than in never-smokers (Fig. 5.1.5). Novel alterations were identified in genes involved in chromatin modification and DNA repair pathways, along with *DACH1*, *CFTR*, *RELN*, *ABCB5*, and *HGF* [23].

Squamous cell lung carcinoma

Squamous cell carcinoma accounts for approximately 20% of all lung cancers in the USA [16]. At diagnosis, most squamous cell carcinomas are located in the central portion of the lung, but in recent years, the frequency of tumours located peripherally appears to have been increasing.

In resection specimens, tumours of this type are subclassified as squamous cell carcinoma, basaloid, clear cell, and small cell variants. Squamous differentiation is identified morphologically as intercellular bridging, squamous pearl formation, and individual cell keratinization (Fig. 5.1.6). In small biopsies or cytology specimens, in poorly differentiated tumours that lack clear squamous morphology, if the tumour is positive for p63 or p40 but negative for TTF-1, the tumour is classified as "NSCLC, favour squamous cell carcinoma".

Genetic alterations in squamous cell carcinoma have been revealed as part of the Cancer Genome Atlas; the data involve genomic and epigenomic alterations in 178 squamous cell lung carcinomas. Most of the previously identified driver mutations were confirmed and several others discovered [24,25]. Although squamous cell carcinomas have been regarded as tumours without specific molecular abnormalities, new discoveries allow most squamous cell lung cancers to be characterized with reference to available targeted therapies (Fig. 5.1.4B). If mutations in *PIK3CA* (20–30%), *FGFR1* (20%), and *DDR2* (4%) are considered,

Table 5.1.1. Molecular targeted therapies for lung cancer

Gene or genetic alteration	Histological type	Therapy
Targeted therapies[a]		
EGFR mutation	Advanced adenocarcinoma	EGFR tyrosine kinase inhibitor Erlotinib, gefitinib
ALK fusion	Adenocarcinoma	Crizotinib
ROS1 fusion	Advanced adenocarcinoma	Crizotinib
Drugs in development		
HER2	Adenocarcinoma	Afatinib (BIBW 2992)
PI3KCA	NSCLC	Trastuzumab, PI3K inhibitor
BRAF	NSCLC	Sorafenib?
MET	NSCLC	Phase 2: rilotumumab (AMG 102), MetMAb
RAS	Adenocarcinoma	PI3K + MEK inhibitors

NSCLC, non-small cell lung carcinoma; PI3K, phosphatidylinositol 3-kinase.
[a] Approved by the United States Food and Drug Administration.

Fig. 5.1.5. Graphical summary of the distinction, including extent of genomic mutation, evident when lung cancer and adjacent normal tissues from smokers and never-smokers are compared. (For details, see [23].)

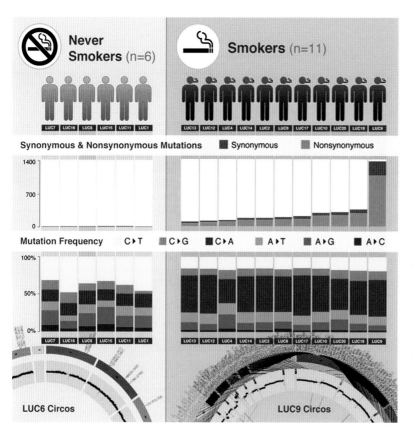

were the oxidative stress response pathway and the squamous differentiation pathway. The oxidative stress response pathway, involving *NFE2L2* and *KEAP1* or *CUL3*, was evident in 30% of the cases, and the alterations described were mutually exclusive. The squamous differentiation pathway was affected by gene alterations in 44% of cases; the affected genes included *SOX2* and *TP63* (which were mutually exclusive in relation to Notch1 or Notch2 *ALSCL4* loss-of-function mutations) and focal deletions of *FOXP1*. Messenger RNA (mRNA) expression profiling indicated altered expression, enhancing the recognition of these alterations as oncogenic driver events. Therapeutic agents for *DDR2* mutation (dasatinib) and *FGFR1* amplification (FGFR1 tyrosine kinase inhibitor) are already available, and United States Food and Drug Administration (FDA) approval is currently anticipated for a target for *PIK3CA*.

Small cell lung carcinoma

Small cell lung cancer accounts for 15% of all lung cancers in the USA

about one half of squamous cell lung carcinomas have genetic alterations that are potential molecular targets. The most frequent mutations in tumours from patients were in *TP53*, *CDKN2A* (*P16*), *PTEN*, *PIK3CA*, *KEAP1*, and *MLL2* [24,25]. Conspicuous regions of somatic copy number alteration, including amplification, were evident, as had been previously detected for *SOX2*, *PI3KCA*, and *FGFR1* [26], together with deletion at *CDKN2A* [24]. Other regions of marked gene copy alteration were discovered on chromosomal segments containing *NFE2L2*, *MYC*, *CDK6*, *MDM2*, *FOXP1*, *PTEN*, and *NF1* [24].

Interestingly, many of the somatic alterations identified in squamous cell carcinoma have been recognized as drivers of initiation and tumour progression. Two pathways affected by genetic alteration

Fig. 5.1.6. Squamous cell carcinoma. The tumour consists of nests of malignant cells with abundant eosinophilic cytoplasm. Abundant extracellular keratin is present.

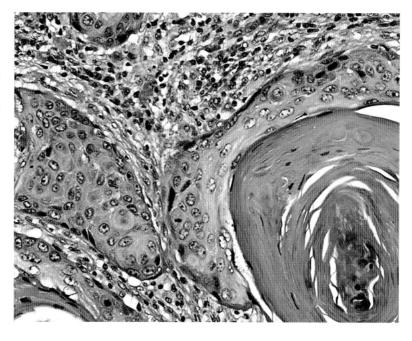

Biomarkers of air pollution

Paolo Vineis

Air pollution can induce cancer (particularly of the lung) through several mechanisms, including damage to DNA. Measurement of biomarkers related to air pollution can improve the investigation of the health effects, by facilitating improved exposure assessment and increased understanding of mechanisms, thereby providing biological plausibility.

Demetriou et al. [1] have reviewed biomarkers for which there is consistent evidence in the literature to support the results of epidemiological studies on the effects of ambient air pollution. Epidemiological evidence from the selected studies has been assessed using a set of criteria that evaluate their credibility. The criteria take into account the total number of subjects investigated, the degree of replication of findings across studies, and potential protection from bias and/or confounding. Overall, 524 papers were evaluated, which described the relationships between ambient air pollution and biomarkers of dose and early response. Studies were ranked from A (strong) to C (weak). The biomarkers that fulfilled the criteria to achieve A or B scores were 1-hydroxypyrene, DNA adducts, chromosomal aberrations, micronuclei, oxidative damage

to nucleobases, and methylation changes. These biomarkers cover the whole spectrum of disease onset and progression, from external exposure to tumour formation, and some have also been suggested as risk predictors of future cancer, reinforcing causal reasoning (Fig. B5.1.2).

Overall, existing biomarkers of dose and effect appear to reinforce the causal nature of the association between air pollution and lung cancer, although the markers in the review were not all specific to lung carcinogenesis. DNA adducts, chromosomal aberrations, micronuclei, and oxidized nucleobase markers have been suggested to be predictive for the risk of cancer. 1-Hydroxypyrene is a marker of internal dose, DNA adducts and oxidized nucleobases are markers of the biologically effective dose, and micronuclei, chromosomal aberrations, and DNA methylation are good markers of early biological effect. The available evidence is stronger for oxidized nucleobase markers, and the mechanisms supported by these biomarkers are likely to be central to the biological process of air pollution-induced lung cancer.

However, certain aspects of biomarkers used in epidemiological

studies need to be clarified. These include their reliability, including inter-laboratory as well as inter-technique variation.

Although chronic inflammation is probably relevant to particle-induced lung carcinogenesis, the overall evidence is still relatively scant. Exposure to air pollutants has been associated with acute inflammation in the airways and to elevated levels of systemic markers of inflammation, such as C-reactive protein and fibrinogen. Recent studies found that medium-term exposure to traffic-related air pollution may induce an increased inflammatory/endothelial response, especially among people with diabetes [2]. So far the inflammatory response has mainly been associated with risk of cardiovascular diseases rather than of cancer [3].

References

1. Demetriou CA et al. (2012). Occup Environ Med, 69:619–627. http://dx.doi.org/10.1136/oemed-2011-100566 PMID:22773658

2. Alexeeff SE et al. (2011). Environ Health Perspect, 119:481–486. http://dx.doi.org/10.1289/ehp.1002560 PMID:21349799

3. Frampton MW (2006). Clin Occup Environ Med, 5:797–815. PMID:17110293

Fig. B5.1.2. Biological markers of exposure and effects of air pollution.

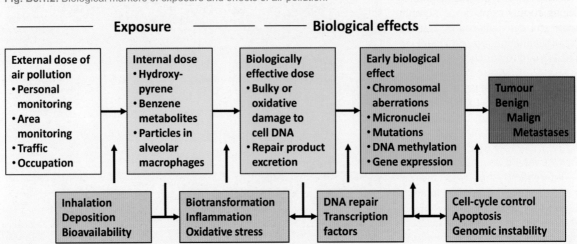

Fig. 5.1.7. Small cell carcinoma. The tumour consists of a cellular sheet of small tumour cells with scant cytoplasm, finely granular nuclear chromatin, and frequent mitoses, and nucleoli are absent.

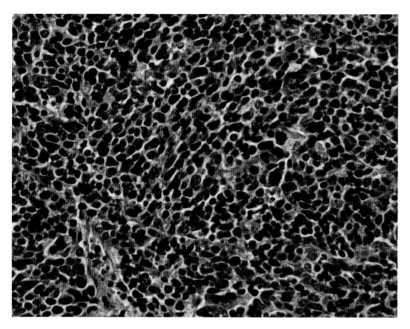

[16]. Most cases of this tumour type are diagnosed on the basis of a peri-hilar mass. Tumour cells are small in size with a round to fusiform shape, scant cytoplasm, finely granular nuclear chromatin, and absent or inconspicuous nucleoli (Fig. 5.1.7) [27]. Necrosis is usually extensive and mitotic rates are high, averaging 80 mitoses per 2 mm² area [27]. Small cell lung cancer is reliably diagnosed in small biopsies and cytology specimens.

Small cell lung cancer typically occurs in heavy smokers and is characterized by the most aggressive growth among lung malignancies. No single molecularly targeted drug has yet shown any clinical activity in small cell lung cancer. Until recently, the relevant molecular genetics was poorly characterized except for the prevalence of inactivating mutations in *TP53* and *RB1*. However, the results of global lung cancer genome research have now been published, including the results of single-nucleotide polymorphism array analysis, transcriptome sequencing, and full-genome sequencing of a total of 63 cases (Table 5.1.2) [28].

In addition to invariable p53/Rb inactivation, mutations were found in *CREBBP*, *EP300*, and *MLL*, which all encode histone modifiers. Also detected were mutations in *PTEN*, *SLIT2*, and *EPHA7*, as well as focal amplification of the *FGFR1* tyrosine kinase gene, thus identifying further oncogenic driver events nominally susceptible to targeted therapy that may be developed. This is an example of how integrative computational genome analysis can provide functionally tractable information in the context of a highly mutated cancer genome, due to the genotoxic effects of tobacco smoke.

Large cell lung carcinoma

Large cell carcinoma accounts for 3% of all lung cancers in the USA [16]. Large cell carcinoma consists of sheets and nests of large polygonal cells with vesicular nuclei and prominent nucleoli and is diagnosed on the basis of exclusion to the extent that the presence of squamous cell or glandular differentiation can be excluded by light microscopy [27]. The diagnosis of large cell carcinoma cannot be made on small biopsies or cytology specimens and requires a resection specimen.

Prospects

Prevention

The primary approach to prevention is smoking cessation, which has been proven effective in both men and women. This subject is not discussed here but is separately addressed in this Report (see Chapter 4.1). Encouragement of smoking cessation by women has yet to make a major impact in Europe, where lung cancer mortality

Table 5.1.2. Genetic alterations in small cell lung carcinoma

Significantly altered (one or more alleles) genes (drivers)	Mode	Percentage
TP53	Inactivation	100
RB1	Inactivation	100
CREBBP	Mutation	18
EP300	Mutation	18
MLL	Mutation	10
PTEN	Mutation	10
SLIT2	Mutation	10
EPHA7	Mutation	5
FGFR1	Amplification	4
MYCL	Amplification	16
E2F2	Amplification	5
CCN2	Amplification	5

rates are still increasing in women. Prevention of occupational cancer and regulatory measures to address air pollution are discussed in Chapter 4.5. In a region of China, decreased risk of lung cancer was associated with improvement of household stoves by adding a chimney to reduce exposure to smoky coal emissions [29].

Screening

Among options to reduce mortality from lung cancer is the introduction of population-based screening. Several small randomized trials of low-dose computed tomography (CT) screening are under way in Europe. From the USA, a decisive outcome was reported for the National Lung Screening Trial [30] conducted from 2002 to 2004 and involving 53 454 individuals screened either with low-dose CT or with chest radiography. The incidence of lung cancer in the two groups was identical. The relative reduction in mortality from lung cancer through low-dose CT screening was 20% (P = 0.004). The rate of death from any cause was reduced in the low-dose CT group by 6.7% (P = 0.02) compared with the radiography group, indicating that the screening was essentially reducing deaths from lung cancer. The United States Preventive Services Task Force has published a recommendation that CT screening

be available to healthy individuals aged 55–79 years with at least a 30 pack-year history of smoking and who have smoked within the past 15 years – estimated at about 10 million people.

Limitations relevant to data from screening trials specifically in Europe are the healthy volunteer effect, which may bias results, the possibility that scanners currently used are technologically more advanced than those used during the trial, and the fact that the United States trial mentioned above was conducted in high-profile medical institutions, recognized for their expertise in radiology diagnosis and treatment of cancer. When the cause of death in the two arms of the trial was reduced to "no death by lung cancer", the reduction in overall mortality was 3.2%, which was not statistically significant. Obviously, the cost-effectiveness of low-dose CT screening must also be considered in the context of competing interventions, particularly smoking cessation.

Other strategies for early detection of lung cancer, including particular molecular markers in blood, sputum, and urine, are being studied in specimens obtained as part of the American College of Radiology Imaging Network and related activity, but are not yet finalized. There is unfortunately no proven biomarker for lung cancer detection [31].

Prognosis

Lung cancer is one of the most aggressive human cancers, with a 5-year survival of 10–15% [16]. Patients with clinical stage IV lung cancer have a 5-year overall survival of 2%, and even for the lowest stage IA, 5-year overall survival is only 50% [32]. Lung cancer accounts for 13% of all cancers and 20% of all cancer deaths. In the USA, lung cancer is the second most common cancer in both men and women, accounting for 14% of cancer cases in each sex, and is the most common cause of cancer mortality in both men and women, accounting for 29% and 26% of cancer deaths, respectively [33]. Poor survival of lung cancer patients is due, at least in part, to 80% of patients being diagnosed with metastatic disease and more than half of patients having distant metastases [16]. Advanced lung cancer has also been resistant to traditional chemotherapy. However, recent advances have led to exciting progress in therapies that are dependent on histology and genetics. The level of scrutiny is exemplified by trials of adjuvant chemotherapy designed to differentiate not only between mutations in codons 12 and 13 of *KRAS*, but also between different amino acid substitutions as determined by particular mutations at codon 12 [34].

References

1. IARC (2012). Personal habits and indoor combustions. *IARC Monogr Eval Carcinog Risks Hum*, 100E:1–575. PMID:23193840

2. Peto J (2012). That the effects of smoking should be measured in pack-years: misconceptions 4. *Br J Cancer*, 107:406–407. http://dx.doi.org/10.1038/bjc.2012.97 PMID:22828655

3. Pesch B, Kendzia B, Gustavsson P *et al.* (2012). Cigarette smoking and lung cancer – relative risk estimates for the major histological types from a pooled analysis of case-control studies. *Int J Cancer*, 131:1210–1219. http://dx.doi.org/10.1002/ijc.27339 PMID:22052329

4. Straif K, Benbrahim-Tallaa L, Baan R *et al.*; WHO International Agency for Research on Cancer Monograph Working Group (2009). A review of human carcinogens – Part C: metals, arsenic, dusts, and fibres. *Lancet Oncol*, 10:453–454. http://dx.doi.org/10.1016/S1470-2045(09)70134-2 PMID:19418618

5. Baan R, Grosse Y, Straif K *et al.*; WHO International Agency for Research on Cancer Monograph Working Group (2009). A review of human carcinogens – Part F: chemical agents and related occupations. *Lancet Oncol*, 10:1143–1144. http://dx.doi.org/10.1016/S1470-2045(09)70358-4 PMID:19998521

6. Brown T, Darnton A, Fortunato L, Rushton L; British Occupational Cancer Burden Study Group (2012). Occupational cancer in Britain. Respiratory cancer sites: larynx, lung and mesothelioma. *Br J Cancer*, 107 Suppl 1:S56–S70. http://dx.doi.org/10.1038/bjc.2012.119 PMID:22710680

7. IARC (2012). Radiation. *IARC Monogr Eval Carcinog Risks Hum*, 100D:1–437. PMID:23189752

8. Yorifuji T, Kashima S (2013). Air pollution: another cause of lung cancer. *Lancet Oncol*, 14:788–789. http://dx.doi.org/10.1016/S1470-2045(13)70302-4 PMID:23849839

9. Loomis D, Grosse Y, Lauby-Secretan B *et al.* (2013). The carcinogenicity of outdoor air pollution. *Lancet Oncol*, 14:1262–1263. http://dx.doi.org/10.1016/S1470-2045(13)70487-X

10. Secretan B, Straif K, Baan R *et al.*; WHO International Agency for Research on Cancer Monograph Working Group (2009). A review of human carcinogens – Part E: tobacco, areca nut, alcohol, coal smoke, and salted fish. *Lancet Oncol*, 10:1033–1034. http://dx.doi.org/10.1016/S1470-2045(09)70326-2 PMID:19891056

11. Barone-Adesi F, Chapman RS, Silverman DT *et al.* (2012). Risk of lung cancer associated with domestic use of coal in Xuanwei, China: retrospective cohort study. *BMJ*, 345:e5414. http://dx.doi.org/10.1136/bmj.e5414 PMID:22936785

12. World Cancer Research Fund/American Institute for Cancer Research (2007). *Food, Nutrition, Physical Activity, and the Prevention of Cancer: A Global Perspective.* Washington, DC: American Institute for Cancer Research.

13. Haraguchi S, Koizumi K, Mikami I *et al.* (2012). Clinicopathological characteristics and prognosis of non-small cell lung cancer patients associated with a family history of lung cancer. *Int J Med Sci*, 9:68–73. http://dx.doi.org/10.7150/ijms.9.68 PMID:22211092

14. Travis WD, Brambilla E, Riely GJ (2013). New pathologic classification of lung cancer: relevance for clinical practice and clinical trials. *J Clin Oncol*, 31:992–1001. http://dx.doi.org/10.1200/JCO.2012.46.9270 PMID:23401443

15. Brennan P, Hainaut P, Boffetta P (2011). Genetics of lung-cancer susceptibility. *Lancet Oncol*, 12:399–408. http://dx.doi.org/10.1016/S1470-2045(10)70126-1 PMID:20951091

16. Howlader N, Noone AM, Krapcho M *et al.* (2012). Lung cancer. In: SEER Cancer Statistics Review, 1975-2009 (Vintage 2009 Populations). Bethesda, MD: National Cancer Institute. Available at http://seer.cancer.gov/csr/1975_2009_pops09/.

17. Travis WD, Brambilla E, Noguchi M *et al.* (2011). International Association for the Study of Lung Cancer/American Thoracic Society/European Respiratory Society international multidisciplinary classification of lung adenocarcinoma. *J Thorac Oncol*, 6:244–285. http://dx.doi.org/10.1097/JTO.0b013e318206a221 PMID:21252716

18. Pao W, Hutchinson KE (2012). Chipping away at the lung cancer genome. *Nat Med*, 18:349–351. http://dx.doi.org/10.1038/nm.2697 PMID:22395697

19. Pao W, Girard N (2011). New driver mutations in non-small-cell lung cancer. *Lancet Oncol*, 12:175–180. http://dx.doi.org/10.1016/S1470-2045(10)70087-5 PMID:21277552

20. Ding L, Getz G, Wheeler DA *et al.* (2008). Somatic mutations affect key pathways in lung adenocarcinoma. *Nature*, 455:1069–1075. http://dx.doi.org/10.1038/nature07423 PMID:18948947

21. Imielinski M, Berger AH, Hammerman PS *et al.* (2012). Mapping the hallmarks of lung adenocarcinoma with massively parallel sequencing. *Cell*, 150:1107–1120. http://dx.doi.org/10.1016/j.cell.2012.08.029 PMID:22980975

22. Paik PK, Johnson ML, D'Angelo SP *et al.* (2012). Driver mutations determine survival in smokers and never-smokers with stage IIIB/IV lung adenocarcinomas. *Cancer*, 118:5840–5847. http://dx.doi.org/10.1002/cncr.27637 PMID:22605530

23. Govindan R, Ding L, Griffith M *et al.* (2012). Genomic landscape of non-small cell lung cancer in smokers and never-smokers. *Cell*, 150:1121–1134. http://dx.doi.org/10.1016/j.cell.2012.08.024 PMID:22980976

24. Hammerman PS, Hayes DN, Wilkerson MD *et al.*; Cancer Genome Atlas Research Network (2012). Comprehensive genomic characterization of squamous cell lung cancers. *Nature*, 489:519–525. http://dx.doi.org/10.1038/nature11404 PMID:22960745

25. Drilon A, Rekhtman N, Ladanyi M, Paik P (2012). Squamous-cell carcinomas of the lung: emerging biology, controversies, and the promise of targeted therapy. *Lancet Oncol*, 13:e418–e426. http://dx.doi.org/10.1016/S1470-2045(12)70291-7 PMID:23026827

26. Weiss J, Sos ML, Seidel D *et al.* (2010). Frequent and focal *FGFR1* amplification associates with therapeutically tractable FGFR1 dependency in squamous cell lung cancer. *Sci Transl Med*, 2:62ra93. http://dx.doi.org/10.1126/scitranslmed.3001451 PMID:21160078

27. Travis WD, Brambilla E, Müller-Hermelink HK, Harris CC, eds (2004). *Pathology and Genetics of Tumours of the Lung, Pleura, Thymus and Heart.* Lyon: IARC.

28. Peifer M, Fernández-Cuesta L, Sos ML *et al.* (2012). Integrative genome analyses identify key somatic driver mutations of small-cell lung cancer. *Nat Genet*, 44:1104–1110. http://dx.doi.org/10.1038/ng.2396 PMID:22941188

29. Lee KM, Chapman RS, Shen M *et al.* (2010). Differential effects of smoking on lung cancer mortality before and after household stove improvement in Xuanwei, China. *Br J Cancer*, 103:727–729. http://dx.doi.org/10.1038/sj.bjc.6605791 PMID:20648014

30. Aberle DR, Adams AM, Berg CD *et al.*; National Lung Screening Trial Research Team (2011). Reduced lung-cancer mortality with low-dose computed tomographic screening. *N Engl J Med*, 365:395–409. http://dx.doi.org/10.1056/NEJMoa1102873 PMID:21714641

31. Hassanein M, Callison JC, Callaway-Lane C *et al.* (2012). The state of molecular biomarkers for the early detection of lung cancer. *Cancer Prev Res (Phila)*, 5:992–1006. http://dx.doi.org/10.1158/1940-6207.CAPR-11-0441 PMID:22689914

32. Goldstraw P, Crowley J, Chansky K *et al.*; International Association for the Study of Lung Cancer International Staging Committee; Participating Institutions (2007). The IASLC Lung Cancer Staging Project: proposals for the revision of the TNM stage groupings in the forthcoming (seventh) edition of the TNM Classification of Malignant Tumours. *J Thorac Oncol*, 2:706–714. http://dx.doi.org/10.1097/JTO.0b013e31812f3c1a PMID:17762336

33. Siegel R, Naishadham D, Jemal A (2012). Cancer statistics, 2012. *CA Cancer J Clin*, 62:10–29. http://dx.doi.org/10.3322/caac.20138 PMID:22237781

34. Shepherd FA, Domerg C, Hainaut P *et al.* (2013). Pooled analysis of the prognostic and predictive effects of *KRAS* mutation status and *KRAS* mutation subtype in early-stage resected non-small-cell lung cancer in four trials of adjuvant chemotherapy. *J Clin Oncol*, 31:2173–2181. http://dx.doi.org/10.1200/JCO.2012.48.1390 PMID:23630215

5.2

Breast cancer

5 ORGAN SITE

Stuart J. Schnitt
Sunil R. Lakhani

Benjamin O. Anderson (reviewer)
Beela Sarah Mathew (reviewer)
Thangarajan Rajkumar (reviewer)

Summary

- Breast cancer is the most common cancer in women worldwide. This chapter is concerned with female breast cancer.

- Well-characterized breast cancer risk factors include age, family history, reproductive factors, mammographic density, and atypia in a prior benign breast biopsy. Agents that cause breast cancer include alcohol consumption, use of combined estrogen–progestogen contraceptives and menopausal therapy, and exposure to X- and γ-radiation.

- A small proportion of breast cancers are due to inherited mutations in high-penetrance breast cancer susceptibility genes (BRCA1 and BRCA2). Several lower-penetrance genes have also been associated with breast cancer, and there are many loci that are linked to an increased risk.

- Recent molecular and genetic studies have emphasized that breast cancer is a highly heterogeneous group of diseases that differ in their prognosis and response to treatment.

- Improved understanding of the molecular pathways and genetic

alterations that underlie the different breast cancer subtypes is leading to a more targeted and personalized approach to breast cancer treatment.

Etiology

The etiology of breast cancer is multifactorial, involving endocrine and reproductive factors including nulliparity, first birth after age 30, and hormonal history; environmental factors such as consumption of alcoholic beverages, use of certain contraceptives and menopausal (hormone replacement) therapy, and exposure to ionizing radiation; and lifestyle factors such as high-calorie diets and lack of exercise (see "Biological mechanisms mediating reduced breast cancer risk through physical activity"). The annual incidence in industrialized countries where such lifestyle factors have existed for some time is 70–90 new cases per 100 000 women. Countries where industrialization is a more recent phenomenon have a rising incidence and higher mortality.

On the basis of a case–control study in Germany, population attributable risk (95% confidence interval) for non-modifiable breast cancer risk factors (age at menarche, age at menopause, parity, benign breast disease, and family history of breast cancer) was 37.2% (27.1–47.2%) for all invasive tumours considered. Of the modifiable risk factors assessed, use of hormone therapy and physical inactivity had the highest impact, with population attributable risks of 19.4% (15.9–23.2%) and 12.8% (5.5–20.8%), respectively, for invasive tumours; all such findings varied depending on the estrogen and progesterone receptor status of tumours [1].

A small proportion of breast cancer is due to a familial predisposition, and two high-risk, high-penetrance genes have been identified: BRCA1 and BRCA2. Mutations in these genes greatly increase the risk of developing breast cancer. Several lower-penetrance genes have also been identified, and there are many loci within the genome that are linked to an increased risk but for which the specific genes have yet to be identified (see Pathology and Genetics sections below).

Hence, for most patients with breast cancer, multiple factors – including personal and family history as well as reproductive and lifestyle factors – are implicated in tumour development.

Pathology

Breast cancer is not a single disease and is heterogeneous both clinically and morphologically. The current *WHO Classification of Tumours of*

Epidemiology

Breast cancer

- Breast cancer is by far the most frequently diagnosed cancer and cause of cancer death among women. There were an estimated 1.7 million new cases (25% of all cancers in women) and 0.5 million cancer deaths (15% of all cancer deaths in women) in 2012.

- Breast cancer is the most common cancer diagnosis in women in 140 countries and the most frequent cause of cancer mortality in 101 countries.

- Age-standardized incidence rates are highest in western Europe and lowest in East Asia. Incidence rates tend to be elevated in countries attaining the highest levels of human development. There is a greater than 2-fold difference between countries categorized as having low versus very high levels of development.

- About 43% of the estimated new cases and 34% of the cancer deaths occurred in Europe and North America.

- Mortality rates vary approximately 2–5-fold worldwide; the case fatality rate is lower in countries with higher levels of human development.

- Whereas incidence has been generally increasing in most areas of the world, it has peaked and declined over the past decade in a number of highly developed countries.

- Mortality rates have been declining in a number of highly developed countries since the late 1980s and early 1990s, a result of a combination of improved detection and earlier diagnosis (through population-based screening) and more effective treatment regimens.

Map 5.2.1. Global distribution of estimated age-standardized (World) incidence rates (ASR) per 100 000, for breast cancer in women, 2012.

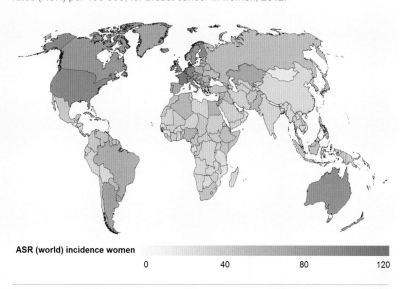

ASR (world) incidence women

| 0 | 40 | 80 | 120 |

Map 5.2.2. Global distribution of estimated age-standardized (World) mortality rates (ASR) per 100 000, for breast cancer in women, 2012.

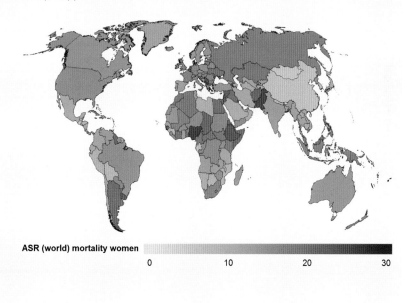

ASR (world) mortality women

| 0 | 10 | 20 | 30 |

For more details about the maps and charts presented in this chapter, see "A guide to the epidemiology data in *World Cancer Report*".

the Breast (4th edition) [2] recognizes more than 20 different subtypes.

Most breast cancers arise from epithelial cells (carcinomas); these tumours are subdivided into in situ and invasive lesions. In situ carcinomas are preinvasive lesions in which the malignant epithelial cells are still confined to the ductal/lobular tree of the breast and the basement membrane surrounding the ducts and lobules is intact to the extent that it has

Chart 5.2.1. Estimated global number of new cases and deaths with proportions by major world regions, for breast cancer in women, 2012.

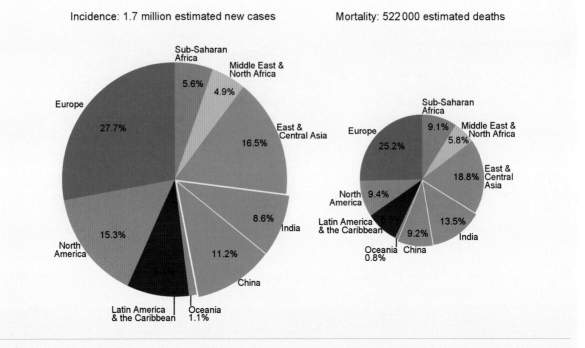

Incidence: 1.7 million estimated new cases

Mortality: 522 000 estimated deaths

Chart 5.2.2. Age-standardized (World) incidence rates per 100 000 by year in selected populations, for breast cancer in women, circa 1975–2012.

Chart 5.2.3. Age-standardized (World) mortality rates per 100 000 by year in selected populations, for breast cancer in women, circa 1975–2012.

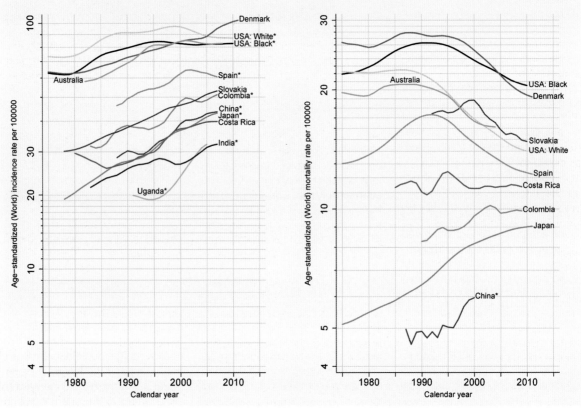

not been penetrated by cancer cells. Preinvasive lesions are further subdivided into ductal carcinoma in situ (DCIS) and lobular carcinoma in situ (LCIS). Despite the "ductal" versus "lobular" terminology, the fact that almost all carcinomas in the breast arise from the structural and functional unit of the breast called the terminal duct lobular unit has been well established for some time [3]. The distinction between DCIS and LCIS is the result not of the microanatomical site of origin (ducts vs lobules) but rather of a difference in the architectural and cytological features of the cells. DCIS and LCIS also differ in their distribution within the breast, in the associated respective risks of bilateral disease, and in their natural history.

Subsets of DCIS and LCIS have also been recognized. DCIS is subclassified according to nuclear grade and architectural features; high-grade DCIS has a greater risk of recurrence and progression to invasive cancer than do lower grades of DCIS [4]. LCIS is often a multifocal and multicentric disease and also carries a risk of bilateral involvement [5]. In its classic form, LCIS presents a small risk of progression to invasive cancer over a period of 20–25 years. Recently, a higher-grade variant, pleomorphic LCIS, has been recognized, but its natural history is unclear at present (Fig. 5.2.1) [6].

Invasive carcinoma characterized as "no special type", also known as ductal carcinoma no special type or invasive ductal carcinoma, makes up the largest subset of invasive breast cancer. This designation identifies a heterogeneous group comprising tumours that are not easily categorized by specific morphological features that characterize the "special subtypes". Hence, it is a default diagnosis for all those tumours (approximately 70%) that cannot be assigned a "special subtype" designation. The most common of the special subtypes include lobular carcinoma, tubular carcinoma, mucinous carcinoma, carcinoma with medullary and apocrine features, micropapillary

Fig. 5.2.1. Ductal carcinoma in situ of low nuclear grade. (A) Classic lobular carcinoma in situ is diagnosed because the characteristic cells distend and distort the acini. (B) Pleomorphic lobular carcinoma in situ. Nuclear enlargement, variability, and prominent nucleoli are associated with abundant cytoplasm. (C) Cribriform pattern. Multiple adjacent ducts are distended by a sieve-like proliferation of monotonous uniform cells. The multiple spaces within the proliferation are rounded and distributed in an organized fashion. (D) This space shows a rim of viable cells with high-grade nuclei. There is comedo-type necrosis and calcification.

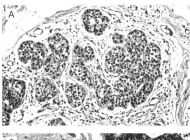
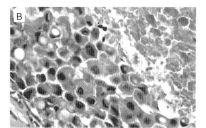
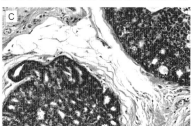
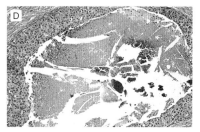

and papillary carcinomas, and metaplastic carcinomas (Fig. 5.2.2).

It is now well recognized that tumours of the breast exhibit both intratumour and intertumour heterogeneity. Histological grade is a measure of how closely a tumour resembles its tissue of origin and is an integral part of a pathology report. The current grading system assesses three parameters of the tumour: (i) the degree of architectural differentiation (tubule formation), (ii) nuclear pleomorphism (nuclear grade), and (iii) proliferation (mitotic count/index). Each parameter is given a score from 1 to 3, and the scores for the three parameters are added together. Tumours with a total score of 3–5 are grade 1 (low grade), those with scores of 6 and 7 are grade 2 (intermediate grade), and those with scores of 8 and 9 are grade 3 (high grade). Although this semiquantitative approach averages the intratumour heterogeneity that exists in many tumours, it remains a powerful indicator of patient prognosis (Table 5.2.1).

Histological grade is also strongly associated with histological type and

with patterns of molecular alterations, such as estrogen receptor (ER) and progesterone receptor (PR) expression and human epidermal growth factor receptor 2 (HER2) protein overexpression and gene amplification.

The histopathological analysis of breast cancers also provides information on stage of disease – meaning the extent of disease involvement. This is determined in two ways: from the size of the cancer and from the assessment of regional lymph node involvement. Both these parameters provide powerful prognostic information for patient management. The overall staging for the patient is recorded with the American Joint Committee on Cancer staging system using the tumour–node–metastasis (TNM) classification. Additional prognostic data, such as lymphovascular permeation and degree of response to neoadjuvant therapy, can also be derived from the histopathological assessment.

The pathological assessment of tumours as described above is inexpensive and quick and can provide useful information on which to base

Fig. 5.2.2. (A) Invasive carcinoma no special type, grade 2. (B) Classic invasive lobular carcinoma with uniform, single-file cells compared with (C). (C) Invasive pleomorphic lobular carcinoma with characteristic pleomorphic, atypical nuclei. (D) Tubular carcinoma. There is a haphazard distribution of rounded and angulated tubules with open lumina, lined by only a single layer of epithelial cells separated by abundant reactive, fibroblastic stroma. (E) The neoplastic cells lining the teardrop-shaped tubules lack significant atypia. (F) Mixed metaplastic carcinoma with spindle, mesenchymal (chondroid), and squamous differentiation. (G) Neuroendocrine carcinoma of the breast. Alveolar pattern with rounded solid nests of spindle cells invading a dense collagenous stroma. (H) Invasive micropapillary carcinoma. Tumour cell clusters with irregular central spaces proliferate within empty stromal spaces. Some clusters have reversed polarity with an "inside-out" morphology.

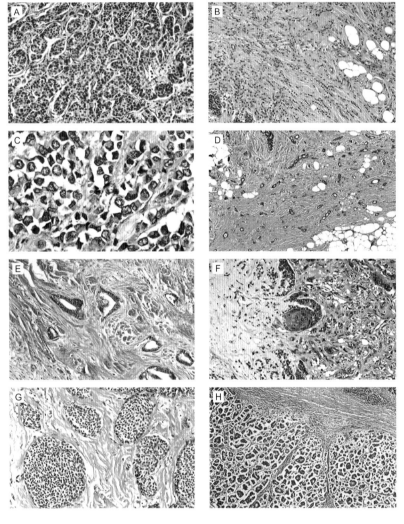

breast cancers, at least in the more developed countries. Such assessment allows prognostication and also provides predictive data with regard to response to anti-estrogen therapy (e.g. tamoxifen) and anti-HER2 therapy (e.g. trastuzumab) [7]. Such therapy is not appropriate for approximately 15% of tumours, which are designated "triple-negative" to indicate lack of expression of ER, PR, or HER2.

DNA microarray technology for gene expression profiling, which allows thousands of genes to be examined simultaneously, has been used to classify breast cancer, develop signatures for "good" versus "poor" prognosis, and identify tumours that may or may not respond to particular therapy [8]. This type of analysis has not only confirmed the two large subsets of breast cancer – ER-positive and ER-negative – but also brought to the fore differences within the ER categories. In ER-positive tumours, the luminal B subset has a worse prognosis than the luminal A subset, probably driven at least in part by higher proliferative activity. Within the ER-negative group, the triple-negative (ER-, PR-, and HER2-negative) and "basal-like" groups are now recognized; these groups are not synonymous but show considerable overlap. The basal-like group comprises tumours that express proteins found in the contractile myoepithelial cell layer of normal breast (e.g. CK14, CK5/6), and a subset of these tumours have a propensity for early recurrence, especially involving metastasis in the brain and lungs [9]. This type of understanding is already determining management strategies and will lead, through clinical trials, to better targeted therapies.

For more than a decade, such gene expression profiling has been applied to define molecular phenotypes of breast cancer. The luminal A and basal-like subtypes mentioned above are the two main subtypes of five that have been identified (Fig. 5.2.4). In an evaluation of differences, signature genes of the luminal A subtype were genes

plans for further management. Nonetheless, limitations are recognized. Patients with a similar type or grade of breast cancer may have very different response to therapy or long-term outcome. There has been considerable progress over the past three decades in understanding the biology of breast cancer and in translating some of the

molecular data into routine clinical practice.

Genetics

The assessment of ER and PR status using immunohistochemistry, and of HER2 status using immunohistochemistry and in situ hybridization, is now routine for all primary

Biological mechanisms mediating reduced breast cancer risk through physical activity

Christine M. Friedenreich

Physical activity has been associated with a 25–30% decrease in breast cancer risk, and research is now focused on understanding the biological mechanisms mediating this association, with the aim of determining the optimal type, dose, and timing of activity needed for maximum risk reduction. Several mechanisms have been hypothesized (Fig. B5.2.1) [1], and intervention trials in postmenopausal, inactive, healthy women have investigated these pathways [2]. These studies have found that exercise decreases endogenous estrogens, adiposity, insulin resistance, leptin, and inflammation, which are all associated independently with increased breast cancer risk. Other emerging hypothesized mechanisms include oxidative stress and genomic instability.

Exercise reduces the endogenous estrogen levels in premenopausal women by inducing anovulatory menstrual cycles or amenorrhea, or through other mechanisms. In postmenopausal women, exercise decreases circulating estrogens directly, and indirectly with exercise-induced weight loss. Obesity, an established risk factor for postmenopausal breast cancer, is decreased with physical activity. Obesity-related effects, notably insulin resistance and altered levels of insulin-like growth factor 1 (IGF-1) and its binding protein IGFBP-3, in addition to altered production of adipokines, specifically leptin and adiponectin, may be important contributors to increasing breast cancer risk. Mechanisms independent of changes in body fat are also relevant. Exercise acutely enhances insulin sensitivity and glucose uptake by skeletal muscle, which can be sustained through prolonged high-intensity activity. With decreased circulating insulin, free IGF-1 levels may also decrease because of lowered growth hormone-mediated hepatic synthesis of IGF-1 and/or increased synthesis of IGFBP-1.

Fig. B5.2.1. Biological mechanisms determining the optimal type, dose, and timing of physical activity needed for maximum reduction in breast cancer risk. IL-6, interleukin-6; SHBG, sex hormone-binding globulin; TNF-α, tumour necrosis factor α.

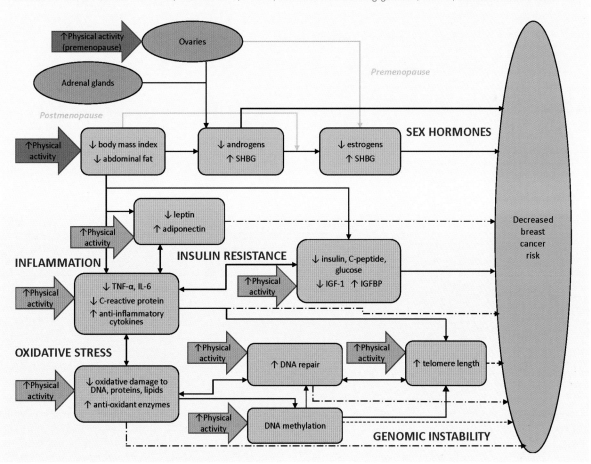

Chronic inflammation is associated with sustained proliferation and oxidative stress, which together promote malignancy. C-reactive protein, a marker of chronic low-grade systemic inflammation, may have a predictive role for breast cancer risk. Exercise may protect against postmenopausal breast cancer by inducing an anti-inflammatory environment and subsequently protecting against chronic low-grade inflammation. Exercise may lower inflammation via reductions in adiposity and other pathways.

Oxidative stress plays an important role in breast cancer carcinogenesis – specifically, the oxidation of DNA in carcinogenesis and tumour promotion. Epidemiological data also suggest associations between oxidative stress and breast cancer. As a part of a favourable biological adaptive response, exercise enhances the capacity of antioxidant and oxidative damage repair enzymes, and subsequently reduces oxidative damage.

Investigators have called for trials of exercise and breast cancer incidence, to provide the ultimate level of evidence about the type, dose, and timing of activity needed for breast cancer prevention, but no studies are currently planned because of the considerable expense and time commitment required [3]. Thus, to date, the epidemiological research performed in healthy populations is restricted to evidence on intermediate end-points for breast cancer. Nonetheless, evidence exists that these pathways are amenable to change by exercise.

References

1. Neilson HK et al. (2009). Cancer Epidemiol Biomarkers Prev, 18:11–27. http://dx.doi.org/10.1158/1055-9965.EPI-08-0756 PMID:19124476

2. Winzer BM et al. (2011). Cancer Causes Control, 22:811–826. http://dx.doi.org/10.1007/s10552-011-9761-4 PMID:21461921

3. Ballard-Barbash R et al. (2009). J Natl Cancer Inst, 101:630–643. http://dx.doi.org/10.1093/jnci/djp068 PMID:19401543

involved in fatty acid metabolism and steroid hormone-mediated signalling pathways, in particular ER signalling, while the corresponding genes for the basal-like subtype were involved in cell proliferation and differentiation, the p21-mediated pathway, and the G1–S cell-cycle checkpoint. A minimal set of 54 genes best discriminated between the two subtypes [10].

Such molecular analyses are also relevant to survival. One study used modelling of messenger RNA (mRNA), copy number alterations, microRNAs, and methylation [11]. For all breast cancers, the strongest predictor of good outcome was acquisition of a gene signature that favoured a high T helper type 1 (Th1)/cytotoxic T lymphocyte response at the expense of Th2-driven immunity.

Next-generation sequencing technology has also been applied to examine the genomes of 100 breast cancers for somatic copy number changes and mutations in the coding exons of protein-coding genes [12]. The number of somatic mutations varied markedly between individual tumours. Strong correlations were evident between number of mutations, age at which cancer was diagnosed, and cancer histological grade, and multiple mutational signatures were observed, including one, present in about 10% of tumours, characterized by numerous mutations of cytosine at TpC dinucleotides. Driver mutations were identified in several new cancer genes, including AKT2, ARID1B, CASP8, CDKN1B, MAP3K1, MAP3K13, NCOR1, SMARCD1, and TBX3 (Fig. 5.2.5). Among the 100 tumours, there were driver mutations in at least 40 cancer genes and 73 different combinations of mutated cancer genes. Overall, one of the most highly contributing genes to development of breast cancer, TP53, is nonetheless probably only involved in 25% of cancers, although its role

Table 5.2.1. Semi-quantitative method for assessing histological grade

Feature	Score
Tubule and gland formation	
Majority of tumour (> 75%)	1
Moderate degree (10–75%)	2
Little or none (< 10%)	3
Nuclear pleomorphism	
Small, regular, uniform cells	1
Moderate increase in size and variability	2
Marked variation	3
Mitotic count	
Dependent on microscope field area	1–3
Final grading	
Add scores for tubule and gland formation, nuclear pleomorphism, and mitotic count:	
Grade 1	Total score, 3–5
Grade 2	Total score, 6 or 7
Grade 3	Total score, 8 or 9

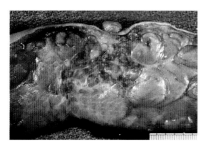

in subsets of breast cancers, such as triple-negative/basal-like, is much higher. A large number of genes appear to be implicated in a small percentage of tumours, and this will provide additional challenges to achieving the dream of a patient-specific targeted and personalized medical intervention.

A better understanding of familial breast cancer due to germline mutations in *BRCA1* and *BRCA2* is determining optimal patient management (see "Treatment determined by *BRCA1/2* mutation"). The

pathology of these tumours is well detailed now, and it is clear that most *BRCA1*-associated breast cancers are high-grade, medullary-like, and triple-negative, and have a basal-like phenotype [13]. There are also data indicating that a proportion of ER-positive tumours in patients with *BRCA1* mutations are also due to inactivation of *BRCA1* and may not be sporadic [14]. The morphological features of *BRCA2*-associated tumours are more heterogeneous, although most are high-grade breast cancers. The pathology has been combined with various personal and family history factors to develop algorithms to predict the risk of carrying a *BRCA1* mutation, and these have been used in the clinic with varying degrees of success.

Prospects

Prevention

To date, most breast cancer prevention strategies have focused on reducing the development of breast cancer in women considered to be at

moderately or greatly increased risk of the disease based on calculated risks determined from prediction models, or in women with germline mutations in high-penetrance breast cancer susceptibility genes (*BRCA1* and *BRCA2*).

Several clinical trials have evaluated the effect on the development of breast cancer of endocrine interventions using selective ER modulators (SERMs) and aromatase inhibitors. The results of the National Surgical Adjuvant Breast and Bowel Project's Breast Cancer Prevention Trial [15] and Study of Tamoxifen and Raloxifene Trial [16] demonstrated that the SERMs tamoxifen and raloxifene are each associated with about a 50% reduction in the development of breast cancer in women considered to be at moderately increased risk of breast cancer based on the Gail risk assessment model. In two other prevention trials, tamoxifen was associated with more modest reductions in the development of breast cancer. However, in both of these trials some of the women received

Fig. 5.2.4. Identification of breast cancer subtypes. (A) Correlation of breast tumour samples with five recognized subtypes of breast tumours. For this analysis, 526 out of 552 previously identified "intrinsic" genes were cross-mapped and subject to hierarchical clustering. (B) Unsupervised hierarchical clustering of 20 breast tumour tissues analysed using the 526 mapped intrinsic genes (the two microarray replicates for each sample are shown). The level of expression of each gene in each sample, relative to the median level of expression of that gene across all the samples, is represented using a colour scale as shown in the key (green, below median; black, equal to median; red, above median). (Left panel) Scaled-down representation of the entire cluster of the 526 intrinsic genes and 20 tissue samples. (Right panel) Experimental dendrogram displaying the clustering of the tumours into three distinct subgroups.

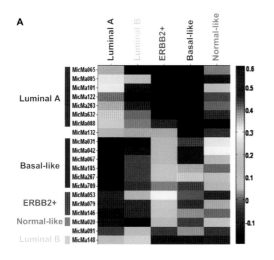

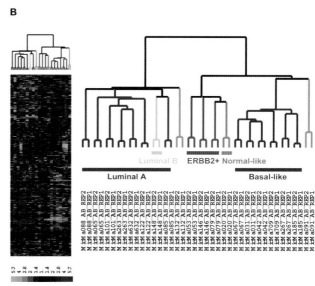

Fig. 5.2.5. Recently identified breast cancer genes and involvement of the JUN kinase signalling pathway. (A) Representations of the protein-coding sequences and major domains in cancer genes relevant to breast cancer. Somatic mutations evident in tumours are shown as circles: truncating (red), essential splice site (blue), missense (green), and in-frame insertion or deletion (yellow). Red lines indicate the positions of large homozygous deletions. aa, amino acids. (B) Pathways regulating the JUN kinases MAP2K7 and MAP2K8, indicating genes with mutations in this series. Genes in green are activated by mutations, whereas genes in purple are inactivated.

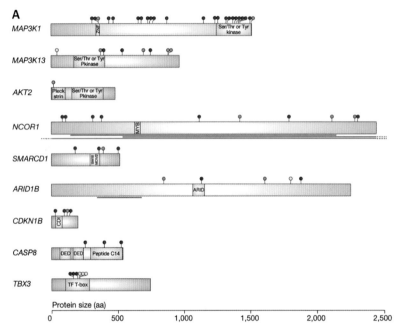

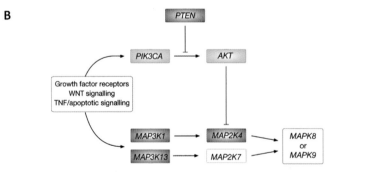

the risk of ER-negative tumours, which account for about 20–30% of breast cancers and are associated with a poorer prognosis [20]. As a result, the potential role in breast cancer prevention of various drugs that target non-endocrine signalling pathways is under active investigation. For example, recent data from the Women's Health Initiative indicated that among postmenopausal women with diabetes, treatment with metformin was associated with a reduced incidence of breast cancer [21]. Other non-endocrine drugs being studied as possible breast cancer prevention agents include cyclooxygenase 2 inhibitors, retinoids, and receptor tyrosine kinase inhibitors, among others. However, clinical trials will be required to evaluate the role of these agents in breast cancer prevention.

Bilateral prophylactic mastectomy is a highly effective strategy to prevent the development of breast cancer in women with *BRCA* mutations. This procedure is associated with a 90% reduction in the development of breast cancer in these

Fig. 5.2.6. Pregnancy before age 30 and breastfeeding reduce a woman's total number of lifetime menstrual cycles, and both factors are associated with lower risk of breast cancer. (For more details, see Chapter 2.5.)

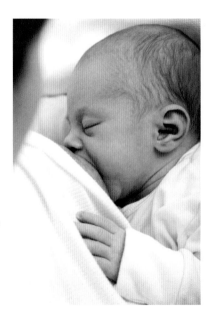

hormone replacement therapy and this may have attenuated the chemopreventive benefit of tamoxifen [17,18]. Despite the demonstrated efficacy of tamoxifen and raloxifene in reducing the development of breast cancer, these SERMs have had limited patient acceptance in the chemoprevention setting.

The role of aromatase inhibitors in breast cancer prevention is also an area of active research. In one recent study, treatment with exemestane was associated with a 65%

relative reduction in the annual incidence of invasive breast cancer in postmenopausal women at moderately increased risk of breast cancer, with no serious toxicity and minimal effect on health-related quality of life [19]. The role of anastrozole in the chemoprevention setting is currently being evaluated. The reduction of breast cancer development associated with these endocrine interventions has been notably limited to ER-positive tumours. These agents have not been effective in reducing

Treatment determined by *BRCA1/2* mutation

Susan M. Domchek

Germline mutations in *BRCA1* and *BRCA2* are associated with an increased lifetime risk of breast and ovarian cancers, as well as other cancers such as male breast cancer, prostate cancer, and pancreatic cancer. The lifetime risk of breast cancer is 60–70% in women harbouring either mutation. Interventions such as prophylactic mastectomy and prophylactic oophorectomy have been demonstrated to reduce the risk of breast and ovarian cancers in several observational cohort studies. Risk-reducing oophorectomy has also been associated with improved overall survival [1]. In women diagnosed with breast cancer, the knowledge that there is an increased risk of developing a second primary breast cancer can factor into decision-making about local therapy with the option of bilateral mastectomy.

Due to the biological functions of BRCA1 and BRCA2 (particularly their roles in DNA damage repair of double-strand breaks), it has been postulated that there may be differential responses of *BRCA1/2*-associated tumours to different types of systemic therapy. In general, BRCA-associated cancers (both breast and ovarian) appear to be more sensitive than sporadic cancers to chemotherapy. Emerging data suggest that specific chemotherapy type may matter clinically. Several small studies have reported high response rates in breast cancer to cisplatin-based chemotherapy given in both the pre-operative and metastatic setting [2]. For example, in a study of 20 patients with *BRCA1*-positive metastatic breast cancer, the objective response rate to cisplatin chemotherapy was 80%. There are no data available from randomized studies comparing cisplatin with other agents, but the reported response rates and progression-free survival data are encouraging.

Novel agents called poly(ADP-ribose) polymerase (PARP) inhibitors are being studied in *BRCA1* and *BRCA2* mutation carriers with both metastatic breast cancer and recurrent ovarian cancer. These drugs, which remain in clinical trials, aim to exploit the fundamental defects in *BRCA1/2*-associated cancers via the concept of synthetic lethality. Synthetic lethality refers to the idea that inhibition or mutation of two pathways leads to cell death when inhibition or mutation of either alone does not. Initial reports have demonstrated high response rates in both *BRCA1/2*-associated metastatic breast cancer and recurrent ovarian cancer [3]. Interestingly, although PARP inhibitors do not appear to have activity in unselected sporadic triple-negative breast cancer, studies have been encouraging in sporadic high-grade serous ovarian cancer.

Mechanisms of resistance to both cisplatin and PARP inhibitors are beginning to be elucidated. One very interesting mechanism is that of secondary or "reversion" mutations, which restore full-length protein. Studies are under way to determine the optimal use of both platinum agents and PARP inhibitors in *BRCA1/2* mutation carriers.

References

1. Domchek SM *et al.* (2010). *JAMA*, 304:967–975. http://dx.doi.org/10.1001/jama.2010.1237 PMID:20810374

2. Byrski T *et al.* (2012). *Breast Cancer Res*, 14:R110. http://dx.doi.org/10.1186/bcr3231 PMID:22817698

3. Tutt A *et al.* (2010). *Lancet*, 376:235–244. http://dx.doi.org/10.1016/S0140-6736(10)60892-6 PMID:20609467

women, and an even higher (95%) reduction in breast cancer among those who have also had their ovaries removed [22]. Bilateral prophylactic mastectomy is associated with an even greater (> 99%) reduction in breast cancer development among women who were considered to be at high risk of the disease and who were cared for in community practices and were therefore not as highly selected as in referral centres [23]. Recent technical improvements in oncoplastic surgery have resulted in better cosmetic outcomes in women who undergo post-mastectomy reconstruction and have, in turn, made the option of prophylactic mastectomy more appealing than in the past. The influence of modifying dietary and lifestyle factors on the prevention of breast cancer is also under active investigation [24].

Screening

Mammography remains the mainstay of population-based breast cancer screening although access to mammographic screening varies widely around the world and the procedure is unavailable in most developing countries. Mammography results in the detection of more in situ lesions than would be identified otherwise and of invasive cancers that are smaller, of lower grade, more often node-negative, and more often of special types (especially tubular carcinomas) than are evident in non-screened populations. Controversies remain about the magnitude of mortality reduction attributable to mammographic screening, the lower and upper age limits of the patients who should be screened, and the most cost-effective screening interval [25]. In addition, mammographic screening can result in overdiagnosis due to the detection of tumours that will never become a threat to life, as well as an excessive number of biopsies, and patient anxiety [25,26].

In recent years, technical advances have improved the sensitivity of mammography for at least a subset of women [25]. In particular, in a

Fig. 5.2.7. A woman undergoing mammography screening. Her breast is being compressed to obtain the optimal mammographic image.

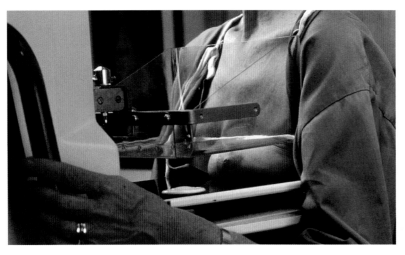

large clinical trial digital mammography was shown to be more sensitive than traditional film mammography in younger women (aged < 50 years, or premenopausal) and in women with dense breasts. Breast tomosynthesis, a variation of digital mammography, produces three-dimensional digital images of the breast but has not been demonstrated to be more sensitive than standard digital mammography. Both ultrasonography and magnetic resonance imaging may be of value as adjuncts to mammography in selected cases. These techniques are associated with high false-positive rates and are not recommended for screening the general population [25]. Magnetic resonance imaging, however, may have a role in the screening of women with *BRCA1* germline mutations. Newer modalities that may ultimately find a role in breast cancer screening include molecular imaging and functional imaging techniques [27]. Alternatives to mammography for breast cancer screening, particularly in developing countries, are being evaluated and include breast awareness and clinical breast examination (see Chapter 4.8).

Targeted agents

Selection of breast cancer treatment, particularly systemic therapy, is currently based primarily on clinical and pathological factors, supplemented by hormone receptor and HER2 status. The standard options for systemic therapy currently include hormone therapy, cytotoxic therapy, and HER2-targeted therapy, singly and in various combinations. Rapidly evolving knowledge of the molecular events and signalling pathways underlying the development and progression of breast cancer has led to the identification of a growing number of new therapeutic targets and to the development of drugs against these targets. Many clinical trials are currently under way worldwide to evaluate the role of these new targeted therapies in the treatment of patients with breast cancer. Newer targeted therapies that have been or are being evaluated, singly and in combination with each other and with traditional cytotoxic agents, include angiogenesis inhibitors, tyrosine kinase inhibitors, inhibitors of mammalian target of rapamycin (mTOR), poly(ADP-ribose) polymerase 1 (PARP1) inhibitors, insulin-like growth factor 1 receptor (IGF-1R) inhibitors, proteasome inhibitors, phosphatidylinositol 3-kinase (PI3K) inhibitors, and others [28]. The ultimate goal of this research is to be able to tailor breast cancer treatment for individual patients based on the particular molecular features of the tumour.

References

1. Barnes BB, Steindorf K, Hein R *et al.* (2011). Population attributable risk of invasive postmenopausal breast cancer and breast cancer subtypes for modifiable and non-modifiable risk factors. *Cancer Epidemiol*, 35:345–352. http://dx.doi.org/10.1016/j.canep.2010.11.003 PMID:21159569

2. Lakhani SR, Ellis IO, Schnitt SJ *et al.*, eds (2012). *WHO Classification of Tumours of the Breast*, 4th ed. Lyon: IARC.

3. Wellings SR, Jensen HM, Marcum RG (1975). An atlas of subgross pathology of the human breast with special reference to possible precancerous lesions. *J Natl Cancer Inst*, 55:231–273. PMID:169369

4. Silverstein MJ, Poller DN, Waisman JR *et al.* (1995). Prognostic classification of breast ductal carcinoma-in-situ. *Lancet*, 345:1154–1157. http://dx.doi.org/10.1016/S0140-6736(95)90982-6 PMID:7723550

5. Beute BJ, Kalisher L, Hutter RV (1991). Lobular carcinoma in situ of the breast: clinical, pathologic, and mammographic features. *AJR Am J Roentgenol*, 157:257–265. http://dx.doi.org/10.2214/ajr.157.2.1853802 PMID:1853802

6. Eusebi V, Magalhaes F, Azzopardi JG (1992). Pleomorphic lobular carcinoma of the breast: an aggressive tumor showing apocrine differentiation. *Hum Pathol*, 23:655–662. http://dx.doi.org/10.1016/0046-8177(92)90321-S PMID:1592388

7. Hammond ME, Hayes DF, Dowsett M *et al.* (2010). American Society of Clinical Oncology/College of American Pathologists guideline recommendations for immunohistochemical testing of estrogen and progesterone receptors in breast cancer. *J Clin Oncol*, 28:2784–2795. http://dx.doi.org/10.1200/JCO.2009.25.6529 PMID:20404251

8. van de Vijver MJ, He YD, van't Veer LJ *et al.* (2002). A gene-expression signature as a predictor of survival in breast cancer. *N Engl J Med*, 347:1999–2009. http://dx.doi.org/10.1056/NEJMoa021967 PMID:12490681

9. Fulford LG, Reis-Filho JS, Ryder K *et al.* (2007). Basal-like grade III invasive ductal carcinoma of the breast: patterns of metastasis and long-term survival. *Breast Cancer Res*, 9:R4. http://dx.doi.org/10.1186/bcr1636 PMID:17217540

10. Sørlie T, Wang Y, Xiao C *et al.* (2006). Distinct molecular mechanisms underlying clinically relevant subtypes of breast cancer: gene expression analyses across three different platforms. *BMC Genomics*, 7:127. http://dx.doi.org/10.1186/1471-2164-7-127 PMID:16729877

11. Kristensen VN, Vaske CJ, Ursini-Siegel J *et al.* (2012). Integrated molecular profiles of invasive breast tumors and ductal carcinoma in situ (DCIS) reveal differential vascular and interleukin signaling. *Proc Natl Acad Sci U S A*, 109:2802–2807. http://dx.doi.org/10.1073/pnas.1108781108 PMID:21908711

12. Stephens PJ, Tarpey PS, Davies H *et al.*; Oslo Breast Cancer Consortium (OSBREAC) (2012). The landscape of cancer genes and mutational processes in breast cancer. *Nature*, 486:400–404. http://dx.doi.org/10.1038/nature11017 PMID:22722201

13. Lakhani SR, Reis-Filho JS, Fulford L *et al.*; Breast Cancer Linkage Consortium (2005). Prediction of *BRCA1* status in patients with breast cancer using estrogen receptor and basal phenotype. *Clin Cancer Res*, 11:5175–5180. http://dx.doi.org/10.1158/1078-0432.CCR-04-2424 PMID:16033833

14. Tung N, Miron A, Schnitt SJ *et al.* (2010). Prevalence and predictors of loss of wild type *BRCA1* in estrogen receptor positive and negative *BRCA1*-associated breast cancers. *Breast Cancer Res*, 12:R95. http://dx.doi.org/10.1186/bcr2776 PMID:21080930

15. Fisher B, Costantino JP, Wickerham DL *et al.* (1998). Tamoxifen for prevention of breast cancer: report of the National Surgical Adjuvant Breast and Bowel Project P-1 Study. *J Natl Cancer Inst*, 90:1371–1388. http://dx.doi.org/10.1093/jnci/90.18.1371 PMID:9747868

16. Vogel VG, Costantino JP, Wickerham DL *et al.*; National Surgical Adjuvant Breast and Bowel Project (NSABP) (2006). Effects of tamoxifen vs raloxifene on the risk of developing invasive breast cancer and other disease outcomes: the NSABP Study of Tamoxifen and Raloxifene (STAR) P-2 trial. *JAMA*, 295:2727–2741. http://dx.doi.org/10.1001/jama.295.23.joc60074 PMID:16754727

17. Cuzick J, Forbes JF, Sestak I *et al.*; International Breast Cancer Intervention Study I Investigators (2007). Long-term results of tamoxifen prophylaxis for breast cancer – 96-month follow-up of the randomized IBIS-I trial. *J Natl Cancer Inst*, 99:272–282. http://dx.doi.org/10.1093/jnci/djk049 PMID:17312304

18. Powles TJ, Ashley S, Tidy A *et al.* (2007). Twenty-year follow-up of the Royal Marsden randomized, double-blinded tamoxifen breast cancer prevention trial. *J Natl Cancer Inst*, 99:283–290. http://dx.doi.org/10.1093/jnci/djk050 PMID:17312305

19. Goss PE, Ingle JN, Alés-Martínez JE *et al.*; NCIC CTG MAP.3 Study Investigators (2011). Exemestane for breast-cancer prevention in postmenopausal women. *N Engl J Med*, 364:2381–2391. http://dx.doi.org/10.1056/NEJMoa1103507 PMID:21639806

20. Cazzaniga M, Bonanni B (2012). Prevention of ER-negative breast cancer: where do we stand? *Eur J Cancer Prev*, 21:171–181. http://dx.doi.org/10.1097/CEJ.0b013e32834c9c26 PMID:21968686

21. Chlebowski RT, McTiernan A, Wactawski-Wende J *et al.* (2012). Diabetes, metformin, and breast cancer in postmenopausal women. *J Clin Oncol*, 30:2844–2852. http://dx.doi.org/10.1200/JCO.2011.39.7505 PMID:22689798

22. Rebbeck TR, Friebel T, Lynch HT *et al.* (2004). Bilateral prophylactic mastectomy reduces breast cancer risk in *BRCA1* and *BRCA2* mutation carriers: the PROSE Study Group. *J Clin Oncol*, 22:1055–1062. http://dx.doi.org/10.1200/JCO.2004.04.188 PMID:14981104

23. Geiger AM, Yu O, Herrinton LJ *et al.* (2005). A population-based study of bilateral prophylactic mastectomy efficacy in women at elevated risk for breast cancer in community practices. *Arch Intern Med*, 165:516–520. http://dx.doi.org/10.1001/archinte.165.5.516 PMID:15767526

24. Willett WC, Tamimi RM, Hankinson SE *et al.* (2010). Nongenetic factors in the causation of breast cancer. In: Harris JR, Lippman ME, Morrow M *et al.*, eds. *Diseases of the Breast*, 4th ed. Philadelphia: Lippincott Williams & Wilkins, pp. 248–290.

25. Warner E (2011). Clinical practice. Breast-cancer screening. *N Engl J Med*, 365:1025–1032. http://dx.doi.org/10.1056/NEJMcp1101540 PMID:21916640

26. Lebovic GS, Hollingsworth A, Feig SA (2010). Risk assessment, screening and prevention of breast cancer: a look at cost-effectiveness. *Breast*, 19:260–267. http://dx.doi.org/10.1016/j.breast.2010.03.013 PMID:20399656

27. Yang WT (2011). Emerging techniques and molecular imaging in breast cancer. *Semin Ultrasound CT MR*, 32:288–299. http://dx.doi.org/10.1053/j.sult.2011.03.003 PMID:21782119

28. Perez EA, Spano JP (2012). Current and emerging targeted therapies for metastatic breast cancer. *Cancer*, 118:3014–3025. http://dx.doi.org/10.1002/cncr.26356 PMID:22006669

5.3 Oesophageal cancer

5 ORGAN SITE

Elizabeth A. Montgomery

Fred T. Bosman (reviewer)
Paul Brennan (reviewer)
Reza Malekzadeh (reviewer)

Summary

- Oesophageal carcinomas are less common than cancers of the colon and stomach but often prove lethal based on diagnosis of predominantly late-stage disease.

- The two main types of oesophageal carcinoma are squamous cell carcinoma and adenocarcinoma.

- Both types are more common in men than women, but squamous cell carcinomas are encountered in individuals from low-resource regions, whereas adenocarcinomas tend to arise in high-resource populations.

- Both types are successfully managed by mucosal ablation strategies if patients present with early-stage lesions, whereas chemoradiation treatment offers limited but slowly improving success in patients presenting with late-stage lesions.

- Screening protocols remain poorly developed for oesophageal carcinomas.

Oesophageal cancer is a malignant, usually epithelial neoplasm most commonly showing squamous, glandular (adenocarcinoma), or neuroendocrine differentiation and arising in the oesophagus. Other, rarer types of malignant neoplasms can be encountered (adenoid cystic carcinoma, adenosquamous carcinoma, muco-epidermoid carcinoma, mixed adenoneuroendocrine carcinoma, various sarcomas, and melanoma). Only squamous cell carcinoma and adenocarcinoma are addressed here as they account for most oesophageal malignant neoplasms.

Oesophageal squamous cell carcinoma

Squamous cell carcinoma of the oesophagus (Fig. 5.3.1) is a malignant epithelial neoplasm with squamous differentiation consisting of keratinocyte cells, often with intercellular bridges or production of keratin.

Etiology

Squamous cell carcinoma of the oesophagus is characterized by great geographical variation. Pockets of high incidence (> 50 per 100 000 people) occur in the Islamic Republic of Iran (e.g. Golestan Province; > 100 per 100 000), parts of China (e.g. Linxian, Henan Province; > 130 per 100 000), and Zimbabwe. Intermediate incidence is seen in East Africa, southern Brazil, the Caribbean, much of China, parts of Central Asia, northern India, and southern Europe; incidence is low in North America, northern Europe, and western Africa. There are some data correlating ethnicity with the risk of squamous cell carcinoma, indicating that Turkish or Mongolian people in Central Asia and African Americans in North America are more likely than other people in those regions to be diagnosed with squamous cell carcinoma.

Alcohol consumption and tobacco smoking and chewing are the strongest risk factors for the development of oesophageal squamous cell carcinoma, although these associations display marked geographical variation. Cessation of smoking substantially reduces the smoking-associated risk. Intake of hot beverages (hot maté in parts of South America; hot tea, hot coffee, or hot soups elsewhere) is similarly

Fig. 5.3.1. Ulcerated oesophageal squamous cell carcinoma.

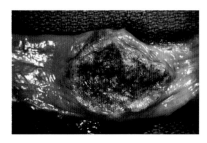

Epidemiology

Oesophageal cancer

- Oesophageal cancer is the eighth most common cancer worldwide, with an estimated 456 000 new cases (3% of all cancers) and 0.4 million cancer deaths (5% of all cancer deaths) in 2012. About 73% of all new cases occurred in countries at low or medium levels of human development, and 49% of all new cases occurred in China.
- Incidence and mortality rates are elevated in Central and East Asia as well as in eastern Africa. Incidence rates tend to be relatively low in western Africa and in some Latin American countries.
- Incidence varies 15-fold between countries worldwide in men and almost 20-fold in women. Incidence and mortality rates are 2–4 times as high in men as in women.
- Due to the high fatality rate, mortality rates are close to incidence rates, regardless of sex differences and human development levels.
- Incidence and mortality trends are variable and reflect the changing prevalence and distribution of the underlying risk factors for oesophageal cancer and its main histological subtypes (adenocarcinoma and squamous cell carcinoma). An increasing tendency to classify cancers located at the gastro-oesophageal junction as adenocarcinoma (rather than gastric cardia cancer) may also have had an impact on the overall trends.

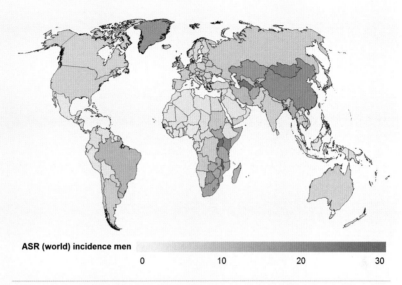

Map 5.3.1. Global distribution of estimated age-standardized (World) incidence rates (ASR) per 100 000, for oesophageal cancer in men, 2012.

ASR (world) incidence men

0   10   20   30

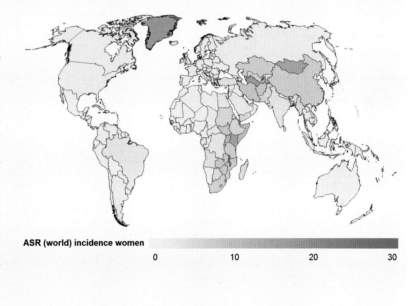

Map 5.3.2. Global distribution of estimated age-standardized (World) incidence rates (ASR) per 100 000, for oesophageal cancer in women, 2012.

ASR (world) incidence women

0   10   20   30

For more details about the maps and charts presented in this chapter, see "A guide to the epidemiology data in *World Cancer Report*".

associated with risk of oesophageal squamous cell carcinoma, as is ingestion of caustic substances (such as occurs in suicide attempts and in accidental swallowing of household toxins by children). Certain dietary habits (low intake of fresh fruits and vegetables, fresh meat or fish, and dairy products, and high intake of barbecued meats and pickled vegetables, which may result in exposure to *N*-nitroso compounds) are associated with a high incidence of oesophageal squamous cell carcinoma. Use of opium, poor oral health, and poor nutrition all interact to affect outcome in oesophageal squamous cell carcinoma in

Chart 5.3.1. Estimated global number of new cases and deaths with proportions by major world regions, for oesophageal cancer in both sexes combined, 2012.

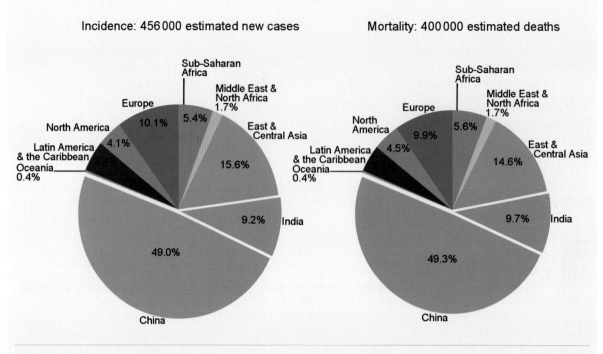

Incidence: 456 000 estimated new cases

Mortality: 400 000 estimated deaths

Chart 5.3.2. Age-standardized (World) incidence rates per 100 000 by year in selected populations, for oesophageal cancer in men, circa 1975–2012.

Chart 5.3.3. Age-standardized (World) incidence rates per 100 000 by year in selected populations, for oesophageal cancer in women, circa 1975–2012.

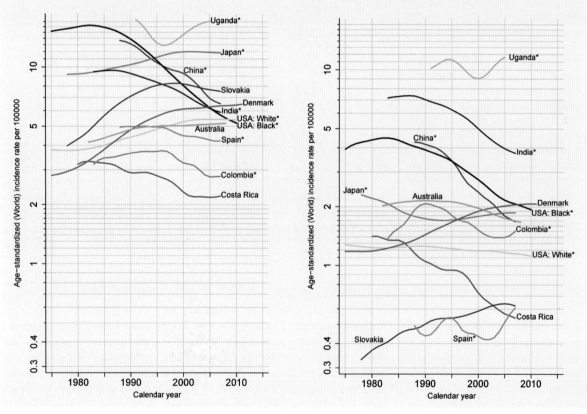

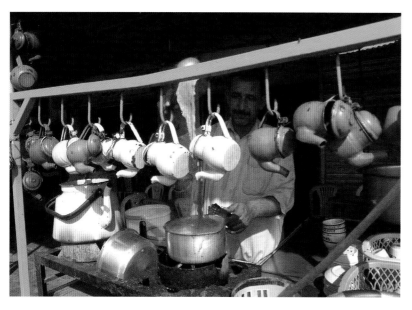

high-risk areas. For example, in the Islamic Republic of Iran, opium intake is associated with poor outcome in univariate analysis but not in adjusted models [1]. Other circumstances mediating increased risk include having Plummer–Vinson syndrome (sideropenic dysphagia, including dysphagia due to oesophageal webs, glossitis, and iron-deficiency anaemia, usually in postmenopausal women), coeliac disease, and achalasia. Finally, exposure to ionizing radiation, often from treatment for breast carcinoma, is a risk factor.

Given that alcohol consumption and tobacco use are the two major known causes of oesophageal squamous cell carcinoma, an Australian study assessed respective population attributable fractions based on 305 cases and 1554 controls. The results were 49% (95% confidence interval [CI], 38–60%) and 32% (95% CI, 25–40%) of oesophageal squamous cell carcinoma cases attributable to smoking and heavy alcohol consumption, respectively. More than 75% of the oesophageal squamous cell carcinoma burden in men could be attributed to smokers with heavy alcohol consumption

[2]. Polymorphisms in acetaldehyde dehydrogenase 2 (*ALDH2*) are key to individual susceptibility to upper aerodigestive tract cancer; patients with inactive ALDH2 are at high risk of oesophageal squamous cell carcinoma [3]. In Asians, polymorphisms in the *ALDH* gene family are associated with altered risk of oesophageal squamous cell carcinoma. The effects of these polymorphisms are synergistic with alcohol consumption and smoking. In addition, the polymorphisms in *ALDH* associated with oesophageal carcinoma also result in accumulation of acetaldehyde, which causes flushing upon ingestion of alcohol (the "Asian flush") in about one third of East Asians (Chinese, Japanese, and Koreans) [4]. Genome-wide association studies in Chinese individuals have identified several susceptibility loci, encompassing 5q11, 6p21, 10q23, 12q24, and 21q22 and including genes related to those encoding ALDH and thereby linked to the association between alcohol consumption and oesophageal squamous cell carcinoma in both Chinese and Japanese people [5,6]. The prevalence of oesophageal squamous dysplasia parallels rates of invasive oesophageal

squamous cell carcinoma; it is typically found in 25% or more of adults older than 35 years in north central China, where the risk of this malignancy is among the highest in the world [7].

Pathology and genetics

Oesophageal squamous cell carcinoma is defined as a squamous neoplasm that invades through the epithelial basement membrane into the lamina propria, submucosa, muscularis propria, or deeper. Variable amounts of keratinization are seen, manifested by cells showing brightly eosinophilic opaque cytoplasm (Fig. 5.3.3A,B). Invasion into the lamina propria begins with the proliferation of rete-like projections of neoplastic squamous epithelium. Both horizontal and vertical spread are observed. Tumours can penetrate vertically through the oesophageal wall and invade the intramural lymphatic channels and veins.

The development of oesophageal squamous cell carcinoma is understood to be a multistep process that progresses from normal squamous epithelium to include intraepithelial neoplasia (dysplasia; Fig. 5.3.3C) and culminates in the growth of invasive carcinoma. Mutation in the *TP53* gene is an early event, sometimes detectable in intraepithelial neoplasia. Amplification of cyclin D1 occurs in 20–30% of these tumours. Inactivation of CDKN2A, either by homozygous deletion or by de novo methylation, appears to be associated with advanced disease.

The scope of molecular analyses applicable to all tumour types is indicated from studies identifying alterations in genes, proteins, and microRNAs in oesophageal squamous cell carcinoma, of which 10 or more studies in each category are available. Epigenetic abnormalities are evident from DNA methylation, histone deacetylation, chromatin remodelling, gene imprinting, and non-coding RNA regulation studies [8]. High-throughput genotyping of metastatic tumours has identified phosphatidylinositol 3-kinase (PI3K) and *BRAF* mutations among the

Fig. 5.3.3. Invasive squamous cell carcinoma and precursor lesions. (A) Nests of carcinoma cells with brightly eosinophilic cytoplasm in keeping with keratinization embedded in desmoplastic stroma from a mucosal biopsy. (B) This squamous cell carcinoma shows a basaloid pattern such that the cells are small and darkly stained owing to their high nuclear-to-cytoplasmic ratio. The clue that this is a squamous cell carcinoma is the overt keratinization at the right side of the field. (C) High-grade squamous dysplasia (intraepithelial neoplasia) of the oesophagus. This lesion has not invaded the basement membrane (Tis) but shows marked cytological alterations. In the oesophagus, such lesions are typically not associated with human papillomavirus.

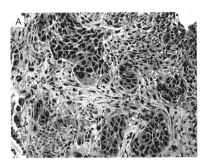
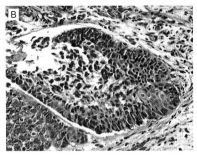
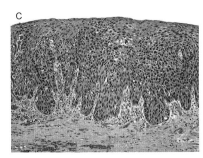

somatic mutations evident [9]. In a separate study, inactivating *NOTCH1* mutations were identified in 21% of oesophageal squamous cell carcinomas from the USA but only rarely in such tumours from China [10].

Familial predisposition to oesophageal cancer has been studied predominantly in association with focal non-epidermolytic palmoplantar keratoderma (also known as tylosis), a rare condition in industrialized countries (low-risk populations). This autosomal dominant inherited disorder of the palmar and plantar skin surfaces is associated with oesophageal cancer. The causative locus, the tylosis oesophageal cancer (*TOC*) gene, maps to 17q25, with missense mutations (c.557T → C [p.Ile186Thr] and c.566C → T [p.Pro189Leu]) in *RHBDF2*, which encodes the inactive rhomboid protease RHBDF2 (also known as iRhom2) [11].

Prospects

The overall prognosis of oesophageal squamous cell carcinoma remains poor based on diagnosis of predominantly late-stage disease. Screening programmes to detect precursor and early-stage lesions have been implemented in some high-risk populations. Radiofrequency ablation therapy and other forms of endoscopic treatments appear promising for eradication of early lesions [12,13].

Oesophageal adenocarcinoma

Adenocarcinoma of the oesophagus is a malignant epithelial neoplasm with glandular differentiation arising predominantly from Barrett mucosa and typically encountered in the lower third of the oesophagus.

Etiology

Oesophageal adenocarcinoma is characterized by a high male-to-female ratio (from 4 to 7), with a higher incidence among Caucasians and among subgroups with a high socioeconomic status [14,15]. The incidence and prevalence of oesophageal adenocarcinoma was reported as rising during the last decades of the 20th century in a number of high-resource countries [14–16]. For example, in the USA, incidence rates for adenocarcinoma have been rising markedly, whereas rates for squamous cell carcinoma are declining steadily. From 1999 to 2008, rates among White men increased substantially (1.8% per year), as among White women (2.1% per year) and Hispanic men (2.8% per year). No significant changes were observed for men or women of other racial/ethnic groups. While rates of oesophageal adenocarcinoma have been increasing among Caucasians in some populations, it is extremely difficult to quantify the rate of increase from analysis of time trends in registry data, due

partly to improvements in recording and capturing histology information (decreasing numbers of tumours without histological confirmation) but also because of changes in the assignment of cancers at the gastro-oesophageal junction, from the gastric cardia (or gastric, other/non-specified) to the oesophagus.

Obesity is a strong risk factor for oesophageal adenocarcinoma, as is gastro-oesophageal reflux disease. The trend of increasing incidence rates of oesophageal adenocarcinoma parallels the growing obesity epidemic and the prevalence of gastro-oesophageal reflux disease [15]. However, in a 2012 study in the USA, incidence rates of oesophageal adenocarcinoma were 7-fold higher among White men than among Black men, despite data indicating that the prevalence of obesity is higher among Black men and women than among White men and women [15].

The countries with the highest incidence of this tumour type are the United Kingdom, Australia, the Netherlands, and the USA. Relatively lower incidence rates are reported from eastern Europe and Scandinavia. In Latin America, Asia, and Africa, oesophageal adenocarcinoma remains uncommon, but it is possibly also underreported (particularly in Latin America).

Although familial association has been reported for patients with

Risk of malignant progression in Barrett oesophagus patients

Liam J. Murray

Barrett oesophagus (BO) is a precursor of oesophageal adenocarcinoma. The magnitude of cancer risk in BO is crucial in determining whether the benefits of screening, surveillance, or treatment of BO outweigh any risks and whether such strategies are cost-effective. The published incidence of malignancy in BO varies widely, from 0 to 35.5 cases per 1000 person-years of risk (pyr) [1]. To date, most studies have been small, and publication bias in favour of studies showing high risks has been demonstrated [2]. Other design issues, such as the inclusion of unrepresentative cohorts of BO patients (e.g. patients from tertiary referral centres), inclusion of those at high risk of progression (e.g. with high-grade dysplasia at baseline), incomplete follow-up of patients, or failure to exclude early incident (most likely prevalent) cancers, have resulted in overestimation of the risks of malignant progression in BO. Differing criteria for diagnosis of BO, for example inclusion of patients without specialized intestinal metaplasia, and differing definitions of malignant progression, for example inclusion/exclusion of incident high-grade dysplasia, have also contributed to the variation in observed rates. The combined risk of oesophageal adenocarcinoma or

high-grade dysplasia may provide a better estimate of malignant progression than risk of oesophageal adenocarcinoma alone, although it will overestimate risk as not all patients with high-grade dysplasia would progress to cancer in the absence of therapeutic intervention [3].

The best estimates of risk of malignant progression in BO are provided by population-based studies with long-term follow-up for a high proportion of patients (excluding those with high-grade dysplasia at baseline) and discounting events occurring soon after diagnosis. Several such studies have recently been published [4–8]. Even in these studies, differing BO definitions, different proportions of patients with low-grade dysplasia at baseline, and differing approaches to, and completeness of, follow-up have resulted in variable estimates of malignant progression. Among patients without low-grade dysplasia at baseline, the incidence of oesophageal adenocarcinoma/high-grade dysplasia ranged from 2.2 per 1000 pyr [4] to 5.2 per 1000 pyr [6,8]; however, the higher estimates were not based on follow-up of all diagnosed cases and may have overestimated risk. Risk of oesophageal adenocarcinoma/high-grade dysplasia was 2–6-fold higher in patients with low-grade

dysplasia at baseline than in those without low-grade dysplasia.

Using currently available data, it is difficult to reach a definite conclusion about the risk of malignant progression in BO, but it is lower than previously thought and, in patients without low-grade dysplasia at baseline, appears to be lower than 5 cases of oesophageal adenocarcinoma/high-grade dysplasia per 1000 pyr.

References

1. Yousef F et al. (2008). Am J Epidemiol, 168:237–249. http://dx.doi.org/10.1093/aje/kwn121 PMID:18550563

2. Shaheen NJ et al. (2000). Gastroenterology, 119:333–338. http://dx.doi.org/10.1053/gast.2000.9302 PMID:10930368

3. Schnell TG et al. (2001). Gastroenterology, 120:1607–1619. http://dx.doi.org/10.1053/gast.2001.25065 PMID:11375943

4. Hvid-Jensen F et al. (2011). N Engl J Med, 365:1375–1383. http://dx.doi.org/10.1056/NEJMoa1103042 PMID:21995385

5. Bhat S et al. (2011). J Natl Cancer Inst, 103:1049–1057. http://dx.doi.org/10.1093/jnci/djr203 PMID:21680910

6. de Jonge PJ et al. (2010). Gut, 59:1030–1036. http://dx.doi.org/10.1136/gut.2009.176701 PMID:20639249

7. Jung KW et al. (2011). Am J Gastroenterol, 106:1447–1455. http://dx.doi.org/10.1038/ajg.2011.130 PMID:21483461

8. Rugge M et al. (2012). Ann Surg, 256:788–794. http://dx.doi.org/10.1097/SLA.0b013e3182737a7e PMID:23095623

oesophageal adenocarcinoma, population-based studies show limited influence of familial risk, consistent with the rapid changes in incidence rates observed in many populations over a very short time period. The epidemiological features of adenocarcinoma of the oesophagus and of the oesophago-gastric junction match those of patients with known intestinal metaplasia in the distal oesophagus, i.e. Barrett oesophagus [15]. Barrett oesophagus has been identified as the single most important precursor lesion and risk factor for oesophageal adenocarcinoma,

irrespective of the length of the segment with intestinal metaplasia. Intestinal metaplasia of the oesophagus develops when the squamous oesophageal epithelium is replaced by columnar epithelium during the process of healing after repetitive injury, typically associated with gastro-oesophageal reflux disease. Intestinal metaplasia can be detected in the majority of patients with oesophageal adenocarcinoma [17].

A meta-analysis of studies in patients with Barrett oesophagus demonstrated an incidence of progression to adenocarcinoma of about

6.1 per 1000 person-years, which reduced to 3.9 per 1000 person-years when only high-quality studies were considered [18], corresponding to a lifetime risk of about 10% in these patients. However, these results may be overestimations that reflect various types of bias in the studies. More recently, an Irish study reported a rate of 3.8 per 1000 person-years [19], whereas a Danish study showed a considerably lower progression rate of only 0.12% per year [20], although obesity is far less prevalent in the Danish population than in the United States or Irish

Fig. 5.3.4. Oesophageal adenocarcinoma and precursor lesions. (A) High-grade columnar epithelial dysplasia in Barrett oesophagus. Note the markedly hyperchromatic nuclei at the surface of the sample (mucosal biopsy). This process in glandular mucosa is a precursor to adenocarcinoma. (B) Oesophageal adenocarcinoma. This gland-forming malignant neoplasm has the appearance of an intestinal-type adenocarcinoma, in the Laurén classification for gastric carcinomas.

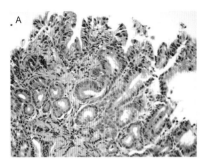 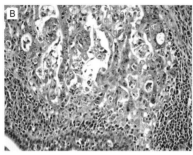

population (see "Risk of malignant progression in Barrett oesophagus patients").

Chronic gastro-oesophageal reflux disease is the usual source of mucosal injury and also provides an abnormal environment during the healing process that predisposes to intestinal metaplasia and adenocarcinoma. In a large Swedish study, individuals with long-standing and severe gastro-oesophageal reflux disease symptoms had a 40-fold increased risk of oesophageal adenocarcinoma [21]. Both experimental and clinical data indicate that combined oesophageal exposure to both gastric acid and duodenal contents (bile acids and pancreatic enzymes) appears to be more carcinogenic than exposure to only gastric juice or duodenal contents. An association between alcohol consumption and oesophageal adenocarcinoma has not been well established. A reduced risk of oesophageal adenocarcinoma is associated with *Helicobacter pylori* infection, and particularly *H. pylori* strains with the CagA protein. A protective effect has been suggested after the use of non-steroidal anti-inflammatory drugs, but not all studies have supported such data.

Pathology and genetics
Adenocarcinoma in Barrett oesophagus develops through a progressive sequence of morphologically

identifiable premalignant lesions termed "dysplasia". Dysplasia is diagnosed by the presence and degree of cytological and architectural atypia [22]. Low-grade dysplasia shows pits with relatively preserved architecture, or minimal distortion, containing cells with atypical nuclei limited to the basal portion of the cell cytoplasm. High-grade dysplasia is diagnosed by the presence of marked cytological abnormalities and/or significant architectural complexity of the glands (Fig. 5.3.4A). Cytological abnormalities include nuclear pleomorphism and loss of polarity, irregularity of nuclear contour, and increased nuclear-to-cytoplasmic ratio. Architectural

abnormalities of high-grade changes include crypt budding, branching, marked crowding, and, rarely, a cribriform growth pattern.

Intramucosal adenocarcinoma (invasion into the lamina propria; T1a) show single cells or small clusters of compact back-to-back glands within the lamina propria, a cribriform or solid pattern of growth with expansion and distortion of the adjacent crypts, and a highly distorted/irregular glandular proliferation not explained by the presence of pre-existing glands. The presence of necrosis and/or desmoplasia is evidence in favour of adenocarcinomas as well, although these features are rarely present in carcinomas limited to the mucosa.

Oesophageal adenocarcinomas are typically papillary and/or tubular. Most cases are of the intestinal type in the Laurén classification (Fig. 5.3.4B), whereas some are of the diffuse type. Multiple genetic alterations are involved in the development and progression of Barrett oesophagus to oesophageal adenocarcinoma, encompassing tumour suppressor genes, oncogenes, growth factor receptors, or enzymes that play important roles in diverse cellular functions such as cell-cycle control, apoptosis, cell signalling, cell adhesion and genetic stability, signal transduction, and DNA repair. Gains in the region of

Fig. 5.3.5. Schematic of protein alterations in DOCK2 and ELMO1 detected by whole-exome sequencing of oesophageal adenocarcinoma. Coding alterations in oesophageal adenocarcinoma are coloured either black (missense) or red (splice site or nonsense); silent mutations are depicted in grey. Conserved domain mapping is from UniProt. DHR, Dlg homologous region, ELMO, engulfment and cell motility; PH, Pleckstrin homology; SH3, SRC homology 3.

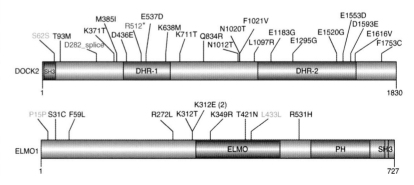

Fig. 5.3.6. Oesophageal cell collection using non-endoscopic devices. (A) The deflated balloon is inserted into the stomach. (B) Once deemed to be in the stomach, the balloon is inflated through the attached catheter and pulled up the oesophagus. Mucosal cells adhere to the balloon, which is then deflated and removed. A similar procedure based on the use of a cytosponge may also be used.

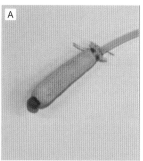
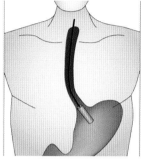
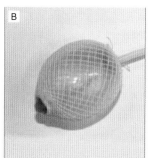
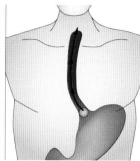

8q (region of *c-myc*) and 20q, and losses at 3p (*FHIT*), 4q, 5q (*APC*) and 18q (*SMAD4*, *DCC*) have all been reported, with an increasing number of chromosomal alterations in the sequence from metaplasia to intraepithelial neoplasia to carcinoma. Gene silencing by promoter hypermethylation has been demonstrated frequently for the *CDH1* gene (which encodes E-cadherin) and the *APC*, *p16*, *MGMT*, and *HPP1* genes. Disorders of *ARID* are also noted.

Exome and whole-genome sequencing of 149 and 15 oesophageal adenocarcinomas has been recently reported [23]. A mutational signature was defined by a high prevalence of A → C transversions at AA dinucleotides. Of 26 significantly mutated genes, *TP53*, *CDKN2*, *SMAD4*, *ARID4*, and *PIK3CA* had been implicated previously. The new significantly mutated genes included chromatin modifying factors and candidate contributors *SPG20*, *TLR4*, *ELMO1*, and *DOCK2* (Fig. 5.3.5). Functional analysis of the relevant mutations in *ELMO1* identified increased cellular invasion.

Prospects

Novel endoscopic techniques for early detection and treatment of oesophageal adenocarcinoma offer promise. Ablation therapy for high-grade dysplasia (the strongest risk factor for adenocarcinoma) is probably cost-effective [24]. Ideal strategies for population-based screening in high-risk patients remain poorly established and inconsistent.

A recent review [25] determined that endoscopic screening is invasive, costly, and error-prone owing to sampling bias and the subjective diagnosis of dysplasia. Non-endoscopic cell sampling methods (Fig. 5.3.6) are less invasive and more cost-effective than endoscopy, but the sensitivity and specificity of cytological assessment of atypia have been disappointing. The use of biomarkers to analyse samples collected using pan-oesophageal cell collection devices may improve diagnostic accuracy.

References

1. Aghcheli K, Marjani HA, Nasrollahzadeh D *et al.* (2011). Prognostic factors for esophageal squamous cell carcinoma – a population-based study in Golestan Province, Iran, a high incidence area. *PLoS One*, 6:e22152. http://dx.doi.org/10.1371/journal.pone.0022152 PMID:21811567

2. Pandeya N, Olsen CM, Whiteman DC (2013). Sex differences in the proportion of esophageal squamous cell carcinoma cases attributable to tobacco smoking and alcohol consumption. *Cancer Epidemiol*, 37:579–584. http://dx.doi.org/10.1016/j.canep.2013.05.011 PMID:23830137

3. Morita M, Kumashiro R, Kubo N *et al.* (2010). Alcohol drinking, cigarette smoking, and the development of squamous cell carcinoma of the esophagus: epidemiology, clinical findings, and prevention. *Int J Clin Oncol*, 15:126–134. http://dx.doi.org/10.1007/s10147-010-0056-7 PMID:20224884

4. Brooks PJ, Enoch MA, Goldman D *et al.* (2009). The alcohol flushing response: an unrecognized risk factor for esophageal cancer from alcohol consumption [Review]. *PLoS Med*, 6:e50. http://dx.doi.org/10.1371/journal.pmed.1000050 PMID:19320537

5. Wu C, Kraft P, Zhai K *et al.* (2012). Genome-wide association analyses of esophageal squamous cell carcinoma in Chinese identify multiple susceptibility loci and gene-environment interactions. *Nat Genet*, 44:1090–1097. http://dx.doi.org/10.1038/ng.2411 PMID:22960999

6. Wu C, Hu Z, He Z *et al.* (2011). Genome-wide association study identifies three new susceptibility loci for esophageal squamous-cell carcinoma in Chinese populations. *Nat Genet*, 43:679–684. http://dx.doi.org/10.1038/ng.849 PMID:21642993

7. Taylor PR, Abnet CC, Dawsey SM (2013). Squamous dysplasia – the precursor lesion for esophageal squamous cell carcinoma. *Cancer Epidemiol Biomarkers Prev*, 22:540–552. http://dx.doi.org/10.1158/1055-9965.EPI-12-1347 PMID:23549398

8. Chen J, Kwong DL, Cao T *et al.* (2013). Esophageal squamous cell carcinoma (ESCC): advance in genomics and molecular genetics. *Dis Esophagus*, http://dx.doi.org/10.1111/dote.12088 PMID:23796192

9. Maeng CH, Lee J, van Hummelen P *et al.* (2012). High-throughput genotyping in metastatic esophageal squamous cell carcinoma identifies phosphoinositide-3-kinase and *BRAF* mutations. *PLoS One*, 7:e41655. http://dx.doi.org/10.1371/journal.pone.0041655 PMID:22870241

10. Agrawal N, Jiao Y, Bettegowda C *et al.* (2012). Comparative genomic analysis of esophageal adenocarcinoma and squamous cell carcinoma. *Cancer Discov*, 2:899–905. http://dx.doi.org/10.1158/2159-8290.CD-12-0189 PMID:22877736

11. Blaydon DC, Etheridge SL, Risk JM *et al.* (2012). *RHBDF2* mutations are associated with tylosis, a familial esophageal cancer syndrome. *Am J Hum Genet*, 90:340–346. http://dx.doi.org/10.1016/j.ajhg.2011.12.008 PMID:22265016

12. Dubecz A, Gall I, Solymosi N *et al.* (2012). Temporal trends in long-term survival and cure rates in esophageal cancer: a SEER database analysis. *J Thorac Oncol*, 7:443–447. http://dx.doi.org/10.1097/JTO.0b013e3182397751 PMID:22173700

13. Bergman JJ, Zhang YM, He S *et al.* (2011). Outcomes from a prospective trial of endoscopic radiofrequency ablation of early squamous cell neoplasia of the esophagus. *Gastrointest Endosc*, 74:1181–1190. http://dx.doi.org/10.1016/j.gie.2011.05.024 PMID:21839994

14. Engel LS, Chow WH, Vaughan TL *et al.* (2003). Population attributable risks of esophageal and gastric cancers. *J Natl Cancer Inst*, 95:1404–1413. http://dx.doi.org/10.1093/jnci/djg047 PMID:13130116

15. Simard EP, Ward EM, Siegel R, Jemal A (2012). Cancers with increasing incidence trends in the United States: 1999 through 2008. *CA Cancer J Clin*, 62:118–128. http://dx.doi.org/10.3322/caac.20141 PMID:22281605

16. Dikken JL, Lemmens VE, Wouters MW *et al.* (2012). Increased incidence and survival for oesophageal cancer but not for gastric cardia cancer in the Netherlands. *Eur J Cancer*, 48:1624–1632. http://dx.doi.org/10.1016/j.ejca.2012.01.009 PMID:22317953

17. Chandrasoma P, Wijetunge S, DeMeester S *et al.* (2012). Columnar-lined esophagus without intestinal metaplasia has no proven risk of adenocarcinoma. *Am J Surg Pathol*, 36:1–7. http://dx.doi.org/10.1097/PAS.0b013e31822a5a2c PMID:21959311

18. Yousef F, Cardwell C, Cantwell MM *et al.* (2008). The incidence of esophageal cancer and high-grade dysplasia in Barrett's esophagus: a systematic review and meta-analysis. *Am J Epidemiol*, 168:237–249. http://dx.doi.org/10.1093/aje/kwn121 PMID:18550563

19. Bhat S, Coleman HG, Yousef F *et al.* (2011). Risk of malignant progression in Barrett's esophagus patients: results from a large population-based study. *J Natl Cancer Inst*, 103:1049–1057. http://dx.doi.org/10.1093/jnci/djr203 PMID:21680910

20. Hvid-Jensen F, Pedersen L, Drewes AM *et al.* (2011). Incidence of adenocarcinoma among patients with Barrett's esophagus. *N Engl J Med*, 365:1375–1383. http://dx.doi.org/10.1056/NEJMoa1103042 PMID:21995385

21. Lagergren J, Bergström R, Lindgren A, Nyrén O (1999). Symptomatic gastroesophageal reflux as a risk factor for esophageal adenocarcinoma. *N Engl J Med*, 340:825–831. http://dx.doi.org/10.1056/NEJM199903183401101 PMID:10080844

22. Montgomery E, Bronner MP, Goldblum JR *et al.* (2001). Reproducibility of the diagnosis of dysplasia in Barrett esophagus: a reaffirmation. *Hum Pathol*, 32:368–378. http://dx.doi.org/10.1053/hupa.2001.23510 PMID:11331953

23. Dulak AM, Stojanov P, Peng S *et al.* (2013). Exome and whole-genome sequencing of esophageal adenocarcinoma identifies recurrent driver events and mutational complexity. *Nat Genet*, 45:478–486. http://dx.doi.org/10.1038/ng.2591 PMID:23525077

24. Hur C, Choi SE, Rubenstein JH *et al.* (2012). The cost effectiveness of radiofrequency ablation for Barrett's esophagus. *Gastroenterology*, 143:567–575. http://dx.doi.org/10.1053/j.gastro.2012.05.010 PMID:22626608

25. Lao-Sirieix P, Fitzgerald RC (2012). Screening for oesophageal cancer. *Nat Rev Clin Oncol*, 9:278–287. http://dx.doi.org/10.1038/nrclinonc.2012.35 PMID:22430857

5.4 Stomach cancer

Fátima Carneiro

Yung-Jue Bang (reviewer)
Takanori Hattori (reviewer)
Elizabeth A. Montgomery (reviewer)

Summary

- Most stomach cancers (90%) are sporadic. In almost all countries, a steady decline in gastric cancer mortality rates has occurred in the past few decades.

- *Helicobacter pylori* is the major environmental cause of gastric cancer development. Other factors contributing to risk include dietary composition – particularly intake of pickled vegetables – and smoking.

- Molecular pathogenesis of gastric cancer is complex. Genes related to receptor tyrosine kinase (RTK)/RAS signalling are frequently amplified, in particular *FGFR2*, *KRAS*, *ERBB2*, *EGFR*, and *MET*. The product of the *HER2* oncogene, when either overexpressed or amplified, is a prognostic factor.

- Hereditary gastric cancer contributes to 1–3% of the burden of stomach cancer. Two syndromes have been identified: hereditary diffuse gastric cancer and gastric adenocarcinoma and proximal polyposis of the stomach.

- Hereditary diffuse gastric cancer is caused by germline alterations of the E-cadherin (*CDH1*) gene; prophylactic gastrectomy is recommended for asymptomatic carriers of pathogenic *CDH1* mutations.

Most stomach cancers are gastric carcinomas, which are malignant epithelial neoplasms. Non-epithelial tumours of the stomach predominantly include lymphomas and mesenchymal tumours. Gastric carcinomas represent a biologically and genetically heterogeneous group of tumours with multifactorial etiologies, both environmental and genetic. They are characterized by broad morphological heterogeneity with respect to patterns of architecture and growth, cell differentiation, histogenesis, and molecular pathogenesis.

Most cases of gastric cancer are sporadic, and familial clustering is observed in about 10% of cases. Hereditary gastric cancer accounts for a very low percentage of cases (1–3%), and two hereditary syndromes have been characterized: hereditary diffuse gastric cancer and gastric adenocarcinoma and proximal polyposis of the stomach. Furthermore, gastric cancer can develop in the setting of other hereditary cancer syndromes.

Etiology

Gastric carcinogenesis is a multistep and multifactorial process that, in many cases, appears to involve a progression from normal mucosa through chronic gastritis (chronic inflammation of the gastric mucosa), atrophic gastritis (with loss of gastric glands), and intestinal metaplasia (substitution of gastric epithelium by intestinal epithelium) to dysplasia (intraepithelial neoplasia) and carcinoma, a sequence of events that may last several years. This sequence has been designated as the Correa cascade of multistep gastric carcinogenesis [1]. However, the Correa model does not explain all carcinogenic steps of gastric cancer. Actually, a proportion of gastric adenocarcinomas arise in non-intestinalized mucosa and retain a gastric phenotype (and gastric differentiation is also observed in gastric dysplasia, the ultimate precursor lesion of gastric adenocarcinoma). Also, in the recently identified syndrome gastric adenocarcinoma and proximal polyposis of the stomach (discussed below), gastric dysplasia and gastric adenocarcinoma develop in fundic gland polyps of the proximal stomach and are related not to intestinal metaplasia but instead to foveolar hyperplasia. Together, this evidence shows that gastric adenocarcinoma can arise

Epidemiology

Stomach cancer

- Stomach cancer is the fifth most common cancer worldwide, with an estimated 952 000 new cases (7% of total cancer incidence) and 723 000 deaths (9% of total cancer mortality) in 2012. Almost three quarters of the new cases occurred in Asia, and more than two fifths occurred in China.
- There is a 10-fold international variation in stomach cancer incidence; rates in men are approximately double those observed in women.
- The highest age-standardized incidence rates are in East Asia and central and eastern Europe. Incidence rates tend to be relatively low in Africa and in North America.
- The case fatality rate is lower in countries with high levels of human development (overall mortality-to-incidence ratio, 0.65) than in countries at low or medium levels of human development (0.83).
- Over the past 50 years, incidence and mortality rates of the non-cardia type of gastric cancer have been uniformly decreasing in almost all countries; rates of gastric cardia cancer have, however, been stable or increasing in the past two to three decades.

Map 5.4.1. Global distribution of estimated age-standardized (World) incidence rates (ASR) per 100 000, for stomach cancer in men, 2012.

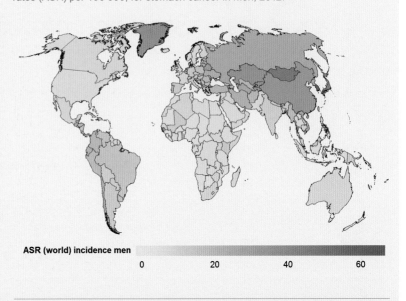

ASR (world) incidence men

Map 5.4.2. Global distribution of estimated age-standardized (World) incidence rates (ASR) per 100 000, for stomach cancer in women, 2012.

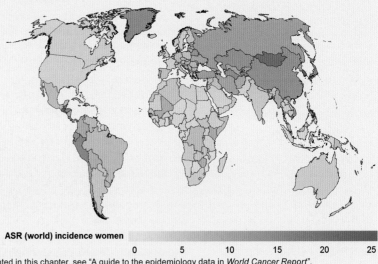

ASR (world) incidence women

For more details about the maps and charts presented in this chapter, see "A guide to the epidemiology data in *World Cancer Report*".

from the gastric epithelium. These findings challenge the classic proposed histogenetic pathway from chronic atrophic gastritis through intestinal metaplasia to adenocarcinoma (with glandular structure), which is frequently designated as intestinal carcinoma (Laurén classification), a misnomer for these cases. Another type of gastric carcinoma, so-called diffuse carcinoma (Laurén classification), probably develops de novo from gastric mucosa. Except for the diffuse carcinomas developing in a hereditary setting (discussed below), no precursor lesions have been well characterized for this type of gastric cancer.

Among environmental factors contributing to increased risk of gastric cancer, *Helicobacter pylori* infection plays a major role. Almost all non-cardia gastric cancers develop from a background of *H. pylori*-infected mucosa [2]. *H. pylori* is a Gram-negative bacterium that colonizes the gastric mucosa. In 1994, IARC categorized

Chart 5.4.1. Estimated global number of new cases and deaths with proportions by major world regions, for stomach cancer in both sexes combined, 2012.

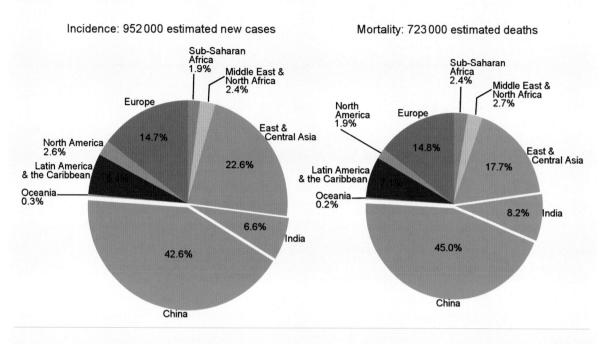

Incidence: 952 000 estimated new cases

- Sub-Saharan Africa 1.9%
- Middle East & North Africa 2.4%
- Europe 14.7%
- North America 2.6%
- Latin America & the Caribbean 5.4%
- Oceania 0.3%
- East & Central Asia 22.6%
- India 6.6%
- China 42.6%

Mortality: 723 000 estimated deaths

- Sub-Saharan Africa 2.4%
- Middle East & North Africa 2.7%
- North America 1.9%
- Europe 14.8%
- Latin America & the Caribbean 7.1%
- Oceania 0.2%
- East & Central Asia 17.7%
- India 8.2%
- China 45.0%

Chart 5.4.2. Age-standardized (World) incidence rates per 100 000 by year in selected populations, for stomach cancer in men, circa 1975–2012.

Chart 5.4.3. Age-standardized (World) incidence rates per 100 000 by year in selected populations, for stomach cancer in women, circa 1975–2012.

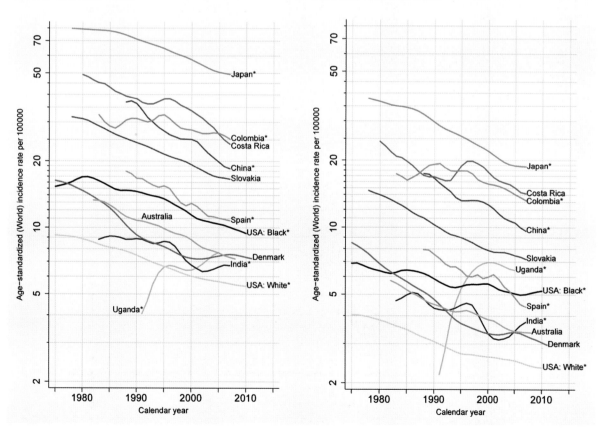

Chart 5.4.2 (men): Japan*, Colombia*, Costa Rica, China*, Slovakia, Australia, Spain*, USA: Black*, Denmark, India*, USA: White*, Uganda*

Chart 5.4.3 (women): Japan*, Costa Rica, Colombia*, China*, Slovakia, Uganda*, USA: Black*, Spain*, India*, Australia, Denmark, USA: White*

Fig. 5.4.1. *Helicobacter pylori* detected in the lumen of gastric glands and adherent to the apical pole of epithelial cells: (A) haematoxylin–eosin (inset: modified Giemsa); (B) Warthin–Starry; (C) immunohistochemistry.

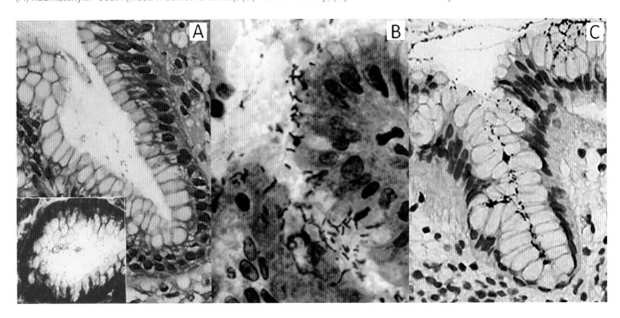

H. pylori as a Group 1 carcinogen for gastric cancer [3] based on results of epidemiological studies that were available at that time; this conclusion was later confirmed. *H. pylori* can be identified in gastric mucosa by routine stains, such as haematoxylin–eosin and modified Giemsa, and other ancillary methods such as Warthin–Starry staining and immunohistochemistry (Fig. 5.4.1). The infection is commonly acquired during early childhood and persists throughout adult life unless eradicated.

Factors associated with colonization and pathogenicity of *H. pylori* include virulence factors – cagA in the *cag* pathogenicity island and the vacuolating cytotoxin vacA [4] – as well as outer membrane proteins of the bacterium. Strains producing the cagA protein that induce a greater degree of inflammation are associated with gastric precancerous lesions and a greater risk of developing cancer of the distal stomach [4]. Although the risk of gastric cancer in some countries of Europe and North America has been related to *vacA* genotype, such relationships have not been observed in countries in East Asia, suggesting that consequences of variation in vacuolating activity are dependent on

geographical region. Corpus-predominant gastritis with multifocal gastric atrophy and hypochlorhydria or achlorhydria is seen in approximately 1% of subjects infected with *H. pylori*. As a direct consequence of elevation in gastric pH, there is a change in gastric flora, with colonization by anaerobic bacteria responsible for the formation of carcinogenic nitrosamines.

Certain dietary habits are associated with an increased risk of gastric cancer [5]. These include high intakes of salt-preserved and/or smoked foods and low intakes of fresh fruit and vegetables. An analysis of 60 relevant studies suggested a potential 50% higher risk of gastric cancer associated with intake of pickled vegetables, and perhaps

Fig. 5.4.2. Food in Seoul, Republic of Korea, typically includes pickled vegetables, the consumption of which is associated with increased risk of gastric cancer.

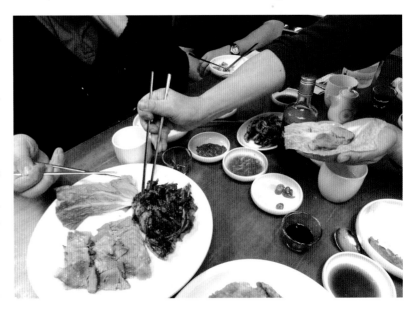

stronger associations in the Republic of Korea and China (Fig. 5.4.2) [6]. Intake of all meat, specifically including red meat and processed meat, is also associated with an increased risk of gastric cancer in the distal stomach. The so-called "Mediterranean diet" was shown to be associated with a significant reduction in the risk of gastric cancer incidence; this diet is characterized as involving high consumption of fruit, vegetables, cereals, legumes, nuts and seeds, and seafood, with olive oil as the main fat source, moderate alcohol consumption (particularly red wine), a low to moderate consumption of dairy products, and a relatively low consumption of red and processed meat.

Tobacco smoking causes stomach cancer; the epidemiological association is not explicable by bias or confounding factors. Smoking also potentiates the carcinogenic effect of infection with cagA-positive *H. pylori*.

Polymorphisms of the interleukin-1β (*IL1B*) gene, which contributes to initiation and amplification of inflammatory response, and of the interleukin-1 receptor antagonist (*IL1RN*) gene, which modulates inflammation, are associated with individual or familial susceptibility to carcinogenesis associated with *H. pylori*. Among individuals with alleles that predispose to inflammation, infection with *H. pylori* may cause increased production of gastric interleukin-1β, leading to severe and sustained inflammation that increases the risk of developing gastric cancer [7].

Pathology

Two major types of gastric carcinoma were described by Laurén in 1965 [8]: the intestinal and diffuse types, which display different clinicopathological profiles and molecular pathogenesis, and often occur in distinct epidemiologic settings. Currently, five major types of gastric cancer are recognized by WHO: tubular (Fig. 5.4.3A), papillary, mucinous, poorly cohesive (with or without signet ring cells) (Fig. 5.4.3B),

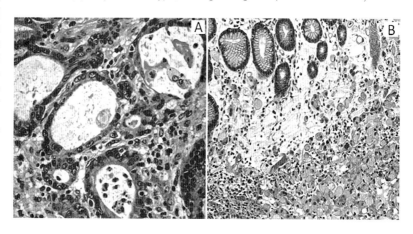

Fig. 5.4.3. Main histological types of gastric carcinoma: (A) intestinal carcinoma (Laurén classification), tubular type (WHO classification); (B) diffuse carcinoma (Laurén classification), poorly cohesive type, with signet ring cells (WHO classification).

and mixed [9]. Tubular and papillary carcinomas roughly correspond to the intestinal type in the Laurén classification, and poorly cohesive carcinomas (encompassing cases constituted, partially or totally, by signet ring cells) correspond to the diffuse type. Furthermore, rare variants account for about 10% of gastric carcinomas.

The gastric antrum (distal stomach) is the most common site of gastric carcinoma. Carcinomas of the oesophago-gastric junction have been most commonly reported in populations in North America and Europe, associated with gastro-oesophageal reflux disease and other characteristics similar to adenocarcinoma arising in Barrett oesophagus, and are unrelated to *H. pylori* infection. However, in parts of Asia, for example in China, but also for a subset of tumours diagnosed in North America and Europe, neoplasms of the proximal stomach arise in a setting of chronic atrophic gastritis with *H. pylori* infection and are similar to distal gastric cancer. Adenocarcinomas located entirely below the oesophago-gastric junction are considered gastric in origin, and for these tumours the use of the ambiguous and often misleading term "carcinoma of the gastric cardia" is discouraged in favour of "carcinoma of the proximal stomach".

Early gastric carcinoma is an invasive carcinoma limited to the mucosa or submucosa, regardless of nodal status. The term "early" does not imply a stage in the genesis of the cancer but means that these are gastric cancers that can often be cured. However, if untreated, 63% of early gastric carcinomas progress to advanced tumours within 5 years. Countries with a high incidence of gastric cancer and in which asymptomatic patients are screened have a high incidence of early gastric carcinomas, ranging from 30% to 50% in Japan and the Republic of Korea, with lower figures for western Europe and North America (16–24%). Lymph-node metastasis occurs in 10–20% of all early gastric carcinomas and correlates with the depth of submucosal invasion and increasing tumour diameter.

Advanced gastric carcinoma invades the muscularis propria of the stomach and beyond. Most patients with advanced carcinoma have lymph-node metastatic disease for which only palliative surgery can be considered. Lymphatic and vascular invasion, often seen in advanced cases, indicate a poor prognosis. Gastric carcinomas can spread by direct extension to adjacent organs, metastasis, or peritoneal dissemination. Carcinomas of the intestinal type preferentially metastasize haematogenously to the liver, whereas

Gastric cancer prevention

Il Ju Choi

Gastric cancer prevention consists of primary prevention (removing possible causes) and secondary prevention (early detection). Primary prevention is a feasible approach considering the marked decrease in gastric cancer incidence during the past century in industrialized countries. This decrease suggests the major effect of environmental factors on stomach cancer development. Dietary intervention, including increased intake of fresh fruit and vegetables and reduced intake of salt and processed or smoked meat, is a main primary prevention strategy.

Helicobacter pylori eradication is another promising strategy. Despite its importance, only two studies have evaluated gastric cancer development as a primary outcome. The first study (of 1630 healthy individuals from a high-risk region of China, in 2004) found that gastric cancer incidence over 7.5 years was similar in *H. pylori* eradication and placebo groups. [1]. From these results, *H. pylori* eradication in the general population is currently not considered to have definite supporting data. Eradication of *H. pylori*, however, may decrease stomach cancer development in the subgroup with no precancerous changes such as atrophy or intestinal metaplasia. The second study (of 544 randomized patients who underwent endoscopic

resection for early gastric cancer in Japan, in 2008) showed at a 3-year follow-up that risk of metachronous gastric carcinoma was reduced to one third in the eradication group [2]. This is the first randomized study showing that *H. pylori* eradication is effective for stomach cancer prevention; however, it has the limitation of not being blinded and of having a short follow-up duration.

Currently, a study recruiting family members of gastric cancer patients, a high-risk population, is under way in the Republic of Korea (ClinicalTrials.gov: NCT01678027). Furthermore, a study with enough statistical power, with recruitment of a larger number of patients from the general population, is also needed before implementation of this strategy in the general population from high-risk regions.

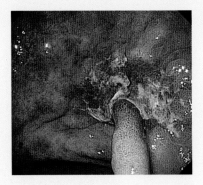

Fig. B5.4.1. Early gastric cancer detected by screening endoscopy.

Secondary prevention is another important aspect of gastric cancer prevention. In the Republic of Korea, where gastric cancer incidence is the highest in the world, the National Cancer Screening Program has been providing biennial gastric cancer screening for people aged 40 years or older since 1999. This is a unique screening programme, which uses endoscopy (which has a much higher sensitivity than radiology with barium meal) as a primary screening tool. Probably owing to the screening effect, the 5-year survival rate of stomach cancer patients in the Republic of Korea has improved, from 46.6% in 1996–2000 to 67.0% in 2006–2010. Furthermore, endoscopic screening at 2-year intervals detects stomach cancer mostly as an early gastric cancer confined to the mucosal or submucosal layers (Fig. B5.4.1), and many such cancers can be cured by endoscopic resection rather than by surgical gastrectomy [3].

References

1. Wong BC *et al.* (2004). *JAMA*, 291:187–194. http://dx.doi.org/10.1001/jama.291.2.187 PMID:14722144

2. Fukase K *et al.* (2008). *Lancet*, 372:392–397. http://dx.doi.org/10.1016/S0140-6736(08)61159-9 PMID:18675689

3. Nam SY *et al.* (2009). *Eur J Gastroenterol Hepatol*, 21:855–860. http://dx.doi.org/10.1097/MEG.0b013e328318ed42 PMID:19369882

carcinomas composed of poorly cohesive cells (the diffuse type) preferentially metastasize to peritoneal surfaces. Mixed carcinomas exhibit the metastatic patterns of both types. When the carcinoma penetrates the serosa, peritoneal implants generally flourish.

Genetic predisposition and hereditary syndromes

First-degree relatives of patients with gastric cancer are almost 3 times as

likely as the general population to develop gastric cancer themselves. This may be partly attributable to *H. pylori* infection being common in families and to the potential role of *IL-1* gene polymorphisms. Susceptibility to carcinogens may play a role as well. For example, polymorphisms of genes encoding for glutathione *S*-transferase enzymes, known to metabolize tobacco-related carcinogens and *N*-acetyltransferase 1, increase the risk of gastric cancer development.

There is evidence also of familial clustering: about 10% of stomach cancers show evidence of a familial component, and approximately 1–3% of gastric cancers are a result of an inherited predisposition, of which the major type is hereditary diffuse gastric cancer [10]. Genomewide association studies have implicated the prostate stem cell antigen (*PSCA*) gene and the mucin 1 (*MUC1*) gene as influencing susceptibility. Approximately 95% of the Japanese population have at least

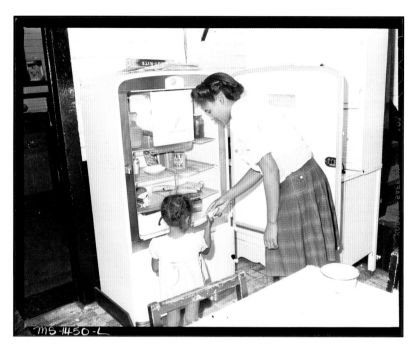

Fig. 5.4.4. A woman gives her daughter a banana from an electrical refrigerator, in a photograph from 1946. Refrigerators have allowed better preservation of food, thus reducing the need for salt preservation.

one of the two risk genotypes, and approximately 56% of the population have both risk genotypes [11].

Hereditary diffuse gastric cancer

On the basis of clinical criteria, the International Gastric Cancer Linkage Consortium defined families with hereditary diffuse gastric cancer syndrome as meeting one of two criteria: (i) two or more documented cases of diffuse gastric cancer in first- or second-degree relatives, with at least one of them diagnosed before the age of 50 years, or (ii) three or more documented cases of diffuse gastric cancer in first- or second-degree relatives, independent of age of diagnosis [12]. Women in these families have an elevated risk of lobular breast cancer. The criteria for genetic testing were updated in 2010 [13].

Alterations of the *CDH1* gene, which encodes E-cadherin, constitute the genetic causal event of hereditary diffuse gastric cancer [14]. In clinically defined hereditary diffuse gastric cancer, *CDH1*

mutations are detected in 30–40% of cases. Most (75–80%) are truncating mutations, and the remainder are missense mutations. In addition to point mutations, large germline deletions have been found in hereditary diffuse gastric cancer families that tested negative for point mutations.

A model of early development of diffuse gastric cancer in *CDH1* mutation carriers has been proposed, encompassing precursor (intraepithelial) lesions (in situ carcinoma and pagetoid spread of signet ring cells), early intramucosal carcinoma, and advanced cancer [15].

Gastric adenocarcinoma and proximal polyposis of the stomach

Recently, a new hereditary syndrome has been identified: gastric adenocarcinoma and proximal polyposis of the stomach, characterized by the autosomal dominant transmission of fundic gland polyposis, including areas of dysplasia or intestinal-type gastric adenocarcinoma, restricted to the proximal stomach, with no evidence of colorectal or duodenal

polyposis or other heritable gastrointestinal cancer syndromes. The genetic defect behind this syndrome has not yet been elucidated [16].

Gastric cancer in other hereditary cancer syndromes

The risk of gastric cancer is also increased in dominantly inherited cancer predisposition syndromes such as familial adenomatous polyposis and Lynch syndrome, and also in Li–Fraumeni syndrome with germline mutation of *TP53*.

Molecular pathology

Gastric carcinoma is the result of accumulated genomic damage affecting cellular functions essential for cancer development: self-sufficiency in growth signals, escape from anti-growth signals, resistance to apoptosis, sustained replicative potential, angiogenesis induction, and invasive or metastatic potential. These genomic changes arise through three genomic instability pathways: microsatellite instability, chromosomal instability, and a CpG island methylation phenotype. Furthermore, genetic and epigenetic changes affect oncogenes and tumour suppressor genes [17].

Some oncogenes are preferentially altered in a specific type of gastric cancer, such as *HER2* and *KRAS* in the intestinal type. Human epidermal growth factor receptor 2 (HER2) overexpression and/or amplification is present in 10–20% of gastric cancers, and it has been suggested that HER2 overexpression and/or amplification may be one of the molecular abnormalities linked to the development of gastric cancer, with a negative impact on prognosis [18]. Recently, a comprehensive survey of genomic alterations in gastric cancer revealed systematic patterns of molecular exclusivity and genes related to receptor tyrosine kinase (RTK)/RAS signalling: *FGFR2* (in 9% of tumours), *KRAS* (9%), *EGFR* (8%), *ERBB2* (7%), and *MET* (4%) [19]. These genes were frequently amplified in gastric cancer in a mutually exclusive manner

Fig. 5.4.5. Mutually exclusive and co-amplified genomic alterations in gastric cancer. (A) Focal regions exhibiting mutually exclusive patterns of genome amplification. Outermost circular track indicates genomic positions by chromosomes (black lines are cytobands, red lines are centromeres). Blue lines indicate pairs of focal regions (genes) exhibiting significant patterns of mutually exclusive genomic amplification. Genes involved in receptor tyrosine kinase (RTK)/RAS signalling are highlighted in red. (B) Focal regions exhibiting patterns of genomic co-amplification. Orange lines indicate pairs of focal regions (genes) exhibiting significant patterns of genomic co-amplification. Genes involved in RTK/RAS signalling are highlighted in red.

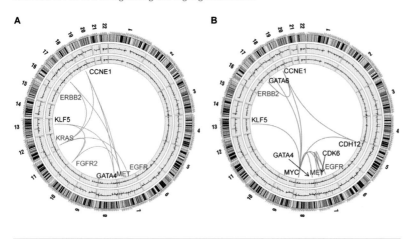

(Fig. 5.4.5), indicating five distinct gastric cancer patient subgroups. Collectively, these subgroups suggest that at least 37% of gastric cancer patients may be potentially treatable by RTK/RAS-directed therapies. A separate study revealed *KRAS* mutations in 4.2% of gastric tumour samples from the United Kingdom, Japan, and Singapore, demonstrating that *KRAS* mutation and DNA mismatch repair deficiency have a role in a small subgroup of these tumours [20].

Some oncogenes are altered preferentially in diffuse carcinoma, such as *BCL2* and *FGFR2* (formerly K-*sam*). Other oncogenes are altered in both intestinal-type and diffuse carcinomas, including *CTNNB1* (encoding β-catenin), *MET*, and *MYC*. Many tumour suppressor genes have been implicated in gastric carcinoma development, including *APC* and *DCC* in intestinal-type carcinomas and *CDH1* and *RB1* in diffuse carcinomas. Other tumour suppressor genes are altered in both

types of gastric carcinoma, such as *PTEN* and *TP53*, although these are more common in intestinal-type carcinoma.

Prevention, screening, and targeted agents

The two major changes that could be made at a population level to reduce gastric cancer incidence are improvement in diet and reduction in the prevalence of *H. pylori*. These changes are already taking place in many populations, as a consequence of economic development, and may explain the decline observed in gastric cancer incidence. Active intervention in a population requires proof that the intervention is effective, and this can only come from randomized trials. Prevention of gastric cancer is a primary public health issue in Japan [21] and the Republic of Korea (see "Gastric cancer prevention").

Radiology with barium meal is used in mass screening protocols in Japan, followed by endoscopy if

an abnormality is detected. In the Republic of Korea, endoscopy is primarily used as a screening procedure. Testing for serum pepsinogen is being evaluated for screening to identify high-risk patients and detect early cancers.

Endoscopy is a sensitive and specific diagnostic test for gastric cancer. Although detection of lesions associated with early gastric cancer can be improved using chromo-endoscopy and narrow-band imaging, a substantial number of such lesions still escape detection. Tumour staging before deciding on a treatment plan involves endoscopic ultrasonography for characterization of the primary tumour but is less useful for lymph-node staging, whereas computed tomography (CT) is used to detect lymph-node and liver metastases. Positron emission tomography in combination with CT imaging may be superior to either alone for preoperative staging. Laparoscopic staging may be the only way to exclude peritoneal seeding.

There is current interest in the immunohistochemical and in situ hybridization detection of HER2 expression in gastric cancer because there is evidence that these tumours may respond well to therapy with the humanized monoclonal antibody trastuzumab [22]. The European Medicines Agency and similar authorities recommend HER2 testing by immunohistochemistry and fluorescence in situ hybridization to identify patients who may benefit from targeted therapy with trastuzumab.

In families fulfilling the criteria for hereditary diffuse gastric cancer, screening for *CDH1* germline alterations is indicated. Asymptomatic carriers of pathogenic changes of the *CDH1* gene are candidates for total prophylactic gastrectomy or annual endoscopic surveillance (in selected groups) as risk reduction strategies.

References

1. Correa P (1992). Human gastric carcinogenesis: a multistep and multifactorial process – First American Cancer Society Award Lecture on Cancer Epidemiology and Prevention. *Cancer Res*, 52:6735–6740. PMID:1458460

2. IARC (2012). Biological agents. *IARC Monogr Eval Carcinog Risks Hum*, 100B:1–441. PMID:23189750

3. IARC (1994). Schistosomes, liver flukes and *Helicobacter pylori*. *IARC Monogr Eval Carcinog Risks Hum*, 61:1–241. PMID:7715068

4. Basso D, Zambon CF, Letley DP *et al.* (2008). Clinical relevance of *Helicobacter pylori cagA* and *vacA* gene polymorphisms. Gastroenterology, 135:91–99. http://dx.doi.org/10.1053/j.gastro.2008.03.041 PMID:18474244

5. World Cancer Research Fund/American Institute for Cancer Research (2007). *Food, Nutrition, Physical Activity, and the Prevention of Cancer: A Global Perspective.* Washington, DC: American Institute for Cancer Research.

6. Ren JS, Kamangar F, Forman D, Islami F (2012). Pickled food and risk of gastric cancer – a systematic review and meta-analysis of English and Chinese literature. *Cancer Epidemiol Biomarkers Prev*, 21:905–915. http://dx.doi.org/10.1158/1055-9965.EPI-12-0202 PMID:22499775

7. El-Omar EM, Carrington M, Chow W-H *et al.* (2000). Interleukin-1 polymorphisms associated with increased risk of gastric cancer. *Nature*, 404:398–402. http://dx.doi.org/10.1038/35006081 PMID:10746728

8. Laurén P (1965). The two histological main types of gastric carcinoma: diffuse and so-called intestinal-type carcinoma. An attempt at a histo-clinical classification. *Acta Pathol Microbiol Scand*, 64:31–49. PMID:14320675

9. Lauwers GY, Carneiro F, Graham DY *et al.* (2010). Gastric carcinoma. In: Bosman FT, Carneiro F, Hruban RH, Theise ND, eds. *WHO Classification of Tumours of the Digestive System*, 4th ed. Lyon: IARC, pp. 48–58.

10. Carneiro F, Charlton A, Huntsman DG (2010). Hereditary diffuse gastric cancer. In: Bosman FT, Carneiro F, Hruban RH, Theise ND, eds. *WHO Classification of Tumours of the Digestive System*, 4th ed. Lyon: IARC, pp. 59–63.

11. Saeki N, Ono H, Sakamoto H, Yoshida T (2013). Genetic factors related to gastric cancer susceptibility identified using a genome-wide association study. *Cancer Sci*, 104:1–8. http://dx.doi.org/10.1111/cas.12042 PMID:23057512

12. Caldas C, Carneiro F, Lynch HT *et al.* (1999). Familial gastric cancer: overview and guidelines for management. *J Med Genet*, 36:873–880. PMID:10593993

13. Fitzgerald RC, Hardwick R, Huntsman D *et al.*; International Gastric Cancer Linkage Consortium (2010). Hereditary diffuse gastric cancer: updated consensus guidelines for clinical management and directions for future research. *J Med Genet*, 47:436–444. http://dx.doi.org/10.1136/jmg.2009.074237 PMID:20591882

14. Guilford P, Hopkins J, Harraway J *et al.* (1998). E-cadherin germline mutations in familial gastric cancer. *Nature*, 392:402–405. http://dx.doi.org/10.1038/32918 PMID:9537325

15. Carneiro F, Huntsman DG, Smyrk TC *et al.* (2004). Model of the early development of diffuse gastric cancer in E-cadherin mutation carriers and its implications for patient screening. *J Pathol*, 203:681–687. http://dx.doi.org/10.1002/path.1564 PMID:15141383

16. Worthley DL, Phillips KD, Wayte N *et al.* (2012). Gastric adenocarcinoma and proximal polyposis of the stomach (GAPPS): a new autosomal dominant syndrome. *Gut*, 61:774–779. http://dx.doi.org/10.1136/gutjnl-2011-300348 PMID:21813476

17. Carneiro F, Oliveira C, Leite M, Seruca R (2008). Molecular targets and biological modifiers in gastric cancer. *Semin Diagn Pathol*, 25:274–287. http://dx.doi.org/10.1053/j.semdp.2008.07.004 PMID:19013893

18. Jørgensen JT, Hersom M (2012). HER2 as a prognostic marker in gastric cancer – a systematic analysis of data from the literature. *J Cancer*, 3:137–144. http://dx.doi.org/10.7150/jca.4090 PMID:22481979

19. Deng N, Goh LK, Wang H *et al.* (2012). A comprehensive survey of genomic alterations in gastric cancer reveals systematic patterns of molecular exclusivity and co-occurrence among distinct therapeutic targets. *Gut*, 61:673–684. http://dx.doi.org/10.1136/gutjnl-2011-301839 PMID:22315472

20. van Grieken NC, Aoyma T, Chambers PA *et al.* (2013). *KRAS* and *BRAF* mutations are rare and related to DNA mismatch repair deficiency in gastric cancer from the East and the West: results from a large international multicentre study. *Br J Cancer*, 108:1495–1501. http://dx.doi.org/10.1038/bjc.2013.109 PMID:23511561

21. Asaka M (2013). A new approach for elimination of gastric cancer deaths in Japan. *Int J Cancer*, 132:1272–1276. http://dx.doi.org/10.1002/ijc.27965 PMID:23180638

22. Bang YJ, Van Cutsem E, Feyereislova A *et al.*; ToGA Trial Investigators (2010). Trastuzumab in combination with chemotherapy versus chemotherapy alone for treatment of HER2-positive advanced gastric or gastro-oesophageal junction cancer (ToGA): a phase 3, open-label, randomised controlled trial. *Lancet*, 376:687–697. http://dx.doi.org/10.1016/S0140-6736(10)61121-X PMID:20728210

5.5 Colorectal cancer

Fred T. Bosman

Stanley R. Hamilton (reviewer)
René Lambert (reviewer)

Summary

- Colorectal cancer is one of the most common cancers in men and women, representing almost 10% of the global cancer incidence.

- Dietary composition, obesity, and lack of physical activity are established as contributing to risk of colorectal cancer, but the underlying causative biological processes are not defined.

- Most colorectal carcinomas develop through an adenoma–carcinoma sequence, underpinning screening colonoscopy for adenomatous polyp removal as a preventive option.

- Three molecular pathways operate: (i) the chromosomal instability pathway, characterized by inactivating mutations of the *APC*, *TP53*, and *TGF-ß* genes, mutations of *KRAS*, and activation of telomerase; (ii) the microsatellite instability pathway, characterized by deficient mismatch repair, arising through mutation of mismatch repair genes or through promoter methylation of *MLH1*, resulting in a hypermutated state; (iii) the CpG island methylation pathway, characterized by a high level of gene promoter methylation, along with typical morphology of the precursor lesions in the form of sessile serrated adenomas.

- Familial colorectal cancer comprises different syndromes, including familial adenomatous polyposis, hereditary non-polyposis colon cancer or Lynch syndrome, *MUTYH*-associated polyposis, and hamartomatous polyp syndromes.

- Inflammatory bowel disease, when long-standing, predisposes to colorectal cancer.

- *KRAS* mutation renders a tumour refractory to anti-EGFR agents, and is therefore predictive.

Colorectal cancer is defined as a carcinoma, usually an adenocarcinoma, in the colon or rectum [1]. The term "colorectal cancer" might suggest a homogeneous disease entity, but this is clearly not the case. The term "colorectal" is customarily used as a topographical indication, but in reality the therapeutic approach for rectal cancer differs significantly from that for colon cancer, primarily due to the quite different anatomical setting of the rectum, which is embedded in a tight space with genitourinary organs nearby. Cancer in the right colon (caecum, ascending colon) is biologically different from that in the left colon (from the splenic flexure down), in terms of both molecular characteristics and response to targeted treatment. Colorectal cancer can develop sporadically, in the context of a familial syndrome, or in the context of inflammatory bowel disease; each of these settings leads to a disease with distinct characteristics. Recent molecular profiling studies suggest that the heterogeneity of colorectal cancer extends beyond these more or less established categories [1–4].

Etiology

An evaluation by the World Cancer Research Fund [2] has determined that the evidence that physical activity protects against colon cancer is convincing; the evidence is convincing that consumption of red meat and processed meat, consumption of alcoholic beverages (for men, and probably for women), body fatness and abdominal fatness, and the factors that lead to greater adult attained height, or its consequences, are causes of colorectal cancer. Consumption of garlic, milk, and calcium probably protects against colorectal cancer.

Therefore, with reference to specifying foods that increase risk

Epidemiology

Colorectal cancer

- Colorectal cancer represents almost 10% of the global cancer incidence burden in 2012, and is the third most common cancer in men (an estimated 746 000 cases) and the second most common in women (614 000 cases). Colorectal cancer is the fourth most common cause of death from cancer worldwide, with an estimated 694 000 deaths.

- More than 65% of new cases occurred in countries with high or very high levels of human development; almost half of the estimated new cases occurred in Europe and the Americas. Colorectal cancer is now the third most common cancer in areas with high human development, and the highest incidence rates are in men in central Europe (Slovakia, Hungary, the Czech Republic) and the Republic of Korea.

- Incidence varies 10-fold between countries worldwide, in both sexes, and rates tend to be relatively low in many African countries. As with incidence, mortality rates are lower in women than in men, except in the Caribbean.

- The scale of the colorectal cancer incidence burden and its temporal development in a given country are key markers of human development transitions, and incidence (and mortality) is increasing in many countries transitioning towards higher levels of human development. In contrast, trends appear to be stabilizing or declining in countries that have attained the highest levels of human development.

Map 5.5.1. Global distribution of estimated age-standardized (World) incidence rates (ASR) per 100 000, for colorectal cancer in men, 2012.

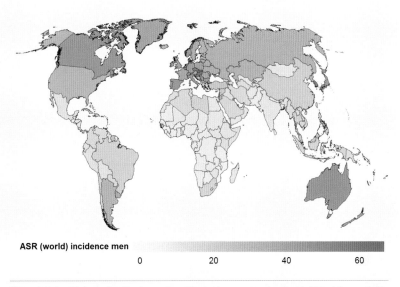

ASR (world) incidence men

0   20   40   60

Map 5.5.2. Global distribution of estimated age-standardized (World) mortality rates (ASR) per 100 000, for colorectal cancer in men, 2012.

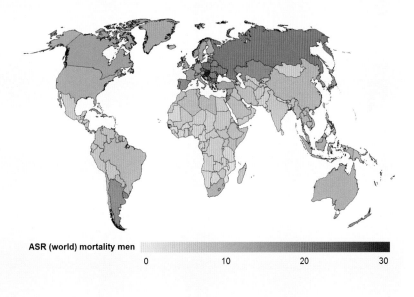

ASR (world) mortality men

0   10   20   30

For more details about the maps and charts presented in this chapter, see "A guide to the epidemiology data in *World Cancer Report*".

of colorectal cancer, the primary focus is on meat. Despite the strength of the epidemiological evidence, relevant biological processes are poorly defined. Cooked meat may contain two classes of carcinogens – heterocyclic amines and polycyclic aromatic hydrocarbons – but these are unlikely to account for the evident risk [3]. An indication of the recognized complexity may be gained from the experimental

Chart 5.5.1. Estimated global number of new cases and deaths with proportions by major world regions, for colorectal cancer in both sexes combined, 2012.

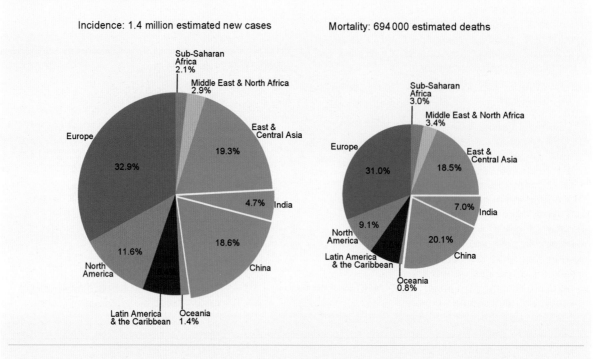

Incidence: 1.4 million estimated new cases

Mortality: 694 000 estimated deaths

Chart 5.5.2. Age-standardized (World) incidence rates per 100 000 by year in selected populations, for colorectal cancer in men, circa 1975–2012.

Chart 5.5.3. Age-standardized (World) mortality rates per 100 000 by year in selected populations, for colorectal cancer in men, circa 1975–2012.

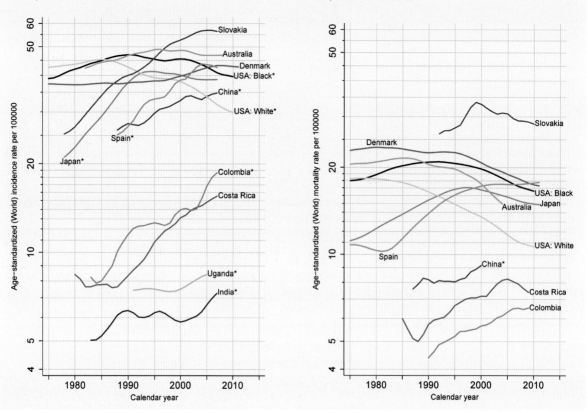

observation that dietary fat can alter the gut microbiota of mice indirectly by affecting bile acids and hence contributing to inflammatory bowel disease (see below) [4]. Such a direct association between diet and carcinogenesis is complemented by current understanding that obesity may play a crucial role in mediating carcinogenesis via inflammation [5]. Obesity-enhanced inflammation is largely orchestrated by increases in adipose tissue macrophages, leading to the secretion of inflammatory cytokines, including tumour necrosis factor α (TNF-α), monocyte chemoattractant protein 1, and interleukin-6 (IL-6), all of which are linked to colorectal cancer [6].

Colorectal cancer is considered primarily as a "lifestyle" disease; its incidence is high in countries with a diet high in calories and animal fat and with a largely sedentary population. One consequence of the lack of precise knowledge as to how multiple factors contribute to risk is that (chemo)preventive measures can only be, and are only, proposed in rather general terms. Solid evidence exists for a role of non-steroidal anti-inflammatory drugs in prevention of the progression from adenoma to carcinoma [7].

Pathogenesis
In the development of colorectal cancer, three distinct pathways operate: the chromosomal instability pathway, the microsatellite instability pathway, and the CpG island methylator pathway [8–10].

Chromosomal instability pathway
The chromosomal instability pathway is found in about 85% of sporadic colorectal cancers and is prototypical for the molecular evolution of this malignancy. Chromosomal abnormalities (mostly a combination of allelic losses and gains) include newly discovered chromosomal translocations [11]. This category of colorectal cancers is characterized by mutations in the Wnt pathway genes *APC* (70%) or *CTNNB* (30%), a crucial element in their molecular carcinogenesis [12]. *KRAS* mutations, usually in codons 12 and 13, occur in 45% of the cases and interfere with anti-epidermal growth factor receptor (EGFR) therapy. *TP53* mutations are found in 70% of cases. Loss of *SMAD4* (which functions downstream of the TGF-β2 receptor) occurs in later stages and confers poor prognosis. In addition to these genes, recent evidence points towards more than 20 genes that are frequently mutated, including

ARID1A, *SOX9*, and *FAM123B/ WXT* [11].

Morphologically, the sequence most likely starts as an aberrant crypt focus, a small focus of mucosa in which the regular crypt architecture is disturbed due to mutations in *KRAS* or *APC*. Aberrant crypt foci with *APC* mutations show morphological signs of dysplasia, signifying a precancerous condition. Subsequent activation of telomerase confers unlimited lifespan to adenoma cells; *TP53* mutations are involved in the progression from a low-grade adenoma to a high-grade adenoma, and other genes, including *SMAD*, in the progression from a non-invasive adenoma to an invasive carcinoma (Fig. 5.5.1).

Microsatellite instability pathway
The microsatellite instability pathway is involved in about 15% of sporadic colorectal cancers. This genetic hallmark is due to an incompetent DNA mismatch repair system, as a result of promoter methylation of *MLH1* (in sporadic microsatellite instability-pathway colorectal cancer) or somatic mutations of the mismatch repair genes (*MLH1, MSH2, MSH6,* or *PMS2*). Also, patients with a germline mutation of one of the mismatch repair genes in Lynch syndrome fall into this category [10,13]. These

Fig. 5.5.1. The chromosomal instability pathway in the development of colorectal cancer (after Vogelstein [8,9]). Morphologically, the adenoma–carcinoma sequence starts with a slight disturbance of crypt architecture and cytonuclear atypia, which is known as an aberrant crypt focus. Activating (+) *KRAS* mutations regularly occur in these lesions. Some of these may show features of epithelial dysplasia (as is shown in the second panel) and go on to develop into an adenoma. In this case, often inactivating (-) *APC* mutations are found. Low-grade adenomas are small and mostly tubular and have limited cytonuclear and architectural features of dysplasia. Once telomerase is activated (+), the lesions often show high-grade features: large, villous architecture and cytonuclear features (loss of polarity, nuclear pleomorphism, mitotic activity) of high-grade dysplasia. Progression towards invasive carcinoma is often accompanied by a *TP53* mutation. Progression towards metastasis (haematogenous metastases most frequently in the liver, as shown in the right panel) is accompanied by further molecular events, such as inactivation (-) of *SMAD4*.

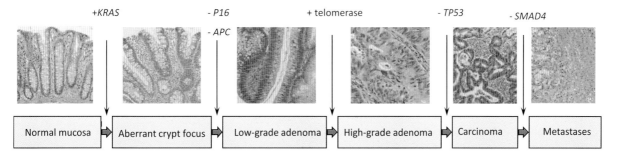

cancers show a relatively high frequency of *BRAF* (V600E) gene mutations. The early phases of development correspond to an adenoma–carcinoma sequence. Adenomas may be of the sessile serrated type with dysplasia, some of which progress to invasive carcinoma. Carcinomas tend to be situated in the right colon, often with a mucinous or medullary histology with a host response characterized by a lymphocytic infiltrate. Cancers that arise through this pathway have a better prognosis but respond differently to standard adjuvant chemotherapy by being less responsive to 5-fluorouracil. When oxaliplatin is added, the survival benefit for cancers with microsatellite instability is maintained, whereas the addition of irinotecan does not seem to improve survival in such patients compared with those with microsatellite stable tumours, but this needs further confirmation [14].

CpG island methylator pathway

The CpG island methylator pathway [15,16] overlaps significantly with the microsatellite instability pathway and is characterized by methylation of the promoter of a variety of genes (CpG island methylator phenotype), including *MLH1*, with resultant microsatellite instability, which contributes to the accumulation of additional genetic abnormalities. Characteristically, an early mutation of the *BRAF* gene (typically the V600E mutation) occurs. The CpG island methylator pathway is characterized by morphologically recognizable precursor lesions. These resemble benign hyperplastic polyps but are large (> 1 cm) and flat, occur notably in the right colon, and show irregular crypt architecture but not necessarily features of dysplasia, as in the conventional adenoma–carcinoma sequence (Fig. 5.5.2). These lesions are known as sessile serrated adenomas or polyps and have an increased risk for the development of colorectal cancer, the extent of which remains to be established.

Pathology and genetics

Colorectal cancer exemplifies stepwise progression [8,9] as it develops initially as a benign precursor lesion (adenoma), which can progress to an invasive lesion (adenocarcinoma) with the capacity to metastasize (metastatic adenocarcinoma). The lesion arises from an intestinal clonogenic precursor cell (crypt base stem cell [17]) through the accumulation of multiple genetic abnormalities, most notably in the Wnt pathway in the form of inactivating mutations of *APC*, activating mutations of *KRAS*, and subsequent mutations of *TP53* and of genes in the TGF-β pathway, which confer invasive and metastatic capacity (see "*Lgr5* stem cells in self-renewal and intestinal cancer").

As outlined above, colorectal cancer comprises many different subtypes, which differ in morphology, genetic background, associated conditions, molecular profile, clinical behaviour, and response to therapy. Categorization of colorectal cancer as sporadic, associated with inflammatory bowel disease, or having familial tendency and associated with familial colorectal cancer syndromes is clinically relevant.

Sporadic colorectal cancer

This is the prototypical cancer type in the colorectum. Histologically, these are adenocarcinomas that as a rule develop from a benign adenomatous polyp, which can be tubular, villous, or tubulovillous in architecture. Only a limited proportion (estimated at 10%) of benign adenomas progress to carcinoma; large adenomas with villous architecture have a high risk of progression [1]. Adenomas are treated by endoscopic polypectomy.

The primary modalities of spread of adenocarcinomas of the colorectum are invasion into the bowel wall and metastasis into the regional lymph nodes. In later stages, liver and lung metastases occur. Colorectal cancer is typically treated by surgery (hemicolectomy), with (adjuvant) chemotherapy depending on the disease stage; rectal cancer is often treated with a neoadjuvant chemo/radiotherapy protocol, followed by surgery. Stage determines prognosis as well as the therapeutic approach (Table 5.5.1), notably as regards the need for adjuvant therapy. For advanced stages, targeted therapy is available, targeting EGFR through monoclonal antibodies (cetuximab, panitumumab), but only in *KRAS* wild-type tumours because *KRAS* mutation renders the tumour insensitive to anti-EGFR therapy [18].

Fig. 5.5.2. Schematic of the CpG island methylator pathway of colorectal carcinoma. An important difference from the chromosomal instability and microsatellite instability pathways is the early occurrence of CpG island methylation together with *BRAF* mutations. Later in the pathway, gene aberrations that frequently occur in the other pathways are also found. SSA/P, sessile serrated adenoma/polyp.

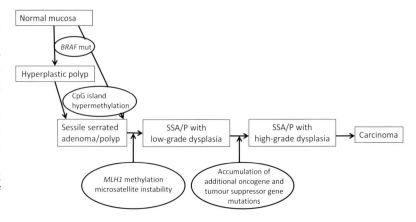

Lgr5 stem cells in self-renewal and intestinal cancer

Hans Clevers

The intestinal epithelium is the most rapidly self-renewing tissue in adult mammals. *Lgr5* was originally identified as a Wnt target gene, transcribed in colon cancer cells. Two knock-in alleles revealed exclusive expression of *Lgr5* in cycling, columnar cells at the crypt base. Using an inducible *Cre* knock-in allele and the Rosa26-*LacZ* reporter strain, lineage tracing experiments were performed in adult mice. The *Lgr5*-positive crypt base columnar cells generated all epithelial lineages throughout life, implying that these cells represent the stem cells of the small intestine and colon. Similar observations were made in hair follicles and stomach epithelium.

Single-sorted *Lgr5*-positive stem cells can initiate ever-expanding crypt–villus organoids in three-dimensional culture. Tracing experiments indicate that the *Lgr5*-positive stem cell hierarchy is maintained in these organoids. The data suggest that intestinal crypt–villus units are self-organizing structures, which can be built from a single stem cell in the absence of a non-epithelial

cellular niche. The same technology has now been developed for the *Lgr5*-positive stomach stem cells.

Intestinal cancer is initiated by Wnt pathway-activating mutations in genes such as *APC*. As in most cancers, the cell of origin has remained elusive. Deletion of *APC* in stem cells, but not in other crypt cells, results in progressively growing neoplasia, identifying the stem cell as the cell of origin of adenomas. Moreover, a stem cell/progenitor cell hierarchy is maintained in early stem cell-derived adenomas, lending support to the "cancer stem cell" concept. Fate mapping of individual crypt stem cells using a multicolour *Cre* reporter revealed that, as a population, *Lgr5* stem cells have a lifelong persistence, yet crypts drift towards clonality within 1–6 months. *Lgr5* cell divisions occur symmetrically. The cellular dynamics are consistent with a model in which the resident stem cells double their numbers every day and stochastically adopt stem or telomerase activator fates after cell division. *Lgr5* stem cells are interspersed between

terminally differentiated Paneth cells that are known to produce bactericidal products. Paneth cells are CD24-positive and express EGF, TGF-α, Wnt3, and the Notch ligand Dll4, all essential signals for stem cell maintenance in culture. Co-culturing of sorted stem cells with Paneth cells dramatically improves organoid formation. This Paneth cell requirement can be substituted by a pulse of exogenous Wnt. Genetic removal of Paneth cells in vivo results in the concomitant loss of *Lgr5* stem cells. In colon crypts, CD24-positive cells residing between *Lgr5* stem cells may represent the Paneth cell equivalents. The data indicate that *Lgr5* stem cells compete for essential niche signals provided by a specialized daughter cell, the Paneth cell.

References

Schepers AG *et al.* (2012). *Science*, 337: 730–735. http://dx.doi.org/10.1126/science.1224676 PMID:22855427

Huch M *et al.* (2013). *Nature*, 494:247–250. http://dx.doi.org/10.1038/nature11826 PMID:23354049

Inflammatory bowel disease

The generic term inflammatory bowel disease refers to two specific entities: Crohn disease and ulcerative colitis. Ulcerative colitis is restricted to the colon and/or rectum and is characterized by a chronic inflammatory reaction restricted to the mucosa and submucosa. Crohn disease is characterized by transmural inflammation and granulomas and can affect any part of the gastrointestinal tract but most commonly affects the terminal ileum. Chronic inflammatory damage to the colon and rectum in both types of inflammatory disease confers an increased risk of malignancy [19]. Some epidemiological evidence exists for an increased incidence of colorectal cancer in chronic colorectal

schistosomiasis [20]. In the connection between inflammation and carcinogenesis, the transcription factor NF-κB is a key mediator, inducing expression of the pro-inflammatory mediators COX-2 and TNF-α, both of which play a role in colorectal carcinogenesis (see "Tumour-elicited inflammation and malignant progression in colorectal cancer"). Genome abnormalities in colorectal cancer in the context of inflammatory bowel disease are similar to those in sporadic colorectal cancer, but *TP53* mutations often occur early. *APC* mutations are less frequent.

Colorectal cancer associated with inflammatory bowel disease develops through a dysplasia–carcinoma sequence (Fig. 5.5.3). Through

endoscopic surveillance, dysplasia can be detected early on and colectomy can then prevent the development of an invasive carcinoma.

Familial colorectal cancer syndromes

Colorectal cancer clusters in families in about 20% of cases, but a familial colorectal cancer syndrome can be pinpointed in less than half of these. When one or more relatives have been diagnosed with this malignancy, the risk of such cancer increases 2–6-fold with an increased number of affected family members and the age at diagnosis of affected relatives. Although a variety of chromosomal loci and, more recently, single-nucleotide polymorphisms

Table 5.5.1. Tumour–node–metastasis (TNM) classifications of carcinoma of the colon and rectum

T – Primary tumour

TX: Primary tumour cannot be assessed

T0: No evidence of primary tumour

Tis: Carcinoma in situ: intraepithelial or invasion of lamina propria

T1: Tumour invades submucosa

T2: Tumour invades muscularis propria

T3: Tumour invades subserosa or into non-peritonealized pericolic or perirectal tissues

T4: Tumour perforates visceral peritoneum and/or directly invades other organs or structures

   T4a: Tumour perforates visceral peritoneum

   T4b: Tumour directly invades other organs or structures

N – Regional lymph nodes

NX: Regional lymph nodes cannot be assessed

N0: No regional lymph-node metastasis

N1: Metastasis in 1–3 regional lymph nodes

   N1a: Metastasis in 1 regional lymph node

   N1b: Metastasis in 2 or 3 regional lymph nodes

   N1c: Tumour deposit(s), i.e. satellites, in the subserosa, or in non-peritonealized pericolic or perirectal soft tissue without regional lymph-node metastasis

N2: Metastasis in 4 or more regional lymph nodes

   N2a: Metastasis in 4–6 regional lymph nodes

   N2b: Metastasis in 7 or more regional lymph nodes

M – Distant metastasis

M0: No distant metastasis

M1: Distant metastasis

   M1a: Metastasis confined to one organ

   M1b: Metastases in more than one organ or the peritoneum

Stage grouping

Stage	T	N	M
Stage 0	Tis	N0	M0
Stage I	T1, T2	N0	M0
Stage II	T3, T4	N0	M0
Stage IIA	T3	N0	M0
Stage IIB	T4a	N0	M0
Stage IIC	T4b	N0	M0
Stage III	Any T	N1, N2	M0
Stage IIIA	T1, T2	N1	M0
	T1	N2a	M0
Stage IIIB	T3, T4a	N1	M0
	T2, T3	N2a	M0
	T1, T2	N2b	M0
Stage IIIC	T4a	N2a	M0
	T3, T4a	N2b	M0
	T4b	N1, N2	M0
Stage IVA	Any T	Any N	M1a
Stage IVB	Any T	Any N	M1b

have been identified (Table 5.5.2) that are associated with increased colorectal cancer risk, the less-penetrant genes and/or gene–environment interactions responsible for such familial disease clusters have yet to be elucidated [12,13].

Familial adenomatous polyposis syndrome accounts for about 1% of all colorectal cancers and is characterized by the development early in life of hundreds to thousands of adenomatous polyps in the colon (Fig. 5.5.4). Mucosal neoplasms higher up in the tubal gut, notably in the stomach, also occur. The syndrome is caused by mutations in the *APC* gene. The APC protein in the Wnt signalling pathway normally binds to β-catenin (in a normal epithelial cell, integrated in the E-cadherin–catenin cell adhesion complex), triggering its degradation in the proteasome [13]. APC loss results in accumulation of β-catenin in the nucleus, where it acts as a transcription factor, promoting transcription of proliferation-stimulating genes, such as *MYC* and cyclin D1. Distinct genotype–phenotype correlations exist [12,13]; some mutations (in codons 1250–1464) are associated with severe polyposis (> 1000 adenomas), while others (before codon 157, after codon 1595, and in the alternatively spliced region of exon 9) are associated with attenuated adenomatous polyposis coli (usually 10–100 adenomas and a 70% lifetime risk of colorectal cancer).

In Gardner syndrome, numerous gastrointestinal polyps occur in combination with other neoplasms, including osteomas, desmoid tumours, epidermoid cysts, and also dental anomalies. *APC* mutations responsible for Gardner syndrome occur in a region encoding for the β-catenin binding site of the protein.

Mismatch repair deficiency syndrome, also known as hereditary non-polyposis colon cancer or Lynch syndrome, is the most common hereditary colorectal cancer predisposition syndrome (about 3% of all such disease), with a lifetime risk of about 80% [13]. The syndrome is autosomal dominant and

Fig. 5.5.3. The dysplasia–carcinoma sequence in colorectal carcinogenesis in inflammatory bowel disease. Chronic inflammation with the continuous liberation of oxygen radicals and inflammatory cytokines creates an environment that is both mutagenic and growth-stimulating. *TP53* mutations occur early in this pathway, associated with the development of low-grade dysplasia. In addition, hypermethylation of CpG islands leads to promoter silencing of *P16* and *P27* among others. Accumulation of such events drives progression towards high-grade dysplasia. Additional events, such as *KRAS* mutations and activation of the Wnt pathway, for example through *APC* mutation, are involved in the progression towards invasive carcinoma. LOH, loss of heterozygosity.

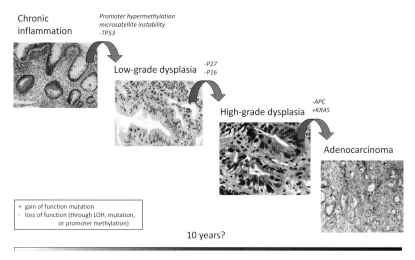

Chronic inflammation

Promoter hypermethylation microsatellite instability -TP53

Low-grade dysplasia *-P27 -P16*

High-grade dysplasia *-APC +KRAS*

Adenocarcinoma

+ gain of function mutation
- loss of function (through LOH, mutation, or promoter methylation)

10 years?

is caused by mutations in one of the DNA mismatch repair genes (*MLH1* on chromosome 3p21, *MSH2* on 2p16, *MSH6* on 2p16, and *PMS2* on 7p22). The mismatch repair protein complex corrects base mismatches or small insertions or deletions that occur during DNA replication. *MLH1* and *MSH2* mutations are the most frequent (about 80%). MSH2 deficiency can also occur through gene silencing by transcriptional read-through of *TACSTD1*, a gene directly upstream of *MSH2* that encodes the Ep-CAM protein. As a result of a germline deletion of the last exons of *TACSTD1*, its transcription is extended into *MSH2*, with functional loss of MSH2 activity.

These cancers exhibit microsatellite instability – increased variability in length of the dinucleotide repeats that occur throughout the genome. These are not necessarily pathogenic but are significant when they occur in key genes in processes such as cell proliferation, apoptosis, or DNA repair. Mismatch repair-deficient cancers are characterized by point mutations (hypermutation) and,

less often, by chromosomal rearrangements and allelic imbalances.

Mismatch repair-deficient cancers develop through an adenoma–carcinoma sequence but not in association with polyposis, typically occur in the right colon, and are often histologically of a mucinous or medullary type, with a striking lymphoid host reaction. The prognosis is better than that of mismatch repair-competent cancers, but mismatch repair-deficient cancers respond less well to adjuvant chemotherapy. These cancers also occur in other organs, including (in decreasing order of frequency) the endometrium, ovary, duodenum, urinary tract, stomach, pancreas, biliary tree, and brain.

The *MUTYH*-associated polyposis (MAP) syndrome has been more recently identified and is estimated to account for about 2% of colorectal cancer. MAP syndrome resembles familial adenomatous polyposis in that multiple adenomatous polyps of the colorectum develop, with a very high lifetime risk of colorectal cancer. The number of adenomas

ranges from very few to hundreds, and therefore MAP resembles attenuated familial adenomatous polyposis. Extracolonic manifestations occur, including duodenal adenomas or adenocarcinomas and various extra-intestinal neoplasms. MAP is an autosomal recessive disorder caused by biallelic mutations in the *MUTYH* gene, located on chromosome 1p. The gene encodes a protein with an important function in the DNA base excision repair pathway.

Prognostic and predictive factors

Currently used criteria for stratification of colorectal cancer patients in view of eventual adjuvant chemotherapy are primarily based on the classic tumour–node–metastasis (TNM) stage parameters tumour extension (T) and lymph-node metastasis (N). However, these lack precision (Table 5.5.1), and better parameters are urgently needed.

Microsatellite instable carcinomas have a better prognosis than those that are microsatellite stable [10]. In addition, patients with microsatellite instable carcinomas might not benefit from 5-fluorouracil-based chemotherapy regimens, but this remains controversial. For microsatellite stable cancers, *BRAF* V600E mutations confer poor prognosis, notably in terms of survival after relapse. *KRAS* mutation status has no prognostic significance for overall survival of patients with stage II/III disease [21]. Recently published tests such as Oncotype DX (based on multiplex reverse transcription polymerase chain reaction) and ColoPrint (microarray-based) might provide additional prognostic value but have not been independently validated [22]. New molecular approaches for prognostic classification are being developed [11, 23–25] but need to be validated in a clinical setting.

KRAS mutation testing has become the mainstay for advanced colorectal cancer because *KRAS*-mutated carcinomas do not respond

Table 5.5.2. Genetic syndromes associated with a possible risk of colorectal carcinoma

Syndrome	Gene (chromosome)	MIM number
Autosomal dominant inheritable colorectal carcinoma		
No or few adenomatous polyps		
Lynch syndrome[a,b]	*MLH1* (3p21-p23) *MSH2* (2p21) *MSH6* (2p21) *PMS2* (7p22)	120435
Adenomatous polyps		
Familial adenomatous polyposis (FAP)[a] and attenuated FAP	*APC* (5q21-q22)	175100
Hamartomatous/mixed/hyperplastic polyps		
Peutz–Jeghers syndrome	*LKB1/STK11* (19p13.3)	175200
Juvenile polyposis syndrome	*SMAD4* (18q21.1) *BMPR1A* (10q22.3)	174900
Hereditary haemorrhagic telangiectasia syndrome[c]	*ENG* (9q33-q34.1) *ACVRL1* (12q11-q14)	187300
Hyperplastic polyposis syndrome[c]	*MUTYH* (1p34.1; autosomal recessive) *MBD4* (3q21.3)	Unassigned
Hereditary mixed polyposis syndrome[c]	*CRAC1* (15q13-q21)	601228
PTEN hamartoma tumour syndrome (Cowden syndrome; Bannayan–Ruvalcaba–Riley syndrome)[c]	*PTEN* (10q23)	158350/153480
Birt–Hogg–Dubé syndrome[c]	*FLCN* (17p11.2)	135150
Autosomal recessive inheritable colorectal carcinoma		
Adenomatous, serrated adenomas and hyperplastic polyps		
MUTYH-associated polyposis[b]	*MUTYH* (1p34.1)	608456

MIM, Mendelian Inheritance in Man (www.omim.org).
[a] Turcot syndrome is a variant of Lynch syndrome, or familial adenomatous polyposis with brain tumours.
[b] Muir–Torre syndrome is a variant of Lynch syndrome, or *MUTYH*-associated polyposis with sebaceous gland tumours.
[c] Risk of colorectal carcinoma is not clear.

to anti-EGFR therapy (cetuximab, panitumumab). This is due to the fact that *KRAS* is downstream of EGFR in the MAPK pathway, which renders approaches targeting the upstream EGFR ineffective. Only about 40% of *KRAS* wild-type colorectal cancers respond to anti-EGFR treatment, implying that other genes are involved, including *PIK3CA*, *BRAF*, *NRAS*, *pTEN*, and others unidentified as yet [21].

Prospects

Screening for colorectal cancer is done through the faecal occult blood test, which has a reasonable sensitivity but low specificity. There is now evidence that screening with flexible sigmoidoscopy can substantially reduce colorectal cancer incidence and mortality. Colonoscopy is increasingly advocated, as colonoscopic polypectomy would, in principle, enable eradication of the disease. Molecular tests for disease-specific DNA abnormalities in faeces or in the blood are currently being developed [26].

The heterogeneity of colorectal cancer continues to challenge clinicians and pathologists. Why cancers of a similar stage that are histologically indistinguishable behave differently in terms of recurrence and response to chemotherapy has long been a mystery. The inclusion of molecular parameters in colorectal cancer classification improves on currently used classification systems [27]. Molecular annotation of large series of colorectal cancers with detailed follow-up data might now lead to new insights into molecular mechanisms that drive this heterogeneity. The Cancer Genome Atlas data [11], along with even more recent approaches towards molecular classification of colorectal cancer [23,24], will in the near future allow the redefinition of colorectal cancer subtypes, with impacts on clinical management. The most recent data point towards at least five molecularly defined subtypes [24] – which partly overlap

Tumour-elicited inflammation and malignant progression in colorectal cancer

Michael Karin

Whereas 2% of colorectal cancer arises in the context of pre-existing inflammatory bowel disease, especially ulcerative colitis, and is known as colitis-associated cancer, most colorectal cancer, including familial and sporadic cases, is found in individuals who do not show any signs of inflammatory bowel disease. Yet expression profiling has revealed the same inflammatory gene signature, which depends on activation of *NF-κB* and *STAT3*, in both colitis-associated cancer and colorectal cancer, findings that pose a question about the origin of the colorectal cancer-elicited inflammatory response.

Early experiments established that activation of *NF-κB*, which leads to production of the pro-inflammatory cytokine interleukin-6 (IL-6), a potent activator of *STAT3*, plays a critical role in the development of colitis-associated cancer. More recently, the origin and role of inflammation in the development and progression of sporadic malignancy, most of which is driven by loss of the tumour suppressor *APC* and activation of the β-catenin signalling pathway, has been investigated. Studies focused on IL-23, a heterodimeric cytokine composed of a unique p19 subunit and a p40 subunit, which it shares with IL-12. IL-23 expression is strongly elevated in colorectal cancer relative to adjacent non-tumour tissue, and these findings have been extended to the *CPC-Apc* mouse model of colorectal tumorigenesis. In *CPC-Apc* mice, the major source of IL-23 expression in colorectal adenomas is tumour-associated macrophages. Importantly, ablation of IL-23 p19, either in all cells or only in bone marrow-derived cells, attenuates the development and slows down the progression of colorectal cancer in *CPC-Apc* mice, and similar results were observed upon ablation of IL-23 receptor (IL-23R). As IL-23R is not expressed on adenoma epithelial cells, IL-23 must exert its pro-tumorigenic effect via an indirect mechanism. Indeed, IL-23 signalling promotes the polarization of IL-17-producing T cells (Th17) and the production of IL-6, both of which contribute to the development and progression of sporadic colorectal tumours in mice.

Importantly, molecular epidemiological studies have revealed an IL-23–Th17 signature that is upregulated in about 10% of human colorectal cancer patients, and have shown that the presence of this signature in stage I/II disease is associated with very poor prognosis and a marked decrease in disease-free survival.

The mechanism responsible for the specific induction of IL-23 in tumour-associated macrophages depends on Toll-like receptor/MyD88 signalling, which appears to be activated in response to components of the colonic microflora that permeate the adenomas. Eubacterial 16S RNA has been detected in both murine and human colon adenomas, as well as increased penetrance of bacterial endotoxin into adenomas relative to surrounding non-cancerous tissue.

The development of colorectal adenomas in both mice and humans is associated with loss of protective mucins and junctional adhesion proteins, and this is likely to be the primary mechanism that accounts for the selective entry of microbial products into the tumour and induction of the tumour-promoting IL-23–Th17 signature. Future studies should focus on the therapeutic value of anti-IL-23 or anti-IL-17 interventions and the genetic or environmental causes of the large variation in the magnitude of IL-17 production among human colorectal cancer patients.

Reference

Grivennikov SI *et al.* (2012). *Nature*, 491:254–258. http://dx.doi.org/10.1038/nature11465 PMID:23034650

with classifications based on well-established classifiers (TNM, microsatellite instability) but do add an additional layer of complexity – that potentially will allow more refined subclassification. In addition, new therapeutic targets and prognostic and predictive biomarkers will emerge.

Fig. 5.5.4. (A) Colon mucosa of a 24-year-old man with familial adenomatous polyposis who underwent total colectomy. (B) Mucosa with multiple adenomatous polyps (haematoxylin–eosin stain).

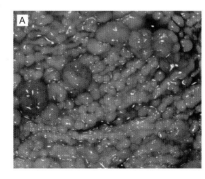

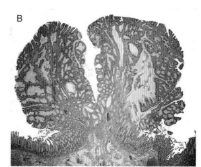

References

1. Hamilton S, Bosman F, Boffetta P *et al.* (2010). Carcinoma of the colon and the rectum. In: Bosman FT, Carneiro F, Hruban RH, Theise ND, eds. *WHO Classification of Tumours of the Digestive System,* 4th ed. Lyon: IARC, pp. 134–146.

2. World Cancer Research Fund/American Institute for Cancer Research (2007). *Food, Nutrition, Physical Activity, and the Prevention of Cancer: A Global Perspective.* Washington DC: American Institute for Cancer Research.

3. Cross AJ, Ferrucci LM, Risch A *et al.* (2010). A large prospective study of meat consumption and colorectal cancer risk: an investigation of potential mechanisms underlying this association. *Cancer Res,* 70:2406–2414. http://dx.doi.org/10.1158/0008-5472.CAN-09-3929 PMID:20215514

4. Devkota S, Wang Y, Musch MW *et al.* (2012). Dietary-fat-induced taurocholic acid promotes pathobiont expansion and colitis in *Il10-/-* mice. *Nature,* 487:104–108. http://dx.doi.org/10.1038/nature11225 PMID:22722865

5. Vazzana N, Riondino S, Toto V *et al.* (2012). Obesity-driven inflammation and colorectal cancer. *Curr Med Chem,* 19:5837–5853. http://dx.doi.org/10.2174/092986712804143349 PMID:23033947

6. Guffey CR, Fan D, Singh UP, Murphy EA (2013). Linking obesity to colorectal cancer: recent insights into plausible biological mechanisms. *Curr Opin Clin Nutr Metab Care,* 16:595–600. http://dx.doi.org/10.1097/MCO.0b013e328362d10b PMID:23743611

7. Thun MJ, Jacobs EJ, Patrono C (2012). The role of aspirin in cancer prevention. *Nat Rev Clin Oncol,* 9:259–267. http://dx.doi.org/10.1038/nrclinonc.2011.199 PMID:22473097

8. Fearon ER, Vogelstein B (1990). A genetic model for colorectal tumorigenesis. *Cell,* 61:759–767. http://dx.doi.org/10.1016/0092-8674(90)90186-I PMID:2188735

9. Kinzler KW, Vogelstein B (1996). Lessons from hereditary colorectal cancer. *Cell,* 87:159–170. http://dx.doi.org/10.1016/S0092-8674(00)81333-1 PMID:8861899

10. Boland CR, Goel A (2010). Microsatellite instability in colorectal cancer. *Gastroenterology,* 138:2073–2087. http://dx.doi.org/10.1053/j.gastro.2009.12.064 PMID:20420947

11. Muzny DM, Bainbridge MN, Chang K *et al.*; Cancer Genome Atlas Network (2012). Comprehensive molecular characterization of human colon and rectal cancer. *Nature,* 487:330–337. http://dx.doi.org/10.1038/nature11252 PMID:22810696

12. Fearon ER (2011). Molecular genetics of colorectal cancer. *Annu Rev Pathol,* 6:479–507. http://dx.doi.org/10.1146/annurev-pathol-011110-130235 PMID:21090969

13. Gala M, Chung DC (2011). Hereditary colon cancer syndromes. *Semin Oncol,* 38:490–499. http://dx.doi.org/10.1053/j.seminoncol.2011.05.003 PMID:21810508

14. Sinicrope FA, Sargent DJ (2012). Molecular pathways: microsatellite instability in colorectal cancer: prognostic, predictive, and therapeutic implications. *Clin Cancer Res,* 18:1506–1512. http://dx.doi.org/10.1158/1078-0432.CCR-11-1469 PMID:22302899

15. Liang JJ, Alrawi S, Tan D (2008). Nomenclature, molecular genetics and clinical significance of the precursor lesions in the serrated polyp pathway of colorectal carcinoma. *Int J Clin Exp Pathol,* 1:317–324. PMID:18787610

16. Snover DC (2011). Update on the serrated pathway to colorectal carcinoma. *Hum Pathol,* 42:1–10. http://dx.doi.org/10.1016/j.humpath.2010.06.002 PMID:20869746

17. Vries RG, Huch M, Clevers H (2010). Stem cells and cancer of the stomach and intestine. *Mol Oncol,* 4:373–384. http://dx.doi.org/10.1016/j.molonc.2010.05.001 PMID:20598659

18. Bohanes P, LaBonte MJ, Winder T, Lenz HJ (2011). Predictive molecular classifiers in colorectal cancer. *Semin Oncol,* 38:576–587. http://dx.doi.org/10.1053/j.seminoncol.2011.05.012 PMID:21810517

19. Xie J, Itzkowitz SH (2008). Cancer in inflammatory bowel disease. *World J Gastroenterol,* 14:378–389. http://dx.doi.org/10.3748/wjg.14.378 PMID:18200660

20. Qiu D-C, Hubbard AE, Zhong B *et al.* (2005). A matched, case-control study of the association between *Schistosoma japonicum* and liver and colon cancers, in rural China. *Ann Trop Med Parasitol,* 99:47–52. http://dx.doi.org/10.1179/136485905X19883 PMID:15701255

21. Roth AD, Tejpar S, Delorenzi M *et al.* (2010). Prognostic role of *KRAS* and *BRAF* in stage II and III resected colon cancer: results of the translational study on the PETACC-3, EORTC 40993, SAKK 60-00 trial. *J Clin Oncol,* 28:466–474. http://dx.doi.org/10.1200/JCO.2009.23.3452 PMID:20008640

22. Kelley RK, Venook AP (2011). Prognostic and predictive markers in stage II colon cancer: is there a role for gene expression profiling? *Clin Colorectal Cancer,* 10:73–80. http://dx.doi.org/10.1016/j.clcc.2011.03.001 PMID:21859557

23. Sadanandam A, Lyssiotis CA, Homicsko K *et al.* (2013). A colorectal cancer classification system that associates cellular phenotype and responses to therapy. *Nat Med,* 19:619–625. http://dx.doi.org/10.1038/nm.3175 PMID:23584089

24. De Sousa E Melo F, Wang X, Jansen M *et al.* (2013). Poor-prognosis colon cancer is defined by a molecularly distinct subtype and develops from serrated precursor lesions. *Nat Med,* 19:614–618. http://dx.doi.org/10.1038/nm.3174 PMID:23584090

25. Merlos-Suárez A, Barriga FM, Jung P *et al.* (2011). The intestinal stem cell signature identifies colorectal cancer stem cells and predicts disease relapse. *Cell Stem Cell,* 8:511–524. http://dx.doi.org/10.1016/j.stem.2011.02.020 PMID:21419747

26. Bosch LJ, Carvalho B, Fijneman RJ *et al.* (2011). Molecular tests for colorectal cancer screening. *Clin Colorectal Cancer,* 10:8–23. http://dx.doi.org/10.3816/CCC.2011.n.002 PMID:21609931

27. Roth AD, Delorenzi M, Tejpar S *et al.* (2012). Integrated analysis of molecular and clinical prognostic factors in stage II/III colon cancer. *J Natl Cancer Inst,* 104:1635–1646. http://dx.doi.org/10.1093/jnci/djs427 PMID:23104212

Websites

American Cancer Society Colorectal Cancer home page: http://www.cancer.org/cancer/colonandrectumcancer/index

MedlinePlus Colorectal Cancer home page: http://www.nlm.nih.gov/medlineplus/colorectalcancer.html

National Cancer Institute Colon and Rectal Cancer home page: http://www.cancer.gov/cancertopics/types/colon-and-rectal

SEER Stat Fact Sheets: Colon and Rectum: http://seer.cancer.gov/statfacts/html/colorect.html

5.6 Liver cancer

5 ORGAN SITE

Neil D. Theise

Chien-Jen Chen (reviewer)
Michael C. Kew (reviewer)

Summary

- The highest incidence rates of hepatocellular carcinoma are in regions with the highest prevalence of predisposing conditions. In Asia and Africa, chronic hepatitis B virus and hepatitis C virus infections are the major causes, and in China and sub-Saharan Africa, exposures to aflatoxins further increase risk.

- Incidence rates of hepatocellular carcinoma in men are more than twice those in women, reflecting greater rates of predisposing chronic liver disease and possibly hormonal influences. In North America and parts of Europe, rates are increasing due to chronic hepatitis C virus infection. Epidemic metabolic syndrome and non-alcoholic fatty liver disease are expected to lead to further increases.

- Universal infant vaccination against hepatitis B virus is recommended by WHO, while antiviral therapy for chronic hepatitis B and C virus infections will lead to reduced incidence of hepatocellular carcinoma in relevant communities. Effective interventions to reduce aflatoxin exposure are also available.

- For individuals with chronic liver disease, routine screening for hepatocellular carcinoma is recommended; individuals without chronic liver disease, or living in areas where such screening is not performed, are likely to present with symptoms of advanced disease.

- The Wnt/β-catenin pathway is commonly disrupted in hepatocellular carcinoma. Mutation of a particular codon in *TP53* may be identified with environmental exposure to aflatoxin.

- Cholangiocarcinoma is uncommon except in South-East Asia where infections with liver flukes, such as *Clonorchis* and *Opisthorchis* species, are endemic. Cholangiocarcinoma remains difficult to treat and is usually lethal.

The most common tumour type occurring in the liver is metastatic disease [1]. Of primary hepatic malignancies, hepatocellular carcinoma, composed of malignant hepatocytes, represents about 80% of tumours. Cholangiocarcinoma, a gland-forming adenocarcinoma deriving from the biliary tree, is the next most common [2]. Other, rare primary tumours include mucinous cystic neoplasm and intraductal papillary biliary neoplasm, the classifications of which have recently been aligned with pancreatic ductal malignancies, tumours of mixed hepatocellular and biliary phenotype, hepatoblastoma in children, and mesenchymal tumours such as angiosarcoma [1].

Etiology

Hepatocellular carcinoma is generally more common in men than in women [1,3]. Men have higher rates of chronic hepatitis B virus (HBV) and hepatitis C virus (HCV) infection and chronic alcohol consumption. Sex hormones may also modulate hepatocarcinogenesis [4]. There are also differences in incidence according to race and ethnic alignment [3]. For example, within the USA, Native Americans and Americans of Asian and Pacific Island descent have higher rates of hepatocellular carcinoma. Intermediate rates are seen in Hispanic/Latino individuals, African Americans, and Native Americans. Caucasians have the lowest rates. These variations are probably indicative of different rates of predisposing conditions and exposures; genetic and epigenetic differences are also probably significant.

The global regions of greatest hepatocellular carcinoma prevalence correspond to those with

Epidemiology

Liver cancer

- Liver cancer represents 6% and 9% of the global cancer incidence and mortality burden, respectively. With an estimated 746 000 deaths in 2012, liver cancer is the second most common cause of death from cancer worldwide.
- Liver cancer is the fifth most common cancer in men (554 000 new cases, 8% of the total) and the ninth most common in women (228 000 cases, 3% of the total). Almost three quarters of the new cases occur in areas with low and medium human development; more than half of the global incidence and mortality is in China.
- Given the high fatality of liver cancer (overall mortality-to-incidence ratio, 0.95), the geographical patterns and trends for mortality are very similar to those observed for incidence.
- By far the highest age-standardized incidence rate is seen in Mongolia. There are elevated incidence rates in East and South-East Asia, in Africa, and in Melanesia. Incidence rates tend to be lower in most highly developed regions.

Map 5.6.1. Global distribution of estimated age-standardized (World) incidence rates (ASR) per 100 000, for liver cancer in men, 2012.

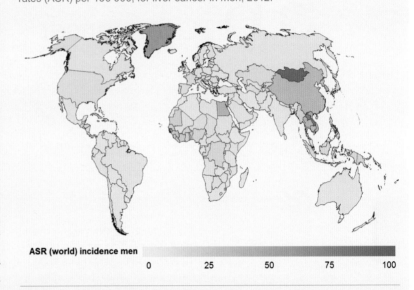

ASR (world) incidence men

0   25   50   75   100

Map 5.6.2. Global distribution of estimated age-standardized (World) incidence rates (ASR) per 100 000, for liver cancer in women, 2012.

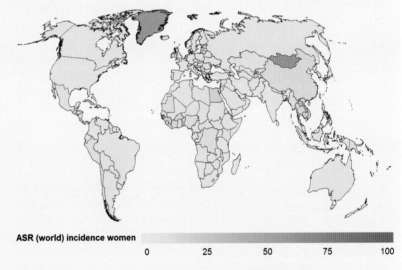

ASR (world) incidence women

0   25   50   75   100

For more details about the maps and charts presented in this chapter, see "A guide to the epidemiology data in *World Cancer Report*".

high rates of predisposing conditions (Maps 5.6.1, 5.6.2; Table 5.6.1) [1,3]. Examples include South and East Asia, where HBV infection is endemic; Egypt, with its high rates of HCV infection from inadequate sterilization during mass vaccination campaigns; and sub-Saharan Africa, South-East Asia, and China, where marked exposure to aflatoxin occurs [3]. In China, the Republic of Korea, Japan, Zimbabwe, and Egypt, incidence rates are more than 20 per 100 000 people [3]. The lowest rates of hepatocellular carcinoma are those reported for North America, South America, and northern Europe, which typically have incidence rates of less than 10 per 100 000 people [3].

Changing incidence rates of hepatocellular carcinoma reflect the changing distribution of predisposing conditions [1,3]. Thus, countries in Europe, North and South America, and Oceania, where HCV-infected populations have expanded, have experienced increasing hepatocellular carcinoma incidence [3]. Non-alcoholic fatty liver disease

Chart 5.6.1. Estimated global number of new cases and deaths with proportions by major world regions, for liver cancer in both sexes combined, 2012.

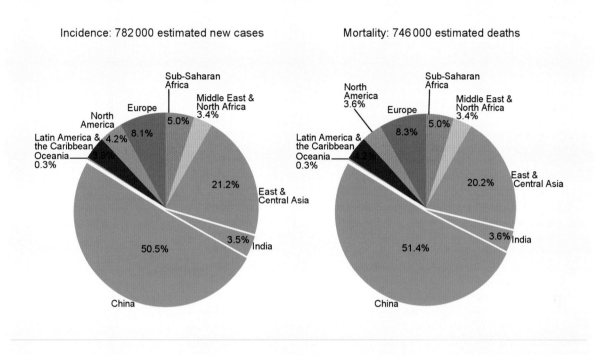

Incidence: 782 000 estimated new cases

Mortality: 746 000 estimated deaths

Chart 5.6.2. Age-standardized (World) incidence rates per 100 000 by year in selected populations, for liver cancer in men, circa 1975–2012.

Chart 5.6.3. Age-standardized (World) incidence rates per 100 000 by year in selected populations, for liver cancer in women, circa 1975–2012.

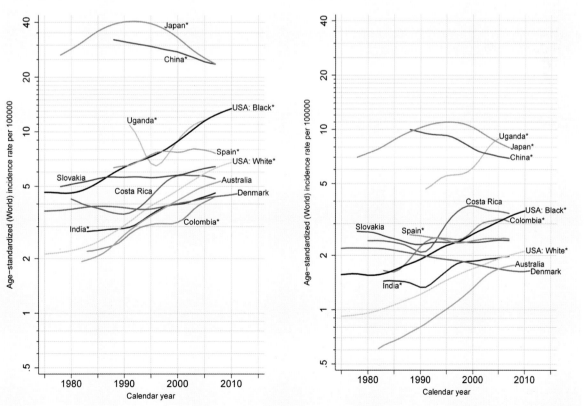

is emerging as a relatively newly understood predisposing condition, and hepatocellular carcinoma incidence rates are likely to increase in affected regions [5]. Increasing survival of individuals with chronic liver disease also may play a role in these upward trends [3].

In contrast, in East Asia incidence rates of hepatocellular carcinoma are declining [1,3]. In Japan, as the cohort of individuals infected by HCV in the first half of the 20th century shrinks, incidence of hepatocellular carcinoma is also declining. In China and Singapore, where HBV infection remains a major predisposing condition, diminished aflatoxin exposure is leading to a decline in HBV-associated disease. Vaccination and treatment for HBV infection and new, more successful treatments for HCV infection will almost certainly lead to diminished rates of hepatocellular carcinoma in places where these are significant risk factors. Indeed, HBV vaccination has been well documented to prevent 70% of hepatocellular carcinoma incidence among vaccinated birth cohorts in a 20-year follow-up study in Taiwan, China [6].

Sporadic cholangiocarcinomas and those associated with HCV, HBV, and primary sclerosing cholangitis are uncommon to rare [1]. However, in regions with endemic liver fluke infestations, such as north-eastern Thailand, incidence is as high as 88 per 100 000 men and 35 per 100 000 women [2].

Hepatocellular carcinoma is most commonly associated with chronic liver disease [1,3,5,7]. Although this malignancy usually occurs in the setting of cirrhosis, cirrhosis per se is not a premalignant lesion [8]. Rather, progression to cirrhosis and hepatocarcinogenesis take place in *parallel* over years to decades [1,9]. Cirrhosis is not, moreover, required for development of hepatocellular carcinoma [1,10]. The most important etiological factors for hepatocarcinogenesis remain viral infections, usually involving HBV or HCV, and toxic injury, typically initiated by ingestion of aflatoxin or consumption of alcohol [1,3]. Where HBV and HCV are endemic, there is a very high incidence of this malignancy. In such chronic infection, viral load is the major driver of the progression of viral hepatitis-related liver disease [10,11]. It should be noted that only about one quarter of patients with chronic HBV and HCV infection will develop hepatocellular carcinoma [2]. Risk calculators that incorporate age, sex, family history of hepatocellular carcinoma, alcohol consumption, serum alanine aminotransferase (ALT) level, and viral factors including HBV e antigen (HBeAg) serostatus, viral load, and genotype have been developed to predict hepatocellular carcinoma caused by chronic HBV infection [12]. Co-infection with both hepatitis viruses further increases risk [13]. HIV infection also appears to be a risk factor for hepatocellular carcinoma [14].

Aflatoxin (specifically, aflatoxin B_1), a mycotoxin produced by moulds of the *Aspergillus* species, contaminates staple food crops in Africa and Asia [15]. Aflatoxin metabolites are present in the urine of affected individuals, as are aflatoxin–albumin adducts in serum [1,15]. These indicators may assist in identifying populations at risk and confirm the important influence of aflatoxin on the development of hepatocellular carcinoma. Risk attributable to aflatoxin acts synergistically with HBV infection and possibly with HCV infection [15]. Alcohol is another toxin that may also act synergistically with other causes, particularly HBV and HCV, and possibly cigarette smoking [16].

Aflatoxin-specific mutations provide a singular relationship between the impact of a carcinogenic agent, the establishment of a biomarker, and inactivation of the relevant tumour suppressor gene [14]. Aflatoxin B_1 is metabolized by members of the cytochrome P450 CYP family, specifically including CYP3A4 and CYP3A5. These isoenzymes metabolize aflatoxin B_1 to its 8,9-*exo*-epoxide, which may react with DNA to form an aflatoxin–N^7-guanine adduct and with protein to generate aflatoxin–albumin adducts. Aflatoxin–albumin adducts may serve as biomarkers for aflatoxin exposure. In hepatocellular carcinomas from areas where exposure to aflatoxin is high, aflatoxin–DNA adducts result in a high prevalence of thymine substitutions at the third guanine in AGG sequences, thereby replacing serine for arginine in expressed proteins. This mutation is specifically recorded at codon 249 of p53 (*TP53*) and has been extensively monitored in hepatocellular carcinoma patients and relevant controls

Table 5.6.1. Risk factors for hepatocellular carcinoma and cholangiocarcinoma

Type of condition	Hepatocellular carcinoma	Cholangiocarcinoma
Epidemic	Chronic HBV infection Chronic HCV infection Aflatoxin exposure	Liver flukes
Common	Chronic alcohol consumption Non-alcoholic fatty liver disease	Primary sclerosing cholangitis Recurrent pyogenic cholangitis
Rare	Hereditary haemochromatosis α-1-Antitrypsin deficiency	Chronic HCV infection Chronic HBV infection Non-alcoholic fatty liver disease

HBV, hepatitis B virus; HCV, hepatitis C virus.

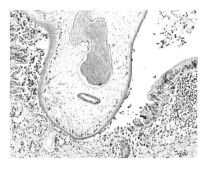

Fig. 5.6.1. Biliary dysplasia related to liver fluke infestation. Low-grade biliary intraepithelial neoplasia (BilIN-1) associated with an intraluminal liver fluke, *Opisthorchis viverrini* (haematoxylin–eosin; 10×).

from many regions, and particularly in studies from China [17].

Metabolic diseases such as hereditary haemochromatosis and α-1-antitrypsin deficiency markedly increase the risk of hepatocellular carcinoma; Wilson disease probably does so with much less frequency [1]. Of probably greater importance is the metabolic syndrome, which is associated with obesity, diabetes, and non-alcoholic fatty liver disease and will become increasingly important as the global epidemics of obesity and diabetes continue to worsen [5]. Moreover, this syndrome is likely to act synergistically for carcinogenesis in people with chronic viral hepatitis [18].

Cholangiocarcinoma is usually sporadic beyond regions characterized by endemic infections with foodborne liver flukes, such as those of the *Clonorchis* and *Opisthorchis* species [1,2]. The feeding, migrating flukes mechanically injure the biliary tree and incite abundant chronic inflammation that contributes to stepwise progression, via increasingly atypical biliary intraepithelial neoplasia, to invasive cholangiocarcinoma (Fig. 5.6.1) [1,2]. Inflammatory cholangiopathies, in particular primary sclerosing cholangitis, hepatolithiasis, and recurrent pyogenic cholangitis, also can lead to biliary intraepithelial neoplasia and cholangiocarcinoma [1,19]. Increased rates of cholangiocarcinoma are also seen associated with non-alcoholic fatty

liver disease, alcoholic liver disease, chronic HBV infection, and chronic HCV infection, although these cholangiocarcinomas remain uncommon [19].

Pathology

Hepatocellular carcinoma may arise from malignant transformation of hepatocytes or of hepatobiliary stem/progenitor cells [1]. In chronic liver disease, with or without cirrhosis, several precursor lesions have been described [20]. Most early lesions are recognized in established cirrhosis since mature hepatocellular carcinoma usually follows the development of such late-stage disease. However, all such lesions are recognized in pre-cirrhotic stages of scarring and regeneration as well [21]. The tumour–node–metastasis (TNM) classifications of hepatocellular carcinoma are shown in Table 5.6.2.

Cellular atypias known as "large cell change" and "small cell change" are related to hepatocarcinogenesis, particularly in patients with chronic viral hepatitis [21]. Large cell change consists of atypical cells with preserved nuclear-to-cytoplasmic ratio. Small cell change consists of small, atypical hepatocytes with increased

nuclear-to-cytoplasmic ratio. These cells appear in microscopic, expansile clusters in the hepatic lobule.

Dysplastic nodules are usually seen in cirrhosis (Fig. 5.6.3) [1,9,20,21]. These are radiologically or grossly distinctive nodules and are further classified as low-grade or high-grade based on the presence of cellular or architectural atypia [9,20,21]. Other high-grade changes include "nodule-in-nodule" lesions in which an expansile subnodule shows cellular and architectural features indicative of, but not yet prominent enough for diagnosis of, malignancy [1,9,20,21].

As premalignant lesions progress towards carcinoma, they initially spread around adjacent vascular and portal structures [9,20]. This can give rise to a radiologically subtle "vaguely nodular" pattern of early hepatocellular carcinoma, sometimes lacking diagnostic features by computed tomography or magnetic resonance imaging (Fig. 5.6.4A) [9,20,21]. With stepwise progression to hepatocellular carcinoma, more highly proliferative and more poorly differentiated subnodules arise, which, with increasingly rapid growth, overtake the pre-existing

Fig. 5.6.2. A young woman arranges maize in a seed house in Dumka, India. Crops stored in a hot and humid environment are particularly susceptible to contamination by strains of *Aspergillus*, resulting in dietary exposure to aflatoxins.

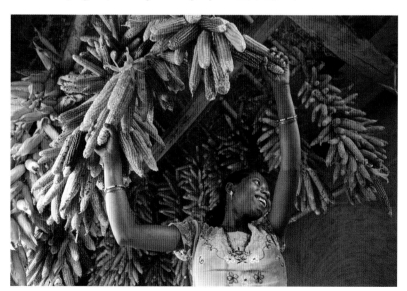

Treating chronic hepatitis with antiviral drugs to prevent liver cancer

Mark R. Thursz

During the past decade there have been major advances in the treatment of chronic viral hepatitis. Replication of hepatitis B virus (HBV) can be suppressed either by induction of immune responses with type 1 interferon or with nucleos(t)ide analogue drugs. Interferon-based therapy succeeds in only about 30% of cases, so nucleos(t)ide analogues are the more popular treatment option. Nucleos(t)ide analogues need to be administered indefinitely to maintain viral suppression, to prevent progression to cirrhosis and from

cirrhosis to decompensated cirrhosis. Furthermore, recent studies show resolution of cirrhosis with long-term treatment. However, the impact of viral suppression on the incidence of hepatocellular carcinoma is more controversial. One randomized placebo-controlled trial demonstrated a reduced incidence of cancer in treated patients. Meta-analysis of subsequent studies comparing successfully treated patients with historical controls or treatment failures now confirms that treatment reduces but does not eliminate the risk of hepatocellular carcinoma.

Chronic hepatitis C virus (HCV) infection can be cured using a combination of pegylated interferon and the nucleoside analogue ribavirin in more than 50% of cases. Combining current treatment with novel protease inhibitors increases the cure rate to about 80%, and there are currently combinations of direct antivirals in trials that, used in the absence of interferon, can cure the infection in more than 95% of cases. As with HBV infection, elimination of HCV infection prevents progression of the disease to cirrhosis and cancer. However, as cirrhosis is an independent risk factor for hepato-

cellular carcinoma, elimination of the infection reduces but does not remove the risk of cancer.

Treatment of viral hepatitis, particularly if it is initiated before the onset of cirrhosis, is an effective method of reducing the burden of hepatocellular carcinoma. However, several barriers prevent the widespread deployment of treatment. First, chronic viral hepatitis is asymptomatic, and it is essential to screen at-risk populations to identify those who need treatment. Second, although some drugs available for treatment of HBV infection are also used to treat HIV infection, The Global Fund to Fight AIDS, Tuberculosis, and Malaria will not supply these drugs for patients with HBV infection. Third, treatment of HCV infection currently requires a high level of medical training, which is not universally available. Finally, in spite of a World Health Assembly resolution in 2010, treatment programmes for viral hepatitis have not been developed for low-resource settings.

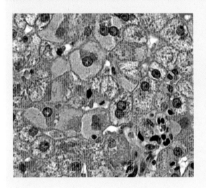

Fig. B5.6.1. High-magnification micrograph of ground-glass hepatocytes, as seen in a chronic hepatitis B virus infection with a high viral load; liver biopsy, haematoxylin–eosin stain.

Reference

Thursz M, Brown A (2011). *Gut*, 60:1025–1026. http://dx.doi.org/10.1136/gut.2010.236521 PMID:21508419

lesion and begin to push adjacent tissues aside to form a pseudocapsule [9,20]. These are features of "progressed" hepatocellular carcinoma (Fig. 5.6.4B). Throughout these processes, there is increasing arterialization, which slowly overtakes the contribution of portal venous blood until it is eventually eliminated in the progressed lesions, a process exploited for radiological assessment (Fig. 5.6.5A) [9,20]. In non-cirrhotic livers, hepatocellular adenomas are also potential precursors of hepatocellular carcinoma [14].

Cholangiocarcinoma is a gland-forming adenocarcinoma usually identified in advanced stages when

the initial, premalignant lesion has been overgrown (Fig. 5.6.1) [1,2]. Extrahepatic spread often occurs through lymphatic and perineural invasion [1]. Cholangiocarcinoma may be mass-forming, have multifocal nodules mimicking metastatic disease, or be a diffusely infiltrative process [1]. Since there is as yet no specific antigenic marker expression to immunohistochemically confirm biliary origin, confirmation of the diagnosis of cholangiocarcinoma requires clinical and radiological exclusion of metastasis from extrahepatic sites, particularly when there is no underlying hepatic disease that predisposes to biliary neoplasia [19].

Molecular and genetic alterations
No single sequence of molecular or genetic alterations contributes to the development of hepatocellular carcinoma [1,22]. The two most common early mutational events lead to activation of β-catenin and inactivation of p53. The former are found in up to 40% of these tumours and are more likely to be unrelated to HBV and to demonstrate genetic instability; the latter are found in up to 60% of hepatocellular carcinoma and are strongly associated with aflatoxin B_1 exposure. However, neither of these alterations is found in pre-malignant, low-grade or high-grade dysplastic nodules.

Table 5.6.2. Tumour–node–metastasis (TNM) classifications of hepatocellular carcinoma

T – Primary tumour

TX: Primary tumour cannot be assessed

T0: No evidence of primary tumour

T1: Solitary tumour without vascular invasion

T2: Solitary tumour with vascular invasion or multiple tumours, none > 5 cm in greatest dimension

T3: Multiple tumours, any > 5 cm, or tumour involving a major branch of the portal or hepatic vein(s)

  T3a: Multiple tumours, any > 5 cm

  T3b: Tumour involving a major branch of the portal or hepatic vein(s)

T4: Tumour(s) with direct invasion of adjacent organs other than the gall bladder or with perforation of visceral peritoneum

N – Regional lymph nodes

NX: Regional lymph nodes cannot be assessed

N0: No regional lymph-node metastasis

N1: Regional lymph-node metastasis

M – Distant metastasis

M0: No distant metastasis

M1: Distant metastasis

Stage grouping

Stage	T	N	M
Stage I	T1	N0	M0
Stage II	T2	N0	M0
Stage IIIA	T3a	N0	M0
Stage IIIB	T3b	N0	M0
Stage IIIC	T4	N0	M0
Stage IVA	Any T	N1	M0
Stage IVB	Any T	Any N	M1

The Wnt/β-catenin pathway is commonly disrupted in hepatocellular carcinoma, mostly as a result of mutations in *CTNNB1* or *AXIN1*, epigenetic silencing of *CDH1*, or changes in the expression of Frizzle receptors. Mutations have also been identified in genes in the interleukin-6 (IL-6)/JAK/STAT pathways [1,22]. The Rb1 pathway may be disturbed by mutation, loss, or silencing of *Rb1* or *CDKN2A*, or by reduced expression of other genes, such as *CDKN1A*.

Recently, a role has been demonstrated for short interfering microRNAs as modulators of these pathways, suppressing HNF4α and resulting in malignant transformation of hepatocytes [23]. This finding links chronic inflammation and hepatic IL-6 directly to malignant transformation without initiating mutations. The elucidation of roles in hepatocarcinogenesis of other microRNAs or other epigenetic mechanisms is likely to be fruitful in the coming years. Other pathways have shown less consistent changes in hepatocellular

carcinoma progression, including the MAPK and PI3K/AKT/mTOR signalling pathways and those moderated by growth factors [22].

Whole-genome sequencing of 88 matched hepatocellular carcinomas and normal pairs, 81 of which were HBV-positive, indicated β-catenin to be the most frequently mutated oncogene (15.9%) and *TP53* the most frequently mutated tumour suppressor gene (35.2%) [24]. The Wnt/β-catenin and JAK/STAT pathways were altered in 62.5% and 45.5% of cases, respectively, and prevalent pathways suggested a basis for categorization of tumours (Fig. 5.6.6).

IL-6 is implicated in the genesis of cholangiocarcinoma; its secretion by tumour cells enhances growth through autocrine mechanisms and may regulate activity of DNA transmethylases and hence alter expression of other genes, including *EGFR*. EGFR expression is a prognostic factor and a risk factor for tumour recurrence. Cholangiocarcinoma displays frequent mutations in cell-cycle regulators (p53, p16) and in

Fig. 5.6.3. Dysplastic nodule in cirrhosis. The distinctive nodule (arrow) in an explanted liver from a patient with end-stage hepatitis B stands out from the surrounding cirrhotic parenchyma in terms of colour and size. Dysplastic nodules, low-grade and high-grade, can be discerned by computed tomography and magnetic resonance imaging based on size, arterialization, and iron content. Histological examination of this lesion revealed a low-grade dysplastic nodule, devoid of cellular or architectural atypia; nonetheless, even low-grade dysplastic nodules in chronic liver disease indicate an increased risk of hepatocellular carcinoma development in the liver as a whole.

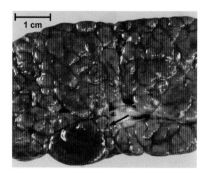

1 cm

MAPK pathways, in particular *KRAS* mutations [1,22]. KRAS in the bile of patients with primary sclerosing cholangitis without cholangiocarcinoma suggests that *KRAS* mutations are probably an early event in cholangiocarcinogenesis. Altered expression of ERRB2/HER2 has been described. Also, SOCS3 inhibition by promoter methylation leads to the constitutive activation of the IL-6/STAT3 pathway. Activation of that pathway, a potent mediator of local inflammatory reactions, provides an avenue for understanding the links between chronic biliary inflammation and carcinogenesis [22].

Detection

For individuals with chronic liver disease, routine screening for hepatocellular carcinoma is recommended; individuals without chronic liver disease, or living in areas where such screening is not performed, are likely to be diagnosed with symptoms of advanced disease [25]. Prospective screening, where possible, takes two forms: assessment of serum markers and repeated radiological examinations. The most widely used serum marker is α-fetoprotein, although it is ineffective for early lesions [1,25]. Other markers have been assessed, such as serum PIVKA and des-gamma-carboxy prothrombin, but none have reached the level of standard of practice [1].

Radiological examination in the course of late-stage (usually cirrhotic) liver disease, in contrast, is informative when possible [9,20,25]. Ultrasonography is generally insensitive for early lesions, but computed tomography and magnetic resonance imaging can often identify dysplastic nodules or early hepatocellular carcinoma [20]. If arterialization is complete, then there will be diagnostic features confirming this malignancy, including arterial enhancement, "washout" appearance, and pseudocapsule (Fig. 5.6.5B) [9,20]. Low-grade, high-grade, and vaguely nodular hepatocellular carcinoma, however, do not consistently show all these features, and

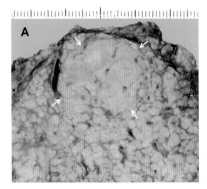 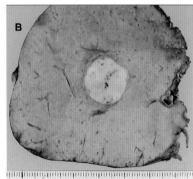

Fig. 5.6.4. Forms of early hepatocellular carcinoma (HCC). (A) The margins of a "vaguely nodular" HCC (arrows) are difficult to distinguish from the surrounding cirrhotic liver. Such lesions may or may not have completely characteristic imaging studies for defining them as HCC. Even biopsy diagnosis in such lesions may be difficult, relying on subtle changes indicative of microscopic stromal invasion. (B) A small but "progressed" HCC will have characteristic imaging features diagnostic of HCC. The pseudocapsule consists of atrophic hepatic tissue compressed by the rapidly expanding tumour.

Fig. 5.6.5. Pathological–radiological correlation of early stages of human hepatocarcinogenesis. (A) International consensus on the classification of small nodular lesions in cirrhotic liver. The diagnosis must consider the context of the lesion, especially the presence of cirrhosis, imaging findings, and growth rate. HCC, hepatocellular carcinoma; H-DN, high-grade dysplastic nodule; hyper, hypervascular; hypo, hypovascular; iso, isovascular; IWP, International Working Party; L-DN, low-grade dysplastic nodule; MD, moderately differentiated; WD, well-differentiated. (B) Liver magnetic resonance image showing a 1.9 cm, well-circumscribed hepatocellular carcinoma in a hepatitis B virus-associated cirrhosis. The lesion is dark to background liver before contrast administration (PRE), avidly enhances immediately after contrast in the hepatic arterial phase (HAP), and displays central "washout" appearance with a peripherally enhancing pseudocapsule in the 3-minute delayed phase imaging (DEL).

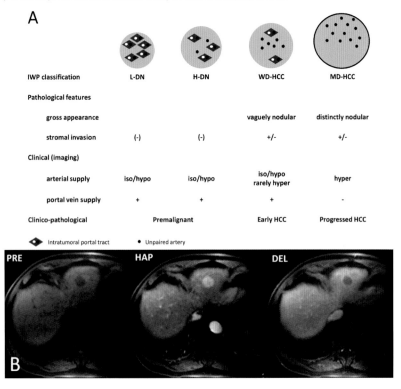

the current practice is to follow up such lesions with greater frequency, awaiting emergence of definitively diagnostic features or rapid increase in size [25]. Diagnosis of early lesions therefore does not depend on biopsy [20,25].

Cholangiocarcinoma has no specific serum markers that are diagnostic; however, in patients with conditions putting them at high risk, rising or high levels of serum markers such as CA19-9 and CEA may be helpful [26]. Repeat elevation of these markers after treatment can also be used to detect disease recurrence.

Prevention

Prevention of hepatic malignancies relies on removing the predisposing causes [26]. In coming decades, vaccination for HBV in endemic regions and screening of blood products for HCV should begin to diminish the incidence of hepatocellular carcinoma [22,25]. Reducing aflatoxin-producing mould in stored food has already resulted in decreased hepatocellular carcinoma incidence, even in HBV-infected populations [3,15]. Antiviral therapies, particularly when virus is eradicated, should also diminish incidence [25] (see "Treating chronic hepatitis with antiviral drugs to prevent liver cancer"). Malignancies associated with non-alcoholic fatty liver disease may prove difficult to prevent [5].

For prevention of cholangiocarcinoma, cooking of infested fish effectively eliminates the possibility of human infection by tumour-causing flukes [2]. However, such a public health intervention may conflict with long-standing cultural practices that include eating raw fish dishes in areas like Thailand. Thus, although prevention is theoretically possible, this goal remains difficult and may be unlikely to be achieved in relevant populations.

Fig. 5.6.6. Molecular subclassification of hepatocellular carcinoma (HCC). (A) Schematic summary of the gene expression, genetic, and clinical profiles of the three HCC subclasses. AFP, α-fetoprotein; HBV, hepatitis B virus integration; mut, mutation (somatic single-nucleotide variant). (B) Kaplan–Meier survival plot for the three HCC subclasses.

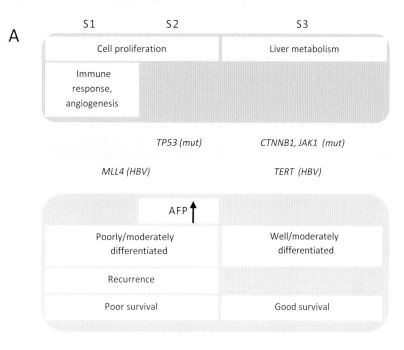

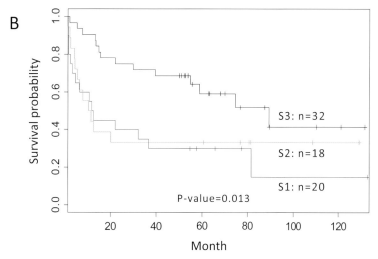

References

1. Bosman F, Carneiro F, Hruban R, Theise ND, eds (2010). *WHO Classification of Tumours of the Digestive System*, 4th ed. Lyon: IARC.

2. Sripa B, Kaewkes S, Sithithaworn P *et al.* (2007). Liver fluke induces cholangiocarcinoma. *PLoS Med*, 4:e201. http://dx.doi.org/10.1371/journal.pmed.0040201 PMID:17622191

3. McGlynn KA, London WT (2011). The global epidemiology of hepatocellular carcinoma: present and future. *Clin Liver Dis*, 15:223–243, vii–x. http://dx.doi.org/10.1016/j.cld.2011.03.006 PMID:21689610

4. Hou J, Xu J, Jiang R *et al.* (2012). Estrogen-sensitive PTPRO expression represses hepatocellular carcinoma progression by control of STAT3. *Hepatology*, 57:678–688. http://dx.doi.org/10.1002/hep.25980 PMID:22821478

5. Baffy G, Brunt EM, Caldwell SH (2012). Hepatocellular carcinoma in non-alcoholic fatty liver disease: an emerging menace. *J Hepatol*, 56:1384–1391. http://dx.doi.org/10.1016/j.jhep.2011.10.027 PMID:22326465

6. Chang MH, You SL, Chen CJ *et al.*; Taiwan Hepatoma Study Group (2009). Decreased incidence of hepatocellular carcinoma in hepatitis B vaccinees: a 20-year follow-up study. *J Natl Cancer Inst*, 101:1348–1355. http://dx.doi.org/10.1093/jnci/djp288 PMID:19759364

7. Lata J (2010). Chronic liver diseases as liver tumor precursors. *Dig Dis*, 28:596–599. http://dx.doi.org/10.1159/000320057 PMID:21088408

8. Theise ND (1996). Cirrhosis and hepatocellular neoplasia: more like cousins than like parent and child. *Gastroenterology*, 111:526–528. http://dx.doi.org/10.1053/gast.1996.v111.agast961110526 PMID:8690221

9. Hytiroglou P, Park YN, Krinsky G, Theise ND (2007). Hepatocarcinogenesis in humans: pathophysiology, radiographic detection and clinical significance. *Gastroenterol Clin North Am*, 36:867–887. http://dx.doi.org/10.1016/j.gtc.2007.08.010

10. Chen CJ, Yang HI, Su J *et al.*; REVEAL-HBV Study Group (2006). Risk of hepatocellular carcinoma across a biological gradient of serum hepatitis B virus DNA level. *JAMA*, 295:65–73. http://dx.doi.org/10.1001/jama.295.1.65 PMID:16391218

11. Lee MH, Yang HI, Lu SN *et al.* (2010). Hepatitis C virus seromarkers and subsequent risk of hepatocellular carcinoma: long-term predictors from a community-based cohort study. *J Clin Oncol*, 28:4587–4593. http://dx.doi.org/10.1200/JCO.2010.29.1500 PMID:20855826

12. Yang HI, Sherman M, Su J *et al.* (2010). Nomograms for risk of hepatocellular carcinoma in patients with chronic hepatitis B virus infection. *J Clin Oncol*, 28:2437–2444. http://dx.doi.org/10.1200/JCO.2009.27.4456 PMID:20368541

13. Huang YT, Jen CL, Yang HI *et al.* (2011). Lifetime risk and sex difference of hepatocellular carcinoma among patients with chronic hepatitis B and C. *J Clin Oncol*, 29:3643–3650. http://dx.doi.org/10.1200/JCO.2011.36.2335 PMID:21859997

14. Bouvard V, Baan R, Straif K *et al.*; WHO International Agency for Research on Cancer Monograph Working Group (2009). A review of human carcinogens – part B: biological agents. *Lancet Oncol*, 10:321–322. http://dx.doi.org/10.1016/S1470-2045(09)70096-8 PMID:19350698

15. Wogan GN, Kensler TW, Groopman JD (2012). Present and future directions of translational research on aflatoxin and hepatocellular carcinoma. A review. *Food Addit Contam Part A*, 29:249–257. http://dx.doi.org/10.1080/19440049.2011.563370 PMID:21623489

16. Grewal P, Viswanathen VA (2012). Liver cancer and alcohol. *Clin Liver Dis*, 16:839–850. http://dx.doi.org/10.1016/j.cld.2012.08.011 PMID:23101985

17. IARC (2012). Chemical agents and related occupations. *IARC Monogr Eval Carcinog Risks Hum*, 100F:1–599. PMID:23189753

18. Chen CL, Yang HI, Yang WS *et al.* (2008). Metabolic factors and risk of hepatocellular carcinoma by chronic hepatitis B/C infection: a follow-up study in Taiwan. *Gastroenterology*, 135:111–121. http://dx.doi.org/10.1053/j.gastro.2008.03.073 PMID:18505690

19. Braconi C, Patel T (2010). Cholangiocarcinoma: new insights into disease pathogenesis and biology. *Infect Dis Clin North Am*, 24:871–884, vii. http://dx.doi.org/10.1016/j.idc.2010.07.006 PMID:20937455

20. International Consensus Group for Hepatocellular Neoplasia (2009). Pathologic diagnosis of early hepatocellular carcinoma: a report of the International Consensus Group for Hepatocellular Neoplasia. *Hepatology*, 49:658–664. http://dx.doi.org/10.1002/hep.22709 PMID:19177576

21. Park YN (2011). Update on precursor and early lesions of hepatocellular carcinomas. *Arch Pathol Lab Med*, 135:704–715. PMID:21631263

22. Nault JC, Zucman-Rossi J (2011). Genetics of hepatobiliary carcinogenesis. *Semin Liver Dis*, 31:173–187. http://dx.doi.org/10.1055/s-0031-1276646 PMID:21538283

23. Hatziapostolou M, Polytarchou C, Aggelidou E *et al.* (2011). An HNF4α-miRNA inflammatory feedback circuit regulates hepatocellular oncogenesis. *Cell*, 147:1233–1247. http://dx.doi.org/10.1016/j.cell.2011.10.043 PMID:22153071

24. Kan Z, Zheng H, Liu X *et al.* (2013). Whole-genome sequencing identifies recurrent mutations in hepatocellular carcinoma. *Genome Res*, 23:1422–1433. http://dx.doi.org/10.1101/gr.154492.113 PMID:23788652

25. El-Serag HB (2011). Hepatocellular carcinoma. *N Engl J Med*, 365:1118–1127. http://dx.doi.org/10.1056/NEJMra1001683 PMID:21992124

26. Razumilava N, Gores GJ (2013). Classification, diagnosis, and management of cholangiocarcinoma. *Clin Gastroenterol Hepatol*, 11:13–21, e1. http://dx.doi.org/10.1016/j.cgh.2012.09.009 PMID:22982100

5.7 Pancreatic cancer

5 ORGAN SITE

Ralph H. Hruban

Günter Klöppel (reviewer)
G. Johan Offerhaus (reviewer)

Summary

- A majority of pancreatic cancers occur in countries with high or very high levels of human development.

- Pancreatic cancer is the seventh most common cause of cancer death worldwide, with a 5-year survival rate of 5%. Infiltrating ductal adenocarcinoma is the most common tumour type (90%).

- The leading identified cause of pancreatic cancer is cigarette smoking. Body fatness is an established risk factor. New-onset diabetes can be an early sign of the disease.

- Exome sequencing of ductal adenocarcinoma has demonstrated 16 significantly mutated genes – those previously recognized (KRAS, CDKN2A, TP53, SMAD4, MLL3, ATM, TGFBR2, ARID1A, and SF3B1) as well as novel genes, including genes involved in chromatin modification (EPC1 and ARID2), DNA damage repair, and other mechanisms (ZIM2, MAP2K4, NALCN, SLC16A4, and MAGEA6).

- Among other pancreatic neoplasms, serous cystadenomas are characterized by VHL mutations, solid-pseudopapillary neoplasms by β-catenin mutations, intraductal papillary mucinous neoplasms by mutations in GNAS, KRAS, and RNF43, and mucinous cystic neoplasms by mutations in RNF43, KRAS, and TP53.

- Inherited mutations in BRCA2, p16/CDKN2A, PRSS1, STK11, PALB2, and ATM and in DNA mismatch repair genes increase risk.

- Personalized therapy is slowly becoming a reality with poly(ADP-ribose) polymerase (PARP) inhibitors or mitomycin C for cancers with BRCA2 or PALB2 mutations, and everolimus for neuroendocrine tumours with mTOR pathway abnormalities.

Pancreatic cancer is not one disease. Several distinct neoplasms with unique clinical and pathological features may arise in the gland. About 95% of all pancreatic cancers develop in the exocrine pancreas, with about two thirds of these in the head of the pancreas. Infiltrating ductal adenocarcinoma is the most common of these neoplasms (accounting for 90% of all pancreatic cancer), and to a large degree the epidemiology of pancreatic cancer reflects the impact of these tumours. Ductal adenocarcinoma is the most aggressive of pancreatic neoplasms [1]. Most patients are diagnosed with metastatic disease, and only 5% survive to 5 years.

Infiltrating ductal adenocarcinoma is an infiltrating epithelial neoplasm with glandular (ductal) differentiation, usually demonstrating luminal and/or intracellular production of mucin, and without a predominant component of any other histological type. An abundant desmoplastic stromal response is a typical feature.

Pancreatic neuroendocrine tumours are less common (1–2% of all pancreatic cancer) but have a significantly better survival rate of 65% at 5 years [1]. In contrast, almost all patients with a serous cystadenoma are cured. Intraductal papillary mucinous neoplasms (IPMNs) and mucinous cystic neoplasms are important because they are curable precursor lesions that, if left untreated, can progress to an incurable invasive carcinoma.

All of the major tumour types of the pancreas have been sequenced. This revolution in our understanding of these neoplasms has opened the door to an understanding of why pancreatic cancer aggregates

Epidemiology

Pancreatic cancer

- Pancreatic cancer is estimated to be the 12th most common cancer in men (178 000 cases) and the 11th most common in women (160 000 cases) worldwide in 2012; 68% of the new cases occurred in countries at high or very high levels of human development.
- There were an estimated 330 000 deaths from pancreatic cancer in 2012, and because of its very high fatality, pancreatic cancer is the seventh most common cause of death from cancer worldwide.
- In 2012, one third of the estimated new cases occurred in Europe. The highest age-standardized incidence rates are found in central and eastern Europe, North America, Argentina, and Uruguay, and among women in Australia. Relatively low incidence rates are observed in most countries in Africa and East Asia.
- Given the overall mortality-to-incidence ratio of 0.98, the geographical patterns and trends for mortality are very similar to those observed for incidence.
- Trends in incidence and mortality rates in both sexes tend to be rather stable over time.

Map 5.7.1. Global distribution of estimated age-standardized (World) incidence rates (ASR) per 100 000, for pancreatic cancer in men, 2012.

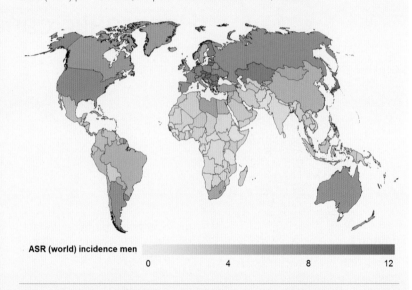

ASR (world) incidence men

Map 5.7.2. Global distribution of estimated age-standardized (World) incidence rates (ASR) per 100 000, for pancreatic cancer in women, 2012.

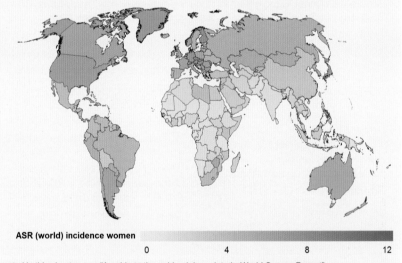

ASR (world) incidence women

For more details about the maps and charts presented in this chapter, see "A guide to the epidemiology data in *World Cancer Report*".

in some families, has helped in the identification of precursor lesions that are likely to progress to invasive cancer, and has created opportunities for personalized therapy.

Etiology

Non-modifiable risk factors for ductal adenocarcinoma of the pancreas include older age (most cases occur after the age of 65 years); race (in the USA, risk for Black populations is ≥ 1.5 that for White populations), and adult attained height. Cigarette smoking causes pancreatic cancer [2]. From meta-analysis, risk is significantly increased, by 74% and 20% for current and former smokers, respectively; pooled analysis indicated a significant elevation of

77% for current smokers and a non-significant increase of 9% for former smokers. Smoking is estimated to cause 20% of pancreatic cancer. Smoking cessation reduces risk, and by 20 years after cessation the risk for former smokers drops to that of never-smokers [3].

World Cancer Research Fund evaluations [4] specify convincing

Chart 5.7.1. Estimated global number of new cases and deaths with proportions by major world regions, for pancreatic cancer in both sexes combined, 2012.

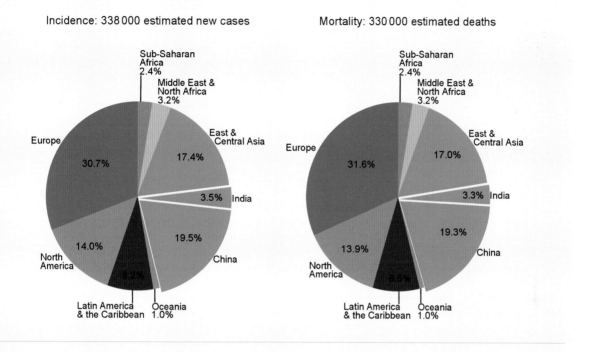

Incidence: 338 000 estimated new cases

Mortality: 330 000 estimated deaths

Chart 5.7.2. Age-standardized (World) incidence rates per 100 000 by year in selected populations, for pancreatic cancer in men, circa 1975–2012.

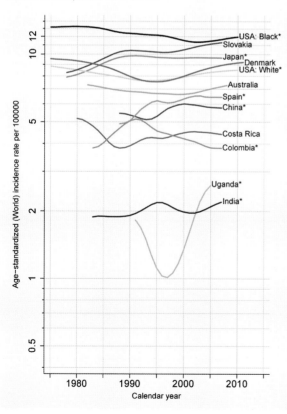

Chart 5.7.3. Age-standardized (World) incidence rates per 100 000 by year in selected populations, for pancreatic cancer in women, circa 1975–2012.

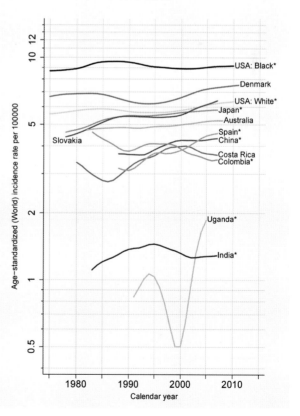

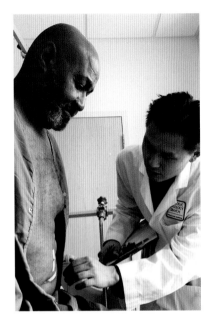

Fig. 5.7.1. A doctor examines a patient in relation to pancreatic disease. Worldwide pancreatic cancer rates are highest for African American men.

evidence that body fatness increases risk and probable evidence in relation to abdominal fatness, whereas evidence is limited for red meat consumption; coffee drinking is unlikely to affect risk. Other risk factors for pancreatic cancer include diabetes and non-O ABO blood type [1,3]. Chronic pancreatitis is an established risk factor for pancreatic ductal adenocarcinoma. However, most patients with this disease do not develop cancer, and most pancreatic cancer patients do not have a history of pancreatitis [5].

Pathology

Infiltrating ductal adenocarcinoma of the pancreas elicits an intense desmoplastic stromal reaction (Fig. 5.7.2) [1]. As a result, the bulk of the tumour is composed of collagen, stromal cells, inflammatory cells, and blood vessels. This dense desmoplastic stroma has two important clinical implications. First, biopsies may miss the neoplastic cells. Second, the dense fibrosis may hinder the delivery of chemotherapeutic agents to the neoplastic cells [6]. Perineural invasion is also

common, and many patients with pancreatic cancer experience pain.

Pancreatic intraepithelial neoplasia lesions are non-invasive microscopic epithelial proliferations in the smaller pancreatic ducts [7]. A growing body of evidence suggests that pancreatic intraepithelial neoplasia can be a precursor to infiltrating ductal adenocarcinoma. These lesions harbour many of the same genetic mutations found in infiltrating ductal adenocarcinomas, and rare clinical cases have been reported of patients with pancreatic intraepithelial neoplasia lesions who later developed an invasive pancreatic cancer. Although most of these precursor lesions are too small to be detected using currently available imaging techniques, they are a potential target for future early detection strategies.

Pancreatic ductal adenocarcinomas comprise a hierarchy of tumour cells that have been hypothesized by some to develop around a population of cancer initiating cells. Primary recognized markers of these cancer initiating cells are CD44, CD24, and ESA [8]. Immune cell infiltrates occur during tumour progression. Infiltration by immune cells with immunosuppressive activities allows for an environment that fosters tumour growth and progression [5]. One contributing factor to the failure of systemic cytotoxic and targeted therapies may be the abundant tumour stromal content that is characteristic of pancreatic ductal adenocarcinoma. The stroma, sometimes referred to as the tumour microenvironment, occupies the majority of the tumour mass and can be targeted in the development of novel therapy [9].

Genetics

The exomes of several ductal adenocarcinomas have been sequenced, and the most commonly mutated genes include an oncogene, *KRAS*, and three tumour suppressor genes, *TP53*, *p16/CDKN2A*, and *SMAD4* (Table 5.7.1) [10]. An understanding of the genes targeted in ductal adenocarcinomas not only provides

insight into the fundamental nature of these neoplasms but also has clinical implications. For example, loss of Smad4 protein expression as assessed by immunolabelling is a surrogate marker for *SMAD4* gene mutations, and can be used to suggest origin in the pancreas for a tumour of unknown origin.

Exome sequencing and copy number analysis have more recently been reported for a prospectively accrued clinical cohort (n = 142) of early (stage I and II) sporadic pancreatic ductal adenocarcinoma [11]. There were 16 significantly mutated genes, reaffirming known mutations (*KRAS*, *TP53*, *CDKN2A*, *SMAD4*, *MLL3*, *ATM*, *TGFBR2*, *ARID1A*, and *SF3B1*) and identifying novel mutated genes, including additional genes involved in chromatin modification (*EPC1* and *ARID2*), DNA damage repair, and other mechanisms (*ZIM2*, *MAP2K4*, *NALCN*, *SLC16A4*, and *MAGEA6*). Also reported were somatic aberrations in genes described as embryonic regulators of axon guidance, particularly SLIT/ROBO signalling. Loss of SLIT/ROBO signalling may be an alternative mechanism for dysregulating pathways downstream of their receptors, and in addition could influence the activity of inhibitors that target these upstream components, such as MET inhibitors (Fig. 5.7.3).

Approximately 10% of pancreatic cancer is believed to have a familial basis, and several genes have been identified that, when mutated in the germline, increase the risk of

Fig. 5.7.2. Photomicrograph of infiltrating ductal adenocarcinoma of the pancreas. Note the haphazard arrangement of the glands and the intense stromal fibrosis.

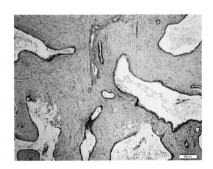

Table 5.7.1. The most common genetic alterations in ductal adenocarcinoma

Gene	Chromosome	Mechanism of alteration	Percentage of cancers
Oncogenes			
KRAS2	12p	Point mutation	95
BRAF	7q	Point mutation	5 (especially those with MSI)
AIB1	20q	Amplification	Up to 60
AKT2	19q	Amplification	10–20
MYB	6q	Amplification	10
Tumour suppressor genes			
p16/CDKN2A	9p	Point mutation plus LOH, HD, promoter methylation	95
TP53	17p	Point mutation plus LOH	75
SMAD4	18q	Point mutation plus LOH, HD	55
USP9X	X	Unclear	50
FAM190A	4q	Internal gene rearrangements	Up to 40
EP300	22q	Point mutation plus LOH	25
ARID1A	1p	Point mutation plus LOH	8
MLL3	7q	Point mutation	6
TGFbetaR2	3p	HD, biallelic intragenic mutations	4–7 (especially those with MSI)
STK11/LKB1	19p	Germline, point mutation plus LOH	4–6
FBXW7	4q	Point mutation plus LOH	< 5
MKK4	17p	Point mutation plus LOH, HD	4
ATM	11q	Point mutation plus LOH	3
TGFbetaR1	9q	HD	2
ACVR1beta	12q	Point mutation plus LOH, HD	2
ACVR2	2q	Point mutation plus LOH, biallelic intragenic mutations	Tumours with MSI

HD, homozygous deletion; LOH, loss of heterozygosity; MSI, microsatellite instability.

pancreatic cancer. These include *p16/CDKN2A, BRCA2, PALB2, PRSS1, STK11*, and *ATM*, and DNA mismatch repair genes (Table 5.7.2) [12].

Prospects

Although ductal adenocarcinomas of the pancreas have seemed to present an impenetrable barrier to progress, several recent advances provide hope. First, although the desmoplastic response may hinder the delivery of chemotherapeutic agents to the neoplastic cells, recent studies in animal models specifically targeting the stroma as a way to improve drug delivery have shown promise [6].

Second, recent studies of the genetic evolution of pancreatic neoplasia suggest that it takes many years for a genetically altered cell in the pancreas to invade and eventually metastasize. This suggests a large window of opportunity for the early detection of curable pancreatic neoplasia. If pancreatic intraepithelial neoplasia and cystic precursor lesions with high-grade dysplasia (discussed below) can be identified early, they can be treated before an infiltrating ductal adenocarcinoma develops.

Third, the discovery of some of the genes responsible for the familial aggregation of pancreatic cancer means that it is now possible to identify a population at risk that would most benefit from early detection. With the exception of *PRSS1*, these germline alterations also increase the risk of extrapancreatic malignancies. Therefore, mortality can be reduced by screening for one of the extrapancreatic malignancies (Table 5.7.2). For example, germline *p16/CDKN2A* mutations increase the risk of both pancreatic cancer and melanoma, and careful skin examinations of carriers of *p16/CDKN2A* mutations can aid early detection [12].

Table 5.7.2. Familial pancreatic cancer syndromes

Hereditary condition	Gene (chromosome)	Increase in lifetime risk of pancreatic cancer	Other cancers
Familial breast cancer, *BRCA2*	*BRCA2* (13q)	3.5–10×	Breast, ovarian, prostate
Hereditary pancreatitis	*PRSS1* (7q)	50–80×	None
Familial atypical multiple mole melanoma	*p16/CDKN2A* (9p)	20–34×	Melanoma
Familial breast cancer, *PALB2*	*PALB2* (16p)	Unknown	Breast
Peutz–Jeghers	*STK11* (19p)	100–132×	Gastrointestinal tract, breast, and others
Hereditary non-polyposis colorectal cancer	*MSH2* (2p) *MLH1* (3p) *PMS2* (7p) *MSH6* (2p)	8–9×	Colorectal, endometrial, ureteral, and others
ATM	*ATM* (11q)	Unknown	Breast?

Finally, a small percentage of the genetic changes identified are targetable with existing therapeutic agents. For example, it has been suggested that infiltrating ductal adenocarcinomas with biallelic inactivation of one of the Fanconi anaemia genes, including *BRCA2* and *PALB2*, are more sensitive to poly(ADP-ribose) polymerase (PARP) inhibitors and to mitomycin C [6]. This suggests a paradigm for personalized therapy in which tumours can be biopsied or resected and the optimal therapy guided by genetic analyses of the neoplastic cells.

Other tumour types

Cystic neoplasms

Intraductal papillary mucinous neoplasms

IPMNs are non-invasive, usually papillary, grossly visible mucin-producing epithelial neoplasms involving the larger pancreatic ducts (Fig. 5.7.4) [1].

Little is known about the epidemiology of these neoplasms, although patients with an IPMN have an increased risk of developing colon cancer. A review of computed tomography scans performed for indications unrelated to the pancreas revealed pancreatic cysts in 2.6% of the patients scanned, and this increased to a prevalence of 8.7% in individuals aged 80–89 years [13]. In individuals with a strong family history

Fig. 5.7.3. SLIT/ROBO signalling in pancreatic ductal adenocarcinoma. SLIT/ROBO signalling normally enhances β-catenin complex formation with E-cadherin and suppresses WNT signalling activity. Loss of ROBO1/2 signalling promotes stabilization of β-catenin, which decreases E-cadherin complex formation and cell adhesion and augments WNT signalling activity through increased nuclear translocation of β-catenin. In addition, SLIT/ROBO signalling can downregulate MET signalling activity; loss of ROBO signalling activity promotes MET signalling downstream and may have an impact on therapeutic strategies aimed at inhibiting MET activity at the receptor level. Aberrations in SLIT2 and/or ROBO1/2 affect 23% of patients.

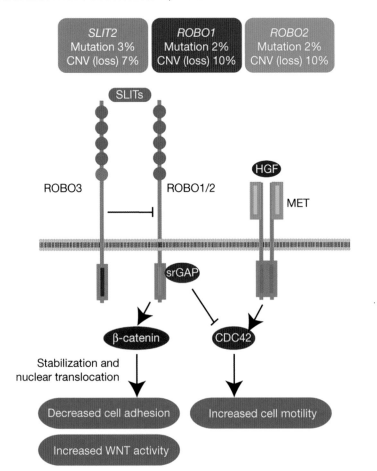

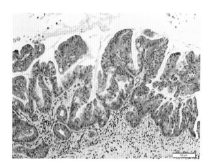

Fig. 5.7.4. Photomicrograph of an intra-ductal papillary mucinous neoplasm with high-grade dysplasia. This neoplasm extensively involved the larger pancreatic ducts. Note the luminal mucin and the non-invasive nature of the lesion.

of pancreatic cancer, the prevalence of these cysts is as high as 40% [14].

IPMNs arise in the larger pancreatic ducts and, in contrast to pancreatic intraepithelial neoplasia, most are grossly visible [1]. IPMNs can have varying grades of dysplasia and can be classified by the predominant direction of differentiation into intestinal, pancreatobiliary, oncocytic, and gastric subtypes. If untreated, as many as one third progress to infiltrating adenocarcinoma. IPMNs that involve the main pancreatic duct are more likely to have an associated invasive carcinoma than are those that involve a smaller branch duct [15]. IPMNs are often multifocal, and multifocality has been established at the genetic level. The exomes of a series of well-characterized IPMNs have recently

been sequenced, and the three genes mutated most frequently in these neoplasms are *KRAS*, *GNAS*, and *RNF43* (Table 5.7.3) [16,17]. The *SMAD4* and *TP53* tumour suppressor genes are inactivated in some high-grade IPMNs.

IPMNs present a unique opportunity to cure pancreatic neoplasia before an invasive carcinoma develops. They are detectable using existing imaging technologies, and some will progress to invasive cancer if left untreated. However, the risk of over-treating patients is significant. Not all cysts in the pancreas are IPMNs. Some are less aggressive serous cystadenomas. In addition, most IPMNs do not progress to infiltrating carcinoma. The Sendai criteria should be used as a guide for deciding which IPMNs to resect and which to observe [15]. These criteria suggest the resection of all main-duct IPMNs and the resection of branch-duct IPMNs that cause symptoms, have an associated mural nodule, or are associated with dilatation of the main duct. Looking forward, it is easy to imagine that an evaluation of the genetic changes in cyst fluid samples will help guide the management of pancreatic cysts.

Mucinous cystic neoplasms
Mucinous cystic neoplasms are non-invasive mucin-producing epithelial neoplasms of the pancreas characterized by a distinctive "ovarian-type" stroma. Most occur in adult women,

with a female-to-male ratio of 20. The etiology is unknown.

In contrast to IPMNs, the cysts of mucinous cystic neoplasms usually do not communicate with the larger pancreatic ducts [1]. Most arise in the tail of the gland. Mucinous cystic neoplasms can show varying grades of dysplasia, and up to one third progress to infiltrating adenocarcinoma. The exomes of a series of mucinous cystic neoplasms have recently been sequenced, and the three genes mutated most frequently in these neoplasms are *KRAS*, *TP53*, and *RNF43* (Table 5.7.3) [17].

As is true for IPMNs, mucinous cystic neoplasms offer an opportunity to detect and treat early curable pancreatic neoplasia before an incurable invasive carcinoma develops. In contrast to IPMNs, mucinous cystic neoplasms do not have a significant risk of multifocal disease. Surgical resection of a non-invasive mucinous cystic neoplasm is therefore almost always curative.

Serous cystadenomas
A serous cystadenoma is a usually cystic neoplasm composed of uniform cuboidal glycogen-rich neoplastic cells. There is a slight female predominance. Most cases are sporadic, but there is an association with von Hippel–Lindau syndrome.

The classic gross appearance of a serous cystadenoma is a neoplasm composed of innumerable small, thin-walled cysts with a central star-shaped scar, often calcified [1]. The cysts are lined by cuboidal neoplastic cells with round, uniform nuclei. The *VHL* gene is inactivated in at least half of these tumours [17].

Since serous cystadenomas are almost always benign, the goal of treatment is not to resect these neoplasms unless they are very large or symptomatic. The challenge is that serous cystadenomas can mimic the more aggressive IPMNs on imaging. It is hoped that preoperative evaluation of cyst fluid for markers of *VHL* inactivation will help guide the management of these lesions in the future.

Table 5.7.3. Genetic alterations in non-ductal neoplasms of the pancreas

Tumour type	Gene (chromosome)
Intraductal papillary mucinous neoplasm	*GNAS* (20q), *RNF43* (17q), *KRAS* (12p), *TP53* (17p), *SMAD4* (18q)
Mucinous cystic neoplasm	*RNF43* (17q), *KRAS* (12p), *TP53* (17p)
Solid-pseudopapillary neoplasm	*CTNNB1* (the β-catenin gene) (3p)
Serous cystic neoplasm	*VHL* (3p)
Pancreatic neuroendocrine tumour	*MEN1* (11q), *ATRX* (X), *DAXX* (6p), *TSC2* (16p), *PTEN* (10q), *PIK3CA*(3q)
Acinar carcinoma	*SMAD4* (18q), *JAK1* (1p), *BRAF* (7q), *RB1* (13q), *TP53* (17p)

**5 ORGAN SITE
CHAPTER 5.7**

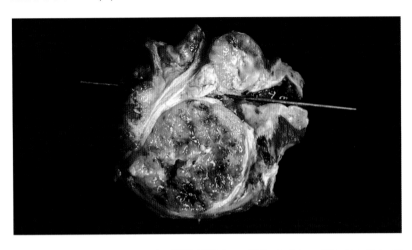

Solid-pseudopapillary neoplasms

A solid-pseudopapillary neoplasm is a low-grade malignant epithelial neoplasm composed of poorly cohesive cells. Most occur in women (with a female-to-male ratio of 10), usually in their twenties. The etiology is unknown.

While solid-pseudopapillary neoplasms can be solid, most undergo cystic degeneration. When they degenerate, the neoplasm has a distinct microscopic appearance with foam cells and the formation of pseudopapillae [1]. Genetically, solid-pseudopapillary neoplasms are characterized by mutations in CTNNB1, the β-catenin gene (Table 5.7.3) [17].

β-Catenin gene mutations result in an abnormal nuclear pattern of expression of the β-catenin protein. Immunolabelling for the β-catenin protein can therefore aid in diagnosis. Most solid-pseudopapillary neoplasms are cured by surgical resection.

Acinar carcinoma

Interestingly, although the normal pancreas largely consists of acinar cells, cancers with acinar differentiation are rare (only 1–2% of the cancers) [1]. Some patients with an acinar cell carcinoma present with the devastating lipase hypersecretion syndrome, in which lipase is released by the neoplasm into the circulation, causing subcutaneous fat necrosis, polyarthralgias, and peripheral blood eosinophilia. Acinar cell carcinomas are fully malignant neoplasms with a 5-year survival rate of only 25–50% [18].

Pancreatic neuroendocrine tumours

Pancreatic neuroendocrine tumours are epithelial neoplasms with significant neuroendocrine differentiation, as can be demonstrated by the expression of synaptophysin or chromogranin. Most occur in individuals aged 30–60 years. Pancreatic neuroendocrine tumours may be sporadic or arise in patients with a genetic syndrome such as multiple endocrine neoplasia type 1 (MEN1) or von Hippel–Lindau syndrome. The etiology is unknown.

Pancreatic neuroendocrine tumours are richly vascular neoplasms usually composed of nests, trabeculae, or sheets of relatively uniform cells with characteristic "salt and pepper" nuclei (Fig. 5.7.6) [1]. They are graded histologically based on the proliferation rate. Grade 1 pancreatic neuroendocrine tumours have a Ki-67 labelling index of 0–2%, grade 2 an index of 3–20%, and grade 3 (which are given the designation neuroendocrine carcinoma) an index of >20%. Grade and stage are important prognosticators. The exomes of a series of these tumours have been sequenced, and three "mountains" were identified (Table 5.7.3). The MEN1 gene is inactivated in about 45% of pancreatic neuroendocrine tumours, ATRX/DAXX in 43%, and one of the mammalian target of rapamycin (mTOR) pathway genes (TSC2, PTEN, or PIK3CA) in 16% [19].

Surgery is the treatment of choice, but most patients have metastatic disease at diagnosis. Somatostatin analogues (including octreotide) have been shown to slow tumour growth, and several significant advances have recently been made in targeted therapy for these tumours. The multiple tyrosine kinase inhibitor sunitinib has shown promise in phase III clinical trials, as has the mTOR pathway inhibitor everolimus. Although it has not been shown clinically, targeting the mTOR pathway may be most beneficial to patients with pancreatic neuroendocrine tumours that harbour mutations in an mTOR pathway gene [19,20].

Conclusions

A better understanding of the precursors to invasive adenocarcinoma of the pancreas may form the basis for improved early detection. Genetic changes can be used to classify neoplasms and thereby guide therapy, and in a small but growing number of cases genetic mutations that produce a therapeutically targetable change offer a promise of advances towards a future of personalized medicine.

Fig. 5.7.6. Photomicrograph of a pancreatic neuroendocrine tumour. Note the nested growth pattern, the absence of a desmoplastic stroma, and the "salt and pepper" chromatin pattern.

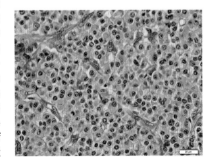

References

1. Hruban RH, Pitman MB, Klimstra DS (2007). *Tumors of the Pancreas (AFIP Atlas of Tumor Pathology* Series 4, Fascicle 6). Washington, DC: American Registry of Pathology and Armed Forces Institute of Pathology.

2. IARC (2012). Personal habits and indoor combustions. *IARC Monogr Eval Carcinog Risks Hum*, 100E:1–575. PMID:23193840

3. Lowenfels AB, Maisonneuve P (2006). Epidemiology and risk factors for pancreatic cancer. *Best Pract Res Clin Gastroenterol*, 20:197–209. http://dx.doi.org/10.1016/j.bpg. 2005.10.001 PMID:16549324

4. World Cancer Research Fund/American Institute for Cancer Research (2007). *Food, Nutrition, Physical Activity and the Prevention of Cancer: A Global Perspective*. Washington, DC: American Institute for Cancer Research.

5. Zheng L, Xue J, Jaffee EM, Habtezion A (2013). Role of immune cells and immune-based therapies in pancreatitis and pancreatic ductal adenocarcinoma. *Gastroenterology*, 144:1230–1240. http://dx.doi.org/10.1053/j.gastro.2012.12.042 PMID:23622132

6. Olive KP, Jacobetz MA, Davidson CJ *et al.* (2009). Inhibition of Hedgehog signaling enhances delivery of chemotherapy in a mouse model of pancreatic cancer. *Science*, 324:1457–1461. http://dx.doi.org/10.1126/science.1171362 PMID:19460966

7. Feldmann G, Beaty R, Hruban RH, Maitra A (2007). Molecular genetics of pancreatic intraepithelial neoplasia. *J Hepatobiliary Pancreat Surg*, 14:224–232. http://dx.doi.org/10.1007/s00534-006-1166-5 PMID:17520196

8. Abel EV, Simeone DM (2013). Biology and clinical applications of pancreatic cancer stem cells. *Gastroenterology*, 144:1241–1248. http://dx.doi.org/10.1053/j.gastro.2013.01.072 PMID:23622133

9. Feig C, Gopinathan A, Neesse A *et al.* (2012). The pancreas cancer microenvironment. *Clin Cancer Res*, 18:4266–4276. http://dx.doi.org/10.1158/1078-0432.CCR-11-3114 PMID:22896693

10. Jones S, Zhang X, Parsons DW *et al.* (2008). Core signaling pathways in human pancreatic cancers revealed by global genomic analyses. *Science*, 321:1801–1806. http://dx.doi.org/10.1126/science.1164368 PMID:18772397

11. Biankin AV, Waddell N, Kassahn KS *et al.*; Australian Pancreatic Cancer Genome Initiative (2012). Pancreatic cancer genomes reveal aberrations in axon guidance pathway genes. *Nature*, 491:399–405. http://dx.doi.org/10.1038/nature11547 PMID:23103869

12. Shi C, Hruban RH, Klein AP (2009). Familial pancreatic cancer. *Arch Pathol Lab Med*, 133:365–374. PMID:19260742

13. Laffan TA, Horton KM, Klein AP *et al.* (2008). Prevalence of unsuspected pancreatic cysts on MDCT. *AJR Am J Roentgenol*, 191:802–807. http://dx.doi.org/10.2214/AJR.07.3340 PMID:18716113

14. Canto MI, Hruban RH, Fishman EK *et al.*; American Cancer of the Pancreas Screening (CAPS) Consortium (2012). Frequent detection of pancreatic lesions in asymptomatic high-risk individuals. *Gastroenterology*, 142:796–804. http://dx.doi.org/10.1053/j.gastro.2012.01.005 PMID:22245846

15. Tanaka M, Fernández-del Castillo C, Adsay V *et al.*; International Association of Pancreatology (2012). International consensus guidelines 2012 for the management of IPMN and MCN of the pancreas. *Pancreatology*, 12:183–197. http://dx.doi.org/10.1016/j.pan.2012.04.004 PMID:22687371

16. Wu J, Matthaei H, Maitra A *et al.* (2011). Recurrent *GNAS* mutations define an unexpected pathway for pancreatic cyst development. *Sci Transl Med*, 3:92ra66. http://dx.doi.org/10.1126/scitranslmed.3002543 PMID:21775669

17. Wu J, Jiao Y, Dal Molin M *et al.* (2011). Whole-exome sequencing of neoplastic cysts of the pancreas reveals recurrent mutations in components of ubiquitin-dependent pathways. *Proc Natl Acad Sci U S A*, 108:21188–21193. http://dx.doi.org/10.1073/pnas.1118046108 PMID:22158988

18. Jiao Y, Yonescu R, Offerhaus GJA *et al.* (2013). Whole exome sequencing of pancreatic neoplasms with acinar differentiation. *J Pathol*, [epub ahead of print]. http://dx.doi.org/10.1002/path.4310 PMID:24293293

19. Jiao Y, Shi C, Edil BH *et al.* (2011). *DAXX/ATRX, MEN1*, and mTOR pathway genes are frequently altered in pancreatic neuroendocrine tumors. *Science*, 331:1199–1203. http://dx.doi.org/10.1126/science.1200609 PMID:21252315

20. Yao JC, Shah MH, Ito T *et al.*; RAD001 in Advanced Neuroendocrine Tumors, Third Trial (RADIANT-3) Study Group (2011). Everolimus for advanced pancreatic neuroendocrine tumors. *N Engl J Med*, 364:514–523. http://dx.doi.org/10.1056/NEJMoa1009290 PMID:21306238

Websites

American Cancer Society Pancreatic Cancer home page: http://www.cancer.org/cancer/pancreaticcancer/index

International Cancer Genome Consortium: http://www.icgc.org/icgc/cgp/68/304/798

Sol Goldman Pancreatic Cancer Research Center: http://pathology.jhu.edu/pc

The Cancer Genome Atlas: http://cancergenome.nih.gov/

5.8 Head and neck cancers

5 ORGAN SITE

Lester D.R. Thompson

Paul Brennan (reviewer)
Luis Felipe Ribeiro Pinto (reviewer)

Summary

- Tobacco smoking, alone and in combination with alcohol, is the most important cause of head and neck cancer.

- Most head and neck cancers are squamous cell carcinoma.

- Infection by human papillomavirus causes cancers of the oropharynx and base of tongue.

- Nasopharyngeal carcinomas are common in parts of South-East Asia and North Africa; their etiology involves Epstein–Barr virus, volatile nitrosamines, and genetic factors.

- Genetic alterations in oral and laryngeal cancer include activation of cyclin D1, *MYC*, *RAS*, *PIK3CA*, and *EGFR* and inactivation of tumour suppressor genes such as *p16*^{INK4A}, *TP53*, and *PTEN*.

- Mutations in PI3K pathway genes are proposed as a predictive biomarker.

- Early-stage tumours of the upper aerodigestive tract can be cured; for late-stage disease, prognosis is poor.

Head and neck cancers are a related group of cancers that involve the oral cavity, pharynx (oropharynx, nasopharynx, hypopharynx), and larynx (Fig. 5.8.1). Most tumours of the oral cavity, larynx, and hypopharynx are squamous cell carcinoma arising from the squamous cells that line these spaces. Other tumours that develop in this area (sinonasal tract, salivary glands) are relatively uncommon. Although related, there are four separate anatomical groups, with distinctly different etiologies but similar metastatic pathways.

Etiology

Cancers of the oral cavity and of the larynx and hypopharynx

The most significant causes of all head and neck cancers are tobacco use and alcohol consumption. These exposures account for the development of approximately 80% of such cancers globally, with some variation for different subsites (65% for oral cavity vs 86% for larynx) [1]. Smoking of cigarettes or bidis poses the most important risk for cancer development, related to the product of smoking rate in packs per day and duration of smoking in years ("pack-years"), and risk is higher for longer duration of smoking, smokers of black tobacco or high-tar cigarettes versus blond tobacco, young age at start of smoking, and deep smoke inhalation. Cigar and pipe smoking also pose a risk, although slightly less [1,2]. The relative risk is higher for glottic than for supraglottic carcinoma. Use of chewing tobacco or smokeless tobacco, and combinations with other substances such as paan or betel

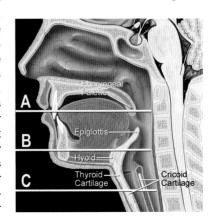

Fig. 5.8.1. The major anatomical sites within the head and neck include the nasal cavity, nasopharynx (A, purple), oral cavity, oropharynx (B, blue), larynx, and hypopharynx (C, green). The pharynx is divided using the junction between the hard and soft palate as the start of the nasopharynx; the inferior surface of the soft palate, uvula, base of tongue, tonsils, and tonsillar pillars within the oropharynx; and the hypopharynx extending from the superior border of the hyoid bone to the inferior border of the cricoid cartilage.

Epidemiology

Laryngeal cancer

- Laryngeal cancer is the 14th most common cancer among men, but it is relatively rare in women: of the 157 000 estimated new cases worldwide in 2012, less than 19 000 occurred in women. The estimated total number of deaths from laryngeal cancer was about 83 000.
- About 53% of the cases occurred in countries at high or very high levels of human development; 49% of the cases occurred in Asia.
- The highest incidence rates in men tend to be observed in eastern Europe and in certain countries in the Caribbean.

Cancer of the lip, oral cavity, and pharynx

- For cancers of the oral cavity and pharynx, an estimated 529 000 new cases occurred worldwide in 2012, with 292 000 deaths. When the main subsites (lip, oral cavity, nasopharynx, and pharynx) are examined separately, they do not rank highly, but combined would rank above cervical cancer as the seventh most frequent type of cancer by incidence and the ninth most common cause of cancer death.
- The highest incidence rates are in Papua New Guinea, Bangladesh, Hungary, and Sri Lanka. The 120 000 new cases and 88 000 deaths occurring in India represent almost one quarter and one third, respectively, of the total burden from these cancers.
- Incidence trends show a decline since the 1990s in populations where the rates were high (India, China, Blacks in the USA, Australia), in both sexes. Conversely, some populations with historically rather low incidence rates show increasing trends (e.g. Denmark, Japan).

Map 5.8.1. Global distribution of estimated age-standardized (World) incidence rates (ASR) per 100 000, for laryngeal cancer in men, 2012.

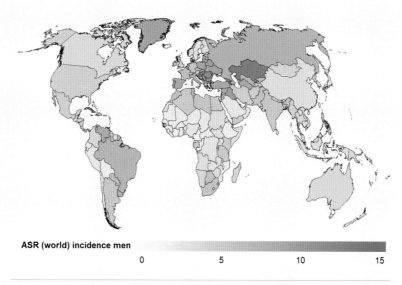

ASR (world) incidence men

0   5   10   15

Map 5.8.2. Global distribution of estimated age-standardized (World) incidence rates (ASR) per 100 000, for pharyngeal cancer in men, 2012.

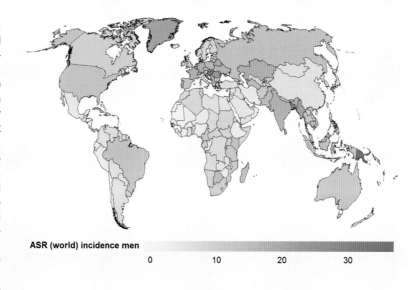

ASR (world) incidence men

0   10   20   30

For more details about the maps and charts presented in this chapter, see "A guide to the epidemiology data in *World Cancer Report*".

Chart 5.8.1. Estimated global number of new cases and deaths with proportions by major world regions, for laryngeal cancer in both sexes combined, 2012.

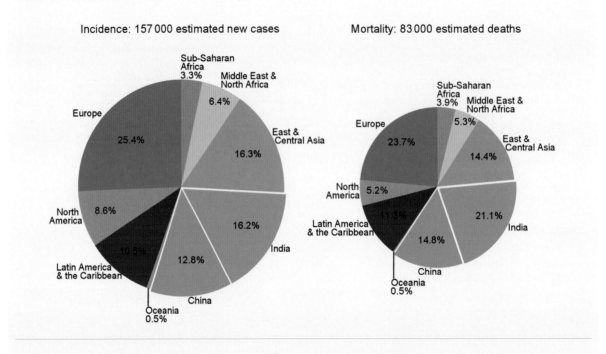

Incidence: 157 000 estimated new cases

Mortality: 83 000 estimated deaths

Chart 5.8.2. Estimated global number of new cases and deaths with proportions by major world regions, for oral and pharyngeal cancer in both sexes combined, 2012.

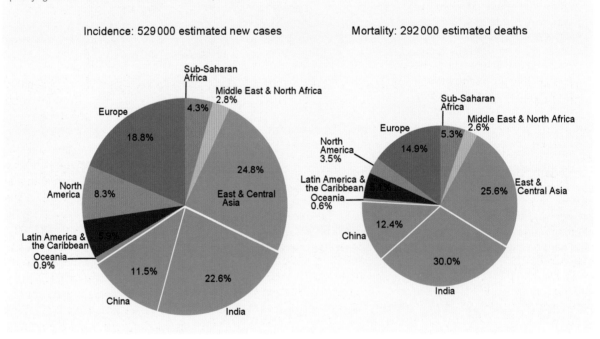

Incidence: 529 000 estimated new cases

Mortality: 292 000 estimated deaths

quid (betel leaf, areca nut, lime, and tobacco) poses an increased risk for oral cancer development, which is highest in India and in Taiwan, China, and especially

affects the floor of the mouth [2]. The risk decreases within 10 years of smoking cessation and is the lowest for groups of never-smokers, such as Seventh-day Adventists and

Mormons. Compared with never-smokers/teetotallers, the relative risk of head and neck cancer is increased between 10- and 100-fold in people who drink and smoke

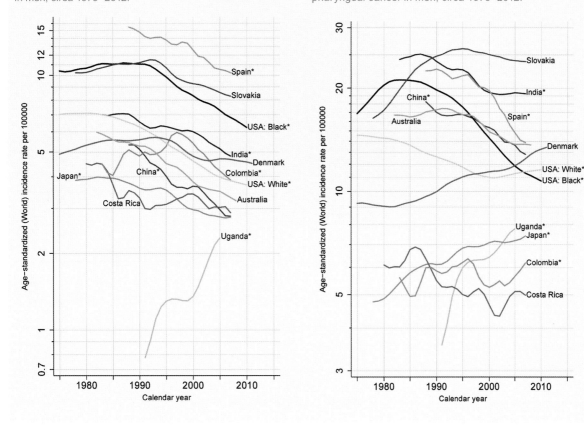

Chart 5.8.3. Age-standardized (World) incidence rates per 100 000 by year in selected populations, for laryngeal cancer in men, circa 1975–2012.

Chart 5.8.4. Age-standardized (World) incidence rates per 100 000 by year in selected populations, for oral and pharyngeal cancer in men, circa 1975–2012.

heavily. If there were total abstinence from drinking and smoking (or quid chewing) worldwide, the risk of oral, pharyngeal, and laryngeal cancers would be extremely low.

Alcohol consumption shows a strong multiplicative effect with tobacco, perhaps related to acetaldehyde, an intermediate metabolite of ethanol and a known carcinogen [3]. There are significant differences between countries in terms of per capita average alcohol consumption and the preferred type of beverage (beer, liquor, or wine). However, even with these differences, the most commonly consumed alcoholic beverage appears to be the one most strongly associated with cancer risk. For increased alcohol consumption, the relative risk is higher for supraglottic and hypopharyngeal carcinoma than for

glottic and subglottic carcinoma. There is a greater risk of pharyngeal and oral cancer related to the number of years of heavy drinking and not the number of drinks per day [1]. There is an increased relative risk of laryngeal carcinoma in patients who are heavy drinkers (> 8 drinks or > 207 ml/day) versus teetotallers or moderate drinkers, even without tobacco use. If individuals are classified as alcoholics, there is an even stronger risk of cancer development. Tumours may develop within a background of field cancerization, with additional tumours arising from the same environmental or epigenetic milieu that gave rise to the first tumour, often in adjacent head and neck sites.

Oral and oropharyngeal carcinomas are also associated with poor oral hygiene, habitual consumption of khat leaves, smoking marijuana,

and drinking maté, but causality with mouthwash use or with coffee drinking is not established [4].

Industrial exposure by working in construction, metal, textile, or ceramic jobs with exposure variously to isopropanol, polycyclic aromatic hydrocarbons, inorganic acid mists containing sulfuric acid and/or mustard gas, and diesel exhausts, and working in the food industry increase the risk of developing laryngeal cancer, after controlling for alcohol consumption and tobacco use. Human papillomavirus (HPV) may play a minor causative role in laryngeal and oral carcinomas [5]. Gastro-oesophageal reflux disease is associated with an increased risk of laryngeal carcinoma, but may also act as a promoter when alcohol and tobacco are used.

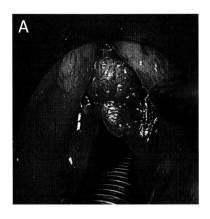

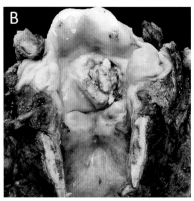

Cancers of the oropharynx and base of tongue

Infection with HPV is one of the major leading causes of cancers of the oropharynx, tonsil, and base of tongue. Due to the relatively high HPV infection rate in sexually active people (> 50%), a significant increase in the incidence of this type of cancer has occurred over the past several decades. This increase is correlated with changes in sexual habits, including the practice of oral sex, lifetime and recent number of sexual partners, the practice of premarital sex, and earlier ages of initial sexual activity, all of which contribute to the likelihood of oral infection. Biologically active HPV prevalence in oropharyngeal cancers ranges from 28% in Europe to 46% in Asia and 47% in North America, although more recent studies show rates of 65–70% [6]. HPV16 accounts for nearly all oropharyngeal cancers, while HPV18 is also a contributor to oral cavity cancers. The odds ratio for oropharyngeal oncogenic type-specific HPV16 E6/E7 antibodies is 72.8 (confidence interval, 16–330), which underscores the causal association of HPV with oropharyngeal carcinoma, along with integration of HPV DNA into the human genome [7], high HPV viral copy numbers [8], and high-level expression of HPV oncogenes (E6 and E7) in tumours. HPV also plays a causative role in selected oral (20.2%, weighted prevalence [WP]), sinonasal (29.6%, WP), laryngeal (23.6%, WP), and nasopharyngeal (31.1%, WP) tumours [5]. Marijuana use is also associated with HPV-positive oropharyngeal cancer development [9].

Nasopharyngeal cancer

Nasopharyngeal carcinoma exhibits a strong association with Epstein–Barr virus (EBV) infection, occupational exposures to wood dusts and formaldehyde, cigarette smoking, radiation exposure, consumption of specific preserved or salted foods, malaria infection, and genetic predisposition, as determined by multivariate-adjusted hazard ratios [10].

EBV is consistently implicated in nasopharyngeal carcinoma oncogenesis. EBV infection seems to be an early initiating event as EBV is found in precursor lesions and shows a clonal episomal form, indicating that the virus entered the tumour cell nucleus before clonal expansion started. This phenomenon results in nearly every tumour cell containing the full length of the EBV genome. Positive serology for the presence of immunoglobulin A antibodies to EBV capsid antigen is present in up to 93% of patients, with an increased titre correlated with high tumour burden. This elevated titre may be used as a marker to screen populations in high-risk areas or to detect tumour recurrence [11]. EBV-encoded early RNA is expressed in nearly all tumour cells. This type of infection shows a type II latency pattern, with expression of EBV nuclear antigen 1 (EBNA1) and latent membrane protein 1 (LMP1). LMP1 can induce squamous hyperplasia, inhibit squamous differentiation, activate NF-κB, and induce expression of epidermal growth factor receptor (EGFR).

Meta-analysis of 16 case–control studies showed that highest-versus-lowest intake of preserved vegetables was associated with a 2-fold increase in the risk of nasopharyngeal cancer, while high intake of non-preserved vegetables was associated with a 36% decrease in the risk of this cancer, irrespective of vegetable type or country of study. It is thought that high levels of volatile nitrosamines in preserved food may be a putative carcinogen. Based on case–control studies, consumption of salt-preserved food (specifically as Cantonese-style salted fish), fermented foods, or foods with related preservation processes, including quaddid (dried mutton stored in oil), and consumption of rancid butter during weaning and early childhood have an adjusted relative risk of up to 7.5, increasing to 37.7 when consumed at least once per week versus less than once per month at age 10 years [12].

Fig. 5.8.3. Tobacco smoking and alcohol consumption are causes of head and neck cancers, specifically cancers of the oral cavity, pharynx, and larynx. People who both smoke and drink alcohol are at markedly greater risk of developing these cancers than those who either smoke or drink alcohol in the absence of the other habit, although both individually increase the likelihood of developing head and neck cancers.

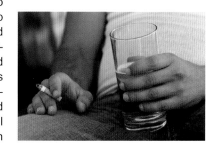

Fig. 5.8.4. The histological progression from normal to invasive squamous cell carcinoma is shown in parallel to genetic and epigenetic events. The accumulation of these genetic changes, and not the exact order, determines the progression to invasive carcinoma.

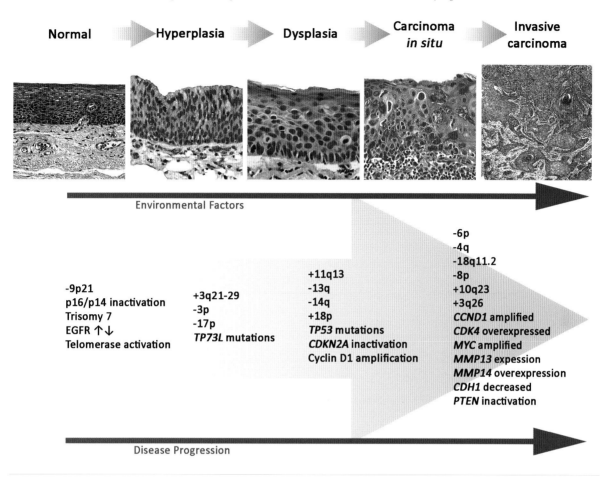

Pathology and genetics

Cancer of the oral cavity and of the larynx and hypopharynx

The squamous cell carcinomas of these two sites are similar one to another. There is in general a progression from epithelial hyperplasia through dysplasia to carcinoma in situ to invasive carcinoma (Fig. 5.8.4), but not all invasive tumours arise from an overlying dysplasia. There is a loss of maturation, architectural disorganization, and increased pleomorphism and cell size with dyskeratosis and increased mitoses to a variable degree with each grade of dysplasia. Although the length of time from dysplasia to invasive carcinoma is quite variable, it is generally measured in years. It is during this interval that disease progression may be altered by changes in habits (smoking, alcohol consumption) or surgical intervention. Tumours are separated into keratinizing and non-keratinizing, in situ versus invasive, and well, moderately, or poorly differentiated (Fig. 5.8.5). Variants are uncommon.

The genetic alterations observed in oral and laryngeal cancer are complex and interrelated. These alterations include activation of proto-oncogenes such as cyclin D1 (*CDKN2A*), *MYC*, *RAS*, *PIK3CA*, and *EGFR* and inactivation of tumour suppressor genes such as *p16*INK4A, *TP53*, and *PTEN*. *TP53* mutations and overexpression are seen in the progression of precursor lesions to invasive carcinomas, although this is reported with greater frequency in developed countries (40–50%) than in developing countries (5–25%). In contrast, tumours in patients from India and South-East Asia are characterized by the involvement of *RAS* oncogenes, including mutation, loss of heterozygosity (*HRAS*), and amplification (*KRAS* and *NRAS*). Mutations may also be seen in genes regulating squamous differentiation (such as *NOTCH1*, *IRF6*, and *TP63*) [13].

Cancers of the oropharynx and base of tongue

HPV-positive oropharyngeal carcinomas are distinct from HPV-negative cancers. HPV-positive cancers tend to be smaller primary tumours but with increased nodal involvement (high N stage), showing a poorly differentiated and non-keratinizing or basaloid histology

Fig. 5.8.5. (A) A moderately differentiated, invasive, keratinizing squamous cell carcinoma of the oral cavity. (B) A poorly differentiated, non-keratinizing squamous cell carcinoma of the larynx.

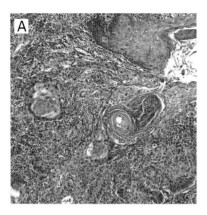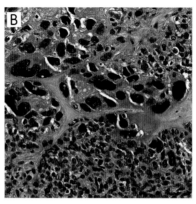

compared with HPV-negative cancers [6]. The tumours can be separated histologically into non-keratinizing, non-keratinizing with maturation, and keratinizing types; the first two types show the strongest association with HPV [14]. The tumours form nests with broad pushing borders and limited stromal response, frequent mitoses, and comedonecrosis. The cells form a syncytium, with indistinct borders, with hyperchromatic nuclei lacking prominent nucleoli. These tumours lack any squamous maturation or keratin pearl formation. Keratinizing squamous cell carcinomas have significant desmoplasia, with polygonal cells that show well-developed cell borders (intercellular bridges) and have abundant eosinophilic cytoplasm. Tumours that are intermediate ("with maturation") are hybrid tumours but are much more closely associated with HPV than the keratinizing type. Although not absolutely correlated, immunohistochemical expression of p16 (> 75% of cells with strong nuclear and cytoplasmic positive reaction) is considered an excellent surrogate marker for biologically active, integrated HPV infection. The interaction of HPV infection with *TP53* mutations and *EGFR* expression requires further investigation as these markers typically show a negative correlation with tumour HPV status.

Nasopharyngeal cancer

WHO classifies nasopharyngeal cancer into three major subtypes: non-keratinizing carcinoma, keratinizing carcinoma, and basaloid squamous cell carcinoma. Non-keratinizing carcinoma is the most common type and is most common in endemic populations, while the keratinizing and basaloid squamous cell carcinoma types tend to be more common in non-endemic populations. Non-keratinizing carcinoma is further separated into two types: differentiated (stratified cells with pleomorphic, hyperchromatic nuclei surrounded by well-defined cell borders, sharply delimited from the stroma but lacking a desmoplastic stromal response) and undifferentiated (a variable growth of cohesive cell nests to more individual dyscohesive cells within a lymphoid stroma) (Fig. 5.8.6). The cells are large with indistinct cell borders, scant cytoplasm, and round nuclei with vesicular chromatin distribution, containing prominent nucleoli. An in situ or precursor lesion is rare. Viral infection works via many interrelated somatic genetic and epigenetic changes that synergistically contribute to the development of nasopharyngeal carcinoma. This pathway is exceedingly complex, but the methylation of several tumour suppressor genes detected by nasopharyngeal brushings or in serum may aid in early detection and diagnosis.

Comprehensive genomic data are not available for nasopharyngeal cancer. One exome study based on biopsies indicated that the EBV-encoded genome maintenance protein EBNA1 along with LMP1, LMP2, and BARF1 were expressed in the majority of specimens studied. Analyses also suggested that loss of the *FHIT* gene may be a driver of tumorigenesis [15]. In another study based on paraffin-embedded specimens, 41 microRNAs were differentially expressed between nasopharyngeal tumour and corresponding non-cancer tissue, and a signature set of five was identified [16].

Prospects

Biomarkers

For oral dysplasia, several biomarkers have been shown to increase the risk of progression to cancer, including loss of heterozygosity, particularly at the 3p ± 9p loci, survivin, matrix metalloproteinase 9 (MMP9), and DNA content. Other markers (p53, p73, *MMP1*, and *MMP2*), did not seem to predict progression [17]. HPV is a significant prognostic biomarker in oropharyngeal squamous cell carcinoma, with the widest risk stratification for survival of any head and neck biomarker yet described, and thus has potential for important therapeutic considerations [18]. Whole-exome sequencing of 151 head and neck squamous cell carcinomas revealed the phosphatidylinositol 3-kinase (PI3K) pathway to be the most frequently mutated oncogenic pathway (30.5%) [19]. In a subset of HPV-positive tumours, *PIK3CA* or *PIK3R1* was the only mutated cancer gene. All tumours with concurrent mutation of multiple PI3K pathway genes were advanced, implicating this pathway in tumour progression and suggesting its use as a predictive biomarker.

Screening

Screening programmes similar to cytology for cervical cancer do not seem to be applicable for oropharyngeal or oral cancer. Cytological abnormalities are rarely detected even when there is known invasive disease, perhaps due to the difficulty of sampling the deep tonsillar crypts and to the lack of an identifiable precursor lesion. Therefore, delayed diagnosis is common. Direct visual inspection of the oral cavity, oropharynx, nasopharynx, and larynx (assisted by endoscopy) or evaluation by imaging studies in high-risk individuals may lead to early diagnosis, although large-scale screening programmes remain to be established on a global or regional scale. Significantly reduced oral cancer mortality has been observed in high-risk individuals in India undergoing repeated rounds of screening by inspection of the oral cavity [20].

Screening for plasma EBV DNA levels might be helpful in detecting nasopharyngeal cancer, based on pooled meta-analysis data sensitivity (91.4%; confidence interval, 89.0–93.4%) and specificity (93.2%; 91.2–95.0%) [11]. Screening of high-risk families (family members of nasopharyngeal carcinoma patients) or patients in endemic areas by EBV serology (for immunoglobulin A viral capsid antigen), EBV DNA, or other techniques (such as nasopharyngoscopy) has a potential benefit (sensitivity of 88.9% and specificity of 87.0%) as it detects cancers at a much earlier stage than symptomatic cancers (by up to 10 years), which yields improved disease-free survival.

Identification of high-risk groups

Patients with certain polymorphisms in enzymes involved in detoxifying alcohol (alcohol and aldehyde dehydrogenases [ADH]), show an increased susceptibility to developing carcinoma [3]. There seems to be a protective effect for patients with the *ADH1B* R48H variant and the *ADH7* A92G variant, with a significant modification based on increasing alcohol consumption; each gene's effect is independent of the other's.

There is an increased risk of upper aerodigestive tract cancers in patients with the *ADH1B* Arg47Arg genotype, much greater than that for patients with a His47His genotype.

Furthermore, there is a modulation of susceptibility when combined with alcohol consumption and interactions with the *ALDH2* 487Lys allele [21]. Additional genetic polymorphisms seen in association with head and neck cancer include those in the *GSTM1*, *GSTT1*, and *EPHX1* genes, *XPD* Lys751Gln, and *P53* codon 72 Pro/Pro.

A family history of head and neck cancer in a first-degree relative increased the risk (odds ratio, 1.7; confidence interval, 1.2–2.3), which was even higher when the relative was a sibling (2.2; 1.6–3.1). This risk was limited to subjects exposed to tobacco and alcohol (7.2; 5.5–9.5) [22]. Hence, if there is a family history of head and neck cancer, avoiding exposure to tobacco and alcohol reduces risk.

There are certain inherited conditions that are associated with an increased risk of developing head and neck cancer, including dyskeratosis congenita and DNA repair pathway disorders, such as Bloom syndrome (helicase gene mutations), Fanconi anaemia (germline mutations in *FAA*, *FAD*, and *FCC* caretaker genes), ataxia telangiectasia (homozygotes), and xeroderma pigmentosum (XP genes). IARC has collected information from 15 centres to study alcohol-related cancer and genetic susceptibility in patients enrolled from these centres, with a clear preponderance of smokers and alcohol drinkers in head and neck cancer cases.

Prevention

Avoiding cigarettes and alcohol could prevent up to 80% of oral cancer and up to 90% of laryngeal and hypopharyngeal cancer. Interventions targeting smoking

Fig. 5.8.6. (A) A non-keratinizing nasopharyngeal carcinoma showing prominent nucleoli and amyloid. (B) Most nasopharyngeal carcinomas have a very heavy inflammatory infiltrate, which can obscure the neoplastic cells. (C) Nearly every one of the neoplastic cells shows a strong nuclear reaction with Epstein–Barr virus-encoded small RNA.

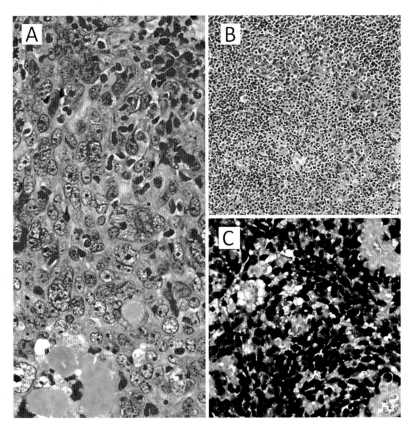

prevention or cessation are most effective when modelled by physicians, individual counsellors, or workplace- and school-based programmes (see Chapter 4.1). Further, national smoke-free policies may have public health benefits for both alcohol- and tobacco-related health problems.

The prophylactic use of the bivalent (HPV16 and 18) or quadrivalent (HPV6, 11, 16, and 18) vaccines in males and females (aged 9–26 years), if proven efficacious, holds great promise for primary prevention of HPV-associated oropharyngeal cancers since such a high proportion of HPV-associated oropharyngeal carcinomas are HPV16-derived [23].

References

1. Lubin JH, Purdue M, Kelsey K *et al.* (2009). Total exposure and exposure rate effects for alcohol and smoking and risk of head and neck cancer: a pooled analysis of case-control studies. *Am J Epidemiol*, 170:937–947. http://dx.doi.org/10.1093/aje/kwp222 PMID:19745021

2. Pednekar MS, Gupta PC, Yeole BB, Hébert JR (2011). Association of tobacco habits, including bidi smoking, with overall and site-specific cancer incidence: results from the Mumbai cohort study. *Cancer Causes Control*, 22:859–868. http://dx.doi.org/10.1007/s10552-011-9756-1 PMID:21431915

3. Xue Y, Wang M, Zhong D *et al.* (2012). *ADH1C* Ile350Val polymorphism and cancer risk: evidence from 35 case-control studies. *PLoS One*, 7:e37227. http://dx.doi.org/10.1371/journal.pone.0037227 PMID:22675424

4. Goldenberg D, Lee J, Koch WM *et al.* (2004). Habitual risk factors for head and neck cancer. *Otolaryngol Head Neck Surg*, 131:986–993. http://dx.doi.org/10.1016/j.otohns.2004.02.035 PMID:15577802

5. Isayeva T, Li Y, Maswahu D, Brandwein-Gensler M (2012). Human papillomavirus in non-oropharyngeal head and neck cancers: a systematic literature review. *Head Neck Pathol*, 6 Suppl 1:S104–S120. http://dx.doi.org/10.1007/s12105-012-0368-1 PMID:22782230

6. Chaturvedi AK (2012). Epidemiology and clinical aspects of HPV in head and neck cancers. *Head Neck Pathol*, 6 Suppl 1:S16–S24. http://dx.doi.org/10.1007/s12105-012-0377-0 PMID:22782220

7. Gillison ML, Koch WM, Capone RB *et al.* (2000). Evidence for a causal association between human papillomavirus and a subset of head and neck cancers. *J Natl Cancer Inst*, 92:709–720. http://dx.doi.org/10.1093/jnci/92.9.709 PMID:10793107

8. Kreimer AR, Clifford GM, Snijders PJ *et al.*; International Agency for Research on Cancer (IARC) Multicenter Oral Cancer Study Group (2005). HPV16 semiquantitative viral load and serologic biomarkers in oral and oropharyngeal squamous cell carcinomas. *Int J Cancer*, 115:329–332. http://dx.doi.org/10.1002/ijc.20872 PMID:15688391

9. Gillison ML, D'Souza G, Westra W *et al.* (2008). Distinct risk factor profiles for human papillomavirus type 16-positive and human papillomavirus type 16-negative head and neck cancers. *J Natl Cancer Inst*, 100:407–420. http://dx.doi.org/10.1093/jnci/djn025 PMID:18334711

10. Hildesheim A, Wang CP (2012). Genetic predisposition factors and nasopharyngeal carcinoma risk: a review of epidemiological association studies, 2000–2011: Rosetta Stone for NPC: genetics, viral infection, and other environmental factors. *Semin Cancer Biol*, 22:107–116. http://dx.doi.org/10.1016/j.semcancer.2012.01.007 PMID:22300735

11. Liu Y, Fang Z, Liu L *et al.* (2011). Detection of Epstein-Barr virus DNA in serum or plasma for nasopharyngeal cancer: a meta-analysis. *Genet Test Mol Biomarkers*, 15:495–502. http://dx.doi.org/10.1089/gtmb.2011.0012 PMID:21410354

12. Jia WH, Qin HD (2012). Non-viral environmental risk factors for nasopharyngeal carcinoma: a systematic review. *Semin Cancer Biol*, 22:117–126. http://dx.doi.org/10.1016/j.semcancer.2012.01.009 PMID:22311401

13. Stransky N, Egloff AM, Tward AD *et al.* (2011). The mutational landscape of head and neck squamous cell carcinoma. *Science*, 333:1157–1160. http://dx.doi.org/10.1126/science.1208130 PMID:21798893

14. Chernock RD (2012). Morphologic features of conventional squamous cell carcinoma of the oropharynx: 'keratinizing' and 'non-keratinizing' histologic types as the basis for a consistent classification system. *Head Neck Pathol*, 6 Suppl 1:S41–S47. http://dx.doi.org/10.1007/s12105-012-0373-4 PMID:22782222

15. Hu C, Wei W, Chen X *et al.* (2012). A global view of the oncogenic landscape in nasopharyngeal carcinoma: an integrated analysis at the genetic and expression levels. *PLoS One*, 7:e41055. http://dx.doi.org/10.1371/journal.pone.0041055 PMID:22815911

16. Liu N, Chen NY, Cui RX *et al.* (2012). Prognostic value of a microRNA signature in nasopharyngeal carcinoma: a microRNA expression analysis. *Lancet Oncol*, 13:633–641. http://dx.doi.org/10.1016/S1470-2045(12)70102-X PMID:22560814

17. Smith J, Rattay T, McConkey C *et al.* (2009). Biomarkers in dysplasia of the oral cavity: a systematic review. *Oral Oncol*, 45:647–653. http://dx.doi.org/10.1016/j.oraloncology.2009.02.006 PMID:19442563

18. Olthof NC, Straetmans JM, Snoeck R *et al.* (2012). Next-generation treatment strategies for human papillomavirus-related head and neck squamous cell carcinoma: where do we go? *Rev Med Virol*, 22:88–105. http://dx.doi.org/10.1002/rmv.714 PMID:21984561

19. Lui VW, Hedberg ML, Li H *et al.* (2013). Frequent mutation of the PI3K pathway in head and neck cancer defines predictive biomarkers. *Cancer Discov*, 3:761–769. http://dx.doi.org/10.1158/2159-8290.CD-13-0103 PMID:23619167

20. Sankaranarayanan R, Ramadas K, Somanathan T *et al.* (2013). Long term effect of visual screening on oral cancer incidence and mortality in a randomized trial in Kerala, India. *Oral Oncol*, 49:314–321. http://dx.doi.org/10.1016/j.oraloncology.2012.11.004 PMID:23265945

21. Cadoni G, Boccia S, Petrelli L *et al.* (2012). A review of genetic epidemiology of head and neck cancer related to polymorphisms in metabolic genes, cell cycle control and alcohol metabolism. *Acta Otorhinolaryngol Ital*, 32:1–11. PMID:22500060

22. Negri E, Boffetta P, Berthiller J *et al.* (2009). Family history of cancer: pooled analysis in the International Head and Neck Cancer Epidemiology Consortium. *Int J Cancer*, 124:394–401. http://dx.doi.org/10.1002/ijc.23848 PMID:18814262

23. D'Souza G, Dempsey A (2011). The role of HPV in head and neck cancer and review of the HPV vaccine. *Prev Med*, 53 Suppl 1:S5–S11. http://dx.doi.org/10.1016/j.ypmed.2011.08.001 PMID:21962471

Websites

American Society of Clinical Oncology Head and Neck Cancer home page:
http://www.cancer.net/cancer-types/head-and-neck-cancer

National Cancer Institute Head and Neck Cancer home page:
http://cancer.gov/cancertopics/types/head-and-neck

National Cancer Institute Throat (Laryngeal and Pharyngeal) Cancer home page:
http://cancer.gov/cancertopics/types/throat

The John Hopkins Medical Institution, Head and Neck Cancer home page:
www.hopkinsmedicine.org/kimmel_cancer_center/centers/head_neck/

5 ORGAN SITE
CHAPTER 5.8

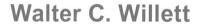

Walter C. Willett

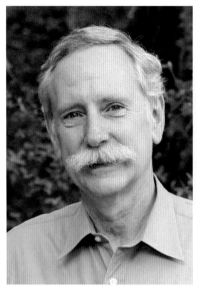

Diet, nutrition, and cancer: where next for public health?

Walter C. Willett is a professor of epidemiology and nutrition at the Harvard School of Public Health and a professor of medicine at Harvard Medical School. His research uses epidemiological approaches to investigate the effects of dietary factors on the cause and prevention of cancer, cardiovascular disease, and other conditions. Dr Willett earned his medical degree from the University of Michigan Medical School and a Doctorate of Public Health in epidemiology from the Harvard School of Public Health. His work emphasizes the long time frames and large cohorts required to obtain reliable data about diseases that may take years to develop. He has applied both questionnaire and biochemical approaches in the Nurses' Health Studies I and II and the Health Professionals Follow-up Study. Dr Willet wrote the classic textbook Nutritional Epidemiology *and also writes books on diet and nutrition for general audiences.*

Summary

Evidence that overweight, obesity, and physical inactivity are causally related to cancer is sufficiently strong to support strong actions to reduce these hazards. Multiple and increasingly intensive strategies will be needed to reverse the obesity epidemic, and actions are needed in many sectors and at all levels of society. Efforts to promote an overall healthy diet, including increases in fruits, vegetables, and whole grains and reductions in red meat, are well justified, but effects on risk of cancer specifically are likely to be modest. Continued research on diet, nutrition, and cancer is needed to expand the scientific basis for future progress to justify public health efforts.

A fundamental goal of research on diet and cancer is to identify constituents of food – including both classic nutrients and other aspects of diet – that increase or decrease the risk of cancer. This quest includes epidemiological investigations, experiments in animals, and in vitro studies. When the weight of evidence becomes sufficiently strong, this knowledge, which has usually been published piecemeal in scientific journals, needs to be translated into actions to prevent cancer. As discussed elsewhere in this Report, the process of research and translation leading to reductions in cancer rates has been highly successful for many types of exposures, including tobacco use, radiation, pharmaceuticals, and occupational hazards. From these experiences, we have learned much about the process of cancer prevention that can be applied to dietary factors. Here, I briefly review our current state of knowledge on diet, nutrition, and cancer, public health approaches to translation of knowledge on diet and cancer, and suggestions for future public health directions.

Current state of knowledge

Research on diet, nutrition, and cancer was limited until the late 1970s, when the large international differences in cancer rates and some animal studies suggested that some aspects of diet might play major roles in the cause and prevention of cancer. In response, many case–control studies were conducted, and large prospective studies were launched and are now producing abundant data. Progress has been more difficult than anticipated by many researchers, partly because of the complexity of human diets but also due to the nature of cancer and its origins.

In particular, we have come to appreciate that many cancers consist of distinct diseases with different causes, and also that the processes that lead to development of cancer can operate over a lifetime, thus making the study of diet and cancer exceedingly challenging. In our own research within several large prospective studies, we have also been investigating dietary factors in relation to risks of cardiovascular disease, diabetes, and many other outcomes, and clear associations between dietary factors and these diseases have emerged much more rapidly than for cancer, probably because the influences of dietary factors on the occurrence of these diseases are more immediate. This experience with other diseases has been important for research on cancer because it has documented that the methodologies to measure diet and to adjust for other factors do work well.

Despite the challenges of studying diet and cancer, several important conclusions have emerged. Most importantly, overweight and obesity have become established causes of many common cancers; this represents a major achievement in cancer research. Although the risks of cancer for an individual who is overweight or obese are not as great as they are for a tobacco smoker, in the USA and some other countries the much higher prevalence of overweight and obesity than of smoking means that the numbers of cancer deaths caused by these two factors are now similar [1]. Because the health consequences of obesity are not manifested immediately, the impact of the recent, rapid increases in the prevalence of obesity on cancer rates will continue to grow even if there is no further increase in prevalence. Physical inactivity is also now well established as a risk factor for several cancers, in part through its contribution to overweight, but also directly. Consumption of red meat, particularly processed red meat, is related to modestly higher risks, and of fruits and vegetables

to modestly lower risks of some forms of cancer.

Given currently available knowledge, control of overweight and obesity must be a high priority for cancer prevention, and increasing physical activity should be part of this effort. The dietary factors related to obesity are many and complex, but sugar-sweetened beverages (e.g. soda) have emerged as a particularly important contributing factor in many places (see Chapter 2.6).

Importantly, overweight or obesity, inadequate physical activity, and low intakes of fruits and vegetables, together with tobacco, are also major risk factors for cardiovascular disease and type 2 diabetes. Thus, programmes for the prevention of cancer should be closely integrated with activities for the prevention of these other diseases.

Public health approaches for cancer prevention through improved diets

To have a substantial impact on cancer rates, specific actions beyond the publication of papers in scattered scientific journals are needed. Knowledge is now often transmitted widely by the general media, such as television and newspapers, and some people will change their diets, become more active, or stop smoking based on this information alone. However, experience from tobacco control suggests that the impact of this will be limited. Also, with the Internet and other new channels of information, the public is being deluged with information on diet and health that is often sensationalist and out of context with other data, leaving many people more confused than they were with earlier, limited sources. Thus, a careful and coordinated public health approach for translation of nutritional knowledge will be needed to have an optimal impact; six levels of action with increasing intensity of intervention are described here [2]. Frieden has noted that, as compared with

individual counselling and clinical interventions, the greatest and most cost-effective public health impact will usually be achieved by changing the context so that the decisions of individuals are by default healthy ones, and by improving underlying socioeconomic factors [3].

1. Education and awareness
This process often begins with systematic reviews and summaries of the scientific literature on a topic, such as those on diet, nutrition, and cancer conducted by the World Cancer Research Fund/American Institute for Cancer Research [4], WHO [5], or national governments [6]. These are often accompanied by dietary guidelines based on the available evidence, and should appropriately consider all health outcomes simultaneously. Although the guidelines are usually developed by committees and are presumably better than judgements of individuals, collective biases and external influences can lead to recommendations that are not optimal. Thus, dietary guidelines are now being evaluated by determining whether adherence to them is actually associated with lower risk of cancer or other health outcomes [7]; this is a practice that should continue, to optimize our guidance. Although education alone often has modest impacts on behaviours, it is fundamentally important, in part because it can provide the foundation of support for more intensive policies, such as taxation.

2. Food and menu labelling
Labelling is currently a topic of much debate and research that requires integration of nutritional and behavioural sciences; the effects can be mediated by changes in consumer choices and by motivating food suppliers to reformulate products or modify serving sizes. Given the importance of overweight and obesity, labelling of energy (caloric) content has been a major focus; the impacts of this are not yet clear, and continued research is needed.

3. Economic strategies

These include taxation and subsidies. Increasing the prices of soda has a clear effect on consumption [8] and for this reason has been fought by the powerful beverage industry. Taxes on soda can be readily justified because the true costs of consumption to others, such as the health consequences, have not been internalized in the price. The scientific evidence base to support soda taxation has become much more solid in the past several years, and this should be pursued vigorously as a public health strategy.

4. Promoting or limiting availability

Limiting sales of tobacco has been an effective strategy, and this intervention is now becoming increasingly used for food and soda. In many places, soda is now no longer available in schools, and the city of Boston, USA, does not allow the sale of soda on any city property. Like tobacco, sale of soda in hospitals and other health-care facilities has become irrational, and is thus increasingly being eliminated in the USA. On the other hand, subsidies for whole grains, fruits, and vegetables can remove an important barrier to access for low-income populations and will promote consumption.

5. Fortification

Fortification has been an effective nutritional strategy to address many conditions, such as rickets, pellagra, goitre, and more recently congenital neural tube defects. Until now, this strategy has not been used specifically for cancer prevention, and concerns have even been raised that folic acid fortification for prevention of neural tube defects may have increased incidence of colorectal cancer. However, the concordance in time between increases in screening for colorectal cancer by colonoscopy and folic acid fortification almost certainly accounts for an apparent increase in incidence [9]. Other evidence suggests that additional folic acid may reduce incidence of colorectal cancer with a latency of more than 10 years. At this time, there is not sufficient evidence to support fortification specifically for cancer prevention, but this might become an option if data suggesting a benefit for vitamin D in reducing cancer risk become stronger.

6. Banning

We have a long regulatory history of banning specific food additives or colouring agents because of potential human carcinogenicity, and more recently partially hydrogenated oils have been banned in many countries, cities, and states because of their effects on cardiovascular disease. Banning whole foods or beverages is more difficult, and the experience of the USA with banning alcohol was notably unsuccessful. Short of absolute bans, a limit on the serving size of soda has been implemented in New York City and is being considered elsewhere, and a proposal to limit the amount of sugar added to beverages has been suggested. These strategies deserve consideration and evaluation.

Multisectoral approach for control of obesity

The rapid increases in obesity globally have led many organizations to develop strategies for controlling the epidemic. Because multiple factors contribute to unhealthy diets and inactivity, it is clear that interventions to address single aspects of the problem will have modest impacts, and multiple approaches will be needed. In most situations actions will be needed in the following sectors:

- schools and childcare settings;
- health-care facilities and systems;
- worksites;
- the food environment (to ensure availability and affordability of healthy food);
- the built environment (to promote physical activity);
- mass media (which is usually used to promote obesogenic foods);
- the economic sector (including taxes and subsidies, but also the analysis of cost and cost-effectiveness of interventions).

Strategic plans encompassing the above-mentioned sectors can be developed at almost every level, from global to national to local communities. The most effective level will vary depending on political realities; many of these actions would be most effective on a national level, but in the USA, political gridlock and the powerful influences of the food and beverage industries often make national actions impossible. Thus, progress is frequently much easier at the city or state levels, where external influences may be less.

Indicators of effectiveness

Unlike smoking, for which some cancers are almost specific, nutritional factors are primarily associated with cancers that have many causes, so it will be difficult to evaluate effectiveness of interventions by declines in cancer incidence. Instead, we will usually need to evaluate interventions by changes in diet or activity or prevalence of overweight and obesity. Some progress has been documented; in the USA, consumption of sugar-sweetened beverages has declined in recent years [8]. Also, in the past several years obesity rates among children have declined slightly in New York City and other cities where multilayered interventions have been developed [10].

Conclusions

Continued research on diet, nutrition, and cancer is needed to expand the scientific basis for future progress. However, evidence that overweight, obesity, and inactivity are causally related to cancer is sufficient to justify strong public health actions to reduce these hazards. These actions are further justified by the many other adverse health effects of these risk factors. Multiple and increasingly intensive strategies will be needed to reverse the obesity epidemic, and actions are needed in many sectors and at all levels of society. We have now begun to see some evidence of success, but sustained efforts will be needed for many years.

References

1. van Dam RM, Li T, Spiegelman D *et al.* (2008). Combined impact of lifestyle factors on mortality: prospective cohort study in US women. *BMJ*, 337:a1440. http://dx.doi.org/10.1136/bmj.a1440. PMID:18796495

2. Willett WC (2013). Policy applications. In: Willett WC, ed. *Nutritional Epidemiology*, 3rd ed. New York: Oxford University Press, pp. 357–379.

3. Frieden TR (2010). A framework for public health action: the health impact pyramid. *Am J Public Health*, 100:590–595. http://dx.doi.org/10.2105/AJPH.2009.185652 PMID:20167880

4. World Cancer Research Fund/American Institute for Cancer Research (2007). *Food, Nutrition, Physical Activity, and the Prevention of Cancer: A Global Perspective*. Washington, DC: American Institute for Cancer Research.

5. Joint WHO/FAO Expert Consultation on Diet, Nutrition and the Prevention of Chronic Diseases (2003). *Diet, Nutrition and the Prevention of Chronic Diseases: Report of a Joint WHO/FAO Expert Consultation*. Geneva: WHO (WHO Technical Report No. 916).

6. U.S. Department of Agriculture and U.S. Department of Health and Human Services (2010). *Dietary Guidelines for Americans, 2010*. Washington, DC: U.S. Government Printing Office.

7. Chiuve SE, Sampson L, Willett WC (2011). The association between a nutritional quality index and risk of chronic disease. *Am J Prev Med*, 40:505–513. http://dx.doi.org/10.1016/j.amepre.2010.11.022 PMID:21496749

8. Brownell KD, Farley T, Willett WC *et al.* (2009). The public health and economic benefits of taxing sugar-sweetened beverages. *N Engl J Med*, 361:1599–1605. http://dx.doi.org/10.1056/NEJMhpr0905723 PMID:19759377

9. Willett WC, Lenart E (2013). Folic acid and neural tube defects. In: Willett WC, ed. *Nutritional Epidemiology*, 3rd ed. New York: Oxford University Press, pp. 468–486. http://dx.doi.org/10.1093/acprof:oso/9780199754038.003.0020

10. Centers for Disease Control and Prevention (2011). Obesity in K-8 students - New York City, 2006-07 to 2010-11 school years. *MMWR Morb Mortal Wkly Rep*, 60:1673–1678. PMID:22169977

5.9 Kidney cancer

5 ORGAN SITE

Holger Moch

Lawrence H. Lash (reviewer)
Ghislaine Scelo (reviewer)

Summary

- Kidney cancer is most common in countries with higher levels of human development.

- Most kidney cancers (70%) are clear cell renal carcinomas; related tumours are papillary (10–15%), chromophobe (about 5%), and collecting duct (< 1%) renal cell carcinomas.

- Tobacco smoking is a cause of kidney cancer.

- Overweight and obesity are established risk factors. Occupational exposure to trichloroethylene causes kidney cancer.

- Hypertension and acquired cystic kidney disease with dialysis increase risk of renal cancer. Some renal cancer subtypes are associated with specific risk factors.

- Mutation or altered expression of the *VHL* gene has been extensively implicated in familial and spontaneous renal cell cancer.

- *PBRM1* has been proposed as a second major clear cell renal carcinoma gene, with truncating mutations in about 40% of cases. Mutations in *PBRM1* and *BAP1* anticorrelate, and PBRM1 and BAP1 apparently regulate different gene expression programmes.

Most renal cancers are renal cell carcinomas, a heterogeneous class of tumours arising from different cell types within the renal parenchyma. Most are clear cell renal carcinomas (about 70% of renal cancer cases), followed by papillary (10–15%), chromophobe (about 5%), and collecting duct (< 1%) renal cell carcinomas. Each of these renal cell tumour subtypes has distinct genetic characteristics [1,2]. Other subtypes in the renal parenchyma include oncocytoma, which is a benign tumour, and nephroblastoma (Wilms tumour), which occurs in children. Mesenchymal, mixed epithelial and mesenchymal, as well as other primary tumours or metastases are rare. The epidemiology of cancers of the renal pelvis differs from that of the renal parenchyma. Cancers of the renal pelvis are urothelial carcinomas and are similar to those of bladder urothelium.

Etiology

Lifestyle factors

Cigarette smoking causes renal cancer. Different meta-analyses confirmed that ever-smoking increases the risk of renal cancer compared with never-smoking [3,4]. There is also a dose-dependent increase in risk related to the number of cigarettes smoked per day. Risk decreases in the 5-year period after smoking cessation.

Using terminology adopted by the World Cancer Research Fund, there is convincing evidence that body fatness is a cause of kidney cancer. It is unlikely that coffee has a substantial effect, or that alcoholic drinks have an adverse effect, on the risk of this cancer [5]. Overweight, especially obesity, is a risk factor for renal cancer in both women and men [6]. The proportion of all cases of renal cancer attributable to overweight and obesity has been estimated to be about 40% in the USA and up

Fig. 5.9.1. The incidence of renal cell carcinoma increases significantly with increasing body mass index, the most common measure of overweight and obesity.

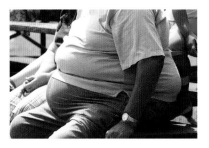

Epidemiology

Kidney cancer

- Kidney cancer is the ninth most common cancer in men (214 000 cases) and the 14th most common in women (124 000 cases) worldwide in 2012; 70% of the new cases occurred in countries with high and very high levels of human development, with 34% of the estimated new cases in Europe and 19% in North America.

- There were an estimated 143 000 deaths from kidney cancer in 2012 (91 000 in men, 52 000 in women); kidney cancer is the 16th most common cause of death from cancer worldwide.

- The highest incidence rates are found in the Czech Republic. Elevated rates are also found in northern and eastern Europe, North America, and Australia. Low rates are estimated in much of Africa and East Asia.

- The case fatality rate is lower in highly developed countries (overall mortality-to-incidence ratio, 0.4) than in countries with low or medium levels of human development (0.5). Only 3.1% of the cases were diagnosed in Africa, but 5.7% of the deaths occurred in this region.

- Incidence and mortality rates have been increasing in many countries, across different levels of human development.

Map 5.9.1. Global distribution of estimated age-standardized (World) incidence rates (ASR) per 100 000, for kidney cancer in men, 2012.

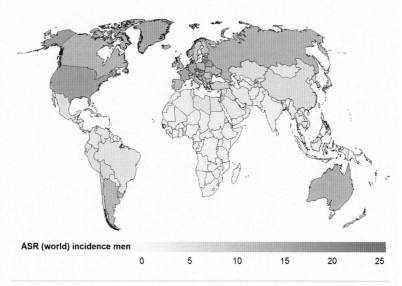

ASR (world) incidence men

0   5   10   15   20   25

Map 5.9.2. Global distribution of estimated age-standardized (World) incidence rates (ASR) per 100 000, for kidney cancer in women, 2012.

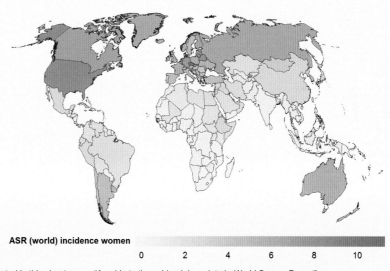

ASR (world) incidence women

0   2   4   6   8   10

For more details about the maps and charts presented in this chapter, see "A guide to the epidemiology data in *World Cancer Report*".

to 40% in European countries [7,8]. The mechanisms by which obesity influences renal carcinogenesis are unclear. Sex steroid hormones may affect renal cell proliferation by direct endocrine receptor-mediated effects. Obesity with the combined endocrine disorders, such as decreased levels of sex hormone-binding globulin and progesterone, insulin resistance, and increased levels of growth factors such as insulin-like growth factor 1 (IGF-1), may contribute to renal carcinogenesis. Recently, a case–control study has reported a stronger association of clear cell carcinoma with obesity.

Some case–control studies support a positive association between red meat intake and risk of renal cancer. The elevated risk of renal cancer is presumably due to the fat and protein content of meat. Several case–control studies found a protective effect of vegetables and fruits. However, the associations of meat and fruit with increased or reduced renal cancer risk are controversial [9]. There are studies showing an inverse association between alcohol intake

Chart 5.9.1. Estimated global number of new cases and deaths with proportions by major world regions, for kidney cancer in both sexes combined, 2012.

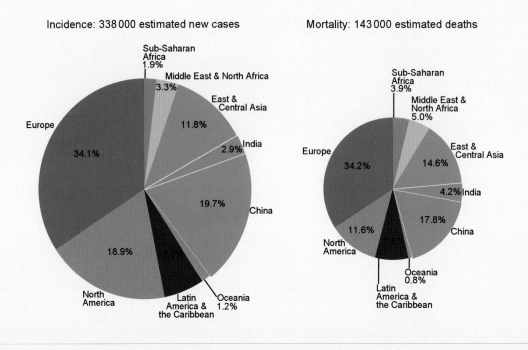

Incidence: 338 000 estimated new cases

Mortality: 143 000 estimated deaths

Chart 5.9.2. Age-standardized (World) incidence rates per 100 000 by year in selected populations, for kidney cancer in men, circa 1975–2012.

Chart 5.9.3. Age-standardized (World) incidence rates per 100 000 by year in selected populations, for kidney cancer in women, circa 1975–2012.

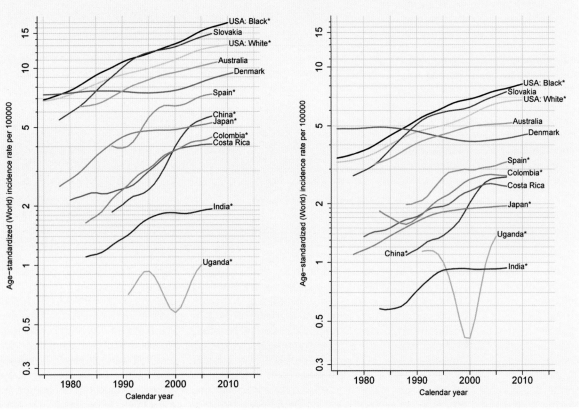

438

and renal cancer risk [10]. Recent analyses of 13 prospective studies from North America and Europe found no association between intakes of red meat, processed meat, poultry, or seafood and renal cell carcinoma risk [9,11]. No histological subtype differences were observed for associations with smoking, hypertension, or family history of kidney cancer [12].

Predisposing medical conditions, use of pharmaceutical drugs, and hormonal and environmental factors

Hypertension or its treatment has been associated with risk of renal cancer [13]. Use of hypertensive medication, including diuretics, has been associated with an elevated risk. The associations between risk of renal cancer and hypertension are independent of obesity. The biological mechanism for the association is not known. A few cohort studies have reported a significantly increased incidence of renal cancer among diabetic patients. However, diabetes may not be an independent risk factor because of its strong relation to obesity and hypertension [14]. Elevated levels of growth factors and growth factor receptors and insulin may mediate the possible relationship between diabetes and renal cancer.

Acquired cystic kidney disease usually develops in patients on long-term haemodialysis due to end-stage renal disease. The incidence of renal cancer is reported to be markedly increased in patients with end-stage disease (3–7%) [15]. Renal cancer occurring in end-stage renal disease has specific characteristics different from those of classic renal cancer. Papillary renal cell carcinoma was believed to be the most common subtype in end-stage renal disease. Currently, renal cancer associated with acquired cystic kidney disease is regarded as its own histological subtype, but all other subtypes (clear cell, papillary, and chromophobe renal cell cancer) also occur in cystic and non-cystic end-stage kidneys. Potentially, renal hyperplastic cysts

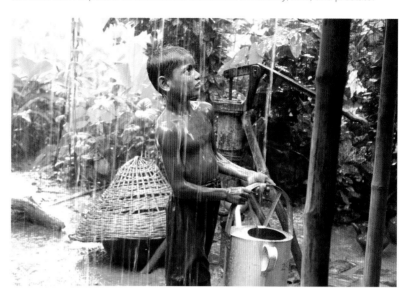

Fig. 5.9.2. A boy collects rainwater for drinking and cooking near an arsenic-contaminated tube well in a village in Rajbari District, Bangladesh. Arsenic in drinking-water causes cancers of the bladder, lung, and skin; a positive association has been observed between such exposure to arsenic and cancers of the kidney, liver, and prostate.

are the precursor lesions of some of these renal tumour types [16].

Phenacetin-containing analgesics are involved in the development of urothelial cancer of the renal pelvis. Several studies have found also an elevated risk of renal cancer with long-term use of phenacetin [17]. Among other analgesics, a few studies have found a positive association between acetaminophen – a metabolite of phenacetin – and renal cancer risk. There is also a potential risk of developing renal cancer for persons using non-aspirin, non-steroidal anti-inflammatory drugs (e.g. ibuprofen and naproxen). Aspirin and acetaminophen use were not associated with renal cell carcinoma risk [18].

Hormone-related factors have been suggested to play a role in renal cancer development, but several studies found no associations with use of oral contraceptives or hormone replacement therapy. Hysterectomy has been associated with increased risk of renal cancer in case–control studies [19]. The possible role of reproductive factors in renal cancer etiology remains poorly understood; certain hormone-related factors are

associated with risk, but these associations cannot explain the lower incidence in women than in men.

Studies in Taiwan (China) and Chile have also linked arsenic in drinking-water with cancer of the kidney.

Occupation

Renal cell cancer is not considered an occupation-related cancer. There are associations with asbestos, gasoline and other petroleum products, lead, cadmium, and trichloroethylene. Trichloroethylene is a solvent that has been widely used as a metal degreaser and chemical additive [20]. A meta-analysis of the association between exposure to trichloroethylene and clear cell renal cancer reported significant relative risks of kidney cancer: 1.3 overall and 1.6 for high-exposure groups [21]. IARC has classified trichloroethylene as Group 1 (carcinogenic to humans) on the basis of causing kidney cancer; the determination involved relevant epidemiological data, together with carcinogenicity of the solvent in both rats and mice. Biotransformation of trichloroethylene, well characterized in humans and animals, occurs

Fig. 5.9.3. Clear cell renal cell carcinoma. Typical cross-section of yellowish, spherical neoplasm in the upper pole of the kidney. Note the tumour in the dilated thrombosed renal vein (arrow). In addition, there is a benign renal angiomyolipoma in the lower pole with a characteristic yellow cut surface due to fat cells (asterisk).

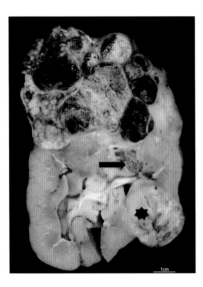

primarily through oxidative metabolism by cytochrome P450 enzymes, resulting in the generation of genotoxic metabolites [22].

Pathology

Clear cell renal cell carcinomas have a very vascular tumour stroma, frequently resulting in haemorrhagic areas [2]. The typical yellow tumour surface is due to the lipid content of the cells; cholesterol, neutral lipids, and phospholipids are also abundant (Figs 5.9.3, 5.9.4). Most renal cell carcinomas have little inflammatory response, but sometimes an intense lymphocytic or neutrophilic infiltrate with natural killer cells is present, and there is an association between a strong lymphocytic infiltration and worse outcome. Clear cell renal cell carcinomas most commonly metastasize haematogenously via the vena cava primarily to the lung.

Papillary renal cell carcinomas are characterized by epithelial cells forming papillae and tubules. Chromophobe renal cell carcinoma is distinguished by large polygonal cells with reticulated cytoplasm and prominent cell membranes. Some cells are irregular and multinucleated. Perinuclear halos are common. Collecting duct renal cell carcinoma is extremely aggressive, with frequent metastasis already at diagnosis. These tumours are usually located in the central region of the kidney. Histologically, collecting duct cancer is characterized by a tubulopapillary architecture with a characteristic desmoplastic stroma reaction.

Genetics

Heritable tumours

Although most renal carcinomas are sporadic, 2–4% have a familial cause. Several genetic diseases are associated with renal cancer [1]. The risk of renal cancer for a first-degree relative of a patient with renal cancer is increased about 2-fold. Each of the common histological subtypes of renal cancer has a corresponding familial cancer syndrome. Table 5.9.1 provides a complete list of syndromes known to be associated with kidney cancer risk. The most common ones include von Hippel–Lindau (VHL) syndrome, hereditary papillary renal cell carcinoma syndrome, hereditary leiomyomatosis and renal cell carcinoma syndrome, and Birt–Hogg–Dubé syndrome.

In VHL syndrome, patients develop haemangioblastoma of the central nervous system, retinal angiomas, and phaeochromocytomas. Renal cancer is found in 40–50% of VHL mutation carriers. The VHL gene produces a protein that targets hypoxia-inducible factor, a transcription factor. Loss of function leads to accumulation of hypoxia-inducible factor and subsequent upregulation of vascular endothelial growth factor and other factors that promote angiogenesis and tumour growth. The risk of developing kidney cancer associated with different germline VHL alleles correlates with the degree to which their protein products are impaired in their ability to regulate hypoxia-inducible factor.

Hereditary papillary renal cell carcinoma is caused by activation of the c-MET proto-oncogene. Mutations lead to constitutive activation of the receptor, which promotes tumour growth. This syndrome is characterized by multifocal papillary renal cell carcinomas. Patients with hereditary leiomyomatosis and

Fig. 5.9.4. Microscopic appearance of clear cell renal cell carcinoma.

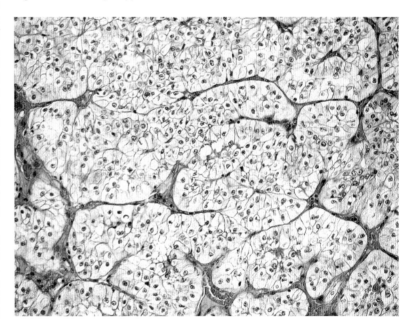

Table 5.9.1. Hereditary renal cell tumours

Syndrome	Gene (chromosome)	Protein	Tumour type	Extrarenal manifestations	
				Dermis	Other organs
von Hippel–Lindau syndrome	*VHL* (3p25)	pVHL	Multiple, bilateral clear cell RCC, renal cysts	–	Haemangioblastoma of retina/central nervous system, phaeochromocytoma, pancreatic/renal cysts, neuroendocrine tumours, epididymal/parametrial cysts, tumours of the inner ear
Hereditary papillary RCC syndrome	*c-MET* (7p31)	HGFR	Multiple, bilateral papillary RCC (type 1)	–	–
Hereditary leiomyomatosis and RCC syndrome	*FH* (1q42)	FH	Papillary RCC (non-type 1)	Leiomyoma	Uterine leiomyoma/leiomyosarcoma
Familial papillary thyroid carcinoma	? (1q21)	?	Papillary RCC, oncocytomas		Papillary thyroid carcinoma
Hyperparathyroidism–jaw tumour syndrome	*HRPT2* (1q25)		Epithelial–stromal mixed tumours, papillary RCC	–	Tumours of the parathyroid glands, fibro-osseous jaw tumours
Birt–Hogg–Dubé syndrome	*BHD* (17p11)	Folliculin	Multiple chromophobe RCC, oncocytomas, papillary RCC	Facial fibrofolliculoma	Pulmonary cysts, spontaneous pneumothorax
Tuberous sclerosis	*TSC1* (9q34)	Hamartin	Multiple, bilateral angiomyolipomas, lymphangioleiomyomatosis	Angiofibroma, subungual fibroma	Cardiac rhabdomyoma, adenomatous polyps of the small intestine, pulmonary/renal cysts, cortical tubers, subependymal giant cell astrocytomas
	TSC2 (16p13)	Tuberin	Rare clear cell RCC		
Constitutional chromosome 3 translocations	? (3p13-14)	?	Multiple, bilateral clear cell RCC	–	–

RCC, renal cell carcinoma.

renal cell carcinoma syndrome frequently have cutaneous leimyomas, and women often have a history of hysterectomy for uterine leimyomas at an early age. These patients show specific papillary renal cell carcinomas. In this syndrome, the *FH* gene shows loss-of-function mutations.

Birt–Hogg–Dubé syndrome is caused by germline loss-of-function mutations of the *BHD* gene and is characterized by fibrofolliculomas, lung cysts, and a spectrum of renal carcinomas including chromophobe renal cell carcinomas and oncocytomas. This syndrome has been correlated also with mutations in the folliculin tumour suppressor gene.

Spontaneous tumours

In sporadic renal cell carcinoma, there is a genotype–phenotype correlation. Clear cell renal carcinoma is characterized by a loss of chromosome 3p and alterations of the *VHL* tumour suppressor gene by mutation or hypermethylation. pVHL is a multifunctional protein and a substrate recognition subunit of a ubiquitin ligase complex that binds directly to hypoxia-inducible factor. Papillary renal cell carcinomas demonstrate frequent trisomy or polysomy of chromosome 7 and 17. Interestingly, activating mutations of the *c-MET* oncogene on chromosome 7 are rare in the sporadic forms of papillary renal cell cancer.

Chromophobe renal cell cancer is characterized by multiple cytogenetic changes, including monosomies of chromosomes 1, 2, 5, 10, 13, 17, and 21.

The role of a particular *VHL* mutation in trichloroethylene-induced malignancy has been highlighted. Model studies suggest that the mutation, P81S, may result in cells less likely to initiate apoptosis in response to a range of stimuli, and hence provide a pro-tumour benefit [23].

Results of exome sequencing are becoming available. One study based on 101 cases identified inactivating mutations in two genes encoding enzymes involved

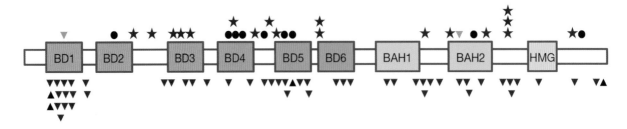

Fig. 5.9.5. *PBRM1* somatic mutations. Representation of PBRM1 transcript; boxes indicate the positions of the bromodomains 1–6 (BD1–BD6), the bromo-adjacent homology domains (BAH1, BAH2), and the high-mobility group domain (HMG). Relative positions of mutations are indicated by symbols: nonsense mutations (stars), missense mutations (dots), frameshift deletions (red triangles), frameshift insertions (black triangles), and in-frame deletions (green triangles). Splice-site mutations are not depicted.

in histone modification – *SETD2*, a histone H3 lysine 36 methyltransferase, and *JARID1C* (also known as *KDM5C*), a histone H3 lysine 4 demethylase – as well as mutations in *UTX* (*KMD6A*), a histone H3 lysine 27 demethylase [24]. A separate investigation resulted in the identification of the SWI/SNF chromatin remodelling complex gene *PBRM1* as a second major clear cell renal carcinoma cancer gene, with truncating mutations in 92 of 227 cases (41%) (Fig. 5.9.5) [25]. More recently, whole-genome and exome sequencing and other investigations have identified several putative two-hit tumour suppressor genes, including *BAP1* [26]. The BAP1 protein, a nuclear deubiquitinase, is inactivated in 15% of clear cell renal cell carcinomas. Mutations in *BAP1* and *PBRM1* are inversely correlated in tumours; BAP1 and PBRM1 regulate seemingly different gene expression programmes.

Recently, a survey of more than 400 clear cell renal cell carcinomas using different genomic platforms identified 19 significantly mutated genes, of which the eight most extreme were *VHL*, *PBRM1*, *SETD2*, *KDM5C*, *PTEN*, *BAP1*, *MTOR*, and *TP53*. The PI3K/AKT pathway was recurrently mutated. Widespread DNA hypomethylation was associated with mutation of *SETD2*; mutations involving the SWI/SNF chromatic remodelling complex were also implicated [27].

Kidney cancer has been characterized as a metabolic disease because many of the known genes associated with kidney cancer – *VHL*, *MET*, *FLCN*, *TSC1*, *TSC2*, *TFE3*, *TFEB*, *MITF*, *FH*, *SDHB*, *SDHD*, and *PTEN* – are involved in the cell's ability to sense oxygen, iron, nutrients, or energy. Understanding the metabolic basis of kidney cancer may enable the development of novel forms of therapy for this disease [28].

Prospects

The main avoidable causes of kidney cancer include cigarette smoking, obesity, and hypertension, representing opportunities for primary prevention [29]. Recent studies have shown associations between specific renal tumour subtypes and established risk factors, for example end-stage kidney disease or specific genetic syndromes. Based on a specific molecular background, novel tumour entities will be recognized as new distinct epithelial tumours within the future WHO classification system [2]. Further reports of these entities are required to better understand the nature and behaviour of rare and highly unusual tumours. The number of biomarkers in renal cell carcinoma is extensive and can range from diagnostic biomarkers, aiding in the classification of different tumour entities, to prognostic biomarkers for use as tools to stratify patient cohorts [30]. Systemic treatment of renal cell carcinoma has changed in the past years, with the development of new agents that target complex molecular pathways regulating tumour angiogenesis, cell proliferation, and survival [31]. Predictive biomarkers allow the choice of the appropriate therapy in patients who present with advanced disease. They provide information on which patients will be responsive or resistant to a targeted therapy. However, there are currently no available renal cancer biomarkers with enough reliability for treatment prediction [32]. Potential candidates for novel prognostic/predictive biomarkers may include microRNA profiles, different proteins, and/or multigene/protein assays. More novel molecular analysis is being used to identify specific molecular pathways involved in various tumour types and may identify potential new therapeutic targets.

References

1. Eble JN, Sauter G, Epstein JI, Sesterhenn IA, eds (2004). Tumours of the kidney. In: *Pathology and Genetics of Tumours of the Urinary System and Male Genital Organs*. Lyon: IARC.

2. Moch H (2013). An overview of renal cell cancer: pathology and genetics. *Semin Cancer Biol*, 23:3–9. http://dx.doi.org/10.1016/j.semcancer.2012.06.006 PMID:22722066

3. Cho E, Adami HO, Lindblad P (2011). Epidemiology of renal cell cancer. *Hematol Oncol Clin North Am*, 25:651–665. http://dx.doi.org/10.1016/j.hoc.2011.04.002 PMID:21763961

4. Hunt JD, van der Hel OL, McMillan GP *et al.* (2005). Renal cell carcinoma in relation to cigarette smoking: meta-analysis of 24 studies. *Int J Cancer*, 114:101–108. http://dx.doi.org/10.1002/ijc.20618 PMID:15523697

5. World Cancer Research Fund/American Institute for Cancer Research (2007). *Food, Nutrition, Physical Activity, and the Prevention of Cancer: A Global Perspective*. Washington, DC: American Institute for Cancer Research.

6. Ljungberg B, Campbell SC, Choi HY *et al.* (2011). The epidemiology of renal cell carcinoma. *Eur Urol*, 60:615–621. http://dx.doi.org/10.1016/j.eururo.2011.06.049 PMID:21741761

7. Renehan AG, Soerjomataram I, Tyson M *et al.* (2010). Incident cancer burden attributable to excess body mass index in 30 European countries. *Int J Cancer*, 126:692–702. http://dx.doi.org/10.1002/ijc.24803 PMID:19645011

8. Renehan AG, Tyson M, Egger M *et al.* (2008). Body-mass index and incidence of cancer: a systematic review and meta-analysis of prospective observational studies. *Lancet*, 371:569–578. http://dx.doi.org/10.1016/S0140-6736(08)60269-X PMID:18280327

9. Lee JE, Männistö S, Spiegelman D *et al.* (2009). Intakes of fruit, vegetables, and carotenoids and renal cell cancer risk: a pooled analysis of 13 prospective studies. *Cancer Epidemiol Biomarkers Prev*, 18:1730–1739. http://dx.doi.org/10.1158/1055-9965.EPI-09-0045 PMID:19505906

10. Lee JE, Hunter DJ, Spiegelman D *et al.* (2007). Alcohol intake and renal cell cancer in a pooled analysis of 12 prospective studies. *J Natl Cancer Inst*, 99:801–810. http://dx.doi.org/10.1093/jnci/djk181 PMID:17505075

11. Lee JE, Spiegelman D, Hunter DJ *et al.* (2008). Fat, protein, and meat consumption and renal cell cancer risk: a pooled analysis of 13 prospective studies. *J Natl Cancer Inst*, 100:1695–1706. http://dx.doi.org/10.1093/jnci/djn386 PMID:19033572

12. Purdue MP, Moore LE, Merino MJ *et al.* (2013). An investigation of risk factors for renal cell carcinoma by histologic subtype in two case-control studies. *Int J Cancer*, 132:2640–2647. http://dx.doi.org/10.1002/ijc.27934 PMID:23150424

13. Weikert S, Boeing H, Pischon T *et al.* (2008). Blood pressure and risk of renal cell carcinoma in the European prospective investigation into cancer and nutrition. *Am J Epidemiol*, 167:438–446. http://dx.doi.org/10.1093/aje/kwm321 PMID:18048375

14. Schlehofer B, Pommer W, Mellemgaard A *et al.* (1996). International renal-cell-cancer study. VI. The role of medical and family history. *Int J Cancer*, 66:723–726. http://dx.doi.org/10.1002/(SICI)1097-0215(19960611)66:6<723::AID-IJC2>3.0.CO;2-1 PMID:8647639

15. Denton MD, Magee CC, Ovuworie C *et al.* (2002). Prevalence of renal cell carcinoma in patients with ESRD pre-transplantation: a pathologic analysis. *Kidney Int*, 61:2201–2209. http://dx.doi.org/10.1046/j.1523-1755.2002.00374.x PMID:12028461

16. Montani M, Heinimann K, von Teichman A *et al.* (2010). VHL-gene deletion in single renal tubular epithelial cells and renal tubular cysts: further evidence for a cyst-dependent progression pathway of clear cell renal carcinoma in von Hippel-Lindau disease. *Am J Surg Pathol*, 34:806–815. http://dx.doi.org/10.1097/PAS.0b013e3181ddf54d PMID:20431476

17. McCredie M, Pommer W, McLaughlin JK *et al.* (1995). International renal-cell cancer study. II. Analgesics. *Int J Cancer*, 60:345–349. http://dx.doi.org/10.1002/ijc.2910600312 PMID:7829242

18. Cho E, Curhan G, Hankinson SE *et al.* (2011). Prospective evaluation of analgesic use and risk of renal cell cancer. *Arch Intern Med*, 171:1487–1493. http://dx.doi.org/10.1001/archinternmed.2011.356 PMID:21911634

19. Lindblad P, Mellemgaard A, Schlehofer B *et al.* (1995). International renal-cell cancer study. V. Reproductive factors, gynecologic operations and exogenous hormones. *Int J Cancer*, 61:192–198. http://dx.doi.org/10.1002/ijc.2910610209 PMID:7705947

20. Kelsh MA, Alexander DD, Mink PJ, Mandel JH (2010). Occupational trichloroethylene exposure and kidney cancer: a meta-analysis. *Epidemiology*, 21:95–102. http://dx.doi.org/10.1097/EDE.0b013e3181c30e92 PMID:20010212

21. Scott CS, Jinot J (2011). Trichloroethylene and cancer: systematic and quantitative review of epidemiologic evidence for identifying hazards. *Int J Environ Res Public Health*, 8:4238–4272. http://dx.doi.org/10.3390/ijerph8114238 PMID:22163205

22. Guha N, Loomis D, Grosse Y *et al.*; International Agency for Research on Cancer Monograph Working Group (2012). Carcinogenicity of trichloroethylene, tetrachloroethylene, some other chlorinated solvents, and their metabolites. *Lancet Oncol*, 13:1192–1193. http://dx.doi.org/10.1016/S1470-2045(12)70485-0 PMID:23323277

23. Desimone MC, Rathmell WK, Threadgill DW (2013). Pleiotropic effects of the trichloroethylene-associated P81S *VHL* mutation on metabolism, apoptosis, and ATM-mediated DNA damage response. *J Natl Cancer Inst*, 105:1355–1364. http://dx.doi.org/10.1093/jnci/djt226 PMID:23990666

24. Dalgliesh GL, Furge K, Greenman C *et al.* (2010). Systematic sequencing of renal carcinoma reveals inactivation of histone modifying genes. *Nature*, 463:360–363. http://dx.doi.org/10.1038/nature08672 PMID:20054297

25. Varela I, Tarpey P, Raine K *et al.* (2011). Exome sequencing identifies frequent mutation of the SWI/SNF complex gene *PBRM1* in renal carcinoma. *Nature*, 469:539–542. http://dx.doi.org/10.1038/nature09639 PMID:21248752

26. Peña-Llopis S, Vega-Rubín-de-Celis S, Liao A *et al.* (2012). BAP1 loss defines a new class of renal cell carcinoma. *Nat Genet*, 44:751–759. http://dx.doi.org/10.1038/ng.2323 PMID:22683710

27. Creighton CJ, Morgan M, Gunaratne PH *et al.*; Cancer Genome Atlas Research Network (2013). Comprehensive molecular characterization of clear cell renal cell carcinoma. *Nature*, 499:43–49. http://dx.doi.org/10.1038/nature12222 PMID:23792563

28. Linehan WM, Ricketts CJ (2013). The metabolic basis of kidney cancer. *Semin Cancer Biol*, 23:46–55. http://dx.doi.org/10.1016/j.semcancer.2012.06.002 PMID:22705279

29. Weikert S, Ljungberg B (2010). Contemporary epidemiology of renal cell carcinoma: perspectives of primary prevention. *World J Urol*, 28:247–252. http://dx.doi.org/10.1007/s00345-010-0555-1 PMID:20390283

30. Eichelberg C, Junker K, Ljungberg B, Moch H (2009). Diagnostic and prognostic molecular markers for renal cell carcinoma: a critical appraisal of the current state of research and clinical applicability. *Eur Urol*, 55:851–863. http://dx.doi.org/10.1016/j.eururo.2009.01.003 PMID:19155123

31. Fisher R, Gore M, Larkin J (2013). Current and future systemic treatments for renal cell carcinoma. *Semin Cancer Biol*, 23:38–45. http://dx.doi.org/10.1016/j.semcancer.2012.06.004 PMID:22705280

32. Algaba F, Akaza H, López-Beltrán A *et al.* (2011). Current pathology keys of renal cell carcinoma. *Eur Urol*, 60:634–643. http://dx.doi.org/10.1016/j.eururo.2011.06.047 PMID:21741159

5.10 Bladder cancer

5 ORGAN SITE

Guido Sauter

Mahul B. Amin (reviewer)
Manolis Kogevinas (reviewer)
Ronald Simon (contributor)

Summary

- Bladder cancer is the ninth most common cancer worldwide, and urothelial carcinoma is the most frequent histological type (> 90%). About 70–80% of patients are diagnosed with non-invasive and low-grade tumours.

- Tobacco smoking remains the most important cause of bladder cancer. Arsenic and some occupational exposures also cause bladder cancer. Chronic infection and inflammation associated with *Schistosoma haematobium* is a cause of squamous cell carcinoma of the bladder.

- Non-invasive and invasive cancers show distinct genetic profiles, reflecting different molecular pathways of development. Low-grade non-invasive tumours frequently show activating mutations of the *FGFR3* gene, which encodes fibroblast growth factor receptor 3, and inactivation of multiple tumour suppressors at chromosome 9. High-grade and invasive disease is accompanied by a high degree of genetic instability, aneuploidy, and alterations of a multitude of tumour suppressor genes and oncogenes, often including *TP53*.

- Despite improvement in diagnosis and therapy, the likelihood of recurrence and progression to invasively growing tumours must be recognized. As many as 50–70% of these tumours recur, and about 10–20% progress to muscle-invasive disease. Only 30–40% of patients with muscle-invasive cancers survive 5 years or longer.

There are five major histological types of bladder cancer, including non-invasive and invasive urothelial carcinoma, as well as squamous cell carcinoma, adenocarcinoma, and small cell carcinoma. All subtypes develop from the urothelium and show characteristic morphological features. Invasive cancers often show mixed features including more than one phenotype.

Etiology

The most important known cause of bladder cancer is tobacco smoking [1]. The risk of developing bladder cancer is increased 2–6-fold in smokers compared with never-smokers. Black tobacco smoke (common in southern Europe and Latin America) contains higher levels of *N*-nitrosamines and aromatic amines and poses a risk that is about twice that posed by the blond tobacco that is typically smoked in the USA and northern Europe. Tobacco smoke contains aromatic amines such as 4-aminobiphenyl and 2-naphthylamine, which are human bladder carcinogens in the context of occupational exposure.

Arsenic contamination in drinking-water is proven to cause bladder

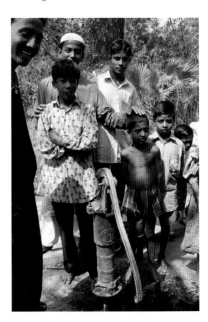

Fig. 5.10.1. Villagers surround a shallow tube well in a village in Comilla District, Bangladesh. The pump is marked with red paint to indicate arsenic-contaminated drinking-water.

Epidemiology

Bladder cancer

- With an estimated 430 000 new cases and 165 000 deaths in 2012, bladder cancer is the ninth most frequent cancer worldwide (in both sexes) and the 13th most common cause of cancer death.
- Incidence and mortality rates are elevated in North America, Europe, North Africa, the Middle East, and Australia and New Zealand. Rates tend to be rather low in many African and Asian countries and some Latin American countries.
- Incidence rates vary 10-fold between geographical regions, and 72% of the new cases occurred in countries that have attained high or very high levels of human development. Incidence and mortality rates in men are commonly 2–4 times those seen in women.
- Trends in bladder cancer incidence are difficult to interpret without precise information on how cancer registries have dealt with papillomas over time. There have generally been declines in incidence and mortality in developed countries, but some rising trends have been observed in eastern Europe and in certain countries in developmental transition.
- While smoking- and occupation-related urothelial bladder cancer tends to be the dominant form of bladder cancer in developed countries, squamous cell carcinomas are common in the Middle East and parts of Africa, as a result of chronic infection with *Schistosoma haematobium*.

Map 5.10.1. Global distribution of estimated age-standardized (World) incidence rates (ASR) per 100 000, for bladder cancer in men, 2012.

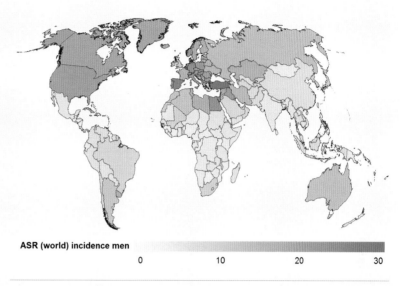

Map 5.10.2. Global distribution of estimated age-standardized (World) incidence rates (ASR) per 100 000, for bladder cancer in women, 2012.

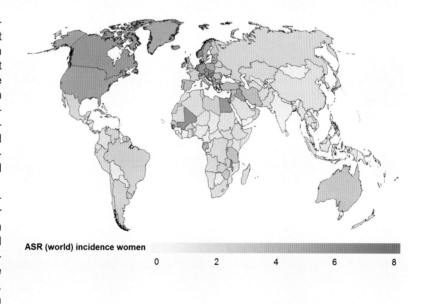

For more details about the maps and charts presented in this chapter, see "A guide to the epidemiology data in *World Cancer Report*".

cancer, particularly in parts of South-East Asia. There is evidence that disinfection by-products – most typically, chemicals generated by water chlorination – could increase the risk of the disease [2]. Bladder cancer, along with cancers of the lung and skin, has been widely recognized as an occupational disease. Male precision metalworkers and metalworking machine operators, automobile mechanics, plumbers, workers in electronic components manufacturing, and landscape industry workers have significantly elevated risks, increasing with the duration of employment. Historically, occupational exposure

Chart 5.10.1. Estimated global number of new cases and deaths with proportions by major world regions, for bladder cancer in both sexes combined, 2012.

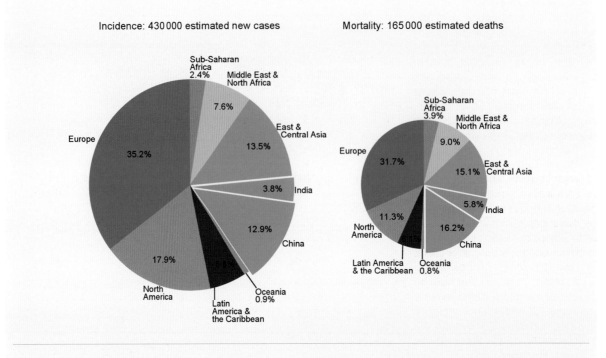

Incidence: 430 000 estimated new cases

Mortality: 165 000 estimated deaths

Chart 5.10.2. Age-standardized (World) incidence rates per 100 000 by year in selected populations, for bladder cancer in men, circa 1975–2012.

Chart 5.10.3. Age-standardized (World) incidence rates per 100 000 by year in selected populations, for bladder cancer in women, circa 1975–2012.

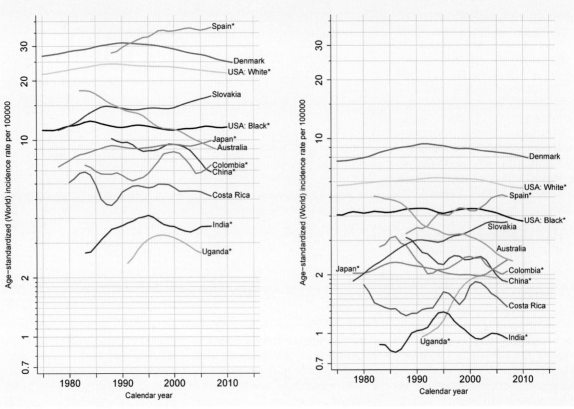

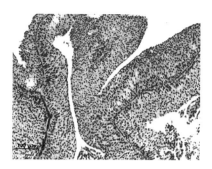

to aromatic amines was established as a causative agent for much occupational bladder cancer; more recently, specific causative agents have been difficult to identify, but exposure to metalworking fluids is strongly implicated [3].

Chronic inflammation of the bladder is a major risk factor, especially for squamous cell carcinomas. Chronic infection with the parasitic trematode *Schistosoma haematobium* causing schistosomiasis has been associated with bladder cancer development in endemic countries, with a 2–15-fold increased risk of cancer in infected compared with non-infected subjects. Continuous mucosal irritation and chronic inflammation from, for example, indwelling catheters or *Schistosoma* infection, can cause squamous metaplasia, dysplasia, and eventually squamous cell carcinomas of the bladder. Patients with long-term paraplegia are at markedly elevated risk for this tumour type due to chronic bladder infection.

Recent genome-wide association studies have identified multiple chromosomal regions of which alterations are linked to the risk of developing bladder cancer [4]. Polymorphisms of the *NAT2* and *GSTM1* metabolic genes have emerged as the most consistent findings; the *NAT2* slow acetylator phenotype is linked with a 2–3-fold increased risk of bladder cancer in former or current heavy smokers, and with a 1.3–1.5-fold increased risk in patients with inactivation of one of two *GSTM1* alleles. Other recurrently identified candidate susceptibility loci include the urea transporter *SLC14A1* and the prostate stem cell antigen (*PSCA*) gene.

Pathology and genetics

The most important element in pathological evaluation of bladder cancer is recognition of the presence and extent of invasion. Non-invasive tumours are restricted to the urothelial cell layers and do not penetrate the lamina propria. The current classification of non-invasive neoplasms of the bladder includes four groups: (i) papillary urothelial neoplasms of low malignant potential, which are characterized by an excellent prognosis and often not identified as "cancer", (ii) non-invasive papillary urothelial carcinomas (low-grade), (iii) non-invasive papillary urothelial carcinomas (high-grade), and (iv) flat carcinoma in situ. Invasive tumours are subdivided according to the depth of invasion.

The nomenclature of bladder cancer was previously confusing because non-invasive and minimally invasive bladder tumours had been combined into the subgroup of "superficial bladder cancers", which was distinguished from the subgroup of "invasive bladder cancers", a term

Fig. 5.10.3. Putative model of bladder cancer development and progression, based on genetic findings. Thick arrows indicate the most frequent pathways, and dotted lines the rarest events. CIS, carcinoma in situ; NIHGC, non-invasive papillary urothelial carcinoma (high-grade); NILGC, non-invasive papillary urothelial carcinoma (low-grade); pT1, primary tumour, stage 1; pT2-4 primary tumour, stage 2–4; PUNLMP, papillary urothelial neoplasm of low malignant potential.

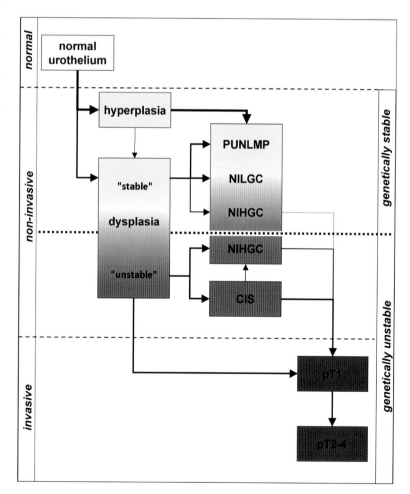

restricted to muscle-invasive tumours. Most non-high-grade non-invasive papillary bladder carcinomas rarely progress to invasive cancer, and most invasive bladder cancers are not preceded by a non-invasive papillary carcinoma.

Bladder urothelial carcinoma

These tumours constitute more than 90% of invasive bladder cancers and can exhibit either a papillary or a solid growth pattern. There is no single characteristic morphological or immunohistochemical feature that is specific for urothelial carcinoma. Therefore, unequivocal diagnosis of urothelial carcinoma relies on identification of precursor lesions such as carcinoma in situ. The histology of invasive urothelial carcinoma is highly variable. These carcinomas often contain areas of divergent differentiation.

Urothelial carcinoma constitutes two genetically distinct subgroups with marked differences in their degree of genetic instability (Fig. 5.10.3). The first category includes the genetically stable tumours: papillary urothelial neoplasms of low malignant potential, non-invasive papillary urothelial carcinomas (low-grade), and probably more than half of non-invasive papillary urothelial carcinomas (high-grade). The second category (genetically unstable cancers) includes carcinoma in situ, about half of non-invasive papillary urothelial carcinomas (high-grade), and invasively growing cancers. Non-invasive papillary urothelial carcinomas account for 70–80% of all bladder cancers and are characterized by a papillary tumour growth pattern and cells showing mild or moderate atypia.

Papillary urothelial neoplasms of low malignant potential and non-invasive papillary urothelial carcinomas (low-grade) are characterized by few genomic alterations, typically including partial or complete deletions of chromosome 9 as well as mutation of the *FGFR3* growth factor receptor [5,6]. Chromosome 9 losses occur in about 50% of tumours, and at comparable frequency also in tumours of all

other grades and stages. Since chromosome 9 deletions are also found in hyperplasia and normal-appearing urothelium, chromosome 9 aberrations are seen as early key events in bladder cancer development. The frequent loss of the entire chromosome 9 suggests that multiple tumour suppressor genes on 9p and 9q might be jointly inactivated by one genetic event. Two tumour suppressor genes have been identified at chromosome 9p21: the cell-cycle control genes *CDKN2A* (*p16/p14*ARF) and *CDKN2B* (also known as *p15*INK4B or *p15*).

Additional tumour suppressor loci have been mapped to 9q, including the tuberous sclerosis 1 (*TSC1*) gene at 9q34 and the deleted in bladder cancer 1 (*DBC1*) gene at 9q32-q33. Deletion and mutation of *TSC1* have been reported to occur in more than 50% and in 15% of bladder cancers, and inactivation of this gene results in the loss of mTOR-mediated control of cell growth. The putative tumour suppressor *DBC1* is often affected by homozygous deletions, although hypermethylation has been suggested as one of the earliest events in bladder cancer development. *FGFR3* mutations occur in 80–90% of papillomas. In neoplastic lesions, the fraction of *FGFR3* mutations is inversely correlated with tumour stage and grade: *FGFR3* mutations are present in more than 60% of low-grade non-invasive tumours, 35% of high-grade non-invasive tumours, 25% of minimally invasive (pT1) cancers, and 16% of muscle-invasive (pT2–4) cancers [7]. Gene amplifications and *TP53* mutations are rare. DNA aneuploidy occurs in less than 50% of cases.

Invasive urothelial carcinomas differ markedly from non-invasive low-grade cancers. They are genetically unstable, often exhibiting high-level amplifications and *TP53* mutations. Aneuploidy is strongly associated with tumour stage and grade and is found in more than 90% of cases. Earlier studies reported frequent deletions involving chromosomes 2q, 5q, 8p, 9p, 9q, 10q, 11p, and 18q and the Y chromosome, as well as gains of 1q, 5p, 8q, and 17q. In addition,

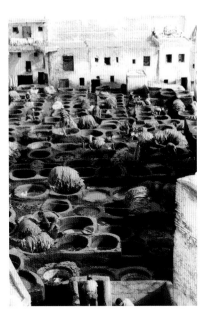

Fig. 5.10.4. An outdoor leather tannery in Fez, Morocco. Men work in the vats curing and dying leather from camels, cattle, and goats. Skins are first dipped in lye, then washed and placed in sulfuric acid. The solvents used in the tanning process have been associated with an increased risk of bladder cancer.

high-level amplifications are frequent in these cancers. The most frequent amplification sites occurring in more than 10% of high-grade/invasive cancers include 11q13, the locus of the cyclin-dependent kinase 1 (*CCND1*) gene; 6p22, with the transcription factor gene *E2F3*; and 17q21, which harbours the human epidermal growth factor receptor 2 (*HER2*) gene (Table 5.10.1).

Methylation studies have revealed – as for other cancers – that invasive bladder cancers exhibit a plethora of differentially methylated areas with hypermethylation in promoter regions and hypomethylation in the gene body [8,9]. Genes suspected to be dysregulated through methylation include 14-3-3 sigma, *SYK*, *CAGE-1*, *PTEN*, *FOXO1*, *MAPK1*, and *PDK1*, as well as various HOX family transcription factors, inactivation of which has been linked to aggressive forms of the disease. Several microRNAs are differentially expressed in urothelial carcinomas, including *miR-10a*, *miR-21*, *miR-30b*,

Table 5.10.1. The most frequent chromosomal aberrations found in larger studies of bladder cancer (≥ 50 tumours analysed)

Aberration	Chromosome arm	Non-invasive		Invasive (pT1–4)	Peak of gain (amplification) or deletion[a]	Candidate gene(s)[b]
		Low-grade	High-grade			
Gains	1q	13%	17%	11%	1q21.2 (35%)	SETDB1
	2p		8–30%	10%	2p25 (10%)	
	3p			10%	3p25 (10–12%)	RAF1
	3q	1%	5%	10–25%	3q26 (10%)	PIK3CA
	4p			5%	4p16 (5%)	
	5p	2%	28%	25%	5p15 (1–25%)	TRIO, SKP2
	6p	1–5%	28%	16–24%	6p22 (3–25%)	E2F3
	7	5%	5%	10–20%		
	8p				8p11-p12 (2–4%)	FGFR1
	8q	5–10%	20%	20–50%	8q21 (4–7%) 8q24 (1–33%)	TPD52 MYC
	10p	3%	5%	10–20%	10p11-p14 (2–15%)	MAP3K8
	11q	5%	15%	20%	11q13 (10%)	CCND1
	12p	1%	5%	5%		
	12q	1–15%	5%	5–30%	12q13-q15 (3–5%)	MDM2 CDK4
	16p			5%	16p13 (5%)	
	16q			5%	16q22 (5%)	
	17q	10–30%	33%	10–50%	17q12-q21 (10–20%)	HER2, TOP2A
	18p			10%	18p11 (1–10%)	YES1
	19q			10%	19q13 (2%)	CCNE
	20q	7–15%	33%	20–30%	20q11 (25%)	BCL2L1
Deletions	2q	4–5%	39%	17–30%	2q36 (25%)	CUL3
	4p	2–5%	22%	10–30%		
	4q	1–10%	17%	10–30%		
	5q	4–20%	33%	16–30%		
	6q	1–10%	33%	19%	6q21-q24 (5%)	
	8p	5–15%	28%	30%	8p11-p12 (30%)	
	9p	36–45%	45%	31–47%	9p21 (30–50%)	CDKN2A
	9q	45%	38%	23–47%	9q34 (30–50%)	DBC1
	10q	5%	28%	18–28%	10q23 (20%) 10q26 (30%)	PTEN
	11p	10%	17%	24–43%		
	11q	6%	23%	22–34%	11q23 (10%)	
	13q	0–20%	17%	19–29%	13q14 (20%)	RB1
	14q	1%		10%	14q23-q24 (10%)	
	15q			8%	15q15 (8%)	
	16p			8%		
	16q			8%	16q13-q21 (8%)	
	17p	1–5%	11%	19–24%	17p13 (24%)	TP53
	18q	7–10%	39%	13–30%	18q21 (10%)	
	Y	10–20%	28%	15–37%		

pT1–4, primary tumour, stage 1–4.
[a] In invasive cancers.
[b] Candidate oncogenes for gains, candidate tumour suppressor genes for deletions.

miR-31, miR-100, miR-141, miR-143, mi-145, miR-192, miR-195, miR-200a/b/c, miR-205, miR-452, and miR-708, and some of these have been linked to invasive growth or poor prognosis. Such findings emphasize the potential of microRNA measurements for diagnostic purposes. Large-scale next-generation sequencing studies are lacking so far, but anecdotal reports on druggable FGFR fusions in bladder cancers have already suggested that these powerful new methods have the potential to significantly advance our knowledge of bladder cancer.

Only few studies have analysed genetic changes in carcinoma in situ and in those high-grade non-invasive papillary urothelial carcinomas with a particularly high degree of atypia (pTaG3). *FGFR3* mutations, which are frequently found in papillomas and papillary urothelial neoplasms of low malignant potential, are virtually absent in carcinoma in situ, whereas *TP53* mutations, a hallmark of muscle-invasive bladder cancer, can frequently be found in carcinoma in situ already. The pattern of deletions and amplifications found was similar to that of invasive cancers [10].

Bladder squamous cell carcinoma

These tumours account for about 2–5% of all bladder cancers and represent a cancer with histologically pure squamous cell phenotype, sometimes accompanied by keratinizing squamous metaplasia in the adjacent flat epithelium. There do not appear to be major differences between muscle-invasive urothelial carcinomas and schistosomiasis-associated squamous cell carcinomas. Frequent cytogenetic alterations include gains of 5p, 6p, 7p, 8q, 11q, 17q, and 20q as well as deletions of 4q, 5q, 8p, 13q, 17p, and 18q. Other key alterations of urothelial carcinoma, such as mutation of *TP53* or overexpression of EGFR and HER2, are also found at comparable frequencies in squamous cell carcinomas.

The genetics of non-schistosomiasis-associated squamous cell carcinomas indicate alterations not markedly different from those in muscle-invasive urothelial carcinomas. Differences may exist in expression levels. One study reported differential expression of keratin-10 and caveolin-1 between the two subtypes [10], and a more recent validation of cytokeratin expression revealed a pattern of CK5/6 positivity and CK5/14 positivity plus CK20 negativity and uroplakin negativity that identifies squamous cell differentiation [11]. A particularly high incidence of 14-3-3 gene methylation, but relatively infrequent methylation of the *SKY* gene, was reported for squamous cell carcinomas compared with urothelial cancers, and loss of expression of both genes has been suggested to contribute to the aggressive clinical behaviour of non-urothelial bladder tumours [12].

Bladder adenocarcinoma

Adenocarcinomas constitute less than 2% of all bladder cancers and are derived from the urothelium, showing a pure glandular phenotype. The growth pattern is variable, with enteric (colonic), signet ring cell, mucinous, clear cell, hepatoid, and mixed types.

Most adenocarcinomas found in bladder biopsies (90%) represent tumours of another origin infiltrating the bladder, such as adenocarcinomas of the prostate, colon, or ovary. Molecular data on pure primary adenocarcinomas of the bladder are rare. Few cases of adenocarcinoma have been analysed cytogenetically, revealing a spectrum of chromosomal alterations that seemed similar to that found in urothelial carcinomas. An early study on 8 schistosomiasis-associated adenocarcinomas reported deletions of 3p, 4p, 4q, 9p, 9q, 17p, 8p, 11p, and 18q [13]. In another series of 13 adenocarcinomas, 4 carried mutations of the *TP53* tumour suppressor [14], an alteration that is also frequently (30–50%) found in invasive urothelial carcinomas. More recently, epigenetic analysis identified frequent promoter methylation

of the 14-3-3 and *CAGE-1* genes in 10 non-schistosomiasis-associated adenocarcinomas and 6 signet ring cell carcinomas [15].

Bladder small cell carcinoma

These tumours, accounting for about 1% and 3% of all bladder cancers in men and women, respectively, are malignant neuroendocrine neoplasms that histologically mimic their pulmonary counterparts. All small cell cancers are invasive at diagnosis and typically appear as a large solid mass of small, uniform cells. About 50% of cancers have areas of urothelial carcinoma and, in rare cases, squamous cell carcinoma and/or adenocarcinoma.

Classic cytogenetic and molecular cytogenetic studies report frequent gains and losses at the same chromosomal loci often affected in muscle-invasive urothelial carcinomas. The most frequent aberrations include deletions at chromosomes 3p25-p26 (*VHL*), 4q, 5q, 9p21 (*p16*), 9q32-q33 (*DBC1*), 10q, 13q, and 17p13 (*TP53*) as well as gains at 5p, 6p, 8q, and 20q. High-level amplifications affect 1p22-p32, 3q26.3 (*PIK3CA*), 8q24 (*MYC*), and 12q14-q21 (*MDM2*, *CDK4*). In addition, promoter methylation and expression studies suggested that silencing of the tumour suppressors *RASSF1*, *MLH1*, *DAPK1*, and *MGMT* might contribute to the malignant behaviour of small cell bladder cancers [16]. Recent genetic studies demonstrate transition from urothelial carcinoma to small cell carcinoma during the course of tumour progression. For example, identical patterns of loss of heterozygosity at five polymorphic loci and inactivation of the same copy of the X chromosome were seen in the urothelial and the small cell component, suggesting a common clonal origin [17]. In addition, identical point mutations of *TP53* were found in the invasive small cell component and in the urothelial in situ carcinoma, suggesting that small cell carcinoma might develop from in situ carcinoma of the bladder [18].

Prospects

Prevention

Cessation of smoking is the most effective measure for prevention of bladder cancer. Intervention in relation to proven or likely workplace exposures will prevent occupational bladder cancer, particularly in relation to work practices in low-income countries. Avoidance of arsenic-contaminated drinking-water should also be implemented. For squamous cell carcinoma, avoidance of infestation with *Schistosoma haematobium* is an effective intervention.

Screening

Attempts to perform population-based screening have not been successful due to the low incidence of bladder cancers and the low specificity (and sensitivity) of tests [19,20].

Targeted therapies

Urothelial carcinoma is one of the most heterogeneous cancer types. Molecular heterogeneity may compromise the efficiency of targeted drugs in this malignancy. Several drugs targeting genes frequently altered in bladder cancer have exhibited disappointing efficacy compared with other cancer types. Thus, in advanced bladder cancer, addition of gefitinib to cisplatin and gemcitabine did not improve response rates or survival [21]. In another phase II study (ClinicalTrials.gov: NCT00380029), neoadjuvant administration of another EGFR inhibitor, erlotinib, showed some beneficial effects. Although mostly heterogeneous, HER2 over expression and amplification is found in about 10–30% of advanced bladder cancers. In a clinical trial investigating the effects of combining chemotherapy (paclitaxel, carboplatin, and gemcitabine) with trastuzumab, there was a 73% response rate and a median survival of 15.2 months [22]. Targeting FGFR3 – which is frequently mutated, particularly in low-grade non-invasive bladder cancers – has

shown encouraging results in multiple myeloma and bladder cancer cell lines [23]. At present, phase II clinical trials are under way for several additional novel targeted agents, including bevacizumab and aflibercept, which target VEGF, and the multiple tyrosine kinase inhibitors sunitinib, sorafenib, and lapatinib.

The prevalence and co-occurrence of actionable genomic alterations in patients with high-grade bladder cancer have been assessed to underpin therapeutic drug discovery [24]. Of the tumours examined,

61% harboured potentially actionable genomic alterations. A core pathway analysis of the integrated data set revealed a non-overlapping pattern of mutations in the RTK/RAS/RAF (Fig. 5.10.5) and PI3K/AKT/mTOR signalling pathways and regulators of G1–S cell-cycle progression. The findings suggested that optimal development of target-specific agents will require pre-treatment genomic characterization.

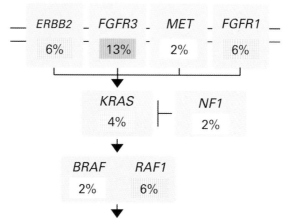

Fig. 5.10.5. Co-occurrence of alterations within the RTK/RAS/RAF signalling pathway in high-grade bladder cancer. Incidence (%) of amplifications, deletions, and mutations of selected receptor tyrosine kinases and downstream targets. The heat map (bottom) compares the distribution of each alteration across tumour samples.

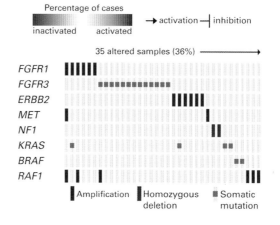

References

1. Freedman ND, Silverman DT, Hollenbeck AR et al. (2011). Association between smoking and risk of bladder cancer among men and women. *JAMA*, 306:737–745. http://dx.doi.org/10.1001/jama.2011.1142 PMID:21846855

2. Costet N, Villanueva CM, Jaakkola JJ et al. (2011). Water disinfection by-products and bladder cancer: is there a European specificity? A pooled and meta-analysis of European case-control studies. *Occup Environ Med*, 68:379–385. http://dx.doi.org/10.1136/oem.2010.062703 PMID:21389011

3. Colt JS, Karagas MR, Schwenn M et al. (2011). Occupation and bladder cancer in a population-based case-control study in Northern New England. *Occup Environ Med*, 68:239–249. http://dx.doi.org/10.1136/oem.2009.052571 PMID:20864470

4. Rothman N, Garcia-Closas M, Chatterjee N et al. (2010). A multi-stage genome-wide association study of bladder cancer identifies multiple susceptibility loci. *Nat Genet*, 42:978–984. http://dx.doi.org/10.1038/ng.687 PMID:20972438

5. Lott S, Wang M, Zhang S et al. (2009). *FGFR3* and *TP53* mutation analysis in inverted urothelial papilloma: incidence and etiological considerations. *Mod Pathol*, 22:627–632. http://dx.doi.org/10.1038/modpathol.2009.28 PMID:19287463

6. Castillo-Martin M, Domingo-Domenech J, Karni-Schmidt O et al. (2010). Molecular pathways of urothelial development and bladder tumorigenesis. *Urol Oncol*, 28:401–408. http://dx.doi.org/10.1016/j.urolonc.2009.04.019 PMID:20610278

7. Knowles MA (2007). Role of FGFR3 in urothelial cell carcinoma: biomarker and potential therapeutic target. *World J Urol*, 25:581–593. http://dx.doi.org/10.1007/s00345-007-0213-4 PMID:17912529

8. Pu RT, Laitala LE, Clark DP (2006). Methylation profiling of urothelial carcinoma in bladder biopsy and urine. *Acta Cytol*, 50:499–506. http://dx.doi.org/10.1159/000326003 PMID:17017434

9. Wolff EM, Chihara Y, Pan F et al. (2010). Unique DNA methylation patterns distinguish noninvasive and invasive urothelial cancers and establish an epigenetic field defect in premalignant tissue. *Cancer Res*, 70:8169–8178. http://dx.doi.org/10.1158/0008-5472.CAN-10-1335 PMID:20841482

10. Zhao J, Richter J, Wagner U et al. (1999). Chromosomal imbalances in noninvasive papillary bladder neoplasms (pTa). *Cancer Res*, 59:4658–4661. PMID:10493521

11. Gaisa NT, Braunschweig T, Reimer N et al. (2011). Different immunohistochemical and ultrastructural phenotypes of squamous differentiation in bladder cancer. *Virchows Arch*, 458:301–312. http://dx.doi.org/10.1007/s00428-010-1017-2 PMID:21136076

12. Kunze E, Wendt M, Schlott T (2006). Promoter hypermethylation of the 14-3-3 sigma, SYK and CAGE-1 genes is related to the various phenotypes of urinary bladder carcinomas and associated with progression of transitional cell carcinomas. *Int J Mol Med*, 18:547–557. PMID:16964403

13. Shaw ME, Elder PA, Abbas A, Knowles MA (1999). Partial allelotype of schistosomiasis-associated bladder cancer. *Int J Cancer*, 80:656–661.http://dx.doi.org/10.1002/(SICI)1097-0215(19990301)80:5<656::AID-IJC4>3.0.CO;2-A PMID:10048962

14. Warren W, Biggs PJ, el-Baz M et al. (1995). Mutations in the *p53* gene in schistosomal bladder cancer: a study of 92 tumours from Egyptian patients and a comparison between mutational spectra from schistosomal and non-schistosomal urothelial tumours. *Carcinogenesis*, 16:1181–1189. http://dx.doi.org/10.1093/carcin/16.5.1181 PMID:7767983

15. Kunze E, Schlott T (2007). High frequency of promoter methylation of the 14-3-3 sigma and CAGE-1 genes, but lack of hypermethylation of the caveolin-1 gene, in primary adenocarcinomas and signet ring cell carcinomas of the urinary bladder. *Int J Mol Med*, 20:557–563. PMID:17786288

16. Zhao X, Flynn EA (2012). Small cell carcinoma of the urinary bladder: a rare, aggressive neuroendocrine malignancy. *Arch Pathol Lab Med*, 136:1451–1459. http://dx.doi.org/10.5858/arpa.2011-0267-RS PMID:23106592

17. Cheng L, Jones TD, McCarthy RP et al. (2005). Molecular genetic evidence for a common clonal origin of urinary bladder small cell carcinoma and coexisting urothelial carcinoma. *Am J Pathol*, 166:1533–1539. http://dx.doi.org/10.1016/S0002-9440(10)62369-3 PMID:15855652

18. Gaisa NT, Tilki D, Losen I et al. (2008). Insights from a whole cystectomy specimen – association of primary small cell carcinoma of the bladder with transitional cell carcinoma in situ. *Hum Pathol*, 39:1258–1262. http://dx.doi.org/10.1016/j.humpath.2007.12.017 PMID:18547617

19. Chou R, Dana T (2010). Screening adults for bladder cancer: a review of the evidence for the U.S. preventive services task force. *Ann Intern Med*, 153:461–468. http://dx.doi.org/10.7326/0003-4819-153-7-201010050-00009 PMID:20921545

20. Kaufman DS, Shipley WU, Feldman AS (2009). Bladder cancer. *Lancet*, 374:239–249. http://dx.doi.org/10.1016/S0140-6736(09)60491-8 PMID:19520422

21. Philips GK, Halabi S, Sanford BL et al.; Cancer and Leukemia Group B (2009). A phase II trial of cisplatin (C), gemcitabine (G) and gefitinib for advanced urothelial tract carcinoma: results of Cancer and Leukemia Group B (CALGB) 90102. *Ann Oncol*, 20:1074–1079. http://dx.doi.org/10.1093/annonc/mdn749 PMID:19168670

22. Hussain MH, MacVicar GR, Petrylak DP et al.; National Cancer Institute (2007). Trastuzumab, paclitaxel, carboplatin, and gemcitabine in advanced human epidermal growth factor receptor-2/neu-positive urothelial carcinoma: results of a multicenter phase II National Cancer Institute trial. *J Clin Oncol*, 25:2218–2224. http://dx.doi.org/10.1200/JCO.2006.08.0994 PMID:17538166

23. Lamont FR, Tomlinson DC, Cooper PA et al. (2011). Small molecule FGF receptor inhibitors block FGFR-dependent urothelial carcinoma growth in vitro and in vivo. *Br J Cancer*, 104:75–82. http://dx.doi.org/10.1038/sj.bjc.6606016 PMID:21119661

24. Iyer G, Al-Ahmadie H, Schultz N et al. (2013). Prevalence and co-occurrence of actionable genomic alterations in high-grade bladder cancer. *J Clin Oncol*, 31:3133–3140. http://dx.doi.org/10.1200/JCO.2012.46.5740 PMID:23897969

5.11 Cancers of the male reproductive organs

5 ORGAN SITE

Peter A. Humphrey

Joachim Schüz (reviewer)

Summary

- Prostate cancer is the second most common cancer in men worldwide. Risk factors for prostate cancer are age, family history, and race.

- Prostate cancers are mainly adenocarcinomas and are indolent in many men, but there is also a lethal form. Gleason histological grade, serum prostate-specific antigen (PSA) level, and stage are significant prognostic indicators.

- Recurrent protein-altering mutations are rare in prostate cancer and are most often seen in the androgen receptor, PTEN, AKT1, and TP53 genes, usually in advanced-stage disease.

- Testicular cancer mostly affects young men. Risk factors include cryptorchidism, a prior testicular germ cell tumour, a family history of germ cell tumour, androgen insensitivity syndrome, and gonadal dysgenesis with a Y chromosome.

- Testicular cancers are typically germ cell neoplasms, with histopathological classification into seminomatous and non-seminomatous types, which has clinical significance. Testicular cancer is a very curable malignancy, even after metastatic spread.

- Single gene mutations are uncommon in testicular germ cell tumours, but KIT, TP53, KRAS/ NRAS, and BRAF are the genes most commonly mutated and implicated in pathogenesis.

Prostate cancer

Prostate cancer in most cases is acinar adenocarcinoma, a glandular malignancy. Primary sarcomas and other types of malignancy do arise in the prostate gland, but are rare.

Etiology

The major identified risk factors for development of prostate cancer are age, family history, and race. Age is strongly related to the detection of prostate cancer, either clinically or at autopsy. The incidence of prostate cancer rises extremely steeply with age. Clinically, carcinoma of the prostate is most often detected in men older than 60 years. The likelihood of detection is nearly 40 times greater for men older than 65 than for men younger than 65. Only about 1% of prostate cancers are detected in men younger than 50 years. Prostate cancer in children is rare and is almost always rhabdomyosarcoma.

A man with a family history of prostate cancer has a significantly higher risk than one without such a history [1]. About 25% of men with prostatic carcinoma have a known family history [2]. The degree of risk is related to the age of the relatives at diagnosis and the number of relatives affected. Men with either a father or a brother with a diagnosis of prostate cancer have an approximately 2–3 times greater risk of developing prostate cancer than men without a family history of the disease. The greatest risk, with an 11-fold increase, is that for the father or the brother of a man diagnosed at about age 40 with prostate cancer, with an additional first-degree relative who has prostate cancer. Genetic factors clearly make a major contribution to prostate cancer susceptibility, as highlighted by a twin cohort study indicating that 42% of prostate cancer cases exhibited heritable risk [3].

The role of race and ethnicity in prostate cancer etiology has been most intensively investigated in the USA, where the African American population is 1.6 times more likely to develop prostate cancer than the Caucasian population. Adjustment for recognized environmental, socioeconomic, and health-care factors does not fully account for this difference.

Epidemiology

Prostate cancer

- Globally, prostate cancer is the second most frequently diagnosed cancer and the fifth most common cause of cancer death among men, with an estimated 1.1 million new cases (15% of all cancers in men) and 0.3 million cancer deaths (7% of all cancer deaths in men) in 2012.
- In 2012, 60% of the estimated new cases and 41% of the deaths occurred in Europe and North America.
- Mortality rates are highest in countries and areas with predominantly Black populations – in the Caribbean and in parts of sub-Saharan Africa – but mortality rates are also high in certain northern European countries, such as the Nordic countries.
- Incidence rates of prostate cancer vary by more than 25-fold in different parts of the world. The highest rates are in Australia and New Zealand (111.6 per 100 000), northern and western Europe, and North America.
- Prostate cancer was the most frequent type of cancer among men in 84 countries worldwide in 2012, largely in countries that have attained high or very high levels of human development, but also in several countries in Central and Southern Africa.
- Incidence rates increased dramatically in the late 1980s in North America as prostate-specific antigen (PSA) testing became available; a similar pattern developed in many of the highest-resource countries during the 1990s. Incidence rates have levelled off in some of these countries but continue to uniformly increase in countries transitioning towards higher levels of human development.

Map 5.11.1. Global distribution of estimated age-standardized (World) incidence rates (ASR) per 100 000, for prostate cancer, 2012.

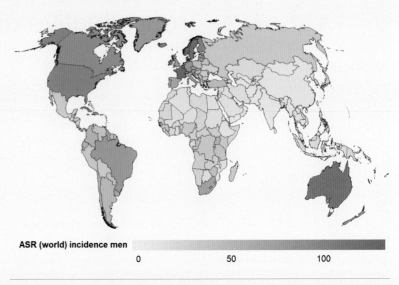

ASR (world) incidence men

0   50   100

Map 5.11.2. Global distribution of estimated age-standardized (World) mortality rates (ASR) per 100 000, for prostate cancer, 2012.

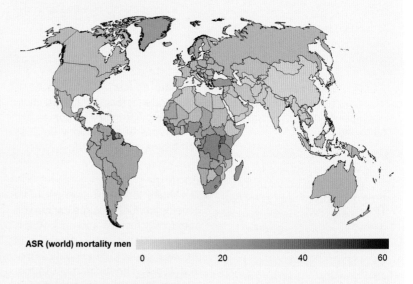

ASR (world) mortality men

0   20   40   60

- Mortality rates, which historically increased with incidence, began to decrease in the 1990s in some of the highest-resource countries, likely as a result of a combination of curative treatment and earlier detection of the disease.

For more details about the maps and charts presented in this chapter, see "A guide to the epidemiology data in *World Cancer Report*".

Chart 5.11.1. Estimated global number of new cases and deaths with proportions by major world regions, for prostate cancer, 2012.

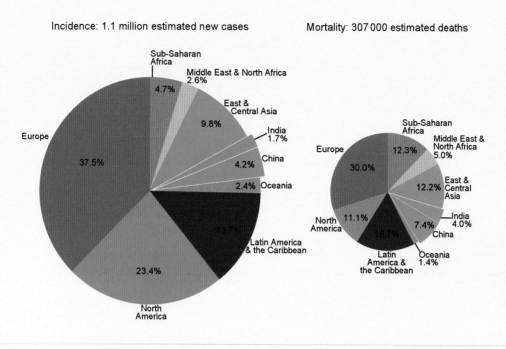

Incidence: 1.1 million estimated new cases

Mortality: 307 000 estimated deaths

Chart 5.11.2. Age-standardized (World) incidence rates per 100 000 by year in selected populations, for prostate cancer, circa 1975–2012.

Chart 5.11.3. Age-standardized (World) mortality rates per 100 000 by year in selected populations, for prostate cancer, circa 1975–2012.

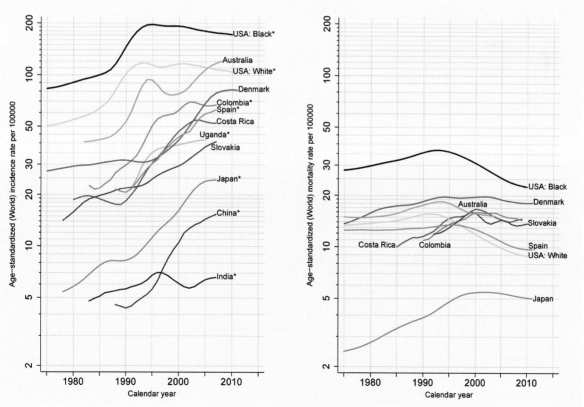

Testicular cancer

- Testicular cancer is a relatively rare cancer overall but a common malignancy among young adult men (aged 15–39 years) in the most developed settings. Hence, while it is the 21th most frequently occurring cancer in men globally, with 55 000 new cases estimated in 2012 for all ages, it is by far the most common cancer in young men in countries that have attained high or very high levels of human development.

- Incidence rates of testicular cancer vary at least 25-fold in different parts of the world. The highest incidence rates are found in Caucasian populations in Europe (notably in Denmark, Norway, and Switzerland), Australia and New Zealand, and North America. Incidence rates are lowest in South-East Asia and throughout Africa.

- In 2012, 55.2% of all new cases of testicular cancer occurred in Europe and North America, but only 20.3% of the deaths. The fatality rate is one of the lowest of all forms of cancer, although it is considerably higher in countries classified as having low or medium levels of human development.

- Over the past 50 years, testicular cancer incidence rates have uniformly increased in many countries with predominantly Caucasian populations, and incidence appears to have peaked in several countries with the highest rates. In contrast, mortality rates have declined in line with improvements in treatment, notably with the introduction of cisplatin therapy.

Map 5.11.3. Global distribution of estimated age-standardized (World) incidence rates (ASR) per 100 000, for testicular cancer, 2012.

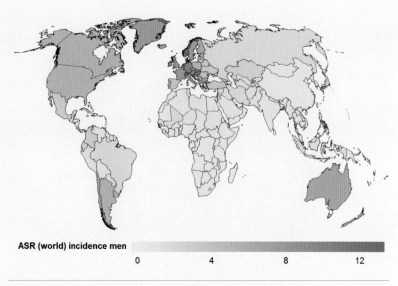

ASR (world) incidence men

0   4   8   12

Map 5.11.4. Global distribution of estimated age-standardized (World) mortality rates (ASR) per 100 000, for testicular cancer, 2012.

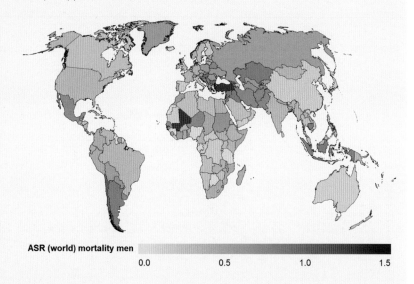

ASR (world) mortality men

0.0   0.5   1.0   1.5

Chart 5.11.4. Estimated global number of new cases and deaths with proportions by major world regions, for testicular cancer, 2012.

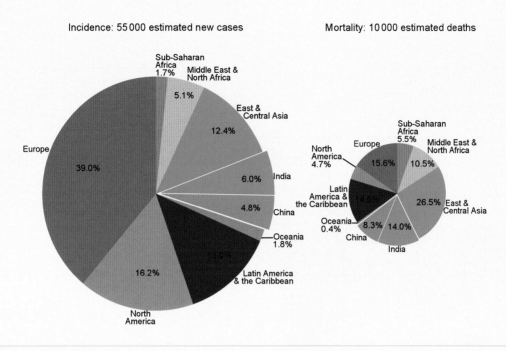

Incidence: 55 000 estimated new cases

Mortality: 10 000 estimated deaths

Chart 5.11.5. Age-standardized (World) incidence rates per 100 000 by year in selected populations, for testicular cancer, circa 1975–2012.

Chart 5.11.6. Age-standardized (World) mortality rates per 100 000 by year in selected populations, for testicular cancer, circa 1975–2012.

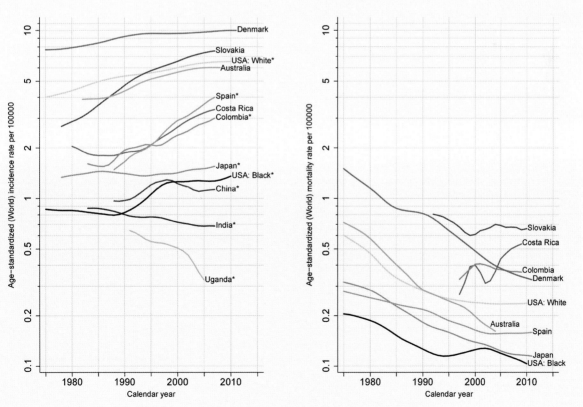

Fig. 5.11.1. Few, if any, exogenous causes of prostate cancer have been clearly established. Accordingly, old age is recognized as one of a very limited number of proven risk factors. Prostate cancer is most common in North America, northern and western Europe, and Australia and New Zealand.

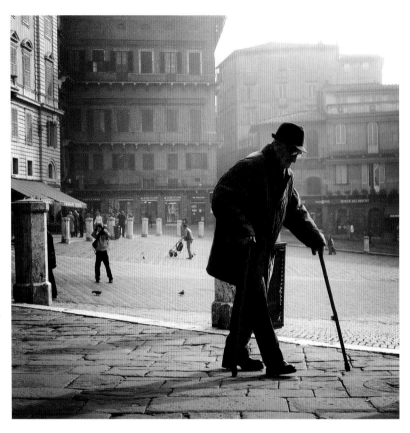

Molecular factors that distinguish between races and are possibly causally related to the difference in incidence include the hormonal milieu of the tumour (with genetic mutations contributing to a higher dihydrotestosterone-to-testosterone ratio), decreased apoptosis due to lower BCL-2 levels, and overexpression of epidermal growth factor receptor [4]. Prostate cancer risk loci at 8q24 and 17q21 appear to be more frequent in men of African descent; together, these two loci could explain up to 60% of the increased risk in men of African descent [4].

Probable risk factors for prostate cancer include diet and nutrition, and hormonal factors [5]. A diet typical of industrialized countries has been proposed to be an important risk factor for prostate cancer, given the large worldwide variation in the incidence of prostate cancer and the increased risk in migrants and their offspring who move from low-risk to high-risk countries. Dietary and saturated fat, red/processed/grilled meat, and milk and dairy products may increase risk, whereas tomatoes/lycopene, fish/marine omega-3 fatty acids, soy, and cruciferous vegetables (such as broccoli, cauliflower, and Brussels sprouts) may decrease risk [5]. Studies on vitamin E are equivocal, and a large randomized intervention trial with vitamin E and selenium, the SELECT trial, did not demonstrate reduced prostate cancer incidence. Data on calcium and zinc are conflicting. Vitamin D intake does not seem to be related to prostate cancer risk. Vitamin A as β-carotene in vegetable sources is not consistently associated with risk.

Hormonal influences on prostate cancer risk include androgens, the androgen receptor, and the insulin-like growth factor axis. The importance of androgens is substantiated by clinical trials on use of 5α-reductase inhibitors (e.g. finasteride, dutasteride), which block the conversion of testosterone to the more active molecule in the prostate, dihydrotestosterone. These trials demonstrated a decrease in low-grade prostate cancer incidence [6]. Circulating testosterone level is not, however, associated with prostate cancer risk. Short CAG repeats in the androgen receptor gene – a structural variation that increases its activity – have been connected in some, but not all, studies with a higher risk of prostate cancer. Finally, circulating levels of insulin-like growth factor, a polypeptide hormone that increases cell proliferation and decreases apoptosis of prostate cells, are associated with increased prostate cancer risk.

Lifestyle factors including physical activity, cigarette smoking, and alcohol consumption have not been definitively linked to prostate cancer risk. Obesity does not appear to be linked to total prostate cancer incidence, but it may be associated with the development of advanced-stage or fatal prostate cancer [5].

No infection has been definitively linked to the development of prostate cancer, although there is a suggestion from two studies that *Trichomonas vaginalis* infection may be associated with an increased risk of prostate cancer, especially more aggressive disease [5]. Findings on the retrovirus XMRV, despite initial excitement, do not support a role for it in the etiology of prostate cancer [7]. Inflammation in the prostate is very common, and several separate lines of research, including epidemiological, genetic, histopathological, molecular pathological, and animal studies, have pointed towards a potential role for inflammation in prostate carcinogenesis [8].

Cholesterol levels may have a role in prostate cancer risk. Lower total cholesterol is associated with a lower risk of high-grade prostate cancer, and use of statins, which lower serum cholesterol, may be related to a lower risk of all prostate cancers and advanced or high-grade prostate cancer.

Pathology

Adenocarcinoma of the prostate is thought to arise most commonly from a precursor proliferation known as high-grade prostatic intraepithelial neoplasia, which is an in situ proliferation of neoplastic prostatic epithelial cells (Fig. 5.11.2) [9]. The initial phase of the natural history of prostatic adenocarcinoma is growth into prostatic stroma. Of note, the prevalence of prostate cancer at autopsy, i.e. latent prostate cancer, is extremely high and increases with age. Rare latent cases are detected in the third decade, and it is of interest that there is a frequency of about 30% in the fourth and fifth decades in the USA. There is variation of the frequency of latent prostate cancer depending on the world region, with the highest frequency in industrialized countries. Pathologically, most of these latent cancers are small and well differentiated, but a small minority of latent prostate cancers are of a similar grade, size, and stage to clinical prostate cancer.

For clinical prostate cancer, a pathological diagnosis of malignancy is most often made based on light microscopic examination of fine-needle aspirates, sections of prostate needle biopsy tissue (Fig. 5.11.3), or sections of prostatic chips from transurethral resection of the prostate. Performance of an 18-gauge needle biopsy of the

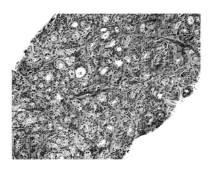

prostate is a common clinical approach when the patient has a palpable prostatic nodule and/or an elevated serum prostate-specific antigen (PSA) level.

Key histological features of malignancy include an abnormal architectural growth pattern of the glands (Fig. 5.11.4), loss of basal cells, and nuclear atypia. The growth patterns depicted in Fig. 5.11.4 indicate the Gleason grade of the tumour, which is one of the most powerful prognostic indicators for men with clinically localized prostate cancer. An additional histopathological finding of clinical importance in needle biopsy tissue is the extent of the cancer. Gleason histological grade, serum PSA level, clinical stage, and extent of cancer in needle core tissue are often used to stratify patients with clinically localized cancer as to risk for aggressive disease and for management/treatment considerations.

The local spread of prostatic adenocarcinoma is into periprostatic adipose tissue, the bladder neck, and the seminal vesicles. Such direct extension of the cancer is diagnosed in radical prostatectomy specimens, and it is the light microscopic examination of these tissue sections that allows for assignment of pathological stage, Gleason grade in the whole gland, and surgical margin status, which are significant indicators of clinical outcome. Metastasis of prostatic adenocarcinoma is mainly to the pelvic lymph nodes and to bone; for bone, the radiological and histological

picture is typically of osteoblastic metastasis.

Genetics

The molecular genetics of prostate cancer may be separated into genetic susceptibility in the germline and the genetics of established sporadic tumours. Susceptibility has been investigated in high-risk men identified with reference to African American heritage or familial disease. Genetic variants associated with prostate cancer susceptibility include more than 30 single-nucleotide polymorphisms identified by genome-wide association studies, with replicated single-nucleotide polymorphisms most often located in the 8q24 region [10]. However, these single-nucleotide polymorphisms together account for only an estimated 25%

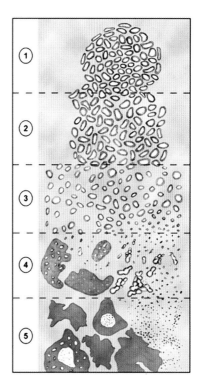

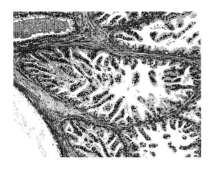

Fig. 5.11.5. Two models of prostate cancer progression: a linear model compared with a molecular diversity model. In the molecular diversity model, not all pathways result in progression. Accumulation of molecular alterations associated with aggressive disease, such as the overexpression of EZH2 or *PTEN* mutations, may lead to invasive disease that progresses to metastatic disease, whereas other lesions, such as those with 5q or 6q gain and overexpression of AZGP1, might be seen most often in indolent disease. Mutations and alterations associated with p53 and the androgen receptor (AR) are probably late events and may play a key role in the development of castration-resistant disease. SNP, single-nucleotide polymorphism.

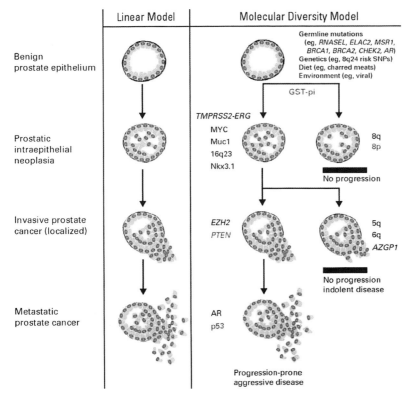

of familial risk. A susceptibility locus that appears to be specific to men of African descent has been identified at 17q21. Mutations in several specific susceptibility genes, including *RNASEL/HPC1*, *ELAC2/HPC2*, *MSR1*, and *HOXB13*, have been identified. These highly penetrant genes from high-risk families likely account for only a small fraction of the genetic predisposition to prostate cancer.

Another approach to susceptibility has involved whole-genome sequencing of 1795 Icelanders. A new low-frequency variant at 8q24 associated with prostate cancer in European populations was identified. This variant was only very weakly correlated with previously reported risk variants at 8q24, and its association remained significant after adjustment for all known risk-associated variants [11].

The molecular genetic profile of established prostate cancer is characterized by structural genomic changes in oncogenes and tumour suppressor genes such as *NKX3.1* and *PTEN*, and amplification of the androgen receptor and *MYC* genes [12]. The prostate cancer genome undergoes frequent large-scale genomic rearrangements, including a common rearrangement producing ETS gene fusions. Although several ETS and non-ETS family members have been observed to be fused with *TMPRSS2* or other 5′ fusion partners, most fusions involve *TMPRSS2-ERG*. In contrast, recurrent protein-altering mutations are

rare in prostate cancer and are most often seen in the androgen receptor, *PTEN*, *AKT1*, and *TP53* genes, usually in advanced-stage disease. A molecular diversity model, where a wide range of possible pathways exist, has been proposed as a basis for pathological and genetic progression of prostate cancer (Fig. 5.11.5) [13].

Metastatic castration-resistant prostate cancer has been the subject of specific investigation. One study [14] reported low overall mutation rates even in such tumours subject to intensive therapy and confirmed the monoclonal origin of lethal disease. The analysis identified disruptions of *CHD1* that defined a subtype of ETS gene family fusion-negative prostate cancer. *ETS2*, which was deleted in approximately one third of metastatic castration-resistant prostate cancers, was also dysregulated through mutation. Furthermore, recurrent mutations in multiple chromatin and histone modifying genes were evident, including *MLL2* (mutated in 8.6% of prostate cancers), as was interaction of the MLL complex with the androgen receptor, which is required for androgen receptor-mediated signalling. There were novel recurrent mutations in the androgen receptor collaborating factor *FOXA1*.

Prospects

The most immediately applicable prevention strategies could include increased physical activity, intake of tomatoes and other foods containing lycopene, intake of foods containing selenium, and avoidance of diets high in calcium. Hence, it would seem beneficial to emphasize a diet consisting of a wide variety of plant-based foods and fish. Chemoprevention with pharmaceutical agents is not recommended at this time.

Screening for prostate cancer is controversial. Screening with serum PSA level has increased detection of all prostate cancers, including indolent prostate cancers. PSA emerged as one of the most-used serum tests to screen for cancer, particularly in the USA but also in Europe. Recent

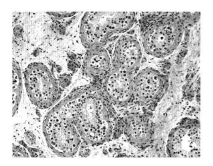

Fig. 5.11.6. Intratubular germ cell neoplasia in the testis. This is a precursor for most testicular cancers.

data from the Prostate, Lung, Colon, and Ovarian Cancer Screening Trial showed no benefit to screening, and the European Randomized Study of Screening for Prostate Cancer showed a 20% reduction in relative risk of cancer-specific mortality, which translated into an absolute reduction of prostate cancer-related deaths of 0.71 per 1000. Each trial has criticisms that may or may not have affected power and outcome, although the rate ratios comparing screening to not screening are similar. Definitive evidence for or against screening is still lacking [15].

The detection via screening of both clinically significant and potentially clinically insignificant prostate cancer has created a dilemma as to which patients should receive aggressive treatment [16]. Overtreatment of screen-detected tumours is a major concern. In the USA, most men with screen-detected cancers undergo aggressive treatment. Such treatment is unlikely to yield a survival benefit in those with indolent disease or in men older than 65 years, but it can result in a considerable decrease in quality of life as a result of potentially persistent urinary, sexual, and bowel dysfunction [16].

Active surveillance of such low-risk disease is one strategy that could potentially counteract some of this overtreatment and has shown favourable outcomes in carefully selected patients. However, the criteria for enrolment into an active surveillance programme are not standardized [17]. Inclusion criteria typically include low serum PSA level, low clinical stage, low Gleason grade (typically, Gleason score 6 or less), and a relatively small amount of cancer in needle core tissue [17]. Molecular markers in needle biopsy tissue hold promise for further refinement in identification of patients with potentially indolent versus aggressive prostate cancer, and could help to stratify patients into active surveillance versus active treatment protocols.

Therapeutic targeting of prostate cancer based on genetic alterations is challenging since there are few recurrent genetic mutations. One promising target is the ETS gene fusions, seen in about one half of all prostate cancers [13].

Prostate cancer clinical biomarkers of benefit are under active investigation. Recent trials in patients with castration-resistant prostate cancer have incorporated the detection of circulating tumour cells, imaging, and patient-reported outcome biomarkers including pain and elevated PSA level [18]. Application of any such putative biomarkers will require a series of prospectively designed studies with adequate statistical support to demonstrate a clinical effect within a well-defined context.

Testicular cancer

Testicular cancer is in most cases a germ cell neoplasm. Sex cord stromal tumours and lymphomas may also involve the testis but are distinctly uncommon.

Etiology

Established risk factors for testicular germ cell tumours include cryptorchidism, a prior testicular germ cell tumour, a family history of germ cell tumour, and various intersex syndromes such as androgen insensitivity syndrome (testicular feminization) and gonadal dysgenesis with a Y chromosome [19,20]. Cryptorchidism carries about a 4-fold increased risk of germ cell tumour development. Patients with a history of testicular germ cell tumour have an increased incidence of contralateral testicular cancer, with an incidence of 2–5%, which translates into a 5–10-fold increased risk.

A small minority of testicular cancers appear to be familial, with approximately 2% of patients having an affected family member. First-degree male relatives of patients with testicular germ cell tumour have a 3–10-fold increased risk of being diagnosed with testicular cancer. The mode of transmission is not known but may be autosomal recessive in nature [20]. Patients with androgen insensitivity syndrome have a 15-fold increased risk of developing a testicular germ cell tumour, while the risk increase is 50-fold for patients with gonadal dysgenesis with a Y chromosome.

Several prenatal factors, including maternal endogenous estrogen levels, and low birth weight have been suggested as risk factors, but the data are inconclusive [20]. One hypothesis is that in utero exposure to exogenous estrogens could result in increased risk of testicular cancer due to increased cryptorchidism and testicular dysgenesis. Several postnatal factors, such as body size (especially height), nutrition, chemical exposure, occupation, infection, and physical activity, have been hypothesized to be potentially associated with testicular cancer, but the data appear mixed [20]. The peak age at diagnosis (twenties and thirties) appears related to sex hormone activity and may reflect promotion of cells initiated during gestation. Finally, migrant studies suggest the importance of as-yet-uncharacterized environmental/dietary factors. For example, the incidence of testicular cancer in Finland is half that found in Sweden, and second-generation Finnish migrants to Sweden have a testicular cancer incidence that approaches that of the Swedish population.

Pathology

The precursor for all types of germ cell tumours that originate in the post-pubertal testis is intratubular germ cell neoplasia. This lesion is seen in about 4% of cryptorchid testes, in approximately 5% of testes

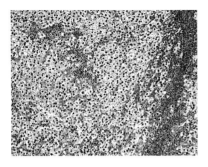

Fig. 5.11.7. Seminoma of the testis, with large primitive neoplastic cells.

contralateral to a testis with a germ cell tumour, and almost always adjacent to an invasive germ cell tumour. Histologically, intratubular germ cell neoplasia is characterized by the presence of large atypical germ cells inside seminiferous tubules (Fig. 5.11.6), which often have a thickened basement membrane. Cytologically, intratubular germ cell neoplasia cells often resemble seminoma cells. Most patients with isolated intratubular germ cell neoplasia develop an invasive germ cell tumour within 7 years. For patients with gonadal dysgenesis with a Y chromosome, gonadoblastoma acts as the in situ precursor proliferation.

Invasive germ cell tumours are broadly classified using histopathological criteria as seminomatous versus non-seminomatous [21]. Microscopically, classic seminoma comprises a solid growth of primitive-appearing cells, separated by fibrous bands infiltrated by lymphocytes (Fig. 5.11.7). In infants and children, yolk sac tumour and teratoma are the most common histological types. Of note, prepubertal teratomas are benign, whereas post-pubertal teratomas are malignant. In adults, pure seminomas account for about 50% of all testicular germ cell tumours. Non-seminomatous germ cell tumour types include embryonal carcinoma, yolk sac tumour, trophoblastic tumours (mainly choriocarcinoma), and teratoma. Mixed malignant germ cell tumours composed of different germ cell types are common, representing 30% of all testicular

cancers. For these mixed tumours, the presence of embryonal carcinoma and the percentage of the tumour that is embryonal carcinoma are important prognostic indicators.

In addition to histological type, important histopathological attributes of germ cell tumours in radical orchiectomy specimens include pathological stage and presence of lymphovascular invasion by the germ cell tumour. Serum tumour marker levels are important in staging and patient management and correlate with specific cell/tumour types. α-Fetoprotein is produced mainly by yolk sac tumours, whereas β-human chorionic gonadotropin is produced by syncytiotrophoblasts in choriocarcinoma and syncytiotrophoblasts seen in seminoma with syncytiotrophoblasts or mixed malignant germ cell tumours.

Testicular germ cell tumours spread by lymphatics, first to retroperitoneal para-aortic lymph nodes and then to mediastinal and supraclavicular lymph nodes. Haematogenous dissemination is primarily to the lungs, but the liver, brain, and bones may be involved. Clinical stage is critical in defining treatment and prognosis.

Genetics

Recently reported genome-wide association studies implicate six gene loci that predispose to testicular germ cell tumour development. These include KIT ligand (*KITLG*; also known as *SCF*), *SPRY4*, *BAK1*, *TERT*, *ATF7IP*, and *DMRT1*. *KITLG*, *SPRY4*, and *BAK1* are involved in KIT signalling, *TERT* and *ATF7IP* maintain telomere length and are reactivated in a range of tumour types, and *DMRT1* is responsible for male sex determination [20,22]. Multiple new susceptibility loci for testicular germ cell tumours continue to be reported [23,24].

The genetics of established paediatric and adult germ cell tumours are distinct [19]. Paediatric tumours are mostly diploid, particularly teratomas, and typically show deletion of 1p, loss of 6q, and structural abnormalities of chromosome 2 and 3p.

In contrast, invasive adult germ cell tumours are consistently aneuploid with gain of chromosomal material on 12p, usually in the form of isochromosome 12p.

Parallels between the origin of testicular germ cell tumours and malignant ovarian germ cell tumours have been considered with reference to germ cell development, endocrinological influences, and pathogenesis [25]. The basis of analysis was genomic aberrations assessed by ploidy, cytogenetic banding, and comparative genomic hybridization.

The development of intratubular germ cell neoplasia may involve an aberrantly activated KITLG/KIT pathway and overexpression of embryonic transcription factors such as NANOG and POU5F1, which leads to suppression of apoptosis, increased proliferation, and accumulation of mutations in gonocytes. Single gene mutations are uncommon in testicular germ cell tumours, but *KIT*, *TP53*, *KRAS/NRAS*, and *BRAF* are the genes most commonly mutated and implicated in pathogenesis. Different histological subtypes of testicular germ cell tumours have different gene expression profiles, which reflect different directions of differentiation. Their distinct gene expression profiles are likely caused by epigenetic regulation, in particular DNA methylation, but not by gene copy number alterations [26].

Prospects

Prevention of testicular germ cell neoplasia is not currently feasible. There are no reliable screening tests for these cancers. Testicular self-examination has not been shown to improve outcomes but is still advocated by some medical professional organizations. Such examination may be more beneficial in men at increased risk of testicular cancer, including men with a history of cryptorchidism, testicular atrophy, or a family history of testicular cancer. Most patients present with a nodule or painless swelling of one gonad, or a painful testis, so these clinical findings should prompt evaluation. A systematic review of options for testicular cancer screening concluded that no published randomized controlled trial of screening compared with no screening had established reduced testicular cancer-specific mortality [27].

There is a high cure rate for testicular germ cell neoplasia, using multidisciplinary management. The 5-year survival rates for men with localized disease, regional spread, and distant metastasis are 99%, 96%, and 72%, respectively. For patients with intermediate- and poor-prognosis germ cell tumours, identification of molecular mechanisms of therapy resistance and development of novel molecularly targeted therapeutic approaches are important goals.

References

1. Johns LE, Houlston RS (2003). A systematic review and meta-analysis of familial prostate cancer risk. *BJU Int*, 91:789–794. http://dx.doi.org/10.1046/j.1464-410X.2003.04232.x PMID:12780833

2. Walsh PC, Partin AW (1997). Family history facilitates the early diagnosis of prostate carcinoma. *Cancer*, 80:1871–1874. http://dx.doi.org/10.1002/(SICI)1097-0142(19971101)80:9<1871::AID-CNCR28>3.0.CO;2-1 PMID:9351562

3. Lichtenstein P, Holm NV, Verkasalo PK *et al.* (2000). Environmental and heritable factors in the causation of cancer – analyses of cohorts of twins from Sweden, Denmark, and Finland. *N Engl J Med*, 343:78–85. http://dx.doi.org/10.1056/NEJM200007133430201 PMID:10891514

4. Henderson BE, Lee NH, Seewaldt V, Shen H (2012). The influence of race and ethnicity on the biology of cancer. *Nat Rev Cancer*, 12:648–653. http://dx.doi.org/10.1038/nrc3341 PMID:22854838

5. Giovannucci E, Platz EA, Mucci L (2011). Epidemiology of prostate cancer. In: Scardino PT, Linehan WM, Zelefsky MJ *et al.*, eds. *Comprehensive Textbook of Genitourinary Oncology*, 4th ed. Baltimore: Lippincott Williams & Wilkins, pp. 1–17.

6. Andriole GL, Bostwick DG, Brawley OW *et al.*; REDUCE Study Group (2010). Effect of dutasteride on the risk of prostate cancer. *N Engl J Med*, 362:1192–1202. http://dx.doi.org/10.1056/NEJMoa0908127 PMID:20357281

7. Sfanos KS, Aloia AL, De Marzo AM, Rein A (2012). XMRV and prostate cancer – a 'final' perspective. *Nat Rev Urol*, 9:111–118. http://dx.doi.org/10.1038/nrurol.2011.225 PMID:22231291

8. Sfanos KS, De Marzo AM (2012). Prostate cancer and inflammation: the evidence. *Histopathology*, 60:199–215. http://dx.doi.org/10.1111/j.1365-2559.2011.04033.x PMID:22212087

9. Epstein JI, Cubilla AL, Humphrey PA (2011). *Tumors of the Prostate Gland, Seminal Vesicles, Penis, and Scrotum* (*AFIP Atlas of Tumor Pathology* Series 4, Fascicle 14). Washington, DC: American Registry of Pathology and Armed Forces Institute of Pathology.

10. Ishak MB, Giri VN (2011). A systematic review of replication studies of prostate cancer susceptibility genetic variants in high-risk men originally identified from genome-wide association studies. *Cancer Epidemiol Biomarkers Prev*, 20:1599–1610. http://dx.doi.org/10.1158/1055-9965.EPI-11-0312 PMID:21715604

11. Gudmundsson J, Sulem P, Gudbjartsson DF *et al.* (2012). A study based on whole-genome sequencing yields a rare variant at 8q24 associated with prostate cancer. *Nat Genet*, 44:1326–1329. http://dx.doi.org/10.1038/ng.2437 PMID:23104005

12. Barbieri CE, Demichelis F, Rubin MA (2012). Molecular genetics of prostate cancer: emerging appreciation of genetic complexity. *Histopathology*, 60:187–198. http://dx.doi.org/10.1111/j.1365-2559.2011.04041.x PMID:22212086

13. Rubin MA, Maher CA, Chinnaiyan AM (2011). Common gene rearrangements in prostate cancer. *J Clin Oncol*, 29:3659–3668. http://dx.doi.org/10.1200/JCO.2011.35.1916 PMID:21859993

14. Grasso CS, Wu YM, Robinson DR *et al.* (2012). The mutational landscape of lethal castration-resistant prostate cancer. *Nature*, 487:239–243. http://dx.doi.org/10.1038/nature11125 PMID:22722839

15. Rove KO, Crawford ED (2012). Randomized controlled screening trials for prostate cancer using prostate-specific antigen: a tale of contrasts. *World J Urol*, 30:137–142. http://dx.doi.org/10.1007/s00345-011-0799-4 PMID:22116599

16. Sandhu GS, Andriole GL (2012). Overdiagnosis of prostate cancer. *J Natl Cancer Inst Monogr*, 2012:146–151. http://dx.doi.org/10.1093/jncimonographs/lgs031 PMID:23271765

17. Buethe DD, Pow-Sang J (2012). Enrollment criteria controversies for active surveillance and triggers for conversion to treatment in prostate cancer. *J Natl Compr Canc Netw*, 10:1101–1110. PMID:22956809

18. Scher HI, Morris MJ, Larson S, Heller G (2013). Validation and clinical utility of prostate cancer biomarkers. *Nat Rev Clin Oncol*, 10:225–234. http://dx.doi.org/10.1038/nrclinonc.2013.30 PMID:23459624

19. Reuter VE (2005). Origins and molecular biology of testicular germ cell tumors. *Mod Pathol*, 18 Suppl 2:S51–S60. http://dx.doi.org/10.1038/modpathol.3800309 PMID:15761466

20. Vaughan DJ, Kanetsky PA, Nathanson KL (2011). The epidemiology and genetics of sporadic and hereditary testicular germ cell tumors. In: Scardino PT, Linehan WM, Zelefsky MJ *et al.*, eds. *Comprehensive Textbook of Genitourinary Oncology*, 4th ed. Baltimore: Lippincott Williams & Wilkins, pp. 509–520.

21. Emerson RE, Ulbright TM (2007). Morphological approach to tumours of the testis and paratestis. *J Clin Pathol*, 60:866–880. http://dx.doi.org/10.1136/jcp.2005.036475 PMID:17307866

22. Gilbert D, Rapley E, Shipley J (2011). Testicular germ cell tumours: predisposition genes and the male germ cell niche. *Nat Rev Cancer*, 11:278–288. http://dx.doi.org/10.1038/nrc3021 PMID:21412254

23. Chung CC, Kanetsky PA, Wang Z *et al.* (2013). Meta-analysis identifies four new loci associated with testicular germ cell tumor. *Nat Genet*, 45:680–685. http://dx.doi.org/10.1038/ng.2634 PMID:23666239

24. Ruark E, Seal S, McDonald H *et al.*; UK Testicular Cancer Collaboration (UKTCC) (2013). Identification of nine new susceptibility loci for testicular cancer, including variants near *DAZL* and *PRDM14*. *Nat Genet*, 45:686–689. http://dx.doi.org/10.1038/ng.2635 PMID:23666240

25. Kraggerud SM, Hoei-Hansen CE, Alagaratnam S *et al.* (2013). Molecular characteristics of malignant ovarian germ cell tumors and comparison with testicular counterparts: implications for pathogenesis. *Endocr Rev*, 34:339–376. http://dx.doi.org/10.1210/er.2012-1045 PMID:23575763

26. Sheikine Y, Genega E, Melamed J *et al.* (2012). Molecular genetics of testicular germ cell tumors. *Am J Cancer Res*, 2:153–167. PMID:22432056

27. Ilic D, Misso ML (2011). Screening for testicular cancer. *Cochrane Database Syst Rev*, 2:CD007853. PMID:21328302

Website

Surveillance, Epidemiology and End Results Program. SEER Cancer Statistics Review, 1975–2009 (Vintage 2009 Populations): http://seer.cancer.gov/csr/1975_2009_pops09/

5.12 Cancers of the female reproductive organs

5 ORGAN SITE

Jaime Prat
Silvia Franceschi

Lynette Denny (reviewer)
Eduardo Lazcano Ponce (reviewer)

Summary

- Cancer of the vulva accounts for 3% of all female genital cancers and it mainly includes two different types of carcinomas. Keratinizing carcinomas predominate in older women and have little association with human papillomavirus (HPV) infection. Conversely, the majority of warty and basaloid carcinomas are caused by HPV.

- Cervical cancer, the fourth most common cancer among women worldwide, with about 70% of the cases occurring in developing countries, is caused by HPV. Precancerous lesions may be detected and treated; HPV vaccination offers the possibility of primary prevention. The most common somatic mutations were found for *PIK3CA*, and are associated with shorter survival.

- More than 80% of endometrial cancers occur as endometrioid carcinomas, a form that is associated with estrogen exposure; obesity is estimated to account for up to 40% of cases worldwide. Principal genetic lesions include microsatellite instability and mutations of the *PTEN*, *PIK3CA*, *ARID1A*, *KRAS*, and *CTNNB1* (β-catenin) genes, whereas *TP53* and *PPP2R1A* mutations, loss of E-cadherin, *HER2/neu* amplification, and loss of heterozygosity at multiple loci occur in non-endometrioid carcinomas.

- Ovarian cancer comprises several tumour types, including the predominant (70%) high-grade serous carcinomas, which exhibit *TP53* mutations and *BRCA* abnormalities and are distinguished from low-grade serous carcinomas (< 5%), which usually exhibit *KRAS* and *BRAF* mutations. Endometrioid and clear cell carcinomas of the ovary have the same genetic abnormalities as their uterine counterparts. Most mucinous carcinomas involving the ovary are metastatic tumours from the gastrointestinal tract.

Vulvar cancer

Cancer of the vulva accounts for 3% of all female genital cancers and occurs mainly in women older than 60 years. Squamous cell carcinoma is the most common type (86%).

Fig. 5.12.1. A patient attends a counselling session with a service provider in the family planning unit at Orolodo primary health centre in Omuaran township in Kwara State, Nigeria.

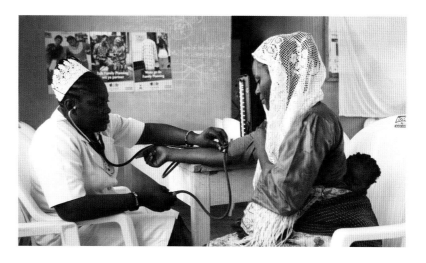

5 ORGAN SITE
CHAPTER 5.12

Epidemiology

Cervical cancer

- Cervical cancer is the fourth most common cancer (528 000 new cases) and the fourth most common cause of cancer death (266 000 deaths) in women worldwide, as estimated in 2012.
- The disease affects predominantly women in lower-resource countries; almost 70% of the global burden occurs in areas with low or medium levels of human development, and more than one fifth of all new cases of cervical cancer are diagnosed in India.
- Incidence rates of cervical cancer vary greatly from country to country. The disease is the most common cancer among women in 39 of the 184 countries worldwide, and is the leading cause of cancer death in women in 45 countries. These countries are mainly in sub-Saharan Africa, parts of Asia, and some countries in Central and South America.
- The lowest incidence rates tend to be in western Europe, North America, Australia and New Zealand, and the eastern Mediterranean.
- Over the past 30 years, cervical cancer rates have declined in many countries that are transitioning towards higher levels of human development. This trend reflects changing societal factors linked to economic

Map 5.12.1. Global distribution of estimated age-standardized (World) incidence rates (ASR) per 100 000, for cervical cancer, 2012.

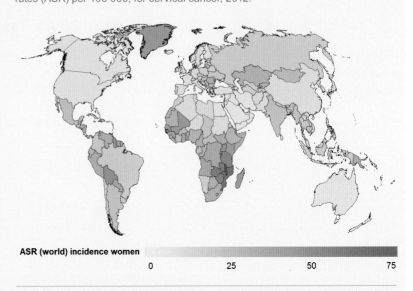

ASR (world) incidence women

0   25   50   75

Map 5.12.2. Global distribution of estimated age-standardized (World) incidence rates (ASR) per 100 000, for cancer of the corpus uteri (endometrial cancer), 2012.

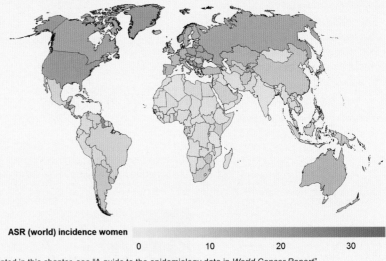

ASR (world) incidence women

0   10   20   30

For more details about the maps and charts presented in this chapter, see "A guide to the epidemiology data in *World Cancer Report*".

These tumours are divided into two groups: keratinizing squamous cell carcinomas, which have little association with human papillomavirus (HPV), and warty and basaloid carcinomas, which are strongly associated with high-risk HPV, mainly HPV16, and are increasingly often diagnosed in younger women in countries in which cervical screening is common.

Etiology

HPV infection causes a subset of squamous cell carcinomas of the vulva and vagina [1]. According to meta-analysis, HPV prevalence was 40.4% in vulvar carcinoma and 69.9% in vaginal carcinoma [2]. Also strongly related to HPV are vulvar intraepithelial and vaginal intraepithelial neoplasias. The meta-analysis

supported the hypothesis that two distinct subsets of carcinomas of the vulva and vagina exist: one that is strongly associated with HPV and that may be preceded by high-grade lesions as cervical carcinoma, and another that arises independently of HPV infection [3].

HPV16 was found in more than three quarters of HPV-positive

progress but also points, in some countries, to the implementation of effective secondary prevention programmes.

- In contrast, rates are increasing in certain countries with high or very high levels of human development, including several eastern European countries and former Soviet states. Recent changes in sexual behaviour have led to an increase in the risk of infection with high-risk human papillomavirus types in these populations, largely in the absence of effective screening programmes.

Cancer of the corpus uteri (endometrial cancer)

- Cancer of the corpus uteri (endometrial cancer) is the sixth most common cancer in women (almost 5% of all cancers in women). There were an estimated 320 000 new cases and 76 000 deaths from the disease in 2012.
- Incidence rates vary 20–30-fold between countries; close to two thirds of the estimated new cases occur in countries with very high or high levels of human development.
- Incidence rates are elevated in northern and eastern Europe and North America, and tend to be low in Africa and West Asia.
- About 48% of the new cases occurred in Europe and North America; 41% of the estimated

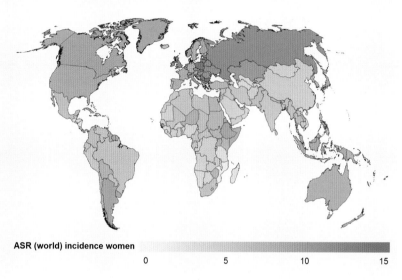

ASR (world) incidence women

0   5   10   15

new cases and 45% of the cancer deaths occurred in Asia.

Ovarian cancer

- With an estimated 239 000 new cases in 2012, ovarian cancer is the seventh most common cancer in women, representing 4% of all cancers in women.
- The fatality rate of ovarian cancer tends to be rather high relative to other cancers of the female reproductive organs, and case fatality is higher in lower-resource settings. As a consequence, ovarian cancer is the eighth most frequent cause of cancer death among women, with 152 000 deaths.

- In 2012, almost 55% of all new cases occurred in countries with high or very high levels of human development; 37% of the new cases and 39% of the deaths occurred in Europe and North America.
- Incidence rates are highest in northern and eastern Europe, North America, and Oceania, and tend to be relatively low in Africa and much of Asia.
- Incidence rates have been declining in certain countries with very high levels of human development, notably in Europe and North America.

carcinomas of the vulva and vagina. Conversely, HPV18 was rarer in carcinomas of the vulva and vagina than in carcinoma of the cervix. HPV6 and 11 were commonly detected in vulvar intraepithelial neoplasias but not in vaginal intraepithelial neoplasias [2].

There is substantial heterogeneity in HPV prevalence in vulvar squamous cell carcinomas. HPV prevalence was 69.4% in warty and basaloid carcinomas but only 13.2% in keratinizing carcinomas. HPV-positive vulvar carcinomas occur in significantly younger women than do

HPV-negative vulvar carcinomas [2], and HPV prevalence in vulvar carcinomas in North America was approximately twice that in other geographical regions [4], possibly attributable to enhanced surveillance of the vulva during cervical screening and some misclassification, together with higher HPV prevalence.

Risk factors for carcinomas of the vulva and vagina other than HPV infection include sexual habits, smoking, and immunosuppression [1]. Current HPV vaccines may prevent

approximately 30% of vulvar carcinomas and 60% of vaginal carcinomas.

Precursor lesions

Two pathogenetic pathways, featuring different precursor lesions, exist for vulvar squamous cell carcinomas, depending on HPV involvement.

Squamous intraepithelial lesions of the vulva are HPV-related in 90% of cases and range from low-grade vulvar intraepithelial neoplasia grade 1 to the severe full-thickness dysplasia of high grade (grade 3) [5]. Patients are usually in their thirties

Chart 5.12.1. Estimated global number of new cases and deaths with proportions by major world regions, for cervical cancer, 2012.

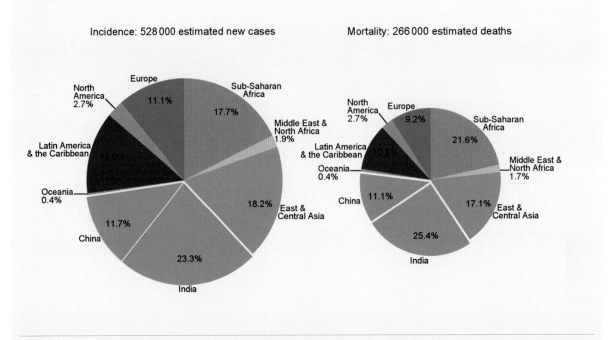

Incidence: 528 000 estimated new cases

Mortality: 266 000 estimated deaths

Chart 5.12.2. Estimated global number of new cases and deaths with proportions by major world regions, for cancer of the corpus uteri (endometrial cancer), 2012.

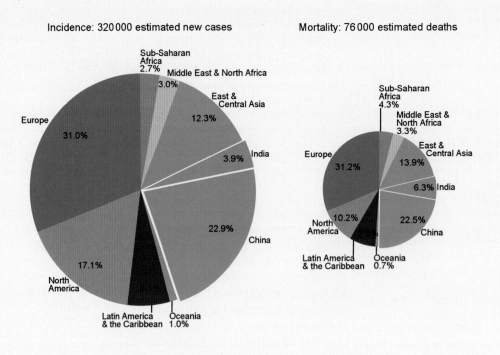

Incidence: 320 000 estimated new cases

Mortality: 76 000 estimated deaths

Chart 5.12.3. Estimated global number of new cases and deaths with proportions by major world regions, for ovarian cancer, 2012.

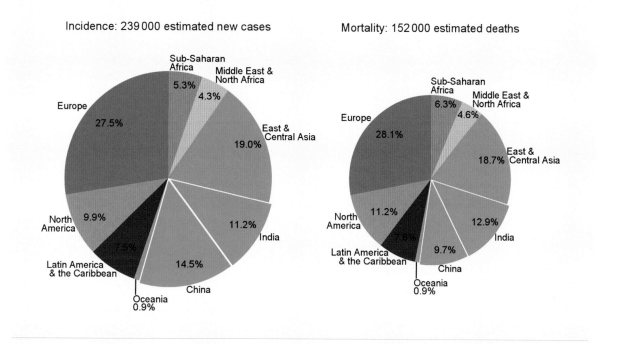

Incidence: 239 000 estimated new cases

Mortality: 152 000 estimated deaths

Chart 5.12.4. Age-standardized (World) incidence rates per 100 000 by year in selected populations, for cervical cancer, circa 1975–2012.

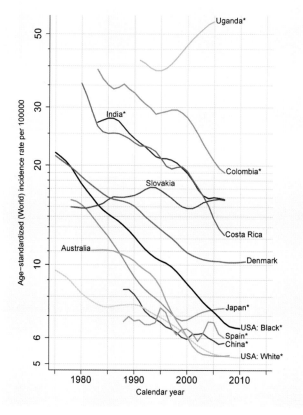

Chart 5.12.5. Age-standardized (World) incidence rates per 100 000 by year in selected populations, for cancer of the corpus uteri (endometrial cancer), circa 1975–2012.

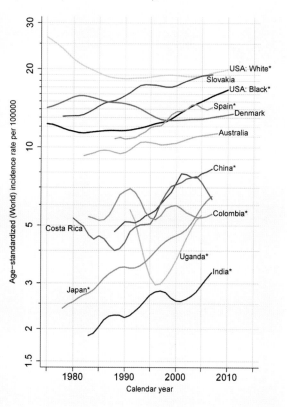

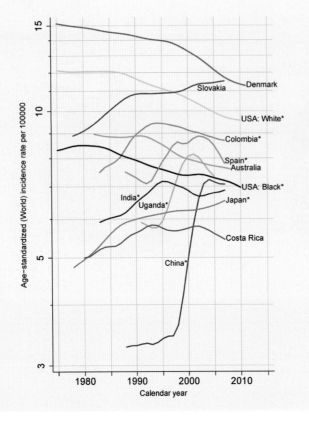

Chart 5.12.6. Age-standardized (World) incidence rates per 100 000 by year in selected populations, for ovarian cancer, circa 1975–2012.

Y-axis: Age-standardized (World) incidence rate per 100000

X-axis: Calendar year

Denmark
Slovakia
USA: White*
Colombia*
Spain*
Australia
USA: Black*
India*
Uganda*
Japan*
Costa Rica
China*

or forties and often have multifocal or multicentric HPV-related disease [6,7]. Most low-grade lesions contain low-risk HPV virus subtypes, whereas high-grade lesions contain high-risk subtypes, most commonly HPV16. The typical progression time from incident infection to clinical disease is 18.5 months [6]. Only about 6% of high-grade lesions progress to invasive carcinomas, except in older or immunosuppressed women [7].

Patients with high-grade vulvar intraepithelial neoplasia of differentiated or simplex type are usually postmenopausal and often have lichen sclerosus or lichen simplex chronicus [8]. Differentiated vulvar intraepithelial neoplasia is more likely (33%) to progress to invasive carcinoma than corresponding HPV-related disease [9]. In one study comparing the association of the two types of vulvar intraepithelial neoplasia with

invasive carcinoma, the rates were 24.2% for HPV-related grade 3 vulvar intraepithelial neoplasia and 83.3% for the corresponding differentiated lesions [6].

Pathology and genetics

Whereas low-grade squamous intraepithelial neoplasia is a rare diagnosis [6], high-grade disease is divided into warty and basaloid subtypes. Warty lesions show a spiky or undulating surface. The thickened epithelium forms wide, deep rete pegs separated by thin dermal papillae. Hyperkeratosis is prominent. In contrast to warty lesions, basaloid lesions show a flat surface and a uniform population of immature cells. Keratinocytes undergo premature keratinization, and rete pegs often contain keratin pearls.

Superficially invasive squamous cell carcinoma is the earliest stage

(stage IA) of invasive vulvar cancer and has an excellent prognosis [10]. Most invasive carcinomas of the vulva arise in a background of lichen sclerosus with or without differentiated vulvar intraepithelial neoplasia. Tumours are frequently exophytic, but some may be ulcerative. Vulvar carcinomas are composed of invasive nests of malignant squamous epithelium with central keratin pearls (Fig. 5.12.2). HPV-related tumours typically occur in younger patients and tend to have a similar morphology [3,6]. Vulvar carcinomas grow slowly, extending to contiguous skin, vagina, and rectum. They metastasize initially to inguinal and femoral lymph nodes, and subsequently to pelvic lymph nodes [11].

Differentiated vulvar intraepithelial neoplasia shows overexpression of p53 in the basal and suprabasal epithelial layers [7]. Cases of lichen sclerosus, differentiated vulval intraepithelial neoplasia, and invasive squamous cell carcinoma with identical *TP53* mutations have been reported [8]. *TP53* mutation, however, is an uncommon and late event in vulvar carcinogenesis. Of greater utility in the diagnosis of high-grade squamous intraepithelial lesions is p16^{INK4A}; as a reliable marker of high-risk HPV [10], it is strongly positive throughout the epithelium [12].

Cervical cancer

Cervical cancer originates at the junction between the columnar epithelium of the endocervix and the squamous epithelium of the ectocervix, a site of continuous metaplastic change, especially at puberty and from after the first pregnancy until menopause. Persistent epithelial infection with one or more oncogenic types of HPV may lead to the development of precancerous lesions, a small proportion of which may progress to invasive cervical cancer over a period of 10–20 years [1].

Etiology

HPV infection is the most common sexually transmitted infection worldwide, and the majority of sexually

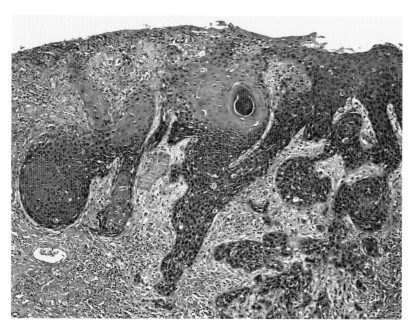

Fig. 5.12.2. Keratinizing squamous cell carcinoma of the vulva. Anastomosing cords of neoplastic squamous cells, some with keratin pearls, are evident.

active individuals of both sexes acquire it at some time during their life. About 291 million women worldwide have HPV infection of the cervix at any time, corresponding to a prevalence of 10.4%, although the prevalence is higher among women younger than 25 years (16.9%) [13].

High HPV prevalence occurs in countries where the burden of cervical cancer is high (Fig. 5.12.3), i.e. in sub-Saharan Africa, Latin America, and India, but also in countries like Mongolia and China. Large differences in age-specific HPV prevalence are evident in several less-developed countries (India, China, and African countries) [14]. More than 90% of new HPV infections at any age regress over 6–18 months [15]. Low-grade squamous intra-epithelial lesions, also known as cervical intraepithelial neoplasia

Fig. 5.12.3. Age-adjusted prevalence (percentage) of cervical human papillomavirus (HPV) DNA in sexually active women aged 15–69 years in various countries.

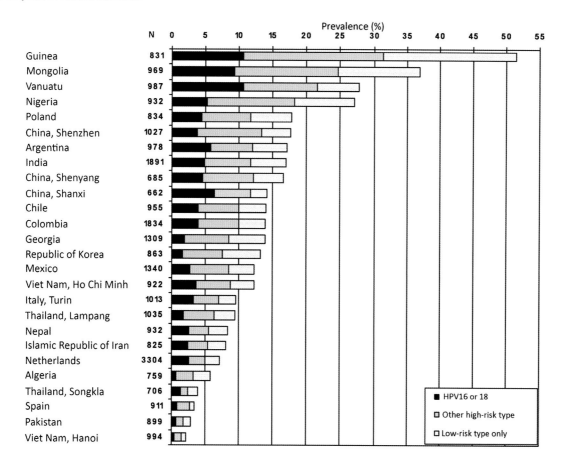

5 ORGAN SITE
CHAPTER 5.12

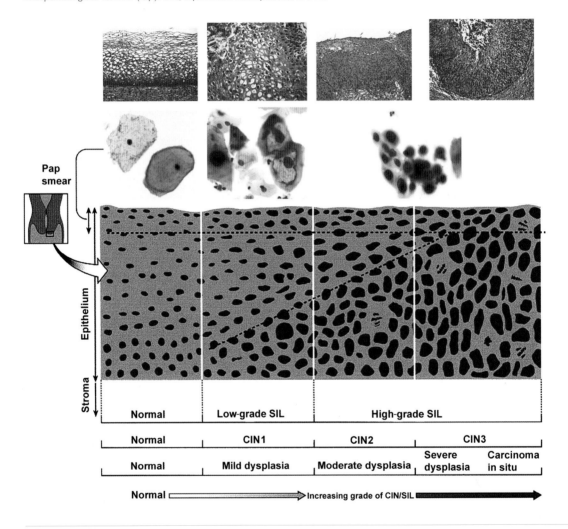

Fig. 5.12.4. Interrelations of naming systems in precursor human papillomavirus (HPV)-related cervical lesions. This chart integrates multiple aspects of the disease. It illustrates the changes in progressively more abnormal disease states and provides terminology for the dysplasia/carcinoma in situ system, the cervical intraepithelial neoplasia (CIN) system, and the Bethesda system. The scheme also illustrates the corresponding cytological smear resulting from exfoliation of the most superficial cells as well as the equivalent histopathological lesions (top). SIL, squamous intraepithelial lesion.

grade 1 (CIN1), is an insensitive proxy of HPV infection and is not precancer. High-grade squamous intraepithelial lesions (CIN grade 2) include a heterogeneous group of lesions that are equivocal in cancer potential. In contrast, grade 3 disease represents the most clinically relevant lesion and is the best surrogate end-point for cervical cancer in screening and vaccination trials. The probability of HPV clearance depends on the duration of the infection [16].

The mean age at which women develop squamous intraepithelial lesions is 24–27 years for low-grade lesions (CIN1) and 35–42 years for high-grade lesions (CIN3). Half of low-grade lesions regress, 10% progress to high-grade lesions, and less than 2% become invasive cancer. The average time for low-grade squamous intraepithelial lesions to progress to high-grade lesions (CIN3) is about 10 years. At least 20% of cases of CIN3 progress to invasive carcinoma in that time.

The strongest risk factors for persistence and progression are immunodeficiency and the type of HPV involved [1]. Of 13 HPV types, HPV16 is by far the likeliest to persist and cause CIN3 and cervical cancer.

The proportion of HPV16 increases among HPV-positive women with the increase in lesion severity [17]. Conversely, the proportion of other high-risk HPV types is diminished in CIN3 and cervical cancer. Women who tested positive twice for HPV16 after a 9–21-month interval had a 3-year cumulative incidence of CIN2 or worse of 40%. The corresponding cumulative incidence was 15% for HPV18 and 8.5% for other high-risk HPV types.

The most commonly detected HPV types in cervical cancer worldwide are HPV16 (57%) and 18 (16%), followed by HPV58, 33, 45, 31, 52, and 35 [17]. Therefore, current vaccines that prevent infection by HPV16 and 18 should prevent about 75% of cervical cancers and 60% of high-grade lesions (that need treatment when detected during screening), with small variations by region [17]. Future confirmation of cross-protection of HPV16 and 18 vaccines against other high-risk types [18] or the introduction of vaccines targeting additional high-risk HPV types would increase prevention (see Chapter 4.6).

Cervical cancer risk factors other than HPV infection are either weak in terms of the magnitude of association (smoking) or represent correlates of the probability of acquisition (number of sexual partners) or, possibly, the likelihood of progression of HPV infection to cancer (age at first sexual intercourse and first birth, parity, and oral contraceptive use) [19].

CIN is a spectrum of epithelial changes that begins with minimal atypia and progresses through stages of greater epithelial abnormalities to invasive squamous cell carcinoma. The terms CIN, dysplasia, carcinoma in situ, and squamous intraepithelial lesion are commonly used interchangeably (Fig. 5.12.4). p16 immunohistochemistry is recommended when the differential diagnosis is between precancer (CIN2 or CIN3) and a mimic of precancer, such as immature squamous metaplasia or reparative changes. Strong and diffuse block-positive p16 results support a diagnosis of precancerous disease [5].

Early phases of infection with *all* HPV types probably show episomal viral propagation throughout a polyclonal epithelial field, with low-grade squamous intraepithelial lesions (CIN1) cytology. These lesions mark a permissive infection, i.e. episomal HPV freely replicates and causes cell death. Huge numbers of virus must accumulate in the cytoplasm before being visible as a koilocyte (Fig. 5.12.4). In contrast, in most cases of CIN2/3, viral DNA integrates into the cell genome. Some 85% of CIN1 lesions, as well as many genital warts, contain low-risk HPV6 or 11. In contrast, cells in CIN2/3 usually have

Fig. 5.12.5. Squamous cell carcinoma, large cell, non-keratinizing type.

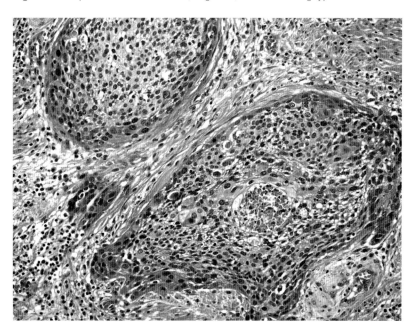

HPV types 16, 18, 58, 33, 45, 31, 52, and 35 [17].

Pathology and genetics

The association with HPV infection is equally strong for the two main histological types of cervical cancer: squamous cell carcinoma and adenocarcinoma. However, since most cervical abnormalities caused by HPV infection are unlikely to progress to high-grade CIN or cervical cancer, other exogenous or endogenous factors acting in conjunction with HPV infection may be necessary for progression of the disease [1].

The normal process by which cervical squamous epithelium matures is disturbed in squamous intraepithelial lesions. In low-grade lesions (CIN1), the most pronounced changes are in the basal third of the epithelium. However, abnormal cells are present throughout the thickness of the epithelium, and nuclei in the upper levels are still abnormal [5]. Thus, the sloughed cells can be detected as abnormal in Pap smears. In high-grade lesions (CIN2), most cellular abnormalities are in the lower and middle thirds of the epithelium. High-grade squamous intraepithelial lesions are often detected

on colposcopic examination. In the case of adenocarcinoma in situ, normal columnar epithelium is replaced by dysplastic glandular epithelium. However, morphological change comparable to CIN1 does not occur in the glandular epithelium.

Superficially invasive or microinvasive squamous cell carcinoma is the earliest stage of invasive cervical cancer. In this setting, stromal invasion usually arises from an overlying squamous intraepithelial lesion. Staging of microinvasive disease is based on width and depth of invasion [11]. The earliest invasive changes, sometimes termed early stromal invasion, appear as tiny irregular epithelial buds emanating from the base of CIN3 lesions. These small (< 1 mm) tongues of neoplastic epithelial cells do not affect the prognosis of CIN3 lesions; hence, both can be treated similarly with conservative surgery.

Histologically, 85–90% of invasive cervical cancers are squamous cell carcinoma, appearing as infiltrating networks of neoplastic cells in the stroma, with varying degrees of differentiation, with or without keratinization (Fig. 5.12.5). Adenocarcinoma and its variants constitute 10–15%

Fig. 5.12.6. Adenocarcinoma, endocervical or usual type.

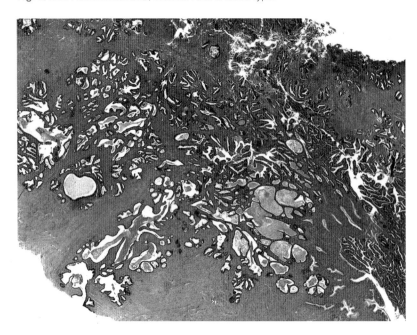

of cervical cancers. The most common type of adenocarcinoma is the endocervical cell type, showing abnormal glands with varying size and shape with budding and branching, infiltrating the stroma (Fig. 5.12.6). Cervical cancer spreads by direct extension, through lymphatic vessels and only rarely by the haematogenous route. Local extension into surrounding tissues (parametrium) results in ureteric compression [11].

Genome-wide association studies have identified loci associated with cervical cancer susceptibility, including those at 4q12 and 17q12 in the Han Chinese population [20] and at 6p21.3 in a Swedish study [21]. A recent genetic analysis examined 80 cervical tumours for 1250 known mutations in 139 cancer genes [22]. Validated mutations were detected in 48 of the 80 tumours (60%). The highest mutation rates were in the *PIK3CA* (31.3%), *KRAS* (8.8%), and *EGFR* (3.8%) genes. *PIK3CA* mutation rates did not differ significantly between adenocarcinomas and squamous cell carcinomas. In contrast, *KRAS* mutations were identified only in adenocarcinomas (17.5% vs 0%), and a novel *EGFR* mutation was detected only in squamous cell carcinomas (0% vs 7.5%). There were no associations between HPV16 or HPV18 and somatic mutations or overall survival. In adjusted analyses, *PIK3CA* mutations were associated with shorter survival.

Prevention

Prophylactic vaccines against HPV currently available include monovalent (HPV16), bivalent (HPV16 and 18), and quadrivalent (HPV6, 11, 16, and 18) virus-like particle vaccines. Furthermore, clinical trials examining the efficacy of a nonavalent vaccine are under way. In large clinical trials, vaccines have shown excellent safety and nearly 100% efficacy in preventing persistent infections and the cervical precancers due to HPV16 and 18 [23,24]. Despite many barriers to implementation of the vaccine in resource-restricted environments, the vaccine has successfully been introduced in several developing countries [23] (see Chapter 4.6).

Early changes in the cervix, specifically squamous intraepithelial lesions, can be detected years before invasive cancer develops by screening tests such as conventional cytology (Pap smear), liquid-based cytology, and HPV testing (Chapter 4.7) [25]. Testing for HPV DNA of oncogenic types is gaining increasing interest and application in cervical cancer screening. It has much greater sensitivity and only slightly lower specificity than Pap cytology. As a primary screening test followed by Pap triage of HPV-positive cases, HPV testing has the potential to improve the overall quality of screening programmes [23]. Women with abnormal screening results are further investigated with colposcopy-directed biopsies.

Endometrial cancer

Endometrial carcinoma is a malignant epithelial tumour, usually exhibiting glandular differentiation (adenocarcinoma), capable of invading the myometrium and spreading outside the uterus. More than 80% of cases are estrogen-related, well- to moderately well-differentiated (endometrioid) adenocarcinomas, which are usually confined to the corpus uteri at diagnosis and can be cured by hysterectomy. The remaining cases, however, are non-estrogen-related high-grade carcinomas (non-endometrioid serous and clear cell adenocarcinomas) associated with poor prognosis.

Etiology

Hormones play an important role in the etiology of endometrial carcinoma. The "unopposed estrogens" hypothesis is widely accepted and explains most of the risk factors for endometrial cancer: early age at menarche, late age at menopause, nulliparity, hormone replacement therapy use, and obesity.

Obesity is the most important risk factor worldwide, estimated to account for 40% of endometrial cancer incidence. In premenopausal women, obesity is associated with anovulatory cycles during which the endometrial tissue receives continuous stimulation. In postmenopausal women, obesity increases the concentration of endogenous estrogens, which are mainly produced by the aromatization of androgens in the adipose tissues.

Excess weight is associated with insulin resistance and chronically elevated insulin concentrations in blood, and with increasing concentrations of sex steroids [26], factors that are associated with increased endometrial cancer risk. Type 2 and type 1 diabetes are strongly associated with an increase in endometrial cancer risk.

The use of oral contraceptives is associated with a long-lasting decrease in endometrial cancer risk, but only when they contain progestogen in addition to estrogens [27]. Use of hormone replacement therapy by postmenopausal women increases the risk of endometrial cancer about 2-fold [28]. Higher endogenous estrogen concentrations in blood are associated with an increase in endometrial cancer risk mainly in postmenopausal women, whereas higher endogenous androgen concentrations are associated with an increase in endometrial cancer risk in both premenopausal and postmenopausal women [26]. Polycystic ovary syndrome – associated with increased blood androgen levels, and with infertility, amenorrhea, hirsutism and diabetes – has been consistently associated with an increase in endometrial cancer risk. Women who develop breast cancer are at increased risk, and are more likely to develop non-endometrioid rather than endometrioid endometrial carcinoma. Although this increase in risk could be explained partly by common risk factors between breast and endometrial malignancies, such as nulliparity or late age at menopause, the use of tamoxifen for the treatment of breast cancer has also been questioned: women under tamoxifen therapy had a more than 2-fold increase in endometrial cancer risk compared with non-users.

Pathology

Endometrial carcinomas are classified into two different clinicopathological types (Fig. 5.12.7) [29]. More than 80% are type I tumours, which are estrogen-related, low-grade endometrioid carcinomas, often preceded by endometrial hyperplasia.

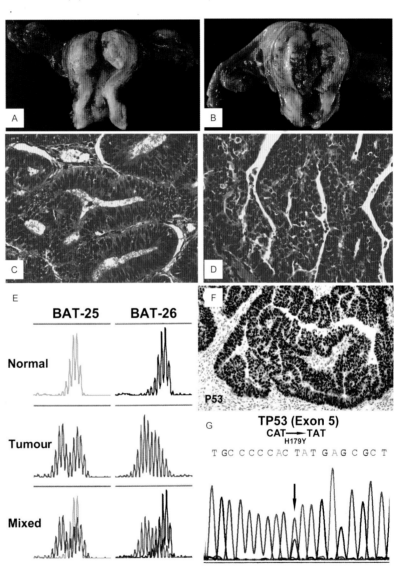

Fig. 5.12.7. Adenocarcinoma of the endometrium. (A) Endometrioid carcinoma (type I). Polypoid endometrial tumour with only superficial myometrial invasion. (B) Non-endometrioid carcinoma (type II). Large haemorrhagic and necrotic tumour with deeper myometrial invasion. (C) Well-differentiated (grade 1) endometrioid adenocarcinoma. The neoplastic glands resemble normal endometrial glands. (D) Non-endometrioid (serous) carcinoma exhibiting stratification of markedly atypical tumour cells with numerous mitoses. (E) Endometrioid carcinoma. *MLH1* inactivation by promoter hypermethylation is the most common cause of the microsatellite instability phenotype in endometrioid endometrial carcinoma. Progressive accumulation of alterations secondary to microsatellite instability affects important regulatory genes and promotes carcinogenesis. (F) Non-endometrioid (serous) carcinoma usually shows a strong p53 immunoreaction as a result of (G) *TP53* mutation.

They are usually confined to the uterus and have a favourable outcome. In contrast, approximately 10% of cases are type II tumours, which are non-endometrioid (mainly serous and, less frequently, clear cell) carcinomas, arising occasionally in endometrial polyps or atrophic endometria. Type II tumours are not associated with estrogen stimulation or hyperplasia; they often, but not always, invade the myometrium and lymphovascular spaces, and they have a high mortality rate.

Table 5.12.1. Hereditary syndromes with lifetime risk of endometrial cancer

Hereditary condition	Gene (chromosome)	Lifetime risk of endometrial cancer
Hereditary non-polyposis colorectal cancer Lynch syndrome II Muir–Torre syndrome	MSH2 (2p21) MLH1 (3p21.3) PMS2 (7p22.2) MSH6 (2p16)	40–60%
Cowden syndrome	PTEN (10q23.3)	5–10%
BRCA1 syndrome	BRCA1 (17q)	2–3%

Key surgical and pathological prognostic indicators include histological type, histological grade, surgical/pathological stage, depth of myometrial invasion, lymphovascular invasion, and cervical involvement [30]. In 2009, a new staging classification of endometrial carcinoma was proposed [12]. Most endometrial cancers are sporadic, but 2–5% are familial (Table 5.12.1). Endometrial carcinoma is the most common extracolonic cancer in women with hereditary non-polyposis colon cancer syndrome, a defect in DNA mismatch repair that is also associated with breast and ovarian cancers.

Genetics

A dualistic model of endometrial carcinogenesis has been proposed (Fig. 5.12.7) [31]. According to this model, normal endometrial cells would transform into endometrioid carcinoma through replication errors, so-called "microsatellite instability", and subsequent accumulation of mutations in oncogenes and tumour suppressor genes. In contrast, alterations of TP53 and loss of heterozygosity on several chromosomes would drive the process of neoplastic transformation into the acquisition of a non-endometrioid carcinoma phenotype.

Molecular genetic alterations in type I, i.e. endometrioid, carcinomas (Table 5.12.2) differ in some respects from those detected in type II (non-endometrioid) carcinomas (Table 5.12.3) [31]. Non-endometrioid carcinomas may also derive from endometrioid carcinoma with microsatellite instability through

tumour progression and subsequent TP53 mutations (Fig. 5.12.8) [31].

In sporadic endometrioid carcinomas, microsatellite instability results from promoter hypermethylation of hMLH1 and leads to mutations in several target genes (containing microsatellites) that are involved in apoptosis, cell proliferation, and cell differentiation. The wide range of mutations would be responsible for tumour heterogeneity. Inactivation of the tumour suppressor gene PTEN may result from microsatellite instability (45%), promoter hypermethylation (16%), or loss of heterozygosity (24%). PTEN

inactivation releases the PI3K/AKT pathway, inhibiting apoptosis and resulting in tumour growth advantage. Recent genomic and related analyses have indicated that most endometrioid tumours have few copy number alterations or TP53 mutations but frequent mutations in PTEN, CTNNB1, PIK3CA, ARID1A, and KRAS, and novel mutations in the SWI/SNF chromatin remodelling complex gene ARID5B [32].

β-Catenin gene mutations occur in 20% of endometrioid carcinomas, correlate with MMP-7 and cyclin D1 overexpression, and are associated with good prognosis. Mutation of the ARID1A gene and loss of the corresponding protein BAF250a have been found in 29–40% of endometrioid carcinomas, 18% of serous carcinomas, and 26% of clear cell carcinomas [33,34]. In contrast, non-endometrioid carcinomas show TP53 and PPP2R1A mutations, inactivation of p16 and E-cadherin, c-erbB2 amplification, STK15 alterations, and

Table 5.12.2. Altered genes in endometrioid endometrial carcinoma

Gene	Chromosome	Mechanism of alteration	Percentage of cancers
Oncogenes			
PIK3CA	3q26.3	Point mutation	24–39%
KRAS	12p12.1	Point mutation	10–30%
CTNNB1 (β-catenin)	3p21	Point mutation	14–44%
PIK3R1	5q13.1	Point mutation	43%
FGFR2	10q26	Point mutation	16%
Tumour suppressor genes			
PTEN	10q23.3	Mutation, loss of heterozygosity	37–61%
ARID1A	1p35.3	Mutation	40%
MLH1 (MSI)	3p21.3	Promoter hypermethylation (epigenetic silencing)	30%
TP53	17p13.1	Mutation	10–20%
CDKN2A (p16)	9p21	Loss of heterozygosity, epigenetic silencing	10%
SPRY2	13q31.1	Epigenetic silencing	20%
RASSF1A	3p21.3	Epigenetic silencing	48%

Fig. 5.12.8. Pathogenesis of endometrial cancer: an alternative to the dualistic model. On the basis of molecular analysis, it has been suggested that non-endometrioid carcinomas may result from tumour progression from pre-existing endometrioid carcinomas. This would explain why these high-grade tumours often retain the molecular alterations of endometrioid carcinomas. Ca, carcinoma; MI, microsatellite instability; NE, normal endometrium.

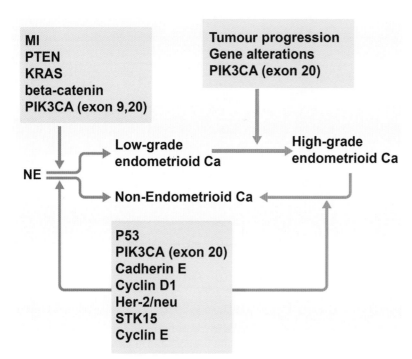

associated with a poor prognosis in endometrial cancer. The role of drugs inhibiting angiogenesis, such as bevacizumab and tyrosine kinase inhibitors, is being studied.

Ovarian cancer

The most common ovarian cancers are ovarian carcinomas, which are also the most lethal gynaecological malignancies. Based on histopathology and molecular genetics, ovarian carcinomas are divided into five main types: high-grade serous (70%), endometrioid (10%), clear cell (10%), mucinous (3%), and low-grade serous carcinomas (< 5%), which together account for more than 95% of cases (Table 5.12.4; Fig. 5.12.9). These types are essentially distinct diseases, as indicated by differences in epidemiological and genetic risk factors, precursor lesions, patterns of spread, molecular events during oncogenesis, response to chemotherapy, and prognosis [39]. Much less common are malignant germ cell tumours (dysgerminomas, yolk sac tumours, and immature

loss of heterozygosity at multiple loci (Table 5.12.3) [29–31].

Targeted therapy

Endometrioid carcinomas with *PTEN* mutations have activation of the PI3K/AKT pathway and genomic instability. Accordingly, these patients are treated with poly (ADP-ribose) polymerase (PARP) inhibitors [35]. Mammalian target of rapamycin (mTOR) is a kinase that regulates cell growth and apoptosis [36]. mTOR inhibitors have recently been developed as potential anticancer agents, and *PTEN*-mutated tumours are particularly susceptible [37]. Angiogenesis is essential to the development and maintenance of any tissue. Increased production of vascular endothelial growth factor (VEGF), frequently observed in hypoxia or inflammation, results in increased endothelial cell proliferation and decreased apoptosis [38]. VEGF overexpression is

Table 5.12.3. Altered genes in non-endometrioid endometrial carcinoma

Gene	Chromosome	Mechanism of alteration	Percentage of cancers
Oncogenes			
PIK3CA	3q26.3	Point mutation and amplification	20–30%
PIK3R1	5q13.1	Point mutation	12%
ERBB2 (HER2/neu)	17q12	Amplification	30%
CCNE1 (cyclin E1)	19q12	Amplification	55%
STK15 (aurora kinase A)	20q13.2	Amplification	60%
CCND1 (cyclin D1)	11q13	Amplification	26%
Tumour suppressor genes			
TP53	17p13.1	Mutation	90%
CDH1 (E-cadherin)	16q22.1	Loss of heterozygosity	80–90%
CDKN2A (p16)	9p21	Loss of heterozygosity, epigenetic silencing	40%
PPP2R1A	19q13.41	Mutation	17–41%

Table 5.12.4. Characteristics of the main types of ovarian carcinoma

Characteristic	Type				
	High-grade serous	**Low-grade serous**	**Mucinous**	**Endometrioid**	**Clear cell**
Usual stage at diagnosis	Advanced	Early or advanced	Early	Early	Early
Presumed tissue of origin/precursor lesion	Fallopian tube or tubal metaplasia in inclusions of ovarian surface epithelium	Serous borderline tumour	Adenoma–border-line tumour–carci-noma sequence; teratoma	Endometriosis, adenofibroma	Endometriosis, adenofibroma
Genetic risk	*BRCA1/2*	?	?	Hereditary non-polyposis colorectal cancer	?
Significant molecular abnormalities	p53 and pRb pathways	*BRAF* or *KRAS*	*KRAS*	*PTEN*, β-catenin, *ARID1A*, *PIK3CA* *KRAS* Microsatellite instability	HNF-1β, *ARID1A*, *PIK3CA*
Proliferation	High	Low	Intermediate	Low	Low
Response to primary chemotherapy	80%	26–28%	15%	?	15%
Prognosis	Poor	Favourable	Favourable	Favourable	Intermediate

teratomas) (3% of ovarian cancers) and potentially malignant sex cord stromal tumours (1–2%), the most common of which are granulosa cell tumours.

Etiology

Ovarian carcinomas most commonly affect nulliparous women and occur least frequently in women with suppressed ovulation, typically by pregnancy or oral contraceptives. These tumours are generally considered to originate from the cells covering the ovarian surface or the pelvic peritoneum. Malignant transformation of this mesothelium has been explained by the "incessant ovulation" theory [40]. Irritants, such as talc or asbestos, have also been implicated, as have hormonal factors. Elevated gonadotropin levels may contribute to malignant transformation. Pregnancy and oral contraceptives are protective factors, and both cause a reduction in pituitary gonadotropins.

Family history of ovarian cancer accounts for 10% of cases; the risk is increased 3-fold when two or more first-degree relatives have been affected. Women with germline mutations in *BRCA1* or *BRCA2* have a 30–70% risk of developing ovarian cancer, mainly high-grade serous carcinomas, by age 70 [41]. *BRCA1* and *BRCA2* are essential components of the homologous recombination DNA repair system, required to repair DNA double-strand breaks [42]. Women with hereditary non-polyposis colon cancer are also at greater risk for ovarian cancer, specifically endometrioid carcinoma.

The cell descriptors used to classify ovarian carcinomas – serous, mucinous, endometrioid, clear cell, transitional, and squamous – do not apply to cells in the normal ovary, and malignancy has long been attributed to Müllerian "neometaplasia" of the ovarian surface epithelium (mesothelium). During embryonic life, the coelomic cavity is lined by mesothelium, which also covers the gonadal ridge and gives rise to Müllerian ducts, from which the fallopian tubes, uterus, and vagina develop. Thus, the tumour cells would resemble morphologically the epithelia of the fallopian tube, endometrium, or endocervix. Although the mesothelial origin cannot be excluded, there is evidence that several primary ovarian cancers have originated in other pelvic organs and involve the ovary secondarily. High-grade serous carcinomas, especially in *BRCA*-positive patients, have been postulated to arise from precursor epithelial lesions in the distal fimbriated end of the fallopian tube, whereas endometrioid and clear cell carcinomas originate from ovarian endometriosis [43].

Pathology and genetics

Serous carcinoma

High-grade serous carcinoma and low-grade serous carcinoma (Fig. 5.12.9, A and B) are fundamentally different tumour types. Low-grade serous carcinomas are usually associated with a non-invasive serous borderline component, carry *KRAS* and *BRAF* mutations, and are unrelated to *TP53* mutations and *BRCA* abnormalities. In contrast, high-grade serous carcinomas are not associated with serous borderline tumours and typically exhibit *TP53* mutations and *BRCA* abnormalities (Table 5.12.4) [44]. Most patients with high-grade serous carcinomas

Fig. 5.12.9. Representative examples of the five main types of ovarian carcinoma, which together account for 98% of cases: (A) high-grade serous carcinoma, (B) low-grade serous carcinoma, (C) endometrioid carcinoma, (D) mucinous carcinoma, and (E) clear cell carcinoma.

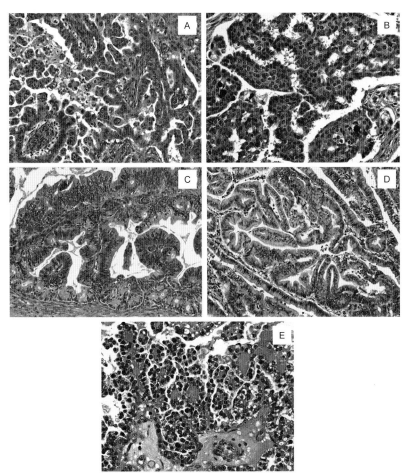

(> 80%) present with advanced disease (stage III).

The genomics of serous ovarian adenocarcinomas has been assessed using DNA sequences of exons from coding genes in 316 of these tumours and other data [45]. High-grade serous ovarian cancer is characterized by *TP53* mutations in almost all tumours (96%); low-prevalence but statistically recurrent somatic mutations in nine further genes, including *NF1*, *BRCA1*, *BRCA2*, *RB1*, and *CDK12*; 113 significant focal DNA copy number aberrations; and promoter methylation events involving 168 genes. Analyses delineated four ovarian cancer transcriptional subtypes, three microRNA subtypes, four promoter methylation subtypes, and a transcriptional signature associated with survival duration. Other data involved the impact that tumours with *BRCA1* or *BRCA2* and *CCNE1* aberrations have on survival. Pathway analyses suggested that homologous recombination is defective in about half of the tumours analysed, and that NOTCH and FOXM1 signalling are involved in serous ovarian cancer pathophysiology.

Consistent patterns of chromosomal change in patient cohorts suggest an underlying interdependency of gains and losses of particular genes in individual tumours [46], for example co-amplification of *CCNE1* and the 20q11 locus involving the cell-cycle regulator *TPX2*, among other genes. Genome-wide association studies continue to identify susceptibility loci for ovarian cancer, specifically including loci at 2q31 and 8q24 [47].

Endometrioid carcinoma

Endometrioid carcinoma, which resembles its endometrial counterpart (Fig. 5.12.9C), is thought to arise by malignant transformation of endometriosis and not from the ovarian surface epithelium. The most common genetic abnormalities in ovarian endometrioid carcinoma are somatic mutations of the *ARID1A*, *CTNNB1* (β-catenin), and *PTEN* genes, and microsatellite instability (Table 5.12.4) [39,48]. Between 15% and 20% of patients with endometrioid carcinoma of the ovary also have endometrial cancer. If ovarian and endometrial cancers coexist, they generally arise independently, although some may be metastases from one or the other, a distinction with important prognostic implications.

Mucinous carcinoma

Mucinous ovarian tumours are often heterogeneous. Benign, borderline, non-invasive, and invasive carcinoma components may coexist within the same tumour. Such a morphological continuum suggests that tumour progression occurs from cystadenoma and borderline tumour to invasive carcinomas. This hypothesis is supported by *KRAS* mutations in mucinous tumours: 56% of cystadenomas and 85% of carcinomas express mutated *KRAS*, and borderline tumours are intermediate (Table 5.12.4) [39]. Mucinous carcinomas are usually large, unilateral cystic masses (Fig. 5.12.9D). The finding of bilateral mucinous tumours should raise suspicion of metastases from a far more frequent mucinous carcinoma elsewhere (e.g. gastrointestinal tract).

Clear cell carcinoma

This enigmatic ovarian cancer is closely related to endometrioid adenocarcinoma, and often occurs in association with endometriosis.

It usually occurs after menopause. The most common genetic abnormalities are somatic mutations of the *ARID1A*, *PTEN*, and *PIK3CA* genes (Table 5.12.4) [39,48]. Clear cell carcinomas of the ovary resemble their counterparts in the vagina, cervix, and corpus uteri; they show sheets or tubules of malignant cells with clear cytoplasm (Fig. 5.12.9E) or tubules lined by "hobnail" cells.

Prognosis

For patients with malignant ovarian tumours, survival is generally poor. The most important prognostic index is the surgical stage of the tumour at the time it is detected. A new staging classification of cancer of the ovary, fallopian tube, and peritoneum has been proposed by the International Federation of Gynecology and Obstetrics [49].

Targeted therapy

The most promising targets in clinical trials are angiogenesis and homologous recombination deficiency. To select patients for trials investigating these targets, predictive biomarkers are required. Other promising targets currently being studied based on ovarian cancer biology include folate receptor, PI3K/AKT, and Ras/Raf/MEK pathways [50].

References

1. IARC (2012). Biological agents. *IARC Monogr Eval Carcinog Risks Hum*, 100B:1–441. PMID:23189750

2. De Vuyst H, Clifford GM, Nascimento MC *et al.* (2009). Prevalence and type distribution of human papillomavirus in carcinoma and intraepithelial neoplasia of the vulva, vagina and anus: a meta-analysis. *Int J Cancer*, 124:1626–1636. http://dx.doi.org/10.1002/ijc.24116 PMID:19115209

3. Kurman RJ, Toki T, Schiffman MH (1993). Basaloid and warty carcinomas of the vulva. Distinctive types of squamous cell carcinoma frequently associated with human papillomaviruses. *Am J Surg Pathol*, 17:133–145. http://dx.doi.org/10.1097/00000478-199302000-00005 PMID:8380681

4. Centers for Disease Control and Prevention (CDC) (2012). Human papillomavirus-associated cancers - United States, 2004–2008. *MMWR Morb Mortal Wkly Rep*, 61:258–261. PMID:22513527

5. Darragh TM, Colgan TJ, Cox JT *et al.*; Members of LAST Project Work Groups (2012). The lower anogenital squamous terminology standardization project for HPV-associated lesions: background and consensus recommendations from the College of American Pathologists and the American Society for Colposcopy and Cervical Pathology. *J Low Genit Tract Dis*, 16:205–242. http://dx.doi.org/10.1097/LGT.0b013e31825c31dd PMID:22820980

6. Skapa P, Zamecnik J, Hamsikova E *et al.* (2007). Human papillomavirus (HPV) profiles of vulvar lesions: possible implications for the classification of vulvar squamous cell carcinoma precursors and for the efficacy of prophylactic HPV vaccination. *Am J Surg Pathol*, 31:1834–1843. http://dx.doi.org/10.1097/PAS.0b013e3180686d10 PMID:18043037

7. van de Nieuwenhof HP, van der Avoort IAM, de Hullu JA (2008). Review of squamous premalignant vulvar lesions. *Crit Rev Oncol Hematol*, 68:131–156. http://dx.doi.org/10.1016/j.critrevonc.2008.02.012 PMID:18406622

8. Pinto AP, Miron A, Yassin Y *et al.* (2010). Differentiated vulvar intraepithelial neoplasia contains *Tp53* mutations and is genetically linked to vulvar squamous cell carcinoma. *Mod Pathol*, 23:404–412. http://dx.doi.org/10.1038/modpathol.2009.179 PMID:20062014

9. van de Nieuwenhof HP, Massuger LF, van der Avoort IA *et al.* (2009). Vulvar squamous cell carcinoma development after diagnosis of VIN increases with age. *Eur J Cancer*, 45:851–856. http://dx.doi.org/10.1016/j.ejca.2008.11.037 PMID:19117749

10. Yoder BJ, Rufforny I, Massoll NA, Wilkinson EJ (2008). Stage IA vulvar squamous cell carcinoma: an analysis of tumor invasive characteristics and risk. *Am J Surg Pathol*, 32:765–772. http://dx.doi.org/10.1097/PAS.0b013e318159a2cb PMID:18379417

11. Report M (2009). The new FIGO staging system for cancers of the vulva, cervix, endometrium and sarcomas. *Gynecol Oncol*, 115:325–328. http://dx.doi.org/10.1016/j.ygyno.2009.10.050

12. McCluggage WG (2009). Recent developments in vulvovaginal pathology. *Histopathology*, 54:156–173. http://dx.doi.org/10.1111/j.1365-2559.2008.03098.x PMID:18637148

13. de Sanjosé S, Diaz M, Castellsagué X *et al.* (2007). Worldwide prevalence and genotype distribution of cervical human papillomavirus DNA in women with normal cytology: a meta-analysis. *Lancet Infect Dis*, 7:453–459. http://dx.doi.org/10.1016/S1473-3099(07)70158-5 PMID:17597569

14. Franceschi S, Herrero R, Clifford GM *et al.* (2006). Variations in the age-specific curves of human papillomavirus prevalence in women worldwide. *Int J Cancer*, 119:2677–2684. http://dx.doi.org/10.1002/ijc.22241 PMID:16991121

15. Schiffman M, Castle PE, Jeronimo J *et al.* (2007). Human papillomavirus and cervical cancer. *Lancet*, 370:890–907. http://dx.doi.org/10.1016/S0140-6736(07)61416-0 PMID:17826171

16. Rodríguez AC, Schiffman M, Herrero R *et al.* (2010). Longitudinal study of human papillomavirus persistence and cervical intraepithelial neoplasia grade 2/3: critical role of duration of infection. *J Natl Cancer Inst*, 102:315–324. http://dx.doi.org/10.1093/jnci/djq001 PMID:20157096

17. Guan P, Howell-Jones R, Li N *et al.* (2012). Human papillomavirus types in 115,789 HPV-positive women: a meta-analysis from cervical infection to cancer. *Int J Cancer*, 131:2349–2359. http://dx.doi.org/10.1002/ijc.27485 PMID:22323075

18. Lehtinen M, Paavonen J, Wheeler CM *et al.*; HPV PATRICIA Study Group (2012). Overall efficacy of HPV-16/18 AS04-adjuvanted vaccine against grade 3 or greater cervical intraepithelial neoplasia: 4-year end-of-study analysis of the randomised, double-blind PATRICIA trial. *Lancet Oncol*, 13:89–99. http://dx.doi.org/10.1016/S1470-2045(11)70286-8 PMID:22075171

19. Veldhuijzen NJ, Snijders PJ, Reiss P *et al.* (2010). Factors affecting transmission of mucosal human papillomavirus. *Lancet Infect Dis*, 10:862–874. http://dx.doi.org/10.1016/S1473-3099(10)70190-0 PMID:21075056

20. Shi Y, Li L, Hu Z *et al.* (2013). A genome-wide association study identifies two new cervical cancer susceptibility loci at 4q12 and 17q12. *Nat Genet*, 45:918–922. http://dx.doi.org/10.1038/ng.2687 PMID:23817570

21. Chen D, Juko-Pecirep I, Hammer J *et al.* (2013). Genome-wide association study of susceptibility loci for cervical cancer. *J Natl Cancer Inst*, 105:624–633. http://dx.doi.org/10.1093/jnci/djt051 PMID:23482656

22. Wright AA, Howitt BE, Myers AP *et al.* (2013). Oncogenic mutations in cervical cancer: genomic differences between adenocarcinomas and squamous cell carcinomas of the cervix. *Cancer*, 119:3776–3783. http://dx.doi.org/10.1002/cncr.28288 PMID:24037752

23. Franco EL, Coutlée F, Ferenczy A (2009). Integrating human papillomavirus vaccination in cervical cancer control programmes. *Public Health Genomics*, 12:352–361. http://dx.doi.org/10.1159/000214925 PMID:19684447

24. Van de Velde N, Boily MC, Drolet M *et al.* (2012). Population-level impact of the bivalent, quadrivalent, and nonavalent human papillomavirus vaccines: a model-based analysis. *J Natl Cancer Inst*, 104:1712–1723. http://dx.doi.org/10.1093/jnci/djs395 PMID:23104323

25. Sankaranarayanan R, Gaffikin L, Jacob M *et al.* (2005). A critical assessment of screening methods for cervical neoplasia. *Int J Gynaecol Obstet*, 89 Suppl 2:S4–S12. http://dx.doi.org/10.1016/j.ijgo.2005.01.009 PMID:15823266

26. Kaaks R, Lukanova A, Kurzer MS (2002). Obesity, endogenous hormones, and endometrial cancer risk: a synthetic review. *Cancer Epidemiol Biomarkers Prev*, 11:1531–1543. PMID:12496040

27. Cogliano V, Grosse Y, Baan R *et al.*; WHO International Agency for Research on Cancer (2005). Carcinogenicity of combined oestrogen-progestagen contraceptives and menopausal treatment. *Lancet Oncol*, 6:552–553. http://dx.doi.org/10.1016/S1470-2045(05)70273-4 PMID:16094770

28. Beral V, Bull D, Reeves G; Million Women Study Collaborators (2005). Endometrial cancer and hormone-replacement therapy in the Million Women Study. *Lancet*, 365:1543–1551. http://dx.doi.org/10.1016/S0140-6736(05)66455-0 PMID:15866308

29. Bokhman JV (1983). Two pathogenetic types of endometrial carcinoma. *Gynecol Oncol*, 15:10–17. http://dx.doi.org/10.1016/0090-8258(83)90111-7 PMID:6822361

30. Prat J (2004). Prognostic parameters of endometrial carcinoma. *Hum Pathol*, 35:649–662. http://dx.doi.org/10.1016/j.humpath.2004.02.007 PMID:15188130

31. Yeramian A, Moreno-Bueno G, Dolcet X *et al.* (2013). Endometrial carcinoma: molecular alterations involved in tumor development and progression. *Oncogene*, 32:403–413.http://dx.doi.org/10.1038/onc.2012.76 PMID:22430211

32. Kandoth C, Schultz N, Cherniack AD *et al.*; Cancer Genome Atlas Research Network (2013). Integrated genomic characterization of endometrial carcinoma. *Nature*, 497:67–73. http://dx.doi.org/10.1038/nature12113 PMID:23636398

33. Guan B, Mao TL, Panuganti PK *et al.* (2011). Mutation and loss of expression of ARID1A in uterine low-grade endometrioid carcinoma. *Am J Surg Pathol*, 35:625–632. http://dx.doi.org/10.1097/PAS.0b013e318212782a PMID:21412130

34. Wiegand KC, Lee AF, Al-Agha OM *et al.* (2011). Loss of BAF250a (ARID1A) is frequent in high-grade endometrial carcinomas. *J Pathol*, 224:328–333. http://dx.doi.org/10.1002/path.2911 PMID:21590771

35. Dedes KJ, Wetterskog D, Mendes-Pereira AM *et al.* (2010). PTEN deficiency in endometrioid endometrial adenocarcinomas predicts sensitivity to PARP inhibitors. *Sci Transl Med*, 2:53ra75. http://dx.doi.org/10.1126/scitranslmed.3001538 PMID:20944090

36. Bansal N, Yendluri V, Wenham RM (2009). The molecular biology of endometrial cancers and the implications for pathogenesis, classification, and targeted therapies. *Cancer Control*, 16:8–13. PMID:19078924

37. Slomovitz BM, Lu KH, Johnston T *et al.* (2010). A phase 2 study of the oral mammalian target of rapamycin inhibitor, everolimus, in patients with recurrent endometrial carcinoma. *Cancer*, 116:5415–5419. http://dx.doi.org/10.1002/cncr.25515 PMID:20681032

38. Ferrara N, Gerber HP, LeCouter J (2003). The biology of VEGF and its receptors. *Nat Med*, 9:669–676. http://dx.doi.org/10.1038/nm0603-669 PMID:12778165

39. Prat J (2012). Ovarian carcinomas: five distinct diseases with different origins, genetic alterations, and clinicopathological features. *Virchows Arch*, 460:237–249. http://dx.doi.org/10.1007/s00428-012-1203-5 PMID:22322322

40. La Vecchia C (2001). Epidemiology of ovarian cancer: a summary review. *Eur J Cancer Prev*, 10:125–129. http://dx.doi.org/10.1097/00008469-200104000-00002 PMID:11330452

41. Risch HA, McLaughlin JR, Cole DE *et al.* (2006). Population BRCA1 and BRCA2 mutation frequencies and cancer penetrances: a kin-cohort study in Ontario, Canada. *J Natl Cancer Inst*, 98:1694–1706. http://dx.doi.org/10.1093/jnci/djj465 PMID:17148771

42. Venkitaraman AR (2009). Linking the cellular functions of BRCA genes to cancer pathogenesis and treatment. *Annu Rev Pathol*, 4:461–487. http://dx.doi.org/10.1146/annurev.pathol.3.121806.151422 PMID:18954285

43. Lee Y, Miron A, Drapkin R *et al.* (2007). A candidate precursor to serous carcinoma that originates in the distal fallopian tube. *J Pathol*, 211:26–35. http://dx.doi.org/10.1002/path.2091 PMID:17117391

44. Singer G, Stöhr R, Cope L *et al.* (2005). Patterns of p53 mutations separate ovarian serous borderline tumors and low- and high-grade carcinomas and provide support for a new model of ovarian carcinogenesis: a mutational analysis with immunohistochemical correlation. *Am J Surg Pathol*, 29:218–224. http://dx.doi.org/10.1097/01.pas.0000146025.91953.8d PMID:15644779

45. Cancer Genome Atlas Research Network (2011). Integrated genomic analyses of ovarian carcinoma. *Nature*, 474:609–615. PMID:21720365

46. Etemadmoghadam D, George J, Cowin PA *et al.*; Australian Ovarian Cancer Study Group (2010). Amplicon-dependent CCNE1 expression is critical for clonogenic survival after cisplatin treatment and is correlated with 20q11 gain in ovarian cancer. *PLoS One*, 5:e15498. http://dx.doi.org/10.1371/journal.pone.0015498 PMID:21103391

47. Goode EL, Chenevix-Trench G, Song H *et al.*; Wellcome Trust Case-Control Consortium; Australian Cancer Study (Ovarian Cancer); Australian Ovarian Cancer Study Group; Ovarian Cancer Association Consortium (OCAC); Ovarian Cancer Association Consortium (OCAC) (2010). A genome-wide association study identifies susceptibility loci for ovarian cancer at 2q31 and 8q24. *Nat Genet*, 42:874–879. http://dx.doi.org/10.1038/ng.668 PMID:20852632

48. Wiegand KC, Shah SP, Al-Agha OM *et al.* (2010). ARID1A mutations in endometriosis-associated ovarian carcinomas. *N Engl J Med*, 363:1532–1543. http://dx.doi.org/10.1056/NEJMoa1008433 PMID:20942669

49. Prat J; for the FIGO Committee on Gynecologic Oncology (2013). Staging classification for cancer of the ovary, fallopian tube, and peritoneum. *Int J Gynecol Obstet*, [epub ahead of print]. http://dx.doi.org/10.1016/j.ijgo.2013.10.001 PMID:24219974

50. Ledermann JA, Marth C, Carey MS *et al.*; Gynecologic Cancer InterGroup (2011). Role of molecular agents and targeted therapy in clinical trials for women with ovarian cancer. *Int J Gynecol Cancer*, 21:763–770. http://dx.doi.org/10.1097/IGC.0b013e31821b2669 PMID:21543938

Websites

Cancer.Net. Uterine Cancer:
http://www.cancer.net/cancer-types/uterine-cancer/

MD Anderson Cancer Center. Endometrial Cancer:
http://www.mdanderson.org/diseases/hereditarygyn

National Cancer Institute. Cervical Cancer:
http://www.cancer.gov/cancertopics/types/cervical

National Cancer Institute. Endometrial Cancer:
http://www.cancer.gov/cancertopics/types/endometrial

National Cancer Institute. Ovarian Cancer:
http://www.cancer.gov/cancertopics/types/ovarian

National Cancer Institute. Vulvar Cancer:
http://www.cancer.gov/cancertopics/types/vulvar

National Institutes of Health. Vulvar Cancer:
http://health.nih.gov/topic/VulvarCancer

Ovarian Cancer Research Program of British Columbia:
http://www.ovcare.ca/

SEER Stat Fact Sheets. Cervix Uteri Cancer:
http://seer.cancer.gov/statfacts/html/cervix.html#risk

SEER Stat Fact Sheets. Vulvar Cancer:
http://seer.cancer.gov/statfacts/html/vulva.html#risk

5.13

Haematopoietic and lymphoid malignancies

Elaine S. Jaffe
Steven H. Swerdlow
James W. Vardiman

Daniel A. Arber (reviewer)
Eve Roman (reviewer)

Summary

- Most non-Hodgkin lymphomas are derived from either mature B or T lymphocytes, and they are morphologically, functionally, and genetically heterogeneous, with lymphoblastic malignancies being derived from precursor lymphoid cells.

- B-cell lymphomas are much more common than T-cell lymphomas, which account for only about 10% of cases.

- Many B-cell lymphomas are characterized by recurrent chromosomal translocations that target the immunoglobulin genes, whereas the molecular pathogenesis of most T-cell lymphomas is as yet undiscovered.

- The classification of acute myeloid leukaemias is largely based on recurrent genetic abnormalities, which have a major impact on prognosis and response to therapy.

- Chronic myeloid leukaemia is a myeloproliferative neoplasm that arises in a pluripotent stem cell and is invariably linked to the BCR-ABL1 fusion.

- The BCR-ABL1-negative myeloproliferative neoplasms are heterogeneous in terms of the cellular targets – for example myeloid, erythroid, or megakaryocytic – and are commonly associated with mutations of JAK2.

Haematological malignancies include all cell types derived from a pluripotent bone marrow stem cell, and as such include neoplasms of the lymphoid, myeloid, mast cell, histiocytic, and dendritic cell lineages. The current approach to the classification of haematopoietic and lymphoid malignancies is based on the integration of morphological, phenotypic, genetic, and clinical features, which allows the identification of distinct disease entities [1]. Most lymphoid malignancies have been related to normal counterparts in the B-cell (Fig. 5.13.1) and T-cell (Fig. 5.13.2) systems. For acute myeloid leukaemias, genetics has taken priority over aspects of cellular differentiation. In recent years there has been great progress in the application of genomic methods, which has advanced our understanding of these neoplasms, led to the recognition of new entities, and pointed the way towards promising new therapies, exploiting the knowledge of molecular pathways of transformation.

Chronic lymphocytic leukaemia/small lymphocytic lymphoma

Chronic lymphocytic leukaemia (CLL), the most common adult leukaemia in industrialized countries, is a small B-cell lymphoid neoplasm composed of monoclonal memory B cells that most typically express CD23 and the T-cell-associated antigen CD5.

Etiology and pathology

CLL/small lymphocytic lymphoma includes a more aggressive subset, with unmutated immunoglobulin heavy-chain genes, and a less aggressive subset, with mutated genes. The diagnosis requires more than 5×10^9 peripheral blood CLL-type cells/l, cytopenias or disease-related symptoms, or extramedullary disease. Individuals who do not fulfil any of these criteria but who have monoclonal CLL-type B cells are now considered to have monoclonal B-cell lymphocytosis (MBL) [2]. MBL can be divided into low-count and high-count MBL; cases of high-count MBL progress to frank CLL at a rate of 1–2% per year [2]. Low-count MBL (< 56 clonal B cells/μl) is found with sensitive techniques at a high frequency among older adults in the general population, and has a minimal propensity to progress. MBL is thought to be secondary to prolonged antigenic stimulation.

Epidemiology

Lymphomas

- There were almost 566 000 new cases of lymphoma worldwide in 2012, and about 305 000 deaths.
- The ICD-10 codes used for lymphomas are: Hodgkin lymphoma (C81); non-Hodgkin lymphoma (C82-85, C96); multiple myeloma and immunoproliferative diseases (C88+C90).
- When the main entities (Hodgkin lymphoma, non-Hodgkin lymphoma, and multiple myeloma) are examined separately, the respective cancer types do not rank highly, yet in combination, lymphomas would rank as the seventh most common form of cancer in terms of cancer incidence.
- Incidence rates for lymphoma tend to be elevated in the most developed areas, including North America, Australia and New Zealand, and northern and western Europe. In global terms, the incidence is greatest in Israel, followed by Australia and the USA.
- Where such data series are available, both incidence and mortality rates of non-Hodgkin lymphoma have tended to increase rather rapidly up until the mid-1990s in both sexes. Subsequently, incidence rates have stabilized, while mortality rates have declined in some settings.

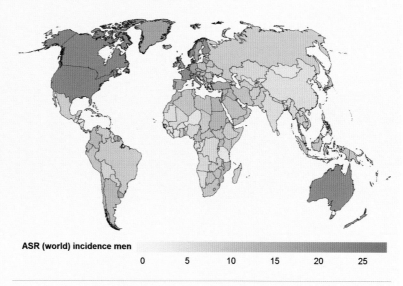

Map 5.13.1. Global distribution of estimated age-standardized (World) incidence rates (ASR) per 100 000, for lymphoma in men, 2012.

ASR (world) incidence men

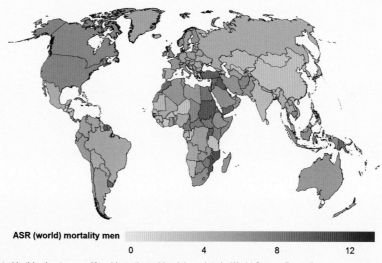

Map 5.13.2. Global distribution of estimated age-standardized (World) mortality rates (ASR) per 100 000, for lymphoma in men, 2012.

ASR (world) mortality men

For more details about the maps and charts presented in this chapter, see "A guide to the epidemiology data in *World Cancer Report*".

MBL with an atypical CLL-type phenotype and a non-CLL phenotype are also recognized. There are no known etiological factors for CLL; however, there is a familial predisposition in 5–10% of cases.

Genetics

Genome-wide association studies have revealed multiple susceptibility loci for CLL, many with proximity to genes involved in apoptosis [3]. There is great interest in prognostication in CLL, which, in addition to mutational status, is based on clinical, phenotypic (CD38, ZAP-70 expression), and molecular/cytogenetic factors, particularly *TP53* deletions and mutations. Recently, next-generation sequencing studies have demonstrated numerous recurrent mutations in genes that are part of varied genetic pathways – each, however, present in only up to about 10–15% of cases. Among those receiving the most attention are activating *NOTCH1* mutations and mutations in the splicing factor *SF3B1*, both adverse prognostic indicators [4,5]. The hope is that this new knowledge may lead to more targeted and effective therapies.

Chart 5.13.1. Estimated global number of new cases and deaths with proportions by major world regions, for lymphoma in both sexes combined, 2012.

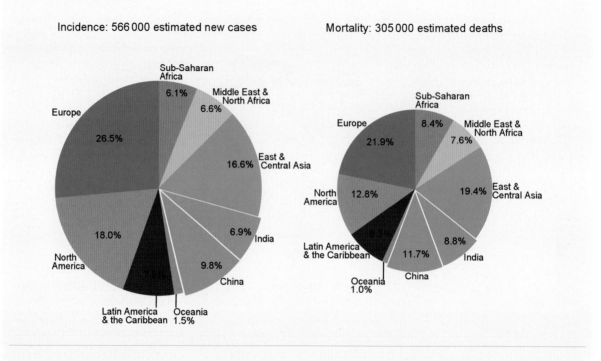

Incidence: 566 000 estimated new cases

Mortality: 305 000 estimated deaths

Chart 5.13.2. Age-standardized (World) incidence rates per 100 000 by year in selected populations, for lymphoma in men, circa 1975–2012.

Chart 5.13.3. Age-standardized (World) mortality rates per 100 000 by year in selected populations, for lymphoma in men, circa 1975–2012.

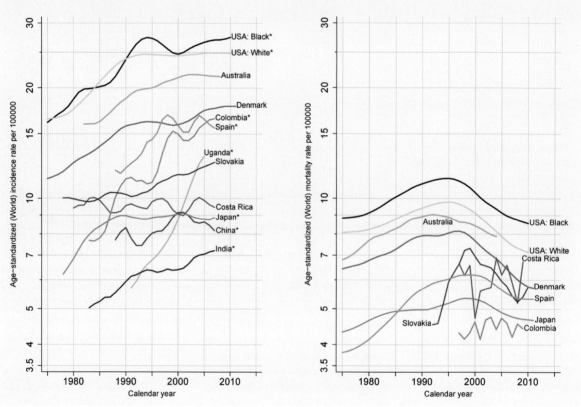

Leukaemias

- There were almost 352 000 new cases of leukaemia globally in 2012, and about 265 000 deaths. The disease ranks as the 11th most frequent in terms of cancer incidence and the 10th most common cause of cancer death.
- The ICD-10 codes used for leukaemias are C91-95.
- As with lymphomas, the incidence rates of leukaemias tend to be highest in countries that have attained the highest levels of human development.
- Incidence rates are elevated in countries with high or very high levels of human development, including Australia and New Zealand, North America, and much of Europe. There is less variation in mortality, although rates are high in certain countries in North Africa and in Central and West Asia.
- Trends are somewhat difficult to decipher for leukaemia, but observed incidence rates are generally stable with time, at least relative to trends in non-Hodgkin lymphoma. Mortality rates have fallen for certain subtypes in higher-income countries due to improving therapeutics.

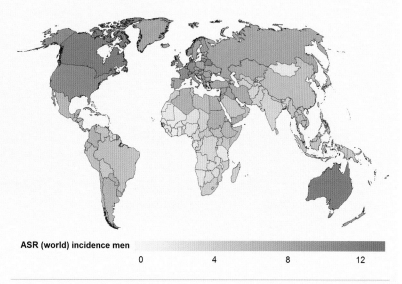

Map 5.13.3. Global distribution of estimated age-standardized (World) incidence rates (ASR) per 100 000, for leukaemia in men, 2012.

ASR (world) incidence men

0   4   8   12

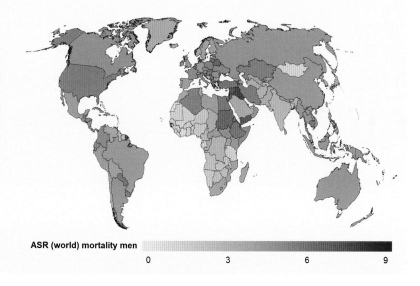

Map 5.13.4. Global distribution of estimated age-standardized (World) mortality rates (ASR) per 100 000, for leukaemia in men, 2012.

ASR (world) mortality men

0   3   6   9

Hairy cell leukaemia

Etiology and pathology

Hairy cell leukaemia is a rare neoplasm, typically of the post-germinal centre B-cell type, characterized by diffuse marrow and splenic red pulp involvement as well as often modest peripheral blood involvement by relatively small B cells with oval to reniform nuclei and prominent "hairy" cytoplasmic projections. Hairy cell leukaemia is diagnosed based on its characteristic morphological appearance and its CD103+, CD25+, CD11c+, annexin A1+ phenotype. The etiology of hairy cell leukaemia is unknown.

Genetics

Virtually all cases have *BRAF* V600E mutations, an abnormality shared with other malignancies such as papillary thyroid carcinoma and melanoma but found in few other B-cell neoplasms (and not in the variant form of hairy cell leukaemia) [6]. This probable driver mutation leads to constitutive activation of the RAF/MEK/ERK mitogen-activated protein kinase pathway. Although most patients with hairy cell leukaemia do well after treatment with purine analogues, *BRAF* V600E mutations provide another therapeutic target with

Chart 5.13.4. Estimated global number of new cases and deaths with proportions by major world regions, for leukaemia in both sexes combined, 2012.

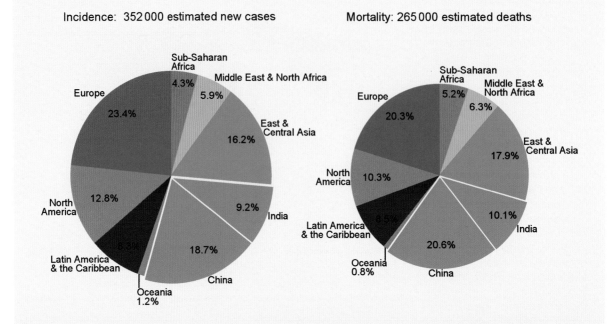

Incidence: 352 000 estimated new cases

Mortality: 265 000 estimated deaths

Chart 5.13.5. Age-standardized (World) incidence rates per 100 000 by year in selected populations, for leukaemia in men, circa 1975–2012.

Chart 5.13.6. Age-standardized (World) mortality rates per 100 000 by year in selected populations, for leukaemia in men, circa 1975–2012.

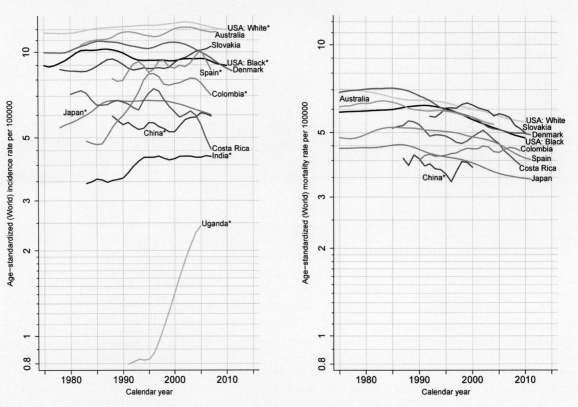

Fig. 5.13.1. Diagrammatic representation of B-cell differentiation. B-cell neoplasms correspond to stages of maturation. Most B cells are activated within the germinal centre, but T-cell independent activation can take place outside the germinal centre. This fact leads to cases of chronic lymphocytic leukaemia (CLL) that may or may not show evidence of somatic hypermutation. AG, antigen; DLBCL, diffuse large B-cell lymphoma; FDC, follicular dendritic cell; HCL, hairy cell leukaemia; GC, germinal centre; Ig, immunoglobulin; MALT, mucosa-associated lymphoid tissue; SLL, small lymphocytic lymphoma.

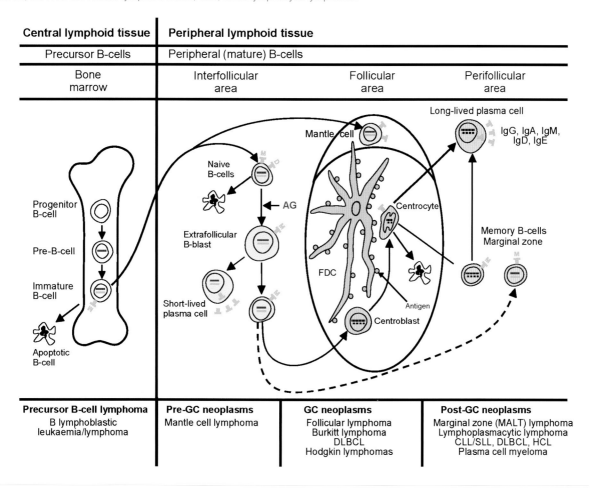

Plasma cell myeloma

Plasma cell myeloma, sometimes referred to as multiple myeloma, is a bone marrow-based, disseminated neoplasm composed of monoclonal post-germinal centre long-lived plasma cells, which must be distinguished from monoclonal gammopathy of undetermined significance and lymphomas with plasmacytic differentiation.

Etiology and pathology

Symptomatic plasma cell myeloma requires a serum and/or urine monoclonal paraprotein, clonal plasma cells in the bone marrow, or a plasmacytoma and related end-organ damage (hypercalcaemia, renal insufficiency, anaemia, bone lesions). Asymptomatic (smouldering) myeloma requires a serum paraprotein level of more than 30 g/l and/or at least 10% clonal bone marrow plasma cells and no myeloma-associated end-organ damage or myeloma-associated symptoms. Other clinical variants include non-secretory myelomas, most of which are still associated with serum-free light-chain abnormalities, and plasma cell leukaemia, in which there are more than 2×10^9 circulating peripheral blood plasma cells/l or they make up more than 20% of all leukocytes. The etiology of plasma cell myeloma is totally unknown in most patients. The disease is more common in African Americans than in Caucasians.

Genetics

Upregulation of one of the cyclin D genes due to hyperdiploidy or translocations involving the immunoglobulin heavy-chain gene and the *CCND1*, *C-MAF*, *FGFR3/MMSET*, *CCND3*, or *MAFB* genes is considered an important early event but is also found in monoclonal gammopathy of undetermined significance. Other important early events seen in a significant minority of patients include monosomy 13 or 13q14

BRAF inhibitors, already explored in other malignancies.

Fig. 5.13.2. Diagrammatic representation of T-cell differentiation. T-cell neoplasms correspond to different stages of maturation. Mature T cells include αβ and γδ T cells, both of which mature in the thymus gland. T-follicular helper (TFH) cells are a recently well-characterized subset of αβ T cells involved in many nodal peripheral T-cell lymphomas. AG, antigen; FDC, follicular dendritic cell; NK, natural killer.

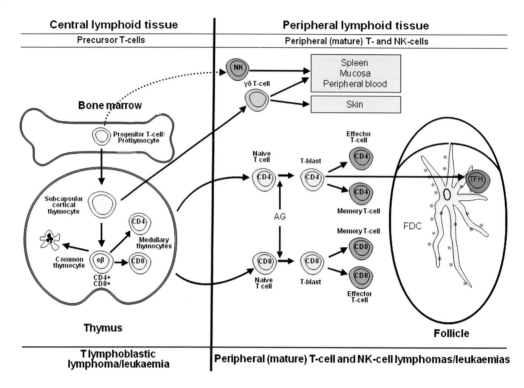

deletion and *K-RAS* or *N-RAS* activating mutations. A variety of other genetic and epigenetic events and pathways are implicated in disease progression, including the recent identification of therapeutically targetable *BRAF* mutations in a small proportion of cases [7].

Follicular lymphoma

Follicular lymphoma, one of the most common adult lymphomas in industrialized countries, is a neoplasm of germinal centre B cells with varying proportions of centrocytes and transformed centroblasts and almost always at least a partially follicular growth pattern.

Etiology, pathology, and genetics

Follicular lymphoma is diagnosed based on its morphological features, phenotype (CD20⁺, usually CD10⁺, BCL6⁺, and usually BCL2⁺), and frequent *IGH/BCL2* translocations or,

much less commonly, *BCL6* translocations. This disease is graded based on the number of centroblasts present. The more common grade 1–2 follicular lymphoma is an indolent but generally widely disseminated and incurable neoplasm, and the grade 3 cases (A and B, based on the presence or absence of centrocytes) are considered more aggressive. The etiology is uncertain, but healthy individuals with pesticide exposure have a greater prevalence of circulating cells with *IGH/BCL2* translocations.

Typical cases need to be distinguished from paediatric follicular lymphoma, a lymphoma that also occurs particularly in younger adults, based on morphological, immunophenotypic, and cytogenetic/molecular differences [8], and from in situ follicular lymphoma/intrafollicular neoplasia/follicular lymphoma-like B cells of uncertain/undetermined significance, where there are scattered follicles with follicular lymphoma-like B cells but with an

intact underlying lymphoid tissue architecture [9]. Primary duodenal follicular lymphoma is also distinctive and often localized. Primary cutaneous follicular lymphoma belongs in the separate category of primary cutaneous follicle centre lymphoma. Most cases have well-recognized secondary cytogenetic/molecular abnormalities, but the critical transformational events required in addition to *BCL2* translocation remain to be established.

Mantle cell lymphoma

Mantle cell lymphoma is a mature B-cell lymphoma believed to be derived from usually naive B cells of the inner mantle zone.

Etiology and pathology

The etiology of mantle cell lymphoma is unknown. In general it is a very aggressive and incurable lymphoma, but the clinical spectrum of mantle cell lymphoma is very broad. Both aggressive (blastoid and pleomorphic) and more indolent variants are recognized. One indolent and very distinctive variant is associated with blood, bone marrow, and sometimes splenic involvement without peripheral adenopathy and typically has mutated immunoglobulin heavy-chain genes and few secondary cytogenetic/molecular abnormalities. The other variant that may not represent an overt malignancy is in situ mantle cell lymphoma/mantle cell lymphoma-like B cells of undetermined/uncertain significance. These cases lack architectural destruction and show partially infiltrated follicular mantle zones, often at the mantle zone/germinal centre interface.

Genetics

Most cases have a *CCND1* translocation and cyclin D1 expression, an early but insufficient pathogenetic event and a useful diagnostic tool. Rare cases are cyclin D1-negative but, like most other MCLs, are SOX11⁺ and usually express cyclin D2 or D3. Otherwise, the diagnosis is made based on a characteristic morphological appearance and a usual CD20⁺, CD5⁺, CD23⁻ phenotype. In addition to CCND1 overexpression, mantle cell lymphoma is characterized by additional abnormalities leading to cell-cycle dysregulation, and assessment of the proliferative fraction is an extremely important prognostic factor [10]. Disruption of the DNA damage response pathways and activation of cell survival mechanisms are also important in the pathogenesis of this disease, with many potentially targetable abnormal signalling pathways. For example, *NOTCH1* mutations similar to those seen in CLL/small lymphocytic lymphoma, and associated with more aggressive disease, were recently reported in 12% of mantle cell lymphomas.

Marginal zone lymphoma and lymphoplasmacytic lymphoma

These diseases are post-germinal centre B-cell neoplasms that show

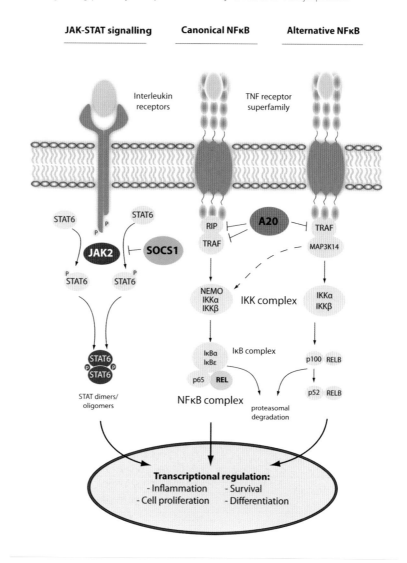

Fig. 5.13.3. The main activation cascades of JAK-STAT and NF-κB signalling are involved in primary mediastinal B-cell lymphoma. Alternative pathway activation exists. Known gene alterations leading to constitutive pathway activity are shown in colour. The NF-κB signalling pathway is implicated in many forms of B-cell lymphoma.

varying degrees of plasmacytoid differentiation.

Etiology, pathology, and genetics

Three distinct forms of marginal zone lymphomas are recognized: extranodal, nodal, and splenic. Extranodal marginal zone lymphomas of mucosa-associated lymphoid tissue (MALT lymphomas) are relatively common; they have been reported in nearly every anatomical site but are most frequent in the stomach, lung, and salivary gland. Antigen drive has

been implicated most clearly in gastric MALT lymphoma, associated with *Helicobacter pylori* infection. The most common translocations identified in MALT lymphoma – t(11;18)(q21;q21), t(1;14)(p22;q32), and t(14;18)(q32;q21) – share a common pathway, which leads to the activation of NF-κB and its downstream targets. Historically, it had been difficult to distinguish lymphoplasmacytic lymphoma from marginal zone lymphomas as both show evidence of plasmacytoid differentiation. Recent studies have identified mutations

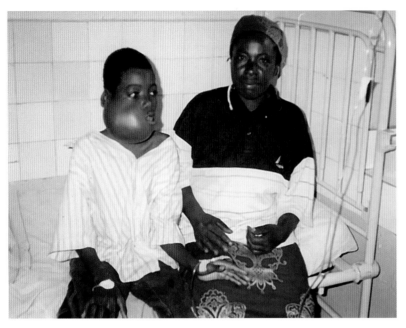

Fig. 5.13.4. A boy with Burkitt lymphoma receives treatment at Banso Baptist Hospital in Cameroon.

in *MYD88* involving L265P in 91% of patients with lymphoplasmacytic lymphoma, nearly all of whom had clinical Waldenström macroglobulinaemia [11]. The mutation was shown to trigger IRAK-mediated NF-κB signalling. Mutations in *MYD88* were rarely encountered in marginal zone lymphomas, facilitating distinction of these groups.

Diffuse large B-cell lymphoma

Diffuse large B-cell lymphomas (DLBCLs) are the most common histological group of lymphoma, representing up to 40% of cases worldwide.

Etiology, pathology, and genetics

DLBCLs are heterogeneous morphologically, clinically, and at the genomic level. To address these issues, DLBCLs were among the first cases to be analysed by complementary DNA array technology, and more recently also by genome-wide analysis [12]. A recent genome-wide association study identified 3q27 as a susceptibility locus for B-cell non-Hodgkin lymphoma, and particularly for DLBCL, in the Chinese population [13]. By gene expression profiling, three groups were identified based on the differential expression of a large set of genes: the germinal centre-like group, the activated B-cell-like group, and primary mediastinal (thymic) large B-cell lymphoma. The third group shares many features with classic Hodgkin lymphoma, showing activation of the NF-κB pathway (Fig. 5.13.3) [14]. More recently, frequent genetic defects have been identified in the B-cell antigen receptor (BCR) signalling and NF-κB pathways in the activated B-cell-like type, providing new insight into the pathogenesis of DLBCL and new potential therapeutic targets [15,16]. In particular, inhibitors of BTK have shown promise in a variety of B-cell lymphomas [17]. Recurrent mutations in the germinal centre-like type of DLBCL appear to target histone-modifying genes [12,18]. Somatic mutations in *EZH2* also have been identified in follicular lymphoma, another tumour of germinal centre derivation.

Burkitt lymphoma

Etiology, pathology, and genetics

Burkitt lymphoma is the first subtype of lymphoma to be associated with a specific genetic aberration: translocations involving *MYC* and one of the immunoglobulin genes, most commonly *IGH*. The translocation is common to all subtypes of Burkitt lymphoma, regardless of the presence of Epstein–Barr virus (EBV) or clinical features. Endemic Burkitt lymphoma is prevalent in equatorial Africa, corresponding in distribution to the malaria belt. It is universally positive for EBV, whereas sporadic and immunodeficiency-associated Burkitt lymphomas are EBV-positive in a smaller proportion of cases (15–30%). Recent studies using genomic sequencing have identified recurrent somatic mutations that provide new insights into the pathogenesis of Burkitt lymphoma (reviewed in [19]). Three independent studies identified mutations in *ID3* in a high proportion of cases, with mutations also seen in the transcription factor 3 (*TCF3*) gene. These studies link Burkitt lymphoma to the cells of the dark zone of the germinal centre. *ID3* mutations were absent in DLBCL. Mutations in this pathway were seen in sporadic and immunodeficiency-associated Burkitt lymphoma, and in a somewhat lesser proportion of endemic cases of this disease.

Peripheral T-cell lymphoma

Peripheral T-cell lymphomas are morphologically, immunophenotypically, and clinically heterogeneous and overall account for only about 10% of all non-Hodgkin lymphomas [20]. Classification schemes generally segregate nodal and extranodal lymphomas of this type; extranodal tumours are more often of cytotoxic origin [21]. Anaplastic large cell lymphoma was the first to be associated with a specific genetic alteration: translocations involving *ALK* and a variety of gene partners, leading to overexpression of ALK. Recently, mutations involving *IDH2* and *TET2* have been identified in

Molecular detection of minimal residual disease in childhood leukaemia

Rosemary Sutton

Minimal residual disease (MRD) is a highly clinically relevant prognostic factor for patients with acute lymphoblastic leukaemia (ALL). Brüggemann et al. [1] cited 27 studies that provided evidence that MRD is important in determining patient outcome in clinical trials for children or adults with newly diagnosed ALL, relapsed ALL, or bone marrow transplants for ALL treatment. Consequently, many current clinical trials for childhood leukaemia patients include the stratification of patients into treatment risk groups based on initial MRD response to therapy measured in bone marrow aspirates using real-time quantitative polymerase chain reaction (PCR) or quantitative flow cytometry methods [1].

In essence, leukaemia patients who relapse usually have a slower response to early therapy than patients who are cured by their treatment (Fig. B5.13.1). PCR MRD techniques can detect residual disease at a sensitivity of about 1 in 100 000 cells (10^{-5}), with quantification to 10^{-4} using definitions and standard procedures established by the EuroMRD group [2].

The molecular detection of submicroscopic residual cancer cells is clinically useful in many malignancies and depends on having specific markers for the disease. The markers most commonly used in ALL are the unique gene rearrangements present in cells of T- and B-cell lineage. The capacity of our immune systems to recognize millions of different antigens depends on the huge diversity of immunoglobulins and T-cell receptors, which results from the genetic rearrangement of numerous alternative gene segments present in the genes coding for these antigen receptor proteins. Each leukaemic clone therefore has one or more unique gene rearrangements that can be used as molecular markers to distinguish the DNA of the leukaemic clone from the patient's normal DNA.

In addition to markers based on antigen receptor genes, several recurrent translocations and microdeletions can be used as markers for smaller subsets of patients with childhood leukaemia to measure MRD in either genomic DNA or RNA samples from blood or marrow. In patients with Philadelphia chromosome-positive leukaemia, the *BCR-ABL* transcripts are measured by reverse-transcriptase PCR to detect disease recurrence at very low levels, allowing immediate intervention to treat molecular disease. Leukaemia in infants often has translocations involving the mixed lineage leukaemia (*MLL*) gene with unique breakpoints, which provide useful MRD markers, particularly in this patient group. MRD markers for ALL based on recurrent deletions in genes implicated in normal lymphoid development, such as *IKZF1* and *CRLF2*, are also likely to be used in the future, especially since they occur in higher-risk patients and their generic PCR MRD assays do not require DNA sequencing for each patient, making MRD diagnostics more accessible [3].

Fig. B5.13.1. Minimal residual disease (MRD) levels in childhood leukaemia patients who relapse compared with patients who are cured by their treatment.

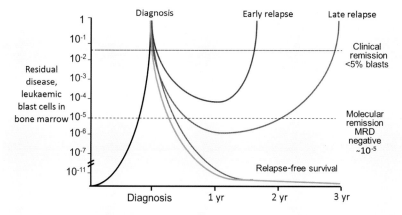

References

1. Brüggemann M et al.; European Working Group for Adult Acute Lymphoblastic Leukemia (EWALL); International Berlin-Frankfurt-Münster Study Group (I-BFM-SG) (2010). *Leukemia*, 24:521–535. http://dx.doi.org/10.1038/leu.2009.268 PMID:20033054

2. van der Velden VH et al.; European Study Group on MRD Detection in ALL (ESG-MRD-ALL) (2007). *Leukemia*, 21:604–611. PMID:17287850

3. Venn NC et al. (2012). *Leukemia*, 26: 1414–1416. http://dx.doi.org/10.1038/leu. 2011.348 PMID:22157735

angioimmunoblastic T-cell lymphomas and other peripheral T-cell lymphomas of T-follicular helper cell origin. However, as yet the molecular pathogenesis of most peripheral T-cell lymphomas remains to be discovered.

Hodgkin lymphoma

Hodgkin lymphomas are divided into classic Hodgkin lymphoma and nodular lymphocyte-predominant Hodgkin lymphoma. Both are derived from B cells, but the B-cell programme is markedly disrupted in classic Hodgkin lymphoma, such that there is downregulation of most B-cell markers and functions. Epigenetic alterations may be responsible in part for loss of the B-cell programme [22]. Studies of the tumour cells implicate the NF-κB

Fig. 5.13.5. Frequency of cytogenetic subtypes of paediatric acute lymphoblastic leukaemia (ALL). Pie chart includes all major B-cell ALLs (shown in green) and T-lineage subtypes of ALL (shown in red), to illustrate the relative frequency of each. The recently described *BCR-ABL1*-like subtype and *BCR-ABL1*-positive ALL are shown in yellow to illustrate the high frequency of childhood B-cell ALL cases with genetic alterations activating tyrosine kinase and cytokine receptor signalling, which may be amenable to targeted therapy. Data are derived from front-line studies of childhood ALL.

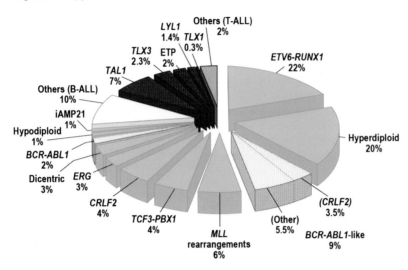

and JAK/STAT signalling pathways. A subset of classic Hodgkin lymphoma, most often mixed cellularity subtype, is positive for EBV, but the viral programme does not appear to primarily drive the neoplastic process.

Acute lymphoblastic leukaemia (ALL)/lymphoblastic lymphoma

Acute lymphoblastic leukaemia (ALL)/lymphoblastic lymphoma are neoplasms of precursor B cells or T cells (lymphoblasts) with features corresponding to stages of B-cell development in the marrow and T-cell development in the thymus (Figs 5.13.1, 5.13.2). They usually involve bone marrow and blood in the case of ALL but can present in extramedullary sites, typically in lymphoblastic lymphoma. Morphology and immunophenotyping suffice to establish the diagnosis, but recurring cytogenetic abnormalities occur in 80% of ALL (Fig. 5.13.5), and many have proven important for risk stratification (see "Molecular detection of minimal residual disease in childhood leukaemia"). However, not all cytogenetic abnormalities are

sufficient to establish a leukaemic clone, and cooperating molecular defects have long been suspected. Recently, whole-genome profiling in ALL has identified several gene mutations and submicroscopic deletions that affect molecules crucial to B- and T-cell maturation, some of which correlate with clinical features. For example, 15% of paediatric B-cell ALL carries deletions or mutations of *IKZF1* that affect transcriptional regulation of lymphoid maturation and confer a poor prognosis. Key genetic alterations in B-cell ALL, in addition to *IKZF1*, involve *PAX5*, *JAK1*, *JAK2*, *CRLF2*, and *CREBBP*. In T-cell ALL, activating mutations of *NOTCH1* are found in about 50% of cases and correlate with a favourable outcome. In the future, whole-genome analyses may allow for better characterization of ALL and identification of abnormalities for targeted therapy [23–25].

Acute myeloid leukaemia

Acute myeloid leukaemia (AML) is a heterogeneous disease characterized by increased blasts (usually ≥ 20% myeloblasts, monoblasts plus

promonocytes, and/or megakaryoblasts) in blood or bone marrow. In recent years, there has been improvement in survival, particularly in younger patients, but AML remains a fatal disease for most patients. The WHO classification of AML assigns patients to categories useful for predicting outcome. Some are classified according to genetic abnormalities that determine morphological and clinical features (AML with recurrent genetic abnormalities), others have morphology and/or genetics that relate them to myelodysplastic syndromes (AML with myelodysplasia-related changes), some are unique because they follow prior cytotoxic therapy (therapy-related myeloid neoplasms), and the remainder are classified by lineage involvement and degree of differentiation.

Currently, karyotype and age are the most powerful predictors of prognosis [26,27]. Whole-genome and exome sequencing have revealed a plethora of gene mutations and submicroscopic genetic defects in this type of leukaemia. Although the prognostic significance of some alterations, particularly mutated *FLT3*, *NPM1*, and *CEBPA*, has been recognized, the significance of many others remains to be determined [28]. A separate study involving 200 cases reported that AML genomes have fewer mutations than those of most other adult cancers, with an average of only 13. A total of 23 genes were significantly mutated, and nearly all samples had at least one non-synonymous mutation in one of nine categories of genes relevant for pathogenesis, including transcription factor fusions (18% of cases), the gene encoding nucleophosmin (*NPM1*) (27%), tumour suppressor genes (16%), DNA methylation-related genes (44%), signalling genes (59%), chromatin modifying genes (30%), myeloid transcription factor genes (22%), cohesin-complex genes (13%), and spliceosome-complex genes (14%) (see "De novo DNA methyltransferases in normal and malignant haematopoiesis") [29].

De novo DNA methyltransferases in normal and malignant haematopoiesis

Margaret A. Goodell

DNA methylation plays a central role in regulating gene expression during development and is known to be disturbed in a variety of malignancies. The mechanisms through which aberrant DNA methylation contributes to malignancy development, and through which hypomethylating agents exert their effects, are poorly understood. De novo DNA methylation in murine haematopoietic stem cells has been studied as a model to address some of these fundamental questions.

Murine haematopoietic stem cells express high levels of both de novo DNA methyltransferases Dnmt3a and Dnmt3b. Using conditional knockout mice, the role of Dnmt3a in murine haematopoiesis has been investigated. The data indicate that in the absence of Dnmt3a, haematopoietic stem cell self-renewal is dramatically enhanced at the expense of differentiation. Serial stem cell transplantation augments this effect, such that phenotypically normal haematopoietic stem cells that fail to differentiate accumulate to high levels. Paradoxically, DNA methylation, examined genome-wide, is both increased and decreased in Dnmt3a knockout haematopoietic stem cells, with CpG islands preferentially hypermethylated, similar to the pattern of DNA methylation alterations in malignancies. The differentiated progeny of Dnmt3a knockout haematopoietic stem cells exhibited aberrant continued expression of stem cell-specific genes that are normally repressed during differentiation. While mutations in *DNMT3A* are prevalent in human acute myeloid leukaemia, no frank leukaemia development was observed in the mice within the time frame initially examined.

Haematopoietic stem cell-specific Dnmt3b knockout mice and Dnmt3a-Dnmt3b double-knockout haematopoietic stem cells have also been examined. In the absence of both de novo DNA methyltransferases, the haematopoietic stem cells accumulate even more dramatically than in the *Dnmt3a* knockout, even though loss of Dnmt3b alone has minimal impact. Introduction of oncogenes into the *Dnmt3a* knockout stem cells decreases the time to malignant transformation compared with the oncogene or *Dnmt3a* knockout alone. These findings are pertinent to understanding the implications of mutations in DNA methyltransferases found in human haematological malignancies.

Reference

Challen GA *et al.* (2012). *Nat Genet*, 44:23–31. http://dx.doi.org/10.1038/ng.1009 PMID:22138693

Chronic myeloid leukaemia, BCR-ABL1-positive

Chronic myeloid leukaemia, *BCR-ABL1* is a myeloproliferative neoplasm arising in a pluripotent haematopoietic stem cell and is always associated with the *BCR-ABL1* fusion gene resulting from the chromosomal translocation t(9;22) (q34;q11.2). *BCR-ABL1* encodes an oncoprotein with constitutively activated tyrosine kinase activity that drives proliferation by interaction with the downstream pathways RAS, RAF, MYC, JUN kinase, and STAT. The natural history includes an initial chronic phase characterized by granulocytic proliferation and granulocytosis, followed by an accelerated phase and/or a myeloid or lymphoid blast phase. The development of tyrosine kinase inhibitors has dramatically improved overall survival, from a 10-year overall survival of 15–20% before these drugs were available to 80–90% subsequent to their use. Point mutations in the tyrosine kinase domain of *BCR-ABL* result in resistance to many tyrosine kinase inhibitors, and disease progression. Most patients refractory to front-line therapy usually respond to newer-generation tyrosine kinase inhibitors, but others may progress to the blast phase, which has a uniformly poor outcome [30].

BCR-ABL1-negative myeloproliferative neoplasms

These diseases, which include polycythaemia vera, essential thrombocythaemia, and primary myelofibrosis, are clonal, stem-cell-derived neoplasms characterized by excessive production of differentiated myeloid cells, which are sometimes difficult to distinguish from reactive marrow proliferations. In 2005, it was found that almost all patients with polycythaemia vera and nearly 50% with essential thrombocythaemia or primary myelofibrosis have an activating somatic mutation, *JAK2* V617F, encoding the cytoplasmic tyrosine kinase JAK2. This discovery proved that these myeloproliferative neoplasms have abnormal cell signalling pathways, providing an important diagnostic tool – the *JAK2* mutation – and raising expectations that tyrosine kinase inhibitors would emulate the successful therapy such agents mediated in chronic myeloid leukaemia. But additional data have shown that the *JAK2* mutation is likely a secondary event and have also uncovered a complex layering of multiple genetic defects, particularly affecting genes such as *TET2*, *EZH2*, and *IDH1/IDH2* involved in epigenetic regulation [31]. These additional abnormalities may account for the only modest success to date using tyrosine kinase inhibitors. Further improvements to understanding of the *BCR-ABL1*-negative myeloproliferative neoplasms will rely on their meticulous classification to enable correlation with the underlying genetic milieu.

References

1. Swerdlow SH, Campo E, Harris NL *et al.*, eds (2008). *WHO Classification of Tumours of Haematopoietic and Lymphoid Tissues*, 4th ed. Lyon: IARC.

2. Scarfò L, Fazi C, Ghia P (2013). MBL versus CLL: how important is the distinction? *Hematol Oncol Clin North Am*, 27:251–265. http://dx.doi.org/10.1016/j.hoc.2013.01.004 PMID:23561472

3. Berndt SI, Skibola CF, Joseph V *et al.* (2013). Genome-wide association study identifies multiple risk loci for chronic lymphocytic leukemia. *Nat Genet*, 45:868–876. http://dx.doi.org/10.1038/ng.2652 PMID:23770605

4. Puente XS, Pinyol M, Quesada V *et al.* (2011). Whole-genome sequencing identifies recurrent mutations in chronic lymphocytic leukaemia. *Nature*, 475:101–105. http://dx.doi.org/10.1038/nature10113 PMID:21642962

5. Wang L, Lawrence MS, Wan Y *et al.* (2011). SF3B1 and other novel cancer genes in chronic lymphocytic leukemia. *N Engl J Med*, 365:2497–2506. http://dx.doi.org/10.1056/NEJMoa1109016 PMID:22150006

6. Tiacci E, Schiavoni G, Forconi F *et al.* (2012). Simple genetic diagnosis of hairy cell leukemia by sensitive detection of the BRAF-V600E mutation. *Blood*, 119:192–195. http://dx.doi.org/10.1182/blood-2011-08-371179 PMID:22028477

7. Egan JB, Shi CX, Tembe W *et al.* (2012). Whole-genome sequencing of multiple myeloma from diagnosis to plasma cell leukemia reveals genomic initiating events, evolution, and clonal tides. *Blood*, 120:1060–1066. http://dx.doi.org/10.1182/blood-2012-01-405977 PMID:22529291

8. Liu Q, Salaverria I, Pittaluga S *et al.* (2012). Follicular lymphomas in children and young adults: a comparison of the pediatric variant with usual follicular lymphoma. *Am J Surg Pathol*, 37:333–343. http://dx.doi.org/10.1097/PAS.0b013e31826b9b57 PMID:23108024

9. Jegalian AG, Eberle FC, Pack SD *et al.* (2011). Follicular lymphoma in situ: clinical implications and comparisons with partial involvement by follicular lymphoma. *Blood*, 118:2976–2984. http://dx.doi.org/10.1182/blood-2011-05-355255 PMID:21768298

10. Jares P, Colomer D, Campo E (2012). Molecular pathogenesis of mantle cell lymphoma. *J Clin Invest*, 122:3416–3423. http://dx.doi.org/10.1172/JCI61272 PMID:23023712

11. Treon SP, Xu L, Yang G *et al.* (2012). MYD88 L265P somatic mutation in Waldenström's macroglobulinemia. *N Engl J Med*, 367:826–833. http://dx.doi.org/10.1056/NEJMoa1200710 PMID:22931316

12. Morin RD, Mendez-Lago M, Mungall AJ *et al.* (2011). Frequent mutation of histone-modifying genes in non-Hodgkin lymphoma. *Nature*, 476:298–303. http://dx.doi.org/10.1038/nature10351 PMID:21796119

13. Tan DEK, Foo JN, Bei J-X *et al.* (2013). Genome-wide association study of B cell non-Hodgkin lymphoma identifies 3q27 as a susceptibility locus in the Chinese population. *Nat Genet*, 45:804–807. http://dx.doi.org/10.1038/ng.2666 PMID:23749188

14. Steidl C, Gascoyne RD (2011). The molecular pathogenesis of primary mediastinal large B-cell lymphoma. *Blood*, 118:2659–2669. http://dx.doi.org/10.1182/blood-2011-05-326538 PMID:21700770

15. Ngo VN, Young RM, Schmitz R *et al.* (2011). Oncogenically active MYD88 mutations in human lymphoma. *Nature*, 470:115–119. http://dx.doi.org/10.1038/nature09671 PMID:21179087

16. Pasqualucci L, Trifonov V, Fabbri G *et al.* (2011). Analysis of the coding genome of diffuse large B-cell lymphoma. *Nat Genet*, 43:830–837. http://dx.doi.org/10.1038/ng.892 PMID:21804550

17. Kenkre VP, Kahl BS (2012). The future of B-cell lymphoma therapy: the B-cell receptor and its downstream pathways. *Curr Hematol Malig Rep*, 7:216–220. http://dx.doi.org/10.1007/s11899-012-0127-0 PMID:22688757

18. Morin RD, Johnson NA, Severson TM *et al.* (2010). Somatic mutations altering EZH2 (Tyr641) in follicular and diffuse large B-cell lymphomas of germinal-center origin. *Nat Genet*, 42:181–185. http://dx.doi.org/10.1038/ng.518 PMID:20081860

19. Campo E (2012). New pathogenic mechanisms in Burkitt lymphoma. *Nat Genet*, 44:1288–1289. http://dx.doi.org/10.1038/ng.2476 PMID:23192177

20. Vose J, Armitage J, Weisenburger D; International T-Cell Lymphoma Project (2008). International peripheral T-cell and natural killer/T-cell lymphoma study: pathology findings and clinical outcomes. *J Clin Oncol*, 26:4124–4130. http://dx.doi.org/10.1200/JCO.2008.16.4558 PMID:18626005

21. Jaffe ES, Nicolae A, Pittaluga S (2013). Peripheral T-cell and NK-cell lymphomas in the WHO classification: pearls and pitfalls. *Mod Pathol*, 26 Suppl 1:S71–S87. http://dx.doi.org/10.1038/modpathol.2012.181 PMID:23281437

22. Küppers R (2012). New insights in the biology of Hodgkin lymphoma. *Hematology Am Soc Hematol Educ Program*, 2012:328–334. PMID:23233600

23. Mullighan CG (2012). Molecular genetics of B-precursor acute lymphoblastic leukemia. *J Clin Invest*, 122:3407–3415. http://dx.doi.org/10.1172/JCI61203 PMID:23023711

24. Iacobucci I, Papayannidis C, Lonetti A *et al.* (2012). Cytogenetic and molecular predictors of outcome in acute lymphocytic leukemia: recent developments. *Curr Hematol Malig Rep*, 7:133–143. http://dx.doi.org/10.1007/s11899-012-0122-5 PMID:22528731

25. Inaba H, Greaves M, Mullighan CG (2013). Acute lymphoblastic leukaemia. *Lancet*, 381:1943–1955. http://dx.doi.org/10.1016/S0140-6736(12)62187-4 PMID:23523389

26. Burnett AK (2012). Treatment of acute myeloid leukemia: are we making progress? *Hematology Am Soc Hematol Educ Program*, 2012:1–6. PMID:23233553

27. Grimwade D (2012). The changing paradigm of prognostic factors in acute myeloid leukaemia. *Best Pract Res Clin Haematol*, 25:419–425. http://dx.doi.org/10.1016/j.beha.2012.10.004 PMID:23200538

28. Patel JP, Gönen M, Figueroa ME *et al.* (2012). Prognostic relevance of integrated genetic profiling in acute myeloid leukemia. *N Engl J Med*, 366:1079–1089. http://dx.doi.org/10.1056/NEJMoa1112304 PMID:22417203

29. Cancer Genome Atlas Research Network (2013). Genomic and epigenomic landscapes of adult de novo acute myeloid leukemia. *N Engl J Med*, 368:2059–2074. http://dx.doi.org/10.1056/NEJMoa1301689 PMID:23634996

30. van Etten RA, Mauro M, Radich JP *et al.* (2013). Advances in the biology and therapy of chronic myeloid leukemia: proceedings from the 6th Post-ASH International Chronic Myeloid Leukemia and Myeloproliferative Neoplasms Workshop. *Leuk Lymphoma*, 54:1151–1158. http://dx.doi.org/10.3109/10428194.2012.745524 PMID:23121619

31. Vakil E, Tefferi A (2011). BCR-ABL1–negative myeloproliferative neoplasms: a review of molecular biology, diagnosis, and treatment. *Clin Lymphoma Myeloma Leuk*, 11 Suppl 1:S37–S45. http://dx.doi.org/10.1016/j.clml.2011.04.002 PMID:22035746

5.14

Skin cancer

5 ORGAN SITE

Christine Guo Lian
Martin C. Mihm Jr

Gérald E. Piérard (reviewer)
Massimo Tommasino (reviewer)

Summary

- Malignant melanoma is an aggressive human cancer; over the past few decades, its incidence has increased dramatically worldwide among Caucasian populations.

- The risk of developing malignant melanoma varies markedly according to racial background (skin pigmentation) and geographical location (sunlight-derived ultraviolet radiation). Ultraviolet-emitting tanning devices increase the risk of malignant melanoma.

- For patients with localized melanoma, prognosis is good with adequate surgical excision; metastatic melanoma is largely resistant to current therapies.

- Non-melanoma skin cancer includes squamous cell carcinoma and basal cell carcinoma, which are malignant epithelial neoplasms that often arise on sun-exposed areas of the skin in fair-skinned populations. These cancers cause local tissue destruction with functional and cosmetic deformity but are rarely a cause of death.

- Avoidance of excessive ultraviolet radiation from sunlight or tanning devices, particularly in young people, is the most effective way to prevent melanoma and non-melanoma skin cancer.

Cutaneous melanoma

Melanoma is the most aggressive form of skin cancer [1,2]. Cutaneous melanoma is a malignant proliferation of melanocytes, the pigment-forming cells of skin.

Etiology

Environmental factors play important roles in melanoma development and progression, including age, sex, degree of sun exposure, and anatomical location, as well as individual susceptibility. Only 20–30% of melanomas arise in association with a melanocytic naevus, but the presence of dysplastic naevi has been shown to be an independent risk factor for the development of multiple primary melanomas [3]. Other risk factors include family history of melanoma and prior melanoma. In addition, rarely germline mutations have been found to confer risk; for example, mutations of the *CDKN2A* gene (on chromosome 9p21) have been found in 20–40% of families with dysplastic naevus syndromes in which at least three first-degree relatives are affected by melanoma [4].

In addition to genetic factors, ultraviolet radiation from sun exposure also contributes to melanoma development. Most melanomas (80%) are caused by ultraviolet damage to sensitive skin, i.e. skin that burns easily, fair or reddish skin, skin with multiple freckles, or skin that does not tan and develops naevi in response to early sunlight exposure. Most damage caused by sunlight occurs in childhood and adolescence. Ultraviolet radiation is particularly hazardous when it involves sporadic intense exposure, especially during childhood and early adolescence, for example through indoor tanning; children and adolescents are thus the most important target group for prevention programmes [5].

Melanoma may occur anywhere on the skin, but in men most melanomas occur on the back, whereas in women most occur on the legs. In addition, patterns of age-specific incidence of melanoma at different anatomical sites in fair-skinned populations show that melanomas arising on intermittently exposed body sites are significantly more common among younger and middle-aged adults, whereas melanomas of the head and neck are most common among older people. The difference in incidence by anatomical site is not completely explained by differential exposure to ultraviolet radiation.

Epidemiology

Melanoma

- There were more than 232 000 new cases of melanoma and about 55 000 deaths estimated in 2012; the relatively low mortality rates are indicative of the reasonable prognosis.
- Incidence varies 100-fold between countries worldwide. Rates are highest in countries with predominantly Caucasian populations, and more than 80% of the estimated new cases and close to 65% of the cancer deaths occurred in Oceania, Europe, and North America.
- Incidence rates in Australia and New Zealand are 2 times those observed in any other country. Incidence rates tend to be rather low in most African, Asian, and Latin American countries.
- Mortality tends to be higher in men than in women, related to sex differences in detection, body location of tumours, and subsequent prognosis.
- Incidence and mortality have been increasing over the past decades in many populations that are predominantly Caucasian. Of note is the (cohort-specific) stabilization and/or recent decline in incidence in certain high-risk populations (e.g. in Australia and among Whites in the USA). In low-risk populations (Asia, Africa, and to some extent Latin America), incidence rates have remained low and stable over time.

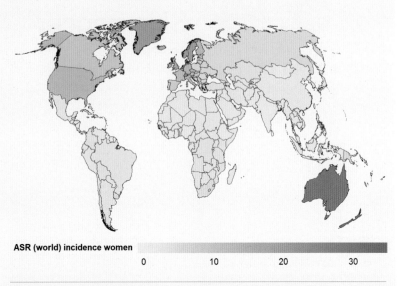

Map 5.14.1. Global distribution of estimated age-standardized (World) incidence rates (ASR) per 100 000, for melanoma in women, 2012.

ASR (world) incidence women

0   10   20   30

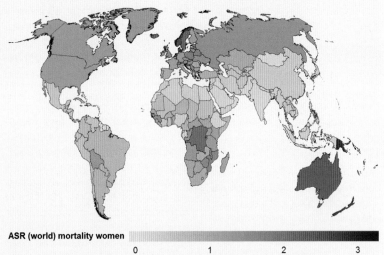

Map 5.14.2. Global distribution of estimated age-standardized (World) mortality rates (ASR) per 100 000, for melanoma in women, 2012.

ASR (world) mortality women

0   1   2   3

For more details about the maps and charts presented in this chapter, see "A guide to the epidemiology data in *World Cancer Report*".

Moreover, melanoma can occur in areas of the body without sun exposure as well as in any ethnic group.

Pathology

Melanomas occur primarily in the skin – more than 95% of cases – but are also found in the mucous membranes of the mouth, nose, anus, and vagina and, to a lesser extent, the intestine; melanocytes are also present in the conjunctiva, the retina, and the meninges. Melanoma can be subtyped histologically into superficial spreading melanoma, nodular melanoma, acral lentiginous melanoma, and lentigo maligna melanoma. A staging system based on the histopathological parameters of the excised lesion, including multiple prognostic factors, is recommended [6]. The most robust independent prognostic factor in melanoma is tumour thickness (Breslow depth), found by measuring the vertical depth from the granular cell layer of the epidermis to the deepest detectable melanoma cell. In recent years, two additional criteria, ulceration and mitosis, have been shown to be important in

Chart 5.14.1. Estimated global number of new cases and deaths with proportions by major world regions, for melanoma in both sexes combined, 2012.

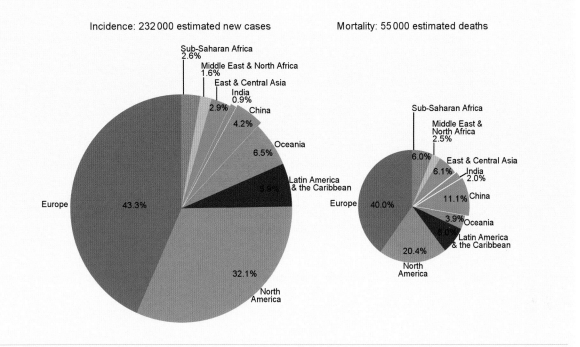

Incidence: 232 000 estimated new cases

Mortality: 55 000 estimated deaths

Chart 5.14.2. Age-standardized (World) incidence rates per 100 000 by year in selected populations, for melanoma in women, circa 1975–2012.

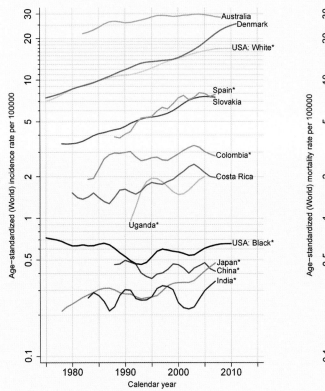

Chart 5.14.3. Age-standardized (World) mortality rates per 100 000 by year in selected populations, for melanoma in women, circa 1975–2012.

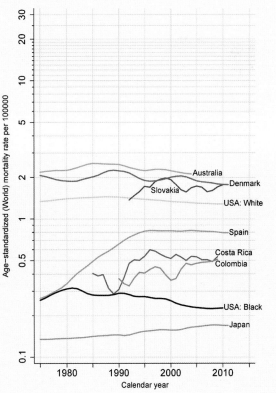

Evaluating sunscreen as a measure to reduce the risk of melanoma

Adèle C. Green

For several decades it was debated whether sunscreen use could prevent melanoma, even though it was biologically plausible that shielding the skin from excessive exposure to solar ultraviolet radiation in the long term would reduce the incidence of melanomas of the skin. Although many studies had examined this issue, human evidence was inconclusive because the studies were not randomized but observational. This means they were unable to distinguish the main drivers of sunscreen use from those of melanoma causation, since they largely overlap: susceptibility to sunburn, high occupational or recreational sun exposure, and family history of melanoma [1]. Arguments against sunscreen as a melanoma preventive were also put forward, such as the example of dedicated sunbathers who misused sunscreen to prolong rather than minimize their sun exposure.

Evidence from a community-based trial has gone a long way towards resolving this debate. The Nambour Skin Cancer Prevention Trial was a randomized controlled trial involving 1621 adults aged 25–75 years who had been randomly selected from all adult residents of Nambour, a subtropical Australian township. In 1992 they were randomized either to apply a freely supplied broad-spectrum sunscreen with a sun protection factor (SPF) of 15+ to the head and arms daily until 1996, or to continue their usual level of sunscreen use or non-use. Trial participants were then followed up for a decade after cessation of the sunscreen intervention, with monitoring of all new melanomas, through pathology laboratories and the Queensland Cancer Registry, and of their ongoing sun behaviour. Ten years after cessation of the sunscreen intervention, the 812 people randomized to daily sunscreen use had half as many new melanomas (11) as the control group of 809 people (22) [2], a difference of borderline statistical significance ($P = 0.051$). The decrease after regular sunscreen use was greater in invasive melanomas than in situ melanomas. During the trial, 75% of the intervention group applied sunscreen at least 3 or 4 days per week, compared with 25% of the control group; the sunscreen group also applied sunscreen more often to the trunk and legs than did the controls. Otherwise, background sun exposure and protection patterns were the same in the intervention and control groups throughout the study period [2].

Use of a sunscreen with a higher SPF or greater ultraviolet A protection may have shown a stronger preventive effect, but increasing the participants' average thickness of sunscreen application would more likely have had an even greater beneficial effect [3]. While this trial showed that regular use of sunscreen could halve people's risk of developing melanoma, replication of the findings in another population would give further weight to the evidence.

References

1. Green AC, Williams GM (2007). *Cancer Epidemiol Biomarkers Prev*, 16:1921–1922. http://dx.doi.org/10.1158/1055-9965.EPI-07-0477 PMID:17932337

2. Green AC *et al.* (2011). *J Clin Oncol*, 29:257–263. http://dx.doi.org/10.1200/JCO.2010.28.7078 PMID:21135266

3. Diffey BL (2001). *Photochem Photobiol*, 74:61–63. http://dx.doi.org/10.1562/0031-8655(2001)074<0061:SAUPAM>2.0.CO;2 PMID:11460538

Table 5.14.1. Classification of melanoma and recommended surgical margins for primary melanoma

Classification	Melanoma thickness	Surgical excision margins
Tis	In situ melanoma/no invasion of the dermis	5 mm
T1	≤ 1 mm	10 mm
T1a	Without ulceration and/or mitosis < 1/mm^2	
T1b	With ulceration and/or mitosis > 1/mm^2	
T2[a]	1.01–2.0 mm	10 mm
T3	2.01–4.0 mm	20 mm
T4	> 4.01 mm	20 mm

[a] Levels T2–4 are classified a if ulceration is present, b if no ulceration is present.

prognosis and have been included in the classification system (Table 5.14.1).

Most acquired naevi feature small round, oval, or spindled melanocytes. Small melanocytes with scant cytoplasm are evident in melanomas in severely sun-damaged skin. Large round or oval epithelioid melanocytes occur both in benign proliferations and in melanoma.

The outcome of melanoma initially depends on the stage at presentation. Excellent prognosis with 5-year survival rates of more than 90% can be achieved for patients who present

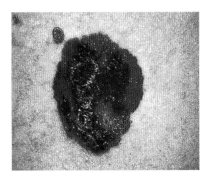

with localized disease and primary tumours less than 1.0 mm in thickness. As recommended in the latest American Joint Committee on Cancer staging manual, melanoma patients are categorized into three groups: localized disease with no evidence of metastases (stage I–II), regional disease (stage III), and distant metastatic disease (stage IV). For localized disease (stage I and II), Breslow tumour thickness, ulceration, and mitotic rate are the three most important characteristics of the primary tumour for predicting outcome [6].

Genetics

Heritable susceptibility is very important in melanoma tumorigenesis. Germline mutations of two genes have been discovered in melanoma-prone families: *CDKN2A* (on chromosome 9p21), which encodes p16^{INK4A}, and *CDK4* (on chromosome 12), which encodes cyclin-dependent kinase 4. A *CDKN2A* mutation causing functional inactivity of p16 has been found in up to 25% of melanoma-prone families worldwide, whereas a *CDK4* mutation causing overexpression of CDK4 protein, which is inhibited by p16, resulting in dysregulation of the cell cycle, has been observed in only a few rare families [7]. In addition, loss-of-function

mutations in the human melanocortin 1 receptor (*MC1R*) gene have been associated with red hair, fair skin, freckles, and decreased ability to tan. However, susceptibility genes identified in melanoma-prone families are rarely mutated in sporadic melanomas. Numerous somatic mutations in melanoma vary between individuals and are different from those in other malignancies. Only 20% of melanomas harbour common *TP53* mutations and inactivation of p16^{INK4A}, associated with a poorer prognosis in melanoma.

Genes identified as playing a role in development of sporadic melanoma include *CDKN2A*, *PTEN*, and *BRAF*, and genes located on chromosomes 1p, 6q, 7p, 9p, and 11q. Mutations in *BRAF* (on chromosome 7q) occur at a high frequency (45%) in melanomas [8], while somatic mutations in *BRAF* have also been detected in 50% of patients with dysplastic naevi. The *BRAF*, *NRAS*, and *KIT* genes, involved in cell-cycle activating pathways, are commonly mutated in melanomas. The current data support a model in which melanoma tumorigenesis requires changes that initiate clonal expansion, overcome cell senescence, and reduce apoptosis. Thus, combination drug therapies with tyrosine kinase inhibitors of multiple components in the mitogen-activated protein kinase pathway, including MEK and ERK, are in clinical trials. Melanoma also is characterized by chromosomal gains, for example at 1q, 3p, 6p, 7, 8q, 11q, 12q14, 17q, and 20q, which encompass the melanoma oncogenes *CDK4*, cyclin D1 (*CCND1*), *MYC*, *MDM2*, and *MITF*, as well as chromosomal losses, for example at 1p, 6q, 9q, 10q, 11q, 17p, and 21q, which harbour the tumour suppressors *p15*^{INK4B}, *p16*^{INK4A}, *p14*^{ARF}, and *PTEN*.

Whole-genome sequence data from 25 metastatic tumours identified *PREX2* – a PTEN-interacting protein and a negative regulator of PTEN in breast cancer – as a significantly mutated gene, with a mutation frequency of approximately 14% in an independent extension cohort of

107 human melanomas [9]. Other genetic changes include microsatellite instability, loss of heterozygosity, and increased activity of the telomerase enzyme.

Changes in gene expression contribute to progression from early benign melanocytic lesions to dysplastic naevi, to primary melanoma with a radial and then a vertical growth pattern, and to the acquisition of metastatic capacities. However, this sequence is challenged by the identification of malignant melanoma stem cells [10]. Stem-like melanoma cells with expression of CD133, ABCB5, CD271, and CD166 are involved in the processes of progression and metastasis and are highly resistant to drugs and toxins [11].

Melanoma development not only requires genetic changes but is also driven by epigenetic alterations. 5-Hydroxymethylcytosine, a further indicator of modified DNA methylation, is lost in melanoma genome-wide [12]. Rebuilding the 5-hydroxymethylcytosine landscape in melanoma cells by reintroducing active TET2 or IDH2 suppresses melanoma growth and increases tumour-free survival in animal models. Tumour suppressor small, non-coding RNAs, including *miR-9*, *miR-34*, *miR-148a*, and *miR-375*, are silenced by promoter hypermethylation [13]. Expression of the histone H3K9 methyltransferase SETDB1 accelerates melanoma formation in zebrafish [14]. In addition, the H3K4 demethylase KDM5B (also called JARID1B) is considered a melanoma stem cell marker [15]. The ability to understand and

Fig. 5.14.2. Malignant melanoma. Micrograph showing a lesion just beneath the epidermis with pigmented and non-pigmented cells.

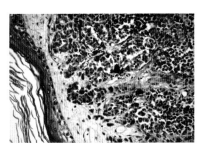

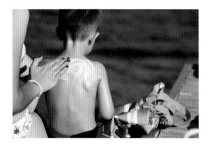

control reversible epigenetic changes before irreversible mutations ensue may play an increasingly important role in further cancer prevention and treatment.

Prospects

Prevention

Prevention of melanoma is based on limiting exposure to ultraviolet radiation, particularly in the first 20 years of life. Sun avoidance behaviour and protection through increased shaded areas and appropriate clothing have been widely adopted as protective measures. Exposure can also be reduced by avoiding artificial sources of ultraviolet radiation like sunbeds. Unequivocal evidence of the melanoma-preventive effects of sunscreen use is lacking (see "Evaluating sunscreen as a measure to reduce the risk of melanoma"). Notwithstanding the inherent uncertainties and assumptions, the available evidence suggests that significant numbers of melanomas might be avoided by regular sunscreen use during recreational summer sun exposure [16]. The matter is of high priority to countries with a large fair-skinned community and strong lifestyle orientation to sun exposure, such as the USA [17] and Australia [18].

Targeted therapy

Ipilimumab, a monoclonal antibody against CTLA-4, was the first immunomodulating antibody approved in the USA, in March 2011, for metastatic melanoma. Vemurafenib [19], a specific inhibitor of signalling by mutated *BRAF*, was approved in August 2011 for patients with stage IV melanoma with documented V600E or V600K mutation of the *BRAF* gene. These targeted agents have significantly changed the treatment regimen of metastatic melanoma. However, the use of these agents is challenged by their side-effects and unique limitations. For example, ipilimumab can achieve durable response but has a low overall response rate of less than 20%; vemurafenib has a higher response rate of 40–50% but with a median duration of only 5–6 months. Recent progress in the understanding of melanoma biology has led to the identification of novel pathways that could serve as targets for novel therapy (Fig. 5.14.4). For example, the PI3K pathway [20] and the p16–cyclin D–CDK4/6–retinoblastoma pathway [21] could be exploited. In addition, some pilot clinical data suggest potential benefits with targeted therapeutic melanoma vaccines, for example infusion of lymphocytes genetically modified to express the MAGE-A3 tumour antigen in patients with advanced melanoma. A consensus statement on tumour immunotherapy for the treatment of cutaneous melanoma has recently been adopted [22].

Non-melanoma skin cancer

Basal cell carcinomas and squamous cell carcinomas are the two malignant epithelial neoplasms and the main forms of non-melanoma skin cancer, accounting for the large majority of all skin cancers.

Etiology

Among several risk factors, sun exposure is the most recognized environmental cause, especially for squamous cell carcinoma. The association between sun exposure and basal cell carcinoma is more complex than that for squamous cell carcinoma [23]. Basal cell carcinoma seems to be associated more with intermittent exposure to high doses of solar radiation compared with similar doses delivered more continuously [24]. Fair-skinned populations who have substantial exposure to

Fig. 5.14.4. (A) Key signalling pathways in melanoma. Potentially druggable targets are indicated by purple shading. Mitogen-activated protein kinase (MAPK) signalling can be constitutively activated through alterations in membrane receptors or through mutations of *RAS* or *BRAF*. *BRAF* is frequently mutated in melanomas, almost invariably by the V600E mutation, which results in an amino acid substitution at position 600, from a valine (V) to a glutamic acid (E), causing constitutive kinase activation. (B) Mechanisms of BRAF inhibitor resistance include reactivation of the MAPK pathway by CRAF, ARAF, or the p61BRAF(V600E) splice variant, mutational activation of *NRAS* or *MEK*, loss of the tumour suppressor *NF1*, and activation of compensatory pathways such as the PI3K network via enhanced receptor tyrosine kinase signalling (particularly through PDGFRβ, IGF1-R, FGFR, HGFR, and EGFR). Therapies approved or pending approval are shown in red. Activating mutations found are indicated by yellow shading, and inactivation by pink shading.

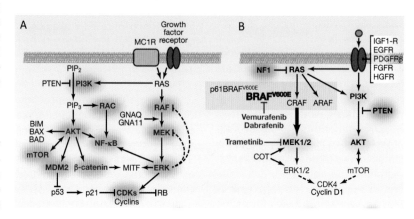

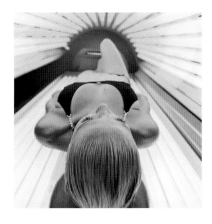

Fig. 5.14.5. A young woman uses a sunbed. Excess exposure to ultraviolet radiation is the most important modifiable risk factor for both malignant melanoma and non-melanoma skin cancer.

ultraviolet radiation from sun exposure as well as indoor tanning, especially at a young age, have an increased risk of developing non-melanoma skin cancers [25,26]. In addition, most of these malignancies develop on sun-exposed skin sites, especially the head and neck area (80%). Actinic keratosis is a precursor with the potential to progress to invasive squamous cell carcinoma, and is considered to be a sun-induced precancerous lesion for these tumours. Besides sun exposure, therapeutic exposure to "psoralen plus ultraviolet A light" therapy for cutaneous disorders is associated with increased risk of non-melanoma skin cancers, particularly squamous cell carcinoma. Ionizing radiation used to treat childhood cancers increases the risk of subsequent development of non-melanoma skin cancers, including basal cell carcinomas. Arsenic exposure, including environmental exposure, has been associated with increased risk of both tumour types.

Immunocompromised individuals – typically organ transplant recipients, patients with a history of long-term steroid use, and people with HIV/AIDS – are at higher risk of non-melanoma skin cancer [27]. Non-melanoma skin cancers in organ transplant recipients are associated with human papillomavirus (HPV)

infection of skin keratinocytes. In addition, detection of beta HPV species in cutaneous squamous cell carcinoma suggests that certain HPV types may be involved in the progression of squamous cell carcinoma in immunocompetent individuals as well. Furthermore, epidermodysplasia verruciformis-associated HPV infection of skin keratinocytes seems to be associated with increased risk of squamous cell but not basal cell carcinomas [28]. This association with HPV remains confined to squamous cell carcinomas arising on chronically sun-exposed areas of the skin.

Development of non-melanoma skin cancer is associated with a range of inherited disorders. Basal cell naevus syndrome (also called naevoid basal cell carcinoma syndrome or Gorlin syndrome) is a rare autosomal dominant disorder due to germline mutations of the *PTCH* gene. Developmental abnormalities, postnatal tumours, and multiple basal cell carcinomas are observed in affected patients. Epidermolysis bullosa syndrome is a heterogeneous group of inherited blistering disorders due to minor trauma. The Dowling–Meara form of epidermolysis bullosa simplex is associated with an increased risk of basal cell carcinoma; squamous cell carcinomas arise primarily in autosomal recessive dystrophic epidermolysis bullosa and are the most serious complication for these patients. Naevus sebaceous is a rare congenital hamartoma of the skin composed of epidermal, follicular, sebaceous, and apocrine elements. While 15% of patients with naevus sebaceous develop some types of appendage tumour, 5% are diagnosed with basal cell carcinoma.

Pathology and genetics
Squamous cell and basal cell carcinomas are the major types of keratinocytic tumours derived from the proliferation of epidermal and adnexal keratinocytes. The multiple variants of basal cell carcinoma have in common lobules, columns, bands, and cords of basaloid cells associated with scant cytoplasm, and a characteristic outer

palisade of cells associated with a surrounding loose fibromucinous stroma. Squamous cell carcinoma is a malignant neoplasm of epidermal keratinocytes in which the component cells show variable squamous differentiation.

Besides the risk factors such as sun exposure, genetic variations of populations also play a role in development of non-melanoma skin cancer. Basal cell and squamous cell carcinomas arise predominantly in sun-sensitive people with fair skin and a history of sunburn [23]. Individuals with albinism, with lack of skin pigmentation, and patients with xeroderma pigmentosum, which causes an extreme sensitivity to sunlight, have a greatly increased risk of developing these tumours because they have little or no ability to repair skin damaged by ultraviolet radiation. In the past decade, significant advances have been made in terms of understanding the molecular pathogenesis of non-melanoma skin cancer. Ultraviolet-induced mutations of the tumour suppressor gene *TP53* are frequently observed in these cancers [29]. The sonic hedgehog signalling pathway plays a critical role in the pathogenesis of basal cell carcinoma. Mutations in the *PTCH* gene, which codes for a receptor of sonic hedgehog, are the underlying cause of naevoid basal cell carcinoma syndrome.

Non-melanoma skin cancers are usually indolent, but certain pathological features indicate high risk of recurrence and the potential for metastasis. In basal cell carcinoma, the histological subtypes of micronodular, infiltrative, and morpheaform basal cell carcinoma are more likely to recur than are the superficial and nodular subtypes. Basosquamous carcinoma, a "collision"-type tumour, is associated with a more aggressive nature, with an increased risk of metastasis [30].

Prospects
The primary approach to preventing skin cancer is protection from sun exposure with various techniques. See the discussion above, at the end of the section on cutaneous melanoma.

References

1. Siegel R, Naishadham D, Jemal A (2012). Cancer statistics, 2012. *CA Cancer J Clin*, 62:10–29. http://dx.doi.org/10.3322/caac. 20138 PMID:22237781

2. Tas F (2012). Metastatic behavior in melanoma: timing, pattern, survival, and influencing factors. *J Oncol*, 2012:647684. http://dx.doi.org/10.1155/2012/647684 PMID:22792102

3. Kang S, Barnhill RL, Mihm MC Jr et al. (1994). Melanoma risk in individuals with clinically atypical nevi. *Arch Dermatol*, 130: 999–1001. http://dx.doi.org/10.1001/arch derm.1994.01690080065008 PMID:8053717

4. Kefford RF, Newton Bishop JA, Bergman W, Tucker MA (1999). Counseling and DNA testing for individuals perceived to be genetically predisposed to melanoma: a consensus statement of the Melanoma Genetics Consortium. *J Clin Oncol*, 17:3245–3251. PMID:10506626

5. Tsao H, Sober AJ (1998). Ultraviolet radiation and malignant melanoma. *Clin Dermatol*, 16:67–73. http://dx.doi.org/10.1016/S0738-081X(97)00191-0 PMID:9472435

6. Balch CM, Gershenwald JE, Soong SJ et al. (2009). Final version of 2009 AJCC melanoma staging and classification. *J Clin Oncol*, 27:6199–6206. http://dx.doi.org/10.1200/JCO.2009.23.4799 PMID:19917835

7. Goldstein AM, Chidambaram A, Halpern A et al. (2002). Rarity of *CDK4* germline mutations in familial melanoma. *Melanoma Res*, 12:51–55. http://dx.doi.org/10.1097/00008390-200 202000-00008 PMID:11828258

8. Davies H, Bignell GR, Cox C et al. (2002). Mutations of the *BRAF* gene in human cancer. *Nature*, 417:949–954. http://dx.doi.org/10.1038/nature00766 PMID:12068308

9. Berger MF, Hodis E, Heffernan TP et al. (2012). Melanoma genome sequencing reveals frequent *PREX2* mutations. *Nature*, 485:502–506. http://dx.doi.org/10.1038/nature11071 PMID:22622578

10. Schatton T, Murphy GF, Frank NY et al. (2008). Identification of cells initiating human melanomas. *Nature*, 451:345–349. http://dx.doi.org/10.1038/nature06489 PMID:18202660

11. Somasundaram R, Villanueva J, Herlyn M (2012). Intratumoral heterogeneity as a therapy resistance mechanism: role of melanoma subpopulations. *Adv Pharmacol*, 65:335–359. http://dx.doi.org/10.1016/B978-0-12-397927-8.00011-7 PMID:22959031

12. Lian CG, Xu Y, Ceol C et al. (2012). Loss of 5-hydroxymethylcytosine is an epigenetic hallmark of melanoma. *Cell*, 150:1135–1146. http://dx.doi.org/10.1016/j.cell.2012.07.033 PMID:22980977

13. Mazar J, Khaitan D, DeBlasio D et al. (2011). Epigenetic regulation of microRNA genes and the role of miR-34b in cell invasion and motility in human melanoma. *PLoS One*, 6:e24922. http://dx.doi.org/10.1371/journal.pone.0024922 PMID:21949788

14. Ceol CJ, Houvras Y, Jane-Valbuena J et al. (2011). The histone methyltransferase SETDB1 is recurrently amplified in melanoma and accelerates its onset. *Nature*, 471:513–517. http://dx.doi.org/10.1038/nature09806 PMID:21430779

15. Roesch A, Fukunaga-Kalabis M, Schmidt EC et al. (2010). A temporarily distinct subpopulation of slow-cycling melanoma cells is required for continuous tumor growth. *Cell*, 141:583–594. http://dx.doi.org/10.1016/j.cell.2010.04.020 PMID:20478252

16. Diffey BL (2009). Sunscreens as a preventative measure in melanoma: an evidence-based approach or the precautionary principle? *Br J Dermatol*, 161 Suppl 3:25–27. http://dx.doi.org/10.1111/j.1365-2133.2009.09445.x PMID:19775353

17. Lazovich D, Choi K, Vogel RI (2012). Time to get serious about skin cancer prevention. *Cancer Epidemiol Biomarkers Prev*, 21:1893–1901. http://dx.doi.org/10.1158/1055-9965.EPI-12-0327 PMID:22962407

18. McCarthy WH (2004). The Australian experience in sun protection and screening for melanoma. *J Surg Oncol*, 86:236–245. http://dx.doi.org/10.1002/jso.20086 PMID:15221930

19. Bollag G, Hirth P, Tsai J et al. (2010). Clinical efficacy of a RAF inhibitor needs broad target blockade in *BRAF*-mutant melanoma. *Nature*, 467:596–599. http://dx.doi.org/10.1038/nature09454 PMID:20823850

20. Kwong LN, Davies MA (2013). Navigating the therapeutic complexity of PI3K pathway inhibition in melanoma. *Clin Cancer Res*, 19:5310–5319. http://dx.doi.org/10.1158/1078-0432.CCR-13-0142 PMID:24089444

21. Sheppard KE, McArthur GA (2013). The cell-cycle regulator CDK4: an emerging therapeutic target in melanoma. *Clin Cancer Res*, 19:5320–5328. http://dx.doi.org/10.1158/1078-0432.CCR-13-0259 PMID:24089445

22. Kaufman HL, Kirkwood JM, Hodi FS et al. (2013). The Society for Immunotherapy of Cancer consensus statement on tumour immunotherapy for the treatment of cutaneous melanoma. *Nat Rev Clin Oncol*, 10:588–598. http://dx.doi.org/10.1038/nrclinonc.2013.153 PMID:23982524

23. Armstrong BK, Kricker A, English DR (1997). Sun exposure and skin cancer. *Australas J Dermatol*, 38 Suppl 1:S1–S6. PMID:10994463

24. Kricker A, Armstrong BK, English DR, Heenan PJ (1995). Does intermittent sun exposure cause basal cell carcinoma? A case-control study in Western Australia. *Int J Cancer*, 60:489–494. http://dx.doi.org/10.1002/ijc.2910600411 PMID:7829262

25. Perkins JL, Liu Y, Mitby PA et al. (2005). Nonmelanoma skin cancer in survivors of childhood and adolescent cancer: a report from the childhood cancer survivor study. *J Clin Oncol*, 23:3733–3741. http://dx.doi.org/10.1200/JCO.2005.06.237 PMID:15923570

26. Wehner MR, Shive ML, Chren M-M et al. (2012). Indoor tanning and non-melanoma skin cancer: systematic review and meta-analysis. *BMJ*, 345:e5909. http://dx.doi.org/10.1136/bmj.e5909 PMID:23033409

27. Grulich AE, van Leeuwen MT, Falster MO, Vajdic CM (2007). Incidence of cancers in people with HIV/AIDS compared with immunosuppressed transplant recipients: a meta-analysis. *Lancet*, 370:59–67. http://dx.doi.org/10.1016/S0140-6736(07)61050-2 PMID:17617273

28. Pfister H (2003). Chapter 8: Human papillomavirus and skin cancer. *J Natl Cancer Inst Monogr*, 2003:52–56. http://dx.doi.org/10.1093/oxfordjournals.jncimonographs.a003483 PMID:12807946

29. Benjamin CL, Melnikova VO, Ananthaswamy HN (2008). p53 protein and pathogenesis of melanoma and nonmelanoma skin cancer. *Adv Exp Med Biol*, 624:265–282. http://dx.doi.org/10.1007/978-0-387-77574-6_21 PMID:18348463

30. Bath-Hextall F, Bong J, Perkins W, Williams H (2004). Interventions for basal cell carcinoma of the skin: systematic review. *BMJ*, 329:705. http://dx.doi.org/10.1136/bmj.38219.515266.AE PMID:15364703

5.15 Thyroid cancer

5 ORGAN SITE

Frank Weber   Dillwyn Williams (reviewer)

Summary

- The incidence of thyroid cancer is increasing worldwide. This trend is attributed predominantly to the improved detection and screening of nodular thyroid disease, particularly involving detection of papillary microcarcinoma.

- Exposure to ionizing radiation, especially during childhood, is a cause of thyroid cancer.

- Multiple endocrine neoplasia type 2 (MEN2)-associated medullary thyroid carcinoma serves as a role model for personalized medicine as *RET* proto-oncogene mutation analysis enables predictive testing and genotype-based, tailored prophylactic treatment.

- Molecular profiling using *BRAF* mutation analysis can allow for risk assessment of papillary thyroid carcinoma.

- Targeted therapy will provide novel options to treat advanced and de-differentiated thyroid cancer.

Thyroid cancer includes a variety of malignancies ranging from the common differentiated thyroid cancers to the very rare but uniformly lethal anaplastic thyroid cancer [1,2]. Thyroid cancers develop either from the follicular epithelial cells – giving rise to papillary thyroid cancer, follicular thyroid cancer, and likely undifferentiated and anaplastic thyroid cancer – or from the parafollicular, calcitonin-producing C cells, which give rise to medullary thyroid cancer (Fig. 5.15.1).

Etiology

Worldwide, thyroid cancer is among the less frequent malignancies. However, in the past decades the incidence has almost doubled – attributed for the most part to the increased diagnosis of papillary thyroid cancer [3]. While the reasons for the increase in thyroid cancer incidence require further elucidation, several lines of evidence indicate that in most circumstances the increase is attributable to optimal diagnostic scrutiny aided by technical advances [3,4]. Overall, the etiology of thyroid cancer is not fully understood.

A clear gender disparity is evident for thyroid cancer; it occurs more frequently in women than in men. In the USA, this tumour type accounts for 1.7% of all malignancies, corresponding to 2.6% of cancers in women and 0.85% of cancers in men, whereas in Japan the female-to-male ratio may be 13

[3]. Reasons for the overall 3-fold higher incidence of thyroid cancers in women than in men remain unclear. A role for female hormonal and reproductive factors as drivers for thyroid cancer development has been shown in vitro but has not been unequivocally established in population-based analysis [5–7]. Thyroid cancer development is strongly associated with a history of benign nodules/adenoma or goitre [7]. Solitary, palpable thyroid nodules can be identified in about 7% of the adult population, and the prevalence of nodules increases with age; the lifetime risk of developing a thyroid

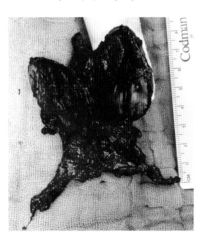

Fig. 5.15.1. Surgical specimen showing thyroidectomy with en bloc central lymphadenectomy for papillary thyroid cancer.

Epidemiology

Thyroid cancer

- With 77% of the cases occurring in women in 2012, thyroid cancer is one of the few non-sex-specific cancers that are more frequent in women. There were 230 000 new cases in women, representing the eighth most frequent cancer among women, compared with 68 000 cases in men, representing the 18th most frequent cancer among men.
- The case fatality of thyroid cancer is very low, most notably in countries with very high levels of human development (mortality-to-incidence ratio, 0.14).
- There were an estimated 40 000 deaths from thyroid cancer in 2012 (27 000 of them in women). Mortality rates are highest in Melanesia, in parts of Africa, and generally in countries with lower levels of human development.
- Although 37% of the estimated new cases occurred in Europe and North America and 48% in Asia, only 21% of the thyroid cancer deaths occurred in Europe and North America, compared with 57% in Asia.
- Elevated incidence rates are found in some European countries and in North America. However, the highest incidence rates globally are in the Republic of Korea, where thyroid cancer is the most frequent cancer among women. Incidence rates tend to be low in many parts of Asia and in Africa.

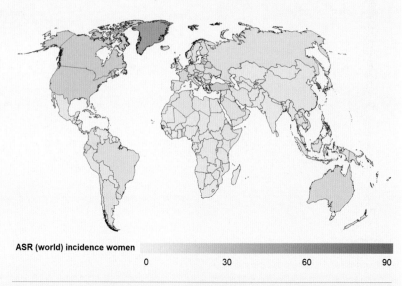

Map 5.15.1. Global distribution of estimated age-standardized (World) incidence rates (ASR) per 100 000, for thyroid cancer in women, 2012.

ASR (world) incidence women

0   30   60   90

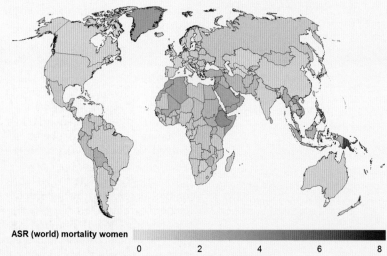

Map 5.15.2. Global distribution of estimated age-standardized (World) mortality rates (ASR) per 100 000, for thyroid cancer in women, 2012.

ASR (world) mortality women

0   2   4   6   8

For more details about the maps and charts presented in this chapter, see "A guide to the epidemiology data in *World Cancer Report*".

nodule is estimated to be 10%. The relative risk of cancer development in patients with thyroid nodules is 3–6 compared with unaffected controls.

Population-based studies suggest that risk of thyroid cancer is associated with several conditions. For instance, height and body mass index are moderately associated with thyroid cancer risk in both men and women [7]. Acromegaly, a rare condition caused by an overproduction of growth hormone, is also associated with increased risk of thyroid cancer. With regard to dietary risk factors for thyroid cancer development, iodine deficiency may induce benign thyroid conditions that predispose for thyroid cancer. Furthermore, iodine deficiency is associated with the prevalence of follicular thyroid cancer [3] because in iodine-deficient countries follicular thyroid cancer accounts for up to 40% of all thyroid cancer, whereas in regions with high iodine supplementation the same tumour type accounts for less than 20% of cases. However, it is uncertain to what extent dietary iodine intake might serve as a risk predictor for thyroid cancer development [7]. Published results

Chart 5.15.1. Estimated global number of new cases and deaths with proportions by major world regions, for thyroid cancer in both sexes combined, 2012.

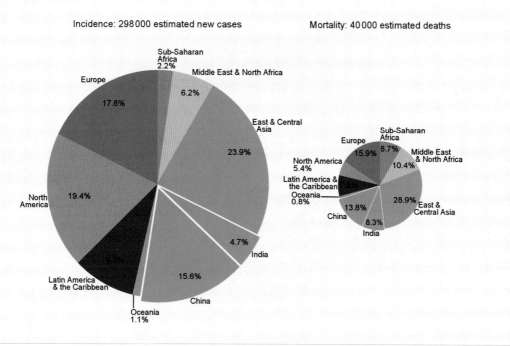

Incidence: 298 000 estimated new cases

Mortality: 40 000 estimated deaths

Chart 5.15.2. Age-standardized (World) incidence rates per 100 000 by year in selected populations, for thyroid cancer in women, circa 1975–2012.

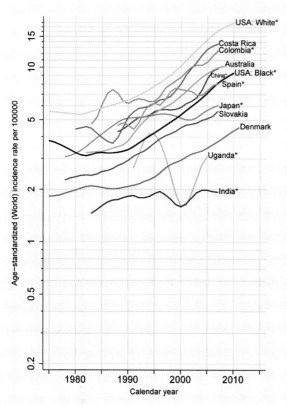

Chart 5.15.3. Age-standardized (World) mortality rates per 100 000 by year in selected populations, for thyroid cancer in women, circa 1975–2012.

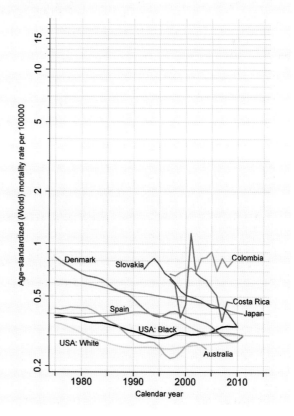

on the contribution of nutritional factors to thyroid cancer development are generally inconsistent and not conclusive.

Among the well-established high-risk factors for thyroid cancer development is exposure to ionizing radiation, especially when this occurs during childhood. Radiation exposure accounts for cancer development in about 5% of patients. Sources of radiation include certain medical treatments as well as radiation fallout from nuclear power plant accidents or nuclear weapons. The Chernobyl nuclear power plant accident took place in 1986, and during the following years an unprecedented rise in papillary thyroid cancer development during childhood was observed. Relevant cases indicated that ionizing radiation leads to chromosomal rearrangements such as *RET/PTC* fusion transcripts that give rise to papillary thyroid cancer development [8,9].

Radiation exposure in the context of medical care has included treatment for acne or enlarged tonsils during the 1960s. While this intervention is no longer used, previously exposed individuals are now in their fifties, the age group for which papillary thyroid cancer occurs most commonly. Other reasons for radiation therapy in childhood are tumour therapy for cancers such as lymphoma, Wilms tumour, or neuroblastoma. Exposure to diagnostic radiation (medical diagnostic radiography) has increased over the past years and currently is the leading source of radiation exposure in the USA. It is not fully established to what extent the repeated exposure to diagnostic radiation leads to an increased risk of thyroid cancer. However, a recent study showed a 13% increase in thyroid cancer risk for every 10 reported dental radiographs; caution should be exercised when requiring repeated radiography – especially during childhood [10].

Several inherited conditions, such as familial adenomatous polyposis syndrome and Cowden syndrome, are associated with different types of thyroid cancer [11]. For

non-syndromic familial non-medullary thyroid cancer, epidemiological data indicate a very high likelihood of familial aggregation and hence a strong genetic component. Indeed, about 10% of all non-medullary thyroid cancers are hereditary, and consequently first-degree relatives of patients with thyroid cancer have an up to 10-fold increased risk compared with the general population. The standardized incidence ratio, an index for estimating familial risk of developing a malignancy, exceeds a notable value of 3.8 for thyroid cancer. Thus, differentiated epithelial thyroid carcinomas have one of the highest familial risks of all cancer sites [11].

Pathology

Thyroid cancer primarily involves the following entities, in decreasing order of frequency: differentiated thyroid cancers, which comprise papillary and follicular thyroid cancer; medullary thyroid cancer; and poorly differentiated thyroid cancer, which includes undifferentiated and anaplastic thyroid cancer [12].

These tumour types are of endodermal origin and arise from the thyroid follicles, except for medullary thyroid cancer, which develops from the parafollicular calcitonin-secreting C cells and is of neuroendocrine origin. In addition, the thyroid stroma contains lymphoid cells as well as connective tissue that might give rise to thyroid lymphomas, which are nearly always non-Hodgkin lymphomas or sarcoma; both, however, are rather rare and account for less than 5% of all thyroid cancers [12].

Differentiated thyroid carcinoma

Papillary thyroid carcinomas are malignant epithelial tumours that show evidence of follicular cell differentiation and display characteristic nuclear features. These are large nuclei that have hypodense chromatin (ground-glass appearance) and show intranuclear inclusions and nuclear grooves. The cellular features of papillary thyroid cancer are amphophilic, finely granular cytoplasm, large pale nuclei, nuclear grooves, and psammoma bodies. On macroscopic inspection, papillary thyroid cancer presents as

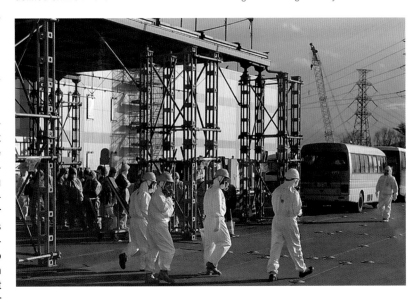

Fig. 5.15.2. More than two years after the accident at Fukushima Daiichi nuclear power plant, work continues to ensure that the damaged units remain stable. Here, workers in protective clothing and masks are shown outside the Emergency Response Centre, the main control hub at the site. Radiation exposure during childhood is the most clearly defined environmental factor associated with benign and malignant thyroid tumours.

Fig. 5.15.3. Fig. 5.15.3. Molecular pathways dysregulated, and putative molecular targets for therapy, in differentiated thyroid carcinoma. The highly complex interaction of protein/lipid phosphatases and protein/lipid kinases indicates that molecular targeted therapy aimed at only one component might not be sufficient to stabilize the dysregulated pathway. Furthermore, molecular targeted therapy will have to be adapted to the genomic make-up of the individual as it interacts with the genome of the tumour. pAKT, phosphorylated protein kinase B; PI3K, phosphatidylinositol 3-kinase; PIP_3, phosphatidylinositol 3,4,5-triphosphate; pMAPK, phosphorylated mitogen-activated protein kinase; PPAR-γ, peroxisome proliferator-activated receptor gamma.

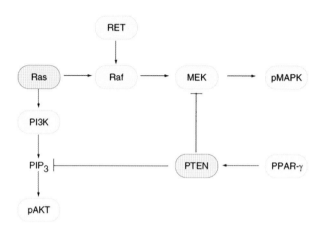

Medullary thyroid carcinoma

On macroscopic examination, medullary thyroid carcinomas are non-encapsulated but well-circumscribed lesions that contain areas of calcification. In a hereditary setting, multifocality is rather common. The unique feature of this cancer is a characteristic deposit of amyloid. Furthermore, staining for calcitonin and carcinoembryonic antigen (CEA) helps to differentiate this cancer from other forms [12].

Poorly differentiated thyroid carcinoma

Poorly differentiated thyroid cancer is a highly aggressive cancer. Based on morphological and clinical criteria, these tumours occupy an intermediate position between differentiated forms (follicular and papillary carcinomas) and anaplastic carcinomas. Most of these cancers develop by de-differentiation from their well-differentiated forms, as described above. Thus, the biology and histology of poorly differentiated thyroid carcinoma show characteristics of follicular or papillary thyroid cancer. Based on the WHO classification of thyroid cancer, poorly differentiated thyroid carcinomas are neoplasms of follicular origin but lack the typical structural presentation of follicular cell differentiation.

Anaplastic thyroid cancers are highly lethal carcinomas derived from the thyroid follicular cells that lack thyroglobulin expression. Most

an invasive neoplasm of whitish colour lacking a tumour capsule [12]. A multifocal manifestation is common. Approximately 50% of these newly detected cancers are papillary microcarcinomas, which measure 1 cm or less in largest diameter [4]. In autopsy studies, these small tumours have been detected in as many as 35% of cases, and meticulous examination of thyroidectomy specimens has revealed micropapillary thyroid cancer in as many as 24% of cases.

There is growing evidence that a subset of these overall apparently indolent micropapillary thyroid cancers are highly aggressive tumours that harbour a tendency to recur, metastasize, and cause death. Thus, it is of great importance to identify prognostic markers. *BRAF* mutation analysis might identify patients at risk. Similarly, histopathological characteristics, such as are indicated by the sclerosing variant, appear to be associated with metastases from these small papillary thyroid cancers (hazard ratio, 11.8) (Fig. 5.15.5) [13].

Follicular thyroid cancers are well-encapsulated lesions that display fibrosis, haemorrhage, and cystic areas. Three types of

follicular thyroid cancer may be distinguished with reference to their clinical relevance: (i) minimally invasive tumours without angioinvasion, which have the best prognosis (disease-free survival, 97%); (ii) minimally invasive follicular thyroid cancers with angioinvasion (disease-free survival, 81%); (iii) widely invasive follicular thyroid cancers, for which distant metastases are found in about 50% of patients [14]. The WHO classification of thyroid cancer defines follicular thyroid carcinoma as a lesion showing evidence of follicular cell differentiation and lacking the diagnostic nuclear features of papillary carcinoma. Thus, the diagnosis of follicular thyroid cancer is based on the exclusion of the typical nuclear features of papillary thyroid cancer [12]. The major challenge for pathology represents those thyroid tumours with a follicular growth pattern that include an array of neoplastic and malignant lesions. In addition, the differentiation of follicular thyroid malignancy from follicular adenoma is based on the identification of vascular and/or capsular invasion [15].

Fig. 5.15.4. Cervical computed tomography image of anaplastic thyroid cancer.

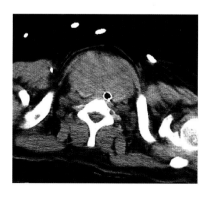

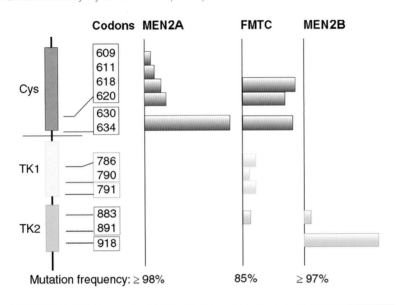

Fig. 5.15.5. Genotype–phenotype correlation in multiple endocrine neoplasia type 2 (MEN2). Germline *RET* mutations are specific for subgroups in MEN2. Codons of the *RET* oncogene affected by germline mutations are depicted in correlation to their physical location within the RET tyrosine kinase (TK) receptor. The horizontal bars indicate the frequency of these mutations in the three clinical subtypes MEN2A, MEN2B, and familial medullary thyroid carcinoma (FMTC).

of these cancers already show local invasion and metastases at the time of diagnosis (Fig. 5.15.4).

Genetics

Thyroid cancer oncogenesis is associated with multiple genetic and epigenetic alterations. The activation of the MAPK and PI3K/AKT signalling pathways appears to be crucial for thyroid cancer initiation and progression (Fig. 5.15.5) [16].

Point mutations of the *BRAF* and *RAS* genes are commonly found in thyroid cancers, as are alterations involving *RET/PTC* and *PAX8/PPAR*-γ chromosomal rearrangements [17,18]. Several lines of evidence indicate that certain etiological factors are associated with specific molecular alterations. For instance, exposure to ionizing radiation leads to chromosomal rearrangements, while exogenous chemicals tend to mediate genomic damage by causing point mutations. The extent to which high iodine intake is associated with the development of *BRAF* point mutations requires clarification as current data are not consistent.

The elucidation of the molecular pathology of thyroid carcinoma has led to the identification of diagnostic and prognostic markers. Among these, a *BRAF* point mutation may be a valuable indicator for the management of patients with thyroid nodules. Growing evidence shows that *BRAF* V600E-positive micropapillary thyroid cancer is more aggressive, and surgical management should be adopted accordingly [19].

Genetic alterations found in undifferentiated and anaplastic thyroid cancer involve the tumour suppressor gene *TP53* and cell-cycle checkpoint genes such as *p27* or *p21*. In addition, the Wnt pathway genes and the PTEN/PI3K/AKT pathway appear to play an important role in advanced thyroid cancer.

Heritable disease

About 25% of all medullary thyroid cancers occur as part of the multiple endocrine neoplasia type 2 (MEN2) syndrome [20]. MEN2 is an autosomal dominant transmitted tumour syndrome caused by germline mutation in the *RET* proto-oncogene and comprises the key endocrine neoplasia components of phaeochromocytoma, hyperparathyroidism, and, importantly, medullary thyroid carcinoma – the life-limiting scenario. MEN2-associated medullary thyroid cancer can be considered the role model for the practice of genomic medicine. The presence of mutations in the *RET* medullary thyroid cancer susceptibility gene has enabled the implementation of a powerful molecular diagnostic test to identify mutation carriers at a premorbid stage (i.e. predictive testing) and the delineation of a genotype–phenotype correlation that allows tailored surgical management based on the distinct amino acid altered (Fig. 5.15.5).

Heritable non-medullary thyroid cancer occurs not as a single entity but as part of different tumour syndromes such as Cowden syndrome, Carney complex, Gardner syndrome (familial adenomatous polyposis syndrome), and Werner syndrome, all of which are transmitted in an autosomal dominant fashion [11]. In these tumour syndromes, differentiated thyroid cancer occurs in up to 20% of patients. A small portion of non-medullary thyroid cancer, termed familial non-medullary thyroid cancer (mostly papillary thyroid cancer), appears to be inherited without other associated pathologies. Non-syndromic familial non-medullary thyroid cancer is characterized by two or more first-degree relatives who are affected by thyroid carcinomas but lack signs of other hereditary syndromes or exposure to other risk factors (i.e. radiation). Despite extensive research over the past 10 years to identify the gene or genes associated with non-syndromic familial non-medullary thyroid cancer, no susceptibility genes have been identified. Nonetheless, at least five putative susceptibility loci have been identified, at 1q21, 2q21, 8p23.1-p22, 14q31, and 19p13.2. Of these, only 14q31 and 19p13.2, which correspond to the location of *NMTC1* and *TCO*, respectively, have been replicated in independent family sets, but the susceptibility genes

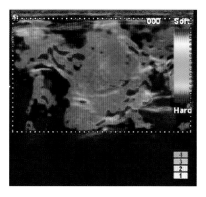

Fig. 5.15.6. Ultrasound elastography image of a suspicious thyroid nodule, indicating a hard nodule (Rago score, 3 or 4).

mapped to these loci have not yet been identified [21–23].

Prospects

Ionizing radiation causes thyroid cancer and, as mentioned above, exposure to such radiation – especially in childhood – should be avoided whenever possible. Since there are no other established causes, one challenge is to identify those patients with benign nodular thyroid disease who have an increased risk of thyroid cancer development. Screening for thyroid cancer in these patients would be optimized by improvement in diagnostic modalities such as ultrasound elastography of the thyroid and molecular classification using fine-needle aspirates (Fig. 5.15.6).

Most types of thyroid cancer are associated with excellent long-term survival: the 10-year overall survival exceeds 90% for papillary thyroid cancer and declines to 85% for follicular thyroid cancer and 70% for medullary thyroid cancer; for anaplastic tumours, the long-term outcome is very poor [1]. Metastasis commonly affects the regional lymph nodes as well as involving spread to the bone, lung, and liver. Tumour recurrence within the thyroid bed and distant recurrence are frequent and occur in about 30% of patients within 10 years after initial diagnosis [2].

Because of the availability of *RET* gene mutation analysis, familial cases of medullary thyroid carcinoma as part of the MEN2 tumour syndrome can be prevented by early, prophylactic resection of the thyroid gland. Elucidation of dysregulated pathways involved in thyroid oncogenesis has enabled the identification of potential new biomarkers and therapeutic targets. Small-molecule therapies targeting receptor tyrosine kinases, as well as their intracellular downstream proteins such as mTOR, BRAF, AKT, or MEK, are being investigated in clinical trials and appear to be promising for the treatment of advanced thyroid cancer [19]. These investigations have opened up a new aspect of cancer therapy and tumour re-differentiation in the setting of advanced tumours that are not amenable to treatment by surgery or radio-iodine therapy.

References

1. Sherman SI (2003). Thyroid carcinoma. *Lancet*, 361:501–511. http://dx.doi.org/10.1016/S0140-6736(03)12488-9 PMID:12583960

2. Mazzaferri EL, Kloos RT (2001). Current approaches to primary therapy for papillary and follicular thyroid cancer. *J Clin Endocrinol Metab*, 86:1447–1463. http://dx.doi.org/10.1210/jc.86.4.1447 PMID:11297567

3. Wartofsky L (2010). Increasing world incidence of thyroid cancer: increased detection or higher radiation exposure? *Hormones (Athens)*, 9:103–108. PMID:20687393

4. Mazzaferri EL (2012). Managing thyroid microcarcinomas. *Yonsei Med J*, 53:1–14. http://dx.doi.org/10.3349/ymj.2012.53.1.1 PMID:22187228

5. Peterson E, De P, Nuttall R (2012). BMI, diet and female reproductive factors as risks for thyroid cancer: a systematic review. *PLoS One*, 7:e29177. http://dx.doi.org/10.1371/journal.pone.0029177 PMID:22276106

6. Rahbari R, Zhang L, Kebebew E (2010). Thyroid cancer gender disparity. *Future Oncol*, 6:1771–1779. http://dx.doi.org/10.2217/fon.10.127 PMID:21142662

7. Dal Maso L, Bosetti C, La Vecchia C, Franceschi S (2009). Risk factors for thyroid cancer: an epidemiological review focused on nutritional factors. *Cancer Causes Control*, 20:75–86. http://dx.doi.org/10.1007/s10552-008-9219-5 PMID:18766448

8. Nikiforov YE (2006). Radiation-induced thyroid cancer: what we have learned from Chernobyl. *Endocr Pathol*, 17:307–317. http://dx.doi.org/10.1007/s12022-006-0001-5 PMID:17525478

9. Gandhi M, Evdokimova V, Nikiforov YE (2010). Mechanisms of chromosomal rearrangements in solid tumors: the model of papillary thyroid carcinoma. *Mol Cell Endocrinol*, 321:36–43. http://dx.doi.org/10.1016/j.mce.2009.09.013 PMID:19766698

10. Neta G, Rajaraman P, Berrington de Gonzalez A *et al.* (2013). A prospective study of medical diagnostic radiography and risk of thyroid cancer. *Am J Epidemiol*, 177:800–809. http://dx.doi.org/10.1093/aje/kws315 PMID:23529772

11. Weber F, Eng C (2008). Update on the molecular diagnosis of endocrine tumors: toward –omics-based personalized healthcare? *J Clin Endocrinol Metab*, 93:1097–1104. http://dx.doi.org/10.1210/jc.2008-0212 PMID:18390809

12. DeLellis RA, Lloyd RV, Heitz PU, Eng C, eds. (2004). *Pathology and Genetics of Tumours of Endocrine Organs*. Lyon: IARC.

13. Pellegriti G, Scollo C, Lumera G *et al.* (2004). Clinical behavior and outcome of papillary thyroid cancers smaller than 1.5 cm in diameter: study of 299 cases. *J Clin Endocrinol Metab*, 89:3713–3720. http://dx.doi.org/10.1210/jc.2003-031982 PMID:15292295

14. O'Neill CJ, Vaughan L, Learoyd DL *et al.* (2011). Management of follicular thyroid carcinoma should be individualised based on degree of capsular and vascular invasion. *Eur J Surg Oncol*, 37:181–185. http://dx.doi.org/10.1016/j.ejso.2010.11.005 PMID:21144693

15. Baloch ZW, Livolsi VA (2002). Follicular-patterned lesions of the thyroid: the bane of the pathologist. *Am J Clin Pathol*, 117:143–150. http://dx.doi.org/10.1309/8VL9-ECXY-NVMX-2RQF PMID:11789719

16. Xing M (2013). Molecular pathogenesis and mechanisms of thyroid cancer. *Nat Rev Cancer*, 13:184–199. http://dx.doi.org/10.1038/nrc3431 PMID:23429735

17. Weber F, Eng C (2005). Gene-expression profiling in differentiated thyroid cancer – a viable strategy for the practice of genomic medicine? *Future Oncol*, 1:497–510. http://dx.doi.org/10.2217/14796694.1.4.497 PMID:16556026

18. Fagin JA, Mitsiades N (2008). Molecular pathology of thyroid cancer: diagnostic and clinical implications. *Best Pract Res Clin Endocrinol Metab*, 22:955–969. http://dx.doi.org/10.1016/j.beem.2008.09.017 PMID:19041825

19. Xing M, Haugen BR, Schlumberger M (2013).). Progress in molecular-based management of differentiated thyroid cancer. *Lancet*, 381:1058–1069. http://dx.doi.org/10.1016/S0140-6736(13)60109-9 PMID:23668556

20. Moline J, Eng C (2011). Multiple endocrine neoplasia type 2: an overview. *Genet Med*, 13:755–764. http://dx.doi.org/10.1097/GIM.0b013e318216cc6d PMID:21552134

21. Eng C (2010). Mendelian genetics of rare – and not so rare – cancers. *Ann N Y Acad Sci*, 1214:70–82. http://dx.doi.org/10.1111/j.1749-6632.2010.05789.x PMID:20946573

22. Eng C (2010). Common alleles of predisposition in endocrine neoplasia. *Curr Opin Genet Dev*, 20:251–256. http://dx.doi.org/10.1016/j.gde.2010.02.004 PMID:20211557

23. Dammann M, Weber F (2012). Personalized medicine: caught between hope, hype and the real world. *Clinics (Sao Paulo)*, 67 Suppl 1:91–97. http://dx.doi.org/10.6061/clinics/2012(Sup01)16 PMID:22584712

Websites

Cancer Research UK thyroid cancer home page:
http://www.cancerresearchuk.org/cancer-help/type/thyroid-cancer/

Online Mendelian Inheritance in Man, Familial Medullary Thyroid Carcinoma:
http://omim.org/entry/155240

5.16 Tumours of the nervous system

5 ORGAN SITE

Paul Kleihues
Jill Barnholtz-Sloan
Hiroko Ohgaki

Webster K. Cavenee (reviewer)
Werner Paulus (reviewer)

Summary

- Tumours of the nervous system account for less than 2% of all cancers but have a marked impact on cancer morbidity and mortality.

- Nervous system tumours occur throughout life. Diffusely infiltrating gliomas manifest predominantly in adults; embryonal malignancies, including medulloblastoma and neuroblastoma, develop typically in children.

- Therapeutic ionizing radiation is the only proven cause of brain cancer. The use of mobile phones remains under investigation.

- Glioblastomas are the most common and most malignant central nervous system neoplasms. Most of them (90%) manifest after a short clinical history in elderly patients (mean age, 60 years). Genetic hallmarks include *EGFR* amplification and *PTEN* mutations.

- Secondary glioblastomas develop in younger patients (mean age, 45 years) through progression from low-grade or anaplastic astrocytoma. Genetic hallmarks include *IDH1* and *TP53* mutations. Distinguishing genetic alterations have been identified for other nervous system tumours, including oligodendroglioma and ependymoma.

- A range of targeted agents have been indicated, but establishment of optimal therapy has not been achieved. At present, the prognosis for most patients with brain cancer is poor.

Brain tumours account for less than 2% of the overall human cancer burden. However, they cause significant morbidity, and for gliomas, the most common histological type of central nervous system neoplasms, the prognosis is still poor. This applies particularly to glioblastomas, the most common and most malignant brain tumours in adults. Malignant embryonal tumours typically manifest in children and occur in the central nervous system in the case of medulloblastoma, and in the sympathetic nervous system and adrenal glands in the case of neuroblastoma. Meningiomas originate in the meninges, the protective coverings of the brain, and are usually benign and are more common in women. The brain is also a common site of metastases, most often due to carcinomas of the breast and lung.

Etiology

With the exception of brain tumours associated with inherited cancer syndromes and causation by therapeutic irradiation, which accounts for very few cases, no causative environmental or lifestyle risk factor has been unequivocally identified.

Environmental factors

Therapeutic irradiation of the head and neck regions is known to have caused brain cancer. In particular,

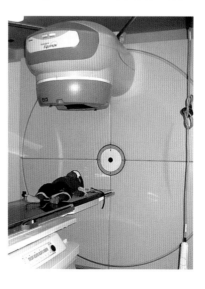

Fig. 5.16.1. Protocols for therapeutic irradiation of children now recognize the inherent risk such radiation presents and are designed to minimize any such risk.

Epidemiology

Nervous system tumours

- Central nervous system tumours represent the 17th most common cancer worldwide, with an estimated 256 000 new cases annually. Rates tend to be higher in more developed countries and therefore, combined with the rather high case fatality rate, these cancers are the 12th most frequent cause of cancer-related death worldwide.

- Comparisons of rates internationally are hampered by under-reporting in many regions, and this may largely explain the low incidence and mortality rates observed in sub-Saharan Africa and some Asian countries.

- Incidence rates are highest in North America, Europe, and Australia, typically 4–8 new cases per 100 000 people annually, but are higher in some Nordic countries. In multi-ethnic communities, adults and children of African or Asian descent have an approximately 2-fold lower risk than people with European ancestry.

- The age distribution of brain tumours is bimodal, with a peak incidence in children and a second, larger peak in adults aged 45–70 years. Glioblastomas are more frequent in men, while benign meningiomas are significantly more common in women.

Map 5.16.1. Global distribution of estimated age-standardized (World) incidence rates (ASR) per 100 000, for tumours of the nervous system in men, 2012.

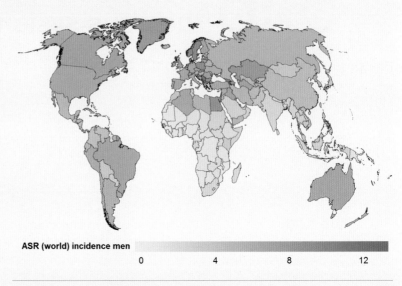

ASR (world) incidence men

0   4   8   12

Map 5.16.2. Global distribution of estimated age-standardized (World) incidence rates (ASR) per 100 000, for tumours of the nervous system in women, 2012.

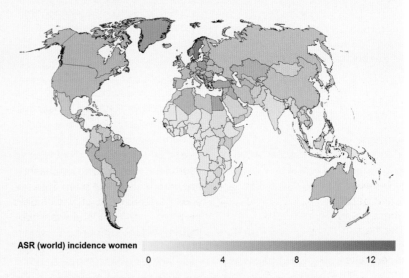

ASR (world) incidence women

0   4   8   12

For more details about the maps and charts presented in this chapter, see "A guide to the epidemiology data in *World Cancer Report*".

children treated with radiotherapy for acute myeloid leukaemia show a significantly elevated risk of developing malignant gliomas, often within 10 years [1]. Radiation-induced meningiomas may follow low-dose irradiation for tinea capitis, a fungal infection of the scalp, and high-dose irradiation for primary brain tumours.

A recent systematic review of eight cohort studies assessing the relationship between ionizing radiation and risk of brain tumours showed that the strength of the association varied between studies and that ionizing radiation was generally more strongly associated with risk of meningioma than with risk of glioma [2].

Electromagnetic fields

Exposure to occupational and residential power-frequency electromagnetic fields has been a subject of public concern. A weak association of brain tumours with occupational exposure to magnetic fields has been observed in some studies [3]; others failed to reveal a significantly

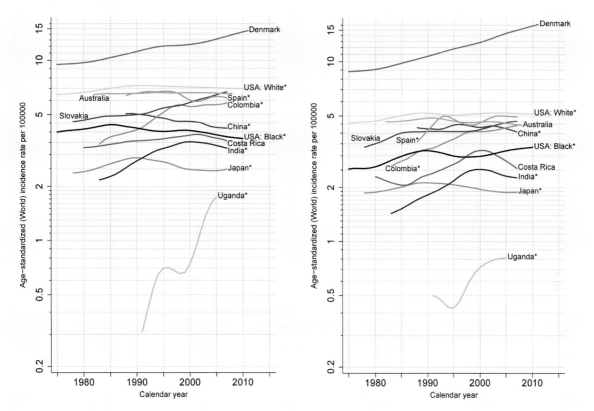

Chart 5.16.1. Age-standardized (World) incidence rates per 100 000 by year in selected populations, for tumours of the nervous system in men, circa 1975–2012.

Chart 5.16.2. Age-standardized (World) incidence rates per 100 000 by year in selected populations, for tumours of the nervous system in women, circa 1975–2012.

elevated risk [4]. The available evidence is insufficient to establish that electromagnetic fields cause brain tumours.

Mobile phones

No consistent association has been found between use of mobile (cell) phones and brain tumours [5–9]. The Interphone study [8] recorded no overall elevated odds ratio 10 years or less after first mobile phone use. In the 10th (highest) decile of recalled cumulative call time, the odds ratio was 1.40 (95% confidence interval [CI], 1.03–1.89) for glioma and 1.15 (95% CI, 0.81–1.62) for meningioma. The odds ratios for glioma were somewhat higher in the temporal lobe. Analysis of United States data indicated possible consistency with the modest excess risks observed in highly exposed people in the Interphone study [9]. In 2011, an IARC Monographs evaluation

determined that the evidence for causation of glioma by mobile phone use was *limited*, resulting in a classification as Group 2B (possibly carcinogenic to humans) [10]. The evidence for this association remains inconclusive because of, among other things, lack of data about long-term mobile phone use [11] (see "An IARC announcement that made waves" in Chapter 2.8).

Allergic conditions

Several studies suggest that having a personal medical history of specific allergic conditions, such as asthma, eczema, and hay fever, has a protective effect against development of glioma [12].

Environmental carcinogens

Several occupational exposures and environmental carcinogens have been reported to be slightly associated

with gliomagenesis. However, many of these reports have not been validated in independent studies, and none of these exposures has been unequivocally identified as causative [1]. Some studies suggest a causal relationship between parental occupational exposure to carcinogens and central nervous system tumours in their offspring, without identifying any specific environmental agent.

Diet

N-nitroso compounds have been detected in nitrite-preserved food and can be formed in the stomach after uptake of their chemical precursors, nitrate/nitrite and secondary amines. Vitamins C and E inhibit the formation of nitroso compounds from these precursors. Since some *N*-nitroso compounds are potent neurocarcinogens in experimental animals, several epidemiological studies have addressed their role in

Fig. 5.16.2. Macroscopic features of frequently occurring brain tumours.

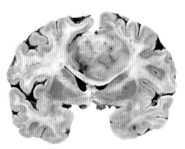

Diffuse astroctyoma

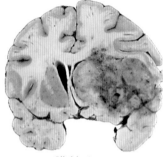

Glioblastoma

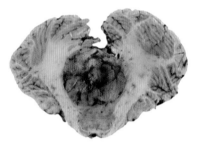

Medulloblastoma

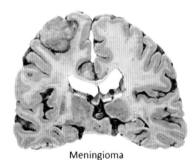

Meningioma

the etiology of human brain tumours. A meta-analysis of nine published studies yielded an elevated risk of glioma among adults frequently consuming cured meat, bacon, and ham, but the data were insufficient to establish a dose–response relationship [13].

Viral infections

JC virus has neuro-oncogenic potential in experimental animals, but JC virus sequences are rarely detectable in human brain tumours [14]. The polyomavirus SV40 was iatrogenically introduced into human populations in 1955–1962 through SV40-contaminated polio vaccines. SV40 sequences have been identified in a variety of human neoplasms, including brain tumours, raising the possibility of an etiological role [15]. SV40 sequences have been reported to be present at variable frequencies in brain tumour biopsies from countries that had used contaminated polio vaccine [14]. However, assays are easily contaminated with plasmids containing SV40 sequences, and recent studies

failed to detect SV40 sequences in brain tumours [16].

Genetic factors

Central nervous system tumours occur in the setting of several inherited cancer syndromes (Table 5.16.1). However, their overall contribution amounts to less than 1% of brain tumour cases.

Genetic basis of non-syndromic familial aggregation

There is a small but significant increased risk of primary brain tumours among relatives of patients with brain tumours. Cohort studies showed a standardized incidence ratio of approximately 2, i.e. a 2-fold increased risk of primary brain tumour or glioma among first-degree relatives of glioma probands, compared with population incidence data [17]. In a population-based study from Sweden and Norway, the standardized incidence ratio for glioma was 1.8 (95% CI, 1.5–2.0) when a parent was a proband, and increased to 11.2 (95% CI, 5.7–19.5) in multiplex families in which a

parent and at least two siblings were affected by a nervous system tumour [18]. A pooled familial aggregation analysis of glioma probands showed an increased risk of gliomas, sarcomas, and melanomas [19]. Genome-wide association studies have identified several low-penetrance susceptibility alleles for glioma [20,21].

Detection

Signs and symptoms of brain tumours largely depend on the location of the neoplasm and include paresis, speech disturbances, and personality changes. Patients with oligodendroglioma often have a long history of epileptic seizures. Eventually, malignant brain tumours cause life-threatening intracranial pressure that ultimately leads to unconsciousness and respiratory arrest. Since the brain does not contain pain receptors, headache is typically present if the tumour infiltrates the meninges. The presence of symptoms usually leads to a detailed neurological examination, using techniques such as computed tomography and magnetic resonance imaging.

Pathology and genetics

The *WHO Classification of Tumours of the Central Nervous System* (4th edition) recognizes more than 50 clinicopathological entities with a great variation in histology, biological behaviour, response to therapy, and clinical outcome [22]. Clinical and genetic data on the most common brain tumours are detailed in Table 5.16.2.

Astrocytic tumours

Tumours of astrocytic origin constitute the largest proportion of gliomas.

Pilocytic astrocytoma

Pilocytic astrocytoma (WHO grade I), the most common central nervous system neoplasm in children, is predominantly located in the cerebellum and midline structures, including the optic tract, brain stem, and spinal cord. It infiltrates adjacent brain structures but grows

Syndrome	Gene (chromosome)	Nervous system tumours	Other lesions
Neurofibromatosis type 1 (MIM no. 162200)	NF1 (17q11.2)	Neurofibroma, malignant peripheral nerve sheath tumour, optic nerve glioma, astrocytoma	Café au lait spots, axillary freckling, iris hamartomas, osseous lesions, phaeochromocytoma, leukaemia
Neurofibromatosis type 2 (MIM no. 101000)	NF2 (22q12)	Schwannoma, meningioma, meningioangiomatosis, spinal ependymoma, astrocytoma	Posterior lens opacities, retinal hamartoma
Tuberous sclerosis TSC1 and TSC2 (MIM no. 191100, 191092)	TSC1 (9q34) TSC2 (16p13.3)	Subependymal giant cell astrocytoma	Cutaneous angiofibroma, peau chagrin, subungual fibroma, cardiac rhabdomyoma, cysts of lung and kidney, renal angiomyolipoma
Li–Fraumeni syndrome (MIM no. 151623, 191170)	TP53 (17p13)	Astrocytoma, secondary glioblastoma, medulloblastoma	Adrenocortical carcinoma, soft tissue and bone sarcomas, leukaemia, breast carcinoma
Turcot syndrome type 1 (MIM no. 276300)	MLH1 (3p21) PMS2 (7p22) MSH2 (2p21)	Astrocytoma, glioblastoma	Café au lait spots Colorectal polyps (< 100) Large polyps (> 3 cm), colorectal cancer
Turcot syndrome type 2 (MIM no. 276300)	APC (5q21)	Medulloblastoma	Small colorectal polyps (> 100) Colorectal cancer
Naevoid basal cell carcinoma syndrome (NBCCS)/Gorlin syndrome (MIM no. 109400)	PTCH (9q22)	Medulloblastoma	Basal cell carcinomas, palmar and plantar pits, jaw cysts, ovarian fibroma, skeletal abnormalities
Rhabdoid tumour predisposition syndrome (RTPS) (MIM no. 609322)	INI1 (22q11.2)	Atypical teratoid/rhabdoid tumour (AT/RT)	Malignant rhabdoid tumour of the kidney

MIM, Mendelian Inheritance in Man (www.omim.org).

slowly and usually has a favourable prognosis, with 5-year survival rates of more than 85%. Some pilocytic astrocytomas occur in the setting of neurofibromatosis type 1 (NF1), particularly those of the optic nerve (optic glioma). Pilocytic astrocytomas typically show BRAF-KIAA1549 fusions [23].

Other types of astrocytoma (WHO grades II–IV) usually develop in the cerebral hemispheres of adults and diffusely infiltrate adjacent brain structures (diffuse astrocytomas).

Low-grade diffuse astrocytoma
Low-grade diffuse astrocytomas (WHO grade II) occur in young adults and grow slowly. However, they infiltrate adjacent brain structures and typically cannot be completely surgically resected. Morphologically, tumour cells resemble differentiated astrocytes. IDH1 or IDH2 mutations (> 80%), TP53 mutations (~65%), and ATRX mutations (65%) are early and frequent genetic events [24,25].

Anaplastic astrocytoma
Anaplastic astrocytomas (WHO grade III) often develop from low-grade astrocytomas, grow relatively quickly, and typically progress to glioblastoma within 2–3 years, accompanied by genetic alterations.

Glioblastoma
Glioblastoma (WHO grade IV) is the most frequent and most malignant nervous system tumour. Glioblastomas diffusely infiltrate the brain, including the opposite hemisphere, and show high cellularity and large areas of necrosis despite excessive vascular proliferation (Fig. 5.16.3).

Secondary glioblastomas develop by malignant progression from low-grade and anaplastic astrocytoma and are characterized by frequent IDH1 or IDH2 mutations, TP53 mutations, ATRX mutations, and loss of heterozygosity on chromosome 10q and 19p [26]. Primary glioblastomas are more frequent, accounting for approximately 90% of glioblastomas, and develop rapidly in older adults, with a short clinical history of usually less than 3 months (Fig. 5.16.4). Their genetic profile includes amplification and overexpression of the EGFR gene, PTEN mutations, TERT promoter mutations, and loss of heterozygosity on chromosome 10p and 10q [26,27].

Glioblastomas have also been classified on the basis of complementary DNA expression profiles, with distinct proneural, neural, classic, and mesenchymal patterns [28]. Secondary glioblastomas with

Table 5.16.2. Clinical and genetic data on the most common tumours of the nervous system

Tumour	Age (years)[a]	5-Year survival	Genetic alterations
Pilocytic astrocytoma (WHO grade I)	< 20	> 85%	*BRAF-KIAA1549* fusion, *NF1* mutation (neurofibromatosis cases)
Diffuse astrocytoma (WHO grade II)	20–45	> 60%	*IDH* mutation, *TP53* mutation, *ATRX* mutation
Secondary glioblastoma (WHO grade IV)	~45	~10%	*IDH* mutation, *TP53* mutation, *ATRX* mutation, LOH 10q, LOH 19q
Primary glioblastoma (WHO grade IV)	~60	< 3%	*EGFR* amplification, *PTEN* mutation, LOH 10p, LOH 10q
Oligodendroglioma (WHO grade II/III)	> 20	> 50%	*IDH* mutation, 1p and 19q co-deletion, *CIC* mutation, *FUBP1* mutation
Ependymoma (WHO grade II)	< 45	< 30%	Chromosome 22 alteration, *NF2* mutation
Medulloblastoma (WHO grade IV)	< 20	> 50%	Isochromosome 17, *TP53* mutation, *PTCH* mutation, β-catenin mutation, *DDX3X* mutation, *SMARCA4* mutation
Neuroblastoma (WHO grade IV)	< 10	> 90%; 20–50%[b]	LOH 1p, LOH 11q, *MYCN* amplification, trisomy 17q, *ALK* mutation

LOH, loss of heterozygosity.
[a] Age range in which 60% or more of the respective tumour types are clinically manifested.
[b] Patients < 1 year old; patients > 1 year old.

IDH1 mutation have a proneural expression profile. Additional genetic changes typical of the proneural type include *PDGFR* amplification or *PIK3CA/PIK3R1* mutations and loss or mutation of *TP53* [29]. The neural subtype is related to the classic expression pattern, which shows chromosome 7 amplification, focal *CDKN2A* deletion, chromosome 10 loss, and *EGFR* amplification or mutation. The mesenchymal subtype has frequent mutation or loss of *NF1*, *TP53*, and *PTEN*, and further chromosomal aberrations at *CDK6*, *MET*, *PTEN*, *CDKN2A*, and *RB1* loci [29].

New drivers of glioblastoma have been identified [30]. *LZTR1* and *CTNND2* mutations and deletions, and *EGFR-SEPT14* gene fusions are proposed to all enhance the self-renewal and transformation of glioblastoma stem cells, thereby contributing to glioblastoma progression.

Key genomic alterations in glioblastoma suggest a range of targeted agents (Fig. 5.16.5). Particular pathways may be identified as a basis for therapy (see "Glioma genomics and its implications in neuro-oncology"). The role of the alkylation-damage DNA repair gene *MGMT* in mediating response of malignant glioma to alkylating agents such as temozolomide has been clarified. Two randomized trials demonstrated that patients with an epigenetically silenced *MGMT* gene fared better when treated with temozolomide, whereas patients with an unmethylated *MGMT* promoter had a longer survival with initial radiotherapy [31].

Oligodendroglial tumours

These neoplasms are assumed to develop from myelin-producing oligodendroglial cells or their precursors and are typically found in the cerebral hemispheres of adults, often including the basal ganglia. Histologically, they are isomorphic, with a typical honeycomb pattern and delicate tumour vessels (a "chicken wire" pattern). Anaplastic oligodendrogliomas show features of anaplasia and high mitotic activity and have a less favourable prognosis. Oligodendrogliomas share with diffuse astrocytomas common and frequent genetic alterations, i.e. *IDH1* or *IDH2* mutations, suggesting that astrocytomas and oligodendrogliomas arise from the same precursor cells. Genetic hallmarks of oligodendrogliomas are frequent *IDH1* or *IDH2* mutations (> 80%), co-deletion of chromosomes 1p and 19q (~70%), *CIC* mutations (~40%), and *FUBP1* mutations (~15%) [26].

Ependymomas

These gliomas develop from the ependymal lining of the cerebral ventricles and the central canal of the spinal cord. They manifest preferentially in children and young adults. Histologically, they are cellular, with typical perivascular rosettes. Spinal ependymomas show a high frequency of mutations in the neurofibromatosis gene *NF2* [22].

Glioneuronal tumours

This group of brain tumours is less frequent and generally has a favourable prognosis. Some manifest preferentially in children (desmoplastic infantile astrocytoma/ganglioglioma, dysembryoplastic neuroepithelial tumour), others preferentially in adolescents and adults (gangliocytoma, central neurocytoma). They often cause a long-term history of epileptic seizures [22].

Embryonal tumours

These neoplasms are derived from embryonal or fetal precursor cells,

Fig. 5.16.3. Typical histological features of glioblastoma, with necrosis (NE) and vascular proliferation (VP).

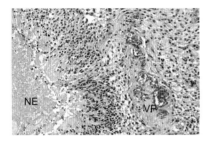

typically manifest in children, and are highly malignant but often respond to radiotherapy or chemotherapy. In the central nervous system, cerebellar medulloblastomas are the most common. The peak incidence age is 3–6 years; these tumours are uncommon in adults. Expression array analysis and DNA sequencing have led to the identification of four distinct subgroups, which differ greatly in clinical outcome [32,33]. The most benign course is seen in medulloblastomas with activation of the WNT pathway, as determined by nuclear β-catenin accumulation, and the presence of *CTNNB1* mutations in most cases [34]. The WNT subtype shows classic medulloblastoma histology and cannot be identified morphologically. The SHH type is biologically characterized by activation of the sonic hedgehog (SHH) signalling pathway, which in about one third of cases is caused by a mutation in the *PTCH* gene [35]. This subtype tends to be associated with the desmoplastic phenotype [36]. Type 3 medulloblastomas are not associated with a distinct signalling pathway, but they typically show NPR3 expression and *MYC* amplification. Type 4 medulloblastomas comprise about one third of all medulloblastomas and have a less favourable clinical outcome. Type 3 and 4 medulloblastomas are characterized by a strong male predominance and a greater tendency to metastasize via cerebrospinal fluid pathways.

Tumours of peripheral nerves

Most of these tumours develop from myelin-producing Schwann cells and are termed neurinomas or schwannomas. Bilateral acoustic schwannomas are diagnostic of inherited neurofibromatosis type 2 (NF2). Acoustic schwannomas are benign (WHO grade I) and rarely recur after surgical resection. Neurofibromas and malignant peripheral nerve sheath tumours represent typical manifestations of the NF1 syndrome [22].

Meningiomas

These are generally benign, slowly growing intracranial tumours attached to the dura mater. They are composed of neoplastic meningothelial (arachnoidal) cells and typically occur in adults, with a marked female predominance, particularly for those located in the spine. Meningiomas do not infiltrate the brain but may cause symptoms of intracranial pressure due to compression of adjacent brain structures. Preferential sites

Fig. 5.16.4. (A) Rapid evolution of a primary glioblastoma. Magnetic resonance image shows a small cortical lesion that within 68 days developed into a full-blown glioblastoma with perifocal oedema and central necrosis. This is in contrast to (B) the development of a secondary glioblastoma through progression from low-grade astrocytoma.

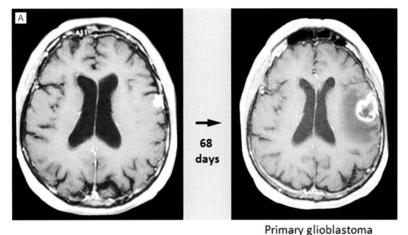

68 days

Primary glioblastoma
WHO grade IV

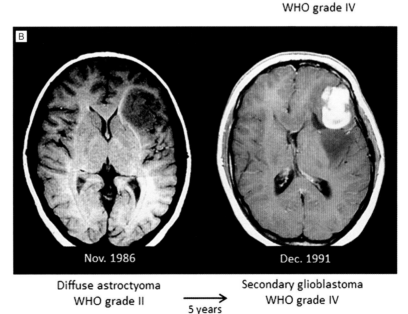

Nov. 1986

Dec. 1991

Diffuse astroctyoma
WHO grade II

5 years

Secondary glioblastoma
WHO grade IV

Glioma genomics and its implications in neuro-oncology

Hai Yan

Mutations in the critical chromatin modifier *ATRX* and mutations in *CIC* and *FUBP1*, which are potent regulators of cell growth, have been discovered in specific subtypes of gliomas, the most common type of primary malignant brain tumour. However, the frequency of these mutations in many subtypes of gliomas, and their association with the clinical features of patients, is poorly understood. These loci were analysed in 363 brain tumours. *ATRX* is frequently mutated in grade II/III astrocytomas (71%), oligoastrocytomas (68%), and secondary glioblastomas (57%), and *ATRX* mutations are associated with *IDH1* mutations and with the alternative lengthening

of telomeres phenotype. *CIC* and *FUBP1* mutations occurred frequently in oligodendrogliomas (46% and 24%, respectively) but rarely in astrocytomas or oligoastrocytomas (< 10%). This analysis enabled the identification of two highly recurrent genetic signatures in gliomas: *IDH1/ATRX* (I-A) and *IDH1/CIC/FUBP1* (I-CF).

Patients with I-CF gliomas had a significantly longer median overall survival (96 months) compared with patients with I-A gliomas (51 months) and patients with gliomas that did not harbour either signature (13 months). The genetic signatures distinguished clinically distinct groups of oligoastrocytoma

patients, who usually present a diagnostic challenge, and were associated with differences in clinical outcome even among individual tumour types. In addition to providing new clues about the genetic alterations underlying gliomas, the results have immediate clinical implications, providing a tripartite genetic signature that can serve as a useful adjunct to conventional glioma classification and that may aid in prognosis, treatment selection, and therapeutic trial design.

Reference

Duncan CG et al. (2012). Genome Res, 22:2339–2355. http://dx.doi.org/10.1101/gr.132 738.111 PMID:22899282

---

are the cerebral hemispheres [22]. Meningiomas can often be cured by surgical resection. Atypical or malignant meningiomas are less frequent (~5% of all meningiomas) (http://www.cbtrus.org) and may infiltrate the brain and often recur locally.

Neuroblastomas

This tumour develops from the primitive neural crest and is the most frequent neoplasm in children younger than 1 year, with an incidence of approximately 1 per 100 000. It is typically located in the adrenal gland and sympathetic nervous system and is responsible for up to 15% of all cancer deaths in children. Neuroblastomas are heterogeneous with respect to the degree of maturation, ranging from highly malignant examples to benign ganglioneuroma.

More than 60% of neuroblastomas are metastatic, often carrying *MYCN* amplification or *ATRX* mutation, and/or *ALK* mutation. Neuroblastoma can evade T cells and natural killer cells. Anti-GD2 antibodies, when combined with

granulocyte-macrophage colony-stimulating factor with or without interleukin-2, offer strategies for

a curative approach to therapy. Neuroblastomas with single copy *MYCN* or similar indicators are

Fig. 5.16.5. Cell-cycle dysregulation in glioblastoma is in part a result of abnormal signalling by several different receptor tyrosine kinases (RTKs), including EGFR, PDGFR, and MET. Genes shown in red may be targeted by agents, including RTK inhibitors. (For details, see [29].)

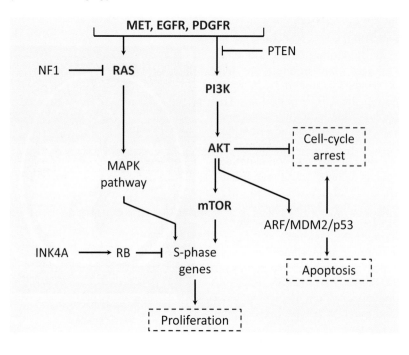

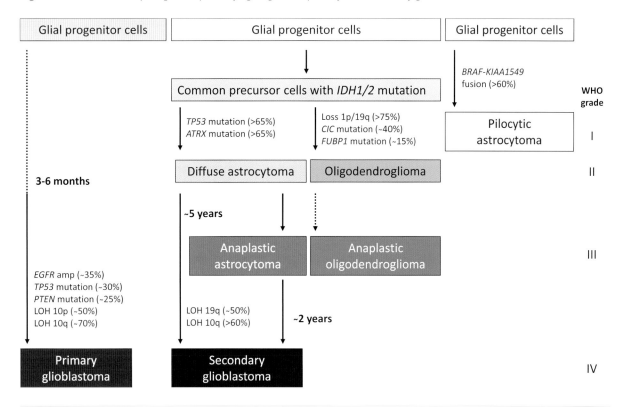

highly curable with surgery alone or with surgery and low-dose chemotherapy [37].

Prospects

Although brain tumours do not occur very frequently, they contribute significantly to morbidity, often affect children, and have an overall poor prognosis. Due to marked resistance to radiation and chemotherapy, the prognosis for patients with glioblastomas, the most common type of malignant brain tumour in adults, is still very poor. Unfortunately no environmental, lifestyle, or genetic risk factor has been discovered that accounts for a significant proportion of newly diagnosed brain tumours. Many genetic alterations involved in the development of nervous system tumours have been identified and may lead to novel targeted therapeutic approaches.

References

1. Ohgaki H, Kleihues P (2005). Epidemiology and etiology of gliomas. *Acta Neuropathol*, 109:93–108. http://dx.doi.org/10.1007/s00401-005-0991-y PMID:15685439

2. Braganza MZ, Kitahara CM, Berrington de González A *et al.* (2012). Ionizing radiation and the risk of brain and central nervous system tumors: a systematic review. *Neuro Oncol*, 14:1316–1324. http://dx.doi.org/10.1093/neuonc/nos208 PMID:22952197

3. Villeneuve PJ, Agnew DA, Johnson KC, Mao Y; Canadian Cancer Registries Epidemiology Research Group (2002). Brain cancer and occupational exposure to magnetic fields among men: results from a Canadian population-based case-control study. *Int J Epidemiol*, 31:210–217. http://dx.doi.org/10.1093/ije/31.1.210 PMID:11914323

4. Thériault G, Goldberg M, Miller AB *et al.* (1994). Cancer risks associated with occupational exposure to magnetic fields among electric utility workers in Ontario and Quebec, Canada, and France: 1970–1989. *Am J Epidemiol*, 139:550–572. PMID:8172168

5. Hardell L, Mild KH, Carlberg M (2002). Case-control study on the use of cellular and cordless phones and the risk for malignant brain tumours. *Int J Radiat Biol*, 78:931–936. http://dx.doi.org/10.1080/09553000210158038 PMID:12465658

6. Inskip PD, Tarone RE, Hatch EE *et al.* (2001). Cellular-telephone use and brain tumors. *N Engl J Med*, 344:79–86. http://dx.doi.org/10.1056/NEJM200101113440201 PMID:11150357

7. Christensen HC, Schüz J, Kosteljanetz M *et al.* (2005). Cellular telephones and risk for brain tumors: a population-based, incident case-control study. *Neurology*, 64:1189–1195. http://dx.doi.org/10.1212/01.WNL.0000156351.72313.D3 PMID:15824345

8. INTERPHONE Study Group (2010). Brain tumour risk in relation to mobile telephone use: results of the INTERPHONE international case-control study. *Int J Epidemiol*, 39:675–694. http://dx.doi.org/10.1093/ije/dyq079 PMID:20483835

9. Little MP, Rajaraman P, Curtis RE *et al.* (2012). Mobile phone use and glioma risk: comparison of epidemiological study results with incidence trends in the United States. *BMJ*, 344:e1147. http://dx.doi.org/10.1136/bmj.e1147 PMID:22403263

10. Baan R, Grosse Y, Lauby-Secretan B *et al.*; WHO International Agency for Research on Cancer Monograph Working Group (2011). Carcinogenicity of radiofrequency electromagnetic fields. *Lancet Oncol*, 12:624–626. http://dx.doi.org/10.1016/S1470-2045(11)70147-4 PMID:21845765

11. Ostrom QT, Barnholtz-Sloan JS (2011). Current state of our knowledge on brain tumor epidemiology. *Curr Neurol Neurosci Rep*, 11:329–335. http://dx.doi.org/10.1007/s11910-011-0189-8 PMID:21336822

12. Chen C, Xu T, Chen J *et al.* (2011). Allergy and risk of glioma: a meta-analysis. *Eur J Neurol*, 18:387–395. http://dx.doi.org/10.1111/j.1468-1331.2010.03187.x PMID:20722711

13. Huncharek M, Kupelnick B, Wheeler L (2003). Dietary cured meat and the risk of adult glioma: a meta-analysis of nine observational studies. *J Environ Pathol Toxicol Oncol*, 22:129–137. PMID:14533876

14. Huang H, Reis R, Yonekawa Y *et al.* (1999). Identification in human brain tumors of DNA sequences specific for SV40 large T antigen. *Brain Pathol*, 9:33–42. http://dx.doi.org/10.1111/j.1750-3639.1999.tb00207.x PMID:9989448

15. Vilchez RA, Kozinetz CA, Arrington AS *et al.* (2003). Simian virus 40 in human cancers. *Am J Med*, 114:675–684. http://dx.doi.org/10.1016/S0002-9343(03)00087-1 PMID:12798456

16. Rollison DE, Utaipat U, Ryschkewitsch C *et al.* (2005). Investigation of human brain tumors for the presence of polyomavirus genome sequences by two independent laboratories. *Int J Cancer*, 113:769–774. http://dx.doi.org/10.1002/ijc.20641 PMID:15499616

17. Malmer B, Adatto P, Armstrong G *et al.* (2007). GLIOGENE – an international consortium to understand familial glioma. *Cancer Epidemiol Biomarkers Prev*, 16:1730–1734. http://dx.doi.org/10.1158/1055-9965.EPI-07-0081 PMID:17855690

18. Hemminki K, Tretli S, Sundquist J *et al.* (2009). Familial risks in nervous-system tumours: a histology-specific analysis from Sweden and Norway. *Lancet Oncol*, 10:481–488. http://dx.doi.org/10.1016/S1470-2045(09)70076-2 PMID:19356978

19. Scheurer ME, Etzel CJ, Liu M *et al.*; GLIOGENE Consortium (2010). Familial aggregation of glioma: a pooled analysis. *Am J Epidemiol*, 172:1099–1107. http://dx.doi.org/10.1093/aje/kwq261 PMID:20858744

20. Wrensch M, Jenkins RB, Chang JS *et al.* (2009). Variants in the *CDKN2B* and *RTEL1* regions are associated with high-grade glioma susceptibility. *Nat Genet*, 41:905–908. http://dx.doi.org/10.1038/ng.408 PMID:19578366

21. Liu Y, Shete S, Hosking FJ *et al.* (2010). New insights into susceptibility to glioma. *Arch Neurol*, 67:275–278. http://dx.doi.org/10.1001/archneurol.2010.4 PMID:20212223

22. Louis DN, Ohgaki H, Wiestler OD, Cavenee WK, eds (2007). *WHO Classification of Tumours of the Central Nervous System*, 4th ed. Lyon: IARC.

23. Korshunov A, Meyer J, Capper D *et al.* (2009). Combined molecular analysis of *BRAF* and *IDH1* distinguishes pilocytic astrocytoma from diffuse astrocytoma. *Acta Neuropathol*, 118:401–405. http://dx.doi.org/10.1007/s00401-009-0550-z PMID:19543740

24. Liu XY, Gerges N, Korshunov A *et al.* (2012). Frequent *ATRX* mutations and loss of expression in adult diffuse astrocytic tumors carrying *IDH1/IDH2* and *TP53* mutations. *Acta Neuropathol*, 124:615–625. http://dx.doi.org/10.1007/s00401-012-1031-3 PMID:22886134

25. Jiao Y, Killela PJ, Reitman ZJ *et al.* (2012). Frequent *ATRX*, *CIC*, *FUBP1* and *IDH1* mutations refine the classification of malignant gliomas. *Oncotarget*, 3:709–722. PMID:22869205

26. Ohgaki H, Kleihues P (2013). The definition of primary and secondary glioblastoma. *Clin Cancer Res*, 19:764–772. http://dx.doi.org/10.1158/1078-0432.CCR-12-3002 PMID:23209033

27. Killela PJ, Reitman ZJ, Jiao Y *et al.* (2013). *TERT* promoter mutations occur frequently in gliomas and a subset of tumors derived from cells with low rates of self-renewal. *Proc Natl Acad Sci U S A*, 110:6021–6026. http://dx.doi.org/10.1073/pnas.1303607110 PMID:23530248

28. Phillips HS, Kharbanda S, Chen R *et al.* (2006). Molecular subclasses of high-grade glioma predict prognosis, delineate a pattern of disease progression, and resemble stages in neurogenesis. *Cancer Cell*, 9:157–173. http://dx.doi.org/10.1016/j.ccr.2006.02.019 PMID:16530701

29. Kotliarova S, Fine HA (2012). SnapShot: glioblastoma multiforme. *Cancer Cell*, 21:710, e1. http://dx.doi.org/10.1016/j.ccr.2012.04.031 PMID:22624719

30. Frattini V, Trifonov V, Chan JM *et al.* (2013). The integrated landscape of driver genomic alterations in glioblastoma. *Nat Genet*, 45:1141–1149. http://dx.doi.org/10.1038/ng.2734 PMID:23917401

31. Stupp R, Hegi ME (2013). Brain cancer in 2012: molecular characterization leads the way. *Nat Rev Clin Oncol*, 10:69–70. http://dx.doi.org/10.1038/nrclinonc.2012.240 PMID:23296110

32. Kool M, Korshunov A, Remke M *et al.* (2012). Molecular subgroups of medulloblastoma: an international meta-analysis of transcriptome, genetic aberrations, and clinical data of WNT, SHH, Group 3, and Group 4 medulloblastomas. *Acta Neuropathol*, 123:473–484. http://dx.doi.org/10.1007/s00401-012-0958-8 PMID:22358457

33. Northcott PA, Korshunov A, Pfister SM, Taylor MD (2012). The clinical implications of medulloblastoma subgroups. *Nat Rev Neurol*, 8:340–351. http://dx.doi.org/10.1038/nrneurol.2012.78 PMID:22565209

34. Ellison DW, Onilude OE, Lindsey JC *et al.*; United Kingdom Children's Cancer Study Group Brain Tumour Committee (2005). β-Catenin status predicts a favorable outcome in childhood medulloblastoma: the United Kingdom Children's Cancer Study Group Brain Tumour Committee. *J Clin Oncol*, 23:7951–7957. http://dx.doi.org/10.1200/JCO.2005.01.5479 PMID:16258095

35. Schwalbe EC, Lindsey JC, Straughton D *et al.* (2011). Rapid diagnosis of medulloblastoma molecular subgroups. *Clin Cancer Res*, 17:1883–1894. http://dx.doi.org/10.1158/1078-0432.CCR-10-2210 PMID:21325292

36. Pietsch T, Waha A, Koch A *et al.* (1997). Medulloblastomas of the desmoplastic variant carry mutations of the human homologue of *Drosophila patched*. *Cancer Res*, 57:2085–2088. PMID:9187099

37. Cheung NK, Dyer MA (2013). Neuroblastoma: developmental biology, cancer genomics and immunotherapy. *Nat Rev Cancer*, 13:397–411. http://dx.doi.org/10.1038/nrc3526 PMID:23702928

Barnett S. Kramer

Controversies in cancer screening and their resolution: a view from the United States "battleground"

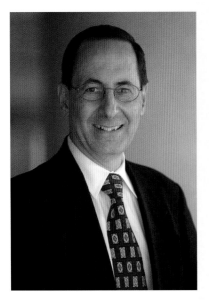

Barnett "Barry" S. Kramer is the director of the Division of Cancer Prevention at the United States National Cancer Institute (NCI) and serves as editor-in-chief of NCI's Physician Data Query (PDQ) Screening and Prevention Editorial Board. Board-certified in internal medicine and medical oncology, Dr Kramer earned his medical degree from the University of Maryland Medical School and also holds a master's degree in public health from Johns Hopkins University's Bloomberg School of Public Health. Dr Kramer has extensive experience in primary cancer prevention studies as well as clinical screening trials of lung, ovarian, breast, and prostate cancers. From 1994 to 2012, he was editor-in-chief of the Journal of the National Cancer Institute. *Dr Kramer's long-standing interest in the challenges of reporting medical research led him to create the Medicine in the Media Workshop to help train journalists to review medical findings critically and to report them accurately.*

Summary

Cancer screening controversies have raged for a long time. However, there are paths forward that could modulate the content and tone of the discussions. They involve use of emerging molecular techniques to help us refine our assessment of screen-detected cancers, professional education, and more nuanced information for the public. Time will tell if such strategies provide resolutions to the controversies.

Cancer screening is one of the most contentious areas in medicine. Debates over the balance of benefits and harms of screening tests play out at national conferences, in the medical literature, in the media, and occasionally in Congress. The intuitive sense that detection of asymptomatic cancers must necessarily be of benefit is strong, sometimes triggering arguments when the benefits of screening are questioned or harms are reported.

The concept that early detection of cancer before clinically evident symptomatic presentation would lead to cure in the majority of cases has its origins more than a century ago. In 1907 Dr Charles Childe, in his book *The Control of a Scourge,*

or How Cancer is Curable, asserted that if people were to only heed the earliest, apparently trivial, symptoms or signs of cancer, "it requires no stretch of the imagination... to say that the majority... would be cured" [1]. In 1924, Dr Joseph Colt Bloodgood of Johns Hopkins Hospital was quoted in the *New York Times* as stating that "deaths from cancer would be practically eliminated" by a careful search for "growths in any part of the body" [2]. (In retrospect, we now know how far off the mark these assertions were.) Nevertheless, the allure of the logic remains strong, and often independent of the actual evidence for several screening tests in common use. But the concept is easy to grasp by health professionals and the public alike. Public health messages have frequently been unequivocal, often at the expense of appropriate nuance [3]. Some cancer advocacy groups have focused on screening as the most important tool in the "war on cancer", sometimes spawning health fairs dedicated to screening as many people as possible [4,5].

The screening message has taken hold, at least in the USA. Data from the United States National Health Interview Survey (NHIS) from 2005 and 2008 indicate that high rates of cancer screening persist even among people aged 80 years and older – a population unlikely to derive substantial benefit from screening but nevertheless at risk for all of the harms. More than 50% of the respondents aged 75 years and older reported that their physician continued to actively recommend screening [6]. Perhaps even more strikingly, an analysis of the Surveillance, Epidemiology and End Results (SEER)-Medicare database showed that a sizeable proportion of patients aged 65 years and older already diagnosed with advanced incurable lung, colorectal, pancreatic, gastrointestinal, or breast cancers (with a median survival time of 4.3–16.2 months) were still being screened with mammography, Pap tests, prostate-specific antigen (PSA) tests, and lower gastrointestinal endoscopy [7]. The assumption of benefit is so strong that the motives of anyone who raises the possibility of screening-associated harms are sometimes attacked. For example, a mammographer recently dismissed a study suggesting that the harms of breast cancer screening due to overdetection of non-life-threatening lesions ("overdiagnosis") have been underestimated [8] as "malicious nonsense" driven simply by a desire to reduce health-care costs [9]. But the genesis of the disagreements goes beyond financial incentives on either side of the argument.

The numerator/denominator problem

Public health is in some sense a science of the denominator (the general population), while clinical medicine is a science of the numerator (people plucked out of the denominator to become patients). Each of the two disciplines has separate training programmes, and the respective trainees acquire distinctly different heuristics and mental shortcuts when interpreting and applying evidence [10]. The target population is usually the relatively healthy general population, but the testing generally takes place in a clinical setting. Cancer screening therefore sits at the interface between these two

worlds, inviting a clash of philosophies that are anchored in totally different worlds.

Health-care professionals are strongly influenced by personal experience, and that is as it should be. Cumulative experience is a core element in the evolution of clinical judgement. However, it has been shown empirically that personal experience can also distort diagnostic reasoning, termed "availability bias" [11]. Cancer specialists, who treat the numerator of cancer patients, witness the suffering of their patients on a daily basis and naturally embrace strategies that could prevent that suffering, even if not based on the strongest achievable evidence. In fact, they may be impatient with public health-oriented professionals, who demand high-quality evidence before making recommendations that affect hundreds of thousands or even millions of healthy people. One of the core principles of cancer screening and prevention is that it is difficult to make healthy people better off than they already are – but not difficult to make them worse off. This numerator/denominator issue also probably accounts for the fact that clinical specialty societies frequently have more aggressive screening recommendations than do general practice specialties [12].

A similar phenomenon occurs in the public. Healthy people inhabit the denominator, not generally knowing which numerator(s) they will ultimately enter. However, the diagnosis of cancer suddenly changes that perspective. Here, availability bias is particularly personal, bringing a desire to benefit others with the newly acquired perspective. Cancer advocacy groups often have more aggressive approaches to screening for cancer than do broad-based health advocacy groups.

Direct experience may distort perceived outcomes of screening

However, there is more than availability bias at work in the clinical setting. Personal experience may

more directly affect a clinician's perceptions of the value of screening, both increasing the magnitude of perceived benefits and decreasing perceived harms [13,14]. Several well-known biases artefactually amplify the apparent benefit of a cancer screening test, and may even make a completely ineffective test appear highly effective in the eyes of an individual clinician. The ultimate benefit of a screening test is determined by its effect on overall or disease-specific mortality, but individual clinicians cannot observe mortality changes in practice. They do, however, directly observe the survival of their patients after diagnosis, and these observations can seriously mislead.

People self-select for screening, introducing confounding factors that are associated both with the propensity to be screened and with favourable health outcomes independent of the actual screening – an effect known as healthy volunteer bias or healthy screenee bias. For example, the number of observed deaths from a variety of causes unrelated to the target cancers was substantially less than expected in participants in a large randomized screening trial for prostate, lung, colorectal, and ovarian cancers [15]. This reduction even extended to deaths from accidents or poisoning, highly unlikely to be affected by the actual screening tests.

Lead-time bias occurs with every screening test because the date of diagnosis of screen-detected cancers is moved up, lengthening the apparent survival time even if the date and cause of death are unaltered. For example, if a cancer killed all of its victims on the fourth anniversary of diagnosis, the 5-year survival would be zero. If a new (but ineffective) screening test advanced the date of diagnosis by 3 years without changing the risk of death, the 5-year survival rate would be 100%. Such a dramatic increase in survival time would make most clinicians true believers in the test.

Most, if not all, cancer screening tests are also associated with length-biased sampling. This occurs because they are better at detecting slow-growing asymptomatic cancers than they are at picking up the most rapidly growing tumours that come to clinical attention between scheduled screenings, even when adjusted for clinical stage and histopathological phenotypic features [16]. An extreme form of length-biased sampling, over-diagnosis, is the detection of tumours that are so slow-growing that they would not have caused any harm during the lifespan of the patient. Without screening, the patient would have gone on to die of a competing cause of death without ever being labelled as a cancer patient. Empirical evidence for detection-related over-diagnosis has been shown for a wide variety of cancers, including melanoma and cancers of the thyroid, prostate, kidney, and breast [8,17]. Since cancer is primarily a disease of ageing, during a period of life in which competing causes of death increase in incidence, cancer screening is particularly prone to overdiagnosis. However, screening has even been shown to produce overdiagnosis in the case of neuroblastoma, a disease of infancy (reviewed in [18]). The effect is not only to increase the survival rate but also to increase the cure rate. After all, it is easiest to "cure" patients who did not need to be treated in the first place.

All of these biases inflate survival rates in association with screening independent of the actual effect of a screening test on mortality. In fact, it has been shown empirically that increasing 5-year survival rates in the USA from 1950 to 1995 and changes in mortality rates for the same cancers had little or no relationship (Pearson $r = 0.00$) [19]. In other words, survival is an unreliable measure of success, whether judged at the individual or population level, when a screening test is involved.

Since survival time after diagnosis, rather than mortality, is the only observation that a physician can directly make, even astute clinicians such as Drs Childe and Bloodgood may be misled by their own careful observations and experience. In fact, surveys show that most primary care physicians erroneously interpret improved survival in association with screening as evidence that screening saves lives [20].

Likewise, patients who undergo screening may interpret observations from their own experience as evidence of benefit, whether or not the screening test is effective. A negative test provides reassurance. A false-positive test brings immense relief when cancer is ruled out. A true-positive test triggers gratitude towards the physician for ordering the test and detecting the cancer early (even if it is nothing more than a case of overdiagnosis). Even severe side-effects of therapy are judged to be worthwhile by both patient and physician. If the patient still goes on to die of cancer, the physician and family alike can feel reassured that everything possible was done. In essence, there is little or no negative feedback [21].

Little wonder that so much scepticism and vitriol is aimed at authors of research papers or media reports that question the net benefits of some screening tests. The reports seem to run counter to personal experience on the part of both the public and physicians. The result is cognitive dissonance, which breeds anxiety, a progenitor of anger.

Are there resolutions to the controversy?

Potential resolutions map to the genesis of the controversies described above: (1) imprecise understanding of the biology of many screen-detected cancers, (2) insufficient training to recognize the powerful biases that affect interpretation of personal experience, and (3) inadequate nuance and framing of messages about screening.

Towards a better understanding of biology

Traditional staging and prognostic systems such as tumour–node–metastasis (TNM) classification and histological grading are crude, providing insufficient guidance in discerning overdiagnosis at the individual level. Therefore, the patient and physician may feel driven to treat all or most screen-detected cancers, even if that means unnecessary treatment or overtreatment in many cases. Some of the controversies would be calmed if there were more reliable ways to distinguish screen-detected cancers that are aggressive from those that would not cause harm, reserving treatment for the former. This approach is implicit in the use of active surveillance for screen-detected prostate cancer and neuroblastoma [22–24]. However, prediction at the individual level for most cancers is too crude for comfort.

One strategy would be to use emerging molecular techniques to characterize screen-detected lesions. This research strategy is under way within the Early Detection Research Network of the United States National Cancer Institute (http://edrn.nci.nih.gov/). An example of a prospective design would be to characterize tumours from patients with screen-detected prostate cancer who are undergoing serial biopsies as part of active surveillance. Cross-sectional designs may also provide initial insights if tumour specimens are accurately annotated with respect to method of diagnosis: screen-detected versus symptomatic interval cancers in people being actively screened. Screen-detected cancers are, on average, less aggressive tumours compared with symptomatic interval cancers, and their molecular patterns can be compared. Finally, rapid autopsy studies to find sub-clinical cancers in people who died of causes unrelated to cancer could be used to characterize the reservoir of cancers that could be overdiagnosed by screening. With better molecular characterization of over-diagnosed cancers, any benefits of screening could be preserved while harms would be minimized.

Improvements in professional training

Formal training that covers the strong screening-related biases that distort clinical observation (and non-randomized screening studies) could better prepare health professionals to judge the value of screening tests and to evaluate published studies, damping down the cognitive dissonance created by personal experience. Such training is best begun early in medical training, before specialty-associated heuristics become imprinted. Additional public health and epidemiology training during medical school could alleviate some of the "numerator/denominator" tension.

Better framing of screening messages

The strength of screening messages should match the strength of evidence. We need to get beyond cancer screening campaigns that oversimplify the complexities of screening [3]. Cancer screening is often a closer call than can be described in sound bites. Informed decision-making, rather than persuasion, should be the goal. Likewise, the benefits of screening are most frequently described in relative terms. Empirical evidence, including randomized trials, has shown that the public develops a better grasp of the efficacy and harms of an intervention when they are presented in terms of absolute rates or frequencies [25,26]. The statement that a screening test for lung cancer has been shown to decrease lung cancer mortality by 20% is roughly equivalent to the statement that if 1000 heavy smokers and former smokers were to be screened annually for three screens, about 4 lung cancer deaths would be avoided over the next 6–7 years (the results of the National Lung Screening Trial comparing low-dose helical computed tomography [CT] with chest radiograph) [27]. However, the "feel" of the two methods of expressing the results is different, and the latter method is generally better incorporated into individual decision-making. An example of this method of presenting the results of the trial can be found at http://www.cancer.gov/newscenter/qa/2002/NLSTstudyGuidePatientsPhysicians.

Opinions expressed in this manuscript are those of the author and do not necessarily represent official positions of the United States federal government or of the Department of Health and Human Services.

References

1. Childe CP (1907). *The Control of a Scourge, or How Cancer Is Curable*. New York: Dutton.

2. [Anonymous]. Cure for cancer in prompt action; Dr. Bloodgood of Johns Hopkins declares elimination almost sure in early stage. *New York Times*, 8 June 1924, p. 25.

3. Woloshin S, Schwartz LM, Black WC, Kramer BS (2012). Cancer screening campaigns–getting past uninformative persuasion. *N Engl J Med*, 367:1677–1679. http://dx.doi.org/10.1056/NEJMp1209407 PMID:23113476

4. Lerner BH (2001). Seek and ye shall find: mammography praised and scorned. In: *The Breast Cancer Wars: Hope, Fear, and the Pursuit of a Cure in Twentieth-Century America*. New York: Oxford University Press, pp. 196–222.

5. Brawley OW, Goldberg P (2011). From the health fair. In: *How We Do Harm: A Doctor Breaks Ranks about Being Sick in America*. New York: St. Martin's Press, pp. 215–224.

6. Bellizzi KM, Breslau ES, Burness A, Waldron W (2011). Prevalence of cancer screening in older, racially diverse adults: still screening after all these years. *Arch Intern Med*, 171:2031–2037. http://dx.doi.org/10.1001/archinternmed.2011.570 PMID:22158573

7. Sima CS, Panageas KS, Schrag D (2010). Cancer screening among patients with advanced cancer. *JAMA*, 304:1584–1591. http://dx.doi.org/10.1001/jama.2010.1449 PMID:20940384

8. Bleyer A, Welch HG (2012). Effect of three decades of screening mammography on breast-cancer incidence. *N Engl J Med*, 367:1998–2005. http://dx.doi.org/10.1056/NEJMoa1206809 PMID:23171096

9. Morin M (2012). To screen or not to screen. *Los Angeles Times*, 21 November 2012.

10. Ferguson JH (1999). Curative and population medicine: bridging the great divide. *Neuroepidemiology*, 18:111–119. http://dx.doi.org/10.1159/000026202 PMID:10202265

11. Mamede S, van Gog T, van den Berge K *et al.* (2010). Effect of availability bias and reflective reasoning on diagnostic accuracy among internal medicine residents. *JAMA*, 304:1198–1203. http://dx.doi.org/10.1001/jama.2010.1276 PMID:20841533

12. Hoffman RM, Barry MJ, Roberts RG, Sox HC (2012). Reconciling primary care and specialist perspectives on prostate cancer screening. *Ann Fam Med*, 10:568–571. http://dx.doi.org/10.1370/afm.1399 PMID:23149535

13. Kramer BS, Croswell JM (2009). Cancer screening: the clash of science and intuition. *Annu Rev Med*, 60:125–137. http://dx.doi.org/10.1146/annurev.med.60.101107.134802 PMID:18803476

14. Croswell JM, Ransohoff DF, Kramer BS (2010). Principles of cancer screening: lessons from history and study design issues. *Semin Oncol*, 37:202–215. http://dx.doi.org/10.1053/j.seminoncol.2010.05.006 PMID:20709205

15. Pinsky PF, Miller A, Kramer BS *et al.* (2007). Evidence of a healthy volunteer effect in the prostate, lung, colorectal, and ovarian cancer screening trial. *Am J Epidemiol*, 165:874–881. http://dx.doi.org/10.1093/aje/kwk075 PMID:17244633

16. Domingo L, Blanch J, Servitja S *et al.* (2013). Aggressiveness features and outcomes of true interval cancers: comparison between screen-detected and symptom-detected cancers. *Eur J Cancer Prev*, 22:21–28. http://dx.doi.org/10.1097/CEJ.0b013e328354d324 PMID:22584215

17. Welch HG, Black WC (2010). Overdiagnosis in cancer. *J Natl Cancer Inst*, 102:605–613. http://dx.doi.org/10.1093/jnci/djq099 PMID:20413742

18. National Cancer Institute. PDQ Neuroblastoma Screening. Bethesda, MD: National Cancer Institute. Date last modified: 23 July 2010. Available at http://www.cancer.gov/cancertopics/pdq/screening/neuroblastoma/HealthProfessional.

19. Welch HG, Schwartz LM, Woloshin S (2000). Are increasing 5-year survival rates evidence of success against cancer? *JAMA*, 283:2975–2978. http://dx.doi.org/10.1001/jama.283.22.2975 PMID:10865276

20. Wegwarth O, Schwartz LM, Woloshin S *et al.* (2012). Do physicians understand cancer screening statistics? A national survey of primary care physicians in the United States. *Ann Intern Med*, 156:340–349. http://dx.doi.org/10.7326/0003-4819-156-5-201203060-00005 PMID:22393129

21. Ransohoff DF, McNaughton Collins M, Fowler FJ (2002). Why is prostate cancer screening so common when the evidence is so uncertain? A system without negative feedback. *Am J Med*, 113:663–667. http://dx.doi.org/10.1016/S0002-9343(02)01235-4 PMID:12505117

22. Ganz PA, Barry JM, Burke W *et al.* (2011). *National Institutes of Health State-of-the-Science Conference Statement: Role of Active Surveillance in the Management of Men with Localized Prostate Cancer*. NIH Consensus and State-of-the-Science Statements, Vol. 28, No. 1, December 5–7, 2011. Bethesda, MD: National Institutes of Health.

23. Nishihira H, Toyoda Y, Tanaka Y *et al.* (2000). Natural course of neuroblastoma detected by mass screening: a 5-year prospective study at a single institution. *J Clin Oncol*, 18:3012–3017. PMID:10944135

24. Yoneda A, Oue T, Imura K *et al.* (2001). Observation of untreated patients with neuroblastoma detected by mass screening: a "wait and see" pilot study. *Med Pediatr Oncol*, 36:160–162. http://dx.doi.org/10.1002/1096-911X(20010101)36:1<160::AID-MPO1039>3.0.CO;2-G PMID:11464874

25. Fagerlin A, Zikmund-Fisher BJ, Ubel PA (2011). Helping patients decide: ten steps to better risk communication. *J Natl Cancer Inst*, 103:1436–1443. http://dx.doi.org/10.1093/jnci/djr318 PMID:21931068

26. Woloshin S, Schwartz LM (2011). Communicating data about the benefits and harms of treatment: a randomized trial. *Ann Intern Med*, 155:87–96. http://dx.doi.org/10.1059/0003-4819-155-2-201107190-00004 PMID:21768582

27. Aberle DR, Adams AM, Berg CD *et al.*; National Lung Screening Trial Research Team (2011). Reduced lung-cancer mortality with low-dose computed tomographic screening. *N Engl J Med*, 365:395–409. http://dx.doi.org/10.1056/NEJMoa1102873 PMID:21714641

6

Cancer
control

Earlier sections of this Report have addressed the worldwide burden of cancer, its causation and prevention, and current understanding of cancer biology as underpinning new approaches to both therapy and prevention, with these various parameters explored in relation to each of the most frequent tumour types. Knowledge about all of these matters, specifically including interventions to reduce cancer incidence and mortality, is

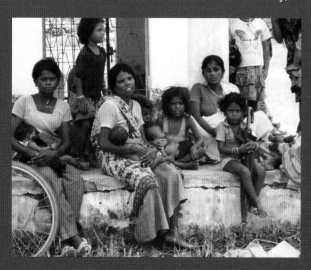

primarily dependent on research; research findings have determined the content of all previous chapters. Section 6 is not primarily a specification of research findings but more a description of the manner and extent to which knowledge of cancer control may be applied at the national level and a consideration of the resources relevant to achieving this end. The focus shifts from the prospect of increased understanding to presently coordinated action predicated on methodologies already known to reduce the burden of cancer. Differences between countries are evident, sometimes usefully expressed in relation to national prosperity, but often extending to other parameters. Development and implementation of an adequately resourced national cancer control plan is now recognized as a fundamental element within the broad scope of population health and clinical services activity. International collaboration provides an opportunity to minimize unnecessary evaluation and to optimize implementation for the benefit of national, or sometimes local, populations. In parallel with the implementation of cancer control measures, infrastructure for continued, locally relevant, implementation research may be adopted and managed, thereby laying the foundation for even more effective cancer control measures consequent to such investigations.

Cancer control in Africa: options for a vulnerable continent

Isaac F. Adewole

Cancer remains a leading noncommunicable disease in Africa, and it is also emerging as a great burden when compared with infections that are ravaging the continent. The triad of ignorance, poverty, and poor health-seeking behaviour makes Africa vulnerable to the cancer burden in both male and female, and young and adult populations [1]. Of the 7.6 million cancer deaths that occur worldwide, 4.8 million occur in developing countries, translating to about 21 000 cancer deaths per day, and Africa shares the highest proportion globally. The rapidly increasing cancer burden is attributable to the transitional demographic profile of several countries in Africa, with increasing proportions of older people in the population and a shift towards lifestyles typical of industrialized countries. Only 17 African countries had operational cancer control policies in 2010, and virtually no African country presently implements a well-funded national cancer control plan. This clearly suggests a lack of political will and commitment across the continent [2]. Addressing this is a continental imperative.

First, each country should produce a blueprint for national cancer control using a framework that is socially and culturally sensitive.

Second, creating awareness about cancer as a complex group of diseases that often have identifiable triggers should be pursued in a systematic manner. This will involve population-wide health promotion strategies focused on diet and exercise, lifestyle modifications, sexuality/family life education programmes, campaigns against cultural norms/practices, and other behavioural change communication strategies that are linkable to cancer risk. In addition, legislative support that promotes healthy living within the household and in communities is imperative. These initiatives are expected to foster a strong primary prevention strategy in a continent where about 33% of cancers are infection-related [3].

Credible evidence abounds that some cancers are preventable with vaccination, and African countries should actively participate in current global efforts using practical approaches that are feasible in their countries, without an overdependence on donor support. Institutionalization of these vaccines into the already existing and successful national immunization programmes provides a true opportunity in the continent [4].

Screening for premalignant and early diseases is another control strategy that has yet to be entrenched in Africa. Priorities should be the establishment of cancer registries as well as centres of excellence, and the training of a critical mass of experts to offer multidisciplinary team care for cancer patients in Africa, through collaboration with cancer centres offering cutting-edge services, professional organizations, and pharmaceutical companies. Tax incentives could be offered for interested foundations, multinational companies, and individuals that are ready to invest in cancer control in Africa.

Cancer control in Africa is feasible, but the focus should be on a control plan that is realistic, sustainable, equitable, and part of a strong health-care system.

References

1. Morhason-Bello IO et al. (2013). Lancet Oncol, 14:e142–e151. http://dx.doi.org/10.1016/S1470-2045(12)70482-5 PMID:23561745

2. Stefan DC et al. (2013). Lancet Oncol, 14:e189–e195. http://dx.doi.org/10.1016/S1470-2045(13)70100-1 PMID:23561751

3. de Martel C et al. (2012). Lancet Oncol, 13:607–615. http://dx.doi.org/10.1016/S1470-2045(12)70137-7 PMID:22575588

4. Sylla BS, Wild CP (2012). Int J Cancer, 130:245–250. http://dx.doi.org/10.1002/ijc.26333 PMID:21796634

6.1

National cancer control plans

6 CONTROL

Simon B. Sutcliffe

Raul Hernando Murillo Moreno (reviewer)

Edward L. Trimble (reviewer)

Summary

- National cancer control plans detail the strategy to address the population burden of cancer through interventions to reduce incidence, mortality, and morbidity and enhance the quality of life of those at risk of, or experiencing, cancer.

- The integrity of these plans is based on current and accurate determination of burden, realistic targets for improvement, and continuous surveillance to document performance and outcomes.

- National cancer control plans define: the purpose of planned activity, the content of interventions to reduce the cancer burden, the context within which activities are adapted to prevailing circumstances, the relationships required between stakeholders, and the resources (internal and external) to execute the plan.

- Adoption and implementation of national cancer control plans has been particular to high-income countries, but progress is now occurring in middle- and low-income countries as strategies appropriate to circumstances and resources are identified.

- Resistance, barriers to implementation, and susceptibility to unplanned modification or revised priorities are an immediate and ever-present reality. Determination, commitment, resolve, and collaboration are mandatory requirements to realize the future gains of population-based interventions to control cancer and other noncommunicable diseases.

A national cancer control plan is a public health programme designed to reduce the number of new cancer cases and cancer-related deaths and to improve the quality of life of cancer patients, through systematic and equitable implementation of evidence-based strategies for prevention, early detection, diagnosis, treatment, and palliation, making the best use of available resources [1].

The population burden of cancer is considerable, with 32.5 million people globally living with cancer [2] and 169.3 million years of healthy life (disability-adjusted life years) lost per year due to cancer [3]. The global burden will only continue to increase in the coming decades due to population growth and ageing. In 2012, there were an estimated 14.1 million new cases of cancer and 8.2 million cancer-related deaths worldwide [2].

Deaths due to cancer are projected to increase to 13 million in 2030. Although incidence rates are lower in lower-resource countries, mortality rates are higher; patterns of disease distribution and survival reflect varying levels of socioeconomic development [2,4,5]. Mortality-to-incidence ratios for cancer vary from less than 0.50 to more than 0.90 across world regions (see Chapter 1.1). This variation reflects less a lack of knowledge of what should be done to control cancer than the level of commitment to implementing effective cancer control interventions population-wide.

The cost of cancer is substantial. In 2009, new cancer cases globally were estimated to cost US$ 286 billion, both in direct – i.e. medical – costs and in indirect costs, principally including lost productivity. Approximately 94% of these costs were incurred in high-resource countries; only 6% were incurred in upper-middle, lower-middle, and low-income countries [6]. Other estimates of the economic cost of cancer are far higher (US$ 1.16 trillion) when taking account of costs of prevention and treatment, and the annual economic cost of disability-adjusted life years (see Chapter 6.7). As the burden of cancer grows, it will unequally and inequitably affect

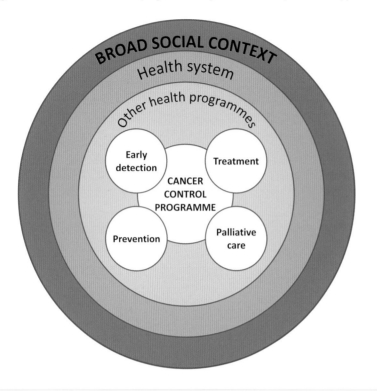

The fundamental role of data

The first step in establishing an NCCP is to understand the scope of the region-specific cancer burden, as patterns of cancer vary by geography. This variation can arise for many reasons, including heterogeneities in etiological risk factors such as tobacco use and chronic infection; geography, as exemplified by climate; social determinants, such as poverty; and health systems, specifically including access to diagnostic, treatment, and care services. These heterogeneities can contribute to variation in pathology and stage, survival, functionality, and quality of life [7]. Given this wide variation, no single NCCP will satisfy the needs of every country or population. Instead, NCCPs must be adapted to national and regional needs and capabilities.

Population data are the foundation for understanding the burden and pattern of cancer. These data can also be used to synthesize and prioritize planned interventions, establish system capacity requirements for care, evaluate population-based cancer control activities, and justify continued investment of resources according to performance and outcomes of plans. Projection

those with the least ability and capability to respond.

To address this growing burden of cancer, population-based cancer control must be recognized as far more than a medical response to cancer. The cancer burden is driven by a complex interaction of changing factors, including social determinants such as poverty, education, the built environment, gender equity, and so on, and population health, including primary prevention/risk factor control and early detection and management of disease and illness. Accordingly, improving cancer control at a population level is a social imperative, which requires a societal response that may be challenging to prevailing social, business, and economic interests.

Addressing the increasing burden of cancer requires a country or population cancer control plan. The WHO strategic definition of a national cancer control plan (NCCP), as specified above, is predicated on evidence-based interventions that need to be implemented for

prevention, early detection, diagnosis, treatment, and palliation. This definition emphasizes the scientific and medical content of a plan, which is the focus of much of the discourse around NCCPs. The success of the plan, however, is dependent not only on its content – what needs to be done – but also on its context, which includes: cultural and circumstance-specific factors influencing implementation; the key actors and stakeholders, and their responsibilities and accountabilities; available resources, including human, technology, facilities, and financing perspectives that influence how the plan will be operationalized; and evaluation of the plan and its impact on cancer control outcomes and the achievement of defined targets. If these elements are not addressed in the NCCP, implementation and sustainability will be difficult to achieve and the impact of the plan on cancer control and the health of the population will be jeopardized regardless of the effectiveness of the interventions outlined within it.

Fig. 6.1.2. A WHO poster for World No Tobacco Day 2010 focuses on the marketing of tobacco to women.

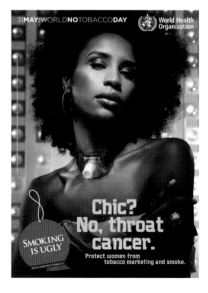

of data can also define future burden, needs, capacity, impact, and required investment.

Cancer registries are the primary source of data for NCCPs. Registries present the population burden of cancer and can do so by time, key population attributes (including age, gender, and recognition of paediatric and adolescent/young adult cases), cancer site/type, impact of interventions as affecting stage distribution, 5-year survival, disability, the presence or absence of health insurance [8], and peer comparison with reference, for example, to geographical, political, economic, ethnic, and heritage status [2,7,9]. In the United Kingdom and the European Union, comparative presentation of data has provided the stimulus for NCCP development, renewal, and implementation. Indeed, increasing recognition of the global variation in incidence, mortality, and 5-year survival, and reasons for this variation – which include access to care, diagnostic and treatment services, and investment in health resources – have provided an important stimulus for viewing NCCPs as a means of improving cancer burden, mitigating variation, and addressing disparities.

However, as fundamental as cancer registries are for cancer control planning, many lower-resource countries are challenged by having neither registries nor a systematic ability to collect data. These challenges result from a lack of medical facilities, low cancer awareness, poor follow-up, poorly maintained records, lack of trained staff, and/or lack of fiscal, medical, and political resolve. Potential solutions include establishing the culture of evidence, supported by data, between clinicians and data registrars; educational meetings to raise awareness; household visits; collection of data on admissions, procedures, and mortality from urban reference centres; and a focus on good data collection from a few, more established centres rather than an entire population survey. Ultimately, efforts to establish reliable population data for programme planning need

to consider comprehensiveness across the disease control spectrum, completeness, accuracy, timeliness, and coverage. Notable examples of approaches by lower-resource countries exist in South and Central America and India.

Once established, registries should not be viewed as static repositories of data. They should be enhanced over time to incorporate more detailed data on diagnosis and treatment. Along with projection and modelling methodologies, these continually updated data will help refine needs, capacity, resources, programme evaluation, and investments, thereby allowing health systems to maintain optimal cancer control outcomes.

The coverage and quality of registry data can vary considerably worldwide. Estimates of the proportion of the population covered by cancer registries range from more than 80% in North America, Europe, and Australia to approximately 30% in the Russian Federation, less than 10% in South America and South-East Asia, and only a few percent in Africa. Regional registries also vary in their comprehensiveness, completeness of information capture, timeliness, accuracy and consistency of terminology, and use of international classifications and recording standards. Irrespective of their coverage and quality, registries are nevertheless useful for informing and refining NCCPs. Thus, even in regions without functioning registries, at least minimal cancer-relevant health surveillance should be developed concurrent with NCCPs to rationalize activities, investments, and performance of cancer control plans [10].

The content of NCCPs

An NCCP is a strategic plan encompassing the spectrum of cancer control measures and is evidence-based, scientifically accurate, and current. Establishing the content of this plan is relatively straightforward as it is based on best practices, the scientific and clinical literature, and

Box 6.1.1. Guiding principles for developing a national cancer control plan.

1. **Comprehensiveness:** The plan should address all members of the population, with attention to addressing inequities and disparities.

2. **Scope:** The plan should address cancer control from the perspectives of human development, risk factor control, and health and disease management.

3. **Evidence base:** The plan should be based on evidence or best practices and should incorporate indicators and metrics of performance, output, and outcomes.

4. **Standards of practice:** The cancer control plan should take into account measures to define standards and ensure consistent application, such as access, timeliness, quality of care, and safety.

5. **Minimization of inappropriate variation of practice and factors influencing compliance with therapy:** The plan should use guidelines or best practices and measures to support adherence and compliance.

6. **Integration and continuity:** The plan should strive for continuity across states of health and illness, and across home, community, and tertiary or specialist environments.

7. **Inclusiveness:** The cancer control plan should be developed with input and support from the public, patients, providers, policy-makers, and payers.

8. **Governance:** The plan should align with population health priorities and outline responsibilities, accountabilities, and reporting.

9. **Sustainability:** The plan should be developed with the intention of being self-sufficient and sustainable.

Box 6.1.2. Elements to be included in a national cancer control plan.

1. **Why a national cancer control plan is necessary:**
- What is the burden of cancer?
- What is the capability and capacity for control?
- What is the imperative for change?
- How important is cancer relative to other health challenges?

2. **What interventions are required:**
- What interventions for cancer are most important: risk factor control, early detection, diagnosis, treatment, and care?
- How will these interventions be prioritized in relation to other elements of cancer and noncommunicable disease control?

3. **How interventions will be implemented, and how the process of implementation will be monitored and evaluated:**
- How will human, technology, facilities, and organizational resources be aligned to the implementation?

4. **Who will be involved:**
- How will collaboration be fostered and managed?
- How will roles and resources be shared?
- How will responsibility and accountability be established?
- How will "buy-in", progress, and performance be communicated and reported?

5. **When activities will be undertaken according to priority, what is the capability and the resource availability (the operational plan).**

6. **How the national cancer control plan and its implementation will be financed (the business plan):**
- What are the contributions of foreign aid, in-kind services, and local financing?
- How are self-sufficiency and sustainability being addressed?

7. **How the plan will be evaluated:**
- How will outputs and outcomes be measured (system performance), linked to a changing burden of cancer, and aligned with resource allocation to determine value?

training and planning manuals [11–13]. Published plans are accessible [14–16]. As NCCPs are about control of disease within the context of a country and the health of its population, each country must adapt the content of its plan to its population and circumstances. A set of core principles have been recognized as guiding acceptance and implementation (Box 6.1.1). The plan must describe how beneficial change in cancer control will occur; address purpose, content, context, relationships, and resources; present a business plan to determine how resource inputs will be acquired, deployed, and accounted for; and include an operational plan to determine how implementation is going to roll out

over time in a coordinated, integrated manner that leads to performance and achievement of results (Box 6.1.2).

Surveys of WHO Member States indicate that elements of functional cancer control plans are present in 35% of low-income countries, 35–60% of countries in the lower-middle and upper-middle income groups, and 75% of high-income countries. However, substantial variation exists within resource settings with respect to the specific components of the plans (see Chapter 6.2).

The context of NCCPs

Critical to the success of the NCCP is its adaptation to its country or

population context. Contextual factors include resources and priorities.

For any country, the level of resources available in the health system is the major determinant for decision-making in health planning and its limitations. Resources include human resources, and specifically qualified personnel; technology, which includes information technology; drugs, and diagnostic and therapeutic equipment; facilities, with reference, for example, to access to transportation and affordable in-patient and ambulatory accommodation; and financial resources, including current and projected annual growth. As interventions move from a population level to a person, tissue, cell, and genome,

Fig. 6.1.3. Poster from the National Research and Safety Institute (INRS), France, advocating the wearing of protective masks by workers exposed to asbestos: "When working on construction sites, I never wore a protective mask against asbestos. Now, I wear a mask every day. With asbestos, don't take chances. Protect yourself!"

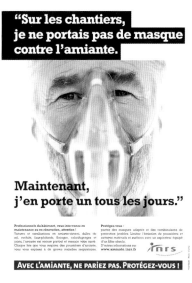

"**Sur les chantiers, je ne portais pas de masque contre l'amiante.**

Maintenant, j'en porte un tous les jours."

Professionnels du bâtiment, vous intervenez en maintenance ou en rénovation, attention !
Tuyaux et canalisations en amiante-ciment, dalles de sol, enduits, faux-plafonds, flocages, colorifugeages et joints, l'amiante est encore partout et menace votre santé. Chaque fois que vous respirez des poussières d'amiante, vous vous exposez à de graves maladies respiratoires.

Protégez-vous :
portez des masques adaptés et des combinaisons de protection jetables. Limitez l'émission de poussières et nettoyez matériels et surfaces avec un aspirateur équipé d'un filtre absolu.
D'autres informations sur www.amiante.inrs.fr

AVEC L'AMIANTE, NE PARIEZ PAS. PROTÉGEZ-VOUS !

the requirements for level of qualifications of personnel, technology, infrastructure, time, and cost increase, while population access commonly decreases. Interventions directed at behaviour change at a community or individual level, while sometimes difficult to achieve, require modest technical support, whereas interventions involving clinical care – such as surgery and provision of radiation and drug-based therapy – require a proficient level of specialist skill and technological capacity.

Recognizing the resource challenges of lower-resource countries, WHO has presented a core set of "best buy" lower-cost intervention strategies for four noncommunicable diseases: cardiovascular disease, chronic respiratory diseases, diabetes, and cancer [17]. These strategies address factors common to more than one such disease, such as tobacco use, alcohol consumption, unhealthy diet, and lack of physical activity. Interventions include tax increases and legislation, as illustrated by measures relating to smoke-free environments, limited retail access, and advertising bans; hepatitis B vaccination and cervical cancer screening programmes; and recommendations for reducing salt intake, substituting trans fats, and using aspirin for myocardial ischaemia.

The annual cost of implementing these interventions for all people in lower-middle-income countries is estimated to be US$ 11.4 billion – an investment of US$ 1 per person in low-income countries to US$ 3 per person in upper-middle-income countries. This contrasts with a current "business as usual" scenario whereby economic losses of US$ 500 billion per year are incurred for the four noncommunicable diseases – a loss equivalent to 4% of annual output of low-income countries and lower-middle-income countries, or US$ 25–50 per person per year. Initial investments, which may be quite modest for many aspects of population health, have a personal, family, community, and economic return on investment based on increased longevity, productivity, societal contribution, and avoidance of health-care costs.

Most of the above-mentioned "best buy" interventions relate to prevention, intuitively considered to be more cost-effective than interventions for early or established disease. A further distinction of disease prevention interventions relates to whether they are environmental (involving measures that affect the whole population) or personal (directed towards changing individual behaviour) and whether they are clinical (delivered in a health-care facility) or non-clinical (delivered outside of the health-care setting). Environmental interventions are generally the most cost-effective as they affect a large proportion of the population. Typically such measures are achieved through policy and regulation – examples are smoke-free laws or food regulations addressing fortification or control of unhealthy food components such as trans fats. In contrast, interventions directed at lifestyle or individual choice, or delivered in clinical settings, are less cost-effective, although not mutually exclusive of environmental interventions [18].

Even though "best buy" interventions are clearly cost-effective, economics is not the sole criterion for NCCP development within limited resources. Other factors, including societal and circumstance-specific factors [19], alternative models of service delivery [20], and priorities within the disease, health, and other sectors will determine ultimate decisions. In low-resource settings, NCCPs may not be feasible as stand-alone plans. The principles underlying NCCPs, however, are also broadly applicable to other noncommunicable diseases, as noted above, even though treatment options may be disease-specific [21].

Enhancing NCCPs

NCCPs commonly define strategies to control cancer. Cancer control measures, however, will be achieved only if the NCCP is implemented within the health system through the

Fig. 6.1.4. Poster from the Iowa Department of Public Health, USA, advocating colorectal cancer screening for Vietnamese Americans: "Life is good, and I'm not letting anything take me away from my family. Asian Americans are at higher risk of colorectal cancer. Treatment is easy if it is detected early through testing. If you are 50 or older, get tested today!"

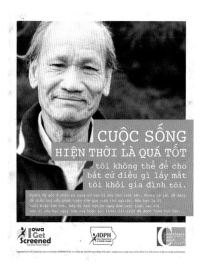

CUỘC SỐNG HIỆN THỜI LÀ QUÁ TỐT
tôi không thể để cho bất cứ điều gì lấy mất tôi khỏi gia đình tôi.

"push" of science and medicine and the "pull" of patients and the public (sociopolitical imperative) [22].

Such an approach involves social mobilization, causing the challenge to be embraced and championed by key constituencies influencing social and political change. There are roles for advocate and stakeholder participation, together with the engagement of relevant networks and coalitions.

Collaboration across networks and coalitions will increase their impact and may extend from information exchange to agreed coordination and cooperation. The latter requires trust, mutual respect, a sensitivity to issues of authority, and understandings about roles, responsibilities, and accountabilities. Examples of such networks include national organizations, such as the Canadian Partnership Against Cancer; regional entities for cancer control, such as the African Organisation for Research and Training in Cancer and the Latin American Network of National Cancer Institutes; and international entities, such as the International Network for Cancer Treatment and Research and the International Cancer Control Congresses. Also key to effective collaboration are well-defined and secure financial commitments through, for example, a business plan, a detailed implementation plan, and an understanding that the NCCP is an integral component of the population health system.

The value of NCCPs

Proof of effectiveness of cancer control measures is hindered by the long time gap between implementation of interventions and changes in incidence and mortality. Other limitations stem from the paucity of data linking intervention and effect directly, the continuous introduction of new technologies and therapeutic advances, and the inability to undertake a controlled study of NCCP versus no-NCCP within a single population over a given time.

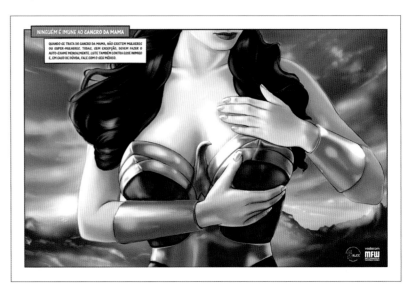

Fig. 6.1.5. The "Nobody's Immune to Breast Cancer" campaign of Associação da Luta Contra o Cancro (Association for the Fight Against Cancer), Mozambique: "When we talk about breast cancer, there are no women or superwomen. Everybody has to do a monthly self-examination. Fight with us against this enemy and, when in doubt, talk with your doctor."

Thus, causality can be approximated and can be discussed; it cannot be assumed [23]. For NCCPs to demonstrate value, they must be implemented and audited.

Although direct evidence of effectiveness is not available, supportive evidence for the benefit of NCCPs exists. This evidence derives from several sources.

The first is programmes addressing specific elements of cancer control. Changes in mortality are evident after the implementation of tobacco control programmes (in Australia, Canada, and Brazil), organized prevention through vaccination (against human papillomavirus in Costa Rica and against hepatitis B virus in Taiwan, China), sun protection campaigns and screening for melanoma (in Australia), and organized early detection programmes for cervical cancer (in Colombia, Ecuador, Chile, the United Kingdom, and Canada).

The second is control of multiple risk factors for noncommunicable diseases, including cancer. In North Karelia, Finland, substantial reductions in cardiovascular disease and cancer – and particularly lung cancer – mortality have been achieved through control of targeted risk factors [24]. In the USA, decreases in coronary heart disease mortality over the past four decades have been achieved through improvements in risk factor control, exemplified by smoking, hypercholesterolaemia, and hypertension, and, more recently, through the introduction and adoption of treatment innovations [25].

The third is treatment improvements. Increased clinical trial enrolment and rigorous definition of benefit and measures to encourage adoption of evidence-based care have led to reduced paediatric cancer mortality in high-income countries and in lower-resource countries such as Argentina. The adoption of professional practice standards to reduce inconsistencies, deficiencies, and variability in clinical practice – including, for example, surgery, pathology assessment, and therapy allocation – has led to decreased mortality for resectable colorectal cancer. Compliance with evidence-based/informed clinical practice guidelines has led to increased breast cancer survival, and implementation and application of evidence-based new therapies have led to reduced mortality for

Box 6.1.3. Conditions underlying the probability of a successful national cancer control plan.

1. Political and professional consistency and resolve to address the population cancer burden.

2. Use of data and a commitment to support and maintain cancer registration and surveillance.

3. Clearly defined vision for cancer control, commonly agreed and supported.

4. Contextual relevance, defined priorities, achievable implementation, and an appropriate time frame to achieve goals.

5. Defined, secure funding commitment.

6. Trust, mutual respect, and willingness to achieve commonly defined goals through collaboration by all key actors.

7. Scalability, incorporation into the health system, self-sufficiency, and sustainability.

8. Applicability to, and coordination and cooperation with, other population disease control plans.

9. Sound governance, evaluation, communication, and ongoing adaptation to meet future needs.

B-cell non-Hodgkin lymphoma. The achievement of surrogate targets of improved health outcomes is illustrated by access to care and treatment, screening rates, and quality and timeliness of diagnostic services [26].

Finally, comparisons have been made of trends in mortality rates in comparable populations with and without NCCPs, as indicated, for example, by survival trends in England versus Wales up to 2007 [27].

Conclusions

Cancer is a major and increasing public health problem and population burden for all countries. An NCCP presents an opportunity to implement effective change at a population level on an ongoing, adaptable basis, using a variety of interventional methods that can be accommodated within the contextual, social, and financial means of even the poorest nations.

The challenge for NCCPs is less the derivation of content than the ability to apply and achieve sustainable change at a population level. If conditions are favourable (Box 6.1.3), with the support and engagement of all key actors and a clear and common vision for cancer control, the plan is more likely to succeed in improving the health of the population.

NCCPs identify why action is necessary and what action is required. To change the population impact of cancer, however, it must be clear how NCCPs will be implemented, adopted, evaluated, and sustained. An NCCP, as defined by WHO, has the potential to change population incidence, suffering, and mortality from cancer through implementation in a contextually aligned manner when supported by all relevant stakeholders in an inclusive and interdisciplinary partnership, and financed and governed to achieve long-term, sustainable improvements in cancer control.

References

1. WHO (2012). *National Cancer Control Programmes: Planning*. Geneva: WHO. Available at http://www.who.int/cancer/nccp/planning/en/.

2. Ferlay J, Soerjomataram I, Ervik M et al. (2013). GLOBOCAN 2012 v1.0, Cancer Incidence and Mortality Worldwide: IARC CancerBase No. 11 [Internet]. Lyon: IARC. Available at http://globocan.iarc.fr.

3. Soerjomataram I, Lortet-Tieulent J, Parkin DM et al. (2012). Global burden of cancer in 2008: a systematic analysis of disability-adjusted life years in 12 world regions. *Lancet*, 380:1840–1850. http://dx.doi.org/10.1016/S0140-6736(12)60919-2 PMID:23079588

4. Bray F, Jemal A, Grey N et al. (2012). Global cancer transitions according to the Human Development Index (2008–2030): a population-based study. *Lancet Oncol*, 13:790–801. http://dx.doi.org/10.1016/S1470-2045(12)70211-5 PMID:22658655

5. Bray F, Ren JS, Masuyer E, Ferlay J (2013). Global estimates of cancer prevalence for 27 sites in the adult population in 2008. *Int J Cancer*, 132:1133–1145. http://dx.doi.org/10.1002/ijc.27711 PMID:22752881

6. Economist Intelligence Unit (2009). *Breakaway: The Global Burden of Cancer – Challenges and Opportunities*. London: The Economist Group. Available at http://www.livestrong.org/pdfs/GlobalEconomicImpact.

7. Coleman MP, Quaresma M, Berrino F et al.; CONCORD Working Group (2008). Cancer survival in five continents: a worldwide population-based study (CONCORD). *Lancet Oncol*, 9:730–756. http://dx.doi.org/10.1016/S1470-2045(08)70179-7 PMID:18639491

8. McDavid K, Tucker TC, Sloggett A, Coleman MP (2003). Cancer survival in Kentucky and health insurance coverage. *Arch Intern Med*, 163:2135–2144. http://dx.doi.org/10.1001/archinte.163.18.2135 PMID:14557210

9. Capocaccia R, Gavin A, Hakulinen T et al.; the EUROCARE Working Group (2009). Survival of cancer patients in Europe, 1995–2002: the Eurocare 4 study. *Eur J Cancer*, 45:901–1094. PMID:19217771

10. Global Initiative for Cancer Registry Development in Low- and Middle-Income Countries (2012). Available at http://gicr.iarc.fr.

11. Planning WHO (2006). *Cancer Control: Knowledge into Action. WHO Guide for Effective Programmes*. Module 1: Planning. Geneva: WHO. Available at http://www.who.int/cancer/publications/cancer_control_planning/en/index.html.

12. Union for International Cancer Control (2012). *Supporting National Cancer Control Planning: A Toolkit for Civil Society Organizations (CSOs)*. Available at http://www.uicc.org/advocacy/advocacy-resources/nccp-toolkit.

13. WHO, International Atomic Energy Agency (2011). *National Cancer Control Programmes Core Capacity Self-Assessment Tool (NCCP core self-assessment tool)*. Geneva: WHO. Available at http://www.who.int/cancer/publications/nccp_tool2011/en/.

14. France: le Plan Cancer 2009–2013. Available at http://www.plan-cancer.gouv.fr/le-plan-cancer/presentation.html.

15. The National Health Service Cancer Plan: a plan for investment, a plan for reform. Available at http://www.dh.gov/uk/en/publicationsandstatistics/publications/publicationspolicyandguidance/dh_4009609.

16. Uruguay: Programa Nacional de Control del Cáncer. Available at http://www.bvsoncologia.org.uy/pdfs/destacados/pronaccan_2005-2010.pdf.

17. WHO (2011). *From Burden to "Best Buys": Reducing the Economic Impact of Non-Communicable Diseases in Low- and Middle-Income Countries*. Geneva: WHO. Available at http://www.who.int/nmh/publications/best_buys_summary/en/.

18. Chokshi DA, Farley TA (2012). The cost-effectiveness of environmental approaches to disease prevention. *N Engl J Med*, 367:295–297. http://dx.doi.org/10.1056/NEJMp1206268 PMID:22830461

19. WHO (2008). *Task Shifting: Global Recommendations and Guidelines*. Available at http://www.who.int/healthsystems/TTR-TaskShifting.pdf.

20. Wools-Kaloustian K, Kimaiyo S (2006). Extending HIV care in resource-limited settings. *Curr HIV/AIDS Rep*, 3:182–186. http://dx.doi.org/10.1007/s11904-006-0014-1 PMID:17032578

21. United Nations (2011). Political Declaration of the High-Level Meeting of the General Assembly on the Prevention and Control of Non-communicable Diseases. New York: United Nations. Available at www.who.int/nmh/events/un_ncd_summit2011/political_declaration_en.pdf.

22. Trubek LG, Oliver TR, Liang C-M, Mokrohisky M (2011). Improving cancer control outcomes through strong networks and regulatory frameworks: lessons from the United States and European Union. *J Health Care Law Policy*, 14:119–151. Available at http://digitalcommons.law.umaryland.edu/jhclp/vol14/iss1/5.

23. Rochester P, Chapel T, Black B et al. (2005). The evaluation of comprehensive cancer control efforts: useful techniques and unique requirements. *Cancer Causes Control*, 16 Suppl 1:69–78. http://dx.doi.org/10.1007/s10552-005-0510-4 PMID:16208576

24. Puska P (2002). Successful prevention of non-communicable diseases: 25 years experience with North Karelia project in Finland. *Public Health Med*, 4:5–7. Available at http://www.who.int/entity/chp/media/en/north_karelia_successful_ncd_prevention.pdf.

25. Ford ES, Capewell S (2011). Proportion of the decline in cardiovascular mortality disease due to prevention versus treatment: public health versus clinical care. *Annu Rev Public Health*, 32:5–22. http://dx.doi.org/10.1146/annurev-publhealth-031210-101211 PMID:21417752

26. Canadian Partnership Against Cancer (2011). *The 2011 Cancer System Performance Report*. Available at http://www.cancerview.ca/idc/groups/public/documents/webcontent/2011_system_performance_rep.pdf.

27. Rachet B, Maringe C, Nur U et al. (2009). Population-based cancer survival trends in England and Wales up to 2007: an assessment of the NHS cancer plan for England. *Lancet Oncol*, 10:351–369. http://dx.doi.org/10.1016/S1470-2045(09)70028-2 PMID:19303813

Cancer control in Canada: challenges and strategies in a high-income country

Heather Bryant and Lee Fairclough

In 2006, the federal government of Canada created the Canadian Partnership Against Cancer, a federally funded nongovernmental organization charged with the implementation of the national cancer control strategy [1,2]. While the development of the strategy was built on many years of collaborative work, there were challenges that needed to be met and lessons to be learned in its implementation.

Many of the initial challenges concerned creating the appropriate measures needed to stimulate and assess the impact of such a strategy. Canada had the same excellent starting point that many high-income countries have: the presence of population-based cancer registries with high-quality data throughout most of the country. However, there were gaps that had not been addressed. The first related to high-quality staging data, which was absent at a pan-Canadian level. Thus, one of the first initiatives of the Canadian Partnership Against Cancer was to work with the provincial registries and clinicians (particularly pathologists) to identify an approach to address this issue. The result was the National Staging Initiative, a large-scale programme designed to catalyse coordinated efforts in all jurisdictions with investments in infrastructure and implementation of standards. The National Staging Initiative has successfully achieved the goal of making collaborative stage information available in a sustainable way for more than 90% of the four major cancers (lung, colorectal, breast, and prostate) starting in the 2010 coding year.

For many years, routine interprovincial comparisons had been done on incidence, mortality, and, to a lesser extent, prevalence and survival. However, none of these measures were able to shine a light on what occurred between the two key time points: diagnosis and death. Some provinces had initiated reporting in this area where limited data existed, but the comparison of this across the country had not occurred. Thus, provincial cancer agencies and health departments were engaged to come to consensus on indicators that would be most useful as initial assessments of concordance of treatment with high-level recommendations. Initially, only a few provinces were able to produce the necessary data. However, over the past few years, the Cancer System Performance Report [3] has evolved from having "proxy" indicators for many variables to a report with an ever-increasing insight into possible areas for improvement in each jurisdiction. These measures are placed with others to provide a view across the cancer control continuum, including population measures of risk factors, of screening, and of patient experience. The report continues to develop, with the joint leadership of senior representatives of each provincial cancer agency and the Canadian Partnership Against Cancer, and has been used by several provinces to target quality initiatives in their own jurisdictions.

References

1. Canadian Partnership Against Cancer (2012). *Sustaining Action Toward a Shared Vision: 2012–2017 Strategic Plan*. Available at http://www.partnership againstcancer.ca/wp-content/uploads/ Sustaining-Action-Toward-a-Shared-Vision-Full-Document.pdf.

2. Fairclough L *et al.* (2012). *Curr Oncol*, 19:70–77. http://dx.doi.org/10.3747/co.19. 1019 PMID:22514493

3. Canadian Partnership Against Cancer (2012). *The 2012 Cancer System Performance Report*. Available at http:// www.cancerview.ca/systemperformance report.

6.2 Current global national cancer control capacity

Andreas Ullrich
Leanne Riley

Robert C. Burton (reviewer)
Folakemi T. Odedina (reviewer)

Summary

- The national capacity of a country for cancer prevention and control may be assessed based on the WHO 2013 Noncommunicable Disease Country Capacity Survey by analysing cancer-specific data. Information is available from 176 countries.

- Although 85% of the participating countries have cancer plans or policies, many of those plans are not operational. Only 38% of countries in Africa and 45% of low-income countries have operational plans with a budget to support implementation.

- Population-based cancer registries were reported to exist in 72% of countries.

- From survey information received by WHO, major gaps in health care for cancer control were identified. Many countries, especially low-income countries, lack a national cancer control policy or plan. Where cancer policies have been developed, such policies are not always comprehensive.

- Because the cancer burden is high and is increasing globally, adoption and implementation,

by each country, of a national cancer policy and plan is an imperative. Political, financial, and technical support is required. Progress could be furthered by making existing cancer plans operational and, in particular, by increasing resources for early detection and treatment capacity.

With increasing awareness by policy-makers of the burden that noncommunicable diseases (NCDs) — including cardiovascular disease, diabetes, and cancer — impose on national health systems and economies, WHO has been asked to provide data indicating the preparedness of national health systems to prevent and control NCDs. Together with monitoring of the cancer burden by cancer registries, cancer capacity assessment is a fundamental requirement for rational cancer control planning. The WHO Global Action Plan for the Prevention and Control of NCDs 2013–2020, endorsed by the 66th World Health Assembly (resolution WHA66.10) in 2013, addresses an urgent requirement to provide the information relevant to national NCD planning. National capacity data from the WHO 2013 Noncommunicable Disease Country Capacity Survey [1] indicate the

current preparedness of countries to undertake cancer control.

A WHO survey of Member States

The WHO 2013 Noncommunicable Disease Country Capacity Survey was a further development of a regular survey conducted periodically to assess responses by individual countries to NCD challenges. Cancer-control-specific items are an integral part of the survey. Those results that are common to all NCDs are published in country profiles [2], which provide an overview of national priority setting for NCDs and the availability of corresponding interventions. The NCD country profiles complement the WHO global report on the burden of these diseases and respective recommended interventions [3].

National NCD capacity is assessed by the dimensions of public health infrastructure and partnerships focused on NCDs, taking account of relevant strategies, programmes, and action plans, health information systems, and health-care capacity. The questionnaire used in the 2013 Noncommunicable Disease Country Capacity Survey included these dimensions in four modules that captured information on cancer. Cancer control capacity is defined as the availability of plans,

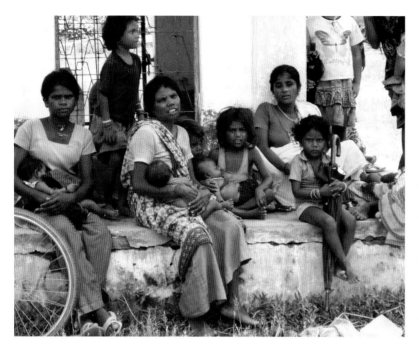

Fig. 6.2.1. Mothers and children at a health-care clinic in Sarlahi District, Nepal. In low-income countries generally, the burden associated with cervical cancer may be markedly reduced by the incorporation of appropriate screening into routine health services.

has the highest coverage of national plans, with 49 of the 50 countries having plans, while the South-East Asia Region has the lowest proportion of national cancer plans, with 7 of the 10 countries so identified. In the African Region, 27 of 37 countries reported having a cancer plan. Overall, cancer control is formally included in national health planning in the majority of countries.

To gain more detailed insight into national cancer control planning processes, several criteria were assessed. These included whether the plan was operational as well as the availability of dedicated funding for the plan. The inclusion of these additional criteria enabled a more differentiated assessment of the status of national cancer plans and policies. In the African and Eastern Mediterranean Regions, in contrast to the high percentage of countries that reported having a formal cancer plan, only 36% of the countries

programmes, and services covering the essential components of a national cancer control programme [4], including prevention, early detection, treatment, and palliative care.

Information to assess the national capacity for prevention and control of cancer was extracted from the 2013 Noncommunicable Disease Country Capacity Survey by using methods that have been previously used and described in detail [1]. The relevant questionnaire was sent in 2012 to appropriate authorities within the ministries of health of all 193 WHO Member States. Detailed information about the situation with respect to NCD control was received from 176 countries.

National cancer plans and their implementation

Ministries of health in the majority of participating countries, specifically 149 of 176, reported having a national cancer policy, strategy, or action plan, hereafter referred to as a "cancer plan". There are, however, regional differences. The European Region

Table 6.2.1. Results from the WHO 2013 Noncommunicable Disease Country Capacity Survey: percentage of countries with cancer policies, strategies, or action plans and their functionality

WHO region[a]	Number of countries	Percentage of countries with cancer policies, strategies, or plans	
		Existing policy	Operational policy with funding
African	37	73%	38%
Americas	31	90%	65%
Eastern Mediterranean	21	76%	43%
European	50	98%	84%
South-East Asia	10	70%	70%
Western Pacific	27	85%	78%
World Bank income group[b]			
Low	29	79%	45%
Lower-middle	43	84%	58%
Upper-middle	49	84%	65%
High	55	91%	78%
Total	176	85%	64%

[a] For a list of countries corresponding to each WHO region, see http://www.who.int/about/regions/en/index.html.

[b] For definitions of World Bank income groups, see http://data.worldbank.org/about/country-classifications.

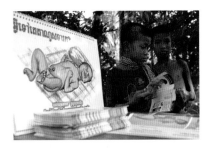

Fig. 6.2.2. The Children's Vaccine Program is working with the Cambodian government and other partners to make hepatitis B vaccines available to all children in the country. Here, health-related brochures are distributed to villagers by the mobile health team in the village of Choumpou in Kampong Cham Province.

reported that the plan was operational and only 43% had dedicated funding available for the implementation of the plan. Similar, but less marked, differences were evident in the other WHO regions, where allocation of resources for implementation of many national plans is lacking. In addition, the specification of a plan does not guarantee that its implementation is monitored or that there is a clear definition of measurable anticipated outcomes.

Approximately 15% of all participating countries did not have a cancer plan. Overall, only 64% of countries reported having cancer control plans that were operational and funded. Analysis of the available findings by World Bank income group revealed a consistent gradient from low-income countries to high-income countries with respect to the specification and completeness of national cancer plans. High-income countries are more likely to have plans that are also funded and monitored with regard to their defined outcomes (Table 6.2.1). However, even within countries in the highest income group, characterized by 90% of countries having a national cancer plan, only a proportion (78%), rather than all countries, confirmed that these plans were operational and funded.

Monitoring the cancer burden

The availability of data establishing the national cancer burden is the basis for any rational cancer planning and the ordering of priorities. Cancer registries therefore play a key role in national cancer planning. In the majority of countries, i.e. in 80% of the

176 countries responding, a registry for cancer was reported, regardless of the type of the registration undertaken (Table 6.2.2). The European Region exhibited the highest proportion of countries with cancer registries (94%), and the South-East Asia Region had the lowest proportion of countries (60%). In 25 of 37 countries in the African Region and in 24 of 27 countries in the Western Pacific Region, there was a monitoring system for cancer.

The various cancer registries were further differentiated from each other by type of registry – some of the key differences are whether the registry is population-based or hospital-based, and whether the population covered is national or is identified at a less comprehensive level. In almost all regions, population-based registries are the predominant type, accounting for 69% in the Eastern Mediterranean Region and 81% in the European Region. The region in which population-based cancer registries are the least common is the South-East Asia Region (50%). There is a consistent link between cancer registration and national

Table 6.2.2. Results from the WHO 2013 Noncommunicable Disease Country Capacity Survey: percentage of countries with cancer registries and type of registry

WHO region[a]	Number of countries	Percentage (number) of countries with cancer registries				
		Existing cancer registries[b]	National registries[c,d]	Subnational registries[c,d]	Population-based registries[d]	Hospital-based registries[d]
African	37	68% (25)	32% (8)	68% (17)	64% (16)	36% (9)
Americas	31	71% (22)	64%	36%	77% (17)	18% (4) (missing 1)
Eastern Mediterranean	21	76% (16)	69%	31%	69% (11)	25% (4) (missing 1)
European	50	94% (47)	81%	19%	81% (38)	15% (7) (missing 2)
South-East Asia	10	60% (6)	17%	83%	50% (3)	50% (3)
Western Pacific	27	89% (24)	75%	25%	58% (14)	42% (10)
World Bank income group[e]						
Low	29	59% (17)	35%	65%	47% (8)	47%
Lower-middle	43	72% (31)	35%	65%	48% (15)	52%
Upper-middle	49	84% (41)	68%	32%	71% (29)	22%
High	55	93% (51)	88%	12%	92% (47)	8%
Total	176	80% (140)	64%	36%	71% (99)	26%

[a] For a list of countries corresponding to each WHO region, see http://www.who.int/about/regions/en/index.html.
[b] Data reporting on the answer "yes" to the overall question "Does your country have a cancer registry (of any kind)?"
[c] Data reporting on the answer to the question "Does your country have a national cancer registry vs a regional registry?" The positive response to this question does not imply that there is national coverage.
[d] Percentage of countries out of the total responding "yes" to the overall question "Does your country have a cancer registry (of any kind)?"
[e] For definitions of World Bank income groups, see http://data.worldbank.org/about/country-classifications.

Cervical cancer prevention in six African countries

Nathalie Broutet

A WHO demonstration programme for cervical cancer prevention began in September 2005 and was completed in May 2009. Training of project coordinators was organized at the University of Zimbabwe, Harare. Training in data management was undertaken at all project sites, with the African Population and Health Research Center (APHRC) and IARC. The project created awareness in communities about cervical cancer and its prevention in six African countries: Madagascar, Malawi, Nigeria, Uganda, the United Republic of Tanzania, and Zambia.

Women were counselled and offered screening using visual inspection with acetic acid (VIA), and patients with a positive screening test were treated using cryotherapy. Patients who were not eligible for cryotherapy were referred to a higher level of health care for further evaluation and treatment (Fig. B6.2.1). Continuous monitoring and

evaluation of the project was carried out by IARC and APHRC, to generate evidence about the acceptability and feasibility in a primary health-care setting, referral site, or district hospital. The project targeted all women resident in the catchment area and aged between 30 and 50 years.

Between September 2005 and May 2009, a total of 19 579 women were screened in the six countries. Overall, 10.1% of screening with VIA results were positive, and 1.7% of women had lesions suspicious of cancer on inspection. A total of 87.7% of all VIA-positive cases were eligible for cryotherapy. The majority of women (63.4%) received cryotherapy within one week of initial screening. The single-visit approach enabled 39.1% of women to be screened and treated on the same day. However, more than 39.1% of all women eligible for cryotherapy did not receive

treatment, for various reasons, including equipment failure and women needing to obtain consent from their spouses before cryotherapy could be done. The VIA and cryotherapy procedures were well tolerated by the women, and almost all of those who underwent these procedures said they would recommend them to other women.

This programme has shown that the "screen and treat" approach can be introduced into existing reproductive health services in low-resource countries. Screening for precancerous lesions using VIA and treatment with cryotherapy is acceptable and feasible at low-level health facilities. VIA is an attractive alternative to cytology-based screening in low-resource settings. The alternative simple and safe cervical cancer prevention techniques simplify the process and render it feasible and acceptable to women and service providers in low-resource settings.

At the final meeting of the project, country teams presented plans on how best to scale up cervical cancer prevention services using the "screen and treat" approach. Training of an adequate number of providers, sustainable supervision, and supply and maintenance of equipment and consumables are key elements of the programme. The country teams noted that funding shortages and limited human resources are some of the factors that may prevent the ministries of health in the six countries from sustaining and scaling up the programme. However, at least four of these six countries now have national cervical cancer prevention programmes.

Fig. B6.2.1. Programme for strengthening cervical cancer prevention: operational framework. VIA, visual inspection with acetic acid.

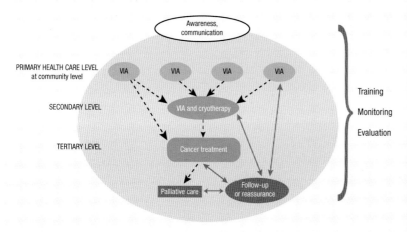

income. In the highest income category, 93% of countries have a monitoring system for cancer, and this proportion falls to 59% for countries in the lowest income group. This gradient in cancer monitoring with the level of prosperity is particularly

dramatic for population-based registries, which are available in only 8 of the 29 countries in the lowest income group compared with 47 of the 55 countries in the highest. Overall, 36 countries reported that they have no cancer-specific registration.

Prevention and early detection policies

Prevention
Certain declared policies to prevent cancer are also amenable to comparison and evaluation. Interventions based on exposure to relevant

Fig. 6.2.3. The World Health Assembly in Geneva, 2011. WHO initiatives, in relation to the global burden of noncommunicable diseases generally, have permitted assessment of national policies for cancer control and their implementation. The data indicate that low-income countries face challenges in implementing proven means to reduce cancer incidence and mortality.

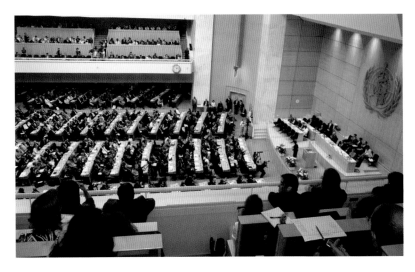

infectious agents and environmental carcinogens, apart from those encountered through lifestyle choice, were not addressed by the survey. Of the 176 responding countries, 92% report having a national policy for tobacco control, 77% have policies on harmful use of alcohol, 84% address unhealthy diet, 77% act on overweight or obesity, and 81% have a policy that focuses on improving physical activity. Although more countries have a policy for tobacco use than have policies in relation to any other NCD-based prevention strategy, only 69% of the responding countries have a tobacco policy that was reported as operational and as having a dedicated budget.

Early detection
Several cancer types of major public health relevance have a high probability of being cured if they are detected early in their clinical course and relevant cases are then referred, in a timely fashion, for definitive diagnosis and treatment at secondary or tertiary levels of care.

Population-based screening for certain cancers is established (see Chapter 4.7) and subject to national survey. Cytology (Pap smear) testing for cervical cancer is the most widely applied detection procedure but requires specialized laboratories and a recall system for test-positive cases. Visual methods, such as inspection of the cervix after acetic acid staining, are options for low-income settings because no sophisticated technology is required (see "Cervical cancer

Table 6.2.3. Results from the WHO 2013 Noncommunicable Disease Country Capacity Survey: percentage of countries where tests and procedures for the early detection of cancer are available

| WHO region[a] | Number of countries | Percentage of countries where available | | | | | |
		Pap smear cervical cytology	VIA	FOBT	DRE	Breast palpation	Mammography
African	37	38%	24%	14%	16%	57%	30%
Americas	31	97%	45%	81%	65%	94%	61%
Eastern Mediterranean	21	38%	24%	38%	24%	81%	43%
European	50	80%	56%	80%	68%	86%	70%
South-East Asia	10	20%	10%	0%	10%	60%	0%
Western Pacific	27	67%	30%	63%	56%	89%	56%
World Bank income group[b]							
Low	29	21%	14%	3%	7%	52%	17%
Lower-middle	43	42%	28%	26%	23%	72%	23%
Upper-middle	49	78%	31%	65%	51%	90%	55%
High	55	91%	62%	93%	80%	91%	85%
Total	176	64%	37%	54%	46%	80%	51%

DRE, digital rectal examination; FOBT, faecal occult blood testing; VIA, visual inspection with acetic acid.
[a] For a list of countries corresponding to each WHO region, see http://www.who.int/about/regions/en/index.html.
[b] For definitions of World Bank income groups, see http://data.worldbank.org/about/country-classifications.

Traditional household cooking: risks and prevention

Majid Ezzati

More than 2 billion people worldwide use biomass fuels (firewood, charcoal, animal dung, and crop residues) and coal for cooking and heating. Biomass use is currently most common in sub-Saharan Africa [1], followed by South Asia. In developing countries, these fuels, which together are called solid fuels, are often burned in open fires or traditional stoves with poor combustion efficiency. Solid-fuel smoke contains many solid (particle) and gaseous pollutants, including known human carcinogens. As a result, people living in homes that use solid fuels, especially women and young children who may spend hours near cooking fires, have high exposures to particles and other pollutants.

There is increasing epidemiological evidence that exposure to biomass and coal smoke is a risk factor for childhood pneumonia, chronic obstructive pulmonary disease, lung cancer, and cataracts, with some evidence of a dose–response relationship. Evidence is also emerging for effects on tuberculosis, low birth weight, and cardiovascular out-

Fig. B6.2.2. A traditional three-stone open fire, as used in many households in developing countries.

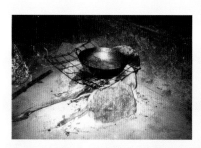

Fig. B6.2.3. The traditional open fire used in many developing counties is associated with high concentrations of pollutants, as seen from the smoke rising from the roof of a house in central Kenya.

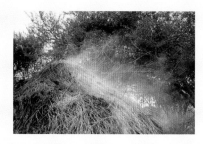

comes. Exposure to air pollution from solid fuels is responsible for an estimated 3.5 million deaths per year and more than 4% of the global disease burden. Importantly, the majority of the burden is now from noncommunicable diseases. The health effects of household air pollution are largest in low-income regions and in poor households.

The large disease burden in poor communities and households has helped make solid fuel use a major global health concern. For example, solid fuel use is an indicator for Goal 7 (ensuring environmental sustainability) of the United Nations Millennium Development Goals. Yet there are several challenges in implementing interventions that reduce exposure by a large amount. Alternative stove technologies, despite having gained support among activists in developed countries, have proven not to be a viable option for intervention in most places because user behaviours modify their

performance and because they require regular maintenance. Clean fuels such as electricity and natural gas will certainly reduce exposure substantially and provide substantial health gains [1,2]. However, widespread use of these clean fuels is restricted by their cost, uncertainty about prices, and the absence of an energy infrastructure that allows households to buy fuels when they need them and without having to travel long distances [3]. In addition to clean fuels, it may be possible to "pre-process" biomass and coal to burn more cleanly, by converting it to gaseous or liquid fuels, charcoal, or briquettes.

In summary, research over the past two decades has helped to establish air pollution from household solid fuel use as an important global health risk, especially among the poor [4]. The increased visibility must be sustained but needs to be accompanied with efforts to reduce the burden of disease, including cancers, caused by emissions from indoor combustion.

References

1. Bailis R et al. (2005). Science, 308:98–103. http://dx.doi.org/10.1126/science.1106881 PMID:15802601

2. Lin HH et al. (2008). Lancet, 372:1473–1483. http://dx.doi.org/10.1016/S0140-6736(08)61345-8 PMID:18835640

3. Ezzati M DM et al. (2004). Annu Rev Environ Resour, 29:383–420. http://dx.doi.org/10.1146/annurev.energy.29.062103.121246

4. IARC (2010). IARC Monogr Eval Carcinog Risks Hum, 95:1–430. PMID:20701241

prevention in six African countries"). Mammography is used to detect early-stage breast cancer. Clinical breast examination by palpation performed by health professionals is a low-cost approach to detect early breast cancer. Rectal cancer can be detected at an early stage by clinical examination

(digital rectal examination). Faecal occult blood testing is in use for early detection of colorectal cancer.

Ministry of health officials were asked whether tests for early detection of cervical, breast, and colorectal cancers were available in the national public system at primary health-care

level. Responses received are summarized in Table 6.2.3. A more detailed assessment of the presence of a specific detection programme (screening programme) was not included in the survey.

Concerning detection of cervical cancer and precancer, 64% of the

Box 6.2.1. Trends in national cancer control capacity.

Of the 176 countries that participated in the WHO 2013 Noncommunicable Disease Country Capacity Survey, responses from those with prior data from a 2010 study were assessed for trends.

Overall, the percentage of countries with a cancer plan increased, from 81% in 2010 to 86% in 2013, as did the percentage with an operational cancer plan (from 61% to 65%). The largest gain in national cancer plans was in low-income countries (from 54% to 79%). However, increases in an operational cancer plan followed an income gradient: high-income countries had the most advancement from 2010 to 2013 (from 74% to 81%), whereas there was little or no gain in lower-middle and low-income countries (remaining at about 56% and 43%, respectively).

The percentage of countries with cancer registries, regardless of their type, remained largely unchanged (80%). Further differentiation found an increase in population-based registries rather than hospital-based registries, from 46% in 2010 to 59% in 2013. While national-level registries among high-income countries remained at a steady 85%, overall this percentage decreased from 64% to 49%, a drop distributed across all other income groups and regions.

The availability of cervical cancer screening by visual inspection after acetic acid staining increased in European countries (from 27% to 56%) and in African countries (from 14% to 24%). The availability of cervical cytology and breast cancer screening by palpation was steady across all countries. Only regional differences were seen: cervical cytology access increased in Africa (from 27% to 38%) and in the Western Pacific Region (from 56% to 67%) while decreasing significantly in Eastern Mediterranean countries (from 57% to 38%). Notably, the South-East Asia Region showed a consistent 20% drop in all survey indicators, including the presence of a cancer plan, an operational cancer plan, cancer registries, and access to cervical cytology and breast cancer screening by palpation.

176 countries reported the availability of a cytology-based screening test at primary care level, a major increase over the corresponding data reported in 2010 (26%) (Box 6.2.1). The presence of cytology services was still low in the African Region (38%) and the South-East Asia Region (20%), as was the availability of visual inspection after acetic acid staining, with 24% of countries in the African Region and 10% in the South-East Asia Region reporting positively. Compared with cytology tests, visual inspection was generally less available in all regions. The availability of breast palpation by a health worker as routine in primary health care was low in the African Region, where 57% of countries reported availability, and in the South-East Asia Region, where the procedure was available in 60% of countries. In Europe, the Eastern Mediterranean, and the Americas, breast examination was reported as generally available in primary health-care facilities in 86%, 81%, and 94% of countries, respectively.

The situations concerning availability of radiotherapy and chemotherapy for cancer treatment in the public health sector, as well as the availability of palliative care services, were also subject to report in the survey but are outside the scope of the present Report.

Imperatives for improvement of cancer control

Analysis of the data collected by the Noncommunicable Disease Country Capacity Survey provides an overview of the extent of national capacity to address the cancer burden in almost all WHO Member States. Although the survey was designed to assess national capacity for NCD control from the perspective of an integrated approach, it is practicable to develop a comparable global picture specifically for cancer control along the continuum from prevention to palliative care. The summation in this chapter has addressed cancer control apart from clinical care.

The recognized limitations of such an analysis arise from the fact that the sources of information were NCD reference points in ministries of health not necessarily closely connected with the cancer control situation. The design of the survey allowed the assessment of key areas of cancer control to inform a global rating, but without any details about, for example, the proportion of the population covered by defined interventions (see "Traditional household cooking: risks and prevention"). The question and response structure of the survey may not have allowed respondents to reflect in detail the na-

Fig. 6.2.4. Cover of WHO Guide for Effective Programmes on cancer control. This publication is a series of six modules on cancer control: Planning, Prevention, Early detection, Diagnosis and treatment, Palliative care, and Policy and advocacy.

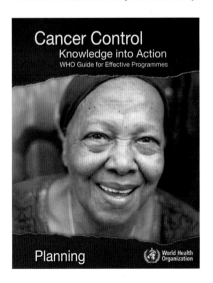

tional particularities of health-care systems and their organizational structures. Finally, although the questionnaire and its instructions were available in almost all WHO official languages (English, French, Spanish, and Russian), there may have been language barriers with regard to the definitions of technical terms and their meaning.

Despite such limitations, the key results available provide evidence of major gaps between what is known about effective cancer control and the implementation of measures to reduce the cancer burden.

• The formal specification of a national cancer control policy or plan does not guarantee implementation. Government officials were very clear in reporting major discrepancies between the endorsement of a formal government policy or plan and its operational status. In only two thirds of all responding countries did a cancer plan or

policy have a specific budget that would allow the necessary organizational arrangements as recommended by WHO (see Chapter 6.1).

• Established cancer prevention policies were far from being implemented universally. Although there is definitive knowledge about the behavioural aspects of cancer causation, such as tobacco use, and there are effective strategies to reduce such use, as outlined in this Report (see Chapter 4.1), national implementation capacity to prevent cancer caused by tobacco and alcohol use, unhealthy diet, obesity, and lack of physical activity is markedly limited.

• Early detection of cancer was generally absent from the public care delivery systems in most countries in the low and lower-middle income groups. Because cervical cancer is of major public health relevance in most of these countries, increasing access to early detection through

organized cervical cancer screening will have a major impact on the cancer burden.

The survey identified major gaps and challenges for national health-care systems to achieve better cancer control. The majority of countries reported the existence of a national policy, strategy, or action plan to address cancer. Even among countries in the lowest income group, where communicable diseases such as HIV/AIDS, tuberculosis, and malaria are the major focus of national health planning and international health aid, national cancer plans are at least formally specified in more than half. However, to be effective, these policies and plans must be further developed and funded. Every country will have to determine national priorities for cancer control in the context of other NCDs and the opportunities that health system reforms will offer.

References

1. WHO (2012). *Assessing National Capacity for the Prevention and Control of Noncommunicable Diseases: Report of the 2010 Global Survey.* Geneva: WHO. Available at http://www.who.int/chp/knowledge/national_prevention_ncds/en/.

2. WHO (2011). *Noncommunicable Diseases Country Profiles 2011.* Geneva: WHO. Available at http://www.who.int/nmh/publications/ncd_profiles2011/en/.

3. WHO (2011). *Global Status Report on Noncommunicable Diseases 2010.* Geneva: WHO. Available at http://www.who.int/chp/ncd_global_status_report/en/.

4. WHO (2002). *National Cancer Control Programmes: Policies and Managerial Guidelines*, 2nd ed. Available at http://www.who.int/cancer/publications/nccp2002/en/index.html.

Websites

WHO Global Action Plan for the Prevention and Control of NCDs 2013–2020:
http://www.who.int/nmh/events/ncd_action_plan/en/

WHO Guide for Effective Programmes – Module 1: Planning:
http://www.who.int/cancer/publications/cancer_control_planning/en/index.html

Cancer control in China: preventive policies and accessible health care

Guiqi Wang

In 2010, cancer accounted for 23.82% of overall deaths and became one of the leading causes of death in China [1]. Most of the cases were diagnosed at a medium or late stage, so the efficacy of treatment was unsatisfactory. The health-care cost of these diseases created a severe economic burden on many individuals and on society, and became a major cause of poverty or returning to poverty for the patients and their families. The Chinese government places great importance on cancer control and carries out active preventive strategies and cancer control projects in collaboration with all sectors of society.

In 2005, China initiated a national programme of early detection and treatment for oesophageal cancer, gastric cancer, colorectal cancer, liver cancer, nasopharyngeal cancer, and lung cancer in high-incidence areas, and in 2009, China started a national screening programme for cervical cancer and breast cancer in rural areas. In both programmes, early detection and treatment has become an effective strategy for cancer control. For example, in some local areas of China, people have had very high rates of oesophageal cancer for a long time. The early detection and treatment programme screens residents in those areas aged 40–69 years by endoscopy with iodine staining and biopsy of early lesions. Patients with early-stage neoplasia, including severe squamous dysplasia, carcinoma in situ, and intramucosal carcinoma, can receive early treatments in a timely manner.

To accumulate experience and optimize techniques for this plan, the national programme first chose eight high-incidence areas as demonstration sites and screened about 13 000 high-risk adults each year. Now, after a step-by-step expansion, 88 high-incidence areas in 26 provinces are participating in this early detection and treatment programme for oesophageal cancer [2]. From 2006 to 2012, 412 641 adults from high-risk areas were screened by endoscopy, and 4011 patients were diagnosed with severe precancerous lesions or early-stage cancer [2]. Most of these patients received timely treatment, with great benefit to health, and an economic analysis of this programme has shown that it is cost-effective [3].

In addition to such early detection and treatment programmes, the Chinese government promotes widespread public education about cancer prevention and treatment, and has conducted interventions to control cancer occurrence, including neonatal vaccination against hepatitis B virus, programmes promoting better nutrition, and targeted programmes to improve occupational safety.

The China National Central Cancer Registry has also improved the national cancer registry system, and since 2008 has reported national cancer registry data annually. In 2012, there were 222 cancer registry sites, covering 200 million people nationwide.

References

1. Yu W (2012). *National Disease Monitoring System 2010: Data Set of Death Causes.* Beijing: Military Medical Science Press.

2. Diseases Prevention and Control Bureau of Ministry of Health, Cancer Foundation of China, Committee of Experts of the Cancer Early Detection and Early Treatment Project (2012). *Report of the Cancer Early Detection and Early Treatment Project 2011/2012.*

3. Dong Z *et al.* (2012). *Chin J Oncol*, 34: 637–640.

6.3

Health systems strengthening for cancer control

6 CONTROL

Massoud Samiei

Benjamin O. Anderson (reviewer)
Eduardo L. Cazap (reviewer)
Nobuo Koinuma (reviewer)

Summary

- Developing countries need stronger health systems to support essential cancer control efforts. The experience in high-income countries has demonstrated that cancer control cannot succeed without well-functioning and flexible health systems.

- In most developing countries, health-related infrastructure and trained human resources are lacking or poorly developed. However, when an infrastructure is established, the availability of treatment services indicates the likelihood of further positive developments within the context of a national cancer control plan.

- Since 2005, WHO and the International Atomic Energy Agency have engaged in demonstration projects using existing radiation medicine capacity in developing countries to initiate multidisciplinary cancer capacity building programmes. These programmes complement and enhance the clinical and public health impact of treatments by concurrently building capacity for all aspects of cancer control, including advocacy, epidemiology, prevention, early detection, diagnosis and treatment, palliative care, and society building.

- Basic strength in the health system, exemplified by a radiotherapy service with adequate personnel and diagnostic facilities, has led to the initiation of a more robust cancer control plan, which in turn tends to further strengthen the health system.

With 8.2 million deaths due to cancer in 2012, cancer remains a leading cause of death and disability worldwide [1]. As highlighted throughout this Report, the pattern of disease has shifted so that an increasing burden now falls on low- and middle-income countries, where healthcare systems are not designed, or prepared, to tackle chronic noncommunicable diseases in general. As population age distributions trend higher [2] and unhealthy lifestyles are increasingly adopted, populations in low- and middle-income countries face an expected rise in annual cancer incidence of nearly 70% by 2030 relative to the 2010 rates [3]. In 2010, there were more than 7.5 million new cases of cancer in low- and middle-income countries, and less than 30% of those patients had access to any reasonable treatment services [4].

For particular malignancies, specific modes of therapy, health technologies, and relevant skills and experience are recognized as the basis for treatment and, in some cases, cure.

All people, including those in low- and middle-income countries, are entitled to means of cancer prevention and appropriate care if they are diagnosed with cancer.

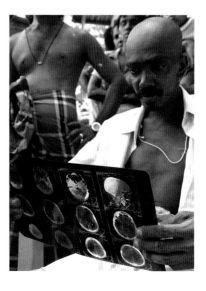

Fig. 6.3.1. In Sri Lanka, a patient with brain cancer looks at his scan. Sri Lanka is one of the WHO-IAEA Programme of Action for Cancer Therapy (PACT) Model Demonstration Sites. The country has implemented a successful comprehensive cancer control plan.

Strengthening national health systems, by providing equitable and affordable access to cancer care for all who require it and making the essential clinical services, such as diagnostic imaging and radiotherapy, available, is an increasingly high priority for most governments in low- and middle-income countries. This is also a priority for WHO and other United Nations agencies, such as IARC and the International Atomic Energy Agency (IAEA), and active nongovernmental organizations such as the Union for International Cancer Control [5] and the International Network for Cancer Treatment and Research [2]. This imperative has been given new emphasis after the resolution approved by all United Nations Member States in September 2011 on the prevention and control of noncommunicable diseases.

In 2012, the World Health Assembly set a global target of a 25% reduction in premature mortality from noncommunicable diseases by 2025, among eight other voluntary targets [6]. As highlighted in the discussion of national cancer control plans (Chapter 6.1), the prevention and control of cancer should be integrated into all major actions for other noncommunicable diseases. Various aspects of cancer control plans – from prevention to management of cancer and related research priorities – should be part of the national initiatives for strengthening each country's health system [7].

Treatment: an essential element of cancer control

As a growing number of cancer patients seek relief from pain and suffering in most developing countries, the traditional focus of attention by health authorities on treatment as the first priority is understandable. Indeed, even with the optimal application of cancer prevention strategies, benefits are evident only after the passage of about 20–30 years, and are not relevant to millions of new cancer patients diagnosed in the interim, specifically in developing

Fig. 6.3.2. The children's cancer ward at Ocean Road Cancer Institute in Dar es Salaam, Tanzania. Despite the crowded conditions, these children are among those fortunate enough to receive treatment.

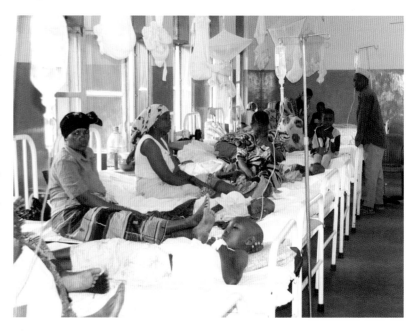

countries. However, early diagnosis and/or screening combined with adequate treatment – often designated as secondary prevention – of certain common cancers has the potential to improve cure rates and to reduce mortality from these cancers in a time frame of 5–10 years. If there is a prospect of effective treatment, people will be motivated to seek screening [8]. Moreover, availability of treatment involves families and different sectors of the community in a common effort to promote health care. The availability of effective treatment also builds public support and motivates a core of professionals who may then campaign for a higher national priority to be accorded to comprehensive cancer control.

Over the past 30 years, a combination of early detection and new treatment modalities has contributed to a modest, but constant, decline in cancer mortality rates in high-income countries [9]. This decline is not only due to the availability of more effective curative drugs, but is also the result of effective national cancer control plans, which have led to better public education and community

access to prompt diagnosis and treatment. Such programmes now result in increased health awareness and prevention, improved cure rates, and improved quality of life for cancer patients in high-income countries [10].

The experience in high-income countries has demonstrated that cancer control cannot succeed without well-functioning, robust, and flexible health systems. More specifically, strengthening health systems to deliver life-saving treatments requires well-developed technical infrastructure and a sufficient number of clinicians trained in treatment delivery. Among other services, pathology services to provide accurate diagnosis and staging of cancers and laboratory facilities, equipment, and technicians to run screening tests and deliver radiotherapy treatments must also be available.

Unfortunately, in most low-income countries and some other countries, such infrastructure and trained human resources are not available or are poorly developed. However, emerging evidence from many developing countries establishes that availability of treatment services can

The first cure of cancer by radiotherapy was reported in 1899, a few years after Röntgen's description of X-rays in 1895 and the discovery of radium in 1898 [16]. The technology has evolved radically since the 1950s, and today knowledge of radiation medicine and the availability of relevant technology are indispensable for cancer diagnosis, cure, and care, where radiation and radioactivity play fundamental roles. Depending on the stage and type of cancer, typically some 50–65% of all cancer patients require radiotherapy during the course of their disease, either as a single modal-ity or in combination with surgery, chemotherapy, hormone therapy, and/or immunotherapy [17].

Worldwide, radiotherapy is a major aspect of investment in health-care systems to treat cancer. Low- and middle-income countries have far to advance if their patients are to have reasonable access to such treatment. Although these countries account for 85% of the world's population, there are only about 4400 megavoltage machines in low- and middle-income countries, less than 35% of the world's radiotherapy facilities, leaving most cancer patients in these countries without any access to potentially life-saving radiotherapy treatment [18].

The International Atomic Energy Agency (IAEA) emphasizes that radiotherapy treatment is most effective when it is linked to a comprehensive national cancer control programme. For this reason, in 2004 IAEA established its Programme of Action for Cancer Therapy to help expand radiotherapy capacity in developing countries and build partnerships with WHO and others to address the huge disparities that exist in cancer control and services [19,20].

create a high probability for further positive developments within the context of a national cancer control plan [11–13]. With proper planning and appropriate strategies, and availability of trained professionals, developing countries can achieve much higher survival rates, in addition to preventing and otherwise controlling cancers. In a comparative study of cancer outcomes across 12 countries in Africa, Asia, and Central America, cancer outcomes correlated with the level of development of health services [14].

The question is to what extent the models from high-income countries can be replicated in low-income settings, and what options are economical and cost-effective in particular situations. For example, which diagnostic and treatment modalities should be developed? The dilemma for policy-makers and health authorities in developing countries is often to determine what comes first. Options may include providing affordable means of treating a portion of the growing number of patients, particularly in terms of medicine and health technology such as diagnostic imaging and radiotherapy, or adapting the most feasible strategies for cancer prevention and screening services.

The development of radiotherapy capacity is evidently a cost-effective and resource-level-appropriate strategy in developing countries to initiate capacity building in treatment [15]. As demonstrated in several countries, radiotherapy can serve as an anchor to develop self-sustaining national cancer control programmes, which in turn could help improve and expand other cancer services and infrastructure. Radiotherapy is fundamental to the optimum management of cancer patients, and provision of radiotherapy services is central to national cancer control strategies (Box 6.3.1) [16–20]. Although it requires long-term planning and appropriate assessment of health-care resources, effective radiotherapy for many cancers can be comprehensively provided at moderate cost, without recourse to sophisticated technologies [21]. Most countries have later expanded their initial radiotherapy capacity to add chemotherapy and other essential capacity, including imaging, pathology, and surgery. Such expanded capacity has often become the focus around which a national cancer centre is established [11].

Health systems strengthened through radiotherapy planning

Experience in many developing countries indicates that cancer control cannot achieve its potential unless the existing health system can sustain and support some key requirements. These include the technical capacity to initiate or manage the national cancer control plan and to deliver certain services. The initiation of a national cancer control plan requires establishing a cancer policy and additional legislative steps, setting or defining some key targets, and/or allocating funds for cancer control activities; this represents a top-down approach. However, quite often, where the leadership of existing cancer clinics or radiotherapy centres is supported by nongovernmental organizations, some members of the community may be particularly active in developing cancer control proposals: a bottom-up approach. For most low- and middle-income countries, a combination of these two approaches is more likely to succeed in initiating cancer control activities [22]. In countries that have been assessed, the initiation of cancer control activities and plans has been prompted by the leadership of an existing radiotherapy centre (often the only one in the country) because such centres are the places that immediately appreciate the severity of the cancer burden. The tragedy in developing countries is that 80%

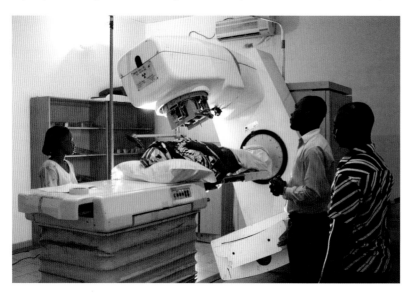

of cancer cases are diagnosed at a very advanced stage of disease.

The burden of late-stage diagnosis of cancer in developing countries provides strong motivation to move such a country towards cancer control planning rather than attempting to expand clinical facilities to treat the large number of patients. Countries that have committed to this option, and initiated some cancer control activities, have been more successful in seeking new funding to acquire additional treatment facilities and resources. Accordingly, basic strength in the health system, exemplified by a radiotherapy centre, can lead to the initiation of a more robust cancer control plan, which in turn can result in further health systems strengthening through improvements in other essential treatment modalities, and most often the establishment of a national cancer centre [11]. The directors of such national cancer centres in more than 40 low- and middle-income countries have prompted the launch of cancer control plans [23]. Arguably, a minimum level of national capacity and infrastructure must be present within the health system of any country before any cancer control activities can be initiated or launched successfully [13].

WHO-IAEA cooperation on cancer control

To build on the premises already described, and after the establishment of the Programme of Action for Cancer Therapy (PACT), WHO and IAEA signed an agreement in March 2009 to launch a cooperation on cancer control, aimed at strengthening and accelerating cancer control in developing countries [24,25]. The formation of a WHO-IAEA cooperation began in May 2005 when the World Health Assembly adopted a far-reaching resolution in response to the marked increase in cancer incidence worldwide. Since then, PACT, WHO, IARC, and other key international cancer organizations have undertaken increasingly productive collaboration. Particular emphasis is placed on providing assistance within a broad, multidisciplinary cancer capacity building programme that complements and enhances the clinical and public health impact of treatment.

The WHO-IAEA cooperation provides the framework for the two organizations to integrate their work, building on their areas of expertise to create a more coordinated and robust approach to combating cancer in low- and middle-income countries. The focus of WHO support within the cooperation is on public awareness, prevention, early detection, and overall care for patients. In particular, WHO emphasizes population-based interventions and the strengthening of public health approaches to prevention and control of cancer, with special attention to primary health care. National cancer control programmes fit into the broader WHO framework to strengthen health systems with a major focus on primary health care, and are part of the implementation of the Action Plan of the Global Strategy for the Preventions and Control of Noncommunicable Diseases, which was endorsed by the World Health Assembly in May 2008 and has been updated to cover the 2013–2020 period [26,27]. Since the launch of PACT, IAEA requires that all of its assistance related to radiation medicine be channelled through ministries of health to ensure an integrated and balanced approach. IAEA recommends that low- and middle-income countries should prepare their national cancer control plans and then specifically examine the need for expansion of diagnostic and treatment services based on local resources, types of cancer, and other relevant conditions.

Cancer control through demonstration projects

Efforts in the WHO-IAEA cooperation on cancer control have been focusing on eight PACT Model Demonstration Sites (PMDS), in Albania, Ghana, Mongolia, Nicaragua, Sri Lanka, the United Republic of Tanzania, Viet Nam, and Yemen [28], most of which have been successful in using their existing radiotherapy programmes to embark on developing cancer control strategies. WHO and IAEA have assisted these countries in needs assessment, evaluation of possible strategies, setting of priorities, and selection of resource-level-appropriate interventions.

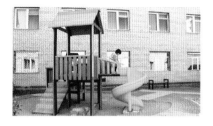

Through the cooperation on cancer control, WHO and IAEA have also responded to requests for cancer control assessment and programme development assistance in more than 45 countries since 2005 [29,30]. Each country has particular features in terms of the cancer burden, cancer risk factors, culture, health system, available financial and human resources, and infrastructure. Careful assessment of these elements helps to establish realistic and achievable priorities for action in a specific context [31]. WHO, IAEA, IARC, and partners assist national authorities in their cancer control endeavours, sharing the experiences of developing countries that have already achieved successes in cancer control. Once a country's most pressing needs are identified and prioritized, partners and donors are approached for adequate response strategies, which may be on the technical and/or financial side. Follow-up missions for monitoring progress are also conducted regularly.

Early evaluation of PMDS

PMDS projects are at different stages of implementation, having started at different baselines. However, they all share very high motivation at the professional and political level. Each of the PMDS projects has worked diligently on developing a national cancer control plan and establishing a national steering committee to oversee the implementation of the plan. With support from partners, PACT has mobilized funds to support countries with expert advice, human resource development, acquisition of radiation medicine equipment, and cancer control capacity building [19].

As reported by a recent evaluation of PMDS [12], it is clear that in each PMDS project, availability of radiation medicine capacity, although still limited, has played a pivotal role as an initial driver of the country's cancer control plan, and in the implementation of elements of each country's national cancer control programme. There are already signs and actions in PMDS projects demonstrating that health authorities have appreciated that health systems strengthening for cancer care and control cannot be achieved without balanced investments in prevention, early detection, diagnosis, treatment, and palliative care.

Hence, the success of national cancer control plans is dependent to a large extent on broader reform measures within the health system of each country to address the inequalities in health care and services. Equally important is the capacity of ministries of health, and their longer-term commitment to implementation and evaluation of the policies and strategies developed. In particular, if there is no commitment towards efforts aimed at prevention, coordination of services, and affordability of, and access to, health services,

then there is unlikely to be an improvement in health systems.

To ensure further progress and sustainability of cancer control programmes already initiated, all developing countries should consider establishing at least one government-supported *cancer centre of excellence* based on existing cancer centres to provide high-quality services and act as a driving force for national cancer control [11,23]. Furthermore, in view of prevailing limitations in workforce capability, for the long-term strengthening and success of cancer control, each country should have a 10–15-year training programme [13]. Cancer registries, health data collection, and health services research in all countries require support [32]. In this context, the IARC Global Initiative for Cancer Registry Development in Low- and Middle-Income Countries and the International Cancer Control Partnership, jointly coordinated by the UICC and the United States National Cancer Institute and involving WHO, IAEA-PACT, IARC, and several key cancer organizations and individual experts, are immediately relevant.

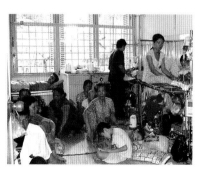

References

1. WHO (2011). United Nations High-Level Meeting on Noncommunicable Disease Prevention and Control. Available at http://www.who.int/nmh/events/un_ncd_summit2011/en/.

2. International Network for Cancer Treatment and Research (2013). Cancer in Developing Countries. Available at http://www.inctr.org/about-inctr/cancer-in-developing-countries/.

3. Ferlay J, Shin HR, Bray F *et al.* (2010). GLOBOCAN 2008 v2.0, Cancer Incidence and Mortality Worldwide: IARC CancerBase No. 10 [Internet]. Lyon: IARC. Available at http://globocan.iarc.fr.

4. IAEA (2011). *Inequity in Cancer Care: A Global Perspective*. IAEA Human Health Reports, No. 3. Available at http://www-pub.iaea.org/books/IAEABooks/8180/Inequity-in-Cancer-Care-A-Global-Perspective.

5. Union for International Cancer Control: http://www.uicc.org.

6. WHO Media Centre (2012). 65th World Health Assembly closes with new global health measures. News release. Available at http://www.who.int/mediacentre/news/releases/2012/wha65_closes_20120526/en/index.html.

7. Sullivan R, Purushottham A (2010). Towards an international cancer control plan: policy solutions for the global cancer epidemic. *INCTR Magazine*, 9:1–8. Available at http://www.inctr.org/network-magazine/past-editions/.

8. World Bank (2013). World Bank in Albania breast cancer campaign. Available at http://web.worldbank.org/WBSITE/EXTERNAL/NEWS/0,,contentMDK:23177166~menuPK:141310~pagePK:34370~piPK:34424~theSitePK:4607,00.html.

9. Abegunde DO, Mathers CD, Adam T *et al.* (2007). The burden and costs of chronic diseases in low-income and middle-income countries. *Lancet*, 370:1929–1938. http://dx.doi.org/10.1016/S0140-6736(07)61696-1 PMID:18063029

10. Levin V, Meghzifene A, Izewska J, Tatsuzaki H (2001). Improving cancer care: increased need for radiotherapy in developing countries. *IAEA Bull*, 43:25–32.

11. Sloan F, Gelband H, eds; Committee on Cancer Control in Low- and Middle-Income Countries (2007). *Cancer Control Opportunities in Low- and Middle-Income Countries*, Washington, DC: National Academies Press.

12. IAEA, PACT (2012). Evaluation of PMDS, 2011–2012. IAEA internal report.

13. Anderson B, Ballieu M, Bradley C *et al.* (2010). Access to cancer treatment in low- and middle-income countries – an essential part of global cancer control. A CanTreat Position Paper. Available at http://ssrn.com/abstract=2055441.

14. Sankaranarayanan R, Swaminathan R, Brenner H *et al.* (2010). Cancer survival in Africa, Asia, and Central America: a population-based study. *Lancet Oncol*, 11:165–173. http://dx.doi.org/10.1016/S1470-2045(09)70335-3 PMID:200005175

15. IAEA (2010). *Planning National Radiotherapy Services: A Practical Tool*. IAEA Human Health Series, No. 14. Available at http://www-pub.iaea.org/books/IAEABooks/8419/Planning-National-Radiotherapy-Services-A-Practical-Tool.

16. Rickwood P (2001). Saving a mother's life. Radiotherapy offers new hope for women of child rearing age suffering cervical cancer in developing countries. Available at http://www.iaea.org/About/Policy/GC/GC45/SciProg/sfradiotherapy.html.

17. IAEA (2008). *Setting up a Radiotherapy Programme: Clinical, Medical Physics, Radiation Protection and Safety Aspects*. Vienna: International Atomic Energy Agency.

18. Burkart W, Chhem RK, Samiei M (2010). Atoms for health: the IAEA's contribution to the fight against cancer. In: *Health G20: A Briefing on Health Issues for G20 Leaders*. Available at http://www-naweb.iaea.org/na/G20-IAEA-article-atoms-for-health.pdf.

19. IAEA-PACT (2013). International Atomic Energy Agency Programme of Action for Cancer Therapy. Available at http://cancer.iaea.org/.

20. Samiei M (2008). Building partnerships to stop the cancer epidemic in the developing world. *UN Special*, No. 676, September 2008. Available at http://www.unspecial.org/UNS676/t31.html.

21. Stewart BW, Kleihues P, eds (2003). *World Cancer Report*. Lyon: IARC.

22. Barton MB, Frommer M, Shafiq J (2006). Role of radiotherapy in cancer control in low-income and middle-income countries. *Lancet Oncol*, 7:584–595. http://dx.doi.org/10.1016/S1470-2045(06)70759-8 PMID:16814210

23. Samiei M (2013). Challenges of making radiotherapy accessible in developing countries. In: *Cancer Control 2013: Cancer Care in Emerging Health Systems*. Global Health Dynamics UK and INCTR Belgium, pp. 85–96.

24. WHO Media Centre (2009). WHO, IAEA join forces to fight cancer in developing countries. News release. Available at http://www.who.int/mediacentre/news/releases/2009/who_iaea_cancer_programme_20090526/en/.

25. WHO, IAEA (2009). Arrangements between the Directors General of the World Health Organization and the International Atomic Energy Agency for the WHO/IAEA Joint Programme on Cancer Control. Available at http://www.who.int/nmh/events/2013/2009arrangements.pdf.

26. WHO (2009). 2008–2013 *Action Plan for the Global Strategy for the Prevention and Control of Noncommunicable Diseases*. Geneva: WHO. Available at http://www.who.int/nmh/publications/9789241597418/en/.

27. WHO (2013). *Global Action Plan for the Prevention and Control of Noncommunicable Diseases 2013–2020*. Geneva: WHO. Available at http://www.who.int/nmh/en/.

28. IAEA-PACT (2013). PACT Model Demonstration Sites (PMDS). Available at http://cancer.iaea.org/pmds.asp.

29. IAEA-PACT (2013). IAEA imPACT (integrated missions of PACT). Available at http://cancer.iaea.org/impact.asp.

30. IAEA-PACT (2012). In Malaysia, IAEA conducts 45th imPACT Cancer Assessment Review Mission. Available at http://www.iaea.org/newscenter/news/2012/impactassessment.html.

31. WHO (2011). *National Cancer Control Programmes: Core Capacity Self-Assessment Tool*. Available at http://www.who.int/cancer/publications/nccp_tool2011/en/index.html.

32. Hanna TP, Kangole ACT (2010). Cancer control in developing countries: using health data and health services research to measure and improve access, quality and efficiency. *BMC Int Health Hum Rights*, 10:24. http://dx.doi.org/10.1186/1472-698X-10-24

Cancer control in France: towards patient-centred precision medicine

Agnès Buzyn

The two successive cancer control plans endorsed by the president of France have helped shape a new era of coordinated and integrated cancer care, centred on the patients' needs and grounded on evidence-based measures. They have helped to build the components of the current organizational cancer care framework in France, which is designed to deliver high-quality services and facilitate the evolution of stratified medicine. This organizational framework bridges both patient-centred and tumour-centred approaches, and encompasses the personalized care programme, specialized structures or organizations (for rare cancers, oncogeriatrics, oncopaediatrics, etc.), and molecular profiling of tumours. The ultimate goal, yet to be attained, is to bring high value to patients and survivors while fighting the roots of health inequities through fair access to innovation.

The personalized care programme offers patients their road map towards completion of their treatment, and helps them to navigate through referral from one point in the process to the next with ease.

The personalized care programme has helped address the fragmentation of the cancer care pathway. As the number of cancer survivors increases in most high-income countries, the next challenge is to further develop a survivorship plan that is fully integrated into the continuum of the person's care, from the onset of the disease.

To strengthen the cancer care framework, specialized networks for rare cancers, and specific organizational frameworks for oncogeriatrics and oncopaediatrics, have been developed based on scientific and clinical excellence, with integrated facilities and dedicated staff. They usually function as a network with a wide geographical coverage. They have close links with biobank resources and molecular genetics infrastructures. The implementation of a quality assurance programme and a collaborative approach warrants that all network centres meet required standards and deliver state-of-the-art cancer care.

Advances in the molecular profiling of tumour tissues have opened up an era of personalized cancer treatment where therapies are matched to the individual tumour. Pivotal to this personalized approach are drugs that have been designed to target a particular molecular pathway affected in a certain cancer type. Targeted therapies have been successfully introduced into clinical practice for breast and stomach cancers (*HER2* overexpression), lung cancer (*EGFR* mutations), and colorectal cancer (*KRAS* mutations). Molecular characterization of tumours has become a decisive factor in the choice of therapeutic strategies for cancer patients. To meet this challenge, a network of molecular genetics centres with nationwide reach was developed. This organizational framework has now been operational for 4 years and is successful in delivering state-of-the-art targeted cancer treatments. Access time to novel therapies has been reduced. The latest genomic knowledge and technologies (next-generation sequencing) should accelerate progress towards precision medicine.

6.4

Research infrastructure –
biobanks, cohorts, registries,
and data linkage

6 CONTROL

Joakim Dillner

Gustavo Stefanoff (reviewer)
Jim Vaught (reviewer)

Summary

- The development and evaluation of effective health services for cancer control is dependent on high-quality prevention and related research, which in turn is reliant on the efficient operation of functional research infrastructures.

- Cohorts, biobanking facilities, and cancer registries play a key role in research and the development and evaluation of cancer control measures.

- From a global perspective, there is an increasing rate of initiation of large population-based cohorts and advanced biobanking facilities. International organizations, including IARC, as well as national and other authorities operate multiple, often large, biobanks. The necessary resources on which cancer research is based are termed the study bases and are formed by longitudinal follow-up of cohorts and biobanks using cancer registry linkages.

- International standardization and networking of infrastructures is required to enable comprehensive investigations and to ensure the standardization and

comparability of research data and results.

Research infrastructure: essential resources for cancer research

Research infrastructure refers to facilities, databases, and collections together with related services used by the scientific community to conduct research [1]. When operated on an international scale, research infrastructure offers unique research services to users from different countries. In addition, a tangential function of research infrastructure is to engage young investigators seeking to establish careers in science and so contribute to the growth of scientific communities. This goal can be achieved when research infrastructure serves as a hub for providing services in essential elements of research such as (i) access to high-quality and standardized data; (ii) access to high-quality, well-documented, and standardized biospecimens; (iii) access to high-performance molecular analysis platforms and/or molecular data generated on demand; (iv) development, implementation, and monitoring of best practices; and (v) education, expertise, and advice.

The concept of the knowledge triangle involves research, education,

and innovation [2]. A high-quality research infrastructure should be at the centre of the knowledge triangle. A successful research infrastructure does not merely serve to provide materials. Research infrastructure should also contribute by having a role in the production of knowledge through research, the diffusion of knowledge through education, and the application of knowledge through innovation.

To enable comparison of health outcomes and research results from different parts of the world [3], collaboration between research infrastructure hubs on an international scale is imperative, specifically in

Fig. 6.4.1. Blood samples are taken from a newborn baby in Sweden for the national phenylketonuria (PKU) registry biobank. In Sweden, such blood samples for the screening of metabolic diseases, including PKU, have been stored since 1974 and comprise about 2.7 million samples.

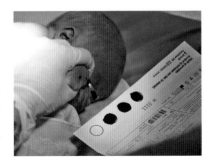

Fig. 6.4.2. Liquid nitrogen containers in the biobank of the Coriell Institute for Medical Research in Camden, New Jersey, USA.

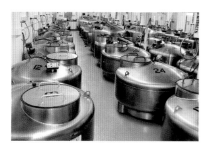

particular areas such as standardization, quality control, and coordinated development. An international infrastructure for cancer research will be required for progress in international cancer control.

There is a growing realization that research is an essential component for delivery of effective healthcare and preventive services in any setting, and is not only relevant to high-income countries. Studies that have affected the development of this concept include the Dartmouth Atlas, a systematic inventory of the different health services delivered in various parts of the USA, their cost, and their effectiveness (www.dartmouthatlas.org). These studies have estimated that if the most cost-effective health services were used throughout, the quality of health care would increase, while provision of health care would be up to 30% less expensive [4].

In health services research, the medical practice under study is in place irrespective of whether there is ongoing research. The purpose of such research is simply to study whether the health services delivered actually work, based on immediate experience. Although there is current political interest in research on the comparative effectiveness of health services, research on the effectiveness of health services has a long tradition in many countries. One of the best known and established traditions of health services research is the activities of cancer registries to evaluate the effectiveness of screening and other cancer

control policies. When new policies are implemented, they are frequently evaluated using randomized study designs, in so-called randomized health services studies [5].

Cohorts: studies of health outcomes and disease etiology

Cohort studies aim to provide a reliable database for investigation of risk factors for the diseases that affect a population. Basic information about the diseases affecting the population and the risk factors that cause these diseases is the foundation for planning of preventive services. A large number of healthy volunteers in the population provide data about living conditions and lifestyle (such as diet, exercise, smoking, and other habits), donate a series of biospecimens, and are followed up longitudinally, specifically in relation to disease development. While it may be inferred that most cancer is attributable to the impact of environmental factors rather than, for example, heritable risk, many causal factors remain to be specifically identified. Cohort studies with comprehensive collection of data

and molecular analysis of biospecimens may clarify – and, in some instances, identify – these factors and the inherent possibility of prevention. This approach was proposed by Doll and Peto more than 30 years ago [6] and has received renewed attention with the emergence of effective and comprehensive resources for molecular analysis of both genetic and environmental risk factors [7].

The Public Population Project in Genomics and Society (www.p3g. org) has a global cohort observatory that lists 15 international cohort networks and 79 individual cohorts. Many of these cohorts are extremely well funded. The best known example is the National Children's Study in the USA, a US$ 200 million/year cohort study that monitors pregnant women and their children to identify factors contributing to healthy childbearing and child development (www.nationalchildrensstudy.gov).

The largest among the comprehensive cohorts is the European Prospective Investigation into Cancer and Nutrition (EPIC), designed to investigate the relationships between diet, nutritional status, lifestyle, and other environmental factors and the incidence of cancer and other chronic

Fig. 6.4.3. Analysis of biological samples, in this case by quantitative micrographic determination, may be undertaken in collaboration with remote investigators where tissues are stored, rather than basing collaboration on the transportation of samples to remote locations.

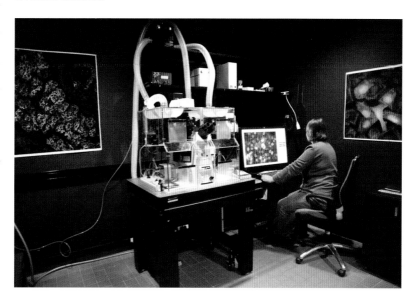

diseases. EPIC recruited more than 520 000 people in 10 European countries: Denmark, France, Germany, Greece, Italy, the Netherlands, Norway, Spain, Sweden, and the United Kingdom [8]. The EPIC cohort has multiple associated working groups, concerned not only with most major cancer types but also with cardiovascular diseases, ageing, and diabetes.

Why are biobanks needed?

Collections of human biological specimens are essential, both for cancer research and for improved clinical diagnosis. The revolutionary development of high-performance molecular analysis platforms in recent years has meant that the rate-limiting step in translating the advances in basic research to cancer control is no longer the molecular analysis, but access to well-characterized specimens with associated follow-up data. Because of biobanking, scientists no longer need to initiate sample collection either individually or within their research groups – relevant samples are already available.

The main advantage of biobanking is that a long follow-up on health outcomes for particular specimens is immediately available without a further requirement for the passage of time. A translational research project need not be restricted to testing new specimens and allowing the passage of a decade or more to determine relevant health outcomes. Rather, the project design may be based on locating specimens that have been stored for decades under circumstances where the health outcomes after specimen donation have been determined by registry linkages [9].

Prevention research may involve the search for novel biomarkers that can be used for early diagnosis and/or as new screening tests. This goal requires specimens taken before diagnosis, and a situation where diagnoses made at a later time are known. Explanations for differences in cancer occurrence worldwide are central to an understanding of cancer etiology. Such research also requires specimens taken before diagnosis, but with data about the later diagnosis of cancer in particular individuals.

The study base and the role of cancer registry linkages

The study base is a term that refers to the specimens and data on which scientific studies are based, i.e. the stored specimens and accessory

Fig. 6.4.4. Map of the Nordic region depicting the enrolment regions for the biobank cohorts that participated in a joint cancer registry linkage that identified more than 2 million sample donors and more than 100 000 prospectively occurring cancer cases.

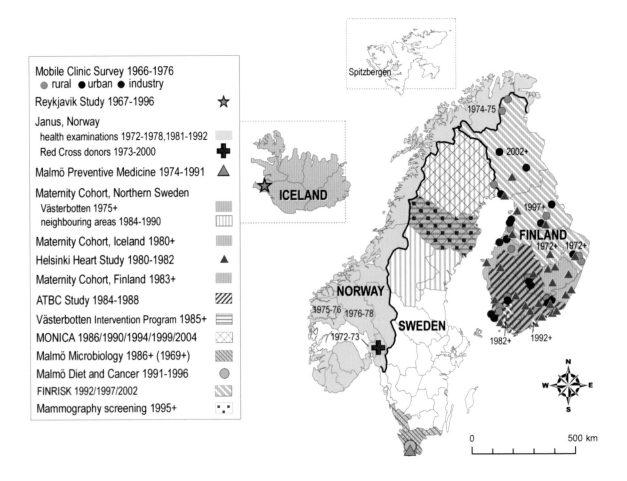

Fig. 6.4.5. Geographical origin of the samples stored at the IARC Biobank (excluding EPIC samples).

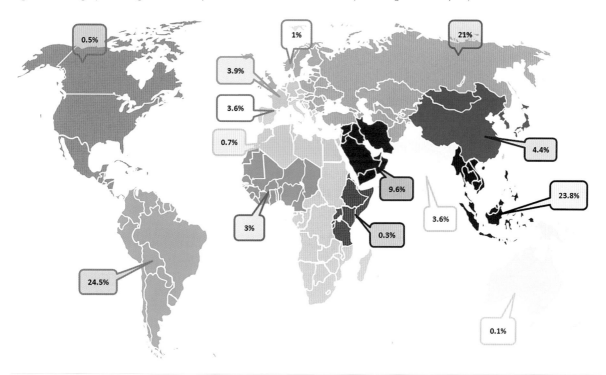

data plus the results of longitudinal follow-up for health outcomes.

A major limitation of biobank-based research is that many biobanks are not regularly linked to the relevant cancer registries and thus the study bases for scientific studies are unknown. Even if the biobanks are regularly followed up, there may be a lack of comprehensive and updated overviews for investigators about which study bases are available. The most advanced presentation of such study bases is currently the Danish National Biobank Register (www.biobanks.dk), which has an online, automated service to determine the study bases by on-demand linkages of the major biobanks in Denmark with the cancer registry and other health data registries. Large-scale and standardized cancer registry linkages for many biobanks in the Nordic countries have also been performed by the Finnish Cancer Registry under the auspices of European Union biobanking projects (Fig. 6.4.4) [10], most recently the FP7 project Eurocourse (Europe

against Cancer: Optimisation of the Use of Registries for Scientific Excellence in Research; www.eurocourse.org). Together with the European Union biobanking platform BBMRI (Biobanking and Biomolecular Resources Research Infrastructure; www.bbmri.eu), Eurocourse has also developed a format for standardized description of available study bases.

The requirement for follow-up to exploit the potential of biobank specimens has important implications. In particular, this has implications for anonymity in respect of specimens. Although scientists who use biobank specimens have access only to coded specimens, the identity of the donors must be known to the agency responsible for the follow-up [11].

In many respects, biobanks are similar to cancer registries. Biobanks constitute research infrastructure responsible for collection and storage of information about patients. Stringent and similar standards are required of biobanks and registries for strict handling of personal data to protect the integrity of individuals.

As linkage to cancer registries is essential for the follow-up of biobank specimens to define the study base, the standardized overview and description of biobanks and biobank-based study bases can be handled by cancer registries. Because cancer registries are the disease registers with the longest follow-up and experience of data handling as well as international networking and standardization of data, it is conceivable that they could drive the excellence in realizing the potential of biobanks for health. A role model for this concept is the Janus Biobank, a population-based biobank with samples from 350 000 donors that is operated entirely by the Cancer Registry of Norway [12].

Biological resource centres
Historically, every research study or diagnostic laboratory developed its own separate system for storing biospecimens. However, this fragmentation resulted in expensive duplication and severely limited the cumulative use of specimens, which had been handled and stored by

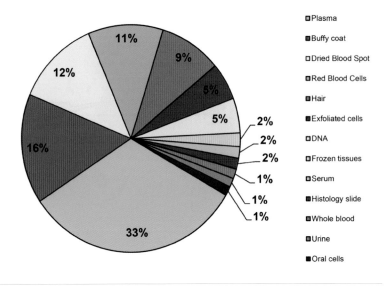

Fig. 6.4.6. An indication of the amount and nature of biological materials that may be subject to collection and storage in a biobank. In this instance, the data refer to samples stored at the IARC Biobank.

Legend:
- Plasma
- Buffy coat
- Dried Blood Spot
- Red Blood Cells
- Hair
- Exfoliated cells
- DNA
- Frozen tissues
- Serum
- Histology slide
- Whole blood
- Urine
- Oral cells

differing procedures. International studies based on samples from several sources were not necessarily valid. With the growing operational complexity of biobanks, investigators are increasingly reliant on specialized service facilities that handle the acquisition, quality control, storage, processing, and distribution of biospecimens [13]. These biobanking facilities are termed biological resource centres. A biological resource centre will provide services for all steps in the scientific study, from contacting study participants to archiving research results.

Most biological resource centres collaborate in international biobanking networks committed to common international standards for collection, labelling, annotation, processing, storage, retrieval, and analysis of the biospecimens, while ensuring biological safety and protection of personal data. Under the auspices of the United States National Cancer Institute, the Cancer Human Biobank (caHUB) is a national biorepository of human tissue, blood, and other biological materials (http://cahub.cancer.gov). In Europe, major networks of biobanks are the above-mentioned Biobanking and Biomolecular Resources Research Infrastructure and the International Society for Biological and Environmental Repositories (www.isber.org). There is increasing emphasis on the view from funding agencies and other stakeholders that publicly funded research materials should be openly accessible.

The IARC Biobank is an international biological resource centre serving more than 50 studies from 30 countries worldwide. As is typical for such centres, study designs include cohorts, case series, prevalence studies, and case–control studies (Fig. 6.4.5). A total of about 5.0 million samples from 1.5 million subjects are stored. Most of the samples are body fluids, including plasma, serum, and urine, as well as extracted DNA samples (Fig. 6.4.6). The IARC Biobank has an access policy to encourage proposals for new collaborative studies on existing biospecimen collections (http://ibb.iarc.fr/).

Cohort and biobanking networks

The Low- and Middle-Income Countries Biobank and Cohort Network (BCNet) is an IARC initiative intended to support the development of cancer control in low- and middle-income countries. Currently, investments in research infrastructure calculated to assist the development of high-quality science, which will underpin effective cancer control measures, are receiving increased attention. Population cohorts can assist countries in providing scientific education, stimulating translational research, and identifying, launching, and evaluating interventions for improving health.

Fig. 6.4.7. Sharing of sample analysis results rather than samples may accelerate research: the concept of the biological expert centre.

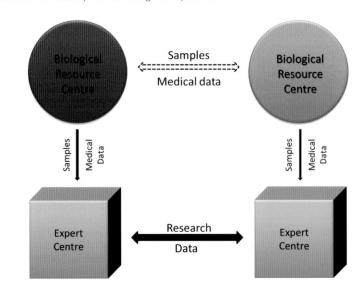

The tools and methodologies used to develop a biobank infrastructure and population cohorts are basically similar. Thus, by comparison with earlier endeavours, lower cost and improved effectiveness in the context of establishing cohorts may be achieved by the operation of international networks. Such networks provide initiating countries with guidance for establishing sustainable infrastructure, often involving procedures that have been tested and optimized in a variety of different settings. Because population cohorts and biobanking facilities are not prevalent in low- and middle-income countries, the development of health sciences and evidence-based cancer control may be affected. BCNet provides an opportunity for these countries to cooperate in a coordinated and effective manner to address local shortfalls in biobanking infrastructure.

A successful biobank is one that fosters successful science. Many current cohort studies are designed to investigate several diseases, with associated disease-specific working groups, as noted above in relation to EPIC. Compared with fragmented studies on a single risk determinant or a single predictive factor, the coordinated approach is necessary to evaluate whether different risk determinants studied represent primary risk factors or are the result of confounding. In the future, many disease working groups will formalize their coordination by publishing open calls for proposals that describe the available study bases, with samples and data relating to different diseases, and invite scientists to apply for access.

Within the Biobanking and Biomolecular Resources Research Infrastructure in the European Union, the concept of the biological expert centre has been developed. This centre offers an alternative to time-consuming and costly sample shipments by providing sample analysis results rather than sending the samples to the investigator (Fig. 6.4.7). This initiative involves the availability of medical and scientific expertise in biobank-based research on issues such as proper sample selection, study design, and data interpretation [14]. At best, such an approach is optimally supported by in-house state-of-the-art analysis platforms that are so standardized and quality-assured that the results of analyses can be shared between centres and used for applications that require stringent quality and documentation of results. It is envisaged that a more rapid, more quality-assured, and less costly delivery of the final data that the customer needs could further advance the central usefulness of biobanks for cancer research.

Conclusion

The continuing quest to understand the causes of cancer and to develop global cancer control requires comparisons between disease patterns in different parts of the world [15]. These research goals may be better achieved through different institutions and countries endorsing the concept that samples and data for research should be openly accessible and that international – rather than national (or even subnational) – standards, rules, and procedures are to be preferred [16,17]. Promoting the adoption of common standards is desirable in high-resource countries as well as in low-resource countries. International collaboration to establish essential research infrastructure, including cohorts, biobanking facilities, and registry linkage systems, is key to promote international cancer research, and is particularly relevant for cancer research in low- and middle-income countries.

References

1. Tunis SR, Benner J, McClellan M (2010). Comparative effectiveness research: policy context, methods development and research infrastructure. *Stat Med*, 29: 1963–1976. http://dx.doi.org/10.1002/sim. 3818 PMID:20564311

2. Maassen P, Stensaker B (2011). The knowledge triangle, European higher education policy logics and policy implementation. *High Educ*, 61:757–769. http://dx.doi. org/10.1007/s10734-010-9360-4

3. Burgers JS, Fervers B, Haugh M *et al.* (2004). International assessment of the quality of clinical practice guidelines in oncology using the Appraisal of Guidelines and Research and Evaluation Instrument. *J Clin Oncol*, 22:2000–2007. http://dx.doi.org/10.1200/JCO.2004.06.157 PMID:15143093

4. Wennberg JE, Fisher ES, Stukel TA *et al.* (2004). Use of hospitals, physician visits, and hospice care during last six months of life among cohorts loyal to highly respected hospitals in the United States. *BMJ*, 328:607. http://dx.doi.org/10.1136/ bmj.328.7440.607 PMID:15016692

5. Hakama M, Malila N, Dillner J (2012). Randomised health services studies. *Int J Cancer*, 131:2898–2902. http://dx.doi. org/10.1002/ijc.27561 PMID:22461063

6. Doll R, Peto R (1981). The causes of cancer: quantitative estimates of avoidable risks of cancer in the United States today. *J Natl Cancer Inst*, 66:1191–1308. PMID:7017215

7. Wild CP, Scalbert A, Herceg Z (2013). Measuring the exposome: a powerful basis for evaluating environmental exposures and cancer risk. *Environ Mol Mutagen*, 54:480–499. http://dx.doi.org/10.1002/em. 21777 PMID:23681765

8. Gonzalez CA, Riboli E (2010). Diet and cancer prevention: contributions from the European Prospective Investigation into Cancer and Nutrition (EPIC) study. *Eur J Cancer*, 46:2555–2562. http://dx.doi. org/10.1016/j.ejca.2010.07.025 PMID: 20843485

9. Riegman PH, de Jong BW, Llombart-Bosch A (2010). The Organization of European Cancer Institutes Pathobiology Working Group and its support of European biobanking infrastructures for translational cancer research. *Cancer Epidemiol Biomarkers Prev*, 19:923–926. http:// dx.doi.org/10.1158/1055-9965.EPI-10-0062 PMID:20332270

10. Pukkala E (2010). Nordic biological specimen bank cohorts as basis for studies of cancer causes and control: quality control tools for study cohorts with more than two million sample donors and 130,000 prospective cancers. In: Dillner J, ed. *Methods in Biobanking*. New York: Springer, pp. 61–112.

11. Langseth H, Luostarinen T, Bray F, Dillner J (2010). Ensuring quality in studies linking cancer registries and biobanks. *Acta Oncol*, 49:368–377. http://dx.doi. org/10.3109/02841860903447069 PMID: 20059313

12. Dillner J, ed. (2009). *The Janus Serum Bank – From Sample Collection to Cancer Research*. Oslo: Cancer Registry of Norway. Available at http://www.kreftregis teret.no/Global/Publikasjoner%20og%20 rapporter/CIN_2008_Special_Issue_ Janus_web.pdf.

13. Massett HA, Atkinson NL, Weber D *et al.* (2011). Assessing the need for a standardized cancer HUman Biobank (caHUB): findings from a national survey with cancer researchers. *J Natl Cancer Inst Monogr*, 2011:8–15. http://dx.doi.org/10.1093/jnci monographs/lgr007 PMID:21672890

14. Watson RW, Kay EW, Smith D (2010). Integrating biobanks: addressing the practical and ethical issues to deliver a valuable tool for cancer research. *Nat Rev Cancer*, 10:646–651. http://dx.doi.org/10.1038/nrc 2913 PMID:20703251

15. Hudson TJ, Anderson W, Artez A *et al.;* International Cancer Genome Consortium (2010). International network of cancer genome projects. *Nature*, 464:993–998. http://dx.doi.org/10.1038/nature08987 PMID:20393554

16. Moore HM, Compton CC, Alper J, Vaught JB (2011). International approaches to advancing biospecimen science. *Cancer Epidemiol Biomarkers Prev*, 20:729–732. http://dx.doi.org/10.1158/1055-9965.EPI-11-0021 PMID:21430299

17. Vaught JB, Henderson MK, Compton CC (2012). Biospecimens and biorepositories: from afterthought to science. *Cancer Epidemiol Biomarkers Prev*, 21:253–255. http://dx.doi.org/10.1158/1055-9965.EPI-11-1179 PMID:22313938

Cancer control in India: cancer care through a four-tier system

G.K. Rath

In 2012, there were an estimated 1.01 million new cancer cases in India (age-standardized incidence, 94.0 per 100 000) and 980 000 cancer-related deaths (age-standardized mortality, 64.5 per 100 000), and the 5-year prevalence was 1.79 million (proportion, 202.9 per 100 000) [1]. The cancer pattern is varied in different parts of the country because of diverse lifestyles. The data from 27 population-based cancer registries in India show that the highest incidence of cancer is in Mizoram state, which is in the north-eastern part of India, compared with the lowest incidence from a rural registry in Barshi, in the western part of the country. There is an increasing trend of incidence rates for all malignancies except for cervical cancer, which has a downward trend.

The government has established the National Centre for Disease Informatics and Research to develop a national research database on cancer, diabetes, cardiovascular diseases, and stroke [2]. India is one of the first countries to initiate a comprehensive national cancer control programme. There are 27 Regional Cancer Centres, including 339 radiotherapy facili-

ties equipped with 481 teletherapy machines. Most Regional Cancer Centres also have medical, surgical, palliative care, imaging, and laboratory facilities. They are actively involved in teaching and research as well.

The government has started a National Programme for Prevention and Control of Cancer, Diabetes, Cardiovascular Diseases, and Stroke. This has been done with the aim of combating the common risk factors for these diseases. The strategies under this programme include prevention through behaviour change, early diagnosis, treatment, capacity building of human resources, surveillance, monitoring, and evaluation.

The cancer care network is envisaged to be a four-tier system. Initially, the programme is being implemented in 100 districts across 21 states. Subsequently, this will be expanded to all 640 districts in the country. District hospitals are being strengthened for prevention, early detection, and management of common cancers, especially oral, breast, and cervical cancers. Tertiary care centres will be the referral for the district hospitals and provide comprehensive cancer care services.

Training will be provided at tertiary care centres/State Cancer Institutes for health-care professionals. State Cancer Institutes will be referral centres for the tertiary care centres and district hospitals, and provide specialized cancer care services. Three apex centres (National Cancer Institutes) will conduct research on the various malignancies that are common and pertinent to our part of the world, i.e. tobacco-related cancers, and cancers of the cervix, gall bladder, and liver. Besides working as referral centres, the National Cancer Institutes will also provide training to generate high-quality human resources. They will help the government in formulating national cancer control policies. State and district noncommunicable disease cells will be established in the selected states/districts for monitoring of the programme's implementation.

References

1. Ferlay J et al. (2013). GLOBOCAN 2012 v1.0, Cancer Incidence and Mortality Worldwide: IARC Cancer Base No. 11 [Internet]. Lyon: IARC. Available at http://globocan.iarc.fr.

2. Indian Council of Medical Research (2013). National Centre for Disease Informatics and Research – National Cancer Registry Programme. Available at http://www.ncdirindia.org/.

6.5 Advocacy for cancer control

Cary Adams
Rebecca Morton Doherty

Bob Chapman (reviewer)
Scott Wittet (reviewer)

Summary

- The 2011 United Nations General Assembly High-Level Meeting on the Prevention and Control of Noncommunicable Diseases presented the cancer community with an unprecedented advocacy opportunity to position cancer as a global health and development issue and to use the momentum generated at the meeting to press for increased efforts to reduce the global cancer burden, particularly in low- and middle-income countries.

- In high-income countries, the role of advocacy in ensuring the provision of optimal clinical care and other benefits is established; advocacy in wider aspects of cancer control is being increasingly specified as a key consideration.

- Comprehensive national cancer control plans, based on knowledge about the cancer burden provided by population-based cancer registries, are fundamental to cancer prevention and control and should be the focus of cancer advocacy efforts.

- Advocacy is about achieving a change that delivers a desired outcome. Advocacy requires a strategic plan, supported by a strong evidence base, emotional appeal, and a convincing financial case, and is most effectively implemented in collaboration with other like-minded organizations.

- Particular roles for advocacy for cancer control are being identified both as contributing to progress in high-income countries and as being developed in the context of local experience in low- and middle-income countries.

Using advocacy to accelerate the fight against cancer

Advocacy is about achieving a change that delivers a desired outcome. Health advocacy aims to raise political awareness and influence public policy decisions in support of an organization's mission. In the context of cancer control, effective advocacy is required to create an engaged political environment conducive to improving the way cancer control knowledge influences policy and practice [1].

In high-income countries particularly, the key role of advocacy in ensuring optimal clinical care is well recognized. Beyond contributing to improving the circumstances of individual patients, such advocacy may serve, for example, to facilitate and encourage participation in clinical trials [2]. Indeed, a role in cancer research is recognized: cancer patient advocates may contribute by offering perspectives different from those derived through government, academic, medical, and scientific approaches [3].

Complementing such perspectives, a role of cancer advocacy in cancer control in its broadest context, including all aspects of prevention, may be recognized. In this context, advocacy has a singular role. Thus, for example, in the prevention of human papillomavirus-related malignancies, a field readily identified with major achievements, more concerted advocacy is encouraged as complementing research and policy initiatives, if progress is to be optimal [4].

In September 2011, the United Nations General Assembly held a historic High-Level Meeting on the Prevention and Control of Noncommunicable Diseases. Only the second such health summit in the history of the United Nations, this meeting represented global recognition of the growing burden of cancer and other noncommunicable diseases, including diabetes and cardiovascular and respiratory diseases,

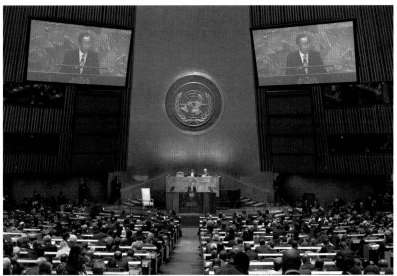

and positioned cancer control as a global health and development imperative. This provided the cancer community with an unprecedented advocacy opportunity to build on the momentum generated at the meeting and by the United Nations Political Declaration on noncommunicable diseases that was adopted [5], to press for increased efforts to reduce the cancer burden, particularly in low- and middle- income countries, where the cancer burden is set to rise by 81% by 2030 [6].

Advocacy for cancer control: what is wanted?

Calling for national cancer control plans

The ultimate goal of advocacy efforts in cancer control is threefold: (i) to ensure that governments develop comprehensive national cancer control plans that span the entire continuum of care; (ii) to ensure that such national plans are informed by population-based cancer registries that provide the necessary knowledge about cancer burden, as well as a means to evaluate the impact of implemented activities; and (iii) to ensure that governments finance

and implement interventions known to be cost-effective and productive.

Even in countries with an existing cancer policy, plan, or strategy, these plans are not always supported by the necessary funds, personnel power, or infrastructure. In a recent survey, only 43% of low-income countries reported having operational national cancer control plans (see Chapter 6.2). Similarly, there are stark disparities in cancer registration between high-income and low- and middle-income countries: the percentage of the population covered by cancer registries in the reference publication *Cancer Incidence in Five Continents*, Vol. X (2013) is 95% in North America and 42% in Europe but only 8% in Latin America, 6% in Asia, and 2% in Africa [7].

Granted circumstances in sub-Saharan Africa, approaches to minimize the cancer burden in the recent past have had little success, among other things because of a poor understanding of the potential for cancer prevention [8]. The situation may be addressed by initiatives in advocacy, research, workforce, care, and funding. Cancer advocates in Africa, for example, may look to

North America and Europe for guidance. However, lessons learned from high-income countries are not necessarily applicable, and relevant resources based on Africa are becoming increasingly available [9].

Population-based cancer registries and national cancer control plans are a vital investment in understanding and responding to the cancer burden in all countries. A well-conceived plan that is based on cancer incidence, prevalence, and survival rate data provided by cancer registries and that outlines evidence-based strategies for prevention, early detection, diagnosis, treatment, and palliation can significantly lower the number of cancer cases and improve the quality of life of cancer patients. In the absence of population-based cancer registries, cancer planners can nevertheless use available data to outline strategies for implementing proven cost-effective interventions for reducing the cancer burden. Given the current economic climate, it is crucial to maximize the population impact of money spent. Investing in the collection of basic cancer information and the development of comprehensive national cancer control plans needs

Fig. 6.5.2. Cover of an advocacy toolkit. This publication from the Union for International Cancer Control provides support to civil society organizations.

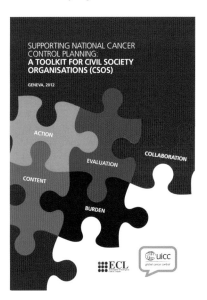

to be clearly specified to ensure that the greatest impact is achieved for the funds allocated.

There are cost-effective evidence-based interventions that can significantly reduce the cancer burden. These include screening for cervical cancer and breast cancer, and vaccination against hepatitis B virus and human papillomavirus to protect against infection-related liver cancer and cervical cancer, respectively. Cervical cancer screening and hepatitis B virus immunization were underscored as priority interventions in the 2011 United Nations Political Declaration on noncommunicable diseases [5] and have also been highlighted by WHO as not only highly cost-effective but also feasible and appropriate to implement within the constraints of health systems in low- and middle-income countries [10].

What does success look like?
Advocacy at a global level was key to adoption of the WHO Framework Convention on Tobacco Control, the first treaty negotiated under the auspices of WHO. The Convention provides a robust framework to confront the efforts of the tobacco industry, which employs lawyers and marketing and communications experts to counter health advocates around the globe. The recent major achievement involving Australia's adoption of legislation for plain packaging of tobacco products highlights the impact that a persistent, united, and vocal civil society may have.

Similarly, the NCD Alliance (www. ncdalliance.org), a global network of more than 2000 civil society organizations from 170 countries addressing the four main noncommunicable diseases (cardiovascular disease, diabetes, cancer, and chronic respiratory disease), played a pivotal role in the lead-up to the United Nations General Assembly High-Level Meeting on the Prevention and Control of Noncommunicable Diseases, pressing governments to recognize that noncommunicable diseases are a global development priority requiring an urgent response. Since then, the NCD Alliance has

sustained global action on noncommunicable diseases and spearheaded remarkable progress, culminating in the adoption of an omnibus resolution on noncommunicable diseases at the 66th World Health Assembly, which will benefit the millions of people worldwide who are at risk of, or living with, noncommunicable diseases.

Advocacy for cancer control: how do we do it?
Effective advocacy for cancer control requires a carefully constructed strategic plan identifying the problem, advocacy goal, key messages and target audiences, activity plan, and evaluation process [1], and is optimally supported by three core components: a comprehensive evidence base, emotional appeal, and a strong financial case. Neglecting both the views of patients and their loved ones and the compelling case for investing in cancer prevention and control now will inevitably result in a rise in the cancer burden and require a significantly greater investment later. In addition to these three core components, effective advocacy for cancer control needs to occur at the local, national, regional, and global levels. These efforts can be enhanced through strong partnerships between local and global advocates, as well as across groups concerned with related diseases, specifically including other noncommunicable diseases, and involving multiple sectors, including the private sector. Thus, in identifying breast cancer control strategies in Asia, Latin America, and the Middle East, a specific role for advocacy was identified [11]. The development of effective strategies may be grounded in the experience of local practitioners, policy-makers, and advocacy leaders.

Evidence-based advocacy
Evidence is critical for influencing public policy decisions; it provides the necessary information for advocates to raise awareness of the nature and extent of a problem and make realistic projections of possible

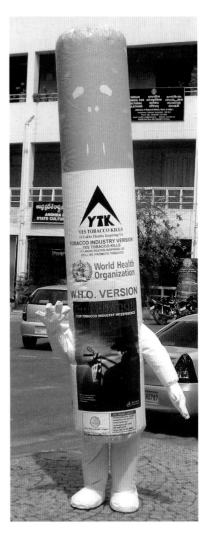

Fig. 6.5.3. This model of a cigarette, an inflated balloon, was displayed in Hyderabad, India, during World No Tobacco Day 2012. World No Tobacco Day is marked on 31 May each year, to create awareness about the harmful effects of tobacco and smoking.

policy outcomes. Screening for cervical cancer is a good example of the links between research, policy, and practice. Over the previous decades, advocacy has helped to drive the research agenda, culminating in large-scale randomized clinical trials to test the "screen and treat" approach using visual inspection with acetic acid. The evidence base generated through these trials, particularly in low-income settings, has resulted in widespread recognition of cervical cancer screening as a proven cost-effective intervention for reducing the global cancer burden, and has enabled the rapid integration of an indicator for cervical cancer screening into the Global Monitoring Framework for the Prevention and Control of Noncommunicable Diseases [12] finalized by United Nations Member States in November 2012. Cervical Cancer Action, a global coalition of organizations including the American Cancer Society, PATH (an international non-profit organization), the Pan American Health Organization, and the Union for International Cancer Control, has been a driving force behind these successful advocacy efforts [13].

The power of the patient voice
Cancer patients, survivors, and their families are not only key to documenting the impact of policies on individuals; these same individuals can also be highly effective and powerful advocates for the adoption of cancer prevention and control policies. Patient participation in cancer advocacy is often hindered by the lack of long-term survivors among those diagnosed with particular malignancies, but as medical advances result in increasing survival rates such situations may change, as highlighted by the rising cohesive body of lung cancer advocacy groups. A good example of this is the Global Lung Cancer Coalition, established in 2001, which now comprises 28 nongovernmental patient organizations from more than 20 countries, and works to improve disease outcomes for lung cancer patients globally [14].

Case study: access to opioids for cancer pain relief
Bringing the patient voice to policy discussions, and emphasizing the need for a rights-based approach to address the global inequities in access to pain relief, has been instrumental in effecting policy changes at the highest level. Since 2009, the Union for International Cancer Control has worked with its members to add the cancer voice

Fig. 6.5.4. A nurse provides pain relief to a cancer patient in Uganda.

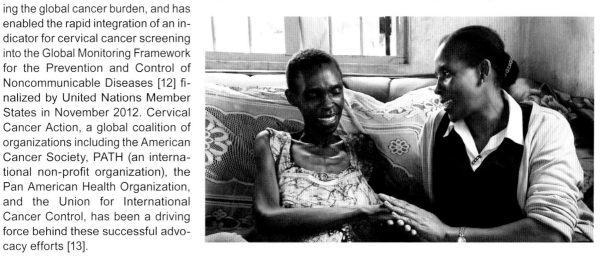

to the human rights and palliative care communities' efforts towards increased access to opioid analgesics. During this period, the United Nations's drug policy-making organ, the Commission on Narcotic Drugs, has adopted two resolutions [15,16], emphasizing that more needs to be done to enhance availability of controlled medications while preventing their diversion and abuse. The 2011 Commission on Narcotic Drugs resolution specifically requested the United Nations Office on Drugs and Crime, in consultation with the International Narcotics Control Board and WHO, to update its model laws to ensure that they reflect an appropriate balance between ensuring adequate access to internationally controlled drugs and preventing diversion and abuse.

In 2012, commendable advocacy efforts led by the palliative care community resulted in the inclusion of an indicator on access to palliative care, assessed by morphine-equivalent consumption of strong opioid analgesics per cancer death, in the Global Monitoring Framework for the Prevention and Control of Noncommunicable Diseases [12].

Building the financial case
The World Economic Forum has identified noncommunicable diseases, including cancer, as the second greatest risk to global economic growth [17]. One half of those who die from noncommunicable diseases are in their most productive years, meaning that the social costs and economic consequences in terms of lost productivity are considerable. The cost of cancer alone is estimated to reach US$ 458 billion in 2030 [10], yet WHO estimates that a basic package of cost-effective strategies to address the common cancer risk factors (tobacco use, alcohol consumption, unhealthy diet, and physical inactivity) would cost only US$ 2 billion a year [18]. Even so, less than 3% (US$ 503 million out of US$ 22 billion) of overall development assistance for health was allocated to noncommunicable diseases in 2007 [19], and only 5% of global spending on cancer is in developing countries. This is despite the fact that nearly 80% of the preventable deaths from these diseases occur in developing countries, with this percentage set to rise [20]. The financial case for investing in cancer is strong, and is one that can and must be used by cancer advocates at all levels to support adequate and sustained resourcing of national cancer control plans.

Multisectoral partnerships
The United Nations Political Declaration on noncommunicable diseases clearly articulated the need for multisectoral partnerships, engaging

Fig. 6.5.5. Cancer Council Australia provides a range of resources related to evidence-based cancer control policy and advocacy on its website.

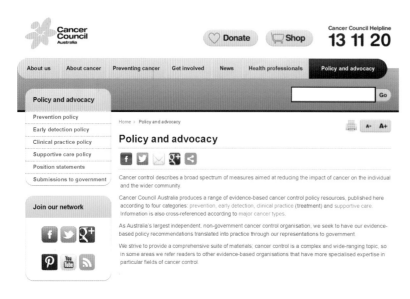

both health and non-health actors, including civil society and the private sector, to promote and support the provision of services for noncommunicable disease prevention and control. In addition to bolstering global and national advocacy efforts, such partnerships are essential for the implementation of cancer interventions at the country level. Given today's financial climate, engagement of parts of the private sector, with appropriate safeguards to manage potential conflicts of interest, is more critical than ever. There is a clear willingness in the private sector to engage at this level; according to a recent survey conducted by Business for Social Responsibility, 40% of companies expect to increase their commitment to global health partnerships focused on noncommunicable diseases in the next 5 years [21]. Global health partnerships could play an important role in improving primary health-care systems, which are the front lines – particularly in low- and middle-income countries – for engaging communities with prevention, diagnosis, and treatment across a range of diseases, including cancer.

Advocacy for cancer control: the road ahead

In May 2013, Member States at the 66th World Health Assembly adopted an omnibus resolution on noncommunicable diseases that combined major decisions and recommendations in a single comprehensive resolution, including (i) adopting a Global Monitoring Framework for the Prevention and Control of Noncommunicable Diseases; (ii) endorsing a Global Action Plan for Noncommunicable Diseases 2013–2020; and (iii) agreeing to establish a Global Coordination Mechanism for Noncommunicable Diseases [22]. This emerging framework for noncommunicable diseases will carve out a new global advocacy space for the cancer community, and an opportunity to ensure that noncommunicable diseases, including cancer, continue to occupy a place on the global health and development agenda. Ensuring that cancer is part of the 2013 Millennium Development Goal review and the emerging debate on universal health coverage, the sustainable development goals, and other development issues will also be vital to ensuring that cancer control remains central to future thinking. Cancer advocates face both new opportunities and challenges as "latecomers" to the development discourse. Now more than ever, innovative partnerships that go beyond traditional health groups and embrace partners in the development sphere, including reproductive, maternal, and child health organizations as well as the AIDS community, are critical if the currently predicted cancer burden for future generations is to be reduced.

References

1. Godfrey E *et al.* (2012). *Cancer Advocacy Training Toolkit for Africa.* Africa Oxford Cancer Foundation (AfrOx), African Organisation for Research and Training in Cancer (AORTIC), European Society for Medical Oncology (ESMO), and Union for International Cancer Control (UICC). Available at http://www.uicc.org/advocacy/advocacy-resources/additional-resources.

2. Katz ML, Archer LE, Peppercorn JM *et al.* (2012). Patient advocates' role in clinical trials: perspectives from Cancer and Leukemia Group B investigators and advocates. *Cancer*, 118:4801–4805. http://dx.doi.org/10.1002/cncr.27485 PMID:22392584

3. Collyar D (2005). How have patient advocates in the United States benefited cancer research? *Nat Rev Cancer*, 5:73–78. http://dx.doi.org/10.1038/nrc1530 PMID:15630417

4. Franco EL, de Sanjosé S, Broker TR *et al.* (2012). Human papillomavirus and cancer prevention: gaps in knowledge and prospects for research, policy, and advocacy. *Vaccine*, 30 Suppl 5:F175–F182. http://dx.doi.org/10.1016/j.vaccine.2012.06.092 PMID:23199961

5. United Nations (2011). Political Declaration of the High-Level Meeting of the General Assembly on the Prevention and Control of Non-communicable Diseases. New York: United Nations. Available at www.who.int/nmh/events/un_ncd_summit2011/political_declaration_en.pdf.

6. WHO (2011). *Global Status Report on Noncommunicable Diseases 2010.* Geneva: WHO. Available at http://www.who.int/nmh/publications/ncd_report2010/en/.

7. Forman D, Bray F, Brewster DH *et al.*, eds (2013). *Cancer Incidence in Five Continents*, Vol. X [electronic version]. Lyon: IARC. Available at http://ci5.iarc.fr.

8. Morhason-Bello IO, Odedina F, Rebbeck TR *et al.* (2013). Challenges and opportunities in cancer control in Africa: a perspective from the African Organisation for Research and Training in Cancer. *Lancet Oncol*, 14:e142–e151. http://dx.doi.org/10.1016/S1470-2045(12)70482-5 PMID:23561745

9. Odedina FT, Rodrigues B, Raja P (2013). Setting the stage for cancer advocacy in Africa: how? *Infect Agent Cancer*, 8 Suppl 1:S6. http://dx.doi.org/10.1186/1750-9378-8-S1-S6 PMID:23902653

10. Bloom DE, Cafiero ET, Jané-Llopis E *et al.* (2011). *The Global Economic Burden of Noncommunicable Diseases.* Geneva: World Economic Forum. Available at www.weforum.org/EconomicsOfNCD.

11. Bridges JF, Anderson BO, Buzaid AC *et al.* (2011). Identifying important breast cancer control strategies in Asia, Latin America and the Middle East/North Africa. *BMC Health Serv Res*, 11:227. http://dx.doi.org/10.1186/1472-6963-11-227 PMID:21933435

12. WHO (2012). *Report of the Formal Meeting of Member States to conclude the work on the comprehensive global monitoring framework, including indicators, and a set of voluntary global targets for the prevention and control of noncommunicable diseases (A/NCD/2).* Available at http://apps.who.int/gb/ncds/pdf/A_NCD 2-en.pdf.

13. Cervical Cancer Action (2012). A Global Coalition to Stop Cervical Cancer. Available at http://www.cervicalcanceraction.org/about/about.php.

14. Global Lung Cancer Coalition (2012) Available at http://www.lungcancercoalition.org/en.

15. The Commission on Narcotic Drugs (2010). *Promoting adequate availability of internationally controlled licit drugs for medical and scientific purposes while preventing their diversion and abuse*, Resolution 53/4. Available at http://www.unodc.org/documents/commissions/CND-Res-2000-until-present/CND53_4e.pdf.

16. The Commission on Narcotic Drugs (2011). *Promoting adequate availability of internationally controlled narcotic drugs and psychotropic substances for medical and scientific purposes while preventing their diversion and abuse*, Resolution 54/6. Available at http://www.unodc.org/documents/commissions/CND-Res-2011to2019/CND54_6e1.pdf.

17. Global Risk Network of the World Economic Forum (2010). *Global Risks 2010: A Global Risk Network Report.* Geneva: World Economic Forum. Available at http://www3.weforum.org/docs/WEF_GlobalRisks_Report_2010.pdf.

18. WHO (2011). *Scaling Up Action Against Noncommunicable Diseases: How Much Will It Cost?* Geneva: WHO. Available at http://www.who.int/nmh/publications/cost_of_inaction/en/.

19. Nugent RA, Feigl AB (2010). *Where Have All the Donors Gone? Scarce Donor Funding for Non-Communicable Diseases.* Center for Global Development Working Paper 228. Available at http://www.cgdev.org/publication/where-have-all-donors-gone-scarce-donor-funding-non-communicable-diseases-working-paper.

20. Knaul FM, Frenk J, Shulman L; for the Global Task Force on Expanded Access to Cancer Care and Control in Developing Countries (2011). *Closing the Cancer Divide: A Blueprint to Expand Access in Low and Middle Income Countries.* Boston, MA: Harvard Global Equity Initiative.

21. Little M, Schappert J (2012). *Working toward Transformational Health Partnerships in Low- and Middle-Income Countries.* Business for Social Responsibility. Available at https://www.bsr.org/en/our-insights/report-view/working-toward-transformational-health-partnerships.

22. Sixty-sixth World Health Assembly (2013). Resolution WHA66.10. Follow-up to the Political Declaration of the High-level Meeting of the General Assembly on the Prevention and Control of Non-communicable Diseases. Available at http://apps.who.int/gb/e/e_wha66.html.

Websites

The NCD Alliance. Putting non-communicable diseases on the global agenda: www.ncdalliance.org

Union for International Cancer Control: www.uicc.org

Cancer control in Jordan: goals for low- and middle-income countries

Omar Nimri

In Jordan, a country with about 6.5 million people, cancer is the second most frequent cause of death, after heart disease. A total of 6820 new cancer cases were registered by the national Jordan Cancer Registry in 2010. Of these, 72% were among Jordanians and 28% were among non-Jordanians.

The rank order of the five most common cancers affecting Jordanians is: breast cancer (19.6% of all cases), colorectal cancer (11.5%), lymphoma (7.9%), lung cancer (7.8%), and prostate cancer (4.5%). The crude annual incidence rate of all cancers among Jordanians is 79.4 per 100 000 (male, 74.0; female, 85.1). The most frequent paediatric cancers (0–14 years) are leukaemias (38%), brain and central nervous system tumours (27%), lymphomas (20%), renal tumours (8%), and soft tissue cancers (7%) [1].

Growing and ageing populations are projected to experience dramatic increases in the number of cancer cases and cancer deaths, particularly in low- and middle-income countries like Jordan. It is imperative that planning begins now to deal not only with those cancers already occurring but also with the larger numbers expected in the future.

A national cancer control plan (NCCP) for Jordan is in the process of being finalized. A simple NCCP existed previously, but the idea of a full, up-to-date NCCP really started in October 2008 at a meeting attended by many parties, including the Jordanian Ministry of Health, the WHO office in Amman, the King Hussein Cancer Center, some nongovernmental organizations, and the King Hussein Institute for Cancer Research and Biotechnology). A draft NCCP was prepared and presented to the minister of health, but unfortunately the draft was not endorsed and the NCCP was shelved.

In January 2012, the International Atomic Energy Agency, upon official request of the Ministry of Health, conducted a mission in close collaboration with the ministry. Based on the findings and recommendations of that mission, a new NCCP is now in preparation. The major partners are the Ministry of Health, the King Hussein Cancer Center, the Jordanian Royal Medical Services, the private medical sector, WHO, nongovernmental organizations such as the Jordan Medical Association and the Jordan Oncology Society, academia and research institutes, smoking cessation programmes, and others. It is hoped that the new, updated NCCP will cover all aspects of cancer, including prevention, early detection, screening, diagnosis and treatment, palliative care, and rehabilitation.

Most people pick up their bad habits at a younger age, leading to unhealthy diet, smoking, poor hygiene, and many other risk factors. The majority of cancers are preventable, by reducing exposure to factors that are known to cause the disease. Hence, education of the youth should be a priority to decrease these risks in the context of cancer control.

In 2001, a national tobacco control programme was started. In 2004, Jordan was the second country in the local region and the 29th in the world to endorse the WHO Framework Convention on Tobacco Control. The prevalence of smoking among adults (18 years and older) was 29% (male, 51%; female, 7%) in 2007. The prevalence among youth (13–15 years) was 11.5% (male, 17.4%; female, 8.3%) in 2009 [2]. In 2008, a law was passed banning smoking in public places; enforcement of this smoke-free legislation is still needed. Also, a repulsive picture of lungs and smoking is required on all cigarette packaging, along with warning statements.

Given that breast cancer is the most common cancer in Jordan, a national programme for breast cancer awareness, early detection, and screening was initiated in 2006, led by the King Hussein Cancer Foundation and Center.

The whole spectrum of cancer treatment is available in Jordan, but the inequality of access is the major obstacle faced.

Palliative care services remain grossly inadequate and represent a further area of priority.

References

1. Jordanian Ministry of Health. Annual Incidence of cancer in Jordan. Available at http://www.moh.gov.jo/EN/Pages/Publications.aspx.

2. WHO (2009). Global Youth Tobacco Survey: Country Fact Sheet – Jordan. Available at http://www.emro.who.int/tobacco/gtss-youth-survey/gyts-factsheets-reports.html.

6.6 Law in cancer control

6 CONTROL

Jonathan Liberman

Marianne Hammer (reviewer)
Roger Magnusson (reviewer)
Anne Lise Ryel (reviewer)

Summary

- The effective application of law is essential to cancer control and requires engagement across such diverse areas as trade law, intellectual property law, investment law, human rights law, drug control law, constitutional law, consumer protection law, negligence law, medical law, and criminal law.

- Current challenges to Australia's world-first plain tobacco packaging legislation have become seminal cases on the intersection between global public health and trade and investment laws and norms, with profound implications for cancer control.

- Overly restrictive laws continue to operate as barriers to the availability of opioid analgesics for the relief of cancer-associated pain. Significant normative progress has recently been made at the international level.

- Efforts to address the unavoidable tensions between the public interests in privacy protection and cancer research should acknowledge the role of the right to health, understood as a collective right of populations, the

fulfilment of which depends on high-quality research.

Law is everywhere in cancer control. Some examples of areas are:
- the regulation of the behaviour of the tobacco, alcohol, food, asbestos, and sunbed industries;
- the regulation of where people can use products that cause harm to third parties, such as laws prohibiting smoking in workplaces, public places, residential facilities, and cars carrying children;
- court challenges to cancer prevention measures such as tobacco product display bans (Norway), graphic health warnings (Uruguay and the USA), and plain packaging (Australia);
- litigation against industries whose products and practices cause cancer;
- the application of occupational health and safety laws to exposure to carcinogens in the workplace;
- the relationship between patent law and pharmaceutical research and the affordability of medicines;
- the effect of laws regulating the trade, prescription, and supply of opioid analgesics on their availability for the treatment of cancer-associated pain;
- the regulation of health professionals, including the protection

of patients from inappropriate or dangerous "treatments";
- the regulation of decision-making in treatment and care, including the end-of-life period;
- the conduct of clinical trials and the relationship between epidemiological research and health information privacy;
- the access of family members to genetic information; and
- intellectual property rights over genetic material and scientific discovery.

In these and a host of other areas, the effective application of law is essential to cancer control.

For each of these areas, law has both domestic and international elements. Domestically, law is constituted by a combination of constitutional arrangements, legislation, regulations, court decisions, regulatory practices and policies, and professional and community understandings of what the law is and how it operates in practice. At the international level, law includes treaties – notably the WHO Framework Convention on Tobacco Control (FCTC); the United Nations Single Convention on Narcotic Drugs; the International Covenant on Economic, Social, and Cultural Rights, which enshrines the right to the highest attainable standard of health; other international human rights treaties;

Fig. 6.6.1. Health warning images and plain packaging designs used in Australia. All brand names are specified in a standard colour, position, font size, and style.

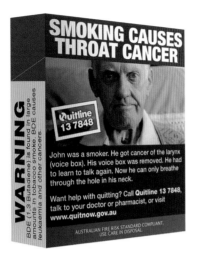 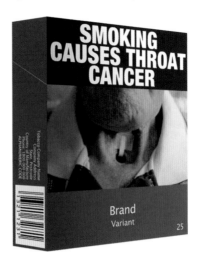

the World Trade Organization (WTO) agreements; and a raft of regional, plurilateral, and bilateral trade and investment treaties – as well as a wide range of "softer" normative instruments, such as declarations, guidelines, and strategies.

Health law and governance – at both domestic and international levels – is an increasingly crowded and fragmented space. The United Nations Political Declaration on the Prevention and Control of Non-communicable Diseases [1] underlines that prevention and control of these diseases require multisectoral approaches, including across such sectors as health, education, energy, agriculture, sports, transport, communication, urban planning, environment, labour, employment, industry and trade, finance, and social and economic development.

Internationally, WHO is the United Nations's specialized agency for health, but it is only one of a large number of international agencies whose work directly or indirectly affects health, including cancer, such as the United Nations Children's Fund, the Food and Agriculture Organization of the United Nations, the United Nations Environment Programme, the United Nations Development Programme, the United Nations Population Fund, the World Bank, the United Nations

Human Rights Council, the WTO, the United Nations Office on Drugs and Crime, the International Atomic Energy Agency, and the International Labour Organization. These agencies have very different mandates, priorities, instruments, and values, meaning that policy and operational coherence in the interests of health is often elusive.

Against this broader backdrop, this chapter focuses on three topical and important areas, relating to prevention, treatment, and research, respectively.

Trade and investment challenges to tobacco control

The foreword to the WHO FCTC [2] describes the treaty as having been "developed in response to the globalization of the tobacco epidemic", the spread of which "is facilitated through a variety of complex factors with cross-border effects, including trade liberalization and direct foreign investment". The WHO FCTC was conceived, in part, as a global response to these dynamics.

Increasingly, the relationship between the WHO FCTC, as an international legal instrument, and the international legal instruments that govern trade, intellectual property, and investment is being played out in the form of legal challenges [3].

As this Report goes to press, challenges to Australia's world-first "plain packaging" laws are the most prominent example.

In November 2011, the Australian Parliament enacted the Tobacco Plain Packaging Act 2011 [4]. As of 1 December 2012, all tobacco products sold in Australia were required to comply with the legislation. The legislation bans the use of logos, brand imagery, symbols, other images, colours, and promotional text on tobacco products and tobacco product packaging, and requires packaging to be a standard drab dark-brown colour in matte finish. Products are differentiated by the brand and product name, displayed in a standard colour, position, font size, and style. Graphic health warnings are required on 75% of the front surface and 90% of the back surface of tobacco packaging. Indeed, the "plain" in "plain packaging" is somewhat of a misnomer.

Plain packaging is supported by two sets of guidelines adopted by the governing body of the WHO FCTC – its Conference of the Parties – in November 2008: one on packaging and labelling (Article 11) [5] and the other on tobacco advertising, promotion, and sponsorship (Article 13) [6]. The guidelines for the implementation of Article 11 state that plain packaging "may increase the noticeability and effectiveness of health warnings and messages, prevent the package from detracting attention from them, and address industry design techniques that may suggest that some products are less harmful than others". The Article 13 guidelines acknowledge that packaging "is an important element of advertising and promotion". The Australian legislation includes as one of its objects "to give effect to certain obligations that Australia has as a party to the Convention on Tobacco Control".

Plain packaging has been challenged both in the WTO and under a bilateral investment treaty between Australia and Hong Kong Special Administrative Region. In the WTO, in which dispute settlement is state–state rather than investor–state,

Ukraine, Honduras, the Dominican Republic, Cuba, and Indonesia have claimed that plain packaging breaches Australia's obligations under the General Agreement on Tariffs and Trade, the Agreement on Technical Barriers to Trade, and the Agreement on Trade-Related Aspects of Intellectual Property Rights. It has been reported that the two multinational tobacco companies, Philip Morris and British American Tobacco, have been providing support to countries to challenge plain packaging [7].

Unlike in the WTO, the bilateral investment treaty between Australia and Hong Kong Special Administrative Region – like many other investment treaties – enables a foreign investor to sue a government directly. Philip Morris Asia – which acquired its interest in Philip Morris Australia on 23 February 2011, i.e. after plain packaging had been announced by the Australian Government, in April 2010 – has brought proceedings against the Australian Government claiming "expropriation" of its investment and denial of "fair and equitable treatment".

The Australian Government is vigorously defending both the WTO and bilateral investment treaty proceedings. These challenges to plain packaging have become seminal cases on the intersection between global public health and trade and investment laws and norms, touching on broader issues relating to the power of governments to regulate in the public interest, the relationship between private intellectual property rights and public health, and the nature and role of evidence in policy-making.

Achieving balance in the regulation of opioids

Opioid analgesics are regulated internationally under the United Nations Single Convention on Narcotic Drugs, 1961, as amended by its 1972 Protocol [8]. The Single Convention seeks to strike a balance between the two aims of ensuring the availability of opioids for medical use for the relief of pain

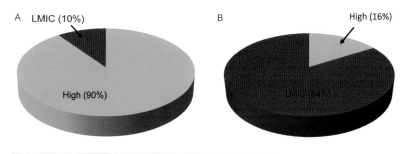

Fig. 6.6.2. Disparity in morphine consumption in high-income countries (High) versus low- and middle-income countries (LMIC). (A) Morphine consumption (as a percentage of the total number of kilograms consumed) in 2010. (B) Total population of countries reporting opioid consumption to the International Narcotics Control Board in 2010.

and suffering – which it describes as "indispensable" – and preventing their diversion and abuse. In practice, this balance has not been achieved, with poor availability in much of the world and great global disparities. In 2011, Australia, Canada, Japan, New Zealand, the USA, and some European countries accounted for more than 93% of total global morphine consumption [9].

The major barriers to the availability of opioid analgesics are well known. They include insufficient training of health-care professionals in the prescription and administration of opioids; misperceptions among health-care professionals, policy-makers, and patients and their families about the safety of opioids; exaggerated fears about the development of dependence; overly restrictive laws and regulations that exceed the requirements of the Single Convention; and unduly harsh sanctions for the unintentional mishandling of opioids by health workers [10].

The Single Convention establishes a regulatory system that includes requirements for: government authorization for participation in the trade and distribution of narcotics; provision by states to the International Narcotics Control Board of estimates of need, and statistical returns covering production, manufacture, consumption, import, and export; export and import licences for international transactions; licensing and record-keeping for trade or distribution; and medical prescriptions for dispensation.

Many states have adopted overly restrictive laws and regulations that exceed the requirements of the Single Convention and that operate as barriers to availability. Examples include limitations on who can prescribe, special prescription procedures, restrictions on doses that may be prescribed or on the number of days' supply that may be provided in a single prescription, arbitrary restrictions on the number of pharmacies that are allowed to dispense opioid medications, and overly burdensome administrative and bureaucratic procedures.

The lack of balance in legal and regulatory approaches to opioid analgesics is increasingly being addressed at the international level. Several important documents have been developed and adopted over the past few years:

- two resolutions of the United Nations's main drug policy-making organ, the Commission on Narcotic Drugs, in 2010 [11] and 2011 [12], with co-sponsorship by countries from different regions and with different levels of income, which have emphasized that more needs to be done to enhance the availability of controlled medications while preventing their diversion and abuse;
- new WHO policy guidelines (2011) [13], which provide guidance on policies and legislation with respect to availability, accessibility, affordability, and control of controlled medicines;
- a special supplement to the 2010 International Narcotics Control

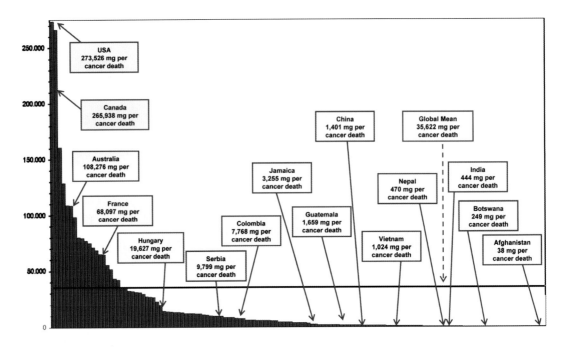

Fig. 6.6.3. Marked differences between countries in relation to medicinal opioid consumption (2010), assessed by morphine-equivalent consumption (in milligrams) of strong opioid analgesics per cancer death.

Board Annual Report [14], which includes recommendations on availability of controlled medicines and their appropriate use, national control systems, and prevention of diversion and abuse;

- a 2011 United Nations Office on Drugs and Crime discussion paper [15], which includes recommendations relating to data collection, laws and policies, and public awareness.

The 2011 Commission on Narcotic Drugs resolution requested the United Nations Office on Drugs and Crime, in consultation with the International Narcotics Control Board and WHO, to update its model laws to ensure that they reflect an appropriate balance between ensuring adequate access to internationally controlled drugs and preventing diversion and abuse. At the 2013 session of the Commission on Narcotic Drugs, the United Nations Office on Drugs and Crime released proposed amendments to its model drug laws [16], including:

- the introduction of substantive objects into the model law (rather than simply compliance with the

relevant conventions): "ensuring the availability of narcotic drugs and psychotropic substances for medical and scientific use, and preventing the non-medical and non-scientific use of narcotic drugs and psychotropic substances".

- the use of neutral terminology to describe drugs that have medical or scientific uses but can cause harm when misused. For example, the proposals describe the Schedule in which morphine is listed as including "drugs and substances having a medical and/ or scientific use which should be subject to control in view of the harms that their non-medical and/ or non-scientific use can cause". This contrasts with the previous wording, which referred to "strictly controlled substances and plants having a medical use" and "substances with a high potential risk to public health *but* having a medical use" (emphasis added). Under the previous formulation, concern about the risk of misuse predominated over the need to ensure appropriate medical treatment.

- an explicit recognition that, as recommended by WHO, the capacity to prescribe controlled medicines should not be restricted to a small number of medical specialties (such as oncologists); controlled medicines should be available at all appropriate levels of care, and the amount of medicine prescribed, the appropriate formulation, and the duration of treatment should be for the health practitioner to decide, based on individual patient needs and sound scientific medical guidance.

Privacy and cancer research

High-quality research – clinical, behavioural, and epidemiological – is key to effective cancer control. Epidemiological research provides a wealth of information that is essential for planning, resource allocation, programme development and delivery, legal and regulatory interventions, therapy development, and care improvement.

In practice, such research cannot be effectively conducted without access to sometimes sensitive personal health information, the disclosure of which can have a range of consequences for individuals. Public health research and surveillance cannot be effectively performed on the basis of fully de-identified data. De-identified data are not sufficient for the individual–data linkages required for epidemiological research designed to investigate more intricate interactions between exposure, lifestyle, preventive interventions, treatment, and outcomes [17]. Even after research has been conducted, data may need to remain re-identifiable to allow for the correction of errors or updating of new data, and for the review of scientific work, thereby guarding against scientific fraud [18].

It is not feasible to condition the use of personal health information in public health research on individual consent in all cases. When information is collected, it is seldom possible to identify all its future valuable uses. When dealing with large data sets, it may not be feasible to obtain consent from each individual whose data is proposed to be used [19]. Further, relying on individual consent can lead to compromised or invalid results because of significant differences between individuals who do and do not grant consent, meaning that research might be conducted on the basis of unrepresentative data [20].

The effect of these research realities is an unavoidable tension between the public interests in privacy protection and cancer research. Many cancer (and other public health) researchers believe that regulation is increasingly privileging privacy protection to the detriment of the conduct of research. One of the striking features of the literature on the relationship between information privacy and public health research – both academic articles and legal and policy documents – is that only one species of right, the right to privacy, seems to feature. There is invariably an "interest" against which the right should be balanced, often expressed as public health. While the point is often made that the "public" consists

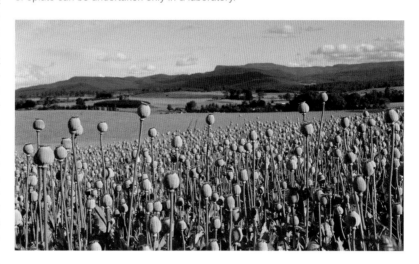

Fig. 6.6.4. An opium poppy field in Tasmania, Australia, where opium is grown for medicinal morphine. The opium poppies are usually genetically modified so that extraction of opiate can be undertaken only in a laboratory.

of individuals, who are the ultimate beneficiaries of public health research [21], it is curious that the right to health seems never to be raised.

This is the case notwithstanding the recognition that fulfilment of the right to health depends on the conduct of research. The International Covenant on Economic, Social, and Cultural Rights is the primary international legal instrument on economic, social, and cultural rights. The United Nations Committee on Economic, Social, and Cultural Rights's General Comment on Article 12 (the right of everyone to the enjoyment of the highest attainable standard of physical and mental health) states that one of the "core obligations" of the article is "to adopt and implement a national public health strategy and plan of action, *on the basis of epidemiological evidence*, addressing the health concerns of the whole population" (emphasis added) [22]. The control of diseases required by Article 12.2(c) necessitates "using and improving epidemiological surveillance and data collection on a disaggregated basis".

Bringing the right to health to bear on matters relating to health information privacy need not entail a disregard, or a downgrading, of the right to privacy or the values it promotes. Rather, it would situate debates in

their proper legal context, and should ultimately influence the way in which public health research is regulated. Too often, public health research appears as an afterthought exception in regimes aimed at strengthening privacy protection, often driven by concerns about such matters as publication of information about celebrities, online security, and identity theft. Acknowledging the role that the right to health has to play here touches on broader debates about the nature of the right to health and the need to conceive of it as not just an individual right but a collective right of populations [23].

Conclusion

Cancer control requires expertise and capacity in law. But there is no single discipline of "cancer control law". Cancer control law requires engagement at both domestic and international levels and across such diverse areas as trade law, intellectual property law, investment law, human rights law, drug control law, constitutional law, consumer protection law, negligence law, medical law, and criminal law. The need for capacity in cancer control law continues to grow. The global cancer control community has begun to recognize and respond to this challenge.

References

1. United Nations (2011). Political Declaration of the High-Level Meeting of the General Assembly on the Prevention and Control of Non-communicable Diseases. New York: United Nations. Available at www.who.int/nmh/events/un_ncd_summit2011/political_declaration_en.pdf.

2. WHO (2003). WHO *Framework Convention on Tobacco Control*. Opened for signature 16 June 2003, 2305 UNTS 166 (entered into force 27 February 2005). Geneva: WHO. Available at http://www.who.int/fctc/text_download/en/index.html.

3. WHO (2012). *Confronting the Tobacco Epidemic in a New Era of Trade and Investment Liberalization*. Geneva: WHO Tobacco Free Initiative. Available at http://www.who.int/tobacco/publications/industry/trade/confronting_tob_epidemic/en/.

4. Australian Government (2011). *Tobacco Plain Packaging Act 2011*. Available at http://www.comlaw.gov.au/Details/C2011A00148.

5. The Conference of the Parties to the WHO FCTC (2008). *Guidelines for Implementation of Article 11 of the WHO Framework Convention on Tobacco Control on Packaging and Labelling of Tobacco Products*, Decision FCTC/COP3(10). Available at http://www.who.int/fctc/guidelines/adopted/article_11/en/.

6. The Conference of the Parties to the WHO FCTC (2008). *Guidelines for Implementation of Article 13 of the WHO Framework Convention on Tobacco Control on Tobacco Advertising, Promotion and Sponsorship*, Decision FCTC/COP3(12). Available at http://www.who.int/fctc/guidelines/adopted/article_13/en/.

7. Thompson C (2012). Big Tobacco backs Australian law opposers. *Financial Times*, 29 April 2012.

8. United Nations (1961). *Single Convention on Narcotic Drugs, 1961, as amended by the 1972 Protocol amending the Single Convention on Narcotic Drugs, 1961*. Opened for signature 25 March 1972, 520 UNTS 204 (entered into force 8 August 1975). New York: United Nations. Available at https://www.unodc.org/unodc/en/treaties/single-convention.html.

9. International Narcotics Control Board (2012). *Estimated World Requirements for 2013 – Statistics for 2011*. New York: United Nations. Available at http://www.incb.org/incb/en/narcotic-drugs/Technical_Reports/narcotic_drugs_reports.html.

10. Hogerzeil HV, Liberman J, Wirtz VJ *et al.*; Lancet NCD Action Group (2013). Promotion of access to essential medicines for non-communicable diseases: practical implications of the UN political declaration. *Lancet*, 381:680–689. http://dx.doi.org/10.1016/S0140-6736(12)62128-X PMID:23410612

11. The Commission on Narcotic Drugs (2010). *Promoting adequate availability of internationally controlled licit drugs for medical and scientific purposes while preventing their diversion and abuse*, Resolution 53/4. Available at http://www.unodc.org/documents/commissions/CND-Res-2000-until-present/CND53_4e.pdf.

12. The Commission on Narcotic Drugs (2011). *Promoting adequate availability of internationally controlled narcotic drugs and psychotropic substances for medical and scientific purposes while preventing their diversion and abuse*, Resolution 54/6. Available at http://www.unodc.org/documents/commissions/CND-Res-2011to2019/CND54_6e1.pdf.

13. WHO (2011). *Ensuring Balance in National Policies on Controlled Substances: Guidance for Availability and Accessibility of Controlled Medicines*. Geneva: WHO. Available at http://www.who.int/medicines/areas/quality_safety/guide_nocp_sanend/en/.

14. International Narcotics Control Board (2011). *Report of the International Narcotics Control Board on the Availability of Internationally Controlled Drugs: Ensuring Adequate Access for Medical and Scientific Purposes*. Available at http://www.incb.org/incb/en/publications/annual-reports/annual-report.html.

15. United Nations Office on Drugs and Crime (2011). *Ensuring Availability of Controlled Medications for the Relief of Pain and Preventing Diversion and Abuse: Striking the Right Balance to Achieve the Optimal Public Health Outcome*. Vienna: United Nations Office on Drugs and Crime. Available at www.unodc.org/docs/treatment/Pain/Ensuring_availability_of_controlled_medications_FINAL_15_March_CND_version.pdf.

16. United Nations Office on Drugs and Crime (2011). Revision of parts of the model law related to availability and accessibility to controlled drugs for medical purposes. Vienna: United Nations Office on Drugs and Crime.

17. Hakulinen T, Arbyn M, Brewster DH *et al.* (2011). Harmonization may be counter-productive – at least for parts of Europe where public health research operates effectively. *Eur J Public Health*, 21:686–687. http://dx.doi.org/10.1093/eurpub/ckr149 PMID:22080476

18. Stenbeck M, Gissler M, Haraldsdóttir S *et al.* (2011). The planned changes of the European Data Protection Directive may pose a threat to important health research, Open Letter to European Decision Makers. Available at http://ki.se/content/1/c6/13/68/01/Appendix3_Open%20letter%20to%20decision%20makers%20data%20protection%20directive.pdf.

19. Xafis V, Thomson C, Braunack-Mayer AJ *et al.* (2011). Legal impediments to data linkage. *J Law Med*, 19:300–315. PMID:22320005

20. Coleman MP, Evans BG, Barrett G (2003). Confidentiality and the public interest in medical research – will we ever get it right? *Clin Med*, 3:219–228. http://dx.doi.org/10.7861/clinmedicine.3-3-219 PMID:12848254

21. Institute of Medicine (2009). *Beyond the HIPAA Privacy Rule: Enhancing Privacy, Improving Health through Research*. Washington, DC: National Academies Press. Available at http://www.iom.edu/Reports/2009/beyond-the-HIPAA-Privacy-Rule-Enhancing-Privacy-Improving-Health-Through-Research.aspx.

22. United Nations Committee on Economic, Social, and Cultural Rights (2000). *The Right to the Highest Attainable Standard of Health (Article 12 of the International Covenant on Economic, Social, and Cultural Rights)*, General Comment No. 14. Available at http://www.ohchr.org/EN/HRBodies/CESCR/Pages/CESCRIndex.aspx.

23. Meier BM, Mori LM (2005). The highest attainable standard: advancing a collective human right to public health. *Columbia Human Rights Law Rev*, 37:101.

Website

McCabe Centre for Law and Cancer: http://www.mccabecentre.org/

Cancer control in Morocco: action in harmony with the socioeconomic and cultural context

Rachid Bekkali

Cancer control in Morocco is a national priority. Created in November 2005, the Lalla Salma Foundation for Cancer Prevention and Treatment has conducted, in collaboration with the Moroccan Ministry of Health, 15 studies to analyse the situation regarding all aspects related to cancer. The findings were the basis for the development of the National Cancer Prevention and Control Plan 2010–2019 (NCPCP), ratified by the government in March 2010. The vision of the NCPCP is to control cancers nationwide through a multisectoral approach, proposing concrete and sustainable actions and making the best use of available resources, while being in harmony with the socioeconomic and cultural context. The values of the NCPCP are equity, solidarity, quality, and excellence. The objective of the NCPCP is to reduce cancer morbidity and mortality, and to improve the quality of life of patients and their relatives.

The NCPCP action strategy consists of 78 operational measures to be undertaken in four strategic fields: prevention, early detection, diagnosis and treatment, and palliative care. These strategic components are supported by the activities of communication, social mobilization, regulation, training, and research. All these components are being integrated around a national and international mobilization and thus constitute the conceptual framework of the NCPCP. Since the creation of the Lalla Salma Foundation, several projects have been accomplished in partnership with the Ministry of Health, national and international nongovernmental organizations, governmental and private agencies, and benefactors. As of the end of 2012, of the 78 measures of the NCPCP, 72 measures had been initiated, among which 51 were well advanced.

In the area of prevention, public awareness campaigns are organized every year, a programme of smoke-free schools and businesses has been implemented, a human papillomavirus vaccination programme is planned to be generalized in 2014, and the strengthening of regulations is ongoing. In the field of health care, several oncology centres were built and equipped, as well as "Houses of Life" to accommodate patients and their families during the treatment period. A programme of access to medication for low-income patients has been established. Human skills have been developed. Therefore, between 2006 and the end of 2012, for example, Morocco improved from two oncology centres to nine, from two accelerators to 22, from one "House of Life" to nine, from 50 oncologists to more than 150, and from 11 500 patients treated to 23 000. In addition, a detection programme for breast and cervical cancers has been implemented, a palliative care network project was initiated, and an ambitious plan to structure cancer research in Morocco has been started.

The situation analysis reports, the NCPCP, and more details about cancer control activities in Morocco can be found at http://www.contrelecancer.ma/en/documents/.

6 CONTROL

Felicia Marie Knaul   Hideyuki Akaza (reviewer)
Héctor Arreola-Ornelas
Oscar Méndez
Marcella Alsan
Janice Seinfeld
Andrew Marx
Rifat Atun

Summary

- The 14 million estimated new cases of cancer worldwide annually inflict a crushing burden of economic costs and human suffering. A significant part of this burden could be avoided by expanding coverage of prevention, early detection, and treatment for specific cancers.

- The estimated total annual economic cost of cancer was approximately US$ 1.16 trillion in 2010 – the equivalent of more than 2% of total global gross domestic product. Even this impressively high figure is a lower bound, as it does not include the substantial longer-term costs to families and caregivers.

- Between one third and one half of cancer deaths could be avoided with prevention, early detection, and treatment – between 2.4 million and 3.7 million avoidable deaths per year, 80% of which occur in low- and middle-income countries.

- Investing strategically in cancer care and control more than pays for itself. A reasonable estimate shows that the world could have saved between US$ 100 billion and US$ 200 billion in 2010 by investing in prevention, early detection, and effective treatment of cancer.

- The ability to prevent, detect, and treat many cancers has improved over time, and many of these advances have led to reductions in costs. Harnessing markets and increasing access can also bring down prices.

Human life and well-being have an intrinsic and immeasurable value. They also have economic value. Viewing health as an investment, rather than a cost, is the philosophy that today inspires human, economic, and environmental global development agendas.

Yet this investment philosophy remains largely ignored in formulating global and national policies to deal with cancer and other chronic illnesses, leaving wide open the agenda for research into the economics of cancer. Impressive opportunities exist to develop and expand the knowledge needed to better understand how to reduce the economic burden of this set of diseases.

This chapter highlights compelling economic arguments for investments to increase global access to cancer care and control, drawing heavily on published research and analysis of the Global Task Force on Expanded Access to Cancer Care and Control [1]. Estimates of the economic value of the avoidable cancer burden are provided, and these are compared with potential savings based on the current costs of cancer care and control. These estimates are illustrative of how economics can contribute to a deeper understanding of the global cancer burden and to more effective strategies for reducing it.

The economics of investing in cancer care and control

The estimated 14 million new cases of cancer worldwide annually lead to enormous economic cost as well as incalculable human suffering [2,3]. The economic consequences of each cancer case include the direct and indirect costs of treatment, the income forgone by patients and their families unable to work during periods of treatment and illness, and, most importantly in economic terms, the productivity lost due to premature death, disability, and suffering. Further, catastrophic health spending undermines the economic stability of families, often generating dynamic losses and forcing families into impoverishment and economic ruin that may extend far beyond the course of the disease. Broader estimates of economic consequences

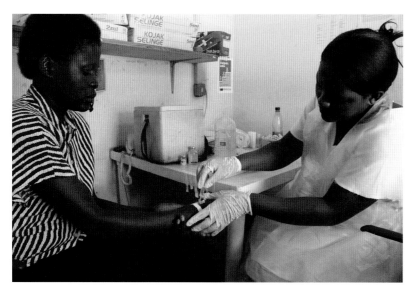

Fig. 6.7.1. A nurse delivers chemotherapy to a patient with Kaposi sarcoma at Neno District Hospital in Malawi. Kaposi sarcoma is among the most common cancers in Malawi, but it is highly treatable – chemotherapy can control Kaposi sarcoma cancer growth and help patients return to normal lives.

also, and appropriately, take into account the perceived costs of human suffering. While a full estimate of the economic burden of cancer would take into account each of these cost components, several of them are difficult to calculate with available data.

A significant part of the economic and health burden of cancer could be avoided by expanding coverage of prevention, early detection, and treatment for specific cancers. Indeed, it is reasonable to consider that the additional financial investments in cancer care and control would be more than counterbalanced by reductions in the economic toll caused by the disease. This hypothesis is analysed below.

The economic cost of cancer

A first approximation of the total annual economic cost of cancer is US$ 1.16 trillion, which is more than 2% of total global gross domestic product. This figure is the sum of the costs of prevention and treatment, plus the annual economic value of disability-adjusted life years (DALYs) lost (a measure that combines years of life lost due to premature mortality

and years of healthy life lost due to disability) as a result of cancer.

The estimate is derived as follows: First, the value of lost productivity due to premature death and disability is taken from a study of DALYs for 17 categories of cancer covering all cancer sites, which produced an estimate of US$ 921 billion for 2010 [3,4]. Second, based on another recent study, the annual global economic cost of treating new (incident) cancer cases was assumed to be US$ 310 billion for 2010 [2,5,6]. Of this, 53% (US$ 163 billion) is due to medical costs, and 23% to the time of caregivers and the cost of transportation to treatment facilities. The remaining 24% is attributed to productivity losses from time in treatment and associated disability; since this portion is also covered in the estimate of DALYs, it was not included in the summation. Finally, the cost of prevention is assumed to be 7% of the cost of treatment. This is a rough estimate that corresponds to the ratio of prevention to health spending in Canada [5,7]. Applied to the global treatment estimate of US$ 163 billion, the cost of prevention of cancer is assumed to be just more than US$ 11.4 billion.

Although impressively high, the figure of US$ 1.16 trillion underestimates the total annual economic cost of cancer, for several reasons. The most important factor is lack of data on the substantial longer-term costs to families and caregivers, which often extend well beyond the first year of treatment. The figure also fails to account for the value that patients and families place on human suffering, which may be far higher than the productivity losses measured by DALYs.

An alternative method for estimating the cost of cancer is to use a value of a statistical life (VSL) approach. This methodology, which includes substantially more of the variety of costs that are incurred by patients and their families, attempts to account for the value individuals themselves place on lost income, out-of-pocket spending on health, and pain and suffering. Based on another recent study, the total 2010 VSL estimate of the global cost of cancer is US$ 2.5 trillion. Of this, close to US$ 1.7 trillion is attributed to high-income countries and the remaining US$ 800 billion to low- and middle-income countries (LMICs) [8].

Working from these estimates of the economic costs of cancer, it is possible to calculate the potential return on investments in expanding cancer care and control by determining values for two other key factors: the economic value of lives that could be saved by expanding access to prevention, early detection, and treatment; and the costs of the expansion of cancer care and control that would be required to achieve these gains.

The "avoidable" cancer burden

A significant proportion of the cancer burden could be avoided through prevention, early detection, and treatment. Calculating the proportion of years of healthy, productive life that could be saved and their value to both the economy and the individual is the key to estimating the economic benefit of investing in cancer care and control.

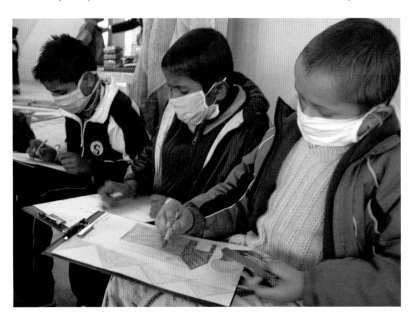

These calculations require an assumption about the proportion of deaths that can be avoided. The literature on avoidable deaths has typically established premature death using an empirical approach to set an upper limit – for example, 64 years. Under this scenario, a death that occurred before the age of 65 years (or any other upper limit) is considered avoidable. The selection of cancers that are considered either preventable or treatable or both preventable and treatable (with or without earlier detection that might have resulted in either a cure or a significant increase in healthy life expectancy) is based on earlier research [9–15].

Each life expectancy scenario is applied to countries' income-group-specific GLOBOCAN estimates of mortality and age at death by cancer type [16,17]. Using a minimum standard of 65 years of life expectancy, an estimated 32% of deaths can be avoided. Setting the standard for life expectancy at the level of the best-performing countries in each income region, 36% of deaths could be avoided. Finally, using life expectancy of 75 years as the standard, an estimated 49% of cancer deaths are considered avoidable with prevention, early detection, and/or treatment.

These estimates suggest, respectively for each scenario, that there are 2.4, 2.7, and 3.7 million avoidable deaths from cancer per year. LMICs account for approximately 80% of this avoidable mortality in each life expectancy scenario.

Costs of treatment and prevention

Another factor that affects the calculations of returns on investments is the dynamic nature of the costs of treatment and prevention. The estimate of the costs of treatment presented above and used as the baseline here – US$ 310 billion – does not account for the possibility of more effective primary and secondary prevention becoming available.

Several of the cancers that generate significant global investment in treatment are preventable, either by reducing exposure to risk factors, such as tobacco, or by vaccination, as for cervical cancer. Preventing the majority of these cancers means avoiding a considerable proportion of treatment costs. For several cancers with a high burden in LMICs – including Kaposi sarcoma and cancers of the cervix, liver, and (most importantly in terms of burden) lung – a considerable proportion of cases could be prevented or detected in precancerous stages, avoiding the far higher costs of treatment. A 90% reduction in cases (through prevention) for Kaposi sarcoma and cancers of the cervix, liver, and lung implies a reduction of at least 20% in the total estimated costs of treating cancer – or approximately US$ 65 billion per year [18]. Prevention can also extend to other cancers with a lower overall burden, such as head and neck cancers, as well as stomach cancers (by treating *Helicobacter pylori*) [5].

Hence, with more effective prevention, the global cost of treatment for cancer would be significantly less than what is currently being spent: rather than the estimated US$ 310 billion, it would be approximately US$ 246 billion. Adding the estimated cost of prevention (US$ 11.4 billion) produces an overall figure of about US$ 257 billion [19].

Fig. 6.7.3. In China, participants in a clinical trial for liver cancer prevention wait to have their blood drawn.

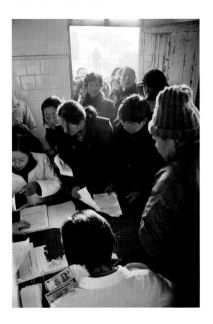

Table 6.7.1. Sensitivity analysis of economic returns to investing in cancer care and control

Cost of care and control[a]	Economic cost of cancer (billions of US dollars)			
	DALYs: valued at US$ 921 billion		VSL less OOP: valued at US$ 2.37 trillion	
	Avoidable deaths		Avoidable deaths	
	49%[b]	36%[c]	49%[b]	36%[c]
Scenario 1. Assuming full cost of treatment based on Bloom *et al.* (2011) [8] + cost of prevention: 310 + 11 = US$ 321 billion	130	10	839	531
Scenario 2. Scenario 1 with reduced costs of treatment based on preventing 90% of Kaposi sarcoma and cancers of the cervix, liver, and lung: (310 − 64) + 11 = US$ 257 billion	194	75	904	596
Scenario 3. Scenario 1 with reduced costs of treatment based on preventing 90% of all potentially preventable cancers: (310 − 100) + 11 = US$ 221 billion[d]	230	110	940	632

DALYs, disability-adjusted life-years; OOP, out-of-pocket health spending by families; VSL, value of a statistical life.

[a] Each cell equals: [(economic cost of cancer) * (% mortality avoided with treatment or prevention)] − (medical and non-medical costs of treating new cancer cases + costs of prevention).

[b] 49% of cancer mortality is assumed avoidable using a scenario of achieving the levels of the best-performing countries – the social justice approach.

[c] 36% of cancer mortality is assumed avoidable using a scenario of achieving the levels of the best-performing country in each income region.

[d] 90% reduction in incidence and hence treatment costs for Kaposi sarcoma and cancers of the cervix, larynx, liver, lung, nasopharynx, other pharynx, and stomach.

Estimating the return on investments in expanding cancer care and control

The estimates in Table 6.7.1 compare the economic value of lives saved in DALYs and VSL to the total costs of treatment and prevention. These estimates provide approximations of what the world could have saved in 2010 by investing in cancer care and control. They range from the most optimistic returns of US$ 230 billion and almost US$ 1 trillion (US$ 940 billion) in terms of DALYs and VSL [18], respectively, to the lower bounds of US$ 10 billion and US$ 531 billion [20], respectively.

A longer-term view

Taking a longer-term, dynamic view of costs and benefits of treatment for cancer provides a more complete vision of the costs and benefits of investing in expanded access to cancer care and control. Existing studies are scarce; this section is restricted to a discussion of issues, and further research in this area is recommended.

Estimates of the total value of lost output from cancer, based on macroeconomic modelling for 2011 to 2030 – an approach that differs from the ones presented above by taking into account accumulated losses over time – suggest substantially higher cumulative economic losses of US$ 2.9 trillion for LMICs and US$ 5.4 trillion for high-income countries [8]. These macroeconomic models show that between 2011 and 2030, noncommunicable diseases – including cancer, cardiovascular disease, chronic respiratory disease, diabetes, and mental health – represent a global cumulative output loss of up to US$ 47 trillion [8].

A further, and significant, consideration in modelling the costs and benefits of investing in cancer care and control is that the dimensions and boundaries of prevention and treatment change over time. Cancers that are considered largely untreatable (liver cancer), or costly to treat (cervical cancer), can now be prevented by applying relatively new medical technologies and vaccines. As science develops, cancers of infectious origin that tend to be more common in LMICs will become increasingly susceptible to prevention, and the global costs of treatment can be expected to decline [1]. Hence, estimates of future global costs of cancer treatment may be overstated as science progresses and identifies new options for prevention that are less costly than treating the cancers that primarily affect people in LMICs.

The cost of producing and delivering drugs and vaccines can fall over time, especially as innovative global financing platforms are developed and implemented [21]. This has been amply demonstrated by the experience with antiretroviral drugs for HIV/AIDS and by huge reductions in the cost of the hepatitis B virus vaccine, achieved in part through the GAVI Alliance, a public–private partnership committed to increasing access to immunization in LMICs. A notable example is the recent GAVI-spurred drop of more than 95% in the price of the human papillomavirus vaccine, from the US$ 130 per dose that prevails in high-income countries to less than US$ 5 per dose in the lowest-income countries. Earlier, the Pan American Health Organization Revolving Fund had garnered an almost 90% reduction, to US$ 14 per dose. Although the vaccine is still unaffordable for

Towards understanding the economics of cancer: priority areas for research

Felicia Marie Knaul

Research in health economics – especially towards a better understanding of the global distribution of costs and the most effective opportunities to achieve impacts – could greatly contribute to reducing both the economic and the health burden of cancer. Yet, economic analysis of cancer is a nascent area of research that to date has focused on high-income countries.

Based on an initial review of the literature, there has never been a comprehensive body of work on the economics of the global cancer burden. Core analysis is, however, being undertaken for an upcoming volume as part of the third round of the Disease Control Priorities project. This is a follow-up volume to the second edition of *Disease Control Priorities in Developing Countries* (published in 2006), which includes several chapters applying economics to cancer care and control [1–3].

Although overall work on the economics of cancer is sparse, a noteworthy exception is the literature on risk factors (or risky behaviour), and especially tobacco consumption and its control [4–8]. Indeed, the existing literature about risky behaviour speaks to the rich array of techniques that economics, and especially health economics, can contribute to reducing the global burden of cancer and closing the cancer divide between rich and poor.

To fully understand the economics of cancer, it will be necessary to analyse each component of the cancer care and control continuum: primary prevention, secondary prevention, diagnostics, treatment, survivorship care, pain control, and palliative care [9]. This is particularly important because cancer covers a complex set of diseases: some are associated with infection or behaviour; others are largely determined by stage at detection; and

yet another, overlapping, subset is susceptible to treatment.

There are a host of opportunities for research on the economics of cancer, based on the field of health economics – an area that has blossomed over the past two to three decades [10]. The research should consider both economics of health (determinants of cancer outcomes) and economics of health care (the market for the provision of cancer care, including global health and health systems), including:

- the economics of global cancer and the relationship between the disease and economic development, using dynamic analysis of the impact on economic growth and the spillover effects on human and social development and the "costs of inaction" [2];
- the analysis of current and future demand for cancer care and control globally, to project global cancer care spending growth under different scenarios for prices and investment in prevention and treatment;
- determinants of cancer incidence and outcomes, the effect of poverty and socioeconomic status, and the social and economic determinants of access to and use of health services;
- spending patterns by families over time on cancer care and control and under different incentive and insurance scenarios, and over time on long-term care;
- analysis of the supply of cancer care and control services globally, and the role of incentives for expanding access, with quality, at the least possible cost and with greatest equity, considering all aspects of service provision and delivery: pharmaceuticals, primary care-based services, hospital-based services, the healthcare workforce, technologies, and so on;

- intellectual property and patent markets for drugs and vaccines, and the role of innovative financing platforms such as the GAVI Alliance [11];
- the economics of pain control and palliation, which spans the global regulatory environment and economics of access;
- the medical workforce and the optimal supply of human resources to respond to current and future needs for cancer care and control;
- health system financing, covering innovations that would optimize the incentive structure for cancer care and control in different resource settings;
- health system reform analysis, including the design, evaluation, and implementation of programmes and policies; and
- other research that could both benefit from and contribute to some of the more novel areas of current health systems work – such as the diagonal approach [9,12,13] and delivery science – and avoid single-intervention analysis by considering value chains to analyse complex processes and diseases and by using the diagonal approach to merge horizontal and vertical interventions to facilitate synergistic investments that generate system-wide improvements [14].

Applying techniques of health economics, and integrating them with novel frameworks in health systems research, would generate new knowledge especially applicable to improving the capacity to respond to the global cancer burden with more appropriate strategies for lower-income settings. Yet to truly improve our understanding of the economic burden of cancer globally and identify the most appropriate ways to face this burden, a multidisciplinary approach is required that links economists to a myriad of other disciplines in health and even in other sectors. The challenge ahead is to both increase economics research and integrate it into efforts to better understand cancer globally.

References

1. Brown ML *et al.* (2006). Health service interventions for cancer control in developing countries. In: Jamison DT *et al.*, eds. *Disease Control Priorities in Developing Countries*, 2nd ed. New York: Oxford University Press, pp. 569–589.

2. Anand S *et al.* (2012). *The Cost of Inaction: Case Studies from Rwanda and Angola*. Cambridge, MA: Harvard University Press.

3. Foley KM *et al.* (2006). Pain control for people with cancer and AIDS. In: Jamison DT *et al.*, eds. *Disease Control Priorities in Developing Countries*, 2nd ed. New York: Oxford University Press, pp. 981–993.

4. Jha P, Chaloupka FJ (2000). *BMJ*, 321:358–361. http://dx.doi.org/10.1136/bmj.321.7257.358 PMID:10926598

5. Jha P, Chaloupka FJ, eds (1999). *Curbing the Epidemic: Governments and the Economics of Tobacco Control*. Washington, DC: World Bank.

6. World Bank (2003). *The Economics of Tobacco Use and Tobacco Control in the Developing World*. Washington, DC: World Bank. Available at http://ec.europa.eu/health/archive/ph_determinants/life_style/tobacco/documents/world_bank_en.pdf.

7. WHO (2011). *Scaling Up Action Against Noncommunicable Diseases: How Much Will It Cost?* Geneva: WHO. Available at http://www.who.int/nmh/publications/cost_of_inaction/en/.

8. Lee K (2008). *PLoS Med*, 5:e189. http://dx.doi.org/10.1371/journal.pmed.0050189 PMID:18798688

9. Knaul FM *et al.* (2012). Health system strengthening and cancer: a diagonal response to the challenge of chronicity. In: Knaul FM *et al.*, eds. *Closing the Cancer Divide: An Equity Imperative*. Based on the work of the Global Task Force on Expanded Access to Cancer Care and Control in Developing Countries. Cambridge, MA: Harvard Global Equity Initiative, pp. 95–122.

10. Pauly MV *et al.* (2012). *Handbook of Health Economics*, Vol. 2. Oxford: North Holland.

11. Atun R *et al.* (2012). *Lancet*, 380:2044–2049. http://dx.doi.org/10.1016/S0140-6736(12)61460-3 PMID:23102585

12. Sepúlveda J *et al.* (2006). *Lancet*, 368:2017–2027. http://dx.doi.org/10.1016/S0140-6736(06)69569-X PMID:17141709

13. Frenk J (2006). *Lancet*, 368:954–961. http://dx.doi.org/10.1016/S0140-6736(06)69376-8 PMID:16962886

14. Kim JY *et al.* (2013). *Lancet*, 382:1060–1069. http://dx.doi.org/10.1016/S0140-6736(13)61047-8 PMID:23697823

many countries, this price reduction marks a huge step forward and was accomplished in only half a decade [22].

Further, the costs of care – and hopes for cure – for several prevalent cancers like breast, colorectal, and cervical cancers depend on the stage at which they are diagnosed. Thus, investing in earlier detection, much of which depends on developing and implementing innovative delivery models, can greatly reduce the cost per year of life saved. At the same time, population-wide screening for cancer can be very costly, making it a priority to develop innovations for earlier detection, many of which will be especially important in LMIC settings.

Many of the dynamic aspects of improving cancer care and control – such as global innovations in financing platforms and country-level innovations in early detection – are part of developing a science of delivery around cancer [23].

Research in health economics, largely unexplored to date, could inform policy and provide recommendations that would help reduce the financial and human burden of cancer. Establishing economic incentives that help change behaviour and increasing the efficacy of services are two avenues (see "Towards understanding the economics of cancer: priority areas for research").

Conclusions

Health is an investment, rather than a cost. Yet this idea has not sufficiently permeated the discussions on cancer care and control. Planning for cancer prevention and management must be integrated in a forward-looking manner into all policy agendas to achieve the most effective investment of health spending. Adopting an investment approach to health reshapes human, economic, social, and sustainable development agendas.

Chronic disease, including cancer, is a leading global economic risk. The drain of tobacco alone on the global economy exceeds the total annual expenditure on health of all LMICs. This makes investment in both prevention and treatment a priority for health and for economic development.

Between one third and one half of cancer deaths can be avoided with prevention, early detection, and treatment. Thus, between 2.4 million and 3.7 million deaths are avoidable per year, 80% of which occur in LMICs.

Given the huge and avoidable suffering caused by cancer, meeting the unmet need for cancer care and control in LMICs is a moral imperative. In addition, and from an economic standpoint, expanding prevention, detection, and treatment of cancer yields benefits that exceed the costs.

The total annual economic cost of cancer – not including longer-term costs to families and caregivers – was approximately US$ 1.16 trillion in 2010, which amounts to more than 2% of total global gross domestic product. By contrast, investing in cancer care and control yields a positive annual return on prevention and treatment because of the number of deaths that are potentially avoidable. Global economic savings of at least US$ 100–200 billion could be achieved by avoiding deaths, and

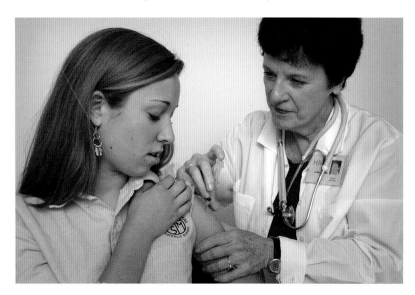

Fig. 6.7.4. A female adolescent receives an intramuscular immunization from a nurse. The availability of vaccines to prevent cervical cancer represents one of the most immediate advances in cancer prevention achieved in the past decade.

hence lost healthy years of productive life, through treatment and prevention. Taking into account the human cost of suffering – the value that individuals place on reduced suffering and illness – the savings are at least US$ 500 billion and could reach almost US$ 950 billion.

Yet, economic analysis of the global cancer burden is a nascent field, and most research to date has focused on high-income countries. Research in this area could greatly contribute to reducing both the economic and health burden. The agenda for this research is ample, and one of the main limiting factors is the lack of adequate data. Indeed,

better data are required to promote a better understanding of the economics of cancer, and any initiative to collect these data could and should be linked to existing initiatives to improve global cancer registries [24].

To truly improve our understanding of the economic burden of cancer globally, a multidisciplinary approach is required that links economists to a myriad of other disciplines. Future efforts should seek to increase economics research and also to integrate it into efforts to better understand cancer globally.

Planning for the future requires harnessing markets in ways that can stimulate innovation, encourage

savings that reduce prices, promote investments that generate system-wide improvements that reduce the impact of cancer and also accrue to other diseases, spread benefits, and reduce costs. These economic benefits could be much greater if the potential cost savings from innovative delivery and financing, combined with more equitable pricing of drugs and other therapies, could be achieved. Adopting a diagonal approach using care delivery value chains can ensure that the potential synergies and shared benefits of interventions are maximized and fully taken into account.

A future where prevention, early detection, and treatment become more accessible to patients and health systems in LMICs is one that builds on the "economics of hope". Neither the costs of prevention nor the potential benefits of extending cancer care and control should be taken as fixed, given the many opportunities that exist to increase access and reduce the global burden of cancer.

This chapter is adapted from Chapter 3 in Knaul FM, Gralow JR, Atun R, Bhadelia A, eds (2012). Closing the Cancer Divide: An Equity Imperative. *Based on the work of the Global Task Force on Expanded Access to Cancer Care and Control in Developing Countries. Cambridge, MA: Harvard Global Equity Initiative. Distributed by Harvard University Press. © 2012 by President and Fellows of Harvard College acting through the Harvard Global Equity Initiative. Reprinted by permission of the Harvard Global Equity Initiative.*

References

1. Knaul FM, Arreola-Ornelas H, Atun R *et al.* (2012). Investing in cancer care and control. In: Knaul FM, Gralow JR, Atun R, Bhadelia A, eds. *Closing the Cancer Divide: An Equity Imperative.* Based on the work of the Global Task Force on Expanded Access to Cancer Care and Control in Developing Countries. Cambridge, MA: Harvard Global Equity Initiative, pp. 71–91.

2. Beaulieu N, Bloom D, Bloom R, Stein R (2009). *Breakaway: The Global Burden of Cancer – Challenges and Opportunities.* A Report from the Economist Intelligence Unit. London: The Economist Group.

3. John RM, Ross H (2008). Economic value of disability-adjusted life years lost to cancers. Available at http://media.marketwire.com/attachments/EZIR/627/18192_Final JournalManuscript.pdf.

4. Shafey O, Eriksen M, Ross H, Mackay J (2009). *The Tobacco Atlas*, 3rd ed. Atlanta, GA: American Cancer Society. Available at http://www.tobaccoatlas.org/.

5. Nikolic IA, Stanciole AE, Zaydman M (2011). *Chronic Emergency: Why NCDs Matter.* Health, Nutrition and Population (HNP) Discussion Paper. Washington, DC: World Bank.

6. Chand S (2012). *Silent Killer, Economic Opportunity: Rethinking Non-Communicable Disease.* Centre on Global Health Security, Briefing Paper. Available at http://www.chathamhouse.org/publications/papers/view/181471.

7. OECD (2010). OECD Stat Extracts database. Paris: Organisation for Economic Co-operation and Development. Available at http://stats.oecd.org/Index.aspx.

8. Bloom DE, Cafiero ET, Jané-Llopis E *et al.* (2011). *The Global Economic Burden of Non-communicable Diseases.* Geneva: World Economic Forum. Available at www.weforum.org/EconomicsOfNCD.

9. Gispert R, Serra I, Barés MA *et al.* (2008). The impact of avoidable mortality on life expectancy at birth in Spain: changes between three periods, from 1987 to 2001. *J Epidemiol Community Health*, 62:783–789. http://dx.doi.org/10.1136/jech.2007.066027 PMID:18701727

10. Gómez-Arias RD, Bonmatí AN, Pereyra-Zamora P *et al.* (2009). Design and comparative analysis of an inventory of avoidable mortality indicators specific to health conditions in Colombia [in Spanish]. *Rev Panam Salud Publica*, 26:385–397. http://dx.doi.org/10.1590/S1020-49892009001100002 PMID:20107689

11. Humblet PC, Lagasse R, Levêque A (2000). Trends in Belgian premature avoidable deaths over a 20 year period. *J Epidemiol Community Health*, 54:687–691. http://dx.doi.org/10.1136/jech.54.9.687 PMID:10942448

12. Weisz D, Gusmano MK, Rodwin VG, Neuberg LG (2008). Population health and the health system: a comparative analysis of avoidable mortality in three nations and their world cities. *Eur J Public Health*, 18:166–172. http://dx.doi.org/10.1093/eurpub/ckm084 PMID:17690129

13. de Martel C, Ferlay J, Franceschi S *et al.* (2012). Global burden of cancers attributable to infections in 2008: a review and synthetic analysis. *Lancet Oncol*, 13:607–615. http://dx.doi.org/10.1016/S1470-2045(12)70137-7 PMID:22575588

14. Knaul FM, Adami HO, Adebamowo C *et al.* (2012). The global cancer divide: an equity imperative. In: Knaul FM, Gralow JR, Atun R, Bhadelia A, eds. *Closing the Cancer Divide: An Equity Imperative.* Based on the work of the Global Task Force on Expanded Access to Cancer Care and Control in Developing Countries. Cambridge, MA: Harvard Global Equity Initiative, pp. 29–70.

15. Gralow GR, Krakauer E, Anderson BO *et al.* (2012). Core elements for provision of cancer care and control in low and middle income countries. In: Knaul FM, Gralow JR, Atun R, Bhadelia A, eds. *Closing the Cancer Divide: An Equity Imperative.* Based on the work of the Global Task Force on Expanded Access to Cancer Care and Control in Developing Countries. Cambridge, MA: Harvard Global Equity Initiative, pp.123–165.

16. WHO (2011). *Global Status Report on Noncommunicable Diseases 2010.* Geneva: WHO. Available at http://www.who.int/nmh/publications/ncd_report2010/en/.

17. World Bank (2010). *World Development Indicators 2010.* Washington DC: World Bank. Available at http://data.worldbank.org/sites/default/files/wdi-final.pdf.

18. Global Risk Network of the World Economic Forum (2010). *Global Risks 2010: A Global Risk Network Report.* Geneva: World Economic Forum. Available at www3.weforum.org/docs/WEF_GlobalRisks_Report_2010.pdf.

19. DeVol R, Bedroussian A (2007). *An Unhealthy America: The Economic Burden of Chronic Disease – Charting a New Course to Save Lives and Increase Productivity and Economic Growth.* Santa Monica, CA: Milken Institute.

20. Stuckler D (2008). Population causes and consequences of leading chronic diseases: a comparative analysis of prevailing explanations. *Milbank Q*, 86:273–326. http://dx.doi.org/10.1111/j.1468-0009.2008.00522.x PMID:18522614

21. Atun R, Knaul FM, Akachi Y, Frenk J (2012). Innovative financing for health: what is truly innovative? *Lancet*, 380:2044–2049. http://dx.doi.org/10.1016/S0140-6736(12)61460-3 PMID:23102585

22. Konduri N, Quick J, Gralow JR *et al.* (2012). Access to affordable medicines, vaccines, and health technologies. In: Knaul FM, Gralow JR, Atun R, Bhadelia A, eds. *Closing the Cancer Divide: An Equity Imperative.* Based on the work of the Global Task Force on Expanded Access to Cancer Care and Control in Developing Countries. Cambridge, MA: Harvard Global Equity Initiative, pp.197–256.

23. Kim JY, Farmer P, Porter ME (2013). Redefining global health-care delivery. *Lancet*, 382:1060–1069. http://dx.doi.org/10.1016/S0140-6736(13)61047-8 PMID:23697823

24. Ferlay J, Soerjomataram I, Ervik M *et al.* (2013). GLOBOCAN 2012 v1.0, Cancer Incidence and Mortality Worldwide: IARC Cancer Base No. 11 [Internet]. Lyon: IARC. Available at http://globocan.iarc.fr.

Cancer control in Peru: "El Plan Esperanza" – the Hope Plan

Carlos Vallejos

Peru has a population of about 30 million people, and the region of Lima (the capital city) is home to about one third of the national population. Peru allocates 5.1% of its gross domestic product to expenditure on health. The growth of the Peruvian economy in the past two decades has led to an increase in life expectancy, from 66.7 years in 1995 to 74.1 years in 2010. Prostate cancer (25.1% of all cases), stomach cancer (15.7%), non-Hodgkin lymphoma (5.8%), and lung cancer (5.4%) are the most frequent malignant tumours in men, and cervical cancer (19.5%), breast cancer (18.9%), stomach cancer (11.5%), and colorectal cancer (5.1%) are the most common in women. Peru's first institution for specialized cancer treatment was the Instituto Nacional de Enfermedades Neoplásicas (INEN), which was founded in 1939 and is supported by government funds. INEN was designated as an autonomous institution in 1985 and is required to formulate, regulate, and advise on the development of health policies in the field of cancer.

Problems frequently faced by oncologists in Peru have been: (i) tumours in advanced stages, mainly because there is a long period between the first signs of cancer and seeking specialist attention; (ii) lack of adherence to treatment, or delay in the treatment, due to costs and because sometimes patients have to travel long distances to receive treatment; and (iii) inadequate follow-up. These three problems are certainly related to the geographical distance between a patient's home and a treatment facility. Until 2000, INEN was the only public centre for cancer care in Peru. The development of new policies for the decentralization of cancer care led to the inauguration of a new specialized centre covering a major population.

In 2007, Peru implemented the first national cancer control plan in Latin America. Priority was accorded to the most relevant cancers in Peru – cancers of the breast, cervix, stomach, lung, and prostate – and beneficial results were obtained. In addition, new policies and strategies were developed to provide access to medical attention for the poorest people under a universal insurance coverage. In 2011, a newly fledged budgetary strategic programme (budget by results) for cancer control was released, which provided US$ 10.3 million, with the benefits being directed mainly to 10 regions (selected according to priorities in terms of population size and cancer incidence). Meeting strategic goals has led to an increase in the budget for nationwide activity to US$ 29.8 million for 2012. These state policies established in the past 10 years have established the foundation for the current "Plan Esperanza" (Hope Plan).

Cancer control in Turkey: an encouraging national cancer control plan for the future

Ezgi Hacikamiloglu, Guledal Boztas, Murat Gultekin, and Murat Tuncer

Turkey's national cancer control programme, which was prepared and initiated in cooperation with national and international organizations to decrease the number of cancer-related deaths, consists of four main pillars: cancer registry activities, cancer prevention, cancer screening and early diagnosis, and cancer treatment and palliative care.

Cancer registry activities

Since 2002, in conjunction with passive registration, active cancer registration has also been implemented. There are 16 active cancer registration centres in 15 cities in Turkey (50% population coverage). Currently, four of the active registration centres are accredited by IARC. The cancer registration centre in the city of İzmir is designated an international training centre (hub) by IARC. The implementation of active registration centres in all 81 cities, with a 100% coverage rate, is planned to be completed by the end of 2015.

Cancer prevention

Cancer prevention in Turkey is managed under certain programmes. The nationwide programmes are the Alcohol Control Programme; the Healthy Nutrition, Obesity Control, and Promotion of Physical Activity Programmes; the Reduction of Excessive Salt Consumption Programme; the Strategic Asbestos Control Programme; the Radon Mapping Programme; and the National Tobacco Control Programme. The National Tobacco Control Programme, which was started in 2008, is extremely successful with excellent outcomes. Tobacco consumption rates decreased from 33.6% to 27.5%, and Turkey became the first country in the world to implement all the tobacco control measures of MPOWER [1–3].

Cancer screening and early diagnosis

A Cancer Early Diagnosis, Screening, and Training Centre has been opened in each city in Turkey. Population-based screening and public training programmes about breast, cervical, and colorectal cancers are being organized within these centres totally free of charge. In 2012, the national cancer screening standards were revised as follows: breast cancer screening every 2 years from the age of 40 years; colorectal cancer screening, by using immunological faecal occult blood testing in conjunction with colonoscopy, for all people aged 51 years and 61 years; and cervical cancer screening implementing human papillomavirus (HPV) DNA testing. Nationwide software packages have been produced to follow European Union quality criteria on screening. By means of 130 new mobile screening units, digitization of mammography, and central mammography reporting units, and by evoking the potential help of family physicians and screening via HPV tests, Turkey aims to raise the population screening rates to 70% by 2015.

Cancer treatment and palliative care

Cancer treatment is free of charge for all citizens in Turkey, and all standard treatments are available in the country. Treatment facilities are implemented according to the 2023 strategic investment plans, according to the disease burden, geographical transportation, and population dynamics. Also, domestic production of some chemotherapeutics and opioids has already started. One of the basic essentials for palliative care, which was started in 2010, is providing health care at home. This service is also being provided for terminal-stage cancer patients. Palliative care legislation has been prepared and is planned to be launched by the end of 2013. In addition, opioid legislation is being evaluated to increase accessibility. Turkey aims to implement a population-based palliative care system based on family physicians and home care teams supported by more than 200 palliative care units within the next 5 years.

References

1. WHO (2012). Global Adult Tobacco Survey. Turkish Statistical Institute. Available at http://www.who.int/tobacco/surveillance/gats_turkey/en/index.html.

2. WHO (2013). *WHO Report on the Global Tobacco Epidemic, 2013: Enforcing Bans on Tobacco Advertising, Promotion and Sponsorship*. Geneva: WHO. Available at http://apps.who.int/iris/bitstream/10665/85380/1/9789241505871_eng.pdf.

3. WHO (2008). *MPOWER: A Policy Package to Reverse the Tobacco Epidemic*. Geneva: WHO. Available at http://www.who.int/tobacco/mpower/mpower_english.pdf.

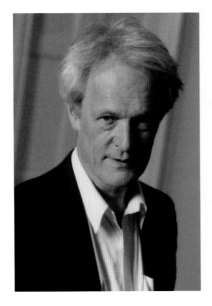

Richard Peto

in collaboration with Alan D. Lopez, Hongchao Pan, and Michael J. Thun

The full hazards of smoking and the benefits of stopping: cancer mortality and overall mortality

Richard Peto is a professor of medical statistics and epidemiology and a co-director of the Clinical Trial Service Unit at the University of Oxford. He studied natural sciences at Cambridge University and obtained his M.Sc. in statistics at the University of London. Dr Peto's work has included studies of the causes of cancer in general, and of the effects of smoking in particular, and the establishment of large-scale randomized trials of the treatment of cancer and various other diseases. He has been instrumental in introducing combined "meta-analyses" of results from diverse studies. Dr Peto is one of the world's most cited medical researchers and was knighted in 1999 for his services to epidemiology and cancer prevention. He devotes much of his energy to advising and providing information on "avoidable death". His work continues to have a direct influence on public policy and adult mortality in many countries.

Summary

Recent studies of the hazards of people in the United Kingdom, USA, or Japan who began smoking in adolescence or early adult life show loss of about 10 years of life expectancy if they continue, and avoidance of more than 90% of the excess risk if they stop before age 40 (and preferably well before age 40). Smokers who did not start in early adult life have much smaller hazards in middle and old age. Hence, when smoking becomes common among a population of young adults, the full eventual effects of tobacco on mortality rates in middle and old age take more than half a century to emerge in that population. For women in many developed countries and men in many other countries, there will be a large increase in tobacco-attributed mortality over the next few decades as a result of increases in smoking that have already happened, unless there is widespread cessation.

Cancer mortality and overall mortality

Taking all countries in the world together, smoking is by far the most important cause of cancer, and although tobacco-attributed cancer mortality is now falling in some populations in developed countries, worldwide it is increasing. Smoking can cause death not only from lung cancer (the main neoplastic hazard) but also from cancer of the mouth, pharynx, larynx, oesophagus, stomach, pancreas, liver, kidney, bladder, or cervix [1]. It also causes more deaths from other diseases (e.g. heart disease, stroke, chronic obstructive lung disease, tuberculosis, and pneumonia) than from cancer.

This Perspective summarizes the full eventual effects on lung cancer mortality, overall cancer mortality, and all-cause mortality of starting to smoke in early adult life and continuing to do so and, conversely, the full eventual effects among smokers who did start when young of cessation at various ages, in comparison with the hazards they would have faced if they had continued smoking.

In general, among cigarette smokers who started in early adult life, those who stop before middle age (here defined as ages 35–69) gain about 10 years of life expectancy. This is now known to be true for both men and women [2–5]. It is likely to be true in any population where the smokers who have not yet reached middle age started smoking cigarettes in early adult life, even if in that population the

The risk is big, if they continue smoking

- At least half are eventually killed by smoking, if they continue. (Among persistent cigarette smokers, male or female, the overall relative risk of death is greater than 2 throughout middle age and well into old age. Thus, among smokers of a given age, more than half of those who die in the near future would not have done so at never-smoker death rates.)

- On average, smokers lose at least 10 years of life. (This average combines a zero loss for those not killed by tobacco with a loss of much more than 10 years for those who are killed by it.)

Those killed in middle age (35–69 years of age) lose many years of life

- Some of those killed in middle age might have died soon anyway, but others might have lived on for another 10, 20, 30, or more years.

- On average, those killed in middle age lose about 20 years of never-smoker life expectancy.

Stopping smoking works

- Those who stop before age 40 (and preferably well before age 40) avoid more than 90% of the excess risk among those who continue to smoke. Those who stop before age 30 avoid more than 97% of the smokers' excess risk.

- Those who have smoked cigarettes since early adult life but stop at 60, 50, 40, or 30 years of age gain, respectively, about 3, 6, 9, or almost the full 10 years of life expectancy, compared with those who continue smoking.

effects of smoking on mortality in middle and old age (i.e. in previous generations) are not yet substantial, because those who started in early adult life will, if they continue smoking, eventually experience substantial hazards in middle and old age.

Effects of smoking cigarettes throughout adult life

Cigarette smokers who start in early adult life are at far greater risk in later adult life than otherwise similar smokers who start somewhat later [6]. This implies a remarkably long delay of half a century or more between cause and full effect. As long as due allowance is made for this delay, reliable quantitative predictions can be made of the substantial hazards that will eventually be faced by those who have been cigarette smokers since early adult life but are still only in their twenties, thirties, or forties if they continue to smoke, and of the substantial benefits for such smokers of stopping at various ages.

Cigarette smoking is extraordinarily destructive (Box P7.1; Figs P7.1, P7.2). It is common in many populations, and where it has been widespread among young adults for many decades, at least half of all persistent cigarette smokers

are eventually killed by it, unless they stop. Bidi smoking (bidis consist of a small amount of tobacco wrapped in the leaf of another plant), which is common in parts of South Asia, can cause similar risks [7–8].

Cigarette smoking causes relatively few deaths before about 35 years of age but causes many deaths in middle and old age. Although some of those killed by tobacco in middle age might have died soon anyway, many would have lived on for another 10, 20, 30, or more years (Box P7.1).

British men, the first severely affected population to be studied

Studies of British men born in the first few decades of the 20th century were particularly informative about the full lifelong hazards of smoking and the benefits of stopping because this was the first large population in which many had begun to smoke cigarettes in early adult life and continued to do so. By 1970, Britain had the worst tobacco-attributed mortality rates in the world [9–11]. The lifelong effects of persistent cigarette smoking, and the corresponding benefits of stopping, can therefore

be illustrated by Doll's study of male British doctors born during the first few decades of the 20th century and followed prospectively throughout the second half of the century (Fig. P7.1) [2].

The doctors who smoked (and those who later stopped smoking) had on average begun at 18 years of age. There were no big differences between smokers, former smokers, and never-smokers in occupation, obesity, or alcohol consumption [12]. As all were doctors, they were easily traced even if they emigrated, and the underlying causes of most deaths were recorded reliably.

Fig. P7.1A compares the cigarette smokers with the never-smokers, showing a 10-year difference in life expectancy. During middle age (35–69), 19% of the never-smokers and 42% of the cigarette smokers died (i.e. the respective probabilities of survival from age 35 to age 70 were 81% and 58%). Much of this absolute difference of 23% in mortality was actually caused by smoking, because it mainly involved differences in the numbers dying from diseases that can be caused by smoking (lung cancer, heart disease, chronic lung disease, etc.).

The full eventual effects of smoking from early adult life in men in the United Kingdom (born 1900–1930), showing the lifelong hazards of smoking and the benefits of stopping at age 40 among male British doctors followed up until old age. (A) Survival from age 35 in continuing smokers and never-smokers, showing 10-year loss. (B) Survival from age 40 in smokers, never-smokers, and those who stopped at age 35–44. Follow-up was from 1951 until 2001, with smoking recorded in 1951 and again every few years until 2001. The smokers and the former smokers had both started at mean age 18 years.

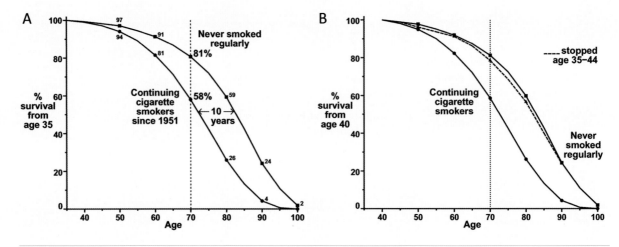

Twenty-first century hazards in women born around 1940 in the United Kingdom and the USA

Among British women, few born early in the 20th century smoked from early adult life, but many born around 1940 did so and were therefore at high risk in later adult life if they continued to smoke. A recent prospective study of 1.3 million such women found hazards comparable to those in men [3].

Fig. P7.2A shows the relationship between daily cigarette consumption and all-cause mortality among these women during the 2000s, when they were in their sixties. On average, smokers had 3 times the overall mortality rate of otherwise comparable never-smokers. This 3-fold relative risk is standardized for age and for many other factors. It therefore means that about two thirds of the deaths of smokers would not have occurred when they did if the smokers had had the same death rates as otherwise similar nonsmokers. Smoking even just a few cigarettes a day was sufficient to double the overall mortality rate.

Similarly extreme smoker versus nonsmoker mortality ratios during the 2000s, and a similar 10-year difference in survival, have recently been reported for men and women in the USA and in Japan [4,5,13].

Cessation, lung cancer mortality, and all-cause mortality in the United Kingdom and the USA

Smokers who stop before age 40 (preferably well before age 40) avoid more than 90% of their risk of being killed by tobacco, gaining on average more than 9 extra years of life expectancy. Fig. P7.1B shows that in Doll's study of British doctors, men who stopped at about 40 (35–44) years of age avoided about 90% of the excess risk they would have suffered if they had continued smoking. Those who stopped at about 60, 50, 40, or 30 years of age gained,

Fig. P7.2. The full eventual effects of smoking from early adult life in women (from the Million Women Study during the 2000s of British women born around 1940): multivariable-adjusted relative risks in never-smokers and in continuing smokers, by daily dose, (A) for all-cause mortality and (B) for lung cancer mortality. The smokers had started at mean age 19 years. For each category, the area of the square is inversely proportional to the variance of the category-specific log risk, which also determines the confidence interval.

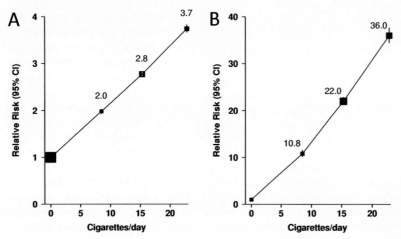

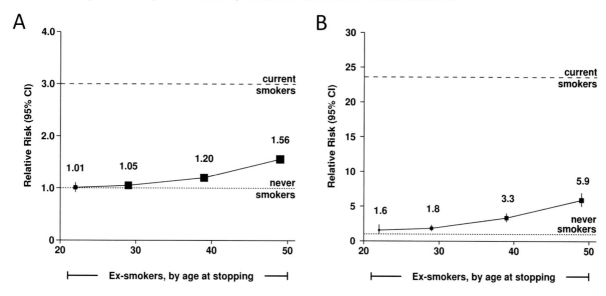

Fig. P7.3. The benefits of stopping at about 30, 40, or 50 years of age in a population where substantial effects of smoking are already apparent (from the Million Women Study during the 2000s of British women born around 1940): multivariable-adjusted relative risks (1.0 for never-smokers) in ex-smokers and in current smokers, (A) for all-cause mortality and (B) for lung cancer mortality. The group of continuing cigarette smokers and the groups who stopped at ages 25–34, 35–44, or 45–54 had all started at mean age about 19 years and all smoked about 15 cigarettes per day. The area of each square is inversely proportional to the variance of the log relative risk (vs never-smokers), which also determines the confidence interval.

respectively, about 3, 6, 9, or almost the full 10 years [2].

Fig. P7.3A shows, based on the much larger Million Women Study, more precise evidence that stopping at age 40 avoids about 90% of the excess mortality among those who continue smoking [3]. Similarly extreme benefits of having stopped at 30 or 40 years of age have been reported from studies of mortality in the USA during the 2000s [4,5].

Lung cancer is one of the main diseases caused by smoking. Even though it accounts for less than half of all smoking-attributed mortality, when the lung cancer death rates among persistent cigarette smokers, former smokers, and never-smokers are compared, the relative risks are so extreme that the long-term hazards of smoking and the benefits of stopping can be seen particularly clearly [3,14,15].

Fig. P7.3B shows the lung cancer findings for smokers by age at cessation in the Million Women Study [3]. Although the former smokers who stopped at about age 30, 40, or 50 still had a highly significant excess lung cancer risk some

decades after stopping, there is a large absolute difference between the risks in those who stopped at these ages and in those who continued smoking.

Those who stopped at 30 avoided 97% of the excess lung cancer risk a few decades later in those who continued (i.e. they had only 3% of the excess risk, with confidence interval 2–4%), and those who stopped at 40 avoided 90% of the excess lung cancer risk in those who continued (i.e. they had only 10% of the smokers' excess risk).

Comparable findings have recently been reported for men and women in the USA [4,5].

Evolution of the epidemic in male and female smokers in the USA

The report by Thun *et al.* [5] is particularly illuminating because it spans a 50-year period (1960–2010) during which there was a more than 10-fold increase in the excess lung cancer mortality among female smokers as the epidemic matured. It describes three separate large studies – one in the 1960s, one in the 1980s, and one

in the 2000s – that recorded each woman's smoking and then monitored lung cancer rates over the next few years among women who were older than 55 years. The age-standardized death rate from lung cancer in women who had never smoked was about the same in all three studies because there has been no big change in nonsmoker lung cancer rates in the USA.

The lung cancer risk ratio comparing current smokers with otherwise similar never-smokers was, however, very different in the three studies (Table P7.1): only 3-fold in the 1960s, 13-fold in the 1980s, and 26-fold in the 2000s (similar to the 24-fold risk ratio in the Million Women Study in the 2000s in the United Kingdom). This is because in the USA women older than 55 who were smokers in the 1960s *had not* been smoking ever since early adult life, whereas most who were smokers in the 2000s *had* been doing so.

Note that in the USA many women who were young smokers in the 1960s (when their mothers and grandmothers were enjoying

Table P7.1. Maturing of the lung cancer epidemic in male and female smokers in the USA from the 1960s to the 2000s: ratio of lung cancer death rates, current smoker versus never-smoker, in three large prospective studies

Sex	Ratio (95% confidence interval)[a]		
	1959–1965	1982–1988	2000–2010
Male	12 (10–16)	24 (21–28)	25 (22–28)
Female	3 (2–4)	13 (11–14)	26 (23–28)

[a] Multivariable-adjusted lung cancer mortality ratio, current smoker versus never-smoker (age > 55 years), and 95% confidence interval. Age-standardized never-smoker lung cancer rates were similar in different time periods (showing no significant trend) and in men and women.

relatively low lung cancer rates in middle and old age) *had* been smoking all their young adult lives, so those of them who kept on smoking for the next 40 years went on to become the older smokers in the 2000s with high lung cancer rates (much higher than those in previous generations of women).

Underestimation of eventual hazards in studies of other populations

Cigarette consumption was low throughout the world in 1900, but among men in many developed countries, such as the United Kingdom and the USA, it increased substantially during the first few decades of the 20th century [1]. In recent decades it has also increased substantially among women in many developed countries and among men in many developing countries, including China [16].

When in a particular population there is an upsurge of cigarette smoking among young adults, it will be 40 or more years before the main upsurge of tobacco-related deaths in middle age is seen, and then another 20 years before the main upsurge of tobacco-related deaths in old age. Thus, even in populations where there is not yet a high death rate from smoking (because relatively few people who are now in middle or old age have been cigarette smokers throughout adult life), many of the young adults who smoke began to do so in adolescence or early adult life, so decades hence they will face substantial risks in middle and old age if they continue, and they have much to gain from prompt cessation.

Many previous studies of smoking and disease were in populations where the middle-aged or, particularly, older smokers had not been smoking cigarettes throughout adult life. The risks found by comparing smokers and never-smokers (or former smokers) in those studies may therefore greatly underestimate the risks that the younger cigarette smokers of today will eventually face if they continue. Hence, in those previous studies the benefits of cessation appear to be substantially less than the benefits that the younger cigarette smokers of today would gain from cessation (in comparison with the risks they would face if they were to continue). Thus, for example, earlier studies that suggested relatively small excess risks among smokers in Japan have been succeeded by a recent study that shows there are now large risks among those in Japan who continue to smoke [13].

In many past studies the proportional excess mortality in middle and old age from smoking was greater among male than among female smokers, but this was chiefly because male smokers had smoked cigarettes more intensively when young than had female smokers. Recent studies of women in the United Kingdom and the USA show, however, that smoking cigarettes throughout adult life eventually produces about as great a proportional increase in female as in male overall death rates, so in terms of years of life expectancy lost, the eventual hazards of persistent cigarette smoking (and the corresponding benefits of cessation) will be about as great for women as for men.

Likewise in China, the hazards that younger cigarette smokers will face in middle and old age may well be substantially greater than the risks now seen among Chinese smokers in middle and old age [17]. Indeed, for any cigarette smoker, male or female, in any part of the world who started smoking substantial numbers of cigarettes when young and has continued, the eventual hazards may well be similar: about half will be killed by smoking unless they stop, and cessation before age 40 (preferably well before 40) would avoid more than 90% of that risk.

In any population in the world, therefore, the prevalence of cigarette (or bidi) smoking among young adults can be used as a proxy to predict reasonably reliably the eventual future impact of smoking on mortality in that population several decades hence if those who now smoke continue to do so, and to predict the importance for those who now smoke of prompt cessation.

Contrasting national trends in tobacco-attributed mortality at ages 35–69

In many countries the trends in overall cancer mortality in the past few decades have been dominated by the delayed effects of long-past increases in cigarette smoking among young adults and, more recently, by the more rapid effects of widespread cessation. The United Kingdom, the USA, and Poland offer contrasting examples of this (Figs P7.4–P7.9).

By 1970, male tobacco-attributed mortality rates in the United Kingdom were the worst in the

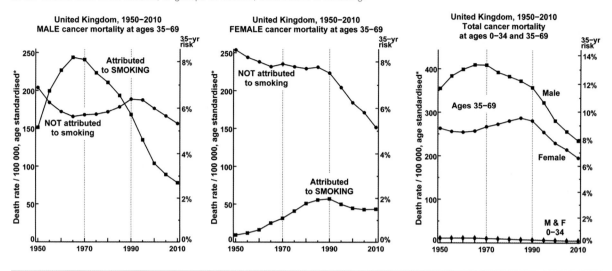

Fig. P7.4. United Kingdom, 1950–2010. Total cancer mortality rates at ages 0–34 and 35–69, with the rates at 35–69 subdivided into parts attributed, and not attributed, to smoking. Rates are calculated from WHO mortality data and UN population estimates. Notes: The rate for a 35-year age range is the mean of the 7 annual death rates in the component 5-year age ranges. (Hence, without other causes of death, a rate of R per 100 000 would imply a 35-year risk of $1 - \exp[-35R/100\,000]$.) The mortality attributed to smoking is estimated indirectly from the national mortality statistics, using the absolute lung cancer rate as a guide to the fraction of the deaths from other causes, or groups of causes, attributable to smoking.

world, with smoking causing well over half of all cancer mortality and almost half of all mortality at ages 35–69, and female tobacco-attributed mortality was rising (Figs P7.4, P7.5). Over the past few decades in the United Kingdom, however, there has been widespread cessation, a substantial decrease in male tobacco-attributed mortality

and, more recently, some decrease in female tobacco-attributed mortality. Had female smokers in the United Kingdom continued smoking, there would have been a major increase in female tobacco-attributed mortality in the United Kingdom throughout the past few decades instead of the moderate decrease actually seen.

In the USA (Figs P7.6, P7.7), a rapid increase in male tobacco-attributed mortality was still in progress when it was halted (well before the cancer or overall death rates from smoking had become as high as they were in the United Kingdom) by a substantial decrease in cigarette consumption over the past few decades. In the USA, male

Fig. P7.5. United Kingdom, 1950–2010. Probabilities of death at ages 0–34 and 35–69, with probabilities of death from smoking at ages 35–69 shaded. Rates are calculated from WHO mortality data and UN population estimates. Notes: Most of those killed by smoking would otherwise have survived beyond age 70, but a minority (shaded area to right of dotted line) would have died by 70 anyway. The mortality attributed to smoking is estimated indirectly from the national mortality statistics.

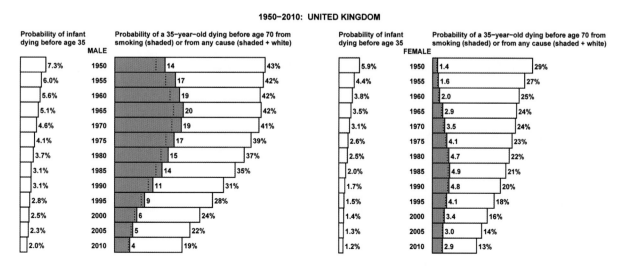

Fig. P7.6. USA, 1950–2010. Total cancer mortality rates at ages 0–34 and 35–69, with the rates at 35–69 subdivided into parts attributed, and not attributed, to smoking. Rates are calculated from WHO (and 2009–2010 United States National Center for Health Statistics) mortality data and UN population estimates. For notes, see Fig. P7.4.

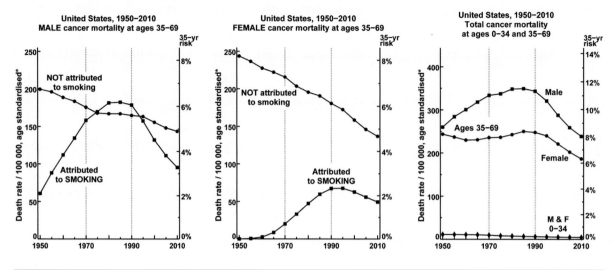

lung cancer mortality in early middle age (35–44; data not shown) has fallen substantially since 1970, and male lung cancer mortality later in middle age is now falling. In the USA, the death rate from smoking among women was still low in 1950, but it rose rapidly and by the 1990s female tobacco-attributed mortality rates in the USA were among the worst in the world, although (as in men in the USA) the rise was eventually halted by a decrease in

cigarette consumption. Again, had female smokers in the USA continued smoking, the steep rise in female death rates from smoking in the USA would still be continuing.

In Poland (Figs P7.8, P7.9), the main increase in cigarette smoking among men took place around the middle of the century and was followed by a large increase in male tobacco-attributed mortality during the second half of the century (to levels comparable with those seen

20 years earlier in the United Kingdom). However, a decrease in smoking since 1990 and changes in the nature of the cigarette have decreased this mortality. In Poland women have thus far been less severely affected than men, but female tobacco-attributed mortality is rising steadily, and young Polish women who now smoke will face substantial hazards if they continue.

The methods used in these three populations to estimate smoking-

Fig. P7.7. USA, 1950–2010. Probabilities of death at ages 0–34 and 35–69, with probabilities of death from smoking at ages 35–69 shaded. Rates are calculated from WHO (and 2009–2010 United States National Center for Health Statistics) mortality data and UN population estimates. For notes, see Fig. P7.5.

1950–2010: UNITED STATES

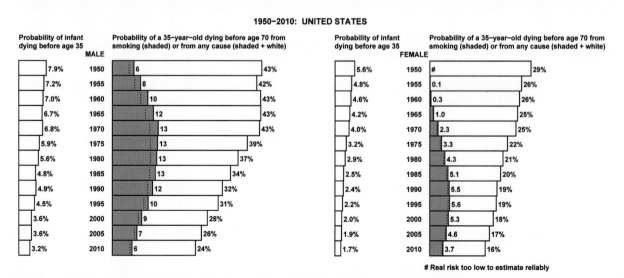

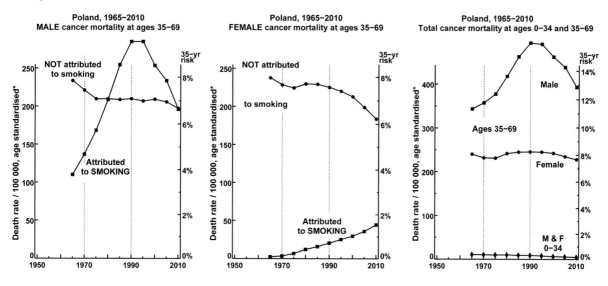

attributed mortality, past and present, are indirect [9,10], but the overall patterns should be reasonably trustworthy, particularly for cancer. The findings demonstrate the enormous potential relevance of smoking cessation to cancer mortality and to overall mortality rates in such countries, and the practicability of substantial changes in tobacco-attributed mortality accumulating over a period of decades. This is true both in populations where smoking is already a major cause of death and in populations where it is not but where it will become so if current smoking patterns persist.

Worldwide trends

Worldwide, about 100 million people a year reach adult life. Based on present smoking patterns, about 30 million (50% of the young men and 10% of the young women) will start to smoke, and more than two thirds will continue because in low- and middle-income countries cessation is uncommon [16]. Of those who continue to smoke cigarettes or bidis, whether in Asia, America, Africa, or Europe, about half will eventually be killed by their habit (unless they die of something else before middle age). Hence, if more than 20 million of these 30 million new smokers a year continue smoking, and do not

Fig. P7.9. Poland, 1955–2010. Probabilities of death at ages 0–34 and 35–69, with probabilities of death from smoking at ages 35–69 shaded. Rates are calculated from WHO mortality data and UN population estimates. For notes, see Fig. P7.5.

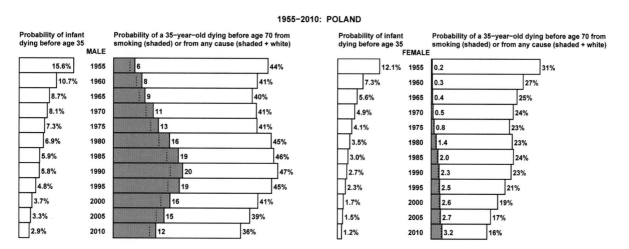

Table P7.2. Projected numbers of deaths from tobacco during the 21st century, if current smoking patterns persist[a]

Period (years)	Deaths from tobacco (millions)
2000–2024	~150
2025–2049	~250–300
2050–2099	> 500
Total, entire 21st century	**~1000**
Total, entire 20th century	~100

[a] Worldwide, about 30% of young adults become smokers, and with the current low cessation rates among smokers in low- and middle-income countries, most who start will not stop.

stop, and half of those who do so are killed by their habit, eventually more than 10 million people per year will be killed by tobacco [18].

Based on current smoking patterns, where 30% start and most who start will not stop, worldwide annual mortality from tobacco is likely to reach 10 million per year (i.e. 100 million per decade) before the middle of this century [10,18,19], and will rise somewhat further in later decades. Tobacco is therefore expected to cause about 150 million deaths in the first quarter of this century (many of which have already happened, as smoking is already causing about 6 million deaths a year worldwide [20]) and 250–300 million in the second quarter. Predictions for the third and, particularly, the fourth quarter of the century are inevitably more speculative. However, due partly to population growth and partly to the maturing of the epidemic, if current smoking patterns persist then the number of tobacco-attributed deaths is likely to exceed 100 million per decade throughout the second half of the century (Table P7.2).

Cessation and not starting

The number of tobacco-related deaths predicted to occur before 2050 cannot be greatly reduced unless a substantial proportion of the adults who have already been smoking for some time give up the habit. A decrease over the next decade or two in the proportion of young people who become smokers will not have its main effects on mortality until the second half of the century. The effects of adult smokers quitting on deaths before 2050 and of young people not starting to smoke on deaths after 2050 will probably be approximately as follows.

Cessation

If many of the adults who now smoke were to give up over the next decade or two, thus halving global cigarette consumption per adult by the 2020s, this would prevent about one third of tobacco-related deaths in the 2020s and almost halve tobacco-related deaths thereafter. Within a decade of their occurrence, such changes could avoid 10 or 20 million tobacco-related deaths per decade, and could avoid 100 million tobacco-related deaths in the second quarter of the century.

Not starting

If, by reduction over the next decade or two in the global uptake rate of smoking by young people, the proportion of young adults who become smokers were to be halved by the 2030s, this would avoid hundreds of millions of deaths from tobacco in the second half of the century. It would, however, avoid almost none of the 150 million deaths from tobacco in the first quarter of the century, and would probably avoid "only" a few million deaths from tobacco in the second quarter of the century.

Thus, using widely practicable ways of helping large numbers of young people not to start smoking could avoid hundreds of millions of tobacco-related deaths in the second half of the century, but not before. In contrast, widely practicable ways of helping large numbers of adult smokers to quit (preferably before middle age, but also in middle age) could well avoid more than 100 million tobacco-related deaths in the first half of this century. Large numbers of deaths during the second half of the century would also be avoided if many of those who, despite everything, still start to smoke in future years could be helped to stop before they are killed by tobacco. Such calculations suggest that the effect of quitting could be more rapidly apparent on a population scale than the effects of not starting to smoke. Both, however, are of great importance.

This Perspective is adapted from IARC (2007) [21]. We are grateful to Jillian Boreham and Kirstin Pirie for help with the figures.

References

1. IARC (2004). Tobacco smoke and involuntary smoking. *IARC Monogr Eval Carcinog Risks Hum*, 83:1–1438. PMID:15285078

2. Doll R, Peto R, Boreham J, Sutherland I (2004). Mortality in relation to smoking: 50 years' observations on male British doctors. *BMJ*, 328:1519–1527. http://dx.doi.org/10.1136/bmj.38142.554479.AE PMID:15213107

3. Pirie K, Peto R, Reeves GK *et al.*; Million Women Study Collaborators (2013). The 21st century hazards of smoking and benefits of stopping: a prospective study of one million women in the UK. *Lancet*, 381:133–141. http://dx.doi.org/10.1016/S0140-6736(12)61720-6 PMID:23107252

4. Jha P, Ramasundarahettige C, Landsman V *et al.* (2013). 21st-century hazards of smoking and benefits of cessation in the United States. *N Engl J Med*, 368:341–350. http://dx.doi.org/10.1056/NEJMsa1211128 PMID:23343063

5. Thun MJ, Carter BD, Feskanich D *et al.* (2013). 50-year trends in smoking-related mortality in the United States. *N Engl J Med*, 368:351–364. http://dx.doi.org/10.1056/NEJMsa1211127 PMID:23343064

6. Doll R, Peto R (1981). The causes of cancer: quantitative estimates of avoidable risks of cancer in the United States today. *J Natl Cancer Inst*, 66:1191–1308. PMID:7017215

7. Gajalakshmi V, Peto R, Kanaka TS, Jha P (2003). Smoking and mortality from tuberculosis and other diseases in India: retrospective study of 43000 adult male deaths and 35000 controls. *Lancet*, 362:507–515. http://dx.doi.org/10.1016/S0140-6736(03)14109-8 PMID:12932381

8. Jha P, Jacob B, Gajalakshmi V *et al.*; RGI-CGHR Investigators (2008). A nationally representative case-control study of smoking and death in India. *N Engl J Med*, 358:1137–1147. http://dx.doi.org/10.1056/NEJMsa0707719 PMID:18272886

9. Peto R, Lopez AD, Boreham J *et al.* (1992). Mortality from tobacco in developed countries: indirect estimation from national vital statistics. *Lancet*, 339:1268–1278. http://dx.doi.org/10.1016/0140-6736(92)91600-D PMID:1349675

10. Peto R, Lopez AD, Boreham J *et al.* (1994). *Mortality from Smoking in Developed Countries 1950–2000: Indirect Estimates from National Vital Statistics.* Oxford: Oxford University Press.

11. Thun M, Peto R, Boreham J, Lopez AD (2012). Stages of the cigarette epidemic on entering its second century. *Tob Control*, 21:96–101. http://dx.doi.org/10.1136/tobaccocontrol-2011-050294 PMID:22345230

12. Doll R, Peto R, Wheatley K *et al.* (1994). Mortality in relation to smoking: 40 years' observations on male British doctors. *BMJ*, 309:901–911. http://dx.doi.org/10.1136/bmj.309.6959.901 PMID:7755693

13. Sakata R, McGale P, Grant EJ *et al.* (2012). Impact of smoking on mortality and life expectancy in Japanese smokers: a prospective cohort study. *BMJ*, 345: e7093. http://dx.doi.org/10.1136/bmj.e7093 PMID:23100333

14. Peto R, Darby S, Deo H *et al.* (2000). Smoking, smoking cessation, and lung cancer in the UK since 1950: combination of national statistics with two case-control studies. *BMJ*, 321:323–329. http://dx.doi.org/10.1136/bmj.321.7257.323 PMID:10926586

15. Brennan P, Crispo A, Zaridze D *et al.* (2006). High cumulative risk of lung cancer death among smokers and non-smokers in Central and Eastern Europe. *Am J Epidemiol*, 64:1233–1241. http://dx.doi.org/10.1093/aje/kwj340

16. Giovino GA, Mirza SA, Samet JM *et al.*; GATS Collaborative Group (2012). Tobacco use in 3 billion individuals from 16 countries: an analysis of nationally representative cross-sectional household surveys. *Lancet*, 380:668–679. http://dx.doi.org/10.1016/S0140-6736(12)61085-X PMID:22901888

17. Peto R, Chen ZM, Boreham J (1999). Tobacco – the growing epidemic. *Nat Med*, 5:15–17. http://dx.doi.org/10.1038/4691 PMID:9883828

18. Peto R, Lopez AD, Boreham J *et al.* (1996). Mortality from smoking worldwide. *Br Med Bull*, 52:12–21. http://dx.doi.org/10.1093/oxfordjournals.bmb.a011519 PMID:8746293

19. Peto R, Lopez AD (2001). Future worldwide health effects of current smoking patterns. In: Koop CE, Pearson C, Schwarz MR, eds. *Critical Issues in Global Health.* New York: Jossey-Bass, pp. 154–161.

20. Lim SS, Vos T, Flaxman AD *et al.* (2012). A comparative risk assessment of burden of disease and injury attributable to 67 risk factors and risk factor clusters in 21 regions, 1990–2010: a systematic analysis for the Global Burden of Disease Study 2010. *Lancet*, 380:2224–2260. http://dx.doi.org/10.1016/S0140-6736(12)61766-8 PMID:23245609

21. IARC (2007). The hazards of smoking and the benefits of stopping: cancer mortality and overall mortality. In: IARC Handbooks of Cancer Prevention, Vol. 11: Tobacco Control: *Reversal of Risk After Quitting Smoking.* Lyon: IARC, pp. 15–27.

Contributors

Jean-Pierre Abastado
Singapore Immunology Network
Singapore
jean-pierre.abastado@fr.netgrs.com

Cary Adams
Union for International Cancer
Control
Geneva, Switzerland
cary.adams@uicc.org

Isaac F. Adewole
University of Ibadan
Ibadan, Nigeria
ifadewole@gmail.com

Hideyuki Akaza
Research Center for Advanced
Science and Technology
The University of Tokyo
Tokyo, Japan
akazah@med.rcast.u-tokyo.ac.jp

Naomi E. Allen
University of Oxford
Oxford, United Kingdom
naomi.allen@ctsu.ox.ac.uk

Marcella Alsan
Stanford University
Stanford, CA, USA
marcella.alsan@gmail.com

Nada Al Alwan
Iraqi National Cancer Research
Center
Baghdad University Medical
College
Baghdad, Iraq
nadalwan@yahoo.com

Mahul B. Amin
Cedars-Sinai Medical Center
Los Angeles, CA, USA
Mahul.Amin@cshs.org

Benjamin O. Anderson
University of Washington School of
Medicine
Fred Hutchinson Cancer Research
Center
Seattle Cancer Care Alliance
Seattle, WA, USA
banderso@u.washington.edu

Ahti Anttila
Mass Screening Registry/Finnish
Cancer Registry
Helsinki, Finland
Ahti.Anttila@cancer.fi

Daniel A. Arber
Stanford University Medical Center
Stanford, CA, USA
darber@stanford.edu

Bruce K. Armstrong
Sydney School of Public Health
The University of Sydney
Sydney, Australia
bruce.armstrong@sydney.edu.au

Héctor Arreola-Ornelas
Fundación Mexicana para la Salud
Mexico City, Mexico
harreola@me.com

Silvina Arrossi
Centro de Estudios de Estado y
Sociedad (CEDES/CONICET)
National Program on Cervical
Cancer Prevention
Ministry of Health/National Cancer
Institute
Buenos Aires, Argentina
silviarrossi2020@gmail.com

Rifat Atun
Imperial College London
London, United Kingdom
and
Harvard School of Public Health
Harvard University
Boston, MA, USA
ratun@hsph.harvard.edu

Robert A. Baan
International Agency for Research
on Cancer
Lyon, France
baanr@visitors.iarc.fr

Yung-Jue Bang
Seoul National University College of
Medicine
Seoul National University Hospital
Seoul, Republic of Korea
bangyj@snu.ac.kr

Emmanuel Barillot
Institut Curie
Paris, France
emmanuel.barillot@curie.fr

Jill Barnholtz-Sloan
Case Comprehensive Cancer
Center
Case Western Reserve University
School of Medicine
Cleveland, OH, USA
and
Central Brain Tumor Registry of the
United States
Hinsdale, IL, USA
jsb42@case.edu

Laura E. Beane Freeman
National Cancer Institute
Bethesda, MD, USA
freemala@mail.nih.gov

Rachid Bekkali
Lalla Salma Foundation for Cancer
Prevention and Treatment
Rabat, Morocco
rachid.bekkali@alsc.ma

Agnès Binagwaho
Ministry of Health
Kigali, Rwanda
agnes_binagwaho@hms.harvard.
edu

Elizabeth H. Blackburn
University of California
San Francisco, CA, USA
Elizabeth.Blackburn@ucsf.edu

Evan Blecher
American Cancer Society
Atlanta, GA, USA
evan.blecher@cancer.org

Ron Borland
Cancer Council Victoria
Carlton, Australia
Ron.Borland@cancervic.org.au

Fred T. Bosman
University Institute of Pathology
Lausanne, Switzerland
fred.bosman@chuv.ch

Peter Bouwman
Netherlands Cancer Institute
Division of Molecular Pathology
Cancer Genomics Centre
Netherlands & Cancer Systems
Biology Center
Amsterdam, Netherlands
p.bouwman@nki.nl

Guledal Boztas
Cancer Control Department
Public Health Institute
Turkish Ministry of Health
Ankara, Turkey
guledal.boztas@thsk.gov.tr

Elisabeth Brambilla
Centre Hospitalier Universitaire
Albert Michallon
Grenoble, France
ebrambilla@chu-grenoble.fr

Freddie Bray
International Agency for Research
on Cancer
Lyon, France
brayf@iarc.fr

Paul Brennan
International Agency for Research
on Cancer
Lyon, France
brennanp@iarc.fr

Louise A. Brinton
National Cancer Institute
Bethesda, MD, USA
brintonl@exchange.nih.gov

Nathalie Broutet
World Health Organization
Geneva, Switzerland
broutetn@who.int

Michael P. Brown
Royal Adelaide Hospital Cancer
Centre
Adelaide, Australia
Michael.Brown@health.sa.gov.au

Heather Bryant
Canadian Partnership Against
Cancer
Toronto, Canada
Heather.bryant@partnershipagainst
cancer.ca

Nikki Burdett
Royal Adelaide Hospital
Adelaide, Australia
Nikki.Burdett@health.sa.gov.au

Robert C. Burton
School of Public Health and
Preventive Medicine
Monash University
The Alfred Centre
Melbourne, Australia
robertcharlesburton@gmail.com

Agnès Buzyn
Institut National du Cancer
Paris, France
abuzyn@institutcancer.fr

Kenneth P. Cantor
National Cancer Institute
Bethesda, MD, USA
kencantor@earthlink.net

Federico Canzian
German Cancer Research Center
Heidelberg, Germany
f.canzian@dkfz-heidelberg.de

Fátima Carneiro
IPATIMUP & Medical Faculty of the
University of Porto
Centro Hospitalar de São João
Porto, Portugal
fcarneiro@ipatimup.pt

Webster K. Cavenee
University of California at San
Diego
La Jolla, CA, USA
wcavenee@ucsd.edu

Eduardo L. Cazap
National Cancer Institute
Ministry of Health
Buenos Aires, Argentina
and
Union for International Cancer
Control
Geneva, Switzerland
ecazap@uicc.org

Frank J. Chaloupka
University of Illinois at Chicago
Chicago, IL, USA
fjc@uic.edu

Stephen J. Chanock
National Cancer Institute
Bethesda, MD, USA
chanocks@mail.nih.gov

Bob Chapman
American Cancer Society Cancer
Action Network
Washington, DC, USA
bob.chapman@cancer.org

Simon Chapman
Sydney School of Public Health
The University of Sydney
Sydney, Australia
simon.chapman@sydney.edu.au

Chien-Jen Chen
Academic Sinica
Taipei, Taiwan, China
chencj@gate.sinica.edu.tw

Il Ju Choi
Centre for Gastric Cancer
National Cancer Centre
Goyang, Republic of Korea
cij1224@ncc.re.kr

Rafael Moreira Claro
Center for Epidemiological Studies
in Health and Nutrition
University of São Paulo
São Paulo, Brazil
rafael.claro@gmail.com

Hans Clevers
Hubrecht Institute
University Medical Center Utrecht
Utrecht, Netherlands
h.clevers@hubrecht.eu

Vincent Cogliano
U.S. Environmental Protection
Agency, Integrated Risk Information
System
Arlington, VA, USA
cogliano.vincent@epa.gov

Aaron J. Cohen
Health Effects Institute
Boston, MA, USA
acohen@healtheffects.org

Carlo M. Croce
Department of Molecular Virology,
Immunology and Medical Genetics
The Ohio State University Medical
Center
Columbus, OH, USA
carlo.croce@osumc.edu

Min Dai
Cancer Hospital
Chinese Academy of Medical
Sciences
Beijing, China
daiminlyon@gmail.com

Sarah C. Darby
Clinical Trial Service Unit
Nuffield Department of Public
Health
University of Oxford
Oxford, United Kingdom
sarah.darby@ctsu.ox.ac.uk

Peter B. Dean
International Agency for Research
on Cancer
Lyon, France
deanp@visitors.iarc.fr

Lynette Denny
University of Cape Town/Groote
Schuur Hospital
Cape Town, South Africa
lynette.denny@uct.ac.za

Ethel-Michele de Villiers
German Cancer Research Center
Heidelberg, Germany
e.devilliers@dkfz.de

John E. Dick
Campbell Family Institute
Ontario Cancer Institute
Princess Margaret Cancer Centre
University Health Network
Toronto, Canada
jdick@uhnres.utoronto.ca

Joakim Dillner
Karolinska Institute
Stockholm, Sweden
joakim.dillner@ki.se

Susan M. Domchek
Basser Research Center
Abramson Cancer Center
University of Pennsylvania
Philadelphia, PA, USA
Susan.Domchek@uphs.upenn.edu

Tandin Dorji
Department of Public Health
Ministry of Health
Thimphu, Bhutan
doj08@yahoo.com

Roland Dray
International Agency for Research
on Cancer
Lyon, France
drayr@iarc.fr

Majid Ezzati
Imperial College London
London, United Kingdom
majid.ezzati@imperial.ac.uk

Lee Fairclough
Canadian Partnership Against
Cancer
Toronto, Canada
Lee.Fairclough@partnership
againstcancer.ca

Jacques Ferlay
International Agency for Research
on Cancer
Lyon, France
ferlayj@iarc.fr

David Forman
International Agency for Research
on Cancer
Lyon, France
formand@iarc.fr

Silvia Franceschi
International Agency for Research
on Cancer
Lyon, France
franceschis@iarc.fr

A. Lindsay Frazier
Dana-Farber Cancer Institute
Boston, MA, USA
lindsay_frazier@dfci.harvard.edu

Christine M. Friedenreich
University of Calgary
Alberta Health Services – Cancer
Care
Calgary, Canada
christine.friedenreich@albertahealth
services.ca

Søren Friis
Danish Cancer Society Research
Center
Danish Cancer Society
Copenhagen, Denmark
friis@cancer.dk

Tamara S. Galloway
College of Life and Environmental
Science
University of Exeter
Exeter, United Kingdom
T.S.Galloway@exeter.ac.uk

Maurice Gatera
Rwanda Biomedical Center
Kigali, Rwanda
gamaurice2003@yahoo.fr

Wentzel C.A. Gelderblom
South African Medical Research
Council
Cape Town, South Africa
Wentzel.Gelderblom@mrc.ac.za

Margaret A. Goodell
Stem Cells and Regenerative
Medicine Center
Baylor College of Medicine
Houston, TX, USA
goodell@bcm.edu

Sharon Lynn Grant
International Agency for Research
on Cancer
Lyon, France
sgrant@imo.org

Mel Greaves
Centre for Evolution and Cancer
Division of Molecular Pathology
The Institute of Cancer Research
Sutton, United Kingdom
greaves@icr.ac.uk

Adèle C. Green
Queensland Institute of Medical
Research
Brisbane, Australia
and
University of Manchester
Manchester Academic Health
Sciences Centre
Manchester, United Kingdom
Adele.Green@qimr.edu.au

Murat Gultekin
Cancer Control Department
Public Health Institute
Turkish Ministry of Health
Ankara, Turkey
mrtgultekin@yahoo.com

Christine Guo Lian
Brigham and Women's Hospital
Harvard Medical School
Boston, MA, USA
cglian@partners.org

Prakash C. Gupta
Healis, Sekhsaria Institute for
Public Health
Navi Mumbai, India
guptapc@healis.org

Ezgi Hacikamiloglu
Cancer Control Department
Public Health Institute
Turkish Ministry of Health
Ankara, Turkey
ezguner@gmail.com

Andrew J. Hall
Senior Visiting Scientist
International Agency for Research
on Cancer
Lyon, France
andrewjhall1@icloud.com

Stanley R. Hamilton
University of Texas MD Anderson
Cancer Centre
Houston, TX, USA
shamilto@mdanderson.org

Marianne Hammer
Norwegian Cancer Society
Oslo, Norway
Marianne.Hammer@kreftforeningen.
no

Curtis C. Harris
National Cancer Institute
Bethesda, MD, USA
curtis_harris@nih.gov

Takanori Hattori
Shiga University of Medical Science
Tokyo, Japan
hattori@belle.shiga-med.ac.jp

Zdenko Herceg
International Agency for Research
on Cancer
Lyon, France
hercegz@iarc.fr

Hector Hernandez Vargas
International Agency for Research
on Cancer
Lyon, France
vargash@iarc.fr

Rolando Herrero
International Agency for Research
on Cancer
Lyon, France
herreror@iarc.fr

David Hill
Melbourne School of Population
and Global Health and Melbourne
School of Psychological Sciences
The University of Melbourne
Melbourne, Australia
DJHill@unimelb.edu.au

Martin Holcmann
Institute of Cancer Research
Medical University of Vienna
Vienna, Austria
martin.holcmann@meduniwien.ac.
at

James F. Holland
Icahn School of Medicine at Mount
Sinai
Mount Sinai Medical Center
New York, NY, USA
james.holland@mssm.edu

Ralph H. Hruban
Johns Hopkins University School of
Medicine
Baltimore, MD, USA
rhruban@jhmi.edu

Thomas J. Hudson
Ontario Institute for Cancer
Research
Toronto, Canada
tom.hudson@oicr.on.ca

Peter A. Humphrey
Washington University School of
Medicine
St. Louis, MO, USA
humphrey@wustl.edu

Elaine S. Jaffe
National Cancer Institute
Bethesda, MD, USA
elainejaffe@nih.gov

Prabhat Jha
St. Michael's Hospital
Dalla Lana School of Public Health
University of Toronto
Toronto, Canada
Jhap@smh.ca

Jos Jonkers
Netherlands Cancer Institute
Division of Molecular Pathology
Cancer Genomics Centre and
Cancer Systems Biology Center
Amsterdam, Netherlands
j.jonkers@nki.nl

Margaret R. Karagas
Norris Cotton Cancer Center
Dartmouth Medical School
Lebanon, NH, USA
Margaret.R.Karagas@dartmouth.edu

Michael Karin
Laboratory of Gene Regulation and
Signal Transduction
Department of Pharmacology and
Pathology
University of California San Diego
School of Medicine
La Jolla, CA, USA
karinoffice@ucsd.edu

Namory Keita
Service de Gynécologie/
Obstétrique
Université de Conakry
Conakry, Guinea
namoryk2010@yahoo.fr

Ausrele Kesminiene
International Agency for Research
on Cancer
Lyon, France
kesminienea@iarc.fr

Michael C. Kew
University of Cape Town
Cape Town, South Africa
michael.kew@uct.ac.za

Tim Key
University of Oxford
Oxford, United Kingdom
tim.key@ceu.ox.ac.uk

Thiravud Khuhaprema
National Cancer Institute
Bangkok, Thailand
tkhuhaprema-v2@hotmail.com

Paul Kleihues
Medical Faculty
University of Zurich
Zurich, Switzerland
kleihues@pathol.uzh.ch

Günter Klöppel
Department of Pathology
Technical University of Munich
Munich, Germany
Guenter.Kloeppel@lrz.tu-muenchen.de

Felicia Marie Knaul
Harvard Global Equity Initiative
Harvard Medical School
Boston, MA, USA
and
Cáncer de mama: Tómatelo a Pecho
Competitividad y Salud, Fundación Mexicana para la Salud
Mexico City, Mexico
and
Global Task Force on Expanded Access to Cancer Care and Control
felicia_knaul@harvard.edu

Manolis Kogevinas
Centre for Research in Environmental Epidemiology
Hospital del Mar Research Institute
Barcelona, Spain
kogevinas@creal.cat

Nobuo Koinuma
Tohoku University School of Medicine
Sendai, Japan
koisan@med.tohoku.ac.jp

Barnett S. Kramer
National Cancer Institute
Rockville, MD, USA
kramerb@mail.nih.gov

Guido Kroemer
Institut national de la santé et de la recherche médicale, Institut Gustave Roussy
University of Paris Descartes
Centre de Recherche des Cordeliers
Hopital Européen George Pompidou
Paris, France
kroemer@orange.fr

James R. Krycer
Garvan Institute
Sydney, Australia
j.krycer@garvan.org.au

Sunil R. Lakhani
University of Queensland Centre for Clinical Research
The Royal Brisbane and Women's Hospital
Brisbane, Australia
s.lakhani@uq.edu.au

René Lambert
International Agency for Research on Cancer
Lyon, France
lambert@iarc.fr

Johanna W. Lampe
Fred Hutchinson Cancer Research Centre
Seattle, WA, USA
jlampe@fhcrc.org

Robert R. Langley
University of Texas MD Anderson Cancer Center
Houston, TX, USA
Rlangley@mdanderson.org

Lawrence H. Lash
Wayne State University School of Medicine
Detroit, MI, USA
l.h.lash@wayne.edu

Mathieu Laversanne
International Agency for Research on Cancer
Lyon, France
laversannem@iarc.fr

Eric Lavigne
Public Health Agency of Canada
Ottawa, Canada
eric.lavigne@hc-sc.gc.ca

Eduardo Lazcano Ponce
Instituto Nacional de Salud Pública
Cuernavaca, Mexico
elazcano@insp.mx

Maria E. Leon
International Agency for Research on Cancer
Lyon, France
leonrouxm@iarc.fr

Alex C. Liber
American Cancer Society
Atlanta, GA, USA
alex.liber@cancer.org

Jonathan Liberman
McCabe Centre for Law and Cancer
Cancer Council Victoria and Union for International Cancer Control
Carlton, Australia
jonathan.liberman@cancervic.org.au

Dongxin Lin
Cancer Institute and Hospital
Chinese Academy of Medical Sciences
Beijing, China
lindx72@cicams.ac.cn

Dana Loomis
International Agency for Research on Cancer
Lyon, France
loomisd@iarc.fr

Alan D. Lopez
Melbourne School of Population and Global Health
The University of Melbourne
Melbourne, Australia
alan.lopez@unimelb.edu.au

Joannie Lortet-Tieulent
International Agency for Research on Cancer
Lyon, France
Joannie.Tieulent@cancer.org

Judith Mackay
World Lung Foundation
Hong Kong Special Administrative Region, China
jmackay1@netvigator.com

Roger Magnusson
Sydney Law School
The University of Sydney
Sydney, Australia
roger.magnusson@sydney.edu.au

Reza Malekzadeh
Tehran University of Medical Sciences
Tehran, Islamic Republic of Iran
malek@tums.ac.ir

Andrew Marx
Harvard Global Equity Initiative
Boston, MA, USA
andrewmarx@mac.com

Beela Sarah Mathew
Regional Cancer Centre
Trivandrum, India
beelasmathew@hotmail.com

James D. McKay
International Agency for Research
on Cancer
Lyon, France
mckayj@iarc.fr

David Melzer
University of Exeter Medical School
Exeter, United Kingdom
D.Melzer@exeter.ac.uk

Oscar Méndez
Fundación Mexicana para la Salud
Mexico City, Mexico
omendez@funsalud.org.mx

Kathryn R. Middleton
Warren Alpert Medical School of
Brown University
The Miriam Hospital
Providence, RI, USA
kathryn_middleton@brown.edu

Martin C. Mihm Jr
Brigham and Women's Hospital
Harvard Medical School
Boston, MA, USA
mmihm@partners.org

Anthony B. Miller
Dalla Lana School of Public Health
University of Toronto
Toronto, Canada
ab.miller@sympatico.ca

J. David Miller
Carleton University
Ottawa, Canada
David.Miller@carleton.ca

Saverio Minucci
Istituto Europeo di Oncologia
Milan, Italy
saverio.minucci@ieo.eu

Holger Moch
University Hospital of Zurich
Zurich, Switzerland
holger.moch@usz.ch

Elizabeth A. Montgomery
Johns Hopkins Medical Institutions
Baltimore, MD, USA
emontgom@jhmi.edu

Rebecca Morton Doherty
Union for International Cancer
Control
Geneva, Switzerland
morton-doherty@uicc.org

Raul Hernando Murillo Moreno
Instituto Nacional de Cancerología
Bogotá, Colombia
rmurillo@cancer.gov.co

Liam J. Murray
Centre for Public Health
School of Medicine, Dentistry and
Biomedical Sciences
Queen's University Belfast
Belfast, United Kingdom
L.Murray@qub.ac.uk

Richard Muwonge
International Agency for Research
on Cancer
Lyon, France
muwonger@iarc.fr

Robert Newton
University of York
York, United Kingdom
Rob.Newton@ecsg.york.ac.uk

Fidele Ngabo
Ministry of Health of Rwanda
Kigali, Rwanda
ngabog@yahoo.fr

Mark J. Nieuwenhuijsen
Center for Research in
Environmental Epidemiology
Barcelona, Spain
mnieuwenhuijsen@creal.cat

Jane R. Nilson
American Cancer Society
Atlanta, GA, USA
janerobinnilson@gmail.com

Omar Nimri
Cancer Prevention Department
Jordan Cancer Registry
Ministry of Health
Amman, Jordan
onimri@gmail.com

Folakemi T. Odedina
Pharmaceutical Outcomes and
Policy
College of Pharmacy
Radiation Oncology, College of
Medicine
Health Disparities, Shands Cancer
Center
University of Florida
Gainesville, FL, USA
Prostate Cancer Transatlantic
Consortium
Seminole, FL, USA
fodedina@cop.ufl.edu

G. Johan Offerhaus
University Medical Center Utrecht
Utrecht, Netherlands
g.j.a.offerhaus@umcutrecht.nl

Hiroko Ohgaki
International Agency for Research
on Cancer
Lyon, France
ohgakih@iarc.fr

Magali Olivier
International Agency for Research
on Cancer
Lyon, France
olivierm@iarc.fr

Jørgen H. Olsen
Danish Cancer Society Research
Center
Danish Cancer Society
Copenhagen, Denmark
jorgen@cancer.dk

Hongchao Pan
Clinical Trial Service Unit and
Epidemiological Studies Unit
University of Oxford
Oxford, United Kingdom
hongchao.pan@ctsu.ox.ac.uk

Pier Paolo Pandolfi
Beth Israel Deaconess Cancer
Center
Harvard Medical School
Boston, MA, USA
ppandolf@bidmc.harvard.edu

Gianpaolo Papaccio
Section of Histology and
Embryology
Tissue Engineering and
Regenerative Medicine Division
Second University of Naples
Naples, Italy
gianpaolo.papaccio@unina2.it

Chris Paraskeva
School of Cellular and Molecular
Medicine
University of Bristol
Bristol, United Kingdom
C.Paraskeva@bristol.ac.uk

Werner Paulus
Institute of Neuropathology
Münster, Germany
paulusw@uni-muenster.de

José Rogelio Pérez Padilla
Instituto Nacional de Enfermedades
Respiratorias
Mexico City, Mexico
perezpad@gmail.com

Richard Peto
Clinical Trial Service Unit and
Epidemiological Studies Unit
University of Oxford
Oxford, United Kingdom
rpeto@ctsu.ox.ac.uk

Paul Pharoah
Department of Public Health and
Primary Care
Department of Oncology
University of Cambridge
Cambridge, United Kingdom
pp10001@medschl.cam.ac.uk

Gérald E. Piérard
University Hospital of Liège
Liège, Belgium
and
University of Franche-Comté
Besançon, France
and
Laboratory of Skin Bioengineering
and Imaging
Department of Dermatopathology
University Hospital Sart Tilman
Liège, Belgium
gerald.pierard@ulg.ac.be

Christopher J. Portier
Senior Contributing Scientist
Environmental Defense Fund
New York, NY, USA
cportier@mac.com

Jaime Prat
Hospital de la Santa Creu i Sant Pau
Autonomous University of
Barcelona
Barcelona, Spain
jprat@santpau.cat

Rachel Purcell
International Agency for Research
on Cancer
Lyon, France
purcellr@iarc.fr

Pekka Puska
National Institute for Health and
Welfare (THL)
Helsinki, Finland
pekka.puska@thl.fi

You-Lin Qiao
Department of Cancer
Epidemiology
Cancer Institute
Chinese Academy of Medical
Sciences
Peking Union Medical College
Beijing, China
qiaoy@cicams.ac.cn

Thangarajan Rajkumar
Cancer Institute
Madras, India
drtrajkumar@gmail.com

Kunnambath Ramadas
Regional Cancer Centre
Trivandrum, India
ramdasrcc@gmail.com

G.K. Rath
Department of Radiotherapy
All India Institute of Medical
Sciences
New Delhi, India
gkrath@rediffmail.com

Cecily S. Ray
Healis, Sekhsaria Institute for
Public Health
Navi Mumbai, India
raycs@healis.org

Jürgen Rehm
Social and Epidemiological
Research Department
Population Health Research Group
Centre for Addiction and Mental
Health
Toronto, Canada
and
Dalla Lana School of Public Health
University of Toronto
Toronto, Canada
and
PAHO/WHO Collaborating Centre
for Mental Health & Addiction
Epidemiological Research Unit
Technische Universität Dresden
Klinische Psychologie &
Psychotherapie
Dresden, Germany
jtrehm@gmail.com

Luis Felipe Ribeiro Pinto
Brazilian National Cancer Institute
(INCA)
Rio de Janeiro, Brazil
lfrpinto@inca.gov.br

Elio Riboli
Imperial College London
London, United Kingdom
e.riboli@imperial.ac.uk

Leanne Riley
World Health Organization
Geneva, Switzerland
rileyl@who.int

Ronald T. Riley
United States Department of
Agriculture – Agricultural Research
Service
Athens, GA, USA
ron.riley@ars.usda.gov

Eve Roman
Epidemiology and Cancer Statistics
Group, Department of Health
Sciences
University of York
Heslington, United Kingdom
eve.roman@york.ac.uk

Isabelle Romieu
International Agency for Research
on Cancer
Lyon, France
romieui@iarc.fr

Hana Ross
American Cancer Society
Atlanta, GA, USA
Hana.Ross@cancer.org

Lesley Rushton
Imperial College London
London, United Kingdom
l.rushton@imperial.ac.uk

Anne Lise Ryel
Norwegian Cancer Society
Oslo, Norway
Anne.Lise.Ryel@kreftforeningen.no

Jonathan M. Samet
University of Southern California
Los Angeles, CA, USA
jsamet@med.usc.edu

Massoud Samiei
International Atomic Energy
Agency-Programme of Action for
Cancer Therapy
Vienna, Austria
massoud.samiei@gmail.com

Rengaswamy Sankaranarayanan
International Agency for Research
on Cancer
Lyon, France
sankar@iarc.fr

Rodolfo Saracci
International Agency for Research
on Cancer
Lyon, France
saraccir@iarc.fr

Guido Sauter
University Medical Center
Hamburg-Eppendorf
Hamburg, Germany
g.sauter@uke.de

Catherine Sauvaget
International Agency for Research
on Cancer
Lyon, France
sauvagetc@iarc.fr

Fabio Savarese
Institute of Cancer Research
Medical University of Vienna
Vienna, Austria
fabio.savarese@boehringer-
ingelheim.com

Augustin Scalbert
International Agency for Research
on Cancer
Lyon, France
scalberta@iarc.fr

Ghislaine Scelo
International Agency for Research
on Cancer
Lyon, France
scelog@iarc.fr

Mark Schiffman
National Cancer Institute
Rockville, MD, USA
schiffmm@exchange.nih.gov

Stuart J. Schnitt
Beth Israel Deaconess Medical
Center
Harvard Medical School
Boston, MA, USA
sschnitt@bidmc.harvard.edu

Joachim Schüz
International Agency for Research
on Cancer
Lyon, France
schuzj@iarc.fr

Janice Seinfeld
Universidad del Pacifico
Lima, Peru
seinfeld_jn@up.edu.pe

Surendra S. Shastri
WHO Collaborating Centre for
Cancer Prevention, Screening and
Early Detection
Tata Memorial Centre
Mumbai, India
surendrashastri@gmail.com

Kevin Shield
Centre for Addiction and Mental
Health
Toronto, Canada
kevin.shield@utoronto.ca

Maria Sibilia
Institute for Cancer Research
Medical University of Vienna
Vienna, Austria
Maria.Sibilia@meduniwien.ac.at

Jack Siemiatycki
University of Montreal
Montreal, Canada
j.siemiatycki@umontreal.ca

Ronald Simon
University Medical Center
Hamburg-Eppendorf
Hamburg, Germany
r.simon@uke.uni-hamburg.de

Pramil N. Singh
Loma Linda University
School of Public Health
Loma Linda, CA, USA
psingh@llu.edu

Rashmi Sinha
National Cancer Institute
Rockville, MD, USA
sinhar@exchange.nih.gov

Nadia Slimani
International Agency for Research
on Cancer
Lyon, France
slimanin@iarc.fr

Avrum Spira
Boston University Medical Centre
Boston, MA, USA
aspira@gmail.com

Gustavo Stefanoff
Brazilian National Cancer Institute
(INCA)
Rio de Janeiro, Brazil
cgstefanoff@inca.gov.br

Eva Steliarova-Foucher
International Agency for Research
on Cancer
Lyon, France
steliarovae@iarc.fr

Bernard W. Stewart
Cancer Control Program
South East Sydney Public Health
Unit
and
School of Women's and Children's
Health
University of New South Wales
Sydney, Australia
Bernard.Stewart@sesiahs.health.
nsw.gov.au

Kurt Straif
International Agency for Research
on Cancer
Lyon, France
straifk@iarc.fr

Simon B. Sutcliffe
Terry Fox Research Institute
Vancouver, Canada
cci-cancercontrol@shaw.ca

Rosemary Sutton
Children's Cancer Institute Australia
Lowy Cancer Research Centre
University of New South Wales
Sydney, Australia
rsutton@ccia.unsw.edu.au

Steven H. Swerdlow
University of Pittsburgh School of
Medicine
Pittsburgh, PA, USA
swerdlowsh@upmc.edu

Neil D. Theise
Beth Israel Medical Center
Icahn School of Medicine at Mount
Sinai
New York, NY, USA
NTheise@chpnet.org

David B. Thomas
Fred Hutchinson Cancer Research
Center
Seattle, WA, USA
dbthomas@fhcrc.org

Lester D.R. Thompson
Woodland Hills Medical Center
Woodland Hills, CA, USA
Lester.D.Thompson@kp.org

Michael J. Thun
American Cancer Society
Atlanta, GA, USA
Michael.Thun@cancer.org

Mark R. Thursz
Imperial College London
London, United Kingdom
m.thursz@imperial.ac.uk

Massimo Tommasino
International Agency for Research
on Cancer
Lyon, France
tommasino@iarc.fr

William D. Travis
Memorial Sloan-Kettering Cancer
Center
New York, NY, USA
travisw@mskcc.org

Edward L. Trimble
NCI Center for Global Health
National Cancer Institute
Rockville, MD, USA
trimblet@ctep.nci.nih.gov

Giorgio Trinchieri
National Cancer Institute
Bethesda, MD, USA
trinchig@mail.nih.gov

Ugyen Tshomo
Jigme Dorji Wangchuck National
Referral Hospital
Thimphu, Bhutan
ugentshomo2000@yahoo.com

Murat Tuncer
Hacettepe University
Ankara, Turkey
mt@hacettepe.edu.tr

Andreas Ullrich
World Health Organization
Geneva, Switzerland
ullricha@who.int

Toshikazu Ushijima
National Cancer Center Research
Institute
Tokyo, Japan
tushijim@ncc.go.jp

Carlos Vallejos
Latin American and Caribbean
Society of Medical Oncology
(SLACOM)
Buenos Aires, Argentina
and
Oncosalud-AUNA
Lima, Perú
cvallejos@oncosalud.pe

Piet van den Brandt
Maastricht University
Maastricht, Netherlands
pa.vandenbrandt@maastricht
university.nl

James W. Vardiman
University of Chicago Medical
Center
Chicago, IL, USA
james.vardiman@uchospitals.edu

Jim Vaught
National Cancer Institute
Bethesda, MD, USA
vaughtj@mail.nih.gov

Cesar G. Victora
Universidade Federal de Pelotas
Rio Grande do Sul, Brazil
cvictora@gmail.com

Paolo Vineis
Imperial College London
London, United Kingdom
p.vineis@imperial.ac.uk

Lawrence von Karsa
International Agency for Research
on Cancer
Lyon, France
karsal@iarc.fr

Melanie Wakefield
Cancer Council Victoria
Carlton, Australia
Melanie.Wakefield@cancervic.org.au

Guiqi Wang
Cancer Hospital/Institute
Chinese Academy of Medical
Sciences
Peking Union Medical College
Beijing, China
wangguiq@126.com

Frank Weber
Medical Faculty
University of Duisburg-Essen
Essen, Germany
frank.weber@uk-essen.de

Elisabete Weiderpass
Cancer Registry of Norway
Oslo, Norway
and
Arctic University of Norway,
University of Tromsø
Tromsø, Norway
and
Karolinska Institute
Stockholm, Sweden
elisabete.weiderpass@ki.se

Zena Werb
University of California
San Francisco, CA, USA
zena.werb@ucsf.edu

Theresa L. Whiteside
University of Pittsburgh Cancer
Institute
Pittsburgh, PA, USA
whitesidetl@upmc.edu

Christopher P. Wild
International Agency for Research
on Cancer
Lyon, France
director@iarc.fr

Walter C. Willett
Harvard School of Public Health
Boston, MA, USA
wwillett@hsph.harvard.edu

Dillwyn Williams
Strangeways Research
Laboratories
Cambridge, United Kingdom
edw1001@medschl.cam.ac.uk

Rena R. Wing
Brown University
Providence, RI, USA
Rena_Wing_PhD@Brown.EDU

Deborah M. Winn
National Cancer Institute
Bethesda, MD, USA
winnde@mail.nih.gov

Martin Wiseman
World Cancer Research Fund
International
London, United Kingdom
m.wiseman@wcrf.org

Scott Wittet
MalariaCare and Cervical Cancer
Prevention Programs, PATH
Seattle, WA, USA
swittet@path.org

Magdalena B. Wozniak
International Agency for Research
on Cancer
Lyon, France
wozniakm@fellows.iarc.fr

Hai Yan
Duke University Medical Center
Durham, NC, USA
hai.yan@duke.edu

Teruhiko Yoshida
National Cancer Center Research
Institute
Tokyo, Japan
tyoshida@ncc.go.jp

Jiri Zavadil
International Agency for Research
on Cancer
Lyon, France
zavadilj@iarc.fr

Harald zur Hausen
German Cancer Research Center
Heidelberg, Germany
zurhausen@dkfz.de

Disclosures of interests

Héctor Arreola-Ornelas reports that his unit at the Mexican Health Foundation benefited from research funding from GlaxoSmithKline, Sanofi S.A., and from Avon Mexico.

Yung-Jue Bang reports that his unit at the Seoul National University College of Medicine benefited from research funding from AstraZeneca, GlaxoSmithKline, Merck, Novartis, Pfizer, Roche, Sanofi-Aventis, Bayer, Bristol-Myers Squibb, Boehringer Ingelheim, Lilly, Otsuka, Hanmi, Green Cross, and from Merrimack; Dr Bang reports receiving personal consultancy fees from AstraZeneca, GlaxoSmithKline, Merck, Novartis, Pfizer, Roche, Sanofi-Aventis, Bayer, Bristol-Myers Squibb, Boehringer Ingelheim, Lilly, Otsuka, Taiho, Macrogenics, Hanmi, and from Green Cross; Dr Bang reports benefiting from support for travel and accommodation from AstraZeneca, GlaxoSmithKline, Merck, Novartis, Pfizer, Roche, Boehringer Ingelheim, and from Lilly; Dr Bang reports receiving personal speaker's fees from GlaxoSmithKline, Pfizer, and from Roche.

Elizabeth H. Blackburn reports owning shares in Telomere Health Inc.

Fred T. Bosman reports benefiting from research funding from Pfizer.

Michael P. Brown reports benefiting from research funding from Novartis; Dr Brown reports receiving personal consultancy fees from Amgen, Bayer, Pfizer, Novartis, GlaxoSmithKline, Bristol-Myers Squibb, and from Roche; Dr Brown reports receiving personal speaker's fees from Bristol-Myers Squibb and from Lilly.

Agnès Buzyn reports receiving personal consultancy fees from Novartis, Bristol-Myers Squibb, and from Amgen; Dr Buzyn reports receiving personal speaker's fees from Novartis, Bristol-Myers Squibb, and from Amgen.

Eduardo L. Cazap reports that his unit at the Latin American and Caribbean Society of Medical Oncology (SLACOM) benefited from research funding from Poniard Pharmaceuticals and from Daiichi Sankyo Pharma; Dr Cazap reports receiving personal consultancy fees from Bayer and from Schering Pharma; Dr Cazap reports receiving personal speaker's fees from Bayer, Bristol-Myers Squibb, and from Fresenius.

Lynette Denny reports benefiting from research funding from MSD and from GlaxoSmithKline; Dr Denny reports receiving personal speaker's fees from MSD and from GlaxoSmithKline.

Joakim Dillner reports that his unit at the Karolinska Institute benefited from research funding from Sanofi Pasteur, MSD and from Merck.

Susan M. Domcheck reports that her unit at the University of Pennsylvania benefited from research funding from Astra Zeneca and from AbbVie.

Adèle C. Green reports that her unit at the Queensland Institute of Medical Research benefited from research funding from L'Oréal Recherche; Dr Green reports benefiting from support for travel and accommodation from L'Oréal Recherche.

James F. Holland reports holding intellectual property rights in two patents owned by his employer, the Icahn School of Medicine at Mount Sinai, on the structure of human mammary tumour virus, and means to detect it.

Ralph H. Hruban reports holding intellectual property rights in a patent owned by Myriad Genetics on PALB2-based diagnostic methods for pancreatic cancer.

Felicia Marie Knaul reports that her unit at the Harvard School of Public Health benefited from research funding from Sanofi S.A., Goldman Sachs Gives, and that her unit at the Mexico Health Foundation benefited from research funding from Sanofi S.A., Avon Mexico, and from GlaxoSmithKline; Dr Knaul reports receiving personal consultancy fees from the Institute for Applied Economics, Global Health and the Study of Business Enterprises, Johns Hopkins University.

Oscar Méndez reports that his unit at the Mexican Health Foundation benefited from research funding from GlaxoSmithKline, Sanofi S.A., and from Avon Mexico.

Fabio Savarese reports being currently employed by Boehringer Ingelheim.

Mark Schiffman reports that his unit at the United States National Cancer Institute benefited from non-financial research support from Qiagen, Roche, and from GlaxoSmithKline.

Kevin Shield reports that his unit at the Centre for Addiction and Mental Health, Toronto, benefited from research funding from Lundbeck A.S.; Dr Shield reports receiving personal consultancy fees from Lundbeck A.S.; Dr Shield reports benefiting from support for travel and accommodation from Lundbeck A.S.

Avrum Spira reports being a founder of and owning shares in Allegro Diagnostics Inc.; Dr Spira reports receiving personal consultancy fees from Allegro Diagnostics Inc.

Mark R. Thursz reports receiving personal consultancy fees from Gilead, Bristol-Myers Squibb, and from Janssen Pharmaceuticals; Dr Thursz reports receiving personal speaker's fees from Gilead, Bristol-Myers Squibb, and from Janssen Pharmaceuticals.

Hai Yan reports benefiting from research funding from Gilead; Dr Yan reports receiving personal consultancy fees from Sanofi; Dr Yan reports holding intellectual property rights in patents owned by Agios Pharmaceuticals, by Eli Lilly, and by Sanofi-Aventis.

Frank J. Chaloupka, **Hans Clevers**, **Fidele Ngabo**, and **Elio Riboli** did not submit a Declaration of Interest.

Sources

Boxes

2.3.1 All relative risk functions obtained from Corrao G, Bagnardi V, Zambon A, La Vecchia C (2004). A meta-analysis of alcohol consumption and the risk of 15 diseases. *Prev Med*, 38:613–619. http://dx.doi.org/10.1016/j.ypmed.2003.11.027 PMID:15066364

P7.1 Compiled from Doll R, Peto R, Boreham J, Sutherland I (2004). Mortality in relation to smoking: 50 years' observations on male British doctors. *BMJ*, 328:1519–1527. http://dx.doi.org/10.1136/bmj.38142.554479.AE PMID:15213107; Pirie K, Peto R, Reeves GK *et al.*; Million Women Study Collaborators (2013). The 21st century hazards of smoking and benefits of stopping: a prospective study of one million women in the UK. *Lancet*, 381:133–141. http://dx.doi.org/10.1016/S0140-6736(12)61720-6 PMID:23107252; Jha P, Ramasundarahettige C, Landsman V *et al.* (2013). 21st-century hazards of smoking and benefits of cessation in the United States. *N Engl J Med*, 368:341–350. http://dx.doi.org/10.1056/NEJMsa1211128 PMID:23343063; Thun MJ, Carter BD, Feskanich D *et al.* (2013). 50-year trends in smoking-related mortality in the United States. *N Engl J Med*, 368:351–364. http://dx.doi.org/10.1056/NEJMsa1211127 PMID:23343064; Sakata R, McGale P, Grant EJ *et al.* (2012). Impact of smoking on mortality and life expectancy in Japanese smokers: a prospective cohort study. *BMJ*, 345:e7093. http://dx.doi.org/10.1136/bmj.e7093 PMID:23100333

Charts

5.1.1 GLOBOCAN 2012[a]

5.1.2 & 5.1.3 *Cancer Incidence in Five Continents*, Vol. X[b]

5.2.1 GLOBOCAN 2012[a]

5.2.2 & 5.2.3 *Cancer Incidence in Five Continents*, Vol. X[b]

5.3.1 GLOBOCAN 2012[a]

5.3.2 & 5.3.3 *Cancer Incidence in Five Continents*, Vol. X[b]

5.4.1 GLOBOCAN 2012[a]

5.4.2 & 5.4.3 *Cancer Incidence in Five Continents*, Vol. X[b]

5.5.1 GLOBOCAN 2012[a]

5.5.2 & 5.5.3 *Cancer Incidence in Five Continents*, Vol. X[b]

5.6.1 GLOBOCAN 2012[a]

5.6.2 & 5.6.3 *Cancer Incidence in Five Continents*, Vol. X[b]

5.7.1 GLOBOCAN 2012[a]

5.7.2 & 5.7.3 *Cancer Incidence in Five Continents*, Vol. X[b]

5.8.1 & 5.8.2 GLOBOCAN 2012[a]

5.8.3 & 5.8.4 *Cancer Incidence in Five Continents*, Vol. X[b]

5.9.1 GLOBOCAN 2012[a]

5.9.2 & 5.9.3 *Cancer Incidence in Five Continents*, Vol. X[b]

5.10.1 GLOBOCAN 2012[a]

5.10.2 & 5.10.3 *Cancer Incidence in Five Continents*, Vol. X[b]

5.11.1 GLOBOCAN 2012[a]

5.11.2 & 5.11.3 *Cancer Incidence in Five Continents*, Vol. X[b]

5.11.4 GLOBOCAN 2012[a]

5.11.5 & 5.11.6 *Cancer Incidence in Five Continents*, Vol. X[b]

5.12.1–5.12.3 GLOBOCAN 2012[a]

5.12.4–5.12.6 *Cancer Incidence in Five Continents*, Vol. X[b]

5.13.1 GLOBOCAN 2012[a]

5.13.2 & 5.13.3 *Cancer Incidence in Five Continents*, Vol. X[b]

5.13.4 GLOBOCAN 2012[a]

5.13.5 & 5.13.6 *Cancer Incidence in Five Continents*, Vol. X[b]

5.14.1 GLOBOCAN 2012[a]

5.14.2 & 5.14.3 *Cancer Incidence in Five Continents*, Vol. X[b]

5.15.1 GLOBOCAN 2012[a]

5.15.2 & 5.15.3 *Cancer Incidence in Five Continents*, Vol. X[b]

5.16.1 & 5.16.2 *Cancer Incidence in Five Continents*, Vol. X[b]

[a] Ferlay J, Soerjomataram I, Ervik M *et al.* (2013). GLOBOCAN 2012 v1.0, Cancer Incidence and Mortality Worldwide: IARC Cancer Base No. 11 [Internet]. Lyon: IARC. Available at http://globocan.iarc.fr.

[b] Forman D, Bray F, Brewster DH *et al.*, eds (2013). *Cancer Incidence in Five Continents*, Vol. X [electronic version]. Lyon: IARC. Available at http://ci5.iarc.fr.

Figures

1.1.1 © 2005 Pierre Thiriet, Courtesy of Photoshare.

1.1.2 Courtesy of Rosss via Wikipedia. License: CC BY-SA 2.05.

1.1.3 Courtesy of Carolina Antunes, www.Morguefile.com.

1.1.4 & 1.1.5 GLOBOCAN 2012[a]

1.1.6 *Cancer Incidence in Five Continents*, Vol. X[b]

1.1.7 GLOBOCAN 2012[a]

1.1.8 *Cancer Incidence in Five Continents*, Vol. X[b]

1.1.9–1.1.13 GLOBOCAN 2012[a]

1.1.14 *Cancer Incidence in Five Continents*, Vol. X[b]

1.1.15–1.1.17 GLOBOCAN 2012[a]

1.1.18 *Cancer Incidence in Five Continents*, Vol. X[b]

1.1.19–1.1.21 GLOBOCAN 2012[a]

1.1.22 *Cancer Incidence in Five Continents*, Vol. X[b]

1.1.23–1.1.25 GLOBOCAN 2012[a]

1.1.26 *Cancer Incidence in Five Continents*, Vol. X[b]

1.1.27–1.1.29 GLOBOCAN 2012[a]

1.1.30 *Cancer Incidence in Five Continents*, Vol. X[b]

1.1.31–1.1.33 GLOBOCAN 2012[a]

1.1.34 *Cancer Incidence in Five Continents*, Vol. X[b]

1.1.35–1.1.37 GLOBOCAN 2012[a]

1.1.38 *Cancer Incidence in Five Continents*, Vol. X[b]

1.1.39 GLOBOCAN 2012[a]

1.1.40–1.1.47 *Cancer Incidence in Five Continents*, Vol. X[b]

1.2.1 © 2006 Vinoth Vijayaraghavan, Courtesy of Photoshare.

1.2.2 Data compiled from the Global Health Observatory Data Repository.

1.2.3 & 1.2.4 Data compiled from the United Nations Development Programme.

1.2.5–1.2.8 GLOBOCAN 2012[a]

1.2.9 & 1.2.10 Data compiled from GLOBOCAN 2012[a] and the United Nations Development Programme.

1.2.11 GLOBOCAN 2012[a]

1.2.12 © 1986 Andrea Fisch, Courtesy of Photoshare.

1.2.13 © 2012 Kyalie Photography, Courtesy of Photoshare.

1.2.14 Freddie Bray.

1.2.15 Data compiled from the Global Health Observatory Data Repository.

1.3.1 GLOBOCAN 2012[a]

1.3.2 Compiled from Moreno F, Loria D, Abriata G, Terracini B; ROHA network (2013). Childhood cancer: incidence and early deaths in Argentina, 2000–2008. *Eur J Cancer*, 49:465–473. http://dx.doi.org/10.1016/j.ejca.2012.08.001 PMID:22980725; Moradi A, Semnani S, Roshandel G *et al.* (2010). Incidence of childhood cancers in Golestan province of Iran. *Iran J Pediatr*, 20:335–342. PMID:23056726; Howlader N, Noone AM, Krapcho M *et al.*, eds (2013). SEER Cancer Statistics Review, 1975–2010. Bethesda, MD: National Cancer Institute. Available at http://www.seer.cancer.gov/csr/1975_2010/browse_csr.php?section=29&page=sect_29_table.02.html; Lacour B, Guyot-Goubin A, Guissou S *et al.* (2010). Incidence of childhood cancer in France: National Children Cancer Registries, 2000–2004. *Eur J Cancer Prev*, 19:173–181. http://dx.doi.org/10.1097/CEJ.0b013e32833876c0 PMID:20361423; Kaatsch P, Spix C (2012). *German Childhood Cancer Registry Annual Report 2011 (1980–2010)*. Mainz: Institute of Medical Biostatistics, Epidemiology and Informatics at the University Medical Center of the Johannes Gutenberg University. Available at http://www.kinderkrebsregister.de/extern/veroeffentlichungen/jahresberichte/aktueller-jahresbericht/index.html?L=1; Wiangnon S, Veerakul G, Nuchprayoon I *et al.* (2011). Childhood cancer incidence and survival 2003–2005, Thailand: study from the Thai Pediatric Oncology Group. *Asian Pac J Cancer Prev*, 12:2215–2220. PMID:22296359; Fajardo-Gutiérrez A, Juárez-Ocaña S, González-Miranda G *et al.* (2007). Incidence of cancer in children residing in ten jurisdictions of the Mexican Republic: importance of the Cancer registry (a population-based study). *BMC Cancer*, 7:68. PMID:17445267; Swaminathan R, Rama R, Shanta V (2008). Childhood cancers in Chennai, India, 1990–2001: incidence and survival. *Int J Cancer*, 122:2607–2611. http://dx.doi.org/10.1002/ijc.23428 PMID:18324630; Baade PD, Youlden DR, Valery PC *et al.* (2010). Trends in incidence of childhood cancer in Australia, 1983–2006. *Br J Cancer*, 102:620–626. http://dx.doi.org/10.1038/sj.bjc.6605503 PMID:20051948; Parkin DM, Ferlay J, Hamdi-Chérif M *et al.* (2003). *Cancer in Africa: Epidemiology and Prevention*. Chapter 5: Childhood cancer. Lyon: IARC (IARC Scientific Publications Series, No. 153), pp. 381–396; Bao PP, Zheng Y, Wang CF *et al.* (2009). Time trends and characteristics of childhood cancer among children age 0–14 in Shanghai. *Pediatr Blood Cancer*, 53:13–16. http://dx.doi.org/10.1002/pbc.21939 PMID:19260104.

1.3.3 & 1.3.4 From Steliarova-Foucher E, O'Callaghan M, Ferlay J *et al.* (2012). European Cancer Observatory: Cancer Incidence, Mortality, Prevalence and Survival in Europe, version 1.0. European Network of Cancer Registries, IARC. Available at http://eco.iarc.fr.

1.3.5 Adapted by permission of Oxford University Press. Stiller CA, Kroll ME, Eatock EM (2007). Survival from childhood cancer. In: Stiller CA, ed. *Childhood Cancer in Britain: Incidence, Survival, Mortality*. Oxford: Oxford University Press, pp. 131–204.

1.3.6 Compiled from GLOBOCAN 2012[a] and *Cancer Incidence in Five Continents*, Vol. X[b]

1.3.7 WHO Mortality Database. Available at http://www.who.int/healthinfo/mortality_data/en/ and http://www-dep.iarc.fr; and adapted from Pritchard-Jones K, Pieters R, Reaman GH *et al.* (2013). Sustaining innovation and improvement in the treatment of childhood cancer: lessons from high-income countries. *Lancet Oncol*, 14:e95–e103. http://dx.doi.org/10.1016/S1470-2045(13)70010-X PMID:23434338, with permission from Elsevier.

1.3.8 Courtesy of Hospital 57357 - Children's Cancer Hospital, Egypt.

1.3.9 Courtesy of the Uganda Child Cancer Foundation.

2.1.1 © 2001 Germain Passamang Tabati, Courtesy of Photoshare.

2.1.2 Reproduced from Thun M, Peto R, Boreham J, Lopez AD (2012). Stages of the cigarette epidemic on entering its second century. *Tob Control*, 21:96–101. http://dx.doi.org/10.1136/tobaccocontrol-2011-050294 PMID:22345230, with permission from BMJ Publishing Group Ltd.

[a] Ferlay J, Soerjomataram I, Ervik M *et al.* (2013). GLOBOCAN 2012 v1.0, Cancer Incidence and Mortality Worldwide: IARC Cancer Base No. 11 [Internet]. Lyon: IARC. Available at http://globocan.iarc.fr.

[b] Forman D, Bray F, Brewster DH *et al.*, eds (2013). *Cancer Incidence in Five Continents*, Vol. X [electronic version]. Lyon: IARC. Available at http://ci5.iarc.fr.

2.1.3 Stephenie Hollyman/WHO.

2.1.4 Courtesy of Wikipedia user Morio. License: CC BY-SA 3.0.

2.1.5 © Massimo Mazzotta. All rights reserved.

2.1.6A Adapted from Jha P (2009). Avoidable global cancer deaths and total deaths from smoking. *Nat Rev Cancer*, 9:655–664. http://dx.doi.org/10.1038/nrc2703 PMID:19693096, by permission from Macmillan Publishers Ltd. © 2009; and adapted from Guérin S, Hill C (2010). Cancer epidemiology in France in 2010: comparison with the USA [in French]. *Bull Cancer*, 97:47–54. http://dx.doi.org/10.1684/bdc.2010.1013 PMID:19995688.

2.1.6B Compiled from ERC (2010). *World Cigarette Reports 2010*. Suffolk, UK: ERC Group; Economist Intelligence Unit (2011). Worldwide Cost of Living Survey. London: The Economist Group; Economist Intelligence Unit (2011). Marlboro cigarette and local cigarette prices, Worldwide Cost of Living Survey. London: The Economist Group; International Monetary Fund (2011). World Economic Outlook Database, April 2011 edition. Available at http://www.imf.org/external/pubs/ft/weo/2011/01/weodata/index.aspx.

2.1.6C Compiled from Blecher EH (2011). *The Economics of Tobacco Control in Low- and Middle-Income Countries* [thesis]. Cape Town, South Africa: School of Economics, University of Cape Town.

2.2.1 Data from Giovino GA, Mirza SA, Samet JM *et al.*; GATS Collaborative Group (2012). Tobacco use in 3 billion individuals from 16 countries: an analysis of nationally representative cross-sectional household survey. *Lancet*, 380:668–679. http://dx.doi.org/10.1016/S0140-6736(12)61085-X PMID:22901888

2.2.2 Data from Eriksen M, Mackay J, Ross H (2012). *The Tobacco Atlas*, 4th ed. Atlanta, GA: American Cancer Society, World Lung Foundation, http://www.tobaccoatlas.org/.

2.2.3 Reprinted from U.S. Department of Health and Human Services (2004). *The Health Consequences of Smoking: A Report of the Surgeon General*. Atlanta, GA: U.S. Department of Health and Human Services, Centers for Disease Control and Prevention, National Center for Chronic Disease Prevention and Health Promotion, Office on Smoking and Health.

2.2.4 © iStockphoto; U.S. Department of Health and Human Services (2004). *The Health Consequences of Smoking: A Report of the Surgeon General*. Atlanta, GA: U.S. Department of Health and Human Services, Centers for Disease Control and Prevention, National Center for Chronic Disease Prevention and Health Promotion, Office on Smoking and Health; and IARC (2012). Personal habits and indoor combustions. *IARC Monogr Eval Carcinog Risks Hum*, 100E:1–575. PMID:23193840

2.2.5 Courtesy of the Library of Congress Prints and Photographs Division, Washington, DC.

2.2.6 Courtesy of Rue & Sue, accessed at www.wedheads.com.

B2.2.1 Adapted from Timofeeva MN, Hung RJ, Rafnar T *et al.*; Transdisciplinary Research in Cancer of the Lung (TRICL) Research Team (2012). Influence of common genetic variation on lung cancer risk: meta-analysis of 14 900 cases and 29 485 controls. *Hum Mol Genet*, 21:4980–4995. http://dx.doi.org/10.1093/hmg/dds334 PMID:22899653, by permission of Oxford University Press.

2.3.1 & 2.3.2 Data from Lim SS, Vos T, Flaxman AD *et al.* (2012). A comparative risk assessment of burden of disease and injury attributable to 67 risk factors and risk factor clusters in 21 regions, 1990–2010: a systematic analysis for the Global Burden of Disease Study 2010. *Lancet*, 380:2224–2260. http://dx.doi.org/10.1016/S0140-6736(12)61766-8 PMID:23245609, © 2012 The Lancet.

2.3.3 © iStockphoto/Webphotographeer.

2.4.1 Reprinted from de Martel C, Ferlay J, Franceschi S *et al.* (2012). Global burden of cancers attributable to infections in 2008: a review and synthetic analysis. *Lancet Oncol*, 13:607–615. http://dx.doi.org/10.1016/S1470-2045(12)70137-7 PMID:22575588, © 2012, with permission from Elsevier.

2.4.2 Courtesy of Flickr user A.J. Cann. License: CC BY-SA 2.0.

2.4.3 Reprinted from Woodman CB, Collins SI, Young LS (2007). The natural history of cervical HPV infection: unresolved issues. *Nat Rev Cancer*, 7:11–22. PMID:17186016, by permission from Macmillan Publishers Ltd. © 2007.

2.4.4 Courtesy of Ed Uthman, MD, American Board of Pathology, accessed at commons.wikimedia.org.

2.4.5 Courtesy of C. Goldsmith, accessed at http://phil.cdc.gov/.

2.4.6 © 2002 Amira Roess, Courtesy of Photoshare.

2.5.1 Reprinted from Collaborative Group on Hormonal Factors in Breast Cancer (2012). Menarche, menopause, and breast cancer risk: individual participant meta-analysis, including 118 964 women with breast cancer from 117 epidemiological studies. *Lancet Oncol*, 13:1141–1151. http://dx.doi.org/10.1016/S1470-2045(12)70425-4 PMID:23084519, © 2012, with permission from Elsevier.

2.5.2 Reprinted from Yang XR, Figueroa JD, Falk RT *et al.* (2012). Analysis of terminal duct lobular unit involution in luminal A and basal breast cancers. *Breast Cancer Res*, 14:R64. http://dx.doi.org/10.1186/bcr3170 PMID:22513288

2.5.3 Reprinted by permission from the American Association for Cancer Research: James RE, Lukanova A, Dossus L *et al.* (2011). Postmenopausal serum sex steroids and risk of hormone receptor-positive and -negative breast cancer: a nested case-control study. *Cancer Prev Res (Phila)*, 4:1626–1635. http://dx.doi.org/10.1158/1940-6207.CAPR-11-0090 PMID:21813404.

2.5.4 Reproduced from Fuhrman BJ, Schairer C, Gail MH *et al.* (2012). Estrogen metabolism and risk of breast cancer in postmenopausal women. *J Natl Cancer Inst*, 104:326–339. http://dx.doi.org/10.1093/jnci/djr531 PMID:22232133

2.5.5 Reproduced from Trabert B, Wentzensen N, Yang HP *et al.* (2013). Is estrogen plus progestin menopausal hormone therapy safe with respect to endometrial cancer risk? *Int J Cancer*, 132:417–426. http://dx.doi.org/10.1002/ijc.27623 PMID:22553145.

2.5.6 Reprinted from Chung SH, Franceschi S, Lambert PF (2010). Estrogen and ERalpha: culprits in cervical cancer? *Trends Endocrinol Metab*, 21:504–511. http://dx.doi.org/10.1016/j.tem.2010.03.005 PMID:20456973, © 2010, with permission from Elsevier.

2.5.7 Compiled from Brinton LA, Richesson DA, Gierach GL *et al.* (2008). Prospective evaluation of risk factors for male breast cancer. *J Natl Cancer Inst*, 100:1477–1481. http://dx.doi.org/10.1093/jnci/djn329 PMID:18840816.

2.5.8 Reproduced from Roddam AW, Allen NE, Appleby P, Key TJ; Endogenous Hormones and Prostate Cancer Collaborative Group (2008). Endogenous sex hormones and prostate cancer: a collaborative analysis of 18 prospective studies. *J Natl Cancer Inst*, 100:170–183. http://dx.doi.org/10.1093/jnci/djm323 PMID:18230794.

2.5.9 © 2011 Joydeep Mukherjee, Courtesy of Photoshare.

2.6.1 © iStockphoto/Fertnig.

2.6.2 © 2012 Thomas Mukoya/REUTERS, Courtesy of Photoshare.

2.6.3 Compiled from Berrington de Gonzalez A, Hartge P, Cerhan JR *et al.* (2010). Body-mass index and mortality among 1.46 million white adults. *N Engl J Med*, 363:2211–2219. http://dx.doi.org/10.1056/NEJMoa1000367 PMID:21121834

---

[a] Ferlay J, Soerjomataram I, Ervik M *et al.* (2013). GLOBOCAN 2012 v1.0, Cancer Incidence and Mortality Worldwide: IARC Cancer Base No. 11 [Internet]. Lyon: IARC. Available at http://globocan.iarc.fr.

[b] Forman D, Bray F, Brewster DH *et al.*, eds (2013). *Cancer Incidence in Five Continents*, Vol. X [electronic version]. Lyon: IARC. Available at http://ci5.iarc.fr.

2.6.4 Compiled from Reeves GK, Pirie K, Beral V *et al.* (2007). Cancer incidence and mortality in relation to body mass index in the Million Women Study: cohort study. *BMJ*, 335:1134 PMID:17986716; and Renehan AG, Tyson M, Egger M *et al.* (2008). Body-mass index and incidence of cancer: a systematic review and meta-analysis of prospective observational studies. *Lancet*, 371:569–578. http://dx.doi.org/10.1016/S0140-6736(08)60269-X PMID:18280327

2.6.5 © 2006 Nengah Kartika, Courtesy of Photoshare.

B2.6.1 Reprinted from Illner AK, Freisling H, Boeing H *et al.* (2012). Review and evaluation of innovative technologies for measuring diet in nutritional epidemiology. *Int J Epidemiol*, 41:1187–1203. http://dx.doi.org/10.1093/ije/dys105 PMID:22933652, by permission of Oxford University Press.

B2.6.2 Reprinted from Gilsing AM, Berndt SI, Ruder EH *et al.* (2012). Meat-related mutagen exposure, xenobiotic metabolizing gene polymorphisms and the risk of advanced colorectal adenoma and cancer. *Carcinogenesis*, 33:1332–1339. http://dx.doi.org/10.1093/carcin/bgs158 PMID:22552404, by permission of Oxford University Press.

2.7.1 © 2006 Adam Scotti, Courtesy of Photoshare.

2.7.2 © 2009 sandipan majumdar, Courtesy of Photoshare.

2.7.3 Courtesy of Álvaro Daniel Gonzalez Lamarque, www.Morguefile.com.

2.7.4 © 2012 Farid Ahmed, Courtesy of Photoshare.

2.7.5 IARC photo library.

2.7.6 Courtesy of Oregon Department of Transportation. License: CC BY 2.0.

2.8.1 Reproduced from European Commission, Research Directorate-General, European Communities (2005). *Health and Electromagnetic Fields: EU-funded research into the impact of electromagnetic fields and mobile telephones on health.*

2.8.2 Reprinted from UN Scientific Committee on the Effects of Atomic Radiation (UNSCEAR) (2010). Annex A: Medical radiation exposures. In: *Sources and Effects of Ionizing Radiation, UNSCEAR 2008 Report to the General Assembly with Scientific Annexes*, Vol. I. New York: UN. Available at http://www.unscear.org/docs/reports/2008/09-86753_Report_2008_Annex_A.pdf

2.8.3 Courtesy of Clare McLean/University of Washington Medicine.

2.8.4 Courtesy of Kræftens Bekæmpelse (The Danish Cancer Society) and TrygFonden – a Danish Foundation. © 2013. All rights reserved.

2.8.5 Reprinted from Schüz J, Exposure to extremely low-frequency magnetic fields and the risk of childhood cancer: update of the epidemiological evidence. *Prog Biophys Mol Biol*, 107:339–342. http://dx.doi.org/10.1016/j.pbiomolbio.2011.09.008 PMID:21946043, © 2011, with permission from Elsevier.

2.8.6 Courtesy of Florentina Kindler.

2.9.1 © 2012 Jerome Salem 05, Courtesy of Photoshare.

2.9.2 Reprinted with permission from Brauer M, Amann M, Burnett RT *et al.* (2012). Exposure assessment for estimation of the global burden of disease attributable to outdoor air pollution. *Environ Sci Technol*, 46:652–660. http://dx.doi.org/10.1021/es2025752 PMID:22148428. © 2012 American Chemical Society.

2.9.3 © Ludolf Dahmen/Greenpeace.

2.9.4 Data source: WHO/Public Health Information and Geographic Information Systems. © WHO 2012. All rights reserved.

2.9.5 © 2006 Rakesh Yogal Shrestha, Courtesy of Photoshare.

2.9.6 U.S. Military, Department of Defense.

B2.9.1 Courtesy of Flickr user Katerha. License: CC BY 2.0.

B2.9.2 Courtesy of Charles O'Rear, U.S. Department of Agriculture.

2.10.1 © iStockphoto/Luca Zola.

2.10.2 © 2004 David Alexander, Courtesy of Photoshare.

2.10.3 Courtesy of Rhoda Baer, U.S. National Cancer Institute, accessed at http://visualsonline.cancer.gov.

2.10.4 Courtesy of Wikipedia user Sauligno. License: CC-BY-SA-3.0

2.10.5 Courtesy of Wikipedia user Mr Hyde, via Wikimedia Commons.

2.11.1 Adapted with permission from Tracy E. Anderson, via www.Flickr.com. All rights reserved. © 2009.

2.11.2 © 1991 Bill Horn, Courtesy of Photoshare.

2.11.3 Reproduced from Pitt JI, Hocking AD (2009). *Fungi and Food Spoilage*, 3rd ed., Fig. 8.13, p. 305; with kind permission from Springer Science+Business Media B.V.

2.11.4 Reproduced from Qian X-Z (1996). *Colour Pictorial Handbook of Chinese Herbs*, by permission from the People's Medical Publishing House.

3.1.1 Thomas J. Hudson.

3.1.2 Reprinted from Zhang J, Baran J, Cros A *et al.* (2011). International Cancer Genome Consortium Data Portal – a one-stop shop for cancer genomics data. *Database* (Oxford), 2011:bar026. http://dx.doi.org/10.1093/database/bar026 PMID:21930502, by permission of Oxford University Press. © 2011.

3.1.3 & 3.1.4 Thomas J. Hudson.

3.1.5 Reprinted from Stratton MR, Campbell PJ, Futreal PA (2009). The cancer genome. *Nature*, 458:719–724. http://dx.doi.org/10.1038/nature07943 PMID:19360079, by permission from Macmillan Publishers Ltd. © 2009.

3.1.6 Joint Genome Institute, U.S. Department of Energy Genomic Science Program, accessed at http://genomicscience.energy.gov/.

B3.1.1 Magali Olivier.

3.2.1 Reprinted from Manolio TA, Collins FS, Cox NJ *et al.* (2009). Finding the missing heritability of complex diseases. *Nature*, 461:747–753. http://dx.doi.org/10.1038/nature08494 PMID:19812666, by permission from Macmillan Publishers Ltd. © 2009; and adapted from McCarthy MI, Abecasis GR, Cardon LR *et al.* (2008). Genome-wide association studies for complex traits: consensus, uncertainty and challenges. *Nat Rev Genet*, 9:356–369. http://dx.doi.org/10.1038/nrg2344 PMID:18398418, by permission from Macmillan Publishers Ltd. © 2008.

3.2.2 Reprinted from Garcia-Closas M, Chanock S (2008). Genetic susceptibility loci for breast cancer by estrogen receptor status. *Clin Cancer Res*, 14:8000–8009. http://dx.doi.org/10.1158/1078-0432.CCR-08-0975 PMID:19088016, by permission from the American Association for Cancer Research.

3.2.3 Stephen J. Chanock.

B3.2.1 Adapted from Hoeijmakers JH (2001). Genome maintenance mechanisms for preventing cancer. *Nature*, 411:366–374. PMID:11357144, by permission from Macmillan Publishers Ltd. © 2001.

3.3.1 Magdalena B. Wozniak and Paul Brennan.

3.3.2 Reprinted from Trollope AF, Gutiérrez-Mecinas M, Mifsud KR *et al.* (2012). Stress, epigenetic control of gene expression and memory formation. *Exp Neurol*, 233:3–11. http://dx.doi.org/10.1016/j.expneurol.2011.03.022 PMID:21466804, © 2012, with permission from Elsevier.

3.3.3A Reprinted from Bastien RR, Rodríguez-Lescure Á, Ebbert MT *et al.* (2012). PAM50 breast cancer subtyping by RT-qPCR and concordance with standard clinical molecular markers. *BMC Med Genomics*, 5:44. http://dx.doi.org/10.1186/1755-8794-5-44 PMID:23035882, © 2012 Bastien *et al.*; licensee BioMed Central Ltd.

a Ferlay J, Soerjomataram I, Ervik M *et al.* (2013). GLOBOCAN 2012 v1.0, Cancer Incidence and Mortality Worldwide: IARC Cancer Base No. 11 [Internet]. Lyon: IARC. Available at http://globocan.iarc.fr.

b Forman D, Bray F, Brewster DH *et al.*, eds (2013). *Cancer Incidence in Five Continents*, Vol. X [electronic version]. Lyon: IARC. Available at http://ci5.iarc.fr.

3.3.3B Reprinted from van 't Veer LJ, Dai H, van de Vijver MJ *et al.* (2002). Gene expression profiling predicts clinical outcome of breast cancer. *Nature*, 415:530–536. http://dx.doi.org/10.1038/415530a PMID:11823860, by permission from Macmillan Publishers Ltd. © 2002.

3.3.4 Reprinted from Esquela-Kerscher A, Slack FJ (2006). Oncomirs – microRNAs with a role in cancer. *Nat Rev Cancer*, 6:259–269. http://dx.doi.org/10.1038/nrc1840 PMID:16557279, by permission from Macmillan Publishers Ltd. © 2006.

3.3.5 Magdalena B. Wozniak and Paul Brennan.

3.3.6 Rhoda Baer, courtesy of U.S. National Institutes of Health (NIH).

B3.3.1 Reprinted from Bouwman P, Jonkers J (2012). The effects of de-regulated DNA damage signalling on cancer chemotherapy response and resistance. *Nat Rev Cancer*, 12:587–598. http://dx.doi.org/10.1038/nrc3342 PMID:22918414, by permission from Macmillan Publishers Ltd. © 2012.

3.4.1 & 3.4.2 Reprinted from Sawan C, Vaissière T, Murr R, Herceg Z (2008). Epigenetic drivers and genetic passengers on the road to cancer. *Mutat Res*, 642:1–13. http://dx.doi.org/10.1016/j.mrfmmm.2008.03.002 PMID:18471836, © 2008, with permission from Elsevier.

3.4.3 & 3.4.4 Toshikazu Ushijima and Zdenko Herceg.

3.5.1 Courtesy of Collectif National des Associations d'Obèses (CNAO, France), www.cnao.fr.

3.5.2–3.5.4 Augustin Scalbert and Isabelle Romieu.

3.6.1 Reprinted from O'Connor TP, Crystal RG (2006). Genetic medicines: treatment strategies for hereditary disorders. *Nat Rev Genet*, 7:261–276. http://dx.doi.org/10.1038/nrg1829 PMID:16543931, by permission from Macmillan Publishers Ltd. © 2006.

3.6.2 Courtesy of Freda Miller, Hospital for Sick Children (Toronto, Canada).

3.6.3 & 3.6.4 Hector Hernandez Vargas.

3.6.5 Courtesy of Johannes Jungverdorben, Life & Brain Center, Bonn, www.eurostemcell.org.

3.6.6 Reprinted from Reya T, Morrison SJ, Clarke MF *et al.* (2001). Stem cells, cancer, and cancer stem cells. *Nature*, 414:105–111. http://dx.doi.org/ 10.1038/35102167 PMID:11689955, by permission from Macmillan Publishers Ltd. © 2001.

3.7.1 Robert R. Langley.

3.7.2 Figure courtesy of Zhi-Yuan Chen, Sun Yat-sen University Cancer Center; reprinted from Qin L, Bromberg-White JL, Qian CN (2012). Opportunities and challenges in tumor angiogenesis research: back and forth between bench and bed. *Adv Cancer Res*, 113:191–239. http://dx.doi.org/10.1016/B978-0-12-394280-7.00006-3 PMID:22429856, © 2012, with permission from Elsevier.

3.7.3 Reprinted from Davis DW, McConkey DJ, Abbruzzese JL *et al.* (2003). Surrogate markers in antiangiogenesis clinical trials. *Br J Cancer*, 89:8–14. http://dx.doi.org/10.1038/sj.bjc.6601035 PMID:12838293, by permission from Macmillan Publishers Ltd on behalf of Cancer Research UK. © 2003.

3.7.4 Reprinted from Langley RR, Fidler IJ (2007). Tumor cell-organ microenvironment interactions in the pathogenesis of cancer metastasis. *Endocr Rev*, 28:297–321. http://dx.doi.org/10.1210/er.2006-0027 PMID:17409287. © 2007, The Endocrine Society.

3.7.5 Robert R. Langley.

3.8.1A & B Image from the RCSB Protein Data Bank, September 2008 Molecule of the Month feature by David Goodsell; http://dx.doi.org/10.2210/rcsb_pdb/mom_2008_9.

3.8.1C Courtesy of Thomas Bauer, Medical University of Vienna.

3.8.2–3.8.4 Courtesy of Thomas Bauer, Medical University of Vienna.

3.9.1 Holger Moch.

3.9.2 Courtesy of Wikipedia user Patho. License: CC-BY-SA-3.0.

3.9.3 Adapted from Pardoll DM (2012). Immunology beats cancer: a blueprint for successful translation. *Nat Immunol*, 13:1129–1132. http://dx.doi.org/10.1038/ni.2392 PMID:23160205, by permission from Macmillan Publishers Ltd. © 2012.

3.9.4 Reprinted from Mellman I, Coukos G, Dranoff G (2011). Cancer immunotherapy comes of age. *Nature*, 480:480–489. http://dx.doi.org/10.1038/nature10673 PMID:22193102, by permission from Macmillan Publishers Ltd. © 2011.

4.1.1 Reproduced with permission from the association Droits des Non-Fumeurs (Paris, France), www.dnf.asso.fr.

4.1.2 Reproduced with permission from The GTSS Atlas: Global Youth Tobacco Survey, 2009 © Myriad Editions www.myriadeditions.com.

4.1.3 Reproduced from IARC (2008). IARC Handbooks of Cancer Prevention, Vol. 12: *Tobacco Control: Methods for Evaluating Tobacco Control Policies.* Lyon: IARC.

4.1.4 Reproduced with permission from the Australian National Preventive Health Agency.

4.1.5 Reproduced with permission from NYC Health and the World Lung Foundation.

4.1.6 WHO © 2013.

B4.1.1 Simon Chapman.

4.2.1 © 2004 Syed Ziaul Habib Roobon, Courtesy of Photoshare.

4.2.2 & 4.2.3 Rena R. Wing and Kathryn R. Middleton.

4.2.4 Courtesy of jusben, www.Morguefile.com.

4.2.5 Crown Copyright 2013, accessed at www.nhs.uk/Change4Life, a website of the National Health Service (NHS).

4.2.6 U.S. Air Force photo by Mike Kaplan, www.defenseimagery.mil.

B4.2.1 Adapted from Pischon T, Boeing H, Hoffmann K *et al.* (2008). General and abdominal adiposity and risk of death in Europe. *N Engl J Med*, 359:2105–2120. http://dx.doi.org/10.1056/NEJMoa0801891 PMID:19005195, with permission from the Massachusetts Medical Society.

4.3.1 Australian National Tobacco Campaign, reproduced with permission from the Australian Government Department of Health and Ageing.

4.3.2 Courtesy of the Asociación Española Contra el Cáncer (Spanish Association Against Cancer), www.aecc.es.

4.3.3 Courtesy of Association Lalla Salma de Lutte contre le Cancer (ALSC, Morocco).

4.3.4 Courtesy of Hong Kong Cancer Fund. All rights reserved (2013).

4.3.5 Courtesy of Breast Cancer Foundation, Singapore. Designed by DDB.

4.3.6 A campaign of the Centers for Disease Control and Prevention, Division of Adolescent and School Health www.VERBnow.com.

4.4.1 Courtesy of Flickr user Cory Doctorow. Permission is granted to copy, distribute and/or modify this image under the terms of the Attribution-Share Alike 2.0 Generic license (http://creativecommons.org/licenses/by-sa/2.0/deed.en).

4.4.2 Reproduced from "BRASIL – Advertências Sanitárias nos Produtos de Tabaco – 2009", accessed at www.inca.gov.br.

4.4.3 A campaign of Children's Healthcare of Atlanta, accessed at www.strong4life.com.

4.4.4 Courtesy of Biswarup Ganguly via Wikimedia Commons. License: CC-BY-SA-3.0.

---

[a] Ferlay J, Soerjomataram I, Ervik M *et al.* (2013). GLOBOCAN 2012 v1.0, Cancer Incidence and Mortality Worldwide: IARC Cancer Base No. 11 [Internet]. Lyon: IARC. Available at http://globocan.iarc.fr.

[b] Forman D, Bray F, Brewster DH *et al.*, eds (2013). *Cancer Incidence in Five Continents*, Vol. X [electronic version]. Lyon: IARC. Available at http://ci5.iarc.fr.

4.4.5 Reproduced with permission from the Drug and Alcohol Office, Western Australia.

4.5.1 Courtesy of Álvaro Daniel Gonzalez Lamarque, www.Morguefile.com.

4.5.2 WHO © 2013.

4.5.3 © State of New South Wales through the Parliament, 2012.

4.5.4 © 2007 Frederick Noronha, Courtesy of Photoshare.

4.5.5 © Greenpeace/Karen Robinson, accessed at www.greenpeace.org/toxics.

B4.5.1 Rafael Moreira Claro.

4.6.1 Courtesy of Matthias Trischler via Wikipedia. License: CC-BY-SA-3.0.

4.6.2 IARC photo library.

4.6.3 Reprinted from WHO/UNICEF coverage estimates, 1980–2005, as of August 2006, 192 WHO Member States.

4.6.4 Reproduced from Tabrizi SN, Brotherton JM, Kaldor JM *et al.* (2012). Fall in human papillomavirus prevalence following a national vaccination program. *J Infect Dis*, 206:1645–1651. http://dx.doi.org/10.1093/infdis/jis590 PMID:23087430, by permission of Oxford University Press.

B4.6.1 Tandin Dorji and the staff of the Jigme Dorji Wangchuck National Referral Hospital.

B4.6.2 © 2004 Eileen Dietrich, Courtesy of Photoshare.

4.7.1 Adapted from de Koning HJ (2009). The mysterious mass(es). [Inaugural address, Professor of Screening Evaluation.] Rotterdam, The Netherlands: Erasmus MC.

4.7.2 Adapted from Vaccarella S, Lortet-Tieulent J, Plummer M *et al.* (2013). Worldwide trends in cervical cancer incidence: Impact of screening against changes in disease risk factors. *Eur J Cancer*, 49:3262–3273. http://dx.doi.org/10.1016/j.ejca.2013.04.024 PMID:23751569, with permission from Elsevier.

4.7.3 & 4.7.4 IARC Screening Group.

4.7.5 Peter B. Dean/IARC.

4.7.6 Rengaswamy Sankaranarayanan/IARC.

4.7.7 IARC Screening Group.

4.7.8 Adapted from von Karsa L (1995). Mammography screening – comprehensive, population-based quality assurance is required! [in German] *Z Allgemeinmed*, 71:1863–1867, with permission of Deutscher Ärzte-Verlag.

4.8.1 Krittika Pitaksaringkarn/IARC.

4.8.2 UNFPA/Omar Gharzeddine.

4.8.3 Courtesy of Mark B. Brown, from the Lutheran World Foundation.

4.8.4 Eric Lucas/IARC.

4.8.5 Courtesy of Osaka Center for Cancer and Cardiovascular Diseases Prevention, Japan.

5.1.1 © 2008 Sandipan Majumdar, Courtesy of Photoshare.

5.1.2 & 5.1.3 Elisabeth Brambilla and William D. Travis.

5.1.4 Reprinted from Heist RS, Engelman JA (2012). SnapShot: non-small cell lung cancer. *Cancer Cell*, 21:448. http://dx.doi.org/10.1016/j.ccr.2012.03.007 PMID:22439939, with permission from Elsevier.

5.1.5 Reprinted from Govindan R, Ding L, Griffith M *et al.* (2012) Genomic landscape of non-small cell lung cancer in smokers and never-smokers. *Cell*, 150:1121–1134. http://dx.doi.org/10.1016/j.cell.2012.08.024 PMID:22980976, with permission from Elsevier.

5.1.6 & 5.1.7 Elisabeth Brambilla and William D. Travis.

B5.1.1 Avrum Spira.

B5.1.2 Figure compiled from Loft S, Voboda P, Kasai H (2005). Prospective study of 8-oxo-7,8-dihydro-20-deoxyguanosine excretion and the risk of lung cancer. *Carcinogenesis*, 27:1245–1250. http://dx.doi.org/10.1093/carcin/bgi313 PMID:16364924

5.2.1A & B & C Sunil R. Lakhani.

5.2.1D Stuart J. Schnitt.

5.2.2A Stuart J. Schnitt.

5.2.2B Puay Hoon Tan, Singapore General Hospital, Singapore.

5.2.2C Sunil R. Lakhani.

5.2.2D Puay Hoon Tan, Singapore General Hospital, Singapore.

5.2.2E Sunil R. Lakhani.

5.2.2F Jorge S. Reis-Filho, The Breakthrough Breast Cancer Research Centre, Institute of Cancer Research, London, United Kingdom.

5.2.2G Gianni Bussolati, University of Turin, Turin, Italy.

5.2.2H Johannes L. Peterse.

5.2.3 From the University of Alabama at Birmingham Department of Pathology PEIR Digital Library © (http://peir.net).

5.2.4 Reprinted from Sørlie T, Wang Y, Xiao C *et al.* (2006). Distinct molecular mechanisms underlying clinically relevant subtypes of breast cancer: gene expression analyses across three different platforms. *BMC Genomics*, 7:127. http://dx.doi.org/10.1186/1471-2164-7-127 PMID:16729877

5.2.5 Reprinted from Stephens PJ, Tarpey PS, Davies H *et al.*; Oslo Breast Cancer Consortium (OSBREAC) (2012). The landscape of cancer genes and mutational processes in breast cancer. *Nature*, 486:400–404. http://dx.doi.org/10.1038/nature11017 PMID:22722201, by permission from Macmillan Publishers Ltd. © 2012.

5.2.6 Courtesy of Petr Kratochvil, accessed at www.publicdomainpictures.net.

5.2.7 Courtesy of Bill Branson, accessed at https://visualsonline.cancer.gov/ (National Cancer Institute).

B5.2.1 From Neilson HK, Friedenreich CM, Brockton NT, Millikan RC (2009). Physical activity and postmenopausal breast cancer: proposed biologic mechanisms and areas for future research. *Cancer Epidemiol Biomarkers Prev*, 18:11–27. http://dx.doi.org/10.1158/1055-9965.EPI-08-0756 PMID:19124476

5.3.1 From the University of Alabama at Birmingham Department of Pathology PEIR Digital Library © (http://peir.net).

5.3.2 © 2008 Khalid Mahmood Raja, Courtesy of Photoshare.

5.3.3 Elizabeth A. Montgomery.

5.3.4 Elizabeth A. Montgomery.

5.3.5 Reprinted from Dulak AM, Stojanov P, Peng S *et al.* (2013). Exome and whole-genome sequencing of esophageal adenocarcinoma identifies recurrent driver events and mutational complexity. *Nat Genet*, 45:478–486. http://dx.doi.org/10.1038/ng.2591 PMID:23525077, by permission from Macmillan Publishers Ltd. © 2013.

5.3.6 Adapted from Lao-Sirieix P, Fitzgerald RC (2012). Screening for oesophageal cancer. *Nat Rev Clin Oncol*, 9:278–287. http://dx.doi.org/10.1038/nrclinonc.2012.35 PMID:22430857, by permission of Macmillan Publishers Ltd. © 2012.

5.4.1 Fátima Carneiro.

5.4.2 Courtesy of Wikipedia user Daderot. This file is made available under the Creative Commons CC0 1.0 Universal Public Domain Dedication (http://creativecommons.org/publicdomain/zero/1.0/deed.en).

ᵃ Ferlay J, Soerjomataram I, Ervik M *et al.* (2013). GLOBOCAN 2012 v1.0, Cancer Incidence and Mortality Worldwide: IARC Cancer Base No. 11 [Internet]. Lyon: IARC. Available at http://globocan.iarc.fr.

ᵇ Forman D, Bray F, Brewster DH *et al.*, eds (2013). *Cancer Incidence in Five Continents*, Vol. X [electronic version]. Lyon: IARC. Available at http://ci5.iarc.fr.

5.4.3 Fátima Carneiro.

5.4.4 Courtesy of Russell Lee, from the U.S. National Archives and Records Administration.

5.4.5 Reproduced from Deng N, Goh LK, Wang H *et al.* (2012). A comprehensive survey of genomic alterations in gastric cancer reveals systematic patterns of molecular exclusivity and co-occurrence among distinct therapeutic targets. *Gut*, 61:673–684. http://dx.doi.org/10.1136/gutjnl-2011-301839 PMID:22315472, with permission from BMJ Publishing Group Ltd.

B5.4.1 Il Ju Choi.

5.5.1 Fred T. Bosman.

5.5.2 Courtesy of Dale C. Snover, Department of Pathology, Fairview Southdale Hospital, Edina, MN, USA.

5.5.3 Reproduced from Bosman FT (2013). Molecular pathology of colorectal cancer. In: Chung L, Eble J, eds. *Molecular Surgical Pathology.* Springer, pp. 1–17, with kind permission from Springer+Business Media B.V.

5.5.4 Courtesy of University of Lausanne Medical Centre, with permission from Fred T. Bosman.

5.6.1 Courtesy of Banchob Sripa, Faculty of Medicine, Khon Kaen University, Khon Kaen, Thailand.

5.6.2 © 2010 Somenath Mukhopadhyay, Courtesy of Photoshare.

5.6.3 Courtesy of Young Nyun Park, Yonsei University College of Medicine, Seoul, Republic of Korea.

5.6.4 Courtesy of Hirohisa Yano, Kurume University School of Medicine, Fukuoka-ken, Japan.

5.6.5A Reproduced with permission International Consensus Group for Hepatocellular Neoplasia (2009). Pathologic diagnosis of early hepatocellular carcinoma: a report of the International Consensus Group for Hepatocellular Neoplasia. *Hepatology*, 49:658–664. http://dx.doi.org/10.1002/hep.22709 PMID:19177576

5.6.5B Courtesy of Alexander Kagen, Albert Einstein College of Medicine, New York NY, USA.

5.6.6 Reproduced from Kan Z, Zheng H, Liu X *et al.* (2013). Whole-genome sequencing identifies recurrent mutations in hepatocellular carcinoma. *Genome Res*, 23:1422–1433. http://dx.doi.org/10.1101/gr.154492.113 PMID:23788652. This article is licensed under a Creative Commons License.

B5.6.1 © 2009 Nephron, Permission is granted to copy, distribute and/or modify this image under the terms of the Attribution-Share Alike 3.0 Unported licence (https://creativecommons.org/licenses/by-sa/3.0/deed.en).

5.7.1 Courtesy of the National Cancer Institute.

5.7.2 Ralph H. Hruban.

5.7.3 Reprinted from Biankin AV, Waddell N, Kassahn KS *et al.*; Australian Pancreatic Cancer Genome Initiative (2012). Pancreatic cancer genomes reveal aberrations in axon guidance pathway genes. *Nature*, 491:399–405. http://dx.doi.org/10.1038/nature11547 PMID:23103869, by permission from Macmillan Publishers Ltd, 2012.

5.7.4 Ralph H. Hruban.

5.7.5 Courtesy of the Armed Forces Institute of Pathology (*AFIP Atlas of Tumor Pathology*).

5.7.6 Ralph H. Hruban.

5.8.1 Used with permission from Amirsys Publishing; Thompson LD, Wenig BM (2011). *Diagnostic Pathology: Head and Neck,* © 2012.

5.8.2 Courtesy of Jason C. Fowler, Meadville Medical Center, Meadville, PA, USA.

5.8.3 iStockphoto: Krakozawr © 2008.

5.8.4 Adapted from Argiris A, Karamouzis MV, Raben D, Ferris RL (2008). Head and neck cancer. *Lancet*, 371:1695–1709, http://dx.doi.org/10.1016/S0140-6736(08)60728-X PMID:18486742, © 2012, with permission from Elsevier.

5.8.5 Lester D.R. Thompson.

5.8.6 Lester D.R. Thompson.

5.9.1 Courtesy of Tony Alter via Flickr. License: CC BY 2.0.

5.9.2 © 2006 Rezaul Haque, Courtesy of Photoshare.

5.9.3 & 5.9.4 Holger Moch

5.9.5 Reprinted from Varela I, Tarpey P, Raine K *et al.* (2011). Exome sequencing identifies frequent mutation of the SWI/SNF complex gene PBRM1 in renal carcinoma. *Nature*, 469:539–542. http://dx.doi.org/10.1038/nature09639 PMID:21248752, by permission from Macmillan Publishers Ltd. © 2011.

5.10.1 © 2001 Jean Sack, Courtesy of Photoshare.

5.10.2 Courtesy of KGH via Wikipedia. License: CC BY-SA 3.0.

5.10.3 Reproduced from Eble JN, Sauter G, Epstein JI, Sesterhenn IA, eds (2004). *Pathology and Genetics of Tumours of the Urinary System and Male Genital Organs.* Lyon: IARC, p. 106.

5.10.4 © 2002 Margaret D'Adamo, Courtesy of Photoshare.

5.10.5 Reprinted with permission from Iyer G, Al-Ahmadie H, Schultz N *et al.* (2013). Prevalence and co-occurrence of actionable genomic alterations in high-grade bladder cancer. *J Clin Oncol*, 31:3133–3140. http://dx.doi.org/10.1200/JCO.2012.46.5740 PMID:23897969. © 2013 American Society of Clinical Oncology. All Rights Reserved.

5.11.1 Courtesy of Jeremy Sheldon ("Pay No Mind") via Flickr. License: CC BY-NC-ND 2.0.

5.11.2 & 5.11.3 Peter A. Humphrey.

5.11.4 Reprinted from Epstein JI, Cubilla AL, Humphrey PA (2011). *Tumors of the Prostate Gland, Seminal Vesicles, Penis, and Scrotum* (*AFIP Atlas of Tumor Pathology* Series 4, Fascicle 14). Washington, DC: American Registry of Pathology and Armed Forces Institute of Pathology.

5.11.5 Reprinted with permission from Rubin MA, Maher CA, Chinnaiyan AM (2011). Common gene rearrangements in prostate cancer. *J Clin Oncol*, 29:3659–3668. http://dx.doi.org/10.1200/JCO.2011.35.1916 PMID:21859993. © 2013 American Society of Clinical Oncology. All rights reserved.

5.11.6 & 5.11.7 Peter A. Humphrey.

5.12.1 © 2012 Akintunde Akinleye/NURHI, Courtesy of Photoshare.

5.12.2 Jaime Prat.

5.12.3 Adapted from Crosbie EJ, Einstein MH, Franceschi S, Kitchener HC (2013). Human papillomavirus and cervical cancer. *Lancet*, 382:889–899. http://dx.doi.org/10.1016/S0140-6736(13)60022-7 PMID: 23618600, © 2013, with permission from Elsevier.

5.12.4 This image was published in Robboy SJ, Mutter GL, Prat J *et al.*, eds (2009). *Robboy's Pathology of the Female Reproductive Tract*, 2nd ed., p. 191, © Elsevier 2009.

5.12.5 & 5.12.6 Jaime Prat.

5.12.7 Jaime Prat.

5.12.8 Reprinted from Catasus L, Gallardo A, Prat J (2009). Molecular genetics of endometrial carcinoma. *Diagn Histopathol*, 15: 554–563, http://dx.doi.org/10.1016/j.mpdhp.2009.09.002, © 2009, with permission from Elsevier.

5.12.9 Jaime Prat.

5.13.1 & 5.13.2 Courtesy of Harald Stein, Pathodiagnostik Berlin, Germany.

---

[a] Ferlay J, Soerjomataram I, Ervik M *et al.* (2013). GLOBOCAN 2012 v1.0, Cancer Incidence and Mortality Worldwide: IARC Cancer Base No. 11 [Internet]. Lyon: IARC. Available at http://globocan.iarc.fr.

[b] Forman D, Bray F, Brewster DH *et al.*, eds (2013). *Cancer Incidence in Five Continents*, Vol. X [electronic version]. Lyon: IARC. Available at http://ci5.iarc.fr.

5.13.3 Reproduced from Steidl C, Gascoyne RD (2011). The molecular pathogenesis of primary mediastinal large B-cell lymphoma. *Blood*, 118:2659–2669. http://dx.doi.org/10.1182/blood-2011-05-326538 PMID:21700770, with permission from the American Society of Hematology.

5.13.4 Courtesy of Peter Hesseling, Faculty of Medicine and Health Sciences, Stellenbosch University, South Africa.

5.13.5 Reproduced from Mullighan CG (2012). Molecular genetics of B-precursor acute lymphoblastic leukemia. *J Clin Invest*, 122:3407–3415. http://dx.doi.org/10.1172/JCI61203 PMID:23023711, with permission from the American Society for Clinical Investigation (ASCI).

B5.13.1 Adapted from Szczepański T, Orfão A, van der Velden VH *et al.* (2001). Minimal residual disease in leukaemia patients. *Lancet Oncol*, 2:409–417. http://dx.doi.org/10.1016/S1470-2045(00)00418-6 PMID:11905735. © 2001 with permission from Elsevier.

5.14.1 Courtesy of CDC/Carl Washington, M.D., Emory Univ. School of Medicine; Mona Saraiya, MD, MPH, accessed at phil.cdc.gov/phil.

5.14.2 From the University of Alabama at Birmingham Department of Pathology PEIR Digital Library © (http://peir.net).

5.14.3 iStockphoto: aydinmutlu © 2011.

5.14.4 Reprinted from Vultur A, Herlyn M (2013). SnapShot: melanoma. *Cancer Cell*, 23:706. http://dx.doi.org/10.1016/j.ccr.2013.05.001 PMID:23680152, © 2013, with permission from Elsevier.

5.14.5 iStockphoto: .shock © 2010.

5.15.1 & 5.15.4 Frank Weber.

5.15.2 Courtesy of Gil Tudor, IAEA Division of Public Information.

5.15.3 & 5.15.5 Reproduced from Weber F, Eng C (2005). Gene-expression profiling in differentiated thyroid cancer – a viable strategy for the practice of genomic medicine? *Future Oncol*, 1:497–510. http://dx.doi.org/10.2217/14796694.1.4.497 PMID:16556026 with permission from Future Medicine Ltd.

5.15.6 Courtesy of Susanne Reger-Tan and Kurt W. Schmid, both of Universitätsklinikum Essen, Germany.

5.16.1 Courtesy of Angela Leuker, IAEA Division of Public Information.

5.16.2–5.16.4 Paul Kleihues.

5.16.5 Reprinted from Kotliarova S, Fine HA (2012). SnapShot: glioblastoma multiforme. *Cancer Cell*, 21:710, e1. http://dx.doi.org/10.1016/j.ccr.2012.04.031 PMID:22624719, © 2012, with permission from Elsevier.

5.16.6 Hiroko Ohgaki.

6.1.1 WHO.

6.1.2 WHO, 2010. All rights reserved.

6.1.3 Courtesy of Institut National de Recherche et de Sécurité (INRS, France; www.inrs.fr).

6.1.4 Courtesy of the Iowa Department of Public Health, accessed at www.idph.state.ia.us.

6.1.5 "Nobody's Immune to Breast Cancer" campaign by DDB MOÇAMBIQUE for the ALCC (Associação da Luta Contra o Cancro; Association for the Fight Against Cancer, Mozambique).

6.2.1 © 2009 Joanne Katz, Courtesy of Photoshare.

6.2.2 © 2004 Philippe Blanc, Courtesy of Photoshare.

6.2.3 Roland Dray/IARC.

6.2.4 WHO (2006). *Cancer Control: Knowledge into Action. WHO Guide for Effective Programmes*. Module 1: Planning. Geneva: WHO.

B6.2.1 Adapted with permission from WHO. WHO/IARC/APHRC (2012). Prevention of cervical cancer through screening using visual inspection with acetic acid (VIA) and treatment with cryotherapy. A demonstration project in six African countries: Malawi, Madagascar, Nigeria, Uganda, the United Republic of Tanzania, and Zambia WHO, Nigeria; Fig. 2, p. 11.

B6.2.2 & B6.2.3 Reprinted from Ezzati M (2004). Indoor air quality in developing nations, In: *Encyclopaedia of Energy*, Vol. 3, pp. 343–350, © 2004, with permission from Elsevier.

6.3.1 © Petr Pavlicek/International Atomic Energy Agency.

6.3.2 © Angela Leuker/International Atomic Energy Agency.

6.3.3 © David Kinley/International Atomic Energy Agency.

6.3.4 Courtesy of the National Cancer Centre of Mongolia.

6.3.5 © Elio Omobono/International Atomic Energy Agency.

6.4.1 © 2012 Wikipedia user Armigo. License: CC-BY-SA-3.0.

6.4.2 NIH/Coriell Institute for Medical Research.

6.4.3 Roland Dray/IARC, with permission from Marie-Pierre Cros.

6.4.4 Reproduced from Pukkala E (2010). Nordic biological specimen bank cohorts as basis for studies of cancer causes and control – quality control of cohorts with more than 2 million sample donors and 100,000 prospective cancers. In: Dillner J, ed. *Methods in Biobanking*. New York: Springer, pp. 61–112, with kind permission from Springer Science+Business Media.

6.4.5 & 6.4.6 IARC, Joakim Dillner.

6.4.7 Courtesy of Kurt Zatloukal (kurt.zatloukal@medunigraz.at) and Biobanking and Biomolecular Resources Research Infrastructure (www.BBMRI.eu).

6.5.1 UN Photo/Marco Castro.

6.5.2 © Union for International Cancer Control (UICC).

6.5.3 © 2012 Srikrishna Sulgodu Ramachandra, Courtesy of Photoshare.

6.5.4 Courtesy www.MoonshineMovies.com.

6.5.5 Courtesy of Cancer Council Australia, www.cancer.org.au.

6.6.1 Health warning images and plain packaging designs used with the permission of the Australian Government.

6.6.2 Figure created by Martha Maurer, copyright Pain & Policy Studies Group, UWCCC/home of WHO Collaborating Center, 2013. Opioid consumption data from International Narcotics Control Board; population data from the United Nations World Population Prospects 2010 Revision; country income level from World Bank Classification of Countries by Income level, http://data.worldbank.org/about/country-classifications/country-and-lending-groups.

6.6.3 Figure created by Martha Maurer, copyright Pain & Policy Studies Group, UWCCC/home of WHO Collaborating Center, 2012. Opioid consumption data from International Narcotics Control Board (values represent the aggregate morphine equivalence consumption of fentanyl, hydromorphone, morphine, oxycodone and pethidine); cancer deaths from Ferlay J, Shin HR, Bray F *et al.* (2010). GLOBOCAN 2008 v1.2, Cancer Incidence and Mortality Worldwide: IARC CancerBase No. 10 [Internet]. Lyon: IARC. Available at http://globocan.iarc.fr (cancer death estimates calculated by applying the 2008 crude death rate per 100 000 to the 2010 population to estimate raw number of cancer deaths for 2010); population data from the United Nations World Population Prospects 2010 Revision.

6.6.4 Courtesy of Barb Gannon, via Flickr. All rights reserved. © 2012.

6.7.1 © 2012 Victoria A Smith, Courtesy of Photoshare.

6.7.2 © 2007 Pradeep Tewari, Courtesy of Photoshare.

[a] Ferlay J, Soerjomataram I, Ervik M *et al.* (2013). GLOBOCAN 2012 v1.0, Cancer Incidence and Mortality Worldwide: IARC Cancer Base No. 11 [Internet]. Lyon: IARC. Available at http://globocan.iarc.fr.

[b] Forman D, Bray F, Brewster DH *et al.*, eds (2013). *Cancer Incidence in Five Continents*, Vol. X [electronic version]. Lyon: IARC. Available at http://ci5.iarc.fr.

6.7.3 © 2003 Justin Fahey, Courtesy of Photoshare.

6.7.4 Courtesy of James Gathany and Judy Schmidt, U.S. Centers for Disease Control and Prevention.

P3.1 Adapted from zur Hausen H, de Villiers EM (2005). Virus target cell conditioning model to explain some epidemiologic characteristics of childhood leukemias and lymphomas. *Int J Cancer*, 115:1–5. http://dx.doi.org/10.1002/ijc.20905 PMID:15688417 This material is reproduced with permission of John Wiley & Sons, Inc.

P4.1 Reproduced with permission from Cambridge University Library.

P4.2 Adapted from Potter NE, Ermini L, Papaemmanuil E *et al.* (2013). Single cell mutational profiling and clonal phylogeny in cancer. *Genome Res*, [epub ahead of print], http://dx.doi.org/10.1101/gr.159913.113 PMID:24056532, with permission from Cold Spring Harbor Laboratory Press.

P4.3 Reproduced from Greaves M (2000). *Cancer: The Evolutionary Legacy.* With permission from Oxford University Press.

P4.4A Mel Greaves.

P4.4B Reproduced from Costanzo M, Baryshnikova A, Bellay J *et al.* (2010). The genetic landscape of a cell. *Science*, 327:425–431. http://dx.doi.org/10.1126/science.1180823 PMID:20093466; with permission from the American Association for the Advancement of Science. All rights reserved.

P4.5 Mel Greaves.

P7.1 Adapted by permission from BMJ Publishing Group Limited. Doll R, Peto R, Boreham J, Sutherland I (2004). Mortality in relation to smoking: 50 years' observations on male British doctors. *BMJ*, 328:1519–1527. http://dx.doi.org/10.1136/bmj.38142.554479.AE PMID:15213107, © 2004.

P7.2 & P7.3 Reprinted from Pirie K, Peto R, Reeves GK *et al.*; Million Women Study Collaborators (2013). The 21st century hazards of smoking and benefits of stopping: a prospective study of one million women in the UK. *Lancet*, 381:133–141. http://dx.doi.org/10.1016/S0140-6736(12)61720-6 PMID:23107252, © 2013, with permission from Elsevier.

P7.4–P7.9 Compiled from Peto R, Lopez AD, Boreham J *et al.* (1992). Mortality from tobacco in developed countries: indirect estimation from national vital statistics. *Lancet*, 339:1268–1278. http://dx.doi.org/10.1016/0140-6736(92)91600-D PMID:1349675; Peto R, Lopez AD, Boreham J *et al.* (1994). *Mortality from Smoking in Developed Countries 1950–2000: Indirect Estimates from National Vital Statistics.* Oxford: Oxford University Press; WHO mortality data and UN population estimates.

page xi Courtesy of Russell E. White, Tenwek Mission Hospital, Kenya.

page 15 GLOBOCAN 2012[a]

page 81 Clockwise from top left: Reproduced from www.pixabay.com; © 2003 Mukunda Bogati, Courtesy of Photoshare; IARC/Roland Dray; Courtesy of Flickr user Didier Vidal. License: CC BY-SA 2.0; Courtesy of Flickr user Alexis O'Toole. License: CC BY-SA 2.0; Courtesy of Aram Dulyan, Wikimedia Commons.

page 183 Clockwise from top left: Rhoda Baer, National Institutes of Health Clinical Centre; Lance Liotta Laboratory, National Cancer Institute; Susan Arnold, provided by Raowf Guirguis, National Cancer Institute; Stanley J. Korsmeyer, Metabolism Branch, Section of Cellular Immunology, National Cancer Institute; National Institutes of Health; Basic Research Laboratory, Frederick Cancer Research Facility, National Cancer Institute.

page 267 Clockwise from top left: © 2005 Emily J. Phillips, Courtesy of Photoshare; Courtesy of Breast Cancer Foundation, Singapore. Designed by DDB; Courtesy of Association Lalla Salma de Lutte contre le Cancer (ALSC, Morocco); Rhoda Baer, National Cancer Institute; WHO © 2013; Courtesy of Flickr user Cory Doctorow, accessed at www.flickr.com.

page 347 Clockwise from top left: Dr Maria Tsokos, National Cancer Institute; Courtesy of Ed Uthman, MD, American Board of Pathology, accessed at http://web2airmail.net/uthman/; Otis Brawley, National Cancer Institute; National Cancer Institute; Courtesy of Department of Clinical Pathomorphology and Cytology, Medical University, Lodz, Poland; Courtesy of Wikipedia user MBq, via Wikimedia Commons.

page 527 © 2009 Joanne Katz, Courtesy of Photoshare.

Maps

[a] Ferlay J, Soerjomataram I, Ervik M *et al.* (2013). GLOBOCAN 2012 v1.0, Cancer Incidence and Mortality Worldwide: IARC Cancer Base No. 11 [Internet]. Lyon: IARC. Available at http://globocan.iarc.fr.

[b] Forman D, Bray F, Brewster DH *et al.*, eds (2013). *Cancer Incidence in Five Continents*, Vol. X [electronic version]. Lyon: IARC. Available at http://ci5.iarc.fr.

Tables

1.3.1 Compiled from Baade PD, Youlden DR, Valery PC *et al.* (2010). Population-based survival estimates for childhood cancer in Australia during the period 1997–2006. *Br J Cancer*, 103:1663–1670. http://dx.doi.org/10.1038/sj.bjc.6605985 PMID:21063404; Bao PP, Zheng Y, Wu CX *et al.* (2012). Population-based survival for childhood cancer patients diagnosed during 2002–2005 in Shanghai, China. *Pediatr Blood Cancer*, 59:657–661. http://dx.doi.org/10.1002/pbc.24043 PMID:22302759; Swaminathan R, Rama R, Shanta V (2008). Childhood cancers in Chennai, India, 1990–2001: incidence and survival. *Int J Cancer*, 122:2607–2611. http://dx.doi.org/10.1002/ijc.23428 PMID:18324630; and Wiangnon S, Veerakul G, Nuchprayoon I *et al.* (2011). Childhood cancer incidence and survival 2003–2005, Thailand: study from the Thai Pediatric Oncology Group. *Asian Pac J Cancer Prev*, 12:2215–2220. PMID:22296359.

2.2.1 Adapted from U.S. Department of Health and Human Services (2004). *The Health Consequences of Smoking: A Report of the Surgeon General*. Atlanta, GA: U.S. Department of Health and Human Services, Centers for Disease Control and Prevention, National Center for Chronic Disease Prevention and Health Promotion, Office on Smoking and Health.

2.3.1–2.3.3 Jürgen Rehm and Kevin Shield.

2.4.1 From IARC (2012). Biological agents. *IARC Monogr Eval Carcinog Risks Hum*, 100B:1–441. PMID:23189750

2.4.2 & 2.4.3 Reprinted from de Martel C, Ferlay J, Franceschi S *et al.* (2012). Global burden of cancers attributable to infections in 2008: a review and synthetic analysis. *Lancet Oncol*, 13:607–615. http://dx.doi.org/10.1016/S1470-2045(12)70137-7 PMID:22575588, © 2012, with permission from Elsevier.

B2.4.1 Reprinted from Schetter AJ, Heegaard NH, Harris CC (2010). Inflammation and cancer: interweaving microRNA, free radical, cytokine and p53 pathways. *Carcinogenesis*, 31:37–49. http://dx.doi.org/10.1093/carcin/bgp272 PMID:19955394

2.5.1 Adapted with permission from Pearce CL, Templeman C, Rossing MA *et al.*; Ovarian Cancer Association Consortium (2012). Association between endometriosis and risk of histological subtypes of ovarian cancer: a pooled analysis of case-control studies. *Lancet Oncol*, 13:385–394. http://dx.doi.org/10.1016/S1470-2045(11)70404-1 PMID:22361336, © 2012, with permission from Elsevier.

2.5.2 Adapted from Trabert B, Wentzensen N, Yang HP *et al.* (2012). Ovarian cancer and menopausal hormone therapy in the NIH-AARP Diet and Health Study. *Br J Cancer*, 107:1181–1187. http://dx.doi.org/10.1038/bjc.2012.397 PMID:22929888, by permission from Macmillan Publishers Ltd on behalf of Cancer Research UK, © 2012.

2.7.1 & 2.7.2 From IARC. Agents Classified by the IARC Monographs: http://monographs.iarc.fr/ENG/Classification/ClassificationsAlphaOrder.pdf.

B2.7.1 Kurt Straif.

B2.7.2 Lesley Rushton.

2.9.1 Kurt Straif.

2.10.1 & 2.10.2 Adapted from Grosse Y, Baan R, Straif K *et al.*; WHO IARC Monograph Working Group (2009). A review of human carcinogens – Part A: pharmaceuticals. *Lancet Oncol*, 10:13–14. http://dx.doi.org/10.1016/S1470-2045(08)70286-9 PMID:19115512, © 2009, with permission from Elsevier.

2.11.1–2.11.4 Ronald T. Riley.

3.1.1 Thomas J. Hudson.

3.6.1 Zdenko Herceg.

3.8.1 Fabio Savarese, Martin Holcmann, and Maria Sibilia.

3.8.2 Adapted from Brown MP, Burdett N (2013). Targeted therapies, aspects of pharmaceutical and oncological management. *Cancer Forum*, 37:70–80, http://www.cancerforum.org.au/Issues/2013/March/Forum/Targeted_therapies.htm, with permission from Cancer Forum.

4.1.1 & 4.1.2 Data compiled from IARC (2008). IARC Handbooks of Cancer Prevention, Vol. 12: *Tobacco Control: Methods for Evaluating Tobacco Control Policies*. Lyon: IARC.

4.5.1 Adapted from Stockwell T (2006). *A Review of Research into the Impacts of Alcohol Warning Labels on Attitudes and Behaviour*. Centre for Addictions Research of BC. University of Victoria, British Columbia, Canada, with permission from Tim Stockwell.

4.5.2 Adapted from IARC (2010). Some aromatic amines, organic dyes, and related exposures. *IARC Monogr Eval Carcinog Risks Hum*, 99:1–658. PMID:21528837. Data compiled from the GESTIS database (Institut für Arbeitsschutz der Deutschen Gesetzlichen Unfallversicherung, IFA).

4.5.3 Adapted from Michaels D, Monforton C (2013). Beryllium's 'public relations problem'. In: Late lessons from early warnings: science, precaution, innovation. EEA report 1/2013. Copenhagen: European Environment Agency, with permission from the European Environment Agency.

4.6.1 Modified with permission from Schiller JT, Castellsagué X, Garland SM (2012). A review of clinical trials of human papillomavirus prophylactic vaccines. *Vaccine*, 30 Suppl 5:F123–F138. http://dx.doi.org/10.1016/j.vaccine.2012.04.108 PMID:23199956, © 2012, with permission from Elsevier.

4.7.1 Lawrence von Karsa.

5.1.1 & 5.1.2 Elisabeth Brambilla and William D. Travis.

5.2.1 Adapted from Elston CW, Ellis IO (1991). Pathological prognostic factors in breast cancer. I. The value of histological grade in breast cancer: experience from a large study with long-term follow-up. *Histopathology*, 19:403–410. http://dx.doi.org/10.1111/j.1365-2559.1991.tb00229.x PMID:1757079, by permission from John Wiley and Sons.

5.5.1 Reproduced from Bosman FT, Carneiro F, Hruban RH, Theise ND, eds (2010). *WHO Classification of Tumours of the Digestive System*, 4th ed. Lyon: IARC, p. 133.

5.5.2 Reproduced from Bosman FT, Carneiro F, Hruban RH, Theise ND, eds (2010). *WHO Classification of Tumours of the Digestive System*, 4th ed. Lyon: IARC, p. 143.

5.6.1 Neil D. Theise.

5.6.2 Reproduced from Bosman FT, Carneiro F, Hruban RH, Theise ND, eds (2010). *WHO Classification of Tumours of the Digestive System*, 4th ed. Lyon: IARC, p. 197.

5.7.1 & 5.7.2 Reproduced from Hruban RH, Pitman MB, Klimstra DS (2007). *Tumors of the Pancreas (AFIP Atlas of Tumor Pathology* Series 4, Fascicle 6). Washington, DC: American Registry of Pathology and Armed Forces Institute of Pathology, with permission from the American Registry of Pathology.

5.7.3 Table adapted from text: Wu J, Matthaei H, Maitra A *et al.* (2011). Recurrent GNAS mutations define an unexpected pathway for pancreatic cyst development. *Sci Transl Med*, 3:92ra66. http://dx.doi.org/10.1126/scitranslmed.3002543 PMID:21775669; and Jiao Y, Shi C, Edil BH *et al.* (2011). *DAXX/ATRX, MEN1*, and mTOR pathway genes are frequently altered in pancreatic neuroendocrine tumors. *Science*, 331:1199–1203. http://dx.doi.org/10.1126/science.1200609 PMID:21252315.

[a] Ferlay J, Soerjomataram I, Ervik M *et al.* (2013). GLOBOCAN 2012 v1.0, Cancer Incidence and Mortality Worldwide: IARC Cancer Base No. 11 [Internet]. Lyon: IARC. Available at http://globocan.iarc.fr.

[b] Forman D, Bray F, Brewster DH *et al.*, eds (2013). *Cancer Incidence in Five Continents*, Vol. X [electronic version]. Lyon: IARC. Available at http://ci5.iarc.fr.

5.9.1 Reprinted from Moch H (2013). An overview of renal cell cancer: pathology and genetics. *Semin Cancer Biol*, 23:3–9. http://dx.doi.org/10.1016/j.semcancer.2012.06.006 PMID:22722066, © 2013, with permission from Elsevier.

5.10.1 Ronald Simon.

5.12.1–5.12.3 Jaime Prat.

5.12.4 Adapted from Prat J (2012). Ovarian carcinomas: five distinct diseases with different origins, genetic alterations, and clinicopathological features. *Virchows Arch*, 460:237–249. http://dx.doi.org/10.1007/s00428-012-1203-5 PMID:22322322, with kind permission from Springer Science+Business Media.

5.14.1 Christine Guo Lian and Martin C. Mihm Jr.

5.16.1 & 5.16.2 Paul Kleihues and Jill Barnholtz-Sloan.

6.2.1–6.2.3 Andreas Ullrich and Leanne Riley.

6.7.1 Reproduced from Knaul FM, Gralow JR, Atun R, Bhadelia A, eds (2012). *Closing the Cancer Divide: An Equity Imperative*. Based on the work of the Global Task Force on Expanded Access to Cancer Care and Control in Developing Countries. Cambridge, MA: Harvard Global Equity Initiative. Distributed by Harvard University Press. © 2012 by President and Fellows of Harvard College acting through the Harvard Global Equity Initiative. Reprinted by permission of the Harvard Global Equity Initiative.

P4.1–P4.3 Mel Greaves.

P7.1 Compiled from Thun MJ, Carter BD, Feskanich D *et al.* (2013). 50-year trends in smoking-related mortality in the United States. *N Engl J Med*, 368:351–364. http://dx.doi.org/10.1056/NEJMsa1211127 PMID:23343064

P7.2 Compiled from Peto R, Lopez AD (2001). Future worldwide health effects of current smoking patterns. In: Koop CE, Pearson C, Schwarz MR, eds. *Critical Issues in Global Health*. New York: Jossey-Bass, pp. 154–161.

Text

page 180 Text quotation reprinted from Richter LM, Victora CG, Hallal PC *et al.* (2012). Cohort profile: the consortium of health-orientated research in transitioning societies. *Int J Epidemiol*, 41:621–626. http://dx.doi.org/10.1093/ije/dyq251 PMID:21224276, by permission of Oxford University Press.

page 262 Text quotation reprinted from Greaves M (2005). In utero origins of childhood leukaemia. *Early Hum Dev*, 81:123–129. PMID:15707724, with permission from Elsevier.

The Editors are grateful to the Charles Rodolphe Brupbacher Stiftung for facilitating inclusion in World Cancer Report 2014 of material based on some contributions to the 2013 Scientific Symposium.

[a] Ferlay J, Soerjomataram I, Ervik M *et al.* (2013). GLOBOCAN 2012 v1.0, Cancer Incidence and Mortality Worldwide: IARC Cancer Base No. 11 [Internet]. Lyon: IARC. Available at http://globocan.iarc.fr.

[b] Forman D, Bray F, Brewster DH *et al.*, eds (2013). *Cancer Incidence in Five Continents*, Vol. X [electronic version]. Lyon: IARC. Available at http://ci5.iarc.fr.

Subject index

β-catenin 420, 476, 479

CCND1 448, 487, 489

CCNE1 479

CDH1 381, 389, 390, 409

CDK4 499

CDKN2A 357, 416, 417, 427, 448, 495, 499

cell surface markers 231

cervical adenocarcinoma 473

cervical cancer 57, 59, 61, 64, 110, 120, 164, 165, 316, 317, 320, 323, 331, 333, 470–474

    screening 323, 324, 326, 332, 333, 474, 541–545, 564

    vaccines 317–320, 474

cervical intraepithelial neoplasia 471–473

cervical squamous cell carcinoma 473

cetuximab 247, 248

chemopreventive agents 165, 166, 167

chemotherapeutic agents 165, 171, 259, 371, 372

chewing tobacco 82, 422

childhood malignancies 69–74, 261, 262

chlorambucil 161

chlorofluorocarbons 156

chloroform 158

cholangiocarcinoma 112, 403, 406–409, 411

cholesterol 458

chromophobe renal cell carcinoma 440, 441

chromosomal instability pathway 395

chromothripsis 185

chronic bladder infection 447

chronic gastritis 383

chronic liver infections 315, 408

chronic lymphocytic leukaemia (CLL) 208, 482, 483

chronic myeloid leukaemia (CML) 184, 185, 493

CIC 516, 518

ciclosporin 162, 171

cigarettes 82–86, 90, 268–278, 350, 354, 422, 426, 429, 436, 586–594

cirrhosis 98, 315, 406–408, 410

cisplatin 371

clear cell renal cell carcinoma 440–442

clonal evolution 339–342

coal combustion 543

coal tar 134, 140

cohort studies 177–180, 555, 558, 559

colectomy 396, 397

colitis 397, 401

collecting duct renal cell carcinoma 440

colon cancer 392–401

colonoscopy 323, 326, 585

colorectal cancer 55, 57, 58, 59, 66, 97, 102, 122, 126, 127, 128, 163, 166, 230, 237, 255, 294, 323, 331, 392–401

    screening 323, 324, 326, 332, 334, 400

colposcopy 473, 474

combined estrogen–progestogen contraceptives 164, 475

combined estrogen–progestogen menopausal therapy 163, 475

combustion emissions 152, 154, 155, 156, 157

competing endogenous RNA (ceRNA) 216

computed tomography (CT) 144, 145, 324, 360, 525

cost-effectiveness of interventions 533

costs of cancer 529, 533, 565, 576–582

Cowden syndrome 506, 508

COX-1 255

COX-2 241, 255, 397

CpG island methylator pathway 396

creosotes 140

crizotinib 355

Crohn disease 397

cryotherapy 323, 541

cryptorchidism 461

CTNNB1 390, 409, 420, 476, 479, 517

cyclophosphamide 161

cystic kidney disease 439

cytokines 254, 257

D

dairy products 126, 458

data linkage 556, 557

DBC1 448

DDR2 356, 357

developmental origins of health and disease 177

diabetes 281, 282, 407, 416, 439, 475

diesel engine emissions 135, 137, 153

fermentation 131, 426

FGFR1 356, 357, 359

FGFR3 448

finasteride 122

fine particles 153–156

5-fluorouracil 396

folate 127

folic acid 127, 434

follicular epithelial cells 503

follicular lymphoma 488

follicular thyroid cancer 504, 507

food 124–132, 171–173, 300, 301, 386, 388, 432–434

food contaminants 171, 172

formaldehyde 156

fruit 126, 433, 434

FUBP1 516, 518

fumonisins 172

fundic gland polyposis 389

fungi 171, 172

Fusarium 172

fusion genes 210

G

Gardner syndrome 398, 508

gastrectomy 390

gastric adenocarcinoma 106

gastric adenocarcinoma and proximal polyposis of the stomach 389

gastric cancer 383–390

    prevention 388, 390

    screening 388, 390

gastric lymphoma 108

gastro-oesophageal reflux disease 378, 379, 380

gefitinib 248, 355

gene–environment interactions 196–198

gene expression 197, 199, 203–212, 214–219

Gene Expression Omnibus 212

gene expression profiling 203–207, 210–212

gene fusions 206

genetic susceptibility 339, 340

    to breast cancer 362, 369

    to cervical cancer 474

    to colorectal cancer 397, 398, 399

    to haematological malignancies 483, 485, 487, 489, 490

    to head and neck cancers 429

    to kidney cancer 440, 441

    to lung cancer 353

    to melanoma 200

    to nervous system tumours 514

    to oesophageal cancer 378

    to ovarian cancer 478

    to pancreatic cancer 416

    to prostate cancer 459

    to skin cancer 499, 501

    to stomach cancer 388

    to testicular cancer 461

    to thyroid cancer 506, 508

    to tobacco-related cancers 91

genital warts 318, 319, 473

genome-wide association studies (GWAS) 91, 193–200

genomics 184–191, 193, 195, 200, 232

genotoxicity 154, 161–163

germ cell tumours 461–463

germline mutations 369, 371

gingivo-buccal cancer 190

glioblastoma 246, 515–518

glioma 148, 512–518

global burden of cancer 16–24, 54–67

Global Burden of Disease study 100

GLOBOCAN 16, 17, 20, 57, 348, 349

glycine 224

glycine decarboxylase 224

glycolysis 222, 223, 224

GNAS 419

gonadal dysgenesis with a Y chromosome 461, 462

Gorlin syndrome 501

granulocyte-macrophage colony-stimulating factor 238, 255

griseofulvin 171

GSTM1 447

insulin 167, 475

interferon 257, 262, 263, 408

interleukins 256, 257, 401

International Atomic Energy Agency 548, 550, 551

International Cancer Genome Consortium 185, 188, 190, 211

intestinal cancer 397

intraductal papillary mucinous neoplasms 418, 419

intratubular germ cell neoplasia 461, 462

involuntary smoking 92, 93, 137, 140, 141, 158, 268, 276, 277, 299

iodine 504

ionizing radiation 144–146, 309, 501, 506, 508, 512

ipilimumab 259, 500

J

JAK2 493

K

Kaposi sarcoma 58, 70, 112

KIAA1549 515

kidney cancer 130, 436–442

KIT 462

KRAS 247, 355, 389, 395, 396, 400, 410, 416, 419, 462, 474, 476, 478, 479

L

lapatinib 248, 451

large cell lung carcinoma 359

laryngeal cancer 97, 422, 425, 427, 429

lasiocarpine 173

law in cancer control 569–573

legislative initiatives 305–312

leukaemia 112, 140, 145, 148, 482, 483, 485, 491–493

Lgr5 397

lichen sclerosus 470

lifestyle intervention 271, 278, 281, 282, 285, 291, 294

linkage disequilibrium 193, 194, 197, 199

liver cancer 57, 59, 97, 100, 108, 122, 164, 172, 314–316, 403–411

    prevention 408, 411

    screening 410

    vaccine 315, 316

liver flukes 112, 406, 407

lobular carcinoma in situ (LCIS) 365

lobular involution 116

lung adenocarcinoma 353, 355, 356

lung cancer 57, 58, 59, 66, 91–94, 134, 135, 137, 142, 145, 146, 152, 155, 156, 158, 350–360, 586–592

    prevention 359

    screening 360

    lycopene 458, 460

lymphoblastic lymphoma 492

lymphoma 105, 108, 482, 488–492

lymphoplasmacytic lymphoma 489

Lynch syndrome 398

M

macrophages 239, 240

magnetic resonance imaging 372

major histocompatibility complex (MHC) 255, 257

MALT lymphoma 489

mammary gland development 256

mammography 164, 324, 325, 332, 371, 372

mantle cell lymphoma 488, 489

marginal zone lymphoma 489

mass media campaigns 277, 290–294

mass spectrometry (MS) 223, 224, 225, 226

mastectomy 370, 371

matrix metalloproteinases 239, 428

mature B-cell lymphoma 488

meat 126, 128, 129, 375, 387, 388, 392, 393, 433, 437, 458, 514

mediastinal large B-cell lymphoma 490

medical radiation 144, 145, 506, 511

medullary thyroid carcinoma 507–509

medulloblastoma 517

melanoma 147, 207, 250, 495–501

melphalan 161

MEN1 420

O

obesity 116, 118, 122, 130–132, 222, 223, 281–284, 287, 309, 367, 378, 395, 407, 433–436, 439, 474

occupational carcinogens 134–142, 310

occupational exposures 134–142, 145, 148, 149, 310, 513

ochratoxin A 172

oesophageal adenocarcinoma 378–381

oesophageal cancer 57, 97, 100, 130, 374–381, 546
  screening 378, 381

oesophageal squamous cell carcinoma 374–378

oligodendroglioma 516, 518

oncogenes 184, 197, 214, 216, 247, 254, 340, 353, 357, 359, 389, 390, 416, 426, 427, 428, 441, 448, 460, 476, 493, 499, 508, 517

oophorectomy 371

opioid analgesics 565, 571, 572

opium 375

optic glioma 515

oral cancer 97, 100, 190, 422–430
  screening 324, 428

oral contraceptives 119, 122, 164, 166, 473, 475, 478

oropharyngeal cancer 100, 110, 111, 317, 320, 422–430

ovarian cancer 119, 120, 163, 164, 166, 371, 477–480

overdiagnosis 324, 325, 326, 371, 523, 524

overtreatment 325, 461, 524

overweight 130, 132, 281, 282, 309, 433, 434, 436

P

p16 416, 417, 427, 448, 450, 476, 499

pancreatic cancer 97, 99, 102, 130, 413–420

pancreatic neuroendocrine tumours 420

pancreatitis 416

papillary renal cell carcinoma 440, 441

papillary thyroid carcinoma 506–508

papillary urothelial neoplasms of low malignant potential 447, 448

Pap smear 324, 473, 474, 542

α-particles 144, 146

β-particles 144, 146

particulate matter 151–156, 353

PBRM1 442

Penicillium 171

penile cancer 110, 316

pentachlorodibenzofuran 136

peripheral T-cell lymphoma 490

pesticides 157

pharmaceutical drugs 161–167, 170, 171, 174, 439

pharyngeal cancer 97, 422, 425–427

phenacetin 165, 439

Philadelphia chromosome-positive leukaemia 491

Philadelphia translocation 184, 185

phosphoglycerate dehydrogenase 223

photosensitivity 165

phylogenetic tree 339, 342

physical activity 132, 281, 282–285, 288, 294, 300, 301, 367, 368, 433, 434

phytochemicals 126, 131

pickled vegetables 375, 386

PIK3CA 356, 357, 427, 428, 474, 476, 480

pilocytic astrocytoma 514

PIVKA 410

plain cigarette packaging 275, 564, 570, 571

plants 173

plasma cell myeloma 487

platelet-derived growth factor receptor β (PDGFR-β) 243

Plummer–Vinson syndrome 377

poly(ADP-ribose) polymerase (PARP) inhibitors 371, 418, 477

polybrominated biphenyls (PBBs) 137

polychlorinated biphenyls (PCBs) 135, 136, 158

polycyclic aromatic hydrocarbons (PAHs) 88, 90, 128, 135, 140, 153, 155, 156

polycystic ovary syndrome 475

polymerase chain reaction (PCR) 204, 218

polypectomy 396, 400

pooled birth cohorts 179, 180

poorly differentiated thyroid carcinoma 507

population attributable fraction (PAF) 105, 109, 111, 112, 113

population-based screening programmes 322–328, 330–334

population-wide prevention campaigns 290–295

single-nucleotide polymorphisms (SNPs) 128, 193, 194, 195, 196, 197, 198, 199

sipuleucel-T 258

skin cancer 147, 156, 158, 162, 246, 495–501

    prevention 500, 501

SMAD4 395, 416, 419

small cell lung carcinoma 353, 357, 359

small lymphocytic lymphoma (SLL) 482

small-molecule inhibitors 237, 247, 248

smoke-free legislation 276, 277, 306–308, 568, 575

smokeless tobacco 82, 85, 86, 88–91, 269, 273, 274, 422

smoking 82–86, 88–94, 268–278, 306, 307, 350, 354, 374, 377, 387, 414, 422, 426, 436, 444, 467, 473, 568, 586–594

smoking-attributed mortality 586–594

smoking cessation 268, 269, 273, 276, 278, 359, 586–594

snuff 89

soil pollution 159

solar radiation 137, 146, 147, 309, 495, 498, 500

solid fuel combustion 543

solid-pseudopapillary neoplasms 420

somatic mutations 186, 188, 200, 368

somatic stem cells 228, 229

soot 135, 140

sorafenib 247, 451

SOX2 357

spinal ependymoma 516

squamous cell carcinoma 165, 246, 356, 357, 422, 427, 428, 465, 466, 500, 501

squamous intraepithelial lesions 467, 470–474

statins 166

stem cells 223, 228–233, 397, 493

sterigmatocystin 172

stomach cancer 57, 58, 59, 106, 158, 383–390

    prevention 388, 390

    screening 388, 390

Streptomyces 170

sugar-sweetened beverages 129, 311, 433, 434

sunburn 147, 294, 498, 501

sunitinib 247, 420, 451

sunlight 146, 147, 309, 495, 498–501

sun protection 147, 309, 498–501

sun protection campaigns 147, 294, 309

sunscreen 498, 500

survivorship 73, 74

susceptibility alleles 193, 194, 197, 199, 200

SV40 514

synthetic lethality 371

T

tamoxifen 165, 166, 369, 475

tanning devices 147, 309, 495, 501

targeted therapy 184, 190, 206, 211, 220, 223, 237, 241, 242, 243, 244–251, 259, 355, 356, 357, 372, 390, 420, 451, 477, 480, 500, 553

taxation 271–273

telomerase 77, 78

telomeres 77–79

telomere syndromes 78

temozolomide 516

TERT 515

testicular cancer 120, 165, 461, 462

testosterone 458

TET2 490, 493

2,3,7,8-tetrachlorodibenzo-*para*-dioxin (TCDD) 136

thiotepa 161

thyroid cancer 146, 503–509

thyroidectomy 507

tissue-specific stem cells 228, 229

TMPRSS2 460

tobacco

    advertising 83, 86, 273, 275, 299

    -attributed mortality 586–594

    control 83, 84, 86, 94, 268–278, 299, 300, 306–308, 568, 570, 571

    economic cost of – 302

    -induced injury 354

    packaging 274–276, 564, 570, 571

    prices 271–273

    -related cancers 90, 91, 586–592

    smoking 82–85, 88, 90, 186, 190, 268–278, 306, 307, 350, 354, 414, 422, 426, 436, 444, 586–594

    -specific nitrosamines 88, 89, 90

    taxation 271–273

    use 82–86, 90, 268–278, 374, 377, 422